Basic
Neurochemistry

Basic
Neurochemistry

Molecular, Cellular, and Medical Aspects

Fourth Edition

Editor-in-Chief

George J. Siegel, M.D.

Professor, Department of Neurology
University of Michigan
Ann Arbor, Michigan

Editors

Bernard W. Agranoff, M.D.

Director of Mental Health Research Institute and
Professor of Biological Chemistry and Psychiatry
University of Michigan
Ann Arbor, Michigan

R. Wayne Albers, Ph.D.

Chief, Section on Enzyme Chemistry
Laboratory of Neurochemistry
National Institute of Neurological
and Communicative Disorders and Stroke
National Institutes of Health
Bethesda, Maryland

Perry B. Molinoff, M.D.

Professor and Chairman
Department of Pharmacology
School of Medicine
University of Pennsylvania
Philadelphia, Pennsylvania

Raven Press   New York

Raven Press, Ltd., 1185 Avenue of the Americas, New York, New York 10036

Made in the United States of America

Library of Congress Cataloging-in-Publication Data

Basic neurochemistry.

Includes bibliographical references and index.
1. Neurochemistry.   I. Siegel, George J.
QP356.3.B27   1981   612'.8042   87-42722
ISBN 0-88167-343-9

9 8 7 6 5 4 3 2 1

Preface

The addition of the phrase, "Molecular, Cellular, and Medical Aspects" to the title of this Fourth Edition of *Basic Neurochemistry* emphasizes our belief that the flourishing of neurochemistry derives from correlations among phenomena that are observed at multiple levels. As discussed in the Preface to the First Edition in 1972, integrating hypotheses are being developed to account for the functioning of the nervous system in terms of molecular events. The current growth of correlative power stems not only from increases in sensitivity and resolution of analytical biochemistry—more data from smaller samples—but equally from technology that permits observing and quantitating molecular events in functioning, complex, and relatively intact biological structures. Examples range from recording the conductance of single ion channels in patches of membrane, to measuring processes in transfected cells or transgenic animals, to imaging receptor-ligand binding, metabolism, and blood flow in brains of awake functioning humans.

Advances in molecular genetics have generated an enthusiastic sense of anticipation among neurobiologists over the past decade. The derivative applications are, on the one hand, revealing more about molecular structures and, on the other, elucidating nervous system development and the bases of genetic diseases affecting human behavior. We are encouraged to believe that increased knowledge of the molecular basis of neurobiology will ultimately lead to an understanding of the coding of experiences that comprise memory and are the substrate of behavior and mind.

This Fourth Edition is nearly a new book. More than half the chapters appear for the first time, while the remainder have been completely revised to include discussions of many significant new developments in neurobiology. A new major section on molecular neurobiology discusses molecular mechanisms, applications of nucleic acid probes for gene expression, and molecular approaches to the elucidation of inherited diseases of the nervous system. Other sections contain new chapters on the molecular structures and mechanisms of membrane channels, neurotransmitter receptors, receptor-activated phosphoinositide turnover, G-proteins, cyclic nucleotides, and phosphorylation in regulation of neuronal signaling functions. There are new chapters on the molecular structure and dynamics of the cytoskeleton of the cell and biochemical changes in brain development, regeneration, plasticity, and aging. Such topics are relevant to our understanding of normal neuronal growth as well as to the elucidation of the pathophysiological basis of neuropsychiatric disease, of biologic repair mechanisms, and of treatment strategies such as tissue transplantation.

Basic Neurochemistry had its origin in the Conference on Neurochemistry Curriculum initiated and organized by R. Wayne Albers, Robert Katzman, and George Siegel under the sponsorship of the National Institute for Neurological Diseases and Stroke, June 19 and 20, 1969, Bronx, New York. At this conference, a group of 30 neuroscientists constructed a syllabus outline delineating the scope of a neurochemistry curriculum appropriate for medical, graduate, and postgraduate neuroscience students. Out of this outline grew the first edition, edited by R. Wayne Albers, George Siegel, Robert Katzman, and Bernard Agranoff. It was anticipated that the book would evolve with the emergence of the field and would stimulate continuing reappraisal of the scientific and educational aspects of neurochemistry. The Editors elected to assign the copyright and all royalties to the American Society for Neurochemistry, the royalties to be used for educational purposes. These funds have been used to sponsor the Annual Basic Neurochemistry Lectureship. With this Fourth Edition, we welcome Perry Molinoff as a coeditor.

The expansion of knowledge has necessitated enlargement of the book. We wished to keep to one volume and to a cost that would encourage its use as a text. This has required us to make difficult decisions regarding the selection and editing of material. The number of authors and quantity of information have increased. In all cases we have attempted to emphasise what is known, to include plausible hypotheses, and to identify areas for future research. Outlines comprised of topic sentences have been introduced to provide a survey of each subject and to emphasize critical points for the student. To save space, the number of references has been restricted to key chapters and reviews that will serve as an entry into the literature. A store of valuable information on the history of development of neurochemistry will be found in the chapter "Neurochemistry in Historical Perspective" by Donald B. Tower in the Third Edition (*Basic Neurochemistry*, Little, Brown & Co., Boston, 1982, pp. 1–16).

Our expanded knowledge of cell metabolism and membrane and organelle biochemistry has enhanced our understanding of brain pathology in ischemia, hypoxia, epilepsy, coma, inherited enzyme defects, metabolic and nutritional disturbances, and brain degenerative disorders. Presentation of these subjects has been correspondingly increased.

The use of new and noninvasive imaging techniques to assess neuronal systems by metabolism, blood flow, and receptor topography in humans has contributed to our understanding of brain function and disease. The relationship between endocrine control of nervous system development and behavior is structured on new data and concepts of peptide synthesis and hormonal regulation of cell biology. Contemporary views of molecular events subserving such integrated brain functions as memory and the control of affect are presented in new chapters.

GEORGE J. SIEGEL
BERNARD W. AGRANOFF
R. WAYNE ALBERS
PERRY B. MOLINOFF

Acknowledgments

We are pleased to acknowledge the enormous contributions of Robert Katzman, who served as one of the Editors of the first three editions of the text. We are grateful to the many colleagues, including participants in the earlier editions, who have generously contributed figures, information, and suggestions for this edition. On behalf of the contributors, we express appreciation to all those investigators whose important work has not been explicitly referenced in the text. We appreciate and acknowledge all the authors whose hard work and genuine cooperation have gone into this book. We also wish to express continued appreciation for the redactory work of Helene Jordan Waddell throughout the first three editions. We thank Catherine Leggieri for her help with typing and correspondence. We would like to acknowledge the assistance of the staff of Raven Press, in particular Kirk Bomont, Nancy Kirkpatrick, Ellen Schwarz, and Beth Weiselberg, in publishing this text. Finally, we wish to thank all of our families whose support in general is crucial for this kind of work.

G. J. S.
R. W. A.
B. W. A.
P. B. M.

Contents

Contributors

Bernard W. Agranoff, M.D.
*Director of Mental Health Research Institute
and
Professor of Biological Chemistry and
Psychiatry
University of Michigan
Ann Arbor, Michigan 48104-1687*

R. Wayne Albers, Ph.D.
*Chief, Section on Enzyme Chemistry
Laboratory of Neurochemistry
National Institute of Neurological and
Communicative Disorders and Stroke
National Institutes of Health
Bethesda, Maryland 20892*

Kevin J. Anderson, Ph.D.
*Assistant Professor
Department of Physiological Sciences
University of Florida
Gainesville, Florida 32610-0144*

Alaric T. Arenander, Ph.D.
*Research Associate
Mental Retardation Research Center
Brain Research Institute, and Departments of
Anatomy and Psychiatry
UCLA School of Medicine
Los Angeles, California 90024*

Jack D. Barchas, M.D.
*Nancy Friend Pritzker Professor
Department of Psychiatry and Behavioral
Sciences
Stanford University School of Medicine
Stanford, California 94305*

Robert L. Barchi, M.D., Ph.D.
*David Mahoney Professor of Neuroscience,
and Director, Mahoney Institute of
Neurological Sciences
University of Pennsylvania School of
Medicine
Philadelphia, Pennsylvania 19104*

A. Lorris Betz, M.D., Ph.D.
*Professor of Pediatrics, Neurology, and
Surgery
University of Michigan
Ann Arbor, Michigan 48109-0718*

John P. Blass, M.D., Ph.D.
*Burke Professor of Neurology and Medicine
Director, Dementia Research Service
Department of Neurology
Cornell University Medical College
White Plains, New York 10605*

Scott T. Brady, Ph.D.
*Assistant Professor
Department of Cell Biology and Anatomy
University of Texas,
Southwestern Medical Center
Dallas, Texas 75235*

Joan Heller Brown, Ph.D.
*Associate Professor
Department of Pharmacology
University of California, San Diego
La Jolla, California 92093*

Michael J. Brownstein, M.D.
Laboratory of Cell Biology
National Institute of Mental Health
National Institutes of Health
Bethesda, Maryland 20892

William A. Catterall, Ph.D.
Professor and Chairman
Department of Pharmacology
University of Washington
Seattle, Washington 98195

Donald D. Clarke, Ph.D.
Professor of Biochemistry
Chemistry Department
Fordham University
Bronx, New York 10458

Arthur J. L. Cooper, Ph.D.
Associate Professor
Departments of Biochemistry and Neurology
Cornell University Medical College
New York, New York 10021

Carl W. Cotman, Ph.D.
Professor of Psychobiology and Neurology
University of California
Irvine, California 92717

Jean de Vellis, Ph.D.
Professor, Neurobiochemistry Group
Mental Retardation Research Center
Brain Research Institute, and Departments of
* Anatomy and Psychiatry*
UCLA School of Medicine
Los Angeles, California 90024

Darryl C. De Vivo, M.D.
Sidney Carter Professor of Neurology
Professor of Pediatrics
College of Physicians and Surgeons
Columbia University
New York, New York 10032

Salvatore DiMauro, M.D.
Co-director, H. Houston Merritt Clinical
* Research Center for Muscular Dystrophy*
* and Professor, Department of Neurology*

College of Physicians and Surgeons
Columbia University
New York, New York 10032

Glen R. Elliott, M.D., Ph.D.
Assistant Professor
Department of Psychiatry and Behavioral
* Sciences*
Stanford University School of Medicine
Stanford, California 94305

S. D. Erulkar, Ph.D., D.Phil.
Professor, Department of Pharmacology
University of Pennsylvania Medical School
Philadelphia, Pennsylvania 19104

A. A. Farooqui, Ph.D.
Research Scientist
Department of Physiological Chemistry
The Ohio State University
Columbus, Ohio 43210

Kym F. Faull, Ph.D
Director Pasarow Analytical Neurochemistry
* Facility*
Department of Psychiatry and Behavioral
* Sciences*
Stanford University School of Medicine
Stanford, California 94305

C. J. Flynn, Ph.D.
Research Scientist
Nathan Kline Institute
Orangeburg, New York 10962

Kirk A. Frey, M.D., Ph.D.
Research Investigator
Mental Health Research Institute
The University of Michigan
Ann Arbor, Michigan 48109

John Gergely, M.D., Ph.D.
Department of Muscle Research
Boston Biomedical Research Institute
Neurology Service
Massachusetts General Hospital, and
* Department of Biological Chemistry and*
* Molecular Pharmacology*

Harvard Medical School
Boston, Massachusetts 02114

Gary W. Goldstein, M.D.
Professor of Neurology and Pediatrics
Johns Hopkins University, and
President, Kennedy Institute
Baltimore, Maryland 21205

Richard H. Goodman, M.D., Ph.D.
Associate Professor of Medicine
Division of Molecular Medicine
New England Medical Center Hospitals
Boston, Massachusetts 02111

Jack Peter Green, M.D., Ph.D.
Professor and Chairman
Department of Pharmacology
Mount Sinai School of Medicine of the City
*   University of New York*
New York, New York 10029-6574

Paul Greengard, Ph.D.
Professor and Head
Laboratory of Molecular and Cellular
*   Neuroscience*
The Rockefeller University
New York, New York 10021

Mark W. Hamblin, M.D., Ph.D.
Postdoctoral Fellow
Department of Psychiatry and Behavioral
*   Sciences*
Stanford University School of Medicine
Stanford, California 94305

Richard Hammerschlag, Ph.D.
Research Scientist
Division of Neurosciences
Beckman Research Institute of the City of
*   Hope National Medical Center*
Duarte, California 91010

Bertil Hille, Ph.D.
Professor of Physiology and Biophysics
University of Washington School of Medicine
Seattle, Washington 98195

Jacob M. Hiller, Ph.D.
Research Associate Professor of Psychiatry
New York University Medical Center
New York, New York 10016

Lloyd A. Horrocks, Ph.D.
Professor
Department of Physiological Chemistry and
*   the Neuroscience Program*
College of Medicine
The Ohio State University
Columbus, Ohio 43210

Yujen Edward Hsia, B.M., F.R.C.P., D.C.H.
Professor of Pediatrics
John A. Burns School of Medicine
University of Hawaii
Honolulu, Hawaii 96826

Robert Katzman, M.D.
Professor and Chairman
Department of Neurosciences
School of Medicine
University of California, San Diego
La Jolla, California 92093

Michel Khrestchatisky, Ph.D.
Research Fellow
Department of Biology
University of California
Los Angeles, California 90024-1606

Abel L. Lajtha, Ph.D.
Director, Center for Neurochemistry
Nathan S. Kline Institute for Psychiatric
*   Research*
Wards Island, New York 10035, and
Research Professor of Psychiatry
New York University School of Medicine
New York, New York 10016

Malcolm J. Low, M.D., Ph.D.
Assistant Professor of Medicine
Division of Molecular Medicine
New England Medical Center Hospitals
Boston, Massachusetts 02111

Howard S. Maker, M.D.
Associate Director of Neurology
Beth Israel Medical Center
New York, New York 10003

Robert C. Malenka, M.D., Ph.D.
Research Fellow
Department of Psychiatry and Behavioral
*   Sciences*
Stanford University School of Medicine
Stanford, California 94305

Gail Mandel, Ph.D.
Assistant Professor of Medicine
Division of Molecular Medicine
New England Medical Center Hospitals
Boston, Massachusetts 02111

Bruce S. McEwen, Ph.D.
Professor and Head
Laboratory of Neuroendocrinology
Rockefeller University
New York, New York 10021

Dale E. McFarlin, M.D.
Chief, Neuroimmunology Branch
National Institute of Neurological and
*   Communicative Disorders and Stroke*
National Institutes of Health,
Bethesda, Maryland 20892

Edith G. McGeer, Ph.D.
Professor and Head
Division of Neurological Sciences
Department of Psychiatry
University of British Columbia
Vancouver, British Columbia,
Canada V6T 1W5

Patrick L. McGeer, M.D., Ph.D.
Professor, Division of Neurological Sciences
Department of Psychiatry
University of British Columbia
Vancouver, British Columbia,
Canada V6T 1W5

Paul McGonigle, Ph.D.
Assistant Professor
Department of Pharmacology
School of Medicine
University of Pennsylvania
Philadelphia, Pennsylvania 19104-6084

Perry B. Molinoff, M.D.
Professor and Chairman
Department of Pharmacology
School of Medicine
University of Pennsylvania
Philadelphia, Pennsylvania 19104-6084

Pierre Morell, Ph.D.
Professor of Biochemistry
Biological Sciences Research Center
University of North Carolina
Chapel Hill, North Carolina 27514

Eric J. Nestler, M.D., Ph.D.
Assistant Professor
Departments of Psychiatry and Pharmacology
Yale University School of Medicine
Connecticut Mental Health Center
New Haven, Connecticut 06508

John K. Northup, Ph.D.
Assistant Professor
Department of Pharmacology
Yale University School of Medicine
New Haven, Connecticut 06510

William Norton, Ph.D.
Professor of Neurology (Neurochemistry) and
*   Neuroscience*
Department of Neurology
Albert Einstein College of Medicine
New York, New York 10461

John P. Perkins, Ph.D.
Professor and Chairman
Department of Pharmacology
Yale University School of Medicine
New Haven, Connecticut 06510

Christine Peterson, Ph.D.
Assistant Research Psychologist
Department of Psychobiology
University of California
Irvine, California 92717

David Pleasure, M.D.
Professor, Neurology and Pediatrics
University of Pennsylvania
Philadelphia, Pennsylvania 19104

Virginia K. Proud, M.D.
Assistant Professor of Child Health
Division of Medical Genetics
University of Missouri–Columbia Medical
*   School*
Columbia, Missouri 65212

William A. Pulsinelli, M.D., Ph.D.
Professor of Neurology, and
Director, Laboratory of Cerebral
*   Metabolism*
Department of Neurology
Cornell University Medical College
New York, New York 10021

Richard H. Quarles, Ph.D.
Chief, Section of Myelin and Brain
*   Development*
National Institute of Neurological and
*   Communicative Disorders and Stroke*
National Institutes of Health
Bethesda, Maryland 20892

Cedric S. Raine, Ph.D., D.Sc.
Professor of Pathology (Neuropathology) and
*   Neuroscience*
Department of Pathology
Albert Einstein College of Medicine
Bronx, New York 10461

Roger N. Rosenberg, M.D.
Professor and Chairman
Department of Neurology
Professor of Physiology
University of Texas, Southwestern Medical
*   Center*
Dallas, Texas 75235

Frederick J. Samaha, M.D.
Albert Barnes Voorheis Professor and
*   Chairman*
Department of Neurology
University of Cincinnati College of Medicine
Cincinnati, Ohio 45267-0525

Hitoshi Shichi, Ph.D.
Professor of Biomedical Sciences
Kresge State Eye Institute
School of Medicine
Wayne State University
Detroit, Michigan 48210

George J. Siegel, M.D.
Professor, Department of Neurology
University of Michigan
Ann Arbor, Michigan 48109

Eric J. Simon, Ph.D.
Professor of Psychiatry and Pharmacology
New York University Medical Center
New York, New York 10016

Louis Sokoloff, M.D.
Chief, Laboratory of Cerebral Metabolism
National Institute of Mental Health
National Institutes of Health
Bethesda, Maryland 20892

Theodore L. Sourkes, Ph.D.
Professor, Departments of Psychiatry and
*   Biochemistry*
Faculty of Medicine
McGill University
Montreal, Quebec, Canada H3A 1A1

William L. Stahl, Ph.D.
Professor, Department of Physiology and
*   Biophysics and Department of Medicine*
*   (Neurology)*
University of Washington School of Medicine,
*   and Veterans Administration Medical*
*   Center*
Seattle, Washington 98108

Kunihiko Suzuki, M.D.
*Director, Biological Sciences Research
    Center*
Professor of Neurology and Psychiatry
*University of North Carolina School of
    Medicine*
Chapel Hill, North Carolina 27599-7250

Palmer Taylor, Ph.D.
Professor and Chairman
Department of Pharmacology
University of California, San Diego
San Diego, California 92093

Leon J. Thal, M.D.
Neurology Service
Veterans Administration Medical Center
San Diego, California 92161, and
Department of Neuroscience
University of California, San Diego
La Jolla, California 92093

Allan J. Tobin, Ph.D.
Professor
Department of Biology
Brain Research Institute and
Molecular Biology Institute
University of California
Los Angeles, California 90024-1606

Claude G. Wasterlain, M.D.
Professor and Vice Chairman
Department of Neurology
UCLA School of Medicine
Los Angeles, California 90024, and
Chief of the Neurology Service
Veterans Administration Medical Center
Sepulveda, California 91343

Norman Weiner, M.D.
Professor and Chairman
Department of Pharmacology
Distinguished Volwiler Research Fellow
University of Colorado School of Medicine
Denver, Colorado 80262

Barry Wolf, M.D., Ph.D.
Professor
Department of Human Genetics, and
Department of Pediatrics, Children's Hospital
Medical College of Virginia
Richmond, Virginia 23298

Leonhard S. Wolfe, M.D., Ph.D.
*Professor, Departments of Neurology and
    Biochemistry*
Montreal Neurological Institute and Hospital
*Donner Laboratory of Experimental
    Neurochemistry*
McGill University
Montreal, Quebec, Canada H3A 2B4

Basic
Neurochemistry

PART ONE

Neural Membranes

CHAPTER 1

Neurocellular Anatomy

Cedric S. Raine

AN UNDERSTANDING OF NEUROANATOMY IS NECESSARY TO THE STUDY OF NEUROCHEMISTRY

Despite the advent of molecular genetics in neurobiology, our understanding of the functional relationships of the components of the central nervous system (CNS) remains in its infancy, particularly in the areas of cellular interaction and synaptic modulation. Nevertheless, the fine structural relationships of most elements of nervous system tissue have been well described [1–5]. (The excellent neuroanatomical atlases of Peters et al. [3] and Palay and Chan-Palay [1] should be consulted for detailed ultrastructural analyses of specific cell types, particularly of neurons with their diverse forms and connections.) This chapter provides a con-

Basic Neurochemistry: Molecular, Cellular, and Medical Aspects, 4th Ed., edited by G. J. Siegel et al. Raven Press, Ltd., New York, 1989.
Correspondence to Cedric S. Raine, Departments of Pathology and Neuroscience, Albert Einstein College of Medicine, 1300 Morris Park Avenue, Bronx, New York 10461.

cise description of the major cytoarchitectural features of the nervous system and gives an entrance into the relevant literature. Although the fine structure of the organelles of the CNS and peripheral nervous system (PNS) is not peculiar to these tissues, the interactions between cell types, such as synaptic contacts between neurons and myelin sheaths around axons, are unique. These specializations and those that allow for the sequestration of the CNS from the outside world, namely, the blood-brain barrier and the absence of lymphatics, become major issues in considerations of normal and disease

processes in the nervous system. For the sake of simplicity, the present section is subdivided first into a section on general organization and then according to major cell types.

Diverse cell types are organized into assemblies and patterns such that specialized components are integrated into a physiology of the whole organ

Central nervous system parenchyma is made up of nerve cells and their afferent and efferent extensions (dendrites and axons), all closely en-

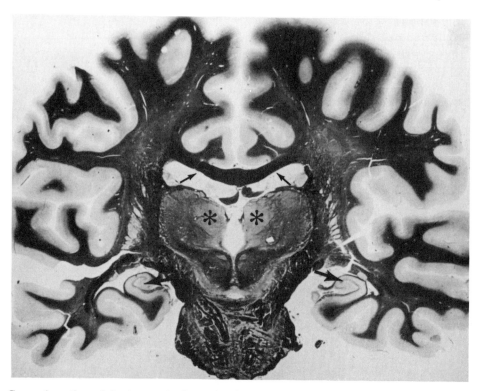

FIG. 1. Coronal section of the human brain at the thalamic level stained by the Heidenhain technique for myelin. Gray matter stains faintly; all myelinated regions are black. The thalamus (∗) lies beneath the lateral ventricles and is separated at this level by the beginning of the third ventricle. The roof of the lateral ventricles is formed by the corpus callosum (*small arrows*). The Ammon's horns are shown at the *large arrows*. Note the outline of gyri and sulci at the surface of the cerebral hemispheres, sectioned here near the junction of the frontal and parietal cortex.

veloped by glial cells. Coronal section of the cerebral hemispheres of the brain reveals an outer convoluted rim of gray matter overlying the white matter (Fig. 1). Gray matter, which also exists as islands within the white matter, contains mainly nerve cell bodies and glia and lacks significant amounts of myelin, the lipid component responsible for the whiteness of white matter. More distally along the neuraxis in the spinal cord, the cerebral situation is reversed. White matter surrounds gray matter, which is arranged in a characteristic H formation (Fig. 2).

A highly diagrammatic representation of the major CNS elements is shown in Fig. 3. The entire CNS is bathed both internally and externally by cerebrospinal fluid (CSF), which circulates throughout the ventricular and leptomeningeal spaces. This fluid, a type of plasma ultrafiltrate, plays a significant role in protecting the CNS from mechanical trauma, balancing electrolytes and protein, and maintaining ventricular pressure (see Chap. 30). The outer surface of the CNS is invested by the triple-membrane system of the meninges. The outermost is the dura mater (derived from the mesoderm), which is tightly adherent to the inner surfaces of the calvaria. The arachnoid membrane is closely applied to the inner surface of the dura mater. The innermost of the meninges, the pia mater, loosely covers the CNS surface. The pia and arachnoid together (derived from the ectoderm) are called the leptomeninges. CSF occupies the subarachnoid space (between the arachnoid and the pia) and the ventricles. The CNS parenchyma is overlaid by a layer of subpial astrocytes, which, in turn, is covered on its leptomeningeal aspect by a basal lamina (see

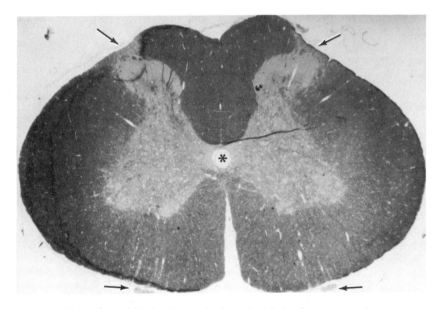

FIG. 2. Transverse section of a rabbit lumbar spinal cord at L-1. Gray matter is seen as a paler staining area in an H configuration formed by the dorsal and ventral horns with the central canal in the center (*). The dorsal horns would meet the incoming dorsal spine nerve roots at the *upper arrows*. The anterior roots can be seen below (*arrows*), opposite the ventral horns from which they receive their fibers. The white matter occupies a major part of the spinal cord and stains darker. Epon section, 1 μm, stained with toluidine blue.

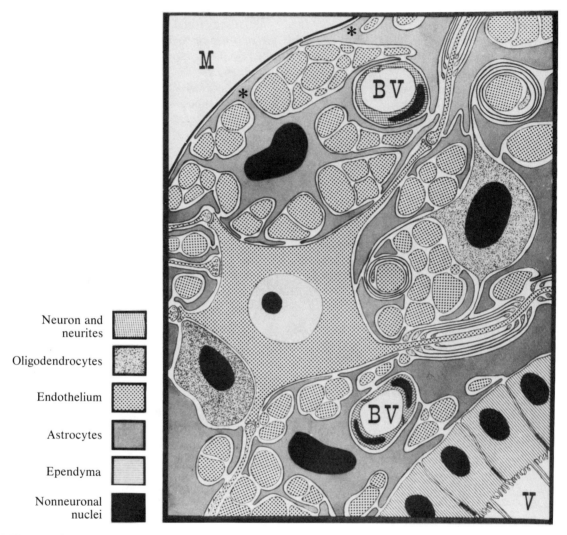

Neuron and neurites

Oligodendrocytes

Endothelium

Astrocytes

Ependyma

Nonneuronal nuclei

FIG. 3. The major components of the CNS and their interrelationships. Microglia are not depicted. In this simplified schema, the CNS extends from its meningeal surface (M); through the basal lamina (*solid black line*) overlying the subpial astrocyte layer of the CNS parenchyma; across the CNS, parenchyma proper (containing neurons and glia) and subependymal astrocytes, to ciliated ependymal cells lining the ventricular space (V). Note how the astrocyte also invests blood vessels (BV), neurons, and cell processes. The pia-astroglia (glia limitans) provides the barrier between the exterior (dura and blood vessels) and the CNS parenchyma. One neuron is seen (*center*), with synaptic contacts on its soma and dendrites. The subarachnoid space of the meninges (M) and the ventricles (V) contain cerebrospinal fluid. Its axon emerges to the right and is myelinated by an oligodendrocyte (*above*). Other axons are shown in transverse section, some of which are myelinated. The oligodendrocyte to the lower left of the neuron is of the nonmyelinating satellite type.

Fig. 3). On the inner (ventricular) surface, the CNS parenchyma is separated from the CSF by a layer of ciliated ependymal cells, which are thought to facilitate the movement of CSF. The production and circulation of CSF are maintained by the choroid plexus, grape-like collections of vascular tissue and cells that protrude into the ventricles (see Chap. 30). Resorption of CSF is effected by vascular structures known as arachnoid villi, located in the leptomeninges over the surface of the brain (see Chap. 30).

Ependymal cells abut layers of astrocytes, which, in turn, envelop neurons, neurites, and vascular components. In addition to neurons and glial cells (astrocytes and oligodendrocytes), the CNS parenchyma contains blood vessels, macrophages (pericytes), and microglial cells.

The PNS and the autonomic nervous system consist of bundles of myelinated and nonmyelinated axons enveloped by Schwann cells, the PNS counterparts of oligodendrocytes. Nerve bundles are enclosed by the perineurium and the epineurium, which are tough, fibrous, elastic sheaths. Between individual nerve fibers are isolated connective tissue (endoneurial) cells and blood vessels. The ganglia (e.g., dorsal root and sympathetic ganglia), located peripherally to the CNS, are made up of large neurons, usually unipolar or bipolar, surrounded by satellite cells that are specialized Schwann cells. A dendrite and an axon, both of which can be of great length (up to several feet), arise from each neuron.

CHARACTERISTICS OF THE NEURON

From an historical standpoint, no other cell type has attracted as much attention or caused as much controversy as the nerve cell. It is impossible in a single chapter to delineate comprehensively the extensive structural, topographical, and functional variation achieved by this cell type. Consequently, despite an enormous literature, the neuron still defies precise definition, particularly with regard to function. It is known that the neuronal population is usually established shortly after birth, that mature neurons do not divide, and that in humans, there is a daily dropout of neurons amounting to approximately 20,000 cells. These facts alone make the neuron unique. (Development and maturation of neurons are discussed in Chap. 25.)

Neurons can be excitatory, inhibitory, or modulatory in their effect; motor, sensory, or secretory in their function. They can be influenced by a large repertoire of neurotransmitters and hormones (see Chap. 8). This enormous repertoire of functions, associated with different developmental influences on different neurons, is largely reflected in the variation of dendritic and axonal outgrowth. Specialization also occurs at axonal terminals, where a variety of junctional complexes (synapses) exist. The subtle synaptic modifications are best visualized ultrastructurally, although immunohistochemical staining also permits distinction among synapses on the basis of transmitter type.

General structural features of neurons are the perikarya, dendrites, and axons

The stereotypic image of a neuron is that of a stellate cell body (soma or perikaryon) with broad dendrites and a fine axon emerging from one pole—an impression gained from the older work of Purkinje, who first described the nerve cell in 1839, and of Deiters, Ramón y Cajal, and Golgi at the end of the nineteenth century and early twentieth century. However, this does not hold true for many neurons. The neuron is the most polymorphic cell in the body and defies formal classification on the basis of shape, location, function, fine structure, or transmitter substance. Although early workers described the neuron as a globular mass suspended between nerve fibers, the teased preparations of Deiters and his contemporaries soon proved this not to be the case. Later work using impregnation staining and culture techniques, elaborated on Deiters' findings. Before Deiters and Ramón y Cajal, neurons were believed to form a syncytium, with no intervening membranes—a postulate also proposed for neuroglia. Today, of course, we are familiar with the specialized membranes and the enormous variety of nerve cell shapes and sizes. They range from the small globular cerebellar granule cells, with a perikaryal diameter of approximately 6 to 8 μm, to the pear-shaped Purkinje cells and star-shaped anterior horn cells, both of which may reach diameters of 60 to 80 μm in humans. Perikaryal size is generally a poor index of total cell volume, however, and it is a general rule in neuroanatomy that neurites occupy a greater percentage of the cell surface area than does the soma. For example, the pyramidal cell of the somatosensory cortex has a cell body that accounts for only 4 percent of the total cell surface area, whereas from its dendritic tree, the dendritic spines alone claim 43 percent (Mungai, quoted by Peters et al. [3]). Hyden [2] quotes Scholl (1956), who calculated that the perikaryon of a "cortical cell" represents 10 percent of the neuronal surface area. In the feline reticular formation, some giant cells possess ratios between soma and dendrites of about 1:5. A single axon is the usual rule, but some cells, like the Golgi cells of the cerebellum, are endowed with several, some of which may show branching.

The extent of the branching displayed by the dendrites is a useful index of their functional importance. Dendritic trees represent the expression of the receptive fields, and large fields can receive inputs from multiple origins. A cell with a less developed dendritic ramification (e.g., the cerebellar granule cell), synapses with a more homogeneous population of afferent sources.

The axon emerges from a neuron as a slender thread and frequently does not branch until it nears its target. In contrast to the dendrite and the soma (with very few exceptions), the axon is frequently myelinated, thus increasing its efficiency as a conducting unit. Myelin, a spirally wrapped membrane (see Chap. 6), is laid down in segments (internodes) by oligodendrocytes in the CNS and by Schwann cells in the PNS. The naked regions of axon between adjacent myelin internodes are known as nodes of Ranvier (see Figs. 20 and 21).

Neurons contain the same intracellular components as do other cells

No unique cytoplasmic inclusions of the neuron serve to distinguish it from any other cell. Neurons have all the morphological counterparts of other cell types, the structures are similarly distributed, and some of the most common, the Golgi apparatus and mitochondria, for example, were first described in neurons (Fig. 4).

The nucleus

A large, usually spherical nucleus containing a prominent nucleolus is typical of most neurons. The nucleochromatin is invariably pale, with little dense heterochromatin. In some neurons (e.g., cerebellar granule cells), the karyoplasm (nucleoplasm) may show more differentiation and dense heterochromatin. The nucleolus is vesiculated and clearly delineated from the rest of the karyoplasm. It usually contains two textures, the pars fibrosa (fine bundles of filaments) and the pars granulosa, in which dense granules predominate. An additional juxtaposed structure, found in neurons of the female of some species, is the nucleolar satellite, or sex chromatin, which consists of dense, but loosely

FIG. 4. A motor neuron from the spinal cord of an adult rat shows a nucleus (N) containing a nucleolus, clearly divisible into a pars fibrosa and a pars granulosa, and a perikaryon filled with organelles. Among these, Golgi apparatus (*arrows*), Nissl substance (S), mitochondria (M), and lysosomes (L) can be seen. An axosomatic synapse (S) occurs below, and two axodendritic synapses abut a dendrite (D). ×8,000.

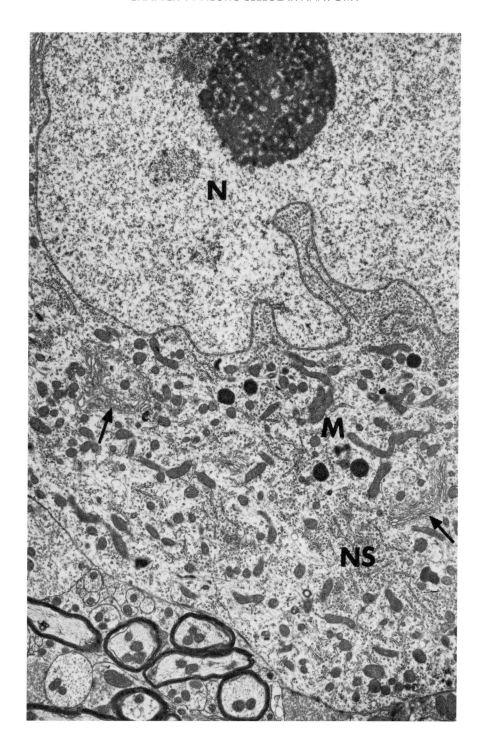

packed, coiled filaments. The nucleus is enclosed by the nuclear envelope, made up on the cytoplasmic side by the inner membrane of the perikaryon (sometimes seen in continuity with the endoplasmic reticulum; Fig. 5) and a more regular membrane on the inner, nuclear aspect. Between the two is a clear channel of between 20 and 40 nm. Periodically, the inner and outer membranes of the envelope come together to form a single diaphragm—a nuclear pore (Fig. 5). In tangential section, nuclear pores are seen as empty vesicular structures, approximately 70 nm in diameter. In some neurons, as in Purkinje cells, that segment of the nuclear envelope which faces the dendritic pole is deeply invaginated.

The perikaryon

The body of the neuron, the perikaryon, is rich in organelles (Fig. 4). It often stands out poorly from a homogeneous background neuropil,

most of which is composed of nonmyelinated neurites (axons and dendrites), synaptic complexes, and glial cell processes. Closer inspection shows that, like all cells, the neuron is delineated by a typical triple-layered unit membrane approximately 7.5 nm wide. Among the most prominent features of the perikaryal cytoplasm is a system of membranous cisternae, divisible into rough endoplasmic reticulum (ER), which forms part of the Nissl substance; smooth (agranular) ER; subsurface cisternae (the hypolemmal system); and the Golgi apparatus. Although these various components are structurally interconnected, each possesses distinct enzymologic properties. Also present within the cytoplasm are abundant lysosomes, lipofuscin granules (aging pigment), mitochondria, multivesicular bodies, neurotubules, neurofilaments and ribosomes. The major neuronal organelles are as follows.

Nissl substance. The intracytoplasmic basophilic masses that ramify loosely through-

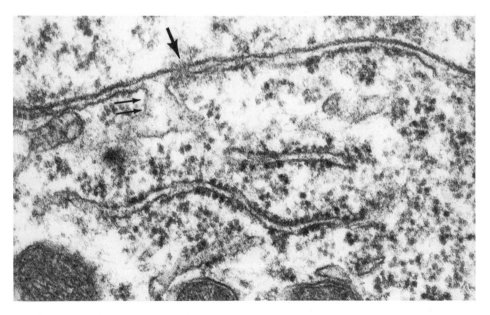

FIG. 5. Detail of the nuclear envelope showing a nuclear pore (*single arrow*) and the outer leaflet connected to smooth ER (*double arrows*). Two cisternae of rough ER with associated ribosomes are also present. ×80,000.

out the cytoplasm and are typical of most neurons are known collectively as Nissl substance (Figs. 4 and 5). The distribution of Nissl substance in certain neurons is characteristic and used as a criterion for identification. By electron microscopy (EM), this substance is seen to comprise regular arrays or scattered portions of flattened cisternae of rough ER, surrounded by clouds of free polyribosomes. The membranes of rough ER are studded with rows of ribosomes. A spacing of 20 to 40 nm is maintained within cisternae. Sometimes, cisternal walls meet at fenestrations. Unlike the rough ER of glandular cells or other protein-secreting cells, such as plasma cells, the rough ER of neurons probably produces most of its proteins for the neuron's own use, a feature imposed by the extraordinary functional demands placed on the cell. Nissl substance does not penetrate axons but does extend along dendrites.

Smooth ER. Most neurons contain at least a few cisternae of smooth (agranular) ER, sometimes difficult to differentiate from rough ER owing to disorderly arrangement of ribosomes. Ribosomes are not associated with these membranes and the cisternae usually assume a meandering, branching course throughout the cytoplasm. In some neurons, smooth ER is quite prominent, for example, in Purkinje cells. Individual cisterns of smooth ER extend along axons and dendrites. Smooth ER within axons has been implicated in protein transport.

Subsurface cisternae. Although not a constant feature, a system of smooth, membrane-bound, flattened cisternae can be found in many neurons. These structures, referred to as hypolemmal cisternae by Palay and Chan-Palay [1], abut the plasmalemma of the neuron and constitute a secondary membranous boundary within the cell. The distance between these cisternae and the plasmalemma is usually 10 to 12 nm, and on occasion, a mitochondrion may be found in close association with the innermost leaflet (e.g., in Purkinje cells). Similar cisternae have been described beneath synaptic complexes, but their functional significance is not known. Some authors have suggested that such a system may play a role in the uptake of metabolites.

Golgi apparatus. Undoubtedly the most impressive demonstration of the Golgi system, a highly specialized form of agranular reticulum, is achieved by using the metal impregnation techniques of Golgi. Ultrastructurally, the Golgi apparatus consists of aggregates of smooth-walled cisternae and a variety of vesicles. It is surrounded by a heterogeneous assemblage of organelles, including mitochondria, lysosomes, and multivesicular bodies. In most neurons, the Golgi apparatus encompasses the nucleus and extends into dendrites but is absent from axons. A three-dimensional analysis of the system reveals that the stacks of cisternae are pierced periodically by fenestrae. Tangential sections of these fenestrations show them to be circular profiles. A multitude of vesicles is associated with each segment of Golgi apparatus, in particular, "coated" vesicles, which proliferate from the lateral margins of flattened cisternae (Fig. 6). Such structures have been variously named, but the term alveolate vesicle seems to be generally accepted. Histochemical staining reveals that these bodies are rich in acid hydrolases, and they are believed to represent primary lysosomes [6]. Acid phosphatase is also found elsewhere in the cisternae but in lesser amounts than in alveolate vesicles.

Lysosomes. The principal organelle responsible for the degradation of cellular waste is the lysosome. It is a common constituent of all cell types of the nervous system and is particularly prominent in neurons, where it can be seen at various stages of development (Fig. 4). It ranges in size from 0.1 to 1 or 2 μm in diameter. The primary lysosome is elaborated from Golgi saccules as a small, vesicular structure (Fig. 6). Its function is to fuse with the membrane of waste-containing vacuoles (phagosomes), into which it releases hydrolytic enzymes. (This is discussed in Chap. 37). The se-

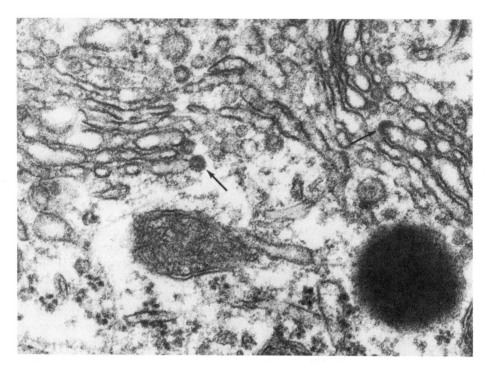

FIG. 6. A portion of a Golgi apparatus. The smooth-membraned cisternae appear beaded. The many circular profiles represent tangentially sectioned fenestrae and alveolate vesicles (primary lysosomes). Two of the latter can be seen budding from Golgi saccules (*arrows*). Mitochondria and a dense body (secondary lysosomes) are also present. ×60,000.

questered material is then degraded within the vacuole, and the organelle becomes a secondary lysosome and is usually electron dense and large. The matrix of this organelle will give a positive reaction when tested histochemically for acid phosphatase. Residual bodies containing nondegradable material are considered to be tertiary lysosomes, and in the neuron, some are represented by lipofuscin granules (Fig. 7). These granules contain brown pigment and lamellar stacks of membrane material and are more common in the aged brain. (For more details on lysosomes, the interested reader is referred to Novikoff and Holtzman [6]).

Multivesicular bodies. Multivesicular bodies are usually found in association with the Golgi apparatus and are visualized by EM as small, single membrane-bound sacs approximately 0.5 μm in diameter. They contain several minute, spherical profiles, sometimes arranged about the periphery. They are believed to belong to the lysosome series (prior to secondary lysosomes) because they contain acid hydrolases and are apparently derived from primary lysosomes.

Neurotubules. The neurotubule has been the subject of intense research in recent years [7]. Neurotubules are usually arranged haphazardly throughout the perikaryon of neurons but are aligned longitudinally in axons and dendrites. Each neurotubule consists of a dense-walled structure enclosing a clear lumen, in the middle of which may be found an electron-dense dot. Sometimes, axonal neurotubules display 5-

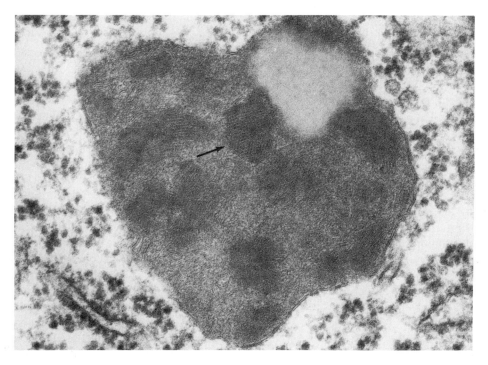

FIG. 7. A lipofuscin granule from a cortical neuron shows membrane-bound lipid (dense) and a soluble component (gray). The denser component is lamellated. The lamellae appear as paracrystalline arrays of tubular profiles when sectioned transversely (*arrow*). The granule is surrounded by a single unit membrane. Free ribosomes can also be seen. ×96,000.

nm filamentous interconnecting side-arms. The diameter of neurotubules varies between 22 and 24 nm. High-resolution studies indicate that each neurotubule wall consists of 13 filamentous subunits arranged helically around a lumen (see also Chap. 24).

Neurofilaments. Neurofilaments are usually found in association with neurotubules. The function of these two organelles has been debated for some time and although it seems reasonable to assume that they play a role in the maintenance of form, their role in axoplasmic transport remains to be clarified [8] (see Chap. 24). Neurofilaments have a diameter of approximately 10 nm, are of indeterminate length, and frequently occur in bundles. They are constant components of axons but are rarer in dendrites.

In the axon, individual filaments can be seen to possess a minute lumen and to be interconnected by proteinaceous side-arms, thereby forming a meshwork. Because of these cross-bridges, they do not form tightly packed bundles in the normal axon, in contrast to filaments within astrocytic processes (see Fig. 14), which lack cross-bridges. Neurofilaments within neuronal somata do not usually display cross-bridges and can be found in tight bundles. A form of filamentous structure finer than neurofilaments is seen at the tips of growing neurites, particularly in the growth cones of developing axons. These structures, known as microfilaments, are 5 nm in size and are composed of actin. They facilitate movement and growth, since it has been shown that axonal extension can be arrested pharmacologically by treatment with compounds that depolymerize these structures. The biochemistry of neurotubules and neurofilaments is dealt with in more detail in Soifer [7] and Wang et al. [8].

Mitochondria. Mitochondria are the centers for oxidative phosphorylation. These organelles occur ubiquitously in the neuron and its processes (Figs. 4 and 6). Their overall shape may change from one type of neuron to another, but their basic morphology is identical to that in other cell types. Mitochondria consist morphologically of double-membraned sacs surrounded by protuberances, or cristae, extending from the inner membrane into the matrix space. (The review by Novikoff and Holtzman [6] discusses in more detail the ultrastructure and enzymatic properties of mitochondria and the above cellular components.)

The axon

As the axon egresses, it becomes physiologically and structurally divisible into distinct regions: the axon hillock, the initial segment, the axon proper, and the axonal termination. (These segments are discussed in detail by Peters and co-workers [3].) Basically, the segments differ ultrastructurally in membrane morphology and the content of rough and smooth ER. The axon hillock may contain fragments of Nissl substance, including abundant ribosomes, which diminish as the hillock continues into the initial segment. Here, the various axoplasmic components begin to align longitudinally. A few ribosomes and smooth ER still persist, and some axoaxonic synapses occur. More interesting, however, is the axolemma of the initial segment, the region for the generation of the action potential, which is underlaid by a dense granular layer similar to that seen at the nodes of Ranvier. Also present in this region are neurotubules, neurofilaments, and mitochondria. The arrangement of the neurotubules in the in-

itial segment, unlike their scattered pattern in the distal axon, is in fascicles; they are interconnected by side-arms [3,8]. Beyond the initial segment, the axon maintains a relatively uniform morphology. It contains the axolemma (without any structural modification, except at nodes and the termination, where submembranous densities are seen); microtubules, sometimes cross-linked; neurofilaments, connected by side-arms; mitochondria; and tubulovesicular profiles, probably derived from smooth ER. Myelinated axons show granular densifications beneath and axolemma at the nodes of Ranvier [9], and synaptic complexes may also occur in the same regions. In myelinated fibers, there is a concentration of sodium channels at the nodal axon, a feature underlying the rapid (saltatory) conduction of such fibers [10] (see Chaps. 4 and 8). The terminal portion of the axon arborizes and enlarges at its synaptic regions, where it might contain synaptic vesicles beneath the specialized presynaptic junction.

The dendrite

The afferent components of neurons, dendrites are frequently arranged around the neuronal soma in stellate fashion. In some neurons, they may arise from a single trunk from which they branch into a dendritic tree. Unlike axons, they generally lack neurofilaments, although they may contain fragments of Nissl substance; however, larger branches of dendrites in close proximity to neurons may contain small bundles of neurofilaments. Some difficulty may be encountered in distinguishing small unmyelinated axons, terminal segments of axons, and small dendrites. In the absence of synaptic data, they can often be assessed by the content of neurofilaments. The synaptic regions of dendrites occur either along the main stems (Fig. 8) or at small protuberances known as dendritic spines or thorns. Axon terminals abut these structures.

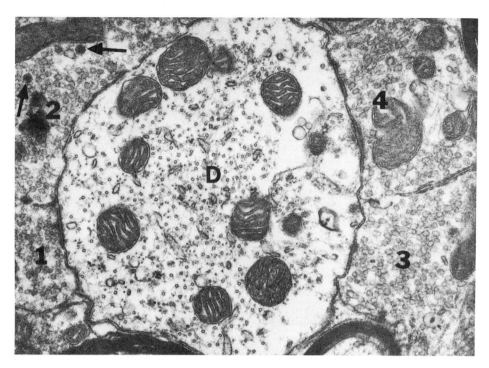

FIG. 8. A dendrite (D) emerging from a motor neuron in the anterior horn of a rat spinal cord is contacted by four axonal terminals. Terminal 1 contains clear spherical synaptic vesicles; terminals 2 and 3 contain both clear spherical and dense-core vesicles (*arrows*); and terminal 4 contains many clear flattened (inhibitory) synaptic vesicles. Note also the synaptic thickenings and, within the dendrite, the mitochondria, neurofilaments, and neurotubules. ×33,000.

The synapse

Axons and dendrites emerging from different neurons intercommunicate by means of specialized junctional complexes known as synapses. This was first proposed by Sherrington in 1897, who also proposed the term synapse. The existence of synapses was immediately demonstrable by EM and can be recognized today in a dynamic fashion by Nomarski optics by light microscopy and by scanning EM. With the development of neurochemical approaches to neurobiology (see Chap. 9), an understanding of synaptic form and function becomes of fundamental importance. As was noted in the first ultrastructural study on synapses (Palade and Palay in 1954, quoted in Mugnaini and Walberg [4]), synapses display interface specialization and are frequently polarized or asymmetrical. The asymmetry is due to the unequal distribution of electron-dense (osmiophilic) material, or thickening, applied to the apposing membranes of the junctional complex and the heavier accumulation of organelles within the presynaptic (usually axonal) component. The closely applied membranes constituting the synaptic site are overlaid on the presynaptic and postsynaptic aspects by an osmiophilic material similar to that seen in desmosomes (see section on ependymal cells, below) and are separated by a gap (cleft) between 15 and 20 nm. The presynaptic component usually contains a collection of clear, 40 to 50-nm synaptic vesicles and several small mitochondria approximately 0.2 to 0.5 μm in diameter (Figs. 8–10). Occasional 24-nm microtubules, coated vesicles, and cisternae of smooth ER are not uncommon in this region. On the postsynaptic side is a density referred to as the subsynaptic web, but apart from an infrequent, closely applied packet of smooth ER (subsurface cisterna) belonging to the hypolemmal system, there are no aggregations of organelles in the dendrite.

At the neuromuscular junction, the morphological organization is somewhat different. Here the axon terminal is greatly enlarged and it is ensheathed by Schwann cells; the postsynaptic (sarcolemma) membrane displays less density and is extensively infolded.

Before elaborating further on synaptic diversity, it might be helpful to outline briefly other ways in which synapses have been classified in the past. Using the light microscope,

Ramón y Cajal [11] was able to identify 11 distinct groups of synapses. Today, most neuroanatomists apply a more fundamental classification schema to synapses, depending on the profiles between which the synapse is formed (i.e., axodendritic, axosomatic, axoaxonic, dendrodendritic, somatosomatic, and somatodendritic). Unfortunately, such a list totally disregards the type of transmission (chemical or electrical) and, in the case of chemical synapses, the neurotransmitter involved.

In terms of physiologic typing, three groups of synapses are recognized: excitatory, inhibitory, and modulatory. Some neuroanatomical studies [11] on excitatory and inhibitory synapses have claimed that excitatory synapses possess spherical synaptic vesicles, whereas inhibitory synapses contain a predominance of flattened vesicles (Fig. 8). Other studies (e.g., Gray [12]) have correlated this synaptic vesicular diversity with physiologic data. In his study on cerebellum, Gray showed that neurons, with a known predominance of excitatory input on

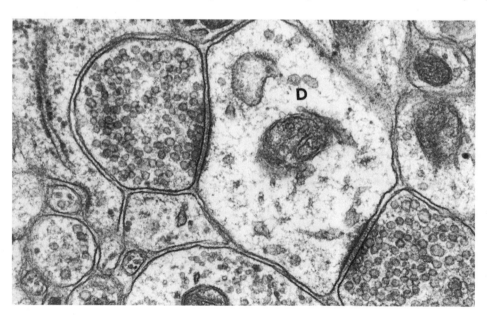

FIG. 9.   A dendrite (D) is flanked by two axon terminals packed with clear spherical synaptic vesicles. Details of the synaptic region are clearly shown. ×75,000.

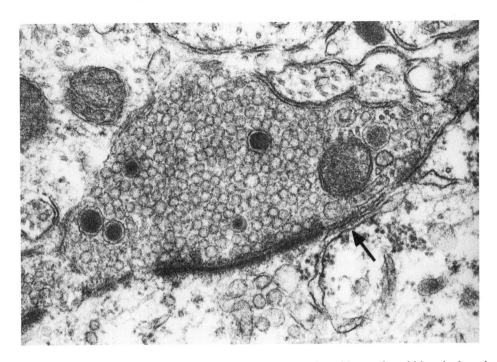

FIG. 10. An axonal terminal at the surface of a neuron from the dorsal horn of a rabbit spinal cord contains both dense-core and clear spherical synaptic vesicles lying above the membrane thickenings. A subsurface cisterna (*arrow*) is also seen. ×68,000.

dendrites and an inhibitory input on the cell body, possessed two corresponding types of synapses; however, although this interpretation fits well in some loci of the CNS, it does not hold true for all regions. Furthermore, some workers feel that the differences between flat and spherical vesicles may reflect an artifact of aldehyde fixation or a difference in physiologic state at the time of sampling. In the light of these criticisms, it is clear that further confirmation as to the correlation between flattened vesicles and inhibitory synapses is required.

Another criterion for the classification of synapses by EM was introduced in 1959 by Gray [12]. Briefly, certain synapses in the cerebral cortex can be grouped into two types, depending on the length of the contact area between synaptic membranes and the amount of postsynaptic thickening. Relationships have been found between type 1—the membranes of which are closely apposed for long distances and have a large amount of associated postsynaptic thickening—and excitatory axodendritic synapses. Type 2 synapses, conversely, are mainly axosomatic, show less close apposition and thickening at the junction, and are believed to be inhibitory. This broad grouping has been confirmed in the cerebral cortex by a number of workers, but it does not hold true for all regions of the CNS.

Most of the data from studies on synapse *in situ* or on synaptosomes (see Section II) have been on cholinergic transmission. Our understanding of the vast family of chemical synapses belonging to the autonomic nervous system that utilize biogenic amines (Chap. 11) as neurotransmitter substances is still in its infancy. Morphologically, catecholaminergic synapses are similar but possess, in addition to clear vesicles, slightly larger dense-core or granular vesicles of variable dimension (Figs. 8 and 10). These vesicles were first identified as synaptic vesicles by Grillo and Palay (see Bloom [13]), who segregated classes of granular vesicles based on vesicle and core size, but no relationship was made between granular vesicles and transmitter substances. About the same time, EM autoradiographic techniques were being employed and, using tritiated norepinephrine, Wolfe and co-workers [14] labeled granular vesicles within axonal terminals. Since this work, other labeling techniques for aminergic synapses have been developed. Several of the methods and requirements for detecting such transmitters have been reviewed by Bloom [13]. Catecholaminergic vesicles are generally classified on a size basis, and not all have dense cores. Another, still unclassified, category of

synapses may be the so-called silent synapses observed in CNS tissue both *in vitro* and *in vivo*. These synapses are morphologically identical to functional synapses but are physiologically dormant.

Finally, with regard to synaptic type, there is the well-characterized electrical synapse [15], where current can pass from cell to cell across regions of membrane apposition that essentially lack the associated collections of organelles present at the chemical synapse. In the electrical synapse (Fig. 11), the unit membranes are closely apposed, and, indeed, the outer leaflets sometimes fuse to form a pentalaminar structure; however, in most places, a gap of approximately 20 nm exists, producing a so-called gap junction. Not infrequently, such gap junctions are separated by desmosome-like regions [3]. Sometimes, electrical synapses exist at terminals that also display typical chemical synapses;

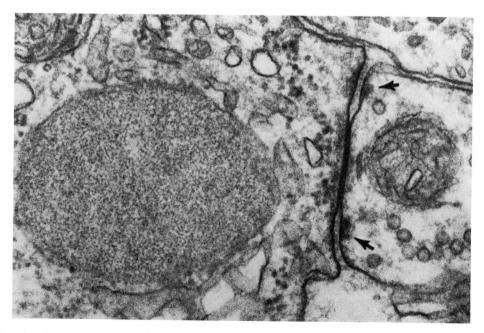

FIG. 11.   An electrotonic synapse is seen at the surface of a motor neuron from the spinal cord of a toadfish. Between the neuronal soma (*left*) and the axonal termination (*right*), a gap junction flanked by desmosomes (*arrows*) is visible. (Photography courtesy of Drs. G. D. Pappas and J. S. Keeter.) ×80,000.

in such cases, the structure is referred to as a mixed synapse. The comparative morphology of electrical and chemical synapses has been reviewed by Pappas and Waxman [15].

CHARACTERISTICS OF NEUROGLIA

In 1846, Virchow first recognized the existence in the CNS of a fragile, nonnervous, interstitial component made up of stellate or spindle-shaped cells, morphologically distinct from neurons, which he named neuroglia ("nerve glue"). It was not until the early part of the twentieth century that this interstitial element was classified as distinct cell types [3,4]. Today, we recognize three broad groups of glial cells: (1) true glial cells (macroglia), such as astrocytes and oligodendrocytes, of ectodermal origin; (2) microglia, of mesodermal origin; and (3) ependymal cells, also of ectodermal origin and sharing the same stem cell as true glia (e.g., the spongioblast). Microglia invade the CNS at the time of vascularization via the pia mater, the walls of blood vessels, and the tela choroidea.

Glial cells differ from neurons in that they possess no synaptic contacts and retain the ability to divide throughout life, particularly in response to injury. The rough schema represented by Fig. 3 demonstrates the interrelationships between the macroglia and other CNS components.

Virtually nothing can enter or leave the CNS parenchyma without passing through an astrocytic interphase

The complex packing achieved by the processes and cell bodies of astrocytes underscores their involvement in brain metabolism. Although astrocytes have traditionally been subdivided into protoplasmic and fibrous astrocytes [4], these two forms probably represent the opposite ends of a spectrum of the same cell type. However, Raff et al. [16] have suggested that the two groups of astrocytes might derive from different progenitors and that the progenitor of the fibrous astrocyte is the same as that of the oligodendrocyte. The structural components of fibrous and protoplasmic astrocytes are identical; the differences are quantitative. In the early days of EM, differences between the two variants were more apparent owing to imprecise techniques but with the development of better procedures, the differences became less apparent.

Protoplasmic astrocytes range in size from 10 to 40 μm, are frequently located in gray matter in relation to capillaries, and have a clearer cytoplasm than do fibrous astrocytes (Fig. 12). Within the perikaryon of both types of astrocytes are scattered 9-nm filaments and 24-nm microtubules (Fig. 13); glycogen granules; lysosomes and lipofuscin-like bodies; isolated cisternae of rough ER; a small Golgi apparatus opposite one pole of the nucleus; and small, elongated mitochondria, often extending together with loose bundles of filaments along cell processes. A centriole is not uncommon. Characteristically, the nucleus is ovoid and the nucleochromatin homogeneous, except for a narrow continuous rim of dense chromatin and one or two poorly defined nucleoli. The fibrous astrocyte occurs in white matter (Fig. 13). Its processes are twig-like, being composed of large numbers of 9-nm glial filaments arranged in tight bundles. The filaments within these cell processes can be distinguished from neurofilaments by their close packing and the absence of side-arms (Figs. 13 and 14). Desmosomes and gap junctions occur between adjacent astrocytic processes.

In addition to protoplasmic and fibrous forms, regional specialization occurs among astrocytes. The outer membranes of astrocytes located in subpial zones and adjacent to blood vessels possess a specialized thickening. Desmosomes and gap junctions are very common in these regions between astrocytic processes. In the cerebellar cortex, protoplasmic astro-

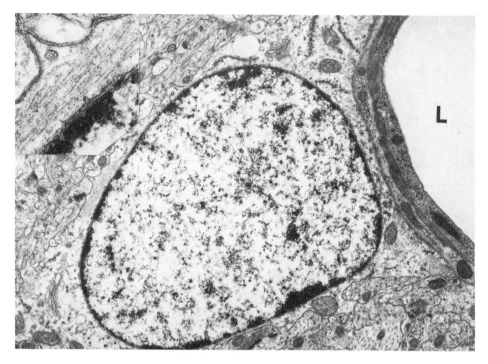

FIG. 12.   A protoplasmic astrocyte abuts a blood vessel (lumen at L) in rat cerebral cortex. The nucleus shows a rim of denser chromatin, and the cytoplasm contains many organelles, including Golgi and rough ER. ×10,000. **Inset:** Detail of perinuclear cytoplasm showing filaments. ×44,000.

cytes can be segregated into three classes—the Golgi epithelial cell, the lamellar or velate astrocyte, and the smooth astrocyte [1]—each ultrastructurally distinct.

Astrocyte function

The functions of astrocytes have long been debated. Their major role is related to a connective tissue or skeletal function, since they invest, possibly sustain, and provide a packing for other CNS components. In the case of astrocytic ensheathment around synaptic complexes and the bodies of some neurons (e.g., Purkinje cells), it may be speculated that the astrocyte serves to isolate these structures.

One well-known function of the astrocyte is concerned with repair. Subsequent to trauma, astrocytes invariably proliferate, swell, accumulate glycogen, and undergo fibrosis by the accumulation of filaments, expressed neurochemically as an increase in glial fibrillary acidic protein (GFAP). This state of gliosis may be total, in which case all other elements are lost, leaving a glial scar, or it may be a generalized response occurring against a background of regenerated or normal CNS parenchyma. Fibrous astrocytosis can occur in both the gray and white matter, thereby indicating common links between protoplasmic and fibrous astrocytes. With age, both fibrous and protoplasmic astrocytes accumulate filaments. In some diseases, astrocytes have been shown to become macrophages. It is interesting to note that the astrocyte is probably the most disease-resistant component in the CNS because very few diseases (one of them, alcoholism) cause depletion of astrocytes.

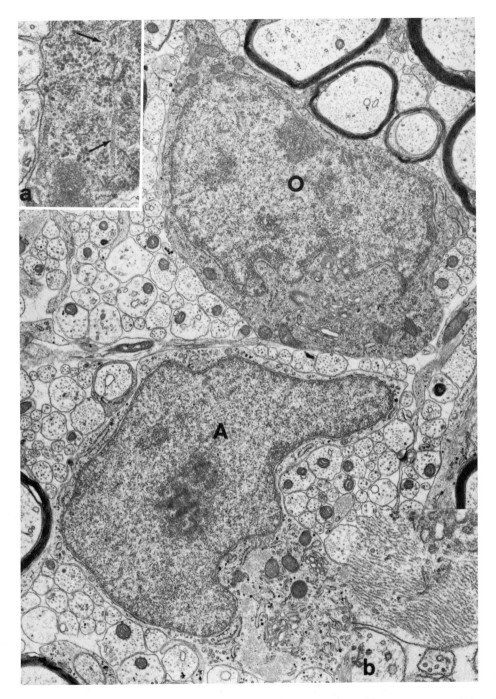

FIG. 13. A section of myelinating white matter from a kitten contains a fibrous astrocyte (A) and an oligodendrocyte (O). The nucleus of the astrocyte (A) has homogeneous chromatin with a denser rim and a central nucleolus. That of the oligodendrocyte (O) is denser and more heterogeneous. Note the denser oligodendrocytic cytoplasm and the prominent filaments within the astrocyte. ×15,000. **Inset a:** Detail of the oligodendrocyte, showing microtubules (*arrows*) and absence of filaments. ×45,000. **Inset b:** Detail of astrocytic cytoplasm showing filaments, glycogen, rough ER, and Golgi apparatus. ×45,000.

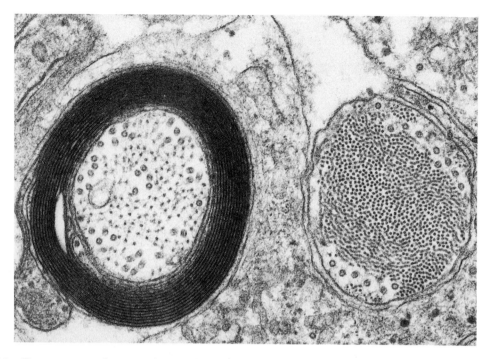

FIG. 14. Transverse sections are shown of a myelinated axon (*left*) and the process of a fibrous astrocyte (*right*) in dog spinal cord. The axon contains scattered neurotubules and loosely-packed neurofilaments interconnected by side-arm material. The astrocytic process contains a bundle of closely-packed filaments with no cross-bridges, flanked by several microtubules. Sometimes, a lumen can be seen within a filament. ×60,000.

Another putative role of the astrocyte is its involvement in transport mechanisms and in the blood-brain barrier system. It was believed for some time that transport of water and electrolytes was effected by the astrocyte, a fact never definitively demonstrated and largely inferred from pathological or experimental evidence. It is known, for example, that damage to the brain vasculature, local injury due to heat or cold, and inflammatory changes produce focal swelling of astrocytes, presumably owing to disturbances in fluid transport. The astrocytic investment of blood vessels might suggest a role in the blood-brain barrier system, but the studies of Reese and Karnovsky [17] and Brightman [18] indicate that the astrocytic end-feet provide little resistance to the movement of molecules and that

blockage of the passage of material into the brain occurs at the endothelial cell-lining blood vessels (see Chap. 30). Finally, it is believed that astrocytes are responsible for the regulation of local pH levels and local ionic balances.

Oligodendrocytes are myelin-producing cells in the CNS

The ultrastructural studies of Schultz and co-workers (1957) and Farquhar and Hartman in 1957 (discussed in Mugnaini and Walberg [4]) were among the first to contrast the EM features of oligodendrocytes with astrocytes (Fig. 12). The study of Mugnaini and Walberg [4] more explicitly laid down the morphological criteria for identifying these cells and, apart from subsequent technical improvements, our EM understanding of these cells has changed little since that time [5,19].

As with the astrocytes, oligodendrocytes are highly variable, differing in location, morphology, and function, but definable by some morphological criteria. The cell soma ranges from 10 to 20 μm and is roughly globular and more dense than that of an astrocyte. The margin of the cell is irregular and compressed against the adjacent neuropil. Few cell processes are seen, in contrast to the astrocyte. Within the cytoplasm, many organelles are found. Parallel cisterns of rough ER and a widely dispersed Golgi apparatus are common. Free ribosomes occur, scattered amid occasional multivesicular bodies, mitochondria, and coated vesicles. Serving to distinguish the oligodendrocyte from the astrocyte is the apparent absence of glial filaments and the constant presence of 24-nm microtubules (Fig. 13), most common at the margins of the cell, in the occasional cell process, and in the cytoplasmic loops around myelin sheaths. Lamellar dense bodies typical of oligodendrocytes are also present [5]. The nucleus is usually ovoid, but slight lobation is not uncommon. The nucleochromatin stains heavily and contains clumps of denser heterochromatin; the whole structure is sometimes difficult to discern from the background cytoplasm. Desmosomes and gap junctions occur between interfascicular oligodendrocytes [5].

Ultrastructural studies on the developing nervous system and labeling studies have demonstrated variability in oligodendrocyte morphology and activity. Mori and Leblond (see Raine [5]) separated oligodendrocytes into three groups based on location, stainability, and DNA turnover. Their three classes correspond to satellite, intermediate, and interfascicular (myelinating) oligodendrocytes. Satellite oligodendrocytes are small (~10 μm), restricted to gray matter, and closely applied to the surface of neurons. They are assumed to play a role in the maintenance of the neuron and are also known

to be potential myelinating cells. Interfascicular oligodendrocytes are large (~20 μm) during myelination but, in the adult, range from 10 to 15 μm, with the nucleus occupying a large percentage of the cell volume. Intermediate oligodendrocytes are regarded as satellite or potential myelinating forms. The nucleus of these cells is small, the cytoplasm occupying the greater area of the soma.

Oligodendrocytes and myelin

Myelinating oligodendrocytes have been studied extensively [5,20]. Examination of the CNS during myelinogenesis (Fig. 15) reveals connections between the cell body and the myelin sheath [21]; however, connections between these elements have never been demonstrated in a normal adult animal, unlike the PNS counterpart, the Schwann cell. In contrast to the Schwann cell (see below), the oligodendrocyte is capable of producing many internodes of myelin simultaneously. It is estimated that oligodendrocytes in the optic nerve might produce between 30 and 50 internodes of myelin [5]. In addition to this heavy structural commitment, the oligodendrocyte is known to possess a slow mitotic rate and a poor regenerative capacity. Damage to only a few oligodendrocytes can therefore be expected to produce an appreciable area of primary demyelination. In most CNS diseases in which myelin is a target, oligodendrocytes are known to be among the most vulnerable elements and the first to degenerate.

Somewhat analogous to the neuron, the relatively small oligodendrocyte soma produces and supports many more times it own volume of membrane and cytoplasm. For example, consider an average 12-μm oligodendrocyte producing 20 internodes of myelin (the lowest number quoted by Peters and Proskauer; see Raine [5]). Each axon has a diameter of 3 μm (small for CNS fibers) and is covered by six lamellae of myelin (a conservative estimate), each lamella representing two fused layers of unit

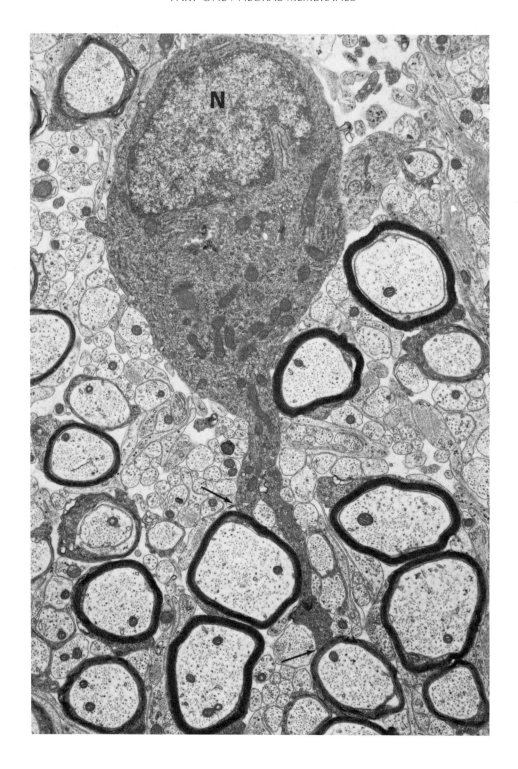

membrane. By statistical analysis, taking into account the length of myelin internode (possibly 500 μm) and the length of the membranes of the cell processes connecting the sheaths to the cell body (~12 μm), the ratio between the surface area of the cell soma and the myelin it sustains is approximately 1:620. In most cases, however, this ratio is probably in the region of 1:3,000. In rare instances, oligodendrocytes have been shown to elaborate myelin around structures other than axons in that myelin has been documented around neuronal somata and nonaxonal profiles. (Myelin formation is discussed in Chap. 6.)

The microglial cell plays a role in phagocytosis and inflammatory responses

Of the few remaining types of CNS cells, the most interesting, and probably the most enigmatic, is the microglial cell, a cell of mesodermal origin, located in the normal brain in a resting state and purported to become a very mobile, active macrophage during disease. Microglia can be selectively stained and demonstrated by light microscopy using Hortega's silver carbonate method, but no comparable technique exists for their ultrastructural demonstration. The cells have spindle-shaped bodies and a thin rim of densely staining cytoplasm difficult to distinguish from the nucleus. The nucleochromatin is homogeneously dense, and the cytoplasm does not contain an abundance of organelles, although representatives of the usual components can be found. During normal wear and tear, some CNS elements degenerate, and microglia phagocytose the debris (Fig. 16). Their identification and numbers (as determined by light microscopy) differ from species to species. The rabbit CNS is known to be richly endowed. In a number of disease instances (e.g.,

trauma), microglia are known to be stimulated and to migrate to the area of injury, where they phagocytose debris. The relatively brief mention of this cell type in the major EM text books [3] and the conflicting EM descriptions [22] are indicative of the uncertainty attached to their identification. Pericytes, the pericapillary macrophages, are believed to be a resting form of microglial cell.

Ependymal cells line the ventricles and the central canal of the spinal cord

Ependymal cells are arranged in single-palisade arrays and line the ventricles of the brain and central canal of the spinal cord. They are usually ciliated, their cilia extending into the ventricular cavity. Their fine structure has been elucidated by Brightman and Palay [23]. They possess several features that clearly differentiate them from any other CNS cell. The cilia emerge from the apical pole of the cell, where they are attached to a blepharoplast, the basal body (Fig. 17), which is anchored in the cytoplasm by means of ciliary rootlets and a basal foot. The basal foot is the contractile component that determines the direction of the ciliary beat. Like all flagellar structures, the cilium contains the common microtubule arrangement of nine peripheral pairs around a central doublet (Fig. 17). In the vicinity of the basal body, the arrangement is one of nine triplets; at the tip of each cilium the pattern is one of haphazardly organized single tubules. Also extending from the free surface of the cell are numerous microvilli containing actin microfilaments (Fig. 17). The cytoplasm stains intensely, having an electron density about equal to that of the oligodendrocyte, whereas the nucleus is similar to that of the astrocyte. Microtubules, large whorls of filaments, coated vesicles, rough ER; Golgi apparatus; lysosomes, and abundant

FIG. 15. A myelinating oligodendrocyte, nucleus (N), from the spinal cord of a 2-day-old kitten extends cytoplasmic connections to a least two myelin sheaths (*arrows*). Other myelinated and unmyelinated fibers at various stages of development, as well as glial processes, are seen in the surrounding neuropil. ×12,750.

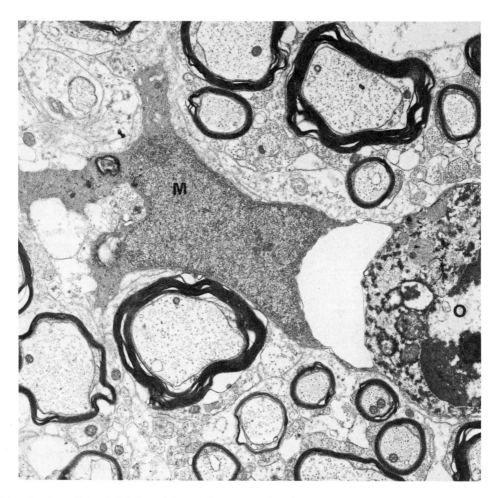

FIG. 16. A microglial cell (M) has elaborated two cytoplasmic arms to encompass a degenerating oligodendrocyte (O) in the spinal cord of a 3-day-old kitten. The microglial cell nucleus is difficult to distinguish from the narrow rim of densely staining cytoplasm, which also contains some membranous debris. × 10,000.

small, dense mitochondria are also present. The base of the cell is composed of involuted processes that interdigitate with the underlying neuropil. The lateral margins of each cell characteristically display long, compound, junctional complexes (Fig. 18) made up of desmosomes (zonulae adhaerentes) and tight junctions (zonulae occludentes).

The biochemical properties of these structures are well known. Desmosomes display protease sensitivity, divalent cation dependency, and osmotic insensitivity, whereas the membranes are mainly of the smooth type. In direct contrast to desmosomes, the tight junction (and also gap junctions and synapses) displays no protease sensitivity, divalent cation dependency, nor osmotic sensitivity, whereas the membranes are complex. These facts have been used in the development of techniques to isolate purified preparations of junctional complexes.

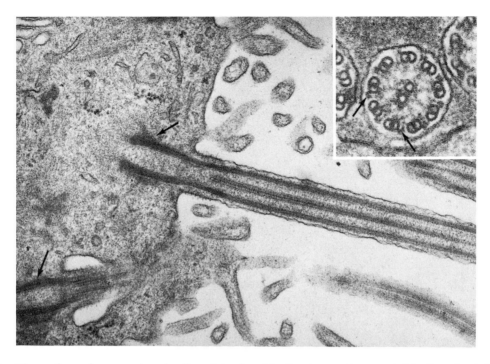

FIG. 17. The surface of an ependymal cell contains basal bodies (*arrows*) connected to the microtubules of cilia, seen here in longitudinal section. Several microvilli are also present. ×37,000. **Inset:** Ependymal cilia in transverse section possess a central doublet of microtubules surrounded by nine pairs, one of each pair having a characteristic hook-like appendage (*arrows*). ×100,000.

The Schwann cell is the myelin-producing cell of the PNS

When axons leave the CNS, they lose their neuroglial interrelationships and traverse a short transitional zone, where they are invested by an astroglial sheath enclosed in the basal lamina of the glia limitans. The basal lamina then becomes continuous with that of axon-investing Schwann cells, at which point the astroglial covering terminates. Schwann cells, therefore, are the axon-ensheathing cells of the PNS, equivalent functionally to the oligodendrocyte of the CNS. Along the myelinated fibers of the PNS, each internode of myelin is elaborated by one Schwann cell and each Schwann cell elaborates one internode. This ratio of one internode of myelin to one Schwann cell is a fundamental distinction between this cell type and its CNS analog, the oligodendrocyte, which is able to proliferate internodes in the ratio of 1:30 or greater. Another distinction is that the Schwann cell body always remains in intimate contact with its myelin internode (Fig. 19), whereas the oligodendrocyte extends processes toward its internodes. Periodically, myelin lamellae open up into ridges of Schwann cell cytoplasm, producing bands of cytoplasm around the fiber, Schmidt-Lanterman incisures, reputed to be the stretch points along PNS fibers. These incisures are usually not present in the CNS. The PNS myelin period is 11.9 nm in preserved specimens (some 30 percent less than in the fresh state), in contrast to the 10.6 nm of central myelin. In

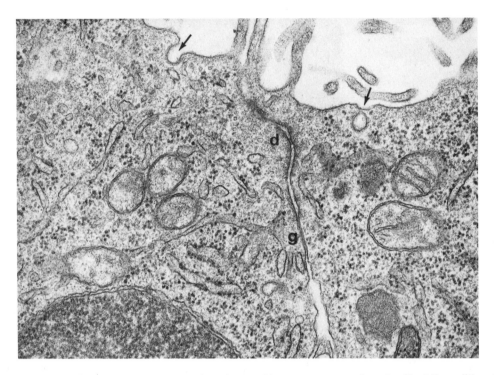

FIG. 18.   A typical desmosome (d) and gap junction (g) between two ependymal cells. Microvilli and coated pits (*arrows*) are seen along the cell surface. ×35,000.

addition to these structural differences, PNS myelin is known to differ biochemically and antigenically from that of the CNS (see Chaps. 6 and 31). Not all PNS fibers are myelinated, but in contrast to nonmyelinated fibers in the CNS, nonmyelineated fibers in the PNS are suspended in groups within Schwann cell cytoplasm, each axon connected to the extracellular space by a short channel, the mesaxon, formed by the invaginated Schwann cell plasmalemma.

Ultrastructurally, the Schwann cell is unique and distinct from the oligodendrocyte. Each Schwann cell is surrounded by a basal lamina made up of mucopolysaccharide approximately 20 to 30 nm thick that does not extend into the mesaxon (Fig. 19). The basal laminae of adjacent myelinating Schwann cells at the nodes of Ranvier are continuous, and Schwann cell processes (''fingers'') interdigi-

tate so that the PNS myelinated axon is never in direct contact with the extracellular space. These nodal Schwann cell fingers display intimate relationships with the axolemma (Figs. 20 and 21), suggesting that the entire nodal complex might serve as an electrogenic pump for the recycling of ions [9]. A similar arrangement between the nodal axon and the fingers of astroglial cells is seen in the CNS. The Schwann cells of nonmyelinated PNS fibers overlap, and there are no nodes of Ranvier.

The cytoplasm of the Schwann cell is rich in organelles. A Golgi apparatus is located near the nucleus, and cisternae of rough ER occur throughout the cell. Lysosomes, multivesicular bodies, glycogen granules, and lipid granules (pi granules) can also be seen. The cell is rich in filaments (in contrast to the oligodendrocyte) and microtubules. The plasmalemma frequently

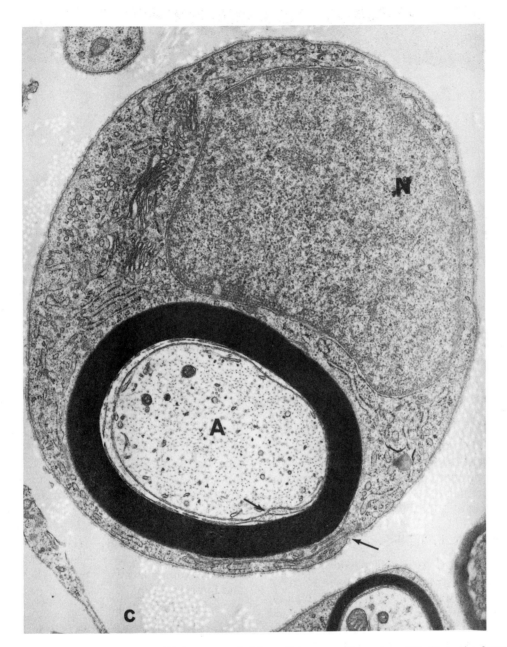

FIG. 19. A myelinated PNS axon (A) is surrounded by a Schwann cell, nucleus (N). Note the fuzzy basal lamina around the cell, the rich cytoplasm, the inner and outer mesaxons (*arrows*), the close proximity of the cell to its myelin sheath, and the 1:1 (cell-myelin internode) relationship. A process of an endoneurial cell is seen (*lower left*), and unstained collagen (c) lies in the endoneurial space (*white dots*). ×20,000.

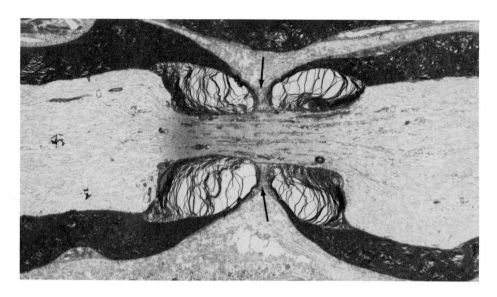

FIG. 20. Low-power electron micrograph of a node of Ranvier in longitudinal section. Note the abrupt decrease in internodal axon diameter where it becomes paranodal and the attendant condensation of axoplasmic constituents. Paranodal myelin is artifactually distorted, a common phenomenon in large-diameter fibers. The nodal gap substance (*arrows*) contains Schwann cell fingers; the nodal axon is bulbous; and lysosomes lie beneath the axolemma within the bulge. Beaded smooth ER sacs are also seen. ×5,000.

shows pinocytic vesicles. Small, round mitochondria are scattered throughout the soma. The nucleus, which stains intensely, is flattened, and oriented longitudinally along the nerve fiber. Aggregates of dense heterochromatin are arranged peripherally. (Additional details concerning the Schwann cells are outlined by Peters et al. [3].)

Schwann cells during disease

In sharp contrast to the oligodendrocyte, the Schwann cell responds vigorously to most forms of injury (see Chap. 36). An active phase of mitosis occurs following traumatic insult, and the cells are capable of local migration. Studies on their behavior after primary demyelination have shown that they are able to phagocytose damaged myelin. They possess remarkable reparatory properties and begin to lay down new myelin approximately 1 week after a fiber loses its myelin sheath. Studies on PNS and CNS remyelination [24] have shown that by 3 months after primary demyelination, PNS fibers are well remyelinated, whereas similarly affected areas in the CNS show relatively little proliferation of new myelin. Under circumstances of severe injury (e.g., transection), axons degenerate, and the Schwann cells form tubes (Bungner bands) containing cell bodies and processes surrounded by a single basal lamina. These structures provide channels along which regenerating axons might later grow. The presence and integrity of the Schwann cell basal lamina is essential for reinnervation.

Other PNS elements

The extracellular space between PNS nerve fibers is occupied by bundles of collagen fibrils, blood vessels, and endoneurial cells [25]. Endoneurial cells are elongated spindle-shaped

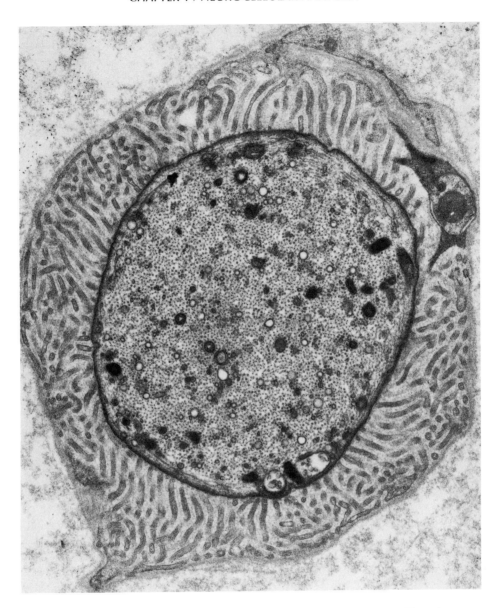

FIG. 21. A transverse section of the node of Ranvier (7–8 μm across) of a large fiber shows a prominent complex of Schwann cell fingers around an axon highlighted by its subaxolemmal densification and closely packed organelles. The Schwann cell fingers arise from an outer collar of flattened cytoplasm and abut the axon at regular intervals of approximately 80 nm. The basal lamina of the nerve fiber encircles the entire complex. The nodal gap substance is granular and sometimes linear. Within the axoplasm, note the transversely sectioned sacs of beaded smooth ER, mitochondria, dense lamellar bodies (which appear to maintain a peripheral location), flattened smooth ER sacs, dense-core vesicles, cross-bridged neurofilaments, and microtubules, which in places run parallel to the circumference of the axon (*above left* and *lower right*), perhaps in a spiral fashion. ×16,000.

cells with tenuous processes relatively poor in organelles except for large cisternae of rough ER. There is some evidence that these cells proliferate collagen fibrils. Sometimes mast cells, the histamine producers of connective tissue, can be seen. Bundles of nerve fibers are arranged in fascicles emarginated by flattened connective tissue cells forming the perineurium, an essential component in the blood-nerve barrier system. Fascicles of nerve fibers are aggregated into nerves and invested by a tough elastic sheath of cells known as the epineurium.

ACKNOWLEDGMENTS

The excellent technical assistance of Everett Swanson, Howard Finch, and Miriam Pakingan is appreciated. I thank Michele Briggs for her secretarial assistance.

The work represented by this chapter was supported in part by USPHS Grants NS 08952 and NS 11920; and NMSS RG 1001-F-6 from the National Multiple Sclerosis Society.

REFERENCES

1. Palay, S. L., and Chan-Palay, V. *Cerebellar Cortex: Cytology and Organization.* New York: Springer, 1974.
2. Hyden, H. The neuron. In J. Brachet and A. E. Mirsky (eds.), *The Cell.* New York: Academic, 1960. Vol. 5, pp. 215–323.
3. Peters, A., Palay, S. L., and Webster, H. de F. *The Fine Structure of the Nervous System: The Cells and Their Processes.* New York: Harper & Row, 1970.
4. Mugnaini, E., and Walberg, F. Ultrastructure of neuroglia. *Ergeb. Anat. Entwicklungsgesch.* 37:194–236, 1964.
5. Raine, S. C. Oligodendrocytes and central nervous system myelin. In R. L. Davis and D. M. Robertson (eds.), *Textbook of Neuropathology.* Baltimore: Williams & Wilkins, 1982, pp. 92–116.
6. Novikoff, A. B., and Holtzman, E. *Cells and Organelles.* New York: Holt, Rinehart and Winston, 1976.
7. Soifer, D. (ed.), Dynamic Aspects of Microtubule Biology. *Ann. N.Y. Acad. Sci.* 466, 1986.
8. Wang, E., Fischman, B., Liem, R. L. and Sun, T.-T. (eds.), Intermediate Filaments. *Ann. N.Y. Acad. Sci.* 455, 1985.
9. Raine, C. S. Differences in the nodes of Ranvier of large and small diameters fibres in the PNS. *J. Neurocytol.* 11:935–947, 1982.
10. Ritchie, J. M. Physiological basis of conduction in myelinated nerve fibers. In P. Morrell (ed.), *Myelin.* New York: Plenum, 1984, pp. 117–146.
11. Bodian, D. Synaptic diversity and characterization by electron microscopy. In G. D. Pappas and D. P. Purpura (eds.), *Structure and Function of Synapses.* New York: Raven, 1972, pp. 45–65.
12. Gray, E. G. Electron microscopy of excitatory and inhibitory synapses: A brief review. *Prog. Brain Res.* 31:141, 1969.
13. Bloom, F. E. Localization of neurotransmitters by electron microscopy. In *Neurotransmitters (Proc. ARNMD).* Baltimore: Williams & Wilkins, 1972, Vol. 50, pp. 25–57.
14. Wolfe, D. E., Potter, L. T., Richardson, K. C., and Axelrod, J. Localizing tritiated norepinephrine in sympathetic axons by electron microscopic autoradiography. *Science* 138:440–442, 1962.
15. Pappas, G. D., and Waxman, S. Synaptic fine structure: Morphological correlates of chemical and electronic transmission. In G. D. Pappas and D. P. Purpura (eds.), *Structure and Function of Synapses.* New York: Raven, 1972, pp. 1–43.
16. Raff, M. C., Miller, R. H., and Noble, M. A. Glial progenitor cell that develops in vitro into an astrocyte or an oligodendrocyte depending on culture medium. *Nature* 303:390–396, 1983.
17. Reese, T. S., and Karnovsky, M. J. Fine structural localization of a blood-brain barrier to exogenous peroxidase. *J. Cell Biol.* 34:207–217, 1967.
18. Brightman, M. The distribution within the brain of ferritin injected into cerebrospinal fluid compartments. II. Parenchymal distribution. *Am. J. Anat.* 117:193–220, 1965.
19. Norton, W. T. (ed.), Oligodendroglia (*Advances*

in Neurochemistry, Vol 5). New York: Plenum, 1984.

20. Raine, C. S. Morphology of myelin and myelination. In P. Morell (ed.), *Myelin*, 2nd ed. New York: Plenum Press, 1984, pp. 1–50.

21. Bunge, R. P. Glial cells and the central myelin sheath. *Physiol. Rev.* 48:197–248, 1968.

22. Fujita, S., and Kitamura, T. Origin of brain macrophages and the nature of the microglia. In Zimmerman, H. (ed.), *Progress in Neuropathology*. New York: Grune and Stratton, 1976, Vol. 2, pp. 1–50.

23. Brightman, M., and Palay, S. L. The fine structure of ependyma in the brain of the rat. *J. Cell Biol.* 19:415–440, 1963.

24. Raine, C. S., Wisniewski, H., and Prineas, J. An ultrastructural study of experimental demyelination and remyelination. II. Chronic experimental allergic encephalomyelitis in the peripheral nervous system. *Lab Invest.* 21:316–327, 1969.

25. Babel, J., Bischoff, A., and Spoendlin, H. Ultrastructure of the peripheral nervous system and sense organs. In *Atlas of Normal and Pathologic Anatomy*. St. Louis: Mosby, pp. 1–171, 1970.

CHAPTER 2

Cell Membrane Structure and Functions

R. Wayne Albers

Basic Neurochemistry: Molecular, Cellular, and Medical Aspects, 4th Ed., edited by G. J. Siegel et al. Raven Press, Ltd., New York, 1989. Correspondence to R. Wayne Albers, Laboratory of Neurochemistry, National Institute of Neurological and Communicative Disorders and Stroke, National Institutes of Health, Bldg. 36, Rm. 4D-20, Bethesda, Maryland 20892.

In addition to the selective detection of environmental inputs, neurons integrate these inputs over both space and time before transmitting the resultant signals to other cells. All of these capabilities are mediated by plasma membrane components. This chapter discusses general principles of membrane organization, some of the experimental techniques used to delineate membrane structures and functions, and some of the unique membrane specializations of nerve cells (Fig. 1).

PHOSPHOLIPID BILAYERS

Cells are separated from their environment by lipid bilayers

The fundamental importance of lipids in membrane structure was established by studies made early in this century that established positive correlations between cell membrane permeabilities to small nonelectrolytes and the oil/

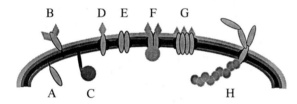

FIG. 1. The generalized structure of plasma membranes can be distinguished from other cellular membranes by the presence of the carbohydrate components of glycolipids and glycoproteins on the outer surface and by the attachment of cytoskeletal proteins to the inner surface. Several different modes of membrane protein interaction are shown: a cytoplasmic protein (A) and an extracellular protein (B), both attached through covalently bonded lipids inserted into the bilayer; a cytoplasmic protein anchored by a hydrophobic peptide segment (C); a monomeric integral membrane protein inserted across the bilayer through hydrophobic transmembrane peptide domains (D); multimeric integral membrane proteins such as those that function as channels and transport proteins (E–G); an integral membrane protein interacting with both cytoskeletal and extracellular proteins (H).

water partition coefficients of these molecules. The high electrical impedance of cells suggested the existence of a hydrocarbon barrier in membranes that was estimated to be approximately 3.3 nm thick. It was originally thought that a membrane containing a lipid monolayer could account for these data. Subsequently, the area of a monolayer formed from total erythrocyte-derived membrane lipids was compared with the surface area of erythrocytes. A ratio of nearly two was found. These studies and other contemporary work on the physical chemistry of lipids made the presence of a continuous lipid bilayer in cell membranes more probable. The reality of the bilayer structure as a principal and universal membrane component has received support from many other studies, including the interpretation of X-ray diffraction data obtained from intact cell membranes [1].

Forces acting between lipids and also between lipids and proteins are primarily noncovalent: electrostatic, hydrogen bonding, and Van der Waals interactions. Although these are individually weak relative to covalent bonds, they can sum to produce associations of considerable stability. Ionic and polar parts of molecules can interact with the dipoles of water to become hydrated. A substance is soluble if its molecules interact with water more strongly than with each other. Large molecules may have surface domains that differ in polarity. Their hydrophobic surfaces may aggregate, forming *micelles* that minimize the exposure of nonpolar surfaces to the aqueous phase. Molecules that have segregated polar and nonpolar surface domains are termed *amphipathic* and include detergents and complex lipids.

Amphipathic molecules that have a comparable extent of polar and nonpolar residues tend to form bilayered lamellar structures

Phospholipids constitute the majority of lipids in most cell membranes (see Chap. 5). They have a polar head group consisting of a glycerophosphoryl ester moiety and a hydrocarbon tail, formed usually of two chains of esterified fatty acids. In the presence of water, the head groups interact with water and other components of the aqueous phase, whereas the nonpolar tails interact principally among themselves to form a separate phase.

Three principal phase structures are formed by most lipids in the presence of water (Fig. 2). Although only the lamellar structure is ordinarily found in cell membranes, hexagonal phases may occur during some membrane transformations. The importance of molecular geometry for bilayer stability is illustrated by the effects of phospholipases, found in certain venoms, which can hydrolyze one of the fatty acid moieties from membrane phospholipids. The resultant lysophosphatides may transform bilayers into hexagonal phase structures, disrupt the membrane continuity, and produce cell lysis. This ability to combine with membrane lipids to form small micelles is characteristic of detergent molecules, which commonly have polar head groups that are somewhat larger than their hydrocarbon domains. In contrast to lysophosphatides and other detergents, cholesterol can stabilize phospholipid bilayers by entering into their structure at the interfaces between the head and tail regions so as to satisfy the bulk requirement for a planar geometry.

Multilamellar structures may form spontaneously if small amounts of water are added to solid- or liquid-phase phospholipids. On dilution, these can be readily dispersed to form vesicular structures called liposomes. Unilamellar liposomes are employed in studies of bilayer properties and may often be combined with membrane proteins to reconstitute functional membrane systems. There are two gen-

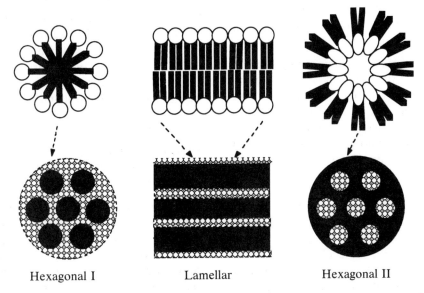

Hexagonal I   Lamellar   Hexagonal II

FIG. 2. Complex lipids interact with water and with each other to form different states of aggregation or "phases." Their structures are generally classified as illustrated in the *lower row*. The hexagonal I and lamellar phases can be dispersed in aqueous media to form the micellar structures shown in the *top row*. Hexagonal II phase lipids will form "reverse micelles" in nonpolar solvents. The stability of lamellar structures relative to hexagonal structures depends on fatty acid chain length, the presence of double bonds, relative sizes of polar head and hydrocarbon tail groups, and temperature.

eral ways to induce proteins to insert into liposomes: One may cause the lipids to form mixed micelles with protein in the presence of a detergent and then transform the micelles into vesicles by removing the detergent; alternatively, one may employ sonication to allow proteins to insert during the disruption of preformed vesicles. Certain proteins may spontaneously insert into preformed vesicles. Another technique for studying the properties of the interaction of proteins with bilayers employs a single bilayer lamella (black lipid membrane) formed across a small aperture in a thin partition between two aqueous compartments. Because pristine lipid bilayers have very low ion conductivities, the modifications of ion-conducting properties produced by membrane proteins can be measured with great sensitivity (see Chap. 4).

Physical states of bilayers vary greatly with composition and may change abruptly with temperature

In aqueous systems containing phospholipids, various phase structures may manifest either crystalline (rigid) or liquid crystalline (two-dimensionally fluid) states. In the case of pure phospholipids, these states interconvert at well-defined transition temperatures. In cell membranes, because of the presence of cholesterol and the heterogeneity of both polar and nonpolar domains, this transition occurs progressively over a broad temperature range. To function normally, cell membrane bilayers must be in the liquid crystalline state, which permits individual phospholipid molecules to have high mobility within the bilayer plane. In contrast, movement of phospholipids transversely between bilayer leaflets rarely occurs. Because of this, the two leaflets of a given membrane can maintain different lipid compositions. For example, most plasma membranes contain substantially more phosphatidyl ethanolamine in the cytoplasmic leaflet than in the outer leaflet; glycolipids, however, are confined to the outer leaflet.

A major fraction of the bilayer phospholipids is physically constrained by association with integral membrane proteins

Although most lipid molecules that interact cooperatively with each other to form the bilayer matrix also rapidly equilibrate with lipids that occur at protein interfaces, several physical measurements indicate that at least a monolayer of lipids immediately surrounding integral membrane proteins is motionally restricted and reoriented relative to the bilayer [2]. This "annulus" fraction may comprise 20 to 90 percent of the total phospholipid. Some membrane proteins preferentially interact with certain lipid species. For example, preferential binding of negatively charged phospholipids to the Na,K-ATPase occurs, and this association increases the enzyme activity. One function of the preferential binding of phospholipids to certain protein surfaces may be to prevent indiscriminate aggregation of integral membrane proteins.

Proton conduction is facilitated in the head-group regions of phospholipid monolayers

In model systems, pH changes are transmitted more rapidly along these interfaces than in bulk solution. This may have particular importance in mitochondrial ATP synthesis and other processes that depend on transmembrane proton gradients [3]. There is no obvious reason that this phenomenon should be restricted to protons, and, in fact, nuclear magnetic resonance (NMR) studies have shown that the mean residence times of metal cations with phospholipid head groups are very short.

MEMBRANE PROTEINS

Membrane proteins may insert through the lipid bilayer ("integral") or bind to other components ("associated") of the membrane

Nearly all proteins fold so as to segregate regions of predominantly nonpolar amino acid residues from more polar regions [1]. Soluble proteins have hydrophobic regions segregated in the interior and more polar regions that form an outer shell of their tertiary or quaternary structures. Integral membrane proteins have some regions with outwardly oriented nonpolar amino acid residues that form hydrophobic surfaces that can insert through the bilayer lipids. In some cases, the membrane-insertion regions may serve only as an anchor for proteins that function wholly on one side of the membrane. An example of this is cytochrome b_5, which can be converted to a wholly active and soluble protein by removing the anchoring domain with trypsin. In contrast, the protomer of bacteriorhodopsin, a photon-driven proton-transporting pump in halophilic bacteria, consists of a single polypeptide chain that crosses the membrane seven times, resulting in residence of 60 to 70 percent of the protein within the bilayer.

Membrane insertion segments nearly always form α helices

Because the peptide backbone of an α helix forms a hydrogen-bonded core, the surface properties of a helical segment can be determined mainly by the amino acid side chains. A length of α helix sufficient to span the usual bilayer requires 18 to 21 residues (Fig. 3). A single segment that serves merely to anchor the protein might be expected to consist largely of hydrophobic amino acid residues. This hypothesis often corresponds to experimental observations. For this reason, the analysis of membrane protein sequences in terms of "hydrophobicity profiles" has become routine (Fig. 4).

Most interactions between a cell and its environment are mediated by integral membrane proteins

To traverse the bilayer functionally, the proteins constituting ion channels, transport pumps, symport and antiport systems, and re-

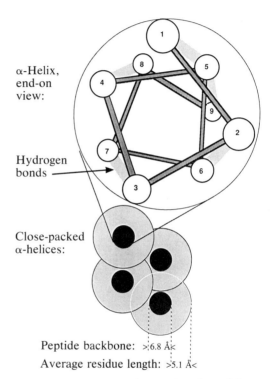

FIG. 3. The transmembrane domains of integral membrane proteins are predominantly α helices. This structure causes the amino acid side chains to project radially. When several parallel α helices are closely packed, their side chains may intermesh as shown, or steric constraints may cause the formation of interchain channels. The outwardly directed residues must be predominantly hydrophobic to interact with the fatty acid chains of lipid bilayers. The bilayer is about 3 nm thick. Each peptide residue extends an α helix by 0.15 nm. Thus, a transmembrane segment must require about 20 residues to span the bilayer. Although local modifications of the bilayer or interactions with other membrane polypeptides could alter this requirement, integral membrane proteins are characterized by the presence of hydrophobic segments approximating this length [see Fig. 4].

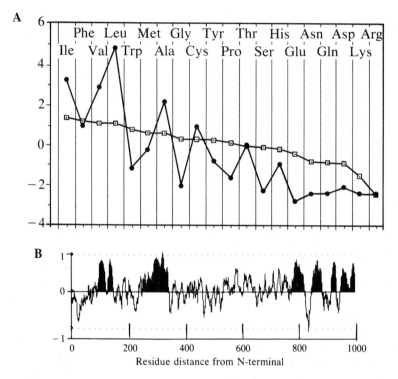

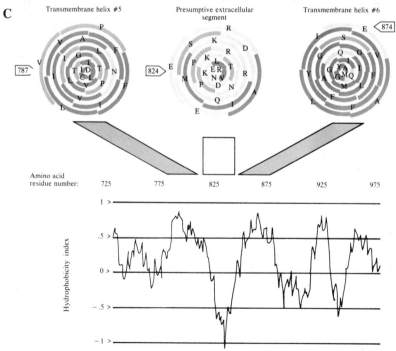

ceptor-effector complexes must have multiple transmembrane segments that interact among themselves as well as with the bilayer lipids to form the walls of aqueous transmembrane paths. In fact, purely hydrophobic transmembrane segments are seldom observed. Instead, polar and helix-destabilizing residues commonly occur within the predominantly hydrophobic segments (Fig. 4). Segments that participate both in the structure of aqueous channels and in hydrophobic interactions may be expected to have polar and nonpolar residues on opposite sides of the helix. Sequences that may permit the formation of such amphipathic helices do occur in membrane proteins, but there is still insufficient data to assess their functional significance.

Fluidity of the bilayer permits specific interactions among different integral membrane proteins

For example, the interaction of certain neurotransmitters and hormones with their receptors can modulate the affinity of the receptor for a transducer protein, which in turn will interact with an effector protein [4] (see Chap. 18). A given effector protein, such as adenylate cyclase, may interact with several different transducers that may affect its activity in different ways. These interactions all require lateral diffusion within the membrane bilayer. Extensive redistribution of membrane proteins can also result from occupation of external receptor sites, as demonstrated by the "patching" and "capping" responses of lymphocyte membrane antibodies subsequent to their binding to membrane-surface antigens.

In contrast to these examples of lateral mobility, the distribution of integral membrane proteins on cell surfaces can be restricted to varying extents by specific interactions with peripheral proteins. Examples are the localization of Na^+ channels and Na^+ pumps of myelinated axons at nodes of Ranvier, and of nicotinic acetylcholine receptors to the postsynaptic membranes of neuromuscular junctions. Some membrane proteins are partitioned into local areas by networks of cytoskeletal proteins. In this way, membrane proteins may have their translational motion restricted, yet exhibit rapid rotational diffusion that is limited only by the bilayer viscosity.

Theoretically, chemical reaction rates can be enhanced simply by constraining diffusion to two dimensions. Particularly dramatic effects are predicted for reactions between membrane proteins because in addition to constrained diffusion, the proteins are oriented relative to the bilayer plane; however, these enhancements can only be realized in a highly fluid membrane [5].

FIG. 4. Evaluation of the distribution of hydrophobic residues in the amino acid sequence of an integral membrane protein may suggest the location of its transmembrane segments. **A:** "Hydrophobicity indices" based on physical properties of the amino acid residues correlate reasonably well with the frequencies of occurrence of these residues in known transmembrane segments of integral membrane proteins. □, theoretical consensus values; ●, observed occurrence. **B:** The hydrophobicity plot of the catalytic subunit of the Na^+ pump suggests seven or more transmembrane segments, as indicated by the *shaded segments* of the plot. **C:** These diagrams show peptide segments schematically as end-on views of the α helical configuration and assigns darker shading to more hydrophobic residues. A characteristic of presumptive transmembrane segments is the occurrence of isolated polar residues in an otherwise hydrophobic environment. For example, presumptive transmembrane helix 5 of the Na^+-pump catalytic subunit contains one asparagine (N), one threonine (T), and two proline (P) residues within a run of 21 otherwise nonpolar residues. These features may have functional and structural significance with respect to the formation of ionophoric pathways across the membrane.

Interactions between integral membrane proteins and other structural proteins are involved in most mechanical cell functions

Mechanical cell functions include cell motility, endo- and exocytosis, formation of cell junctions, and regulation of cell shape. Several peripheral membrane proteins are known that mediate specific interactions among integral membrane proteins, cytoskeletal proteins, and contractile proteins (Fig. 5.)

The manner in which cytoskeletal proteins associate with membranes has been best studied in erythrocytes. In these cells, the major structural link of plasma membrane to cytoskeleton is mediated by an interaction between the anion antiporter (see Chap. 3) and *ankyrin*, a 215-kilodalton (kDa) monomeric protein. Ankyrin links the anion antiporter with a rod-shaped 225-kDa subunit of the tetrameric protein, spectrin. Spectrin, in turn, self-associates to form a network parallel to the membrane. Spectrin has further links to actin polymers that form the principal microfilamentous component. Neurons contain spectrin and an additional variant called fodrin. Fodrin is found throughout neurons, whereas spectrin occurs only in the soma and dendrites. These associations are undoubtedly subject to complex regulation. For example, phosphorylation of ankyrin can alter its affinity for spectrin. Brain contains a protein that

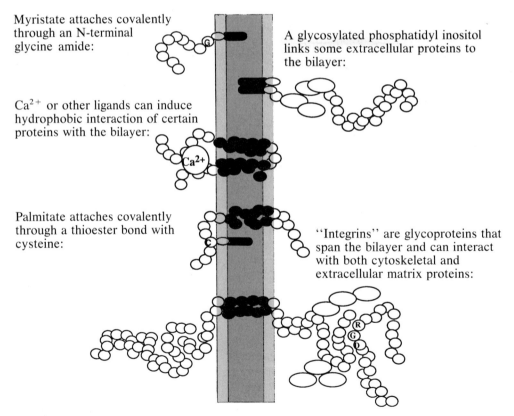

Myristate attaches covalently through an N-terminal glycine amide:

A glycosylated phosphatidyl inositol links some extracellular proteins to the bilayer:

Ca^{2+} or other ligands can induce hydrophobic interaction of certain proteins with the bilayer:

Palmitate attaches covalently through a thioester bond with cysteine:

"Integrins" are glycoproteins that span the bilayer and can interact with both cytoskeletal and extracellular matrix proteins:

FIG. 5. Proteins may associate with membranes either through several types of direct interactions with the bilayer lipids or by associating with specific sites on integral membrane proteins.

is immunoreactively similar to erythrocyte ankyrin and that has binding sites for spectrin, actin, and microtubules. Cytoskeletal interactions with neuronal membranes may occur in forming and modifying synaptic junctions (see Chap. 48). Endo- and exocytotic processes such as neurotransmitter release probably also involve interactions of membrane and cytoskeletal components. In support of this, intracellular injection of an antibody to fodrin has been shown to interfere with catecholamine release from chromaffin cells.

Electrostatic coupling of peripheral membrane proteins to the bilayer lipids may occur

Spectrin interacts strongly with monolayers of phosphatidyl serine despite the large net negative charge (~300 per dimer) of the protein [7]. Evidently, there are negatively charged domains of spectrin that are favorably disposed to these interactions and that may participate in stabilizing the shape of the cell.

Certain transmembrane glycoproteins can mediate interactions between the cytoskeleton and the extracellular matrix

Certain transmembrane glycoproteins possess specific receptors both for sites found on extracellular matrix proteins or other cell surfaces and for sites on cytoskeletal proteins [8]. In some cases, the dual specificity is (a) for the Arg-Gly-Asp or "RGD" site found on extracellular proteins such as fibronectin [9]; and (b) for a cytoskeletal protein, talin, which can further interact with the intermediate filament protein, vinculin (Fig. 5). Talin occurs postsynaptically at neuromuscular junctions [10].

Since these transmembrane glycoproteins mediate diverse functions, they vary widely with respect to internal and external receptor specificities. One group, the "integrins," is characterized by their size (200–300 kDa) and

by their structure in that they are all transmembrane heterodimers with subunits linked by disulfide bonds [8].

Neuronal cell adhesion molecules (N-CAMs) belong to another family of cell-surface glycoproteins of wide distribution. They have been studied intensively with respect to their role in neuronal development [11,12]. There appears to be a single N-CAM gene from which several differently spliced mRNAs can result in the expression of at least three different polypeptides. Two of these (130 and 160 kDa) are transmembrane glycoproteins characterized by identical extracellular domains and differing "small" and "large" cytoplasmic domains. A third form is not a transmembrane peptide; rather, its extracellular domain is anchored to the membrane by a covalent attachment involving phosphatidyl inositide (see below).

The N-terminal extracellular domains of N-CAMs are heavily glycosylated and uniquely contain long, unbranched polysialic acid chains. Increased sialylation suppresses the adhesive properties of the extracellular domains. Variations in polysialic acid content apparently influence cell and axon migrations (see Chap. 25). The extracellular binding sites of N-CAMs have been described as homotypic, meaning that they can bind to each other; however a heparin-binding site is also present [13].

Covalently attached lipids frequently participate in binding proteins to membranes

Three different types of covalent lipid attachments have been identified (Fig. 5). Myristate can be added cotranslationally to N-terminal glycines of a number of peripheral proteins, thus participating in their binding to the cytoplasmic surface of plasma membranes [14]. These proteins include the catalytic subunit of cyclic AMP (cAMP)-dependent protein kinase, calcineurin B, and NADH-cytochrome b_5 reductase.

Fatty acids, primarily palmitate, can be

linked as thioesters to a cysteine usually located near a membrane-binding domain of the protein. Rhodopsin, ankyrin, and transferrin receptor are known to become post-translationally acylated in this manner. Vinculin, a protein involved in the attachment of actin microfilaments to adhesion plaques at the cytoplasmic surface of plasma membranes, appears to do so by means of one or more covalently bound palmitates. In this case, the interaction with membranes is probably reversible [16].

Proteins that are bound to complex glycosylated phosphoinositides on the external surface of plasma membranes [15] can be converted from membrane-bound to water-soluble forms by exposure to phosphoinositide-specific phospholipase C. They include alkaline phosphatase, 5′-nucleotidase, one form of acetylcholinesterase (see Chap. 10), and one form of N-CAM. A single diacylglycerol moiety appears to be sufficient, in these cases, to produce a stable membrane anchor.

Several proteins interact with membranes in consequence of reversible noncovalent interactions with lipids

These proteins include α-actinin (16) and protein kinase C; diacyl glycerol and phorbol esters promote membrane binding [17] (see Chap. 16).

Allosteric regulation of the hydrophobicity of protein-binding surfaces frequently occurs

One of the best known cases is the Ca^{2+}-dependent binding of calmodulin to other proteins (see Chap. 3). Several families of proteins exhibit Ca^{2+}-dependent associations with cell membranes [18,19]. Several proteins have been shown to bind to membranes with increased affinity in the presence of Ca^{2+}. In most cases, their functions are unknown; however, one group has been defined in terms of its association with chromaffin secretory granules in the presence of Ca^{2+} and is hypothesized to have a function in exocytosis. In the cases of "lipocortins" or "calpactins" and related proteins, Ca^{2+} binding increases the affinity of the protein for direct interaction with phospholipids, and, conversely, interactions with phospholipids increase their affinity for Ca^{2+}. These proteins can also interact with actin microfilaments and may thus link cytoskeletal components to the membrane [20].

Mechanisms for insertion of newly synthesized integral membrane proteins into the endoplasmic reticulum bilayer and secretory protein transport into the endoplasmic reticulum lumen appear to be related

Since the same ribosomal machinery is used for synthesizing both soluble and membrane proteins, targeting and insertion through the bilayer must require additional mediators.

The information that targets a polypeptide to the endoplasmic reticulum (ER) membrane is contained in a segment called the signal sequence [21]. These sequences are highly variable but consist of a hydrophobic segment of nine or more residues bracketed by basic residues at the N-terminal and a mixture of acidic and basic residues at the C-terminal (Fig. 6). Proteins destined for import into mitochondria have distinctly different signal peptide patterns of charged and polar residues.

In many cases, targeting to the ER begins with an interaction of a signal-recognition particle (SRP) with the nascent signal sequence as it emerges from the mRNA-ribosome complex (Fig. 6). SRP is an 11S ribonucleoprotein consisting of six different peptides and one 7S RNA [22]. Binding of the SRP to the complex in the absence of ER membrane arrests the translation process. Only after the ribosome-SRP complex interacts with a component of the ER membrane, the SRP receptor, or docking protein,

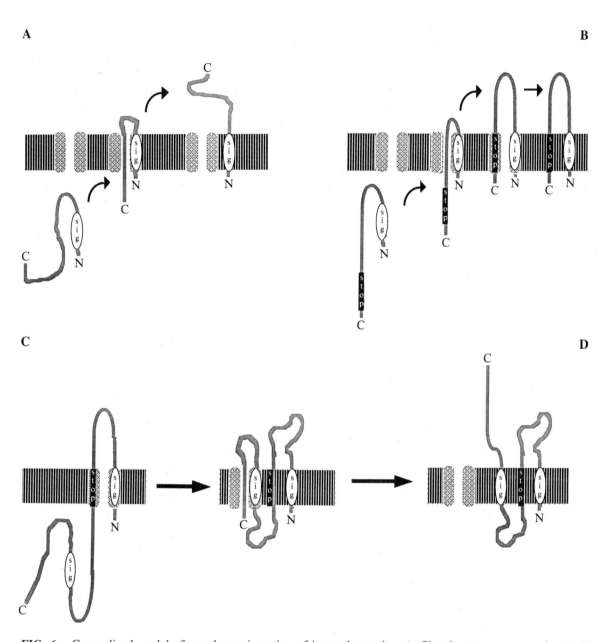

FIG. 6. Generalized model of membrane insertion of integral proteins. **A:** Signal sequences are orientated N → C outward as they insert through a membrane. As long as the succeeding sequence is unable to interact with the translocator proteins, the peptide chain continues to pass through the lumen of the channel. **B:** If a transmembrane or stop segment is encountered, an interaction with the translocator proteins shunts it into the bilayer. **C,D:** Dissociation of this segment from the translocator proteins makes them available for possible interaction with a following *internal signal sequence* and translocation of another domain of the growing peptide chain.

can synthesis continue. This interaction causes the SRP to dissociate from the ribosome and the signal sequence to initiate insertion into the ER membrane, and permits the mRNA translation to continue. Once a conjunction of the ribosomal complex with the ER membrane is established, the growing peptide passes through the membrane. This mechanism is called cotranslational insertion.

Most secreted proteins are synthesized in this manner as a "pro-protein" with an N-terminal signal sequence. After the rest of the peptide has been exported, the signal sequence is cleaved from the secreted product by a signal peptidase, itself a membrane protein with its active site within the ER lumen. Some integral membrane proteins, having a single anchoring segment near the NH_2-terminal, may insert by a similar mechanism involving an uncleaved signal sequence (Fig. 6a). However, other proteins have a single anchor near the COOH-terminal, and their insertion would seem to require in addition (a) a stop-transfer sequence to form a permanent transmembrane segment, and (b) cleavage of the initial signal peptide (Fig. 6b).

Some integral membrane proteins are known to have more than one uncleaved signal sequence. An example is opsin, which traverses the membrane seven times. Since it has four intraluminal domains, as many as four uncleaved signal sequences may be required. By the use of selectively deleted cDNA and subsequent translation of the corresponding RNA transcripts, evidence has been obtained that in fact the first and sixth transmembrane segments contain signal sequences that are necessary for proper membrane insertion [23]. Even these variations are not sufficient to account for all the complexities of membrane protein insertion. Ribosomal synthesis of some integral membrane proteins is not inhibited by SRP. For example, the Ca^{2+}-pump ATPase contains one or more uncleaved signal sequences, and although SRP is required for membrane insertion, the absence of membranes containing the docking protein does not arrest its synthesis [24].

Other integral membrane proteins, such as cytochrome b_5, can be synthesized on free ribosomes and subsequently insert into membranes in the absence of the SRP. The spontaneous insertion hypothesis attempts to account for the occurrence of post-translational insertion by postulating that two hydrophobic peptide segments associate to form a hairpin configuration that can insert into a lipid bilayer independently of facilitating proteins. This mechanism does not solve the problem of providing a pathway for the transport of hydrophilic sequences that form the extracytoplasmic domains of many integral membrane proteins and for which the bilayer constitutes a large energy barrier.

To circumvent this objection and to account for all possible configurations of integral membrane proteins, a unitary hypothesis has been proposed [25]. It assumes that all insertions can be post-translational. There is some experimental support for this. In one case, the inability for post-translational insertion of an integral membrane protein into ER was found to result from the formation of internal disulfide bonds as the newly synthesized peptide chains folded; a more reducing environment, however, permitted post-translational insertion. A further assumption of this model is that there are translocator proteins in the ER membrane that can interact with the signal sequences to form a hydrophilic channel that traverses the bilayer (Fig. 6). Alternation of hydrophobic stop sequences with uncleaved signal sequences and appropriate responses by the translocator proteins to these signals can account for most of the observed transmembrane dispositions of polypeptide segments.

Neuronal membranes are specialized to detect, integrate, and transmit signals

The functional specializations that permit neurons to detect environmental signals selectively, to integrate these signals temporally and spatially over their dendritic trees, to transmit action potentials, and to release neurotransmitters are all properties of neuronal membranes. Moreover, there are multiple regulatory mechanisms acting on most of these systems. Neither the basic processes nor their regulation are adequately understood at the molecular level, although a few beginnings have been made. Perhaps the most studied are the receptor-transducer-effector systems that are activated by neurotransmitters (see Chaps. 10–20) and by photons (see Chap. 7). The proteins of postsynaptic densities from CNS neurons receive considerable attention, particularly by investigators interested in factors that may regulate synaptic plasticity (see Chap. 48). Presynaptic vesicle membranes and the membranes of axon terminals are under investigation in an effort to understand neurotransmitter release mechanisms (see Chap. 8). Studies of the factors that control the localization of the nicotinic receptor, acetylcholine esterases, and other specific components of the neuromuscular junction have also led to some insights with respect to both physiological and pathological mechanisms (see Chap. 32). An understanding of the molecular organization of the channels, pumps, and structural elements at axonal nodes is necessary to understand adequately conduction mechanisms (see Chap. 4) and their pathologies (see Chap. 35).

REFERENCES

1. Tanford, C. *The Hydrophobic Effect: Formation of Micelles and Biological Membranes*, 2nd ed. New York: Wiley, 1980.
2. Jost, P. C., and Griffith, O. H. The lipid-protein interface in biological membranes. *Ann. N.Y. Acad. Sci.* 348:391–407, 1980.
3. Prats, M., Teissie, J., and Tocanne, J.-F. Lateral proton conduction at lipid-water interfaces and its implications for the chemiosmotic-coupling hypothesis. *Nature* 322:756–758, 1986.
4. Poo, M. Mobility and localization of proteins in excitable membranes. *Annu. Rev. Neurosci.* 8:369–406, 1985.
5. Grasberger, B., Minton, A. P., DeLisi, C., Metzger, H. Interaction between proteins localized in membranes. *Proc. Natl. Acad. Sci. U.S.A.* 83:6258–6262, 1986.
6. Adam, G., and Delbruck, M. Reduction of dimensionality in biological diffusion processes. In A. Rich and N. Davidson (eds.), *Structural Chemistry and Molecular Biology.* New York: Freeman, 1968.
7. Maksymiw, R., Sui, S., Gaub, H., and Sackmann, E. Electrostatic coupling of spectrin dimers to phosphatidylserine-containing lipid lamellae. *Biochemistry* 26:2983–2990, 1987.
8. Hynes, R. O. Integrins: A family of cell surface receptors. *Cell* 48:549–554, 1987.
9. Ruoslahti, E., and Pierscbacher, M. D. Arg-Gly-Asp: A versatile cell recognition signal. *Cell* 44:517–518, 1986.
10. Sealock, R., Paschal, B., Beckerle, M., and Burridge, K. Talin is a post-synaptic component of the rat neuromuscular junction. *Exp. Cell Res.* 163:143–150, 1986.
11. Rutishauser, U. Differential cell adhesion through spatial and temporal variation of NCAM. *Trends Neurosci.* 9:374–378, 1986.
12. Edelman, G. M. Cell adhesion and the molecular process of morphogenesis. *Annu. Rev. Biochem.* 54:135–140, 1985.
13. Cole, G. J., et al. Topographic localization of the heparin-binding domain of the neural cell adhesion molecule N-CAM. *J. Cell Biol.* 103:1739–1744, 1986.
14. Sefton, B. M., and Buss, J. E. The covalent modification of eukaryotic proteins with lipid. *J. Cell Biol.* 104:1449–1453, 1987.
15. Low, M. G., et al. Covalently attached phosphatidylinositol as a hydrophobic anchor for membrane proteins. *Trends Behav. Sci.* 11:212–215, 1986.
16. Burn, P., and Burger, M. The cytoskeletal protein vinculin contains transformation-sensitive, covalently bound lipid. *Science* 235:476–478, 1987.
17. Nishizuka, Y. Studies and perspectives of protein kinase C. *Science* 233:305–312, 1986.
18. Owens, R. J., and Crumpten, M. J. *Biochem. Essays* 1:61–63, 1984.
19. Geisow, M. J., et al. A consensus amino-acid sequence repeat in *Torpedo* and mammalian Ca^{2+}-dependent membrane-binding proteins. *Nature* 320:636–38, 1986.

20. Davidson, F. F., Dennis, E. A., Powell, M., and Glenney, J. R. Inhibition of phospholipase A2 by "lipocortins" and calpactins. *J. Biol. Chem.* 262:1698–1705, 1987.

21. Wickner, W. T., and Lodish, H. F. Multiple mechanisms of protein insertion into and across membranes. *Science* 230:400–07, 1985.

22. Walter, P., and Blobel, G. Signal recognition particle contains a 7S RNA essential for protein translocation across the endoplasmic reticulum. *Nature* 299:691, 1982.

23. Friedlander, and Blobel, G. Bovine opsin has more than one signal sequence. *Nature* 318:338, 1985.

24. Anderson, D. J., Mostov K. E., and Blobel G. Mechanisms of integration of *de novo*-synthesized polypeptides into membranes. *Proc. Natl. Acad. Sci. U.S.A.* 80:7249–7253, 1983.

25. Singer, S. J., Maher, P. A. A., and Yaffe, M. P. On the translocation of proteins across membranes. *Proc. Natl. Acad. Sci. U.S.A.* 84:1015–1019, 1987.

CHAPTER 3

Membrane Transport

R. Wayne Albers, George J. Siegel, and William L. Stahl

Basic Neurochemistry: Molecular, Cellular, and Medical Aspects, 4th Ed., edited by G. J. Siegel et al. Raven Press, Ltd., New York, 1989. Correspondence to R. Wayne Albers, Laboratory of Neurochemistry, National Institute of Neurological and Communicative Disorders and Stroke, National Institutes of Health, Bldg. 36, Rm. 4D-20, Bethesda, Maryland 20892.

TRANSPORT PROCESSES

Cells modify their environment by means of membrane transport processes

Membrane transport mechanisms selectively control the concentrations of ions and molecules within the cell and, often, in the immediate extracellular environment. Transmembrane ion gradients constitute a major store of potential energy that is drawn on for many different purposes. The electrical potential derived from ion gradients is central to the primary function of neurons; that is, to the generation of signals that may be propagated as transmembrane ion currents. Other uses of the potential energy stored in ion gradients include

1. synthesis of ATP by proton gradients in mitochondria;
2. concentrative acquisition of nutrients and recovery of metabolites that commonly use Na^+ or H^+ gradients; and
3. regulation of other processes via control of intracellular pH and ionic environments.

These are all mediated by specific integral membrane proteins. Examples could be cited in each category for which the relevant protein has been isolated, purified, and sequenced. In most cases, however, there is still much to be learned about the detailed mechanisms of membrane transport.

Concentration gradients across membranes are analyzed in terms of two components: Diffusion and active transport

The Gibbs free energy (ΔG) involved in the diffusion of each molecule of solute is calculated from the equation

$$\Delta G = RT \ln(C_2/C_1) \qquad (1)$$

where R = 1.99 cal/degree Kelvin (K); T is temperature (K); C_2 and C_1 are concentrations of solute on opposite sides of a permeable membrane. Cell membranes separate electrical charge. Therefore, translocation of charged solutes produces electrical potentials as well as chemical concentration gradients. (Electrical potentials and their generation are discussed in detail in Chapter 4.) For our purposes, the energy related to electrical potential is given by

$$\Delta G = ZFV \qquad (2)$$

where Z is valence; F is the Faraday constant (23,500 cal $V^{-1}mol^{-1}$); and V represents the transmembrane potential difference in volts. The minimal amount of total free energy change related to the movement of 1 mol of a solute with respect to the combined electrochemical gradient is the sum of Eqs. 1 and 2:

$$\Delta G = RT \ln(C_2/C_1) + ZFV \qquad (3)$$

If the chemical and electrical components are not equal and opposite, then ΔG is not equal to zero, and work is performed by some other exergonic process to maintain a steady state. The amount of work needed per unit time (power) is proportional to the rate of diffusion down the electrochemical gradient.

The work performed in cells to maintain a steady-state electrochemical gradient for Na^+ and K^+ can be calculated as follows. The sum of ΔG for both Na^+ and K^+ gradients is

$$\Delta G_{total} = RT \ln([Na^+]_e/[Na^+]_i) + ZFV$$
$$+ RT \ln([K^+]_i/[K^+]_e) - ZFV$$
$$= RT \ln([Na^+]_e[K^+]_i/[Na^+]_i[K^+]_e) \quad (4)$$

where e is the extracellular and i the intracellular concentration. Assuming typical values for Na^+ and K^+ concentration gradients ($[Na^+]_e/[Na^+]_i = 12$; $[K^+]_i/[K^+]_e = 50$), ΔG is about

3.8 kcal/mol Na^+ exchanged for K^+. The hydrolysis of a high-energy phosphate bond of ATP may yield about 12 kcal/mol, thus permitting the exchange of about 3 mol cation/mol ATP hydrolyzed to ADP and P_i. Actually, a ratio of 3 Na^+:2 K^+:1 ATP is most often observed in various tissue preparations.

Processes mediated by transport proteins and by channel proteins are distinct

Channels provide aqueous pathways through membranes for the diffusion of ions or molecules down prevailing electrochemical gradients (Chap. 4) and conduct several thousand ions per millisecond. Since they do not interact strongly with these ions or molecules, their selectivity is limited to discrimination by size and electrical charge, and their conductance is proportional to the electrochemical gradient. In contrast, transport proteins form highly specific complexes with their substrates. Typically, these interactions initiate a cycle of conformational transitions of the proteins that release the substrate on the opposite face of the membrane. Transport processes may require several milliseconds to transport only a few substrate ions or molecules. The relationship of rate of transport to substrate concentration is described by saturation kinetics, as in the case of enzymes.

Selective transport of molecules or ions through membranes may occur without coupling to any other substrate. Such a process is termed facilitative or uncoupled transport, an example of which is the stereoselective entrance of D-glucose into neurons. Binding of an appropriate transport substrate is sufficient to initiate an uncoupled transport cycle in which the substrate is conveyed across the membrane and the unoccupied transport binding site is restored to its original orientation (Fig. 1).

Secondary, or flux-coupled, transport processes obligatorily couple the transport of one molecular or ionic species to the transport of

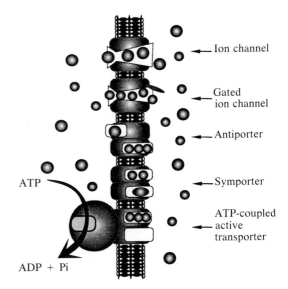

FIG. 1. Types of channels and transporters. Channel proteins provide diffusion paths across cell membranes. They display selectivity with respect to the size and charge of their substrate molecules or ions but do not interact strongly with them. Gated channels can exist in open, closed, or inactivated states, and these states may be regulated by membrane potential, by interaction with regulator ligands, or by covalent modification. Transport proteins regulate the distribution of ions and molecules across membranes and possess binding sites with relatively high affinity for their substrates. Transport occurs consequent to a change in the conformation of the protein-substrate complex. Simultaneous or sequential complexing with two or more substrates may be required to initiate the conformational transitions, resulting in the coupling of these substrate fluxes in the same (symport) or opposite (antiport) directions. The conformational transitions may be coupled to a chemical reaction that supplies the metabolic energy that is required to generate concentration gradients across cell membranes (active transport).

another. The coupled processes are termed symport or antiport according to the relative direction of the two transport events (Fig. 1). Many essential nutrients are accumulated by symport systems. Several specific neurotransmitter re-uptake systems are symporters coupled to Na^+ flux into neurons. In coupled transport, both substrates must be available, either simultaneously or sequentially. The binding is on the same side of the membrane, in the case of a symporter, or on opposite sides, in the case of an antiporter. Substrate velocity kinetics for these systems are analogous to those of multi-substrate enzymes. More than two substrates are involved in some secondary transport systems, as exemplified by the bumetanide-sensitive $(Na^+, K^+, 2 Cl^-)$-symporter.

Primary active transport processes comprise those in which one or more substrates are transported in concert with a chemical reaction that provides the free energy for concentrative substrate accumulation. All of the known primary active transport processes in animals transport cations: H^+, Na^+, K^+, and Ca^{2+}. The principal function of primary Na^+ and K^+ transport in most cells is to store metabolic energy; however, H^+ and Ca^{2+} pumps often act as regulators of intracellular pH and $[Ca^{2+}]$, which in turn control the rates of other cell functions (see below).

Biochemical terminology is curiously inadequate to describe proteins that have energy transducing functions. In addition to proteins that execute primary active transport, members of this group include proteins that produce contractile forces (myosins, dyneins); those that transport macromolecules and organelles intracellularly (kinesins; see Chap. 24); and some that transform the shapes or relative positions of other macromolecules (peptidyl transferases, DNA helicases, topoisomerases). Most of these proteins catalyze ATP or GTP hydrolysis; however these catalytic activities are only by-products of their primary energy transducing functions, which in each case produce some form of local ordering of cellular structure. This transcends the usual definition of an enzyme as catalyst. For this reason, it is preferable to refer to the primary active transport systems as pumps rather than as ATPases. On the other hand, the concept of substrate is usually restricted to the ligands that are chemically transformed as a result of forming a transient complex with enzymes. In the case of membrane pumps, the bound molecules or ions are transported rather than transformed, but because in every other way they behave as substrates, the term will be so applied in the following discussion.

THE ATP-DEPENDENT Na^+, K^+-PUMP

The principal primary active transport system in neurons, as in most other animal cells, is a pump that extrudes Na^+ and simultaneously accumulates K^+

This process requires ATP and is specifically inhibited by cardiac glycosides such as ouabain. The protein that constitutes this molecular machinery can be measured as an ATPase activity and, for brevity, is termed the Na,K-ATPase. Different tissues have vastly different requirements for pumping Na^+ and K^+, depending on their functions. Despite an enormous range in the absolute values of Na,K-ATPase activity and the Na^+ and K^+ fluxes, the constant ratio of the ouabain-sensitive fluxes and of these fluxes to ouabain-sensitive ATPase activity strongly support the conclusion that the fluxes are produced by the ATPase (Fig. 2). This has been established conclusively by experimentally reconstituting the pump activity in artificial vesicles composed only of lipids and the purified protein components of the ATPase [1]. In the reconstituted system, as in intact erythrocytes, the measured stoichiometry is 3 Na^+ ions and 2 K^+ ions pumped per molecule of ATP hydrolyzed.

The purified Na,K-ATPase consists of equimolar ratios of two different polypeptide subunits and a minimal amount of associated lipid. The probable oligomeric structure is $\alpha_2\beta_2$, with a protein molecular weight of about 270,000. Ion-transporting ATPases generally require phospholipids for optimum activity (see Chap. 2). The Na,K-ATPase needs 100 to 200 molecules of phospholipid per molecule of enzyme, and the activity can also be modulated

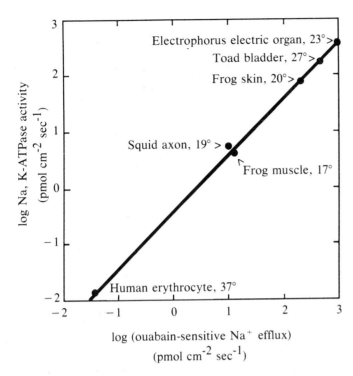

FIG. 2. Correlation of ouabain-sensitive Na^+ efflux with ouabain-sensitive ATPase activities in a variety of tissues. Note that although the absolute values vary over four orders of magnitude, the ratio remains nearly constant. (Data adapted from S. L. Bonting and L. L. Caravaggio, *Arch. Biochem. Biophys.* 101:37, 1963.)

by the fluidity of the acyl chains of the lipids and is promoted by negatively charged lipid head groups.

Na,K-ATPase exists in multiple forms

At least two forms of the catalytic subunit exist in brain: (a) High-resolution sodium deodecyl-sulfate (SDS)-polyacrylamide gels show a doublet in preparations from brain; and (b) in preparations from rodent brain, inhibition of Na,K-ATPase activity by cardiotonic steroids is biphasic [2]. The amino acid sequences of multiple forms of both subunits have been deduced from cDNA clones [3], and the tissue distribution of the isoforms and the corresponding mRNAs have been examined. The major form in kidney has been designated α_1, and three forms appear to be expressed in rodent brains. The three forms show about 85 percent sequence similarity, with the most substantial dif-

ferences occurring in the N-terminal region (Fig. 3A). The regions including the catalytic phosphorylation site are identical for a length of 85 residues, and there are major hydrophobic domains with 94 to 96 percent similarity.

The isoforms are expressed to varying extents in different tissues and at different stages of development. There is evidence that at least five different genes can specify an α subunit and that the β-subunit gene can be transcribed in alternative ways. The extent to which these multiple forms specify different functions is presently under investigation: Glia appear to have the α_1 form exclusively, whereas multiple forms are associated with neurons. There is a current hypothesis that α_1 has a relatively low affinity for cardiac glycosides. An intriguing possibility is that one of the isoforms may be uniquely adapted for clearing extracellular K^+ (see below) and that some of the forms may be subject to post-translational regulation.

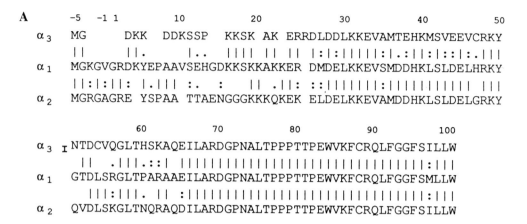

A

```
        -5   -1  1           10          20          30          40          50
 α₃   MG      DKK  DDKSSP  KKSK AK ERRDLDDLKKEVAMTEHKMSVEEVCRKY
      ||      ||.         |..  |||| || || |:|:|||||:|.:||:|::|:.|||
 α₁   MGKGVGRDKYEPAAVSEHGDKKSKKAKKER DMDELKKEVSMDDHKLSLDELHRKY
      ||:|:||: |.||| :.  :     || .||: ::|||||||:|||||||||||| |||
 α₂   MGRGAGRE YSPAA TTAENGGGKKKQKEK ELDELKKEVAMDDHKLSLDELGRKY

                 60          70          80          90         100
 α₃ ᵢNTDCVQGLTHSKAQEILARDGPNALTPPPTTPEWVKFCRQLFGGFSILLW
      ||  .|||.::| ||||||||||||||||||||||||||||||||||:|||
 α₁  GTDLSRGLTPARAAEILARDGPNALTPPPTTPEWVKFCRQLFGGFSMLLW
      |||:|||. || :||||||||||||||||||||||||||||||||||:|||
 α₂  QVDLSKGLTNQRAQDILARDGPNALTPPPTTPEWVKFCRQLFGGFSILLW
```

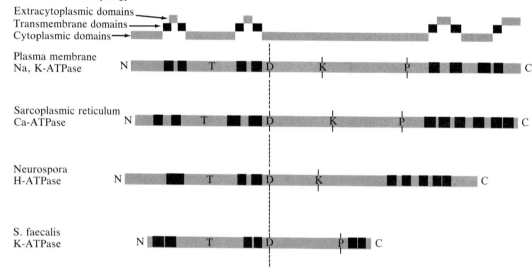

B Probable membrane topology:

FIG. 3. **A:** Multiple forms of Na,K-ATPase α subunit. N-terminal amino acid sequences of the catalytic subunit isoforms were deduced from the sequences of cDNA derived from rat brain mRNA [3]. The residue numbering refers to the α_1 sequence. The sequences have been aligned to maximize their similarities. The extent of conservation is indicated by the symbols between the lines as follows: (|) identity, (:) two or more shared properties, (·) shared polarities. The number of residues in the complete peptides are α_1, 1018; α_2, 1015; α_3, 1013. The one-letter amino acid code is described in the Glossary. **B:** Conservation of structure and sequence in type 2 transport ATPases. The probable topological distribution of peptide segments with respect to the plane of the membrane bilayer has been deduced from hydropathy plots, determinations of accessibility to proteases, and to other probe molecules. The candidate transmembrane segments are indicated by *black bar* segments. Loci of certain highly conserved sequences are indicated by *capital letters within the bars*: In terms of the single-letter amino acid code, (T) TGES; (D) DKTGTLT; (K) KGAP; (P) PXL, where X is S or A; D is the active site aspartyl residue that is transiently phosphorylated in each catalytic cycle. The K and P sites probably participate in ATP binding. The functional role of the T site may relate to energy transduction. Note the apparent conservation of structure in the left half of the map across species and functional diversities.

Na$^+$ and K$^+$ concentration gradients are controlled by the Na$^+$,K$^+$-pump

Gradients for a number of ions are shown in Chap. 4, Table 1. Energy for the work of producing the gradients for Na$^+$ and K$^+$ is provided by the hydrolysis of ATP to ADP and P$_i$. Where other ions are found in concentrations removed from their electrochemical equilibria, transport also must be linked to metabolism directly or indirectly.

Under steady-state conditions, the rate of ATP hydrolysis by the Na$^+$,K$^+$-pump is, by definition, equal to the sum of the rates of the Na$^+$ entry processes. The pump rate can be regulated by both [Na$^+$]$_i$ and [K$^+$]$_e$; however, under physiological conditions, [Na$^+$]$_i$ is usually less than that required for 50 percent occupation of the pump internal Na$^+$ sites, whereas [K$^+$]$_e$ is sufficient to occupy the external K$^+$ sites maximally. Thus, the pump rate is more responsive to [Na$^+$]$_i$ than to [K$^+$]$_e$. Other pump properties that can influence the pump rate include the structure of its binding sites and their sensitivity to other ligands, such as Mg^{2+}, ATP, ADP, and P$_i$, which can modify their reactivities with Na$^+$ and K$^+$. Changes in intracellular pH and [Ca^{2+}] may also modify pump rates. The capacity of the cell to keep pace with processes that dissipate cation gradients and the rate at which it can respond to perturbations in the gradients are determined by these factors as well as by the number of pumps in the cell membrane.

Endogenous regulators, such as hormones and peptides, may produce shifts in the Na$^+$,K$^+$-pump affinity for regulatory ligands and substrates by combining directly with the enzyme; by leading to receptor-activated post-translational modifications, such as phosphorylation; or by regulating biosynthesis of some other regulatory factor. In addition, hormones produce long-acting effects by regulating Na$^+$,K$^+$-pump biosynthesis (see below).

A major fraction of cerebral energy production is required for Na$^+$ extrusion

The energy demands for the cation pump in brain are related to three major factors: electrical activity, geometry of the cellular elements, and myelination. Cation flux during action potentials is two to three orders of magnitude greater than in the resting state. The Na$^+$ entry and K$^+$ efflux from a squid giant axon during a single action potential (duration, ~1 msec) is about 3×10^{-12} mol cm^{-2} membrane [4]. The resting membrane flux in this tissue is 12×10^{-12} mol cm^{-2} sec^{-1} (see Chap. 4). Therefore, it would take the pump about 0.25 sec to discharge the flux of one spike at the pump rate in the resting membrane. Based on these estimates, the Na$^+$,K$^+$-pump rate would have to respond through a range of 2.5 to 25 times in order to maintain a steady state when the neuron is conducting at frequencies of 10 to 100 impulses per second.

The electrical currents associated with postsynaptic membrane excitatory or inhibitory potentials (~10 mV) may produce ion flux densities about one-tenth of those produced during an action potential, but these postsynaptic depolarizations may last 10 to 1,000 times longer than action potentials and may occupy much larger membrane areas. Slow plateau depolarizations dependent on inward Na$^+$ currents are found in some neuronal somata. These may last several seconds and reach amplitudes of 10 to 30 mV. While producing ion flux that leads to increased pump activity, these postsynaptic and plateau depolarizations can, depending on their extent, either activate repetitive action potentials or block them. In this situation, the total ion flux and the pump rate necessary to maintain a steady state cannot be simply correlated with neuronal activity.

Considering the energetics of cation flux, the geometry of the cellular elements is significant. Because the ratio of membrane area to volume for cylinders or spheres increases as the radius decreases, ΔG for a given flux per unit membrane area is relatively greater for smaller axons and cells. Myelination is a third factor. In myelinated axons, only the axolemma underlying the node of Ranvier is completely depolarized by action potentials. Thus the total ion flux per unit length associated with action potentials is lower for myelinated axons than for unmyelinated fibers of the same radius (see Chaps. 4 and 6).

In summary, the energy utilized to maintain cation gradients in a volume of heterogeneous nerve tissue such as cortex will be determined by

1. the distribution of cellular elements with differing geometries and extent of myelination; and
2. the superimposed distribution of differing action potential frequencies, postsynaptic potentials, and resting and plateau potentials.

An important principle derived from these considerations is that although energy utilization may be directly related to cation flux, the latter has a complex relationship to neuronal activity in heterogeneous tissue such as cortex.

It is variously estimated from ouabain-sensitive increments in O_2 consumption related to K^+ uptake in brain slices after depolarization that 25 to 40 percent of brain energy utilization is related to Na,K-ATPase activity. Another approach to this question is to calculate brain ATP utilization based on Na,K-ATPase activity *in vitro*. In mature rat brain, this is reported to be 4 to 7 μmol mg^{-1} hr^{-1}, which corresponds to 6.5 to 11.5 mM min^{-1}, or 25 to 50 percent total brain high-energy phosphate production. The Na^+,K^+-pump transports Na^+ at less than 0.5 Na^+ per millisecond, whereas the conductance through voltage-dependent channels is 4,000 to 5,000 Na^+ per millisecond. Estimates of the number of Na^+,K^+-pump sites (from ouabain

binding or Na^+-dependent phosphorylation) and of voltage-dependent Na^+ channels (from tetrodotoxin binding) indicate a ratio of 10:1. This relationship suggests that were an average of more than 0.1 percent of voltage-dependent Na^+ channels in the open state, the Na^+,K^+-pump even at full capacity would not maintain a steady state. Thus, the above values for energy utilization by the Na^+,K^+-pump are probably underestimates.

It can be calculated that the energy expenditure for most known biochemical processes in brain, including osmotic work, protein and lipid synthesis in the mature brain, and turnover of neurotransmitters, is relatively small, probably less than 10 percent of total ATP utilization. The energy utilized by other processes, such as axoplasmic transport, Ca^{2+} transport, receptor-mediated P_i turnover, phosphorylation reactions, and vesicle recycling, may be of significant proportions; however, it is evident that cation transport is the single enzymatic reaction accounting for the largest share of energy flux.

Coupled active transport of Na^+ and K^+ results from a cycle of conformational transitions of the transport protein

The ATPase activity that is associated with the Na^+,K^+-pump is actually the sum of Na^+-dependent phosphorylation of an aspartyl residue of the pump protein and subsequent K^+-dependent hydrolysis of enzyme acyl phosphate (Fig. 4). These are the molecular events that direct metabolic energy into the pumping process. The initial phosphorylation of an enzyme molecule by ATP occurs only after 3 Na^+ have bound to sites accessible from the cytoplasmic side of the plasma membrane. In this $E_1{\sim}P$ conformation, the phosphorylation is readily reversible; that is, the energy state of the protein acyl phosphate is comparable to that of the ATP phosphate bond. However, the phosphorylation initiates a rapid transition of the pump to the $E_2{-}P$ state, from which Na^+ is discharged extracellularly;

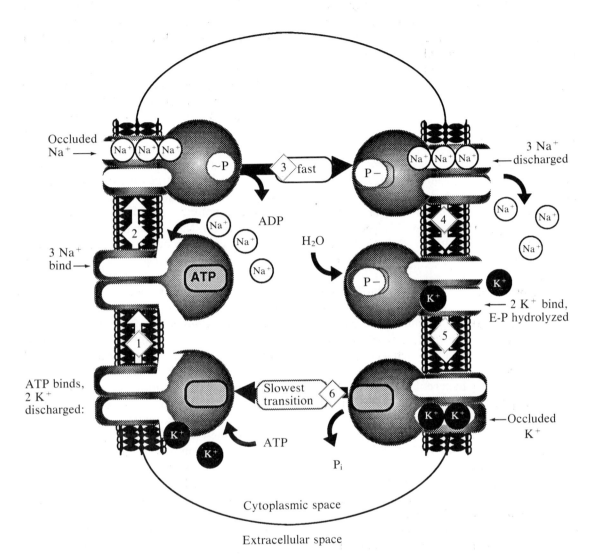

FIG. 4. The mechanism of the ATP-dependent Na^+,K^+-pump. The sequence of reaction steps is indicated by the *large arrows*. On the left, pump molecules are in the E_1 conformation with high affinity for Na^+ and for ATP and low affinity for K^+: Ionophoric sites are accessible only from the cytoplasmic side. *Step 1:* K^+ is discharged as metabolic energy is added to the system by ATP binding. *Step 2:* Na^+ binds, and the enzyme is reversibly phosphorylated. *Step 3:* The conformational transition from $E_1\sim P$ to E_2—P, shown at the top, is normally the "power stroke" of the pump during which the ionophoric sites with their three bound Na^+ become accessible to the extracellular side and decrease their affinity for Na^+. Part of the free energy of the enzyme acylphosphate has been dissipated in this process. *Step 4:* Na^+ dissociates from E_2—P. *Step 5:* K^+ binds, and more free energy is dissipated as the enzyme acylphosphate is hydrolyzed. At this point, K^+ becomes tightly bound ("occluded"). *Step 6:* E_2 reverts to E_1, carrying K^+ to the cytoplasmic side.

K^+ then binds to E_2—P, initiating hydrolysis of the acyl phosphate. This destabilizes E_2, which spontaneously reverts to E_1, carrying K^+ into the cell. The cycle is completed as the K^+ dissociates in concert with initiation of the next cycle by ATP binding.

The Na^+,K^+-pump and the cell membrane potential are interactive

The ratio of Na^+ to K^+ exchanged is greater than unity in almost all model systems studied and is usually given as 3:2 per mol ATP. In nerve and muscle, various studies have yielded estimates ranging from 4:3 to 5:1. The net outward flux of positive charge tends to hyperpolarize the membrane. Therefore, the pump is termed electrogenic.

The proportion of the membrane potential that is produced by the pump has been estimated from the extent of immediate depolarization that results from application of metabolic poisons or pump inhibitors, such as ouabain, or by acutely lowering the temperature. Alternatively, the extent of hyperpolarization produced by the pump has been estimated as the ouabain-sensitive increase in potential resulting either from acutely increased $[Na^+]_i$ or from increased $[K^+]_e$. $[Na^+]_i$ can be rapidly raised by transmitter- or electrically-induced depolarization, by injection of Na^+ through intracellular recording pipettes, or by producing intracellular acidosis, which raises $[Na^+]_i$ because of the increased rate of H^+/Na^+ exchange.

Depolarization due to action potentials and neurotransmitter effects and increases in $[H^+]_i$ may all participate in modifying membrane potential via secondary stimulation of the pump *in vivo*. Estimates of the pump-related potential vary to 10 mV, but under certain conditions may be 30 percent of the resting membrane potential. The electrogenic effects of the pump may shorten the duration of the action potential, contribute to negative afterpotentials, and in heart cells, may produce the hyperpolarization observed after sustained increases in firing rate. The latter is a possible cause of cardiac arrhythmia.

If the pump produces net current and electrical potential, then it is expected that the membrane potential affects both ATPase activity and pump rate. A complete equilibrium expression for the pump *in situ* must include the electrical potential as well as the ion gradients and the chemical equilibria for ATP and its products. The net positive charge efflux produced by the pump is the common "reactant" linking membrane potential and the hydrolysis of ATP utilized by the Na^+,K^+-pump.

An increase in membrane potential, or hyperpolarization, is expected to reduce the net positive charge efflux. This might be effected through reductions in the rate of pump cycling or in the ratio of Na^+ to K^+ exchanged. Opposite effects would be produced by depolarization, thus facilitating return to the resting potential. A key question is, Which step of the pump cycle is sensitive to membrane voltage?

The Na^+,K^+-pump that is reconstituted into liposomes can be subjected to a membrane potential [5]. If the potential is created by filling the liposomes with KCl in the presence of valinomycin, the imposed potential accelerates Na^+/K^+ exchange up to 30 percent at saturating cytoplasmic Na^+ and ATP concentrations but not when ATP is rate limiting. Under the latter condition, the rate-limiting enzyme reaction is $E_2[K^+]_e \rightarrow E_1[K^+]_i$ (Fig. 4, step 6). Since no effect is seen when step 6 is rate-limiting, it is excluded from being voltage sensitive. Also, no effect of diffusion potential is observed on (ATP + P_i)-dependent Rb^+/Rb^+ exchange, which also corresponds to step 6. In contrast, the accelerating effect of potential is relatively greater at low external, "cytoplasmic," Na^+ concentrations, indicating an increase in the apparent affinity for Na^+. Thus, it is suggested that the membrane potential has an effect on a

Na^+-dependent enzyme reaction in which there is net transport of one positive charge. The most likely candidate for the voltage-sensitive step is step 3:

$$(3Na^+)_iE_1{\sim}P \to (3Na^+)_eE_2{-}P$$

The potential has an effect on Na^+ affinity analogous to the effects produced by sulfhydryl-binding reagents that are known to block step 3: Na^+ affinity is increased, and the rate of step 3 is reduced. This would be the situation approached in a resting cell with low $[Na^+]_i$. At the onset of an action potential, membrane depolarization will have the effects of increasing the rate of step 3 as well as increasing $[Na^+]_i$; however, the pump rate could be transiently suppressed by the reduced Na^+ affinity consequent to depolarization.

Activity of Na,K-ATPase increases about tenfold during the development of fetal to adult rat brain

The activity of rat brain Na,K-ATPase expressed as units per milligram of microsomal protein increases about 10 times from fetal to adult stages [6]. The stage of most rapid increase in Na,K-ATPase begins just prior to rapid myelination. This corresponds to the time of glial cell proliferation, intricate elaboration of neuronal and glial processes, and increasing excitability. It is a stage during which membranes become specialized for cation transport.

Subcellular localization of Na,K-ATPase is consistent with the known cellular physiology in most cases

In almost all epithelial cells adapted for secretion or reabsorption, such as kidney tubules and exocrine glands, Na,K-ATPase is concentrated asymmetrically on the basolateral or antiluminal surfaces. The two known exceptions are the retinal pigment epithelium and choroid plexus ependyma, where the enzyme is concentrated on the apical or luminal surface (Fig. 5). It is believed that the concentration of the enzyme within a subcellular membrane domain subserves a specific transport function of the tissue and that disposition to that domain is regulated by specific routing and membrane assembly processes in the cell [7].

In the nervous system, Na,K-ATPase is concentrated in membrane regions associated with high ionic flux, including the nodes of Ranvier, and fine axonal processes, dendrites, and glial membranes that comprise the neuropil of cerebral, cerebellar, and spinal gray matter (Fig. 6). Within the retina, heavy concentrations are found in the retinal photoreceptor inner segments, moderate amounts in inner and outer plexiform, and large amounts in the ganglion cell and optic nerve fiber layers. Na,K-ATPase is also localized in astrocytes and Schwann cells [7–10]. The precise distribution of Na,K-ATPase isoforms among these neuronal and glial membranes is under active investigation.

Hormones may regulate both biosynthesis and activity of the Na^+,K^+-pump

It is known that thyroid hormone increases the metabolic rate of various muscle and epithelial tissues but not of mature brain. In adult rat kidney and heart, but not brain, it induces increased synthesis of mRNA for Na,K-ATPase [11]. It is believed that the resulting increased cation flux in target tissues contributes to the thermogenic responses to thyroid hormone.

Adrenal corticosteroids increase Na,K-ATPase activity levels in a number of tissues, including kidney, intestine, and other osmoregulatory tissues, such as fish gills. These hormones serve adaptive functions related to salt and water balance. Glucocorticoid stimulation of enzyme activity in isolated kidney thick ascending limb tubules can be observed within an

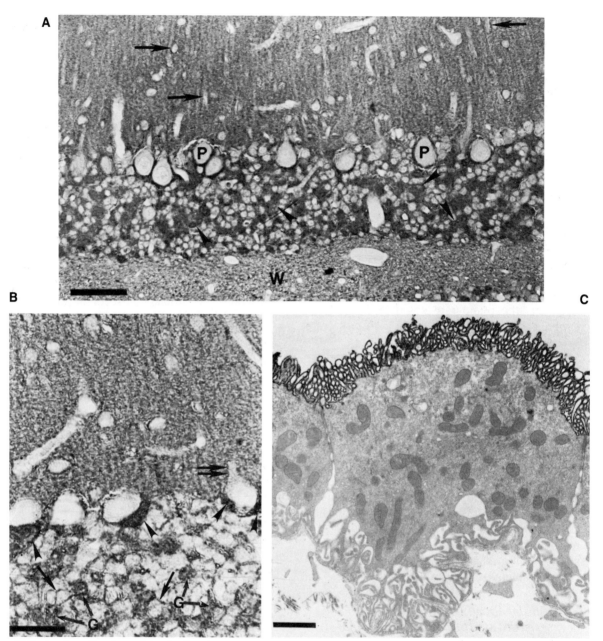

FIG. 5. Localization of the Na^+,K^+-pump in cerebellum and choroid plexus. Immunocytochemical localization in mouse tissues with the peroxidase-conjugated antibody method. **A:** The cerebellum shows stain along the surfaces of Purkinje cell bodies (P) and within synaptic glomeruli of the granular layer (*arrowheads*). The neuropil of the molecular layer is stained more diffusely, with distinct vertical striations (*arrows*) that extend to the cortical surface. White matter (W), although stained weakly, has punctate deposits throughout. Original magnification, ×315; bar, 50 μm. **B:** The cerebellar cortex shows intensely stained basket regions adjacent to Purkinje cells and little staining along the apical dendrites (*double arrows*) of Purkinje cells. Although reaction product is dense over glomeruli (G), a fine deposition outlines the plasmalemma of granule cell bodies (*arrows*). ×620 before 10% reduction; bar, 45 μm. (From ref. 7.) **C:** Choroid plexus contains epithelial cells with intensely stained microvillar and inter microvillar plasma membranes. The basal and lateral plasma membrane surfaces are not stained. ×8000 before 20% reduction; bar, 1.6 μm. (From Ernst, Palacios, and Siegel, *J. Histochem. Cytochem.* 34:189, 1986.)

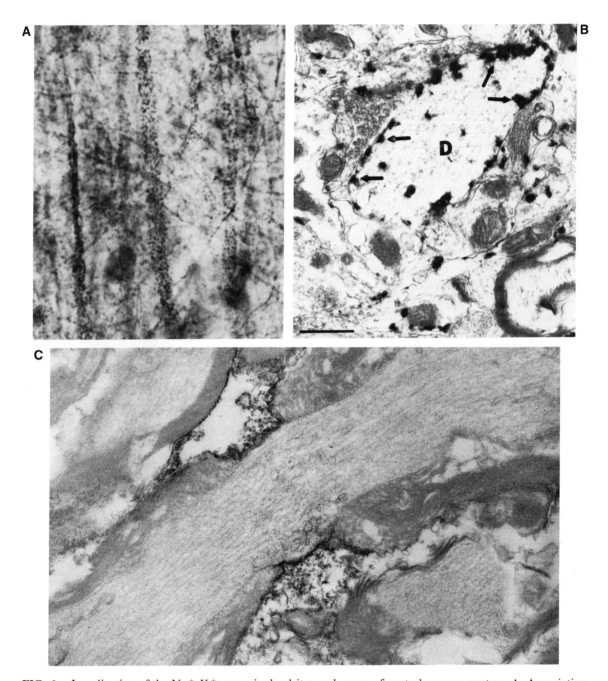

FIG. 6. Localization of the Na^+,K^+-pump in dendrites and axons of central nervous system. **A:** Association of K^+-p-nitrophenylphosphatase activity with dendrites in layer 4 of rat somatosensory cortex. $\times 1600$ before 34% reduction. (From ref. 9.) **B:** EM localization of K^+-p-nitrophenylphosphatase in a dendrite (D) shows that the reaction product is associated with the cytoplasmic aspect (*arrows*) of the plasmalemma. Bar, 0.5 μm. (From Broderson, Patton, and Stahl, *J. Cell Biol.* 77:R13, 1978.) **C:** EM immunocytochemical localization of Na,K-ATPase in goldfish optic nerve with the peroxidase-antiperoxidase method. Reaction product (*dark precipitate*) is found at the axolemma only at the nodes of Ranvier and at the outer lamellae of myelin. $\times 41,000$ before 30% reduction. (From Schwartz, Ernst, Siegel, and Agranoff, *J. Neurochem.* 36:107, 1981.)

hour. This corresponds to glucocorticoid stimulation of Na^+ reabsorption related to urine dilution in this segment. The increase in Na,K-ATPase activity is blocked by actinomycin D and cycloheximide, indicating involvement of nuclear DNA and protein synthesis [12].

The inductive effect of adrenal hormones on Na,K-ATPase may be even more prominent in the developing animal. Maternal adrenalectomy almost completely prevents the normal rise in kidney enzyme activity in the fetus. Significant stimulation of immature kitten and rat cerebral Na,K-ATPase, but not that of adult brain, has been produced by administration of cortisol, methylprednisolone or ACTH to the intact animals. Norepinephrine released from nerve endings in proximity to renal tubules may participate in renal nerve regulation of Na^+ reabsorption in the proximal tubule. Norepinephrine in the bathing medium of proximal tubules increases ouabain-sensitive O_2 consumption and Na,K-ATPase activity. Since no effect of norepinephrine is seen in purified membranes, a receptor-mediated mechanism is presumed [13].

Insulin has the effect of reducing K^+ efflux and $[Na^+]_i$ in muscle. This effect is not completely understood, but there is evidence that insulin *in vitro* stimulates Na,K-ATPase activity and both ouabain-sensitive and insensitive components of Na^+ efflux in some muscle preparations. Increased Na^+/H^+ exchange may be the basis for Na,K-ATPase stimulation under some conditions. In rat adipocytes, insulin increases the Na^+ affinity of a cardiac glycoside-sensitive isoform [14]. In addition, Na,K-ATPase in membranes from frog skeletal muscle treated with insulin is increased even after ouabain inhibition, and this increase is blocked by monensin but not by actinomycin in the bathing medium. Since monensin inhibits translocation of proteins from the Golgi apparatus, insulin may act on transport of protein to the membrane [15].

Hormonal or other growth factors may induce enzyme biosynthesis directly or indirectly through effects on neuronal excitability. In rat brain, regional changes associated with sexual differentiation have been correlated with estrogen and androgen effects on excitability [16].

Neurotransmitter action may alter Na^+, K^+-pump activity

A functional link between neurotransmitter release and the Na^+, K^+-pump has been postulated. Stimulation of Na,K-ATPase activity in synaptosomes by biogenic amines has often been reported and is sometimes associated with reduced neurotransmitter release. Conversely, ouabain has been shown to stimulate acetylcholine release from synaptosomes [17]. It is speculated that a physiological influx of Ca^{2+} could inhibit the Na^+, K^+-pump, which could promote a further increase in $[Ca^{2+}]_i$, which can trigger neurotransmitter release. Proposed mechanisms for Na,K-ATPase stimulation by biogenic amines include (a) direct coupling of a receptor to the pump; (b) complexing of pump inhibitors; (c) inhibition of membrane lipid peroxidation; and (d) unmasking of latent enzyme activity. The experimentally observed modulation of ATPase by these agents probably involves a combination of these processes. A functional link between the Na^+, K^+-pump and neurotransmitter release *in situ* remains inconclusive [1].

Post-translational modifications may regulate Na,K-ATPase activity

Various secretagogues, including adrenergic and muscarinic neurotransmitters and peptide hormones, affect secretory tissues, leading to both Na^+-pump activation and secretion, which can be inhibited by ouabain. Thus, activation of the pump may mediate secretion. Pump activation may be caused by increased $[Na^+]_i$ or $[K^+]_e$ following depolarization; opening of cation-specific channels; depolarization; or second-messenger effects, such as protein phosphorylation mediated by cyclic nucleotide-dependent protein kinase, Ca^{2+}-calmodulin-kinase, or protein kinase C (see Chaps. 16 and 19). These mechanisms are the subject of current investigation.

In rat submandibular gland, carbachol stimulation leads to phosphorylation of a $96,000\text{-}M_r$ protein apparently identical to the Na,K-ATPase α subunit [18]. In pancreatic acinar cells, phorbol esters, which stimulate protein kinase C, were found to increase Na,K-ATPase activity [19]; however, the exact reactions or sites of secretagogue effects are not known.

In rabbit aortic tunica intima-media incubated *in vitro*, about 60 percent of the O_2 uptake that is dependent on adding *myo*-inositol and arachidonic acid to depleted incubation media is sensitive to ouabain. These data suggest that phosphatidyl-inositol turnover is linked to regulation of the Na^+,K^+-pump, possibly via protein kinase C [20].

Regulation of Na,K-ATPase may be disturbed in diabetes mellitus

Experimentally induced pancreatic acinar cell destruction leads to reduced Na,K-ATPase activity in sciatic nerve perineurium and dorsal root ganglia of rats and in certain retinal layers of rabbits. Elevated tissue glucose concentrations, as in diabetes mellitus, cause a decline in intracellular *myo*-inositol. Rabbit peripheral nerve shows reduced ouabain-sensitive O_2 utilization when the animal is made diabetic by alloxan administration. The O_2 consumption is increased in this preparation by the addition of phorbol esters that stimulate protein kinase C. These observations also suggest that protein kinase C links inositol phospholipid turnover and Na,K-ATPase and, furthermore, that diabetic neuropathy and other tissue pathology may be caused by a failure of kinase C activa-

tion of the Na^+-pump [21]. Biochemical demonstration of Na,K-ATPase regulation by any of these proposed mechanisms remains to be shown. Na,K-ATPase activity is likely to be reduced nonspecifically in pathologic tissue with cell loss or destruction due to various causes.

OTHER TRANSPORT SYSTEMS

There are several classes of ATP-dependent transport systems

The type 1 ATPases occur in prokaryote plasma membranes, chloroplasts, and mitochondria. They couple the synthesis of ATP to energy derived from the flow of protons. They are assemblages of five or more different subunits containing several nucleotide-binding sites. A phosphorylated enzyme is not an intermediate in the synthesis of ATP by these systems.

There are structural similarities among several cation transport ATPases that are designated type 2 (Fig. 3B). Well-characterized examples include the sarcoplasmic reticulum Ca^{2+}-ATPase and gastric H^+,K^+-ATPase in addition to the Na^+,K^+-pump. In each case examined, the transport mechanism appears to be analogous to that of Fig. 4—a conformational cycle in which an aspartyl residue is alternately phosphorylated and dephosphorylated at different stages. These transport proteins occur in plasma membranes, and some may function in endoplasmic reticulum.

A third class is represented by the ATP-dependent proton transporters that occur in membranes of Golgi cisternae; lysosomes; clathrin-coated vesicles, including presynaptic vesicles; peptide hormone storage vesicles; and catecholamine-storage vesicles, i.e., organelles related to either secretion or endocytosis. Synaptic plasma membranes may also contain a proton pump, which has not been well characterized. In each case, protons are pumped out of the cytoplasm into the vesicle. The subunit structures and sensitivities to inhibitors of these proton pumps differ from those of both type 1 and type 2 transport ATPases [22].

Numerous secondary active transport systems are important for neural functions

Active transport via specific carriers linked to the transmembrane Na^+ gradient is the primary mechanism responsible for transporting a variety of molecules in the nervous system, including Ca^{2+}, choline, catecholamines, γ-aminobutyric acid (GABA), glutamate, and other amino acids (Fig. 1). High-affinity transport processes are particularly important for terminating the action of neurotransmitters by their reuptake into nerve terminals. The precise distribution of the relevant carriers has not been determined, but these processes can be demonstrated in subcellular synaptosome preparations as well as in isolated and cultured neurons and glia. Both high- and low-affinity transport systems have been described. Typically, these systems have high affinity ($K_m < 10 \ \mu M$) for their ligands and are inhibited noncompetitively by ouabain because of discharge of the Na^+ gradient. Individual carriers may often be blocked by specific inhibitors. Examples include inhibition of biogenic amine uptake by cocaine and the tricyclic antidepressants and inhibition of high-affinity choline transport by hemicholinium-3. Generally, high-affinity transport systems for amino acids and neurotransmitters (see Chaps. 8–15) in the nervous system are Na^+ symporters, whereas important antiporters include Na^+/Ca^{2+} and Na^+/H^+ exchange proteins.

In several Na^+ symport systems, Na^+ binding to the carrier increases its affinity for the second ligand. The complex with filled external sites can then transit to the form with internally oriented sites. Because of the Na^+ gradient, association is favored at extracellular sites and dissociation is favored at internally oriented sites, leading to transport of both Na^+ and the ligand. Even though several symporters have been partially purified and functionally reconstituted into lipid vesicles, the molecular events that achieve these ligand movements are poorly understood.

Intracellular free Ca^{2+} is regulated by Ca^{2+}-ATPase and the Na^+/Ca^{2+} antiporter

The concentration of intracellular free Ca^{2+} ($[Ca^{2+}]_i$) is between 10^{-8} and 10^{-7} M, which is several orders of magnitude lower than the concentration of $[Ca^{2+}]_e$. Regulation of $[Ca^{2+}]_i$ is vital to functions of all cells but is particularly important in the regulation of intraneuronal signals; $[Ca^{2+}]_i$ regulates certain cation channels (see Chap. 4), acts in second-messenger systems (see Chaps. 16 and 19), and participates in neurotransmitter release (see Chap. 8).

Buffering of $[Ca^{2+}]_i$ is accomplished by an efficient but complex system that involves several pumps located in the plasma membrane and in intracellular organelle membranes (Fig. 7). The two major systems for regulating $[Ca^{2+}]_i$ are Ca^{2+}-ATPase, which is most efficient at low $[Ca^{2+}]_i$, and the Na^+/Ca^{2+} antiporter [23], which has a higher pumping capacity. Both are located in the plasma membrane and probably operate in parallel; however, there is still debate about their relative contributions to Ca^{2+} homeostasis. Different parts of the cell, for example, the plasma membrane of the cell body compared to that of synaptic terminals, probably vary in terms of the relative contributions made by these systems. The predominant form of Ca^{2+}-ATPase in brain appears to have a calmodulin receptor. It has a high affinity ($K_m < 1 \ \mu M$) but relatively low activity in brain. The main regulator, quantitatively, appears to be the Na^+/Ca^{2+} antiporter [24]. Direct studies of Na^+/Ca^{2+} fluxes suggest there is a transport

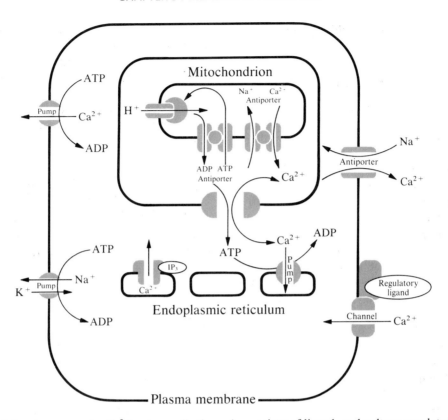

FIG. 7. Calcium homeostasis. Ca^{2+} enters cells through a variety of ligand- and voltage-regulated channels, but intracellular free Ca^{2+} is normally maintained at less than micromolar levels. Intracellular Ca^{2+} is probably regulated coordinately by a Na^+/Ca^{2+} antiporter in plasma membranes and by several different Ca-ATPases in plasma membranes and endoplasmic reticulum. The driving force for Na^+/Ca^{2+} antiporter exchange is the inwardly directed Na^+ gradient that is maintained by Na,K-ATPase. Mitochondria may participate transiently in Ca^{2+} homeostasis if the capacities of these other systems are exceeded. Internal stores of Ca^{2+} may be released from endoplasmic reticulum through the action of inositol-(1,4,5)-trisphosphate (IP_3) acting as a second messenger in response to various receptor systems (see Chap. 16).

ratio of about 3:1 and that under physiological conditions, this exchange pump is responsible for 30 to 50 percent of total Ca^{2+} efflux.

There is growing evidence that endoplasmic reticulum also contains an ATP-dependent Ca^{2+}-pump and participates in the Ca^{2+} buffering process [25]. Mitochondria also may function as a temporary buffer if the capacities of the higher affinity plasma membrane and endoplasmic reticulum systems are exceeded. In

mitochondria, Ca^{2+} may enter and exit by different pathways. The Ca^{2+} is transported into respiring mitochondria by a secondary transport process driven by the membrane potential; Ca^{2+} uptake is compensated by extrusion of 2 H^+ produced by the respiratory chain. Extrusion occurs primarily by a separate Na^+/Ca^{2+} antiporter, similar to that present in plasma membrane. Other participants in $[Ca^{2+}]_i$ buffering are the Ca^{2+}-binding proteins, which include calmodulin, paralbumin, calbindin, and calcineurin [24].

Glia contribute to K^+ homeostasis

Neuronal activity can readily lead to elevations of 1 to 3 mM in $[K^+]_e$ and during epileptogenesis, levels may be three to four times higher [26]. Elevated $[K^+]_e$ increases neuronal excitability, so that clearance of K^+ from the extracellular space is critical. Both neurons and astroglia are likely to be involved, and both active and passive transport are probably important. The relative contributions of the two cell types and of the two cell processes remain controversial. It is clear that neurons reaccumulate K^+ almost exclusively by means of active transport, but the Na^+,K^+-pump is slow relative to the channel-mediated K^+ release from neurons and to the rates of K^+ increase in the extracellular space. Moreover, the neuronal Na^+,K^+-pump is saturated at low $[K^+]_e$. If a Na^+,K^+-pump has a special role in clearing elevated $[K^+]_e$, its activity should increase at the higher levels of $[K^+]_e$. There is some evidence that the pump in astroglia may have such a response [27], since it appears to have a higher K_m for K^+ than does the pump in neurons.

In addition, astroglia passively transport K^+ by spatial buffering. In this case, K^+ is taken up by the perineuronal processes of glia, and an equal amount of K^+ exits from distal processes of these astroglia or from cells electrically coupled to them in regions where K^+ is lower. The K^+ is thereby transferred away from the site where the initial increase has occurred and K^+ can then be reaccumulated by neurons at the slower pace consistent with normal Na^+,K^+-pump activity. The process of spatial buffering has received strong support in the case of Müller cells, which are a form of glia that extend from the pigment epithelium to the vitreous surface of the retina. Most of the K^+-conductance channels of Müller cells are localized to the cell endfeet, which contact the vitreous surface so that high concentrations of K^+ at the basal surface lead to K^+ efflux at the endfeet [28]. In retina and brain it appears that this passive buffering by glial cells is more efficient than simple diffusion of K^+ through the narrow extracellular spaces. Its role relative to active transport of K^+ is more difficult to assess.

Intracellular pH can be regulated by ATP-dependent proton pumps, Na^+/H^+ antiporters, and anion antiporters

Cerebral metabolic energy is primarily derived from the oxidation of glucose to CO_2, which, in the steady state, could enter the circulation without disturbing the ionic balance. However, to the extent that oxidation is incomplete, i.e., that there is lactate or ketoacid production (see Chap. 28) or that CO_2 equilibrates to $H^+ + HCO_3^-$, local pH will decrease. *In vivo* cerebral respiration is profoundly sensitive to pH, decreasing with decreasing pH so that without adequate pH control, local metabolic deficits may be intensified and propagated [29].

Many epithelial cells can extrude protons via a transport ATPase in their plasma membranes. The best characterized mammalian enzyme of this type is the type 2 H^+,K^+-ATPase from gastric epithelia. Its occurrence in neural tissue has not been reported.

A Na^+/H^+ antiporter occurs in synaptosomes and in glia [30] and neuroblastoma cells [31] (Fig. 8). It is relatively inactive at neutral pH; however, a decrease in intracellular pH produces an efflux of protons at the expense of the Na^+ gradient. Although the antiporter has an Na^+/H^+ stoichiometry of 1:1, it is allosterically regulated by the internal pH: Protonation of a cytoplasmic site increases the affinity of the proton ionophoric site, thus amplifying its sensitivity to changes in intracellular pH.

The Na^+/H^+ antiporter is also regulated by receptor mechanisms in some cells. Several growth factors and hormones produce transient

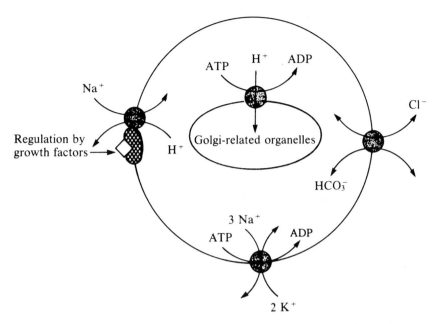

FIG. 8. Intracellular pH regulation. Protons can be secreted from cells in exchange for Na^+, mediated by a Na^+/H^+ antiporter. Many secretory granules, lysosomes, and endocytic vesicles contain inwardly directed ATP-dependent proton pumps. Metabolically generated bicarbonate can be exchanged for chloride through a ubiquitous plasma membrane anion antiporter.

cytoplasmic alkalinization, perhaps by mediating a protein kinase phosphorylation of the antiporter to increase its internal proton affinity. Other mechanisms may also be important for local pH control. The combined activities of a HCO_3^-/Cl^- antiporter and carbonic anhydrase mediate CO_2 transport in erythrocytes. A similar system may play a role in pH regulation in brain [32].

Cell volumes are controlled by means of ion transport mechanisms

Inadequate control of cell volume in the brain can lead to the cytotoxic form of cerebral edema (see Chap. 40). The phenomenon of spreading depression that occurs during seizures includes complex changes in both pH and cell volume that may involve the Na^+/H^+ antiporter [29]. Astrocytes rapidly swell when ATP is depleted if the Na^+,K^+-pump is inhibited by ouabain or exposed to high $[K^+]_e$. This swelling is a consequence of an uptake of salts that can be blocked by furosemide and bumetanide. Sensitivity to these drugs is characteristic of a transporter that links the symport of 1 Na^+, 1 K^+, and 2 Cl^- [33]. The mechanism of recovery, called regulatory volume decrease, is better understood in several other cell types (Fig. 9) and results from opening K^+ and Cl^- channels. A mechanism of regulatory volume increase is initiated in response to hyperosmotic cell shrinking that seems to involve protein phosphokinase activation of the Na^+/H^+ antiporter. [34].

Glucose crosses the blood-brain barrier and the plasma membranes of most cells via a facilitated diffusion process

The glucose transporter that mediates this process has been best characterized in erythro-

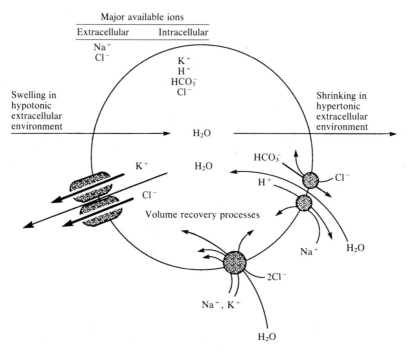

FIG. 9. Ionic regulation of cell volume. Many cells respond to external osmotic changes by an initial swelling or shrinking followed by a return toward their initial "normal" volumes. These secondary responses result from osmotic activation of ion transport pathways that may vary with cell type. Regulatory volume decreases after swelling in hypotonic media can occur by outflow of KCl through the opening of channels. Regulatory volume increases subsequent to hypertonic shrinking may occur by NaCl influx through symporters, either with or without coupling to K^+ influx. (From ref. 35.)

cytes. The unliganded transporter appears to exist primarily in two conformations characterized by inward- and outward-facing glucose-binding sites. Transport appears to involve transitions between these two states, perhaps involving intermediate forms that transiently open an aqueous channel through the protein [36]. The structural unit is a 55-kilodalton (kDa) glycoprotein. It is noteworthy that despite the vital dependence of the brain on an adequate supply of glucose, the brain has no mechanism at the cellular level for coupling glucose transport to its metabolic requirements. Instead, normal brain metabolism is closely coupled to local blood flow (see Chap. 29).

REFERENCES

1. Stahl, W. L. The Na,K-ATPase of nervous tissue. *Neurochem. Int.* 8:449–476, 1986.
2. Sweadner, K. J. Two molecular forms of (Na$^+$ + K$^+$)-stimulated ATPase in brain. *J. Biol. Chem.* 254:6060–6067, 1979.
3. Shull, G. E., Greeb, J., and Lingrel, J. B. Molecular cloning of three distinct forms of the Na,K-ATPase α-subunit from rat brain. *Biochem.* 25:8125–8132, 1986.
4. Hodgkin, A. L., and Keynes, R. D. Active transport of cations in giant axons from *Sepia* and *Loligo*. *J. Physiol.* 128:28–60, 1955.
5. Goldshlegger, R., Karlish, S. J. D., Rephaeli, A., and Stein, W. D. The effect of membrane po-

tential on the mammalian Na^+,K^+-pump reconstituted into phospholipid vesicles. *J. Physiol. (Lond.)* 387:331–355, 1987.

6. Bertoni, J. M., and Siegel, G. J. Development of Na,K-ATPase in rat cerebrum: Correlation with Na^+-dependent phosphorylation and K^+-*p*-nitrophenylphosphatase. *J. Neurochem.* 31:1501–1511, 1978.

7. Siegel, G. J., Holm, C., Schreiber, J. H., Desmond, T. J., and Ernst, S. A. Purification of mouse brain Na,K-ATPase catalytic unit, characterization of antiserum, and immunocytochemical localization in cerebellum, choroid plexus and kidney. *J. Histochem. Cytochem.* 32:1309–1318, 1984.

8. Ariyasu, R., and Ellisman, M. H. The distribution of Na,K-ATPase is continuous along the axolemma of unensheathed axons from spinal roots of 'dystrophic' mice. *J. Neurocytol.* 16:239–248, 1987.

9. Stahl, W. L., and Broderson, S. H. Localization of Na,K-ATPase in brain. *Fed. Proc.* 35:1260–1265, 1976.

10. McGrail, K. M., and Sweadner, K. J. Immunofluorescent localization of two different Na,K-ATPases in the rat retina and in identified dissociated retinal cells. *J. Neurosci.* 6:1272–1283, 1986.

11. Chaudhury, S., Ismail-Beigi, F., Gick, G. G., Levenson, R., and Edelman, I. Effect of thyroid hormone on the abundance of Na,K-adenosine triphosphatase α-subunit messenger ribonucleic acid. *Mol. Endocrinol.* 1:83–89, 1987.

12. Doucet, A., Hus-Citharel, A., and Morel, F. *In vitro* stimulation of Na,K-ATPase in rat thick ascending limb by dexamethasone. *Am. J. Physiol.* 251:F851–F857, 1986.

13. Beach, R. E., Schwab, S. J., Brazy, P. C., and Dennis, W. W. Norepinephrine increases Na,K-ATPase and solute transport in rabbit proximal tubules. *Am. J. Physiol.* 252:F215–F220, 1987.

14. Lytton, J. Identification of two molecular forms of Na,K-ATPase in rat adipocytes. *J. Biol. Chem.* 260:4052–4058, 1986.

15. Kanbe, M., and Kitasato, H. Stimulation of Na,K-ATPase activity of frog skeletal muscle by insulin. *Biochim. Biophys. Res. Commun.* 134:609–616, 1986.

16. Guerra, M., Del Castillo, A. R., Battaner, E., and Mas, M. Androgens stimulate preoptic area Na,K-ATPase activity in male rats. *Neurosci. Lett.* 78:97–100, 1987.

17. Cooper, J. R., and Meyer, E. M. Possible mechanisms involved in the release and modulation of release of neuroactive agents. *Neurochem. Int.* 6:419–433, 1984.

18. Collins, S. A., Pon, D. J., and Sen, A. K. Phosphorylation of the α-subunit of Na,K-ATPase by carbachol in tissue slices and the role of phosphoproteins in stimulus-secretion coupling. *Biochim. Biophys. Acta* 927:392–401, 1987.

19. Hootman, R. R., Brown, M. E., and Williams, J. A. Phorbol esters and A23187 regulate Na^+-pump activity in pancreatic acinar cells. *Am. J. Physiol.* 252:G499–G505, 1987.

20. Simmons, D. A., Kern, E. F., Winegrad, A. I., and Martin, D. B. Basal phosphatidylinositol turnover controls aortic Na,K-ATPase activity. *J. Clin. Invest.* 77:503–512, 1986.

21. Greene, D. A., and Lattimer, S. A. Protein kinase C agonists acutely normalize decreased ouabain-inhibitable respiration in diabetic rabbit nerve. *Diabetes* 35:242–245, 1986.

22. Rudnick, G. ATP-driven H^+ pumping into intracellular organelles. *Annu. Rev. Physiol.* 48:403–413, 1986.

23. Carafoli, E., and Zurini, M. The Ca^{2+}-pumping ATPase of plasma membranes. *Biochim. Biophys. Acta* 683:279–301, 1982.

24. McBurney, R. N., and Neering, I. R. Neuronal calcium homeostasis. *Trends Neurosci.* 10:164–169, 1987.

25. Shah, J., Cohen, R. S., and Pant, H. C. Inositol trisphosphate-induced calcium release in brain microsomes. *Brain Res.* 419:1–6, 1987.

26. Katzman, R., and Grossman, R. Neuronal activity and potassium movement. In D. H. Invar and H. Lassen (eds.), *Brain Work: The Coupling of Function, Metabolism and Blood Flow in Brain.* Copenhagen: Munkesgaard, pp. 149–156, 1975.

27. Franck, G., Grisar, T., and Moonen, G. Glial and neuronal Na^+,K^+ pump. *Adv. Cell Neurobiol.* 4:133–159, 1983.

28. Newman, E. A. Distribution of potassium conductance in mammalian Müller (glial) cells: A

comparative study. *J. Neurosci.* 7:2423–2432, 1987.

29. Siesjo, B. K., et al. Extra- and intra-cellular pH in the brain during seizures and in the recovery period following the arrest of seizure activity. *J. Cereb. Blood Flow Metab.* 5:47–57, 1985.

30. Kimelberg, H. K., Biddlecomb, S., and Bourke, R. S. SITS-inhibitable Cl^- transport and Na^+-dependent H^+ production in primary astroglial cultures. *Brain Res.* 173:111–124, 1979.

31. Jean T., Frelin, C., Vigne, P., Barbry, P., and Lazdunski, M. Biochemical properties of the Na^+/H^+ exchange system in rat brain synaptosomes. *J. Biol. Chem.* 260:9678–9684, 1985.

32. Lowe, A. G., and Lampert, A. Chloride-bicarbonate exchange and related transport processes. *Biochim. Biophys. Acta* 694:353–374, 1983.

33. Kimelberg, H. K., and Frangakis, M. V. Furosemide- and bumetanide-sensitive ion transport and volume control in primary astrocyte cultures from rat brain. *Brain Res.* 361:125–134, 1985.

34. Grinstein, S., Goetz-Smith, J. D., Stewart, D., Beresford, B. J., and Mellors, A. Protein phosphorylation during activation of Na^+/H^+ exchange. *J. Biol. Chem.* 261:8009–8016, 1986.

35. Sarkadi, B., Attisani, L., Grinstein, S., Buchwald, M., and Rothstein, A. Volume regulation of Chinese hamster ovary cells in anisoosmotic media. *Biochim. Biophys. Acta* 774:159–168, 1984.

36. Alvarez, J., Lee, D. C., Baldwin, S. A., Chapman, D. Fourier transform infrared spectroscopic study of the structure and conformational changes of the human erythrocyte glucose transporter. *J. Biol. Chem.* 262:3502–3509, 1987.

CHAPTER 4

Electrical Excitability and Ionic Channels

Bertil Hille and William A. Catterall

Basic Neurochemistry: Molecular, Cellular, and Medical Aspects, 4th Ed., edited by G. J. Siegel et al. Raven Press, Ltd., New York, 1989.
Correspondence to Bertil Hille, Department of Physiology and Biophysics SJ-40, University of Washington Medical School, Seattle, Washington 98195.

The nervous system enables animals to receive and act on internal and external stimuli with speed and in a coordinated manner. Activity of the nervous system is reflected in a variety of electrical and chemical signals that arise in the receptor organs, the nerve cells, and the effector organs, including the muscles and secretory glands. Consider, for example, a simple reflex arc mediating reflex withdrawal of the hand from a hot surface. Four cell types are involved in a network shown diagrammatically in Fig. 1. The message travels from skin receptors through the network as a volley of electrical disturbances, terminating in the contraction of some muscles. This chapter concerns the origin of electrical potentials in such excitable cells. As we shall see, potentials are generated by the passive diffusion of ions such as Na^+, K^+, Ca^{2+}, and Cl^-, through highly selective molecular pores in the cell surface membrane called ionic channels. Ionic channels play a role in membrane excitation as central as the role of

enzymes in metabolism. The opening and closing of specific channels shapes the membrane potential changes and gives rise to characteristic electrical messages. (The interested reader is referred to Hodgkin [1], Armstrong [2], Kuffler et al. [3] and Hille [4,5] for more detailed treatment of this subject.)

ELECTRICAL PHENOMENA IN EXCITABLE CELLS

All excitable cells have a membrane potential

At rest, the entire cytoplasm is electrically more negative than the external bathing fluid by 30 to 100 mV. All of this potential drop appears across the extremely thin external cell membrane, as may be ascertained by recording with an electrolyte-filled glass pipette microelectrode. When such an electrode is used to probe potentials around an excitable cell, a sudden negative drop appears at the moment the thin tip of the pipette penetrates the cell surface. By convention, the membrane potential is always reported in terms of "inside" minus "outside," so the resting potential is a negative number; for example, -70 mV in a myelinated nerve fiber. Signals that make the cytoplasm more positive are said to depolarize the membrane, and those making it more negative are said to hyperpolarize the membrane.

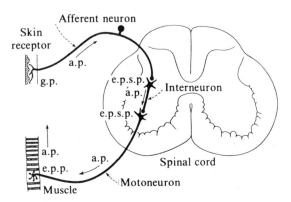

FIG. 1. Path of excitation in a simplified spinal reflex that mediates withdrawal of the arm from a painful stimulus. In each of the three neurons and in the muscle cell, excitation starts with a localized slow potential and is propagated via an action potential (a.p.). The slow potentials are generator potential (g.p.) at the skin; excitatory postsynaptic potentials (e.p.s.p.) at the interneuron and the motoneuron; and end-plate potential (e.p.p.) at the neuromuscular junction. Each neuron makes additional connections to other pathways that are not shown.

Electrical signals recorded from cells are basically of two types: stereotyped action potentials characteristic of each cell type, and a variety of slow potentials

The action potential of axons is a brief, spike-like depolarization that propagates regeneratively as an electrical wave without decrement and at a high, constant velocity from one end of the axon to the other [3]. It is used for all rapid signaling over a distance. For example, in the reflex arc of Fig. 1, action potentials in motor axons might carry the message from spinal cord to arm, telling the muscle fibers of the biceps to contract. In large mammalian axons at body temperature, the action potential at any one patch of membrane may last only 0.4 msec as it propagates at a speed of 100 m/sec. The action potential is normally elicited when the cell membrane is depolarized by some type of stimulus to beyond a threshold level; and it is said to be produced in an all-or-nothing manner because a subthreshold stimulus gives no propagated response, whereas every suprathreshold stimulus elicits the stereotyped propagating wave. Underlying the propagated action potential is a regenerative wave of opening and closing of voltage-gated ionic channels that sweeps along the axon. Action potentials are also frequently referred to as spikes, or impulses. Most nerve cell and muscle cell membranes can make action potentials and are said to be electrically excitable, but a few cannot.

By contrast, slow potentials are localized membrane depolarizations and hyperpolarizations, with the time courses ranging from several milliseconds to minutes. They are associated with a variety of transduction mechanisms. For example, slow potentials arise at the membrane site of action of neurotransmitter molecules and of some hormones, and also in sensory endings of chemosensors, mechanosensors, and other receptor cells. These electrical signals in sensory endings are frequently called generator, or receptor, potentials, and the signals arising postsynaptically at chemical synapses are called postsynaptic potentials. Slow potentials are graded in relation to their stimulus and sum with each other both spatially and temporally while decaying passively over a distance of no more than a few millimeters from their site of generation. Underlying the slow potential is a graded and local opening or closing of ionic channels reflecting the intensity of the stimulus. The natural stim-

ulus for the initiation of propagated action potentials is a depolarizing slow potential exceeding the firing threshold. Thus, impulses in a wide variety of presynaptic cells often give rise to a barrage of excitatory (depolarizing) and inhibitory (hyperpolarizing) postsynaptic potentials in the dendrites of a postsynaptic neuron. These slow potentials sum in the cell body to provide the drive stimulating or suppressing the initiation of action potentials at the axon hillock, which then propagate down the axon. In each of the four cell populations involved in the reflex arc in Fig. 1, depolarizing slow potentials give rise to propagating action potentials as the message moves forward.

THE IONIC HYPOTHESIS AND THE MEMBRANE THEORY

In the late nineteenth century, such scientific giants as Kohlrausch, Arrhenius, Ostwald, Nernst, and Planck elucidated the nature of ionic dissociation and movement in aqueous solution, and physiologists realized that the currents and potentials in excitable cells might be due to the diffusion of ions. This view was put in a clear form as early as 1902 by Julius Bernstein in his "membrane theory." He postulated that

1. Electrical potentials arise across a semipermeable plasma membrane that completely envelops each cell.
2. The potential arises because of concentration gradients of ions such as K^+ across the membrane and because the membrane is not equally permeable to all ions.
3. The potentials change when some chemical alteration in the membrane changes the ionic permeability.

Although 50 more years of electrophysiological work were required to complete the proof, the membrane theory is now fully tested and is no longer a hypothesis. Before we can discuss its consequences in further detail, we must review the physical chemistry of electrodiffusion.

RULES OF IONIC ELECTRICITY

How do membrane potentials arise?

Consider the electrolyte system represented in Fig. 2 (left), where a porous membrane separates aqueous solutions of unequal concentrations of a fictitious salt KA. Two electrodes permit the potential difference between the two solutions to be measured. Now, assume that the membrane pores are permeable exclusively to K$^+$ so that K$^+$ begins to diffuse across the membrane but A$^-$ does not. For simple statistical reasons, the movement of K$^+$ from the concentrated side to the dilute side will initially

exceed the movement in the reverse direction, and we speak of a net flux of K$^+$ down the concentration gradient. However, this process does not continue long since K$^+$ carries a positive charge from one compartment to the other and leaves a net negative charge behind. Separation of the charge creates an electrical potential difference (the membrane potential) between the two solutions, and a positive charge appears on the side into which the K$^+$ ions diffuse, thereby setting up an electrical force that tends to oppose further net movement of K$^+$.

Equilibrium potential is membrane potential at which there are no net ionic movements

The membrane potential reached in a system with only one permeant ion and no perturbing forces is called the equilibrium, or Nernst, potential for that ion; that is, the final membrane potential for the system in Fig. 2 is the potassium equilibrium potential E_K. At that potential, there is no further net movement of K$^+$, and unless otherwise disturbed, the membrane potential and ionic gradient will remain stable indefinitely. The value of the Nernst potential is derived from thermodynamics by recognizing that the change of electrochemical potential $\triangle\mu_j$ for moving the permeant ion j^{+z} across the membrane must be zero at equilibrium:

$$\triangle\mu_j = 0 = RT \ln \frac{[j]_o}{[j]_i} - zFE \qquad (1)$$

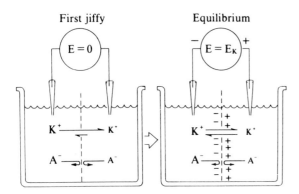

FIG. 2. Origin of the membrane potential in a purely K$^+$-permeable membrane. The porous membrane separates unequal concentrations of the dissociated salt K$^+$A$^-$. In the first "jiffy," the membrane potential E, recorded by the electrodes above, is zero, and K$^+$ diffuses to the right down the concentration gradient. The anion A$^-$ cannot cross the membrane, so a net positive charge builds up on the right-hand side and a negative charge on the left. At equilibrium, the membrane potential, caused by the charge separation, has built up to the Nernst potential E_K, and the fluxes of K$^+$ become equal in the two directions.

where R is the gas constant [8.31 joules (J)/deg/mol], T is absolute temperature in degrees Kelvin ($^\circ$C + 273.2), and F is Faraday's constant [96,500 coulombs (C)/mol]. Using terms appropriate to biology, $[j]_o$ and $[j]_i$ represent activities of ion j^{+z} outside and inside a cell; z is the ionic valence, and E the membrane potential defined as "inside minus outside." Solving for E and calling it E_j to denote the ion at equilibrium gives the Nernst equation for ion j:

$$E_j = \frac{RT}{zF} \ln \frac{[j]_o}{[j]_i} \qquad (2)$$

For practical use at 20° C, the Nernst equation can be rewritten

$$E_j = \frac{58 \text{ mV}}{z} \log \frac{[j]_o}{[j]_i} \qquad (3)$$

showing that for a 10:1 transmembrane gradient, a monovalent ion can give 58 mV of membrane potential. Table 1 gives approximate intracellular and extracellular concentrations of the four electrically most important ions in a mammalian skeletal muscle cell and the Nernst potentials calculated from these numbers at 37°C (neglecting possible activity coefficient corrections). Experimentally, it is found that the resting muscle membrane is primarily permeable to K^+ and Cl^-, and therefore the resting potential in muscle is -90 mV, close to the equilibrium potentials E_K and E_{Cl}. During a propagated action potential, ionic channels permeable to Na^+ open, some Na^+ enters the fiber, and the membrane potential swings transiently toward E_{Na}. When these pores close again, the membrane potential returns to near E_K and E_{Cl}. To summarize, membrane potentials arise by diffusion of a small number of ions down their concentration gradient across a permselective membrane.

Fluxes and nonequilibrium potentials are found in real cells

Although the concept of equilibrium potentials is essential to understand and predict the membrane potentials generated by ionic permeability, real cells are actually never at equilibrium, because different ionic channels open and close during excitation and, even at rest, several types of channels are open simultaneously. Under these circumstances, the ionic gradients are dissipated constantly, albeit slowly, and ionic pumps are always needed in the long run to maintain a steady state (see Chap. 3). The net passive flux M_j of each ion is proportional to the permeability P_j for that ion and is often given, at least approximately, by an empirical formula called the Goldman-Hodgkin-Katz flux equation [4,6]:

$$M_j = P_j z_j \frac{EF}{RT} \frac{[j]_o - [j]_i \exp(z_j EF/RT)}{1 - \exp(z_j EF/RT)} \qquad (4)$$

Experimentally, these fluxes may be measured as an electric current or by using radioactive tracers or with sensitive indicator substances responding to the ion in question by fluorescence or other optical changes. In most cases, the fluxes are too small to detect by the less sensitive classical method of chemical analysis for the total amount of an ion.

When the membrane is permeable to several ions, the steady-state potential is given by

TABLE 1. Approximate free ion concentrations in mammalian skeletal muscle

Ion	Extracellular concentration (mM)	Intracellular concentration (mM)	$\frac{[Ion]_o}{[Ion]_i}$	Nernst potential[a] (mV)
Na^+	145	12	12	$+66$
K^+	4	155	0.026	-97
Ca^{2+}	1.5	$<10^{-3}$	$>1,500$	>97
Cl^-	120	4^b	30^b	-90^b

[a] Equilibrium potentials calculated at 37°C from the Nernst equation.
[b] Calculated assuming a -90 mV resting potential for the muscle membrane and assuming that chloride ions are at equilibrium at rest.

the sum of contributions of the permeant ions, weighted according to their relative permeabilities [4,6]:

$$E = \frac{RT}{F} \ln \frac{P_{Na}[Na^+]_o + P_K[K^+]_o + P_{Cl}[Cl^-]_i}{P_{Na}[Na^+]_i + P_K[K^+]_i + P_{Cl}[Cl^-]_o} \quad (5)$$

This Goldman-Hodgkin-Katz voltage equation is often used to determine the relative permeabilities to ions from experiments where the bathing-ion concentrations are varied and changes in the membrane potential are recorded. It has the same form as the equation usually used to describe the responses of ion-selective electrodes in analytical work in the laboratory.

During excitation, ionic channels open or close, ions move, and the membrane potential changes

The extra ionic fluxes during activity act as an extra load on the Na^+-K^+ pump and the Ca^{2+} pump, consuming ATP and stimulating an extra burst of cellular oxygen consumption until the original gradients are restored. How large are these fluxes? The physical minimum, calculated from the rules of electricity, is a very small number. Only 10^{-12} equivalents of charge need be moved to polarize 1 cm² of membrane by 100 mV, meaning that, ideally, the movement of 1 pmol/cm² of monovalent ion would be enough to depolarize the membrane more than fully. This quantity, related to the electrical capacitance of the membrane, is a constant throughout the animal and plant kingdoms, as would be the case were the effective thickness and dielectric constant of the insulating (hydrophobic) part of all cell plasma membranes similar. In practice, unmyelinated axons gain about 4 to 8 pmol of Na^+ and lose about the same amount of K^+ per square centimeter for one action potential. The figure is higher than the physical ideal because the oppositely directed fluxes of Na^+ and K^+ overlap considerably in time, working against each other. With this kind of Na^+ gain, a squid

unmyelinated giant axon of 1 mm diameter could be stimulated 10^5 times, and a mammalian fiber of 0.2-µm diameter only 10 to 15 times before the internal Na^+ concentration would be doubled, assuming that the Na^+-K^+ pump had been blocked. In myelinated nerve, the Na^+ gain in one impulse is very small, amounting to only 2×10^{-7} mol/kg of nerve because of the special low-capacitance properties of myelin.

Transport systems may also produce membrane potentials

The equations just discussed are those for passive electrodiffusion in ionic channels where the only motive forces on ions are thermal and electrical, and they do indeed explain almost all the potentials of excitable cells. However, there is another type of electric current source in cells that can generate potentials: the ion pumps and other membrane devices that couple ion movements to the movements of other molecules. In excitable cells, the most prominent is the Na^+-K^+ pump (see Chap. 3), which gives a net export of positive charge and hence tends to hyperpolarize the cell-surface membrane in proportion to the rate of pumping [7]; but hyperpolarization from this electrogenic pumping is typically only a modest few millivolts. By contrast, mitochondria (and plant, algal, and fungal cells) have powerful current sources in their proton transport systems. Their membrane potentials are at times dominated by this electrogenic system and would then not be describable in terms of diffusion in simple passive channels.

ELECTRICALLY EXCITABLE CELLS

Permeability changes of the action potential

Given the rules of ionic electricity, the major biological problem in understanding action potentials is to describe and explain the ionic permeability mechanisms in the membrane. The opening and closing of ionic channels involves passive conformational changes driven by electric field changes or ligand binding but not by direct consumption of metabolic energy. The independence of immediate metabolic input can be demonstrated in studies with internally perfused cells and with channels reconstituted into lipid bilayers. For example, the great majority of the axoplasm may be squeezed from one cut end of a squid giant axon, and then the axon may be reinflated with a continuously flowing column of salt solution that enters at one end and leaves at the other, and excitability can still be preserved. A giant axon perfused with isotonic potassium sulfate can continue to fire several hundred-thousand impulses. Analogous experiments using dialysis techniques or diffusion of ions through holes sucked in cell membranes or using excised patches of membrane have been done with other axons, skeletal muscle, and invertebrate and vertebrate neuronal cell bodies. These experiments prove that ATP and other intracellular, small molecules of metabolism are not required either for many cycles of opening and closing of Na^+, K^+, or Ca^{2+} channels or for the resulting depolarizing and repolarizing ionic current flows. They also show, however, that ATP, guanosine cyclic $3',5'$ phosphate (cGMP) and Ca^{2+}, as well as phosphorylation by a variety of protein kinases, can be intracellular modulators of channel activities. In the long term, ATP and other molecules are also needed to fuel the Na^+-K^+ and Ca^{2+} pumps and to maintain the biochemical structure and integrity of the membrane and its channels. We must emphasize that channels differ from pumps in their structure, mechanism of ionic flux, function, and regulation.

Gating mechanisms for Na^+ and K^+ channels in the axolemma are voltage dependent

In a classic series of experiments, Hodgkin, Huxley, and Katz [1,3–5,8] measured the ki-netics of ionic permeability changes in squid giant-axon membranes by a direct electrical method called the voltage clamp. As the name implies, the method controls the membrane voltage electrically (usually to follow step changes of potential) while ionic movements are recorded directly as electric current flowing across the membrane. The recorded current may be resolved into individual ionic components by changing the ions in the solutions that bathe the membrane. The voltage clamp is a rapid and sensitive assay for studying the opening and closing of ionic channels. A modern and now widely used version of the voltage clamp is the patch clamp, a technique with sufficient sensitivity to study the current flow in a single ionic channel [9]. A glass micropipette with a tip diameter <1 μm is fire polished at the tip and then pressed against the membrane of a cell. Because the tip is smoothed rather than having sharp edges, it seals to the membrane in the annular zone of contact rather than piercing the membrane and defines a tiny patch of the cell surface whose few ionic channels can readily be detected by the currents flowing through them. With the patch clamp a flux of as little as 10^{-20} mol of ion in less than 1 msec can readily be measured.

By using the voltage clamp, Hodgkin and Huxley [8] discovered that the processes underlying gating (the opening and closing conformational changes) of axonal Na^+ and K^+ channels are controlled by the membrane potential and therefore derive their energy from the work done by the electric field on charges or dipolar groups associated with the channel macromolecule. Hodgkin and Huxley [8] identified currents from two types of ion-selective channels—Na^+ channels and K^+ channels—which account for almost all of the current in axon membranes, and they made a kinetic model of the opening and closing steps, which may be simplified as shown in Fig. 3. Depolarization of the membranes is sensed by the channels and causes the conformational reactions to proceed to the right. Repolarization or hyper-

Na⁺ Channels

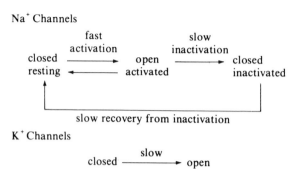

K⁺ Channels

FIG. 3. Simplified kinetic model for opening and closing steps of Na⁺ and K⁺ channels. (Adapted from Hodgkin and Huxley [8].)

polarization causes them to proceed to the left. We can understand the action potential in these terms. The action potential, caused by a depolarizing stimulus, begins with a transient, voltage-gated opening of Na⁺ channels that allows Na⁺ to enter the fiber and depolarize the membrane fully, followed by a transient, voltage-gated opening of K⁺ channels that allows K⁺ to leave and repolarize the membrane. Figure 4 shows a calculation of the temporal relation between channel-opening and membrane-potential changes in an axon at 18.5°C, using the model of Hodgkin and Huxley [8].

The action potential is propagated by local spread of depolarization

If there are no chemical or mechanical signals for voltage-gated channels to open, how does the action potential propagate smoothly down an axon, bringing new ionic channels into play ahead of it? Any electrical depolarization or hyperpolarization of a cell membrane spreads a small distance in either direction from its source by a purely passive process often called cable, or electrotonic, spread. The spread occurs because the intracellular and extracellular media are much better conductors than is the membrane, so any charges injected at one point across the membrane repel each other and dis-

perse over the membrane surface. Electrophysiologists usually describe this process formally in terms of current flow in an electrical equivalent circuit, with resistors and capacitors representing the geometry of the cell and its membranes. One of the common resulting equations is called the cable equation in analogy to the similar description of how signals spread in electrical cables. The lower part of Fig. 4 shows diagrammatically the so-called local circuit currents that spread the depolarization forward. In this way, an excited depolarized membrane area smoothly depolarizes the next unexcited region ahead of the action potential, bringing it above firing threshold, opening Na⁺ channels there, and advancing the wave of excitation. The action potential in the upper part of Fig. 4 is calculated by combining the known "cable properties" of the squid giant axon with the rules of ionic electricity and the kinetic equations (Hodgkin-Huxley equations) for the voltage-dependent gating of Na⁺ and K⁺ channels. The success of the calculations means that the factors described are sufficient to account for action-potential propagation.

Membranes at nodes of Ranvier are characterized by high concentrations of Na⁺ channels

A wide variety of cells have now been studied by voltage clamp methods, and quantitative descriptions of their permeability changes are available. All axons, whether vertebrate or invertebrate, operate on the same principles: They have a small background permeability, primarily to K⁺, which sets the resting potential, and display brief, dramatic openings of Na⁺ and K⁺ channels in sequence to shape the action potentials. Chapter 6 describes myelin, a special adaptation of large (1–20-μm diameter) vertebrate nerve fibers for higher conduction speed. In myelinated nerves, like unmyelinated ones, the depolarization spreads from one excitable membrane patch to another by

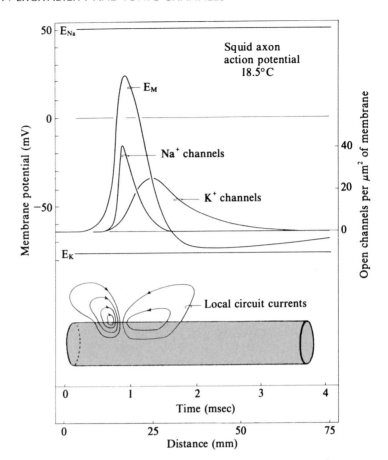

FIG. 4. Events of the propagated action potential calculated from the Hodgkin-Huxley [8] kinetic model. Because the action potential is a nondecrementing wave, the diagram shows equivalently the timecourse of events at one point in the axon, or the spatial distribution of events at one time as the excitation propagates to the left. *Upper:* Action potential (E_M) and the opening and closing of Na^+ and K^+ channels. The Nernst potentials for Na^+ and K^+ are indicated by E_{Na} and E_K. *Lower:* Local circuit currents. The intense loop on the left spreads the depolarization to the left into the unexcited membrane.

local circuit currents; but because of the insulating properties of the coating myelin, the excitable patches of axon membrane (the nodes of Ranvier) may be more than 1 mm apart, so the rate of progression of the impulse is faster. The wavelength of an action potential is such that 20 to 40 nodes of Ranvier are active at one time, and every 15 to 20 μsec, a new node in front begins to depolarize, and an old one behind finishes repolarizing. Nodes of Ranvier have the same type of Na^+ channels as do other axon membranes, but nodal membranes have at least ten times as many channels per unit area to depolarize the long, passive, internodal myelin. The Na^+-K^+ pump may be distributed similarly (see Chap. 3). The internodal axon membrane

has K^+ channels but few Na^+ channels [10]; however, hidden underneath the myelin, these K^+ channels are not in a position to contribute to action potentials. After experimental demyelination by diphtheria toxin (a process taking several days), and probably in the course of several demyelinating diseases (see Chap. 36), Na^+ channels and excitability can develop in a formerly internodal section of axon [11].

A wide repertoire of voltage-sensitive conductance channels are found among cell types

In seeking diversity among types of channels, we need not look to evolution, for channels seem to be conservative and quite similar among animals with nervous systems. Rather, diversity is found in the different cell types in any one organism, where the repertoire of functioning channels is adapted to the special role each cell plays in the body. All axons have only to transmit brief action potentials that code a message by their frequency, so their channels are similar. However, the action potential of a variety of muscles and secretory cells may serve instead to time the duration or fix the intensity of a contraction or a secretory response, and their action potentials are never as brief and rarely as invariant as those of axons. Their activities may require more than ten types of channels, several of which are subject to modulatory influences, often phosphorylation, that regulate the overall behavior of the cell. A neuron cell body also has many more channel types than does the axon coming from it. In all of these cell types, it is not uncommon to find Ca^{2+} channels that open with depolarization, supplementing the depolarizing effect of Na^+ channels by adding a slower, depolarizing Ca^{2+} influx or sometimes even acting alone to depolarize the membrane without Na^+ channels [12,13]. Ca^{2+} channels have a special importance, because the entering Ca^{2+} often plays the role of a chemical messenger to activate exocytosis (secretion), contraction, gating of other channels, ciliary reorientation, metabolic pathways, etc. Indeed, whenever an electrical message activates any nonelectrical event, a change of the intracellular free Ca^{2+} concentration acts as an intermediary. In addition, muscles, secretory cells, and neuron cell bodies usually have many types of K^+ channels, some opened by depolarization, as in axons, some also opened by raised intracellular free Ca^{2+}, and some turned off by depolarization. Several of these K^+ channels may be modulated by neurotransmitters and hormones. The electric eel electroplax has a high density of conventional Na^+ channels to generate the strong currents of the electric discharge and resting K^+ channels that turn off

with depolarization to avoid opposing the effect of the Na^+ channels.

PROPERTIES OF VOLTAGE-GATED IONIC CHANNELS

Ionic channels are macromolecules or macromolecular complexes that form aqueous pores in the lipid membrane

Much of what we know about ionic channels comes from functional studies with voltage clamp and patch clamp methods on channels still imbedded in the cell membrane [2,4,5]. Figure 5A summarizes the major functional properties of a voltage-gated macromolecular channel in terms of a fanciful cartoon. The pore is narrow enough in one place, the ionic selectivity filter, to "feel" each ion and to distinguish among Na^+, K^+, Ca^{2+}, and Cl^-. The channel also contains charged or dipolar components that sense the electric field in the membrane and drive conformational changes that, in effect, open and close gates controlling the permeability of the pore. In Na^+, K^+, and Ca^{2+} channels, the gates seem to close the axoplasmic mouth of the pore, and the selectivity filter seems to be near the outer end of the pore.

How do we know that a channel is a pore? By far the most convincing evidence is the large ionic flux a single channel can handle. It is not unusual in patch clamp work to measure ionic currents of 2 to 10 pA flowing each time one channel in the patch is open. This would correspond to 12 to 60 $\times$ 10^6 monovalent ions moving per second. Such a turnover number is several orders of magnitude faster than known enzymatic or carrier mechanisms and agrees well with the theoretical properties of a pore of atomic dimensions. Similar fluxes have been observed with pore-forming antibiotic peptides in model systems. These substances, including gramicidin A, alamethicin, and monazomycin, spontaneously form pores permeable to water

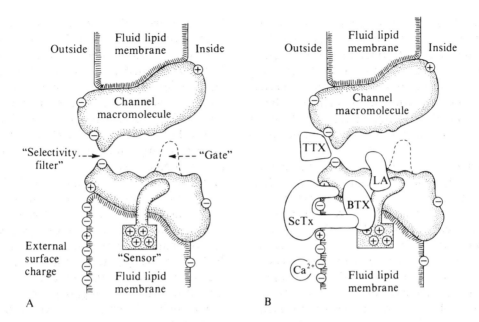

FIG. 5. Diagram of the functional units of an ionic channel (**A**) and the hypothesized binding sites for several drugs and toxins affecting Na^+ channels (**B**). The drawing is fanciful, and the dimension and shapes of the parts are not known. Drug receptors: (TTX) tetrodotoxin and saxitonin; (ScTx) scorpion toxins and anemone toxins; (BTX) batrachotoxin, aconitine, veratridine, and gray-anotoxin; (LA) local anesthetics; (Ca^{2+}) divalent ions screening and associating with surface negative charge.

and small ions in lipid bilayer membranes, as well as in biological membranes. Their antibiotic effect can be attributed to the collapsing of ionic gradients across membranes. They are small enough to be synthesized in many variants in the laboratory and are an excellent model system for elucidating structure-function relations in ionic pores. Several of the antibiotic substances even have very steeply voltage-dependent gating; however, none of the pore-forming agents characterized so far can discriminate between small cations to the degree that Na^+ channels or K^+ channels can.

Water molecules break and make hydrogen bonds with other waters 10^{11} to 10^{12} times per second, and alkali ions exchange water molecules or other oxygen ligands at least 10^9 times per second. In these terms, the progress of an ion across the membrane is not the movement

of a fixed hydrated complex; rather it is a continual exchange of oxygen ligands as the ion dances through the sea of relatively free water molecules and of polar groups that form the wall of the pore. It is generally assumed that polar and charged groups are in the pore to provide stabilization energy to the permeating ion, compensating for those water molecules that must be left behind as the ion enters into the pore. Evidence for important negative charges at the mouth or in the selectivity filter of Na^+ and K^+ channels comes from a block of their permeability as the pH of the external medium is lowered below pH 5.5 [5].

The minimum size of ionic channels has been determined from the van der Waals dimensions of ions that will go through them [5]. For example, Na^+ channels will pass at least ten ions other than Na^+, many of them organic ions. The largest is aminoguanidinium, which requires an orifice of somewhat more than 3 × 5 Å in the selectivity filter of the channel. A sodium ion (ionic diameter 1.90 Å) crossing such a narrow region would have to be partly, but not fully, dehydrated. It might still be in contact with three water molecules (diameter 2.80 Å) at the moment of maximum dehydration.

Because channels are narrow and neither geometrically nor chemically uniform along their length, ionic fluxes cannot be perfectly described by the equations of free diffusion already discussed, and models capable of describing temporary binding to attractive sites and jumps over barriers are frequently used instead. Formally, the kinetics of flux through channels are construed similarly to enzyme kinetics. It is assumed that the channel passes through a sequence of "channel-ion complexes" as it catalyzes the progression of an ion across the membrane. Such theories also can describe other properties of ionic channels, such as selectivity, saturation, competition, and block by permeant ions [5].

Voltage-dependent gating requires voltage-dependent conformational changes in the protein component(s) of ionic channels

The molecular basis of gating is unknown. On theoretical grounds, a membrane protein that responds to a change in membrane potential must have charged or dipolar amino acid residues, or both, located within the membrane electrical field, as illustrated in Fig. 5A. Changes in the membrane potential then exert a force on these protein-bound dipoles and charges. If the energy of the field-charge interactions is great enough, the protein may be induced to undergo a change to a new stable, conformational state in which the net charge or the location of charge within the membrane electrical field has been altered. For such a voltage-driven change of state,

the steepness of the state function versus membrane potential curve defines the equivalent number of charges that move according to a Boltzmann distribution. On this basis, Hodgkin and Huxley [8] predicted that activation of sodium channels would require the movement of six positive charges from the intracellular to the extracellular side of the membrane. The movement of a larger number of charges through a proportionately smaller fraction of the membrane electrical field would be equivalent.

Such a movement of membrane-bound charge gives rise to a capacitative current that can be detected electrophysiologically. Capacitative currents associated with activation of Na^+ channels (gating currents) were first detected in studies of the squid giant axon [14]. The observed outward-gating currents are approximately 0.3 percent as large as the sodium current during an action potential and reach a maximum in 80 μsec as the inward sodium current begins to increase. Their voltage and time dependence are consistent with the multistep changes of channel state from resting to active. Inactivation of channels during a depolarizing prepulse blocks gating currents with the same time and voltage dependence as it blocks sodium currents. In all probability, the moving charged groups are amino acids whose position in the protein structure is altered in the conformational change leading to activation.

In contrast to activation, inactivation of Na^+ channels from the open state does not seem to be a strongly voltage-sensitive process [14]. This inactivation can be blocked irreversibly by proteolytic enzymes and amino acid-modifying reagents that attack tyrosine, lysine, and arginine [15] acting from the intracellular side of the channel. For some Ca^+ channels, intracellular calcium itself plays an important role in inactivation [16]. It seems from these results that regions of ionic channels that are exposed at the intracellular surface of the membrane may be important in mediating the process of inactivation.

Pharmacological agents acting on ionic channels help define their functions

The Na^+ channel is so essential to successful body function that it has become the target in the evolution of several potent poisons. The pharmacology of such agents has provided important insights to the further definition of functional regions of the channel [2,4,5,17]. Figure 5B shows the supposed sites of action of the four most prominent classes of Na^+ channel agents. At the outer end of the channel is a site where the puffer fish poison, tetrodotoxin (TTX), a small, lipid-insoluble charged molecule binds with a K_i of 1 to 10 nM and blocks Na^+ permeability. An analogous substance, saxitoxin (STX), also called paralytic shellfish poison, has the same action. Both of these molecules have been tritiated and are widely used to count the number of sodium channels in a tissue, as diagnostic tools in physiological experiments, and as markers for chemical isolation of the channels. For example, there are 200 to 500 toxin-binding sites per square micrometer of membrane in squid giant axons and in frog skeletal muscle. A second important class of Na^+ channel blockers includes such clinically useful local anesthetics as lidocaine and procaine and related antiarrhythmic agents. They are lipid-soluble amines with a hydrophobic end and a polar end, and they bind to a hydrophobic site on the channel protein where they also interact with the inactivation gating machinery. The relevant clinical actions of local anesthetics are fully explained by their mode of blocking Na^+ channels. Two other classes of toxins either open Na^+ channels spontaneously or prevent them from closing normally once they have opened. These are lipid-soluble steroids, such as the frog skin poison used on arrows, batrachotoxin (BTX), the plant alkaloids aconitine and veratridine, both acting at a site within the membrane, and peptide toxins from scorpion and anemone venoms, which act at two sites on the outer surface of the membrane. Most scorpion

and anemone toxins block the inactivation gating step specifically. All of these reagents play an important role in studies of the molecular properties of Na^+ channels. It is interesting to note that the affinity of the channel for each of these classes of toxins depends on the gating conformational state of the channel.

Fewer specific agents are known that affect K^+ channels or Ca^{2+} channels; K^+ channels can be blocked by tetraethylammonium ion, Cs^+ and Ba^{2+}, and 4-aminopyridine. Except for 4-aminopyridine, there is good evidence that these ions become lodged within the channel at a narrow place from which they may be dislodged by K^+ coming from the other side [2]. In addition, certain K^+ channels are inhibited by polypeptide toxins from scorpion and bee venoms; Ca^{2+} channels can be blocked by the phenylalkylamine verapamil and the related substance D-600, by the benzothiazepine diltiazem, and by many divalent ions applied externally, including particularly Mn^{2+}, Co^{2+}, Cd^{2+}, and Ni^{2+}. In addition, calcium channels may be either activated or inhibited by reversible binding of diverse members of the dihydropyridine class of drugs (e.g., nifedipine) at a single site on the channel. The three classes of organic Ca^{2+} channel blockers have widespread use in the treatment of cardiovascular disorders. It is expected that such organic reagents will play an important role in future studies of the molecular properties of Ca^{2+} and K^+ channels.

MOLECULAR COMPONENTS OF VOLTAGE-SENSITIVE IONIC CHANNELS

Why should we study the biochemical properties of the channel macromolecules themselves? Although biophysical techniques define the functional properties of voltage-sensitive ionic channels clearly, we cannot yet relate those functional properties to the structure of the channel proteins. Understanding the structural basis for function should help to establish the basic physical and chemical principles underlying electrical excitation and signal transmission in excitable cells.

More is known about the structural and functional properties of voltage-sensitive Na^+ channels than about any of the other voltage-gated channels. The protein components have been identified, isolated in pure form, and shown to function in the purified state. Moreover, the amino acid sequence of the principal functional component of the Na^+ channel is now known, allowing specific hypotheses to be made concerning the structural basis of channel function. Thus, we focus almost entirely on the Na^+ channel here. Since the structural basis of selective ion transport and voltage-dependent gating may be conserved among different channels, we anticipate that the information derived from studies of Na^+ channels will be applicable to understanding the function of the numerous types of voltage-gated Ca^{2+} and K^+ channels as well.

Radiolabeled neurotoxins that act on Na^+ channels are used as molecular probes to tag the channel proteins, allowing their identification and purification

Photoreactive derivatives of the polypeptide toxins of scorpion venom have been covalently attached to Na^+ channels in intact cell membranes, allowing direct identification of channel components without purification. Reversible binding of STX and TTX to their common receptor has been used as a biochemical assay for the channel protein. Solubilization of excitable membranes with nonionic detergents releases the Na^+ channel in association with detergent in a form that retains the ability to bind STX and TTX with high affinity. Once released from the membrane in this way, the channel can be purified by chromatographic techniques that separate glycoproteins by size, charge, and composition of covalently attached carbohydrate. Using this general strategy, Na^+ channels have been purified from the electric organ of the electric eel and from mammalian brain and skeletal muscle [18–20].

Covalent labeling of Na^+ channels in intact excitable cells or membranes and purification of channels solubilized by nonionic detergents result in identification of a large glycoprotein with a molecular weight of 260,000 as the principal component. In eel electroplax, it appears to be the only protein component, but in mammalian brain this large α-subunit is associated with two additional polypeptides: $β_1$, with a molecular weight of 36,000, and $β_2$, with a molecular weight of 33,000. In skeletal muscle, the α-subunit is associated with a single polypeptide with a molecular weight of 38,000 that is similar in properties to the $β_1$ subunit from the brain.

Figure 6A illustrates the most probable arrangement of the subunits of the Na^+ channel from brain. The α-subunit is a transmembrane polypeptide, because it has sites on the external surface of the channel for attachment of carbohydrate chains and for binding of neurotoxins and sites on the intracellular surface for phosphorylation by cAMP-dependent protein kinase. Since this single polypeptide may suffice to form a channel by itself (see below), a transmembrane orientation is essential to its function.

The $β_1$- and $β_2$-subunits are placed at the extracellular surface of the membrane because they are heavily glycosylated. The $β_1$-subunit must also lie near the binding site for scorpion toxins, since it can be covalently labeled. The $β_2$-subunit is covalently attached to the α-subunit via a disulfide bond. The β-subunits are integral membrane proteins that interact with the phospholipid bilayer, but it is not known whether either of them penetrates to the intracellular surface of the membrane.

All three subunits of the channel contain a large amount of covalently attached carbohydrate. Approximately 25% of the mass of the α-

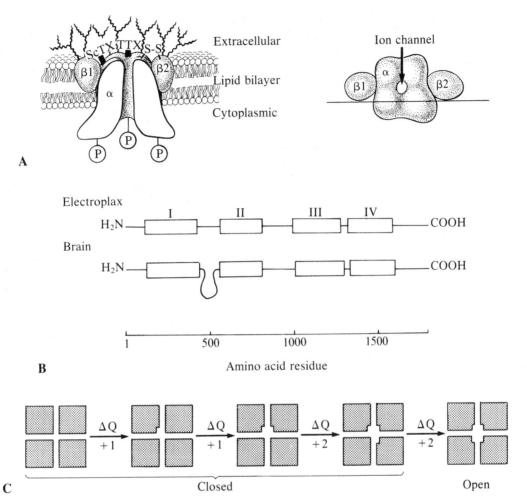

FIG. 6. Structural model of the sodium channel. **A:** (*Left*): Topological model of the rat brain sodium channel illustrating the probable transmembrane orientation of the three subunits, the binding sites for tetrodotoxin (TTX) and scorpion toxin (ScTX), oligosaccharide chains (*wavy lines*), disulfide bond (*S—S*), and cAMP dependent phosphorylation (P). (*Right*) *En face* view of the protein from the extracellular side illustrating the formation of a transmembrane ion pore in the midst of a square array of four transmembrane domains of the α-subunit. **B:** Linear representation of the amino acid sequence of the α-subunits from electroplax and brain illustrating the four internally homologous domains in each polypeptide. **C:** Sequential gating of the sodium channel. A reaction pathway from closed to open sodium channels is depicted. Each square represents one homologous domain of the α-subunit. Each domain undergoes a conformational change initiated according to the sliding helix model illustrated in Fig. 7.

subunit and approximately 30% of the mass of β_1- and β_2-subunits are carbohydrate. Much of this carbohydrate is sialic acid, which contributes to the strong net negative charge of the channel subunits. It is not known whether these extensive carbohydrate moieties play a role in channel function; however, they are required for normal biosynthesis and assembly of the functional channel in neurons. If glycosylation is inhibited, newly synthesized α-subunits are rapidly degraded and are not inserted into the cell surface membrane.

Functional reconstitution of purified Na$^+$ channel has been accomplished in two ways

In the first approach, purified channels were incorporated into vesicles of pure phospholipid. Activation of the reconstituted channels by treatment with the neurotoxins veratridine or BTX markedly increased the permeability of the vesicles to Na$^+$. The purified channels retain the ion selectivity and pharmacologic properties of native channels. In the second approach, ion conductance mediated by single purified channels was measured electrically. Channels reconstituted in phospholipid vesicles were studied directly using patch clamp methods or incorporated into planar phospholipid bilayer membranes by fusion. The individual purified channels observed retained the single-channel conductance, ion selectivity and voltage dependence of activation and inactivation that are characteristic of native channels. Hence, purified Na$^+$ channels seem to contain all the functional components necessary for electrical excitability.

What are the functional roles of the various components of the purified channel? All evidence points to a dominant role for the large α-subunit. The β_2-subunit can be removed from the Na$^+$ channel of mammalian brain without a major effect on the functional properties of the purified channel. Although the β_1-subunit is

required to maintain a functional state of the purified channel from brain, it is not found in the electroplax. The basic functions of ion conductance and voltage-dependent gating are likely to be mediated by the α-subunit with the β_1- and β_2-subunits serving secondary or modulatory functions, perhaps in a tissue-specific manner.

How does the primary structure carry out the function of the Na$^+$-channel α-subunit?

The amino acid sequence of the Na$^+$-channel α-subunits from eel electroplax and mammalian brain have been determined by cloning and sequencing DNA (cDNA) complementary to the mRNA encoding them [21,22]. The primary structures are illustrated diagrammatically in Fig. 6B. The large α-subunit is composed of 1,800 to 2,000 amino acids and contains four repeated domains having greater than 50 percent internal sequence identity, as indicated by the open rectangles in Fig. 6B. This structure implies that this polypeptide arose during evolution from a smaller precursor through two cycles of gene duplication. Sequence similarity implies similar secondary and tertiary structures for the four domains. Each domain contains six segments that are predicted to form transmembrane α-helices. All of these predicted transmembrane segments are in the four homologous domains that are connected by relatively hydrophilic amino acid sequences. This arrangement of amino acid sequences is similar for electroplax and brain Na$^+$ channels, except that an additional segment of approximately 200 amino acid residues is inserted between domains I and II of the brain α-subunit (Fig. 6B). The four homologous transmembrane domains are probably connected by hydrophilic regions that protrude from the membrane.

The cloning of the cDNA encoding the Na$^+$-channel α-subunit permits alternative tests of the functional properties of that polypeptide. cDNA clones can be used to synthesize mRNA encoding the α-subunit or to isolate the natural mRNA by specific hybridization. When injected into appropriate recipient cells such as frog oocytes, isolated mRNAs can be translated to yield functional proteins. In such experiments, mRNA encoding only the α-subunit of the channel is capable of directing the synthesis of functional channels in oocytes [23,24]. The α-subunits therefore seem sufficient to carry out the basic functions of the channel.

Transmembrane pore

How does the structure of the α-subunit allow it to mediate selective ion transport and voltage-dependent gating? The answer remains unknown, but two working hypotheses have been developed that help to guide current research on this problem. The structures of two other high-conductance ionic channels are known in more detail than that of the Na$^+$ channel, and they provide useful models for consideration of mechanisms of ion transport. The gap-junction channel, which connects adjacent cells, is formed by symmetrical hexagonal arrays of six identical subunits in the surface membrane of each cell. The approximately cylindrical subunits of each hexameric connexon are oriented perpendicularly to the plane of the membrane [25]. Electron diffraction and image reconstruction show that a transmembrane channel is formed at the center of each hexagonal array of subunits. The nicotinic acetylcholine receptor consists of a pseudosymmetric pentagonal array of five homologous subunits (see Chap. 10). As in the gap-junction channel, a transmembrane channel is formed in the center of this symmetrical array of subunits with their long axes perpendicular to the membrane. These two examples suggest the generalization that high-conductance ionic channels will form their transmembrane pore at the center of symmetrical arrays of homologous structural units.

   As we have discussed, the amino acid sequence of the α-subunit of the Na$^+$ channel contains four internally homologous transmembrane domains. The Na$^+$ channel may accomplish with homologous domains in a single polypeptide what the gap-junction channel and the nicotinic acetylcholine receptor do with arrays of homologous subunits. Thus, the transmembrane pore of the Na$^+$ channel may be formed at the center of a square array of the four transmembrane domains (Fig. 6). The suggestion that this polypeptide can form a functional channel by itself is supported by its transmembrane orientation, by reconstitution studies on the purified Na$^+$ channel from electroplax, and by expression studies of mRNA encoding the α-subunits.

Voltage sensors

Structural models for voltage-dependent gating must identify the voltage sensors or gating charges (Fig. 5A) within the channel structure and suggest a plausible mechanism for transmembrane movement of gating charge and its coupling to the opening of a transmembrane pore. The S4 segments of the homologous domains have been proposed as voltage sensors [22,26,27]. These segments, which are nearly fully conserved in structure in electroplax and brain, consist of repeated triplets of two hydrophobic amino acids followed by a positively charged residue (Fig. 7). In the α-helical configuration, these segments would form a spiral staircase of positive charge across the membrane, a structure well suited for transmembrane movement of gating charge. Each positive charge is proposed to be neutralized by a negative charge in one of the surrounding transmembrane segments to form a spiral array of ion pairs (Fig. 7). At the resting membrane potential, the force of the electric field pulls the positive charges inward and pushes the negative charges outward to stabilize one set of ion-pair interactions. Depolarization abolishes this force and allows a spiral outward movement of the

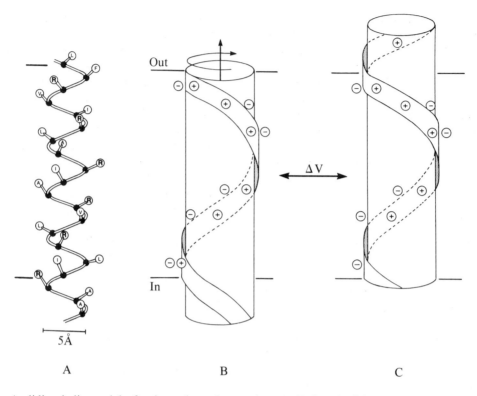

FIG. 7. A sliding helix model of voltage-dependent gating. **A:** Ball-and-stick, three-dimensional representation of the transmembrane S4 helix of domain IV: (●) α-carbon of each amino acid residue; (○) direction of projection of the side chain of each residue away from the core of the helix. For single letter code, See Glossary. **B** and **C:** Movement of the proposed transmembrane S4 helix in response to membrane depolarization. The spiral path made by the positively charged arginine residues (R) is illustrated in the form of a ribbon wrapped around the central core of the helix. At the resting membrane potential (**B**), all positively charged residues are paired with fixed negative charges on other transmembrane segments of the channel and the transmembrane segment is held in that position by the negative internal membrane potential. Depolarization (**C**) reduces the force holding the positive charges in their inward position. The S4 helix is then proposed to undergo a screw-like motion through a rotation of approximately 60° and an outward displacement of approximately 5Å. This movement leaves an unpaired negative charge on the inward surface of the membrane and reveals an unpaired positive charge on the outward surface to give a net charge transfer of +1. (Adapted from Catterall, [26].)

S4 helix to take up new ion-pair partners. This spiral movement would have the net effect of transferring one positive charge across the membrane permeability barrier to yield a total of at least four gating charges transferred in the four homologous domains. The spiral movement of the S4 helix in each domain is proposed to initiate a more general conformational change

in that domain. After conformational changes have occurred in all four domains, the transmembrane pore can open as illustrated diagrammatically in Fig. 6C.

Although the models for formation of a voltage-gated transmembrane pore by the Na⁺ channel α-subunit are speculative at this time, they illustrate a general scientific method: New data, such as the amino acid sequences of the Na^+-channel α-subunits, inevitably lead to the formulation of specific hypotheses. These hypotheses then spawn a new generation of experiments designed to test their merit. The next phase of research on the molecular properties of Na^+ channels should give us clearer insight into two of the critical functions of ionic channels: selective ion conductance and voltage-dependent gating.

Voltage-sensitive K^+ and Ca^{2+} channels are studied with the same strategy used for the Na^+ channel

Drugs and neurotoxins that act on these channels have been used to identify some of their protein components and experiments to restore their function in purified form and to determine their primary and secondary structures are in progress. Since voltage-gated ionic channels are likely to have evolved from common ancestor proteins, comparison of the conserved structural features among the many different channels will sharpen our view of the molecular basis of their function.

CHEMICAL AND MECHANICAL GATING OF IONIC CHANNELS

The channels used in the action potential, by having strongly voltage-dependent gating, contrast with those generating slow potentials at synapses and sensory receptors. The latter channels have gates controlled by chemical transmitters, intracellular messengers, or by other energies, such as mechanical deformations in touch and hearing. In general, less is known about these channels than about Na^+ and K^+ channels of action potentials, with the exception of the nicotinic acetylcholine receptor channel of the neuromuscular junction (see Chap. 10). The ionic selectivity of these channels include a very broad monovalent anion

permeability at inhibitory synapses; a cation permeability (about equal for Na^+ and K^+) at several excitatory synapses, at the neuromuscular junction, and at many sensory transducers; and other more selective K^+ and Na^+ permeabilities in other synapses. The acetylcholine receptor of the neuromuscular junction has been solubilized and chemically purified, and the amino acid sequences of its subunits have been determined by methods of molecular genetics (see Chap. 10). Work on other transmitter-gated channels, such as the γ-aminobutyric acid ($GABA_A$) receptor and the glycine receptor, is well under way.

It should be emphasized that there is great diversity among ionic channels and they play many roles in cells throughout the body. We can speculate that hundreds of genes code for structural components of the channels. Channel activity in endocrine cells regulates the episodes of secretion of insulin from the pancreas and epinephrine from the adrenal gland. Channels form part of the regulated pathway for the ion movements underlying absorption and secretion of electrolytes by epithelia. Thus, although they are especially prominent in the function of the nervous system, channels are actually a basic component of all animal cells, indeed of all eukaryotic cells [5].

ACKNOWLEDGMENT

The preparation of this chapter was supported by Grants NS-08174 and NS-15751 from the National Institutes of Health.

REFERENCES

1. Hodgkin, A. L. *The Conduction of the Nervous Impulse.* Springfield, Illinois: Charles C Thomas, 1964.
2. Armstrong, C. M. Ionic pores, gates, and gating currents. *Q. Rev. Biophys.* 7:179–210, 1975.

3. Kuffler, S. W., Nicholls, J. G., and Martin, A. R. *From Neuron to Brain*. Sunderland, Massachusetts: Sinauer Associates, 1984.

4. Hille, B. Ionic Basis of Resting and Action Potentials. In J. M. Brookhart et al. (eds.). *Handbook of Physiology*, Washington, D.C.: American Physiological Society, 1977, Vol. 1, pp. 99–136.

5. Hille, B. *Ionic Channels in Excitable Membranes*. Sunderland, Massachusetts: Sinauer Associates, 1984.

6. Hodgkin, A. L., and Katz, B. The effect of sodium ions on the electrical activity of the giant axon of the squid. *J. Physiol. (Lond.)* 108:37–77, 1949.

7. Thomas, R. C. Electrogenic sodium pump in nerve and muscle cells. *Physiol. Rev.* 52:563–594, 1972.

8. Hodgkin, A. L., and Huxley, A. F. A quantitative description of membrane current and its application to conduction and excitation in nerve. *J. Physiol. (Lond.)* 117:500–544, 1952.

9. Hamill, O. P., Marty, A., Neher, E., Sakmann, B., and Sigworth, F. J. Improved patch-clamp techniques for high-resolution current recording from cells and cell-free membrane patches. *Pflugers Arch.* 391:85–100, 1981.

10. Chiu, S. Y., and Ritchie, J. M. Evidence for the presence of potassium channels in the internode of frog myelinated nerve fibres. *J. Physiol. (Lond.)* 322:485–501, 1982.

11. Bostock, H., and Sears, T. A. The internodal axon membrane: Electrical excitability and continuous conduction in segmental demyelination. *J. Physiol. (Lond.)* 280:273–301, 1978.

12. Hagiwara, S., and Byerly, L. Calcium channel. *Annu. Rev. Neurosci.* 4:69–125, 1981.

13. Tsien, R. W. Calcium channels in excitable cell membranes. *Annu. Rev. Physiol.* 45:341–158, 1983.

14. Armstrong, C. M. Sodium channels and gating currents. *Physiol. Rev.* 61: 644–683, 1981.

15. Brodwick, M. S., and Eaton, D. C. Chemical modification of excitable membranes. In B. Haber, J. R. Perez-Polo, and J. D. Coulter (eds.). *Proteins in the Nervous System: Structure and Function*. New York: Alan R. Liss, 1982, pp. 51–72.

16. Eckert, R., and Chad, J. E. Inactivation of Ca channels. *Prog. Biophys. Molec. Biol.* 44:215–267, 1984.

17. Catterall, W. A. Neurotoxins acting on sodium channels. *Annu. Rev. Pharmacol. Toxicol.* 20:15–43, 1980.

18. Agnew, W. S. Voltage-regulated sodium channel molecules. *Annu. Rev. Biochem.* 46:517–530, 1984.

19. Barchi, R. L. Voltage-sensitive sodium ion channels. Molecular properties and functional reconstitution. *Trends Biochem. Sci.* 9:358–361, 1984.

20. Catterall, W. A. Molecular properties of voltage-sensitive sodium channels. *Annu. Rev. Biochem.* 55:953–985, 1986.

21. Noda, M., Shimizu, S., Tanabe, T., Takai, T., Kayano, T., et al. Primary structure of *Electrophorus electricus* sodium channel deduced from cDNA sequence. *Nature* 312:121–127, 1984.

22. Noda, M., Ikeda, T., Kayano, T., Suzuki, H., Takeshima, H., Kurasaki, M., Takahashi, H., and Numa, S. Existence of distinct sodium channel messenger RNAs in rat brain. *Nature* 320:188–192, 1986.

23. Noda, M., Ikeda, T., Suzuki, H., Takeshima, H., Takahashi, T., Kuno, M., and Numa, S. Expression of functional sodium channels from cloned cDNA. *Nature* 322:826–828, 1986.

24. Goldin, A. L., Snutch, T., Lubbert, H., Dowsett, A., Marshall, J., et al. Messenger RNA coding for only the alpha subunit of the rat brain Na channel is sufficient for expression of functional channels in *Xenopus oocytes*. *Proc. Natl. Acad. Sci. U.S.A.* 83:7503–7507, 1986.

25. Unwin, P. N. T., and Zampighi, G. Structure of the junction between communicating cells. *Nature* 283:545–549, 1980.

26. Catterall, W. A. Voltage-dependent gating of sodium channels: Correlating structure and function. *Trends Neurosci.* 9:7–10, 1986.

27. Guy, H. R., and Seetharamulu, P. Molecular model of the action potential sodium channel. *Proc. Natl. Acad. Sci. U.S.A.* 83:508–512, 1986.

CHAPTER 5

Lipids

Bernard W. Agranoff

Lipid biochemistry and neurochemistry have evolved together. This interrelationship continues because, relative to other organs, the brain has a high content of lipids, including some, such as gangliosides and galactocerebrosides, that are not found in as high quantities elsewhere. Phospholipids account for the high total phosphorous content of brain, which in the past, led to an alchemical mystique that associated phosphorescence and thought and, in the nine-teenth century, to the apocryphal claim that fish are good "brain food," since fish, too, are rich in phosphorous.

PROPERTIES OF LIPIDS

Lipids can be defined as apolar biomolecules in the main, serving one of two functions: as re-

Basic Neurochemistry: Molecular, Cellular, and Medical Aspects, 4th Ed., edited by G. J. Siegel et al. Raven Press, Ltd., New York, 1989. Correspondence to Bernard W. Agranoff, Neuroscience Laboratory, University of Michigan, 1103 East Huron, Ann Arbor, Michigan 48104-1687.

positories of chemical energy (''depot fat,'' primarily triglycerides) or as structural components of membranes. Brain contains virtually no triglyceride, and it is as membrane components that brain lipids have received the continued attention of neurochemists. The brain is enriched in a highly specialized membrane, myelin, which to a large extent accounts for the brain's high lipid content (see Chap. 6). In addition to the two principal functions, there are lipids with specific physiological effects. For example, a number of trace lipids are known to be cellular messengers in the brain, as well as in other tissues. In this category can be included the steroid hormones, the prostanoids (see Chap. 20), and platelet-activating factor, a naturally occurring ether lipid that has vasoactive properties.

Lipids were originally defined operationally, on the basis of their extractability from tissues with apolar solvents such as a chloroform/methanol mixture, but this is no longer the sole criterion. For example, the myelin component proteolipid protein is extractable into lipid solvents but is not considered to be a lipid, since its structure is that of a polypeptide. We now know that many proteins contain apolar ''membrane-spanning'' regions. Conversely, gangliosides are considered to be lipids on the basis of their structure, even though they are more polar than apolar. It is apparent then that lipids are defined not only by their physical properties, but also on the basis of their chemical structure.

MAJOR BRAIN LIPIDS

Lipids can be classified into three main categories: isoprenoids (or terpenoids), glycerolipids, and sphingolipids. Other lipids, such as fatty acids and alcohols, are also present in brain lipid extracts, but are not quantitatively significant.

The isoprenoid family is formed from the polymerization of isoprenoid units

Isoprenoid units have the formular composition C_5H_8 and the structure

$$\underset{\underset{\text{H}}{|}}{\overset{\overset{\text{H}}{|}}{-\text{C}}} - \overset{\overset{\text{CH}_3}{|}}{\text{C}} = \overset{\overset{\text{H}}{|}}{\text{C}} - \underset{\underset{\text{H}}{|}}{\overset{\overset{\text{H}}{|}}{\text{C}}} -$$

The most abundant of these by far is cholesterol (Fig. 1). As in other eukaryotic tissues, cholesterol is a major component of brain membranes. Unlike other tissues, however, adult brain contains virtually no cholesterol ester, except in pathological conditions. Desmosterol, the immediate biosynthetic precursor of cholesterol, is found in developing brain and in some brain tumors. Other isoprenoid substances present in brain are the dolichols, very long branched-chain alcohols, and the carotenoids, including retinal and retinoic acid.

Synthesis and degradation

Brain cholesterol appears to be biosynthesized *in situ* by the pathway: β-hydroxy-β-methylglutaryl (HMG)-CoA → mevalonate → isopentenyl pyrophosphate. The latter product is the active isoprene polymerizing unit. Linear polymerization up to C_{100} can occur, as in the dolichols. Condensation of two trimeric units (farnesyl pyrophosphate) forms squalene ($C_{30}H_{50}$). This hydrocarbon then condenses oxidatively to form lanosterol, which, following three demethylations, leads to cholesterol. Although cholesterol esters are normally absent, the enzyme that cleaves them, cholesterol esterase, is present in brain and is a convenient marker of oligodendroglial membranes (see Chap. 6). Labeled mevalonic acid is a convenient tool for the measurement of cholesterol synthesis, since it is committed to terpene synthesis and enters cells readily (as mevalonolactone). Once formed, brain cholesterol turns over very

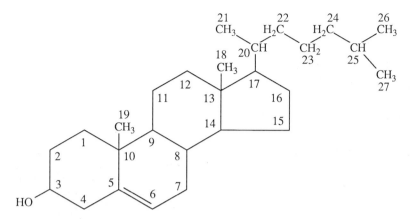

FIG. 1. Cholesterol. In cholesterol esters, long-chain fatty acids are esterified at C-3. The esters are present in developing brain and in pathological conditions but not in normal brain. Cholesterol esters with very long fatty acid chains (C_{22}–C_{26}) accumulate in white matter in adrenoleukodystrophy. The enzyme cholesterol esterase is a good marker of oligodendroglial membranes. Desmosterol, the metabolic precursor of cholesterol, differs by the presence of a double bond at C-24 to C-25.

slowly, and there is both metabolic and analytic evidence to indicate an accretion of brain cholesterol with age.

Brain glycerolipids are mainly phosphorylated and are considered derivatives of sn-glycerol-3-phosphate

The notation *sn* refers to stereochemical numbering, with the secondary hydroxyl or glycerol shown on the left of C-2. The phosphate is on C-3 of glycerol in naturally occurring lipids. As shown in Fig. 2, the hydroxyl groups on C-1 and C-2 of glycerolipids are esterified with fatty acids. The substituent at *sn*-1 is usually saturated, whereas that at *sn*-2 is unsaturated. In addition, there are species in which *sn*-1 is either linked to an aliphatic alcohol (alkyl) or to an α,β-unsaturated ether (alkenyl: alk-1′-enyl). The latter lipids are referred to as plasmalogens. Although glycerophospholipids are generally alkali labile, or saponifiable, the alkenyl ethers are alkali stable and acid labile. Alkyl ethers are stable to both acids and bases. A useful general term that includes these various aliphatic sub-

stituents—acyl, alkenyl, and alkyl—is "radyl," for example, 1,2-diradyl-*sn*-glycerol-3-phosphate.

If positions 1 and 2 are acylated and the *sn*-3 hydroxyl group is free, the lipid is a diacylglycerol (DG). The DGs play a cellular regulating role in that they activate protein kinase C (see Chap. 16). In addition, DGs are known to be fusogenic and may play a role in altering cell morphology, for example, in fusion of synaptic vesicles. Other nonphosphorous-containing glycerides of interest are DG-galactoside and its sulfate [1]. These minor glyceroglycolipids are found primarily in white matter and appear to be analogous to their sphingosine-containing counterparts, the cerebrosides, described below.

Glycerophospholipid classes are defined on the basis of the substituent at *sn*-3 of the diacylglycerophosphoryl (phosphatidyl) function (Fig. 2). In quantitatively decreasing order in brain they are phosphatidylethanolamine (PE), phosphatidylcholine (PC), and phosphatidylserine (PS). The phosphoinositides—phosphatidylinositol (PI), phosphatidylinositol-4-phos-

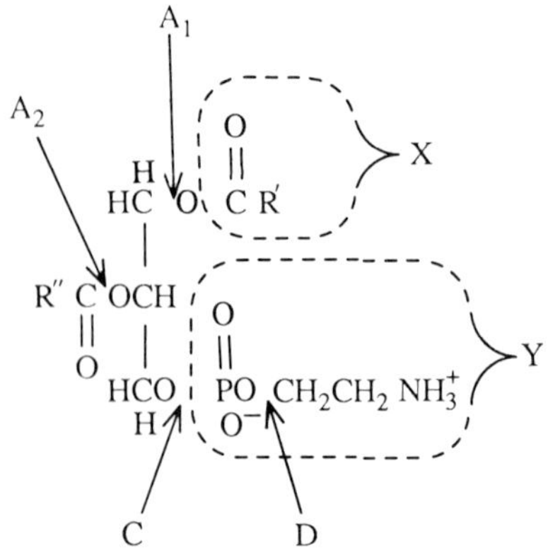

FIG. 2. The structure of a phosphoglycerolipid. Phosphatidylethanolamine is shown with various possible substitutions. Those at X indicate the structures of alkyl and alkenyl ethers. They are prominent in brain PE. Diacylglycerylgalactoside, phosphatidylinositol, and phosphatidylglycerol may be further substituted. Arrows indicate sites of enzymatic degradation of the phosphoglycerolipids, as described in the text.

X

—CH$_2$R	(Alkyl ether)
—CH=CHR	(Alkenyl ether)

Y

—H	Diacylglycerol (DG)
—Galactose	DG-galactose
—PO$_3$	Phosphatidate
—POCH$_2$CH$_2$NH$_3$$^+$	Phosphatidyl ethanolamine (PE)
—POCH$_2$CH$_2$N(CH$_3$)$^+$	Phosphatidyl choline (PC)
—POCH$_2$CHNH$_3$COO$^-$	Phosphatidyl serine (PS)
—Inositol	Phosphatidyl inositol (PI)
—Glycerol	Phosphatidyl glycerol (PG)

phate (PIP), and phosphatidylinositol-4,5-bisphosphate (PIP$_2$)—are quantitatively minor phospholipids but play an important role in signal transduction (see Chap. 16). The phosphatidylglycerols of brain, as in other tissues, are present in mitochondrial membranes. Of these, cardiolipin (bisphosphatidylglycerol) is the most prevalent.

The phospholipid class in a given tissue has a characteristic fatty acid composition. The composition of a given phospholipid class can be quite different in gray and white matter. This is exemplified by comparison of an analysis of PE from both gray and white matter of human brain (Table 1). It can be further seen from Table 1 that brain lipids contain some unusually long and polyunsaturated fatty acids. They are in both the ω6 and ω3 (counting from the methyl end to the first double bond) families of essential fatty acids; that is they cannot be biosynthesized in the animal body *de novo* (Figs. 3 and 4; also see Chap. 34). This also means that there are mechanisms for transporting essential fatty acids across the blood-brain barrier. There is considerable interest in the role of the polyunsaturated fatty acids and their metabolites in brain following breakdown of their parent phospholipids in conditions such as ischemia and anoxia (see Chap. 40).

Biosynthesis of the glycerophospholipids

Phosphatidylethanolamine is synthesized from DG and CDP-ethanolamine (Fig. 5). As shown in Fig. 5, dihydroxyacetone phosphate

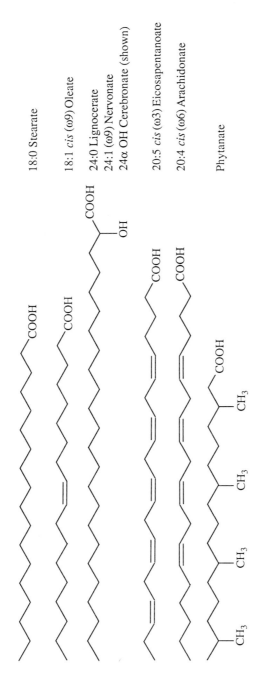

18:0 Stearate

18:1 *cis* (ω9) Oleate

24:0 Lignocerate
24:1 (ω9) Nervonate
24α OH Cerebronate (shown)

20:5 *cis* (ω3) Eicosapentanoate

20:4 *cis* (ω6) Arachidonate

Phytanate

FIG. 3. Structures of some fatty acids of neurochemical interest. (See also Fig. 4 legend and text.)

95

TABLE 1. Fatty acid composition of phosphatidylethanolamine[a]

Fatty acid	Gray matter	White matter
14:0	0.2	0.5
16:0	6.7	6.7
16:1	0.4	1.4
18:0	26.0	9.0
18:1 ω9	11.9	42.4
18:2 ω6	Tr	Tr
20:1 ω9	1.5	7.9
20:2 ω9	Tr	2.4
20:3 ω9	0.5	1.6
20:3 ω6	Tr	Tr
20:4 ω6	13.8	6.4
22:4 ω6	Tr	Tr
22:5 ω6	14.3	13.7
22:5 ω3	Tr	0.5
22:6 ω3	24.3	3.4

[a] PE was isolated from a 55-year-old human brain. Methyl esters were identified by GLC. (Adapted from O'Brien and Sampson [2].)

(DHAP) produced during glycolysis can be reduced to furnish glycerophosphate, a precursor of diacylglycerophosphate (DGP), also termed phosphatidate (PA). (The abbreviation recommended by the International Union of Biochemistry Nomenclature Committee is Ptd.) Note that, alternatively, DHAP may first be acylated. It can then be reduced to acyl-GP, or the acyl group can be exchanged enzymatically for an alkyl group. This is the only known pathway for ether biosynthesis [3]. The alkyl, acyl-DHAP, then goes on to form the alkyl derivative of PE, which may then be oxidized to form PE plasmalogen, also referred to as phosphatidylethanolamine, which is relatively enriched in brain. The enzymes of the acyl-DHAP pathway are localized in brain peroxisomes (see Chap. 37). An inherited metabolic defect called Zellweger syndrome is characterized by lack of peroxisomes and thus of the enzymes of the acyl-DHAP pathway [4]. It is associated with mental retardation. The pathogenesis of the retardation is not yet understood.

Phosphatidylcholine can be formed from CDP-choline and DG or by sequential methylation of PE, the methyl donor being S-adenosyl methionine. The latter pathway is the predominant one. Although the older literature indicates that brain lacks the enzymatic activity for the methylation of PE, there is good evidence that it indeed occurs [5].

The inositol- and the glycerol-containing phospholipids are each formed by a completely different pathway, employing the liponucleotide CDP-diglyceride (Fig. 5). CDP-DG and inositol, or glycerophosphate, in the presence of their specific synthases, form PI (or phosphatidylglycerophosphate), respectively (see also Chap. 16).

Phosphatidylserine biosynthesis is less straightforward. In bacterial systems, it is formed via the CDP-DG pathway, whereas in animal systems it appears to be formed by exchange of serine with PE, with release of ethanolamine. PS can be decarboxylated to reform PE [5].

FIG. 4. Pathways of brain fatty acid synthesis. The elongations and desaturations outlined all occur as the CoA thioesters. **A:** Fatty acids totally biosynthesized in brain. Note that desaturation does not occur in brain or other eukaryotic tissues for the first nine carbons starting at the methyl end; that all double bonds are *cis*; and that once a double bond is in place, subsequent desaturations proceed toward the carboxyl end at C_2 intervals. Elongation occurs by C_2 units added at the COOH end. The ω10 acids are found only in developing brain and are not seen in other tissues. Also shown as possible fates of the 24:0 and 26:0 acids are hydroxylation at C-2 and subsequent decarboxylation at C-1, leading to an odd-carbon (C_{23} or C_{25}) fatty acid. **B and C:** Formation of the major polyunsaturated fatty acid substituents of phosphoglycerides, starting with dietary linoleic acid (18:2 ω6) and linolenic acid (18:3 ω3), respectively. Various possible elongation and desaturation products shown, such as 22:5 (ω3; "EPA"), also may be ingested directly.

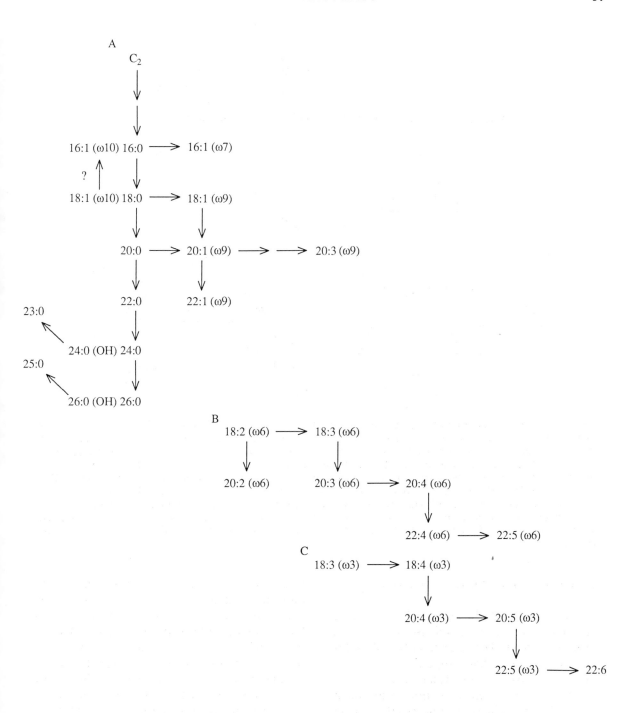

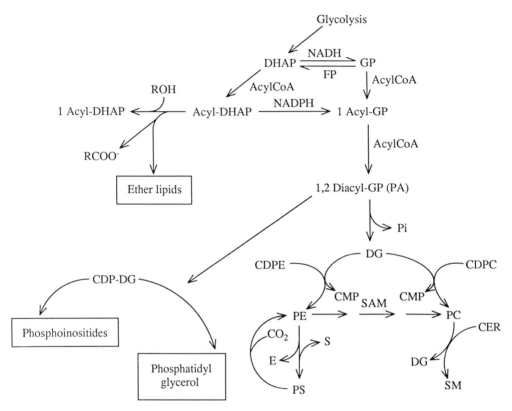

FIG. 5. Schematic representation of glycerophospholipid biosynthesis. Note that dihydroxyacetone phosphate (DHAP) may be reduced to glycerolphosphate or may first be acylated and can then serve as precursors of the lipid ethers. Lysophosphatidate is acylated to phosphatidate (PA), which can be converted to the liponucleotide cytidine diphosphodiacylglycerol (CDP-DG) and then to the inositol or cardiolipin series. Alternatively, PA can be dephosphorylated by PA phosphatase to yield DG, which may then react with CDPE (or CDPC) to form PE (or PC). PE may then be converted to PS by base exchange with L-serine. PE also serves as the major source of PC via three methylation steps using *S*-adenosylmethionine (SAM). PC serves as precursor for sphingomyelin (SM) via a reaction with ceramide. In plasmalogen synthesis, alkyl acyl DG reacts with CDPE, and the results of alkyl acyl PE may then be oxidized to the alkenyl acyl derivative (not shown).

Degradation of glycerophospholipids

As shown in Fig. 2, the fatty acid at position 2 may be cleaved by phospholipase A_2, releasing a free fatty acid. The remaining lysophospholipid has detergent-like properties and if produced excessively *in situ*, destabilizes the membrane, leading to cell disruption. Subsequent action of phospholipase A_1 releases the remaining fatty acid, leaving a glycerophosphoryl ester. The existence of phospholipase B, thought to attack the acyl group directly at either position 1 or 2, is questionable and certainly not quantitatively significant. Glycerophosphodiesters, representing the backbone of the parent phospholipids, are normally present in small amounts in tissues and can be readily identified *in vivo* by their characteristic ^{31}P nuclear magnetic resonance (NMR) signal [6]. Alternatively, phospholipids may be initially cleaved at the phosphodiester locus to release diacylglycerol and a phosphate ester, such as phosphoethanolamine. Phosphodiesterases cleaving lipids by this mechanism are referred to as phospholipase C, and some have considerable substrate specificity, acting on only one phospholipid class (see also Chap. 16). Phospholipase D action refers to distal cleavage of the phosphodiester of glycerophospholipids to yield PA and a base such as ethanolamine. Base exchange reactions also occur to some extent among the phosphoglyceride classes [7].

In sphingolipids, the C_{18} aminoalcohol sphingosine serves as the lipid backbone rather than glycerol

To some extent, sphingosine resembles a monoradyl glycerol molecule, and when *N*-acylated at the amino group on C-2, the resultant ceramide (Fig. 6) corresponds roughly to DG, since it has two aliphatic tails: that of the fatty acid and that of sphingosine itself. The various sphingolipid classes are substituted on the oxygen at C-1. The C-3 hydroxyl is not known to be acylated.

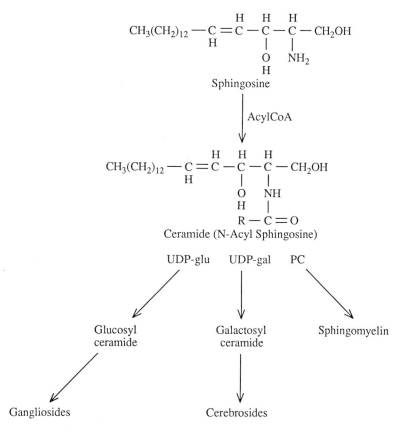

FIG. 6. Biosynthesis of sphingolipids. Sphingosine is acylated to ceramide. Ceramide may then react with UDP-glu to initiate ganglioside synthesis, with UDP-gal to form galactosylceramides (cerebrosides), or with PC, as indicated in Fig. 5, to form SM.

Substitution with phosphocholine on C-1 yields sphingomyelin (SM), the sole phosphorus-containing sphingolipid in brain. It is found in all eukaryotic membranes. Fatty acid substituents in SM are bimodal in distribution: They are either C_{16} and C_{18} (short, in this context) or C_{22} to C_{26} (long), including 24:1 (OH) and odd-carbon fatty acids.

The cerebrosides, consisting primarily of galactosyl ceramide (galactocerebroside; ceramide $\xrightarrow{\beta 1-1'}$ gal); and the cerebroside sulfates (sulfatides), in which galactosyl ceramide is sulfated on the 3'OH of galactose, are characteristic of myelin and are not found in other organs in significant amounts. In the case of the cerebrosides, fatty acid substituents may be odd carbon, such as C_{25}, or may be α-hydroxylated. They are enriched in lignoceric, nervonic, and cerebronic acids (see Fig. 3). Glucocerebrosides are present in brain but in very small amounts. They are also found in other tissues.

In the gangliosides, ceramide is conjugated to a complex oligosaccharide moiety. They contain N-acetylneuraminic (sialic) acid (Fig. 7) and a specific β-glycosodically linked tetrasaccharide configuration, or fraction thereof (Figs. 8 and 9), consisting of glucosylceramide to which galactose, N-acetylgalactosamine, and galactose are sequentially linked. The number of sialic acid substituents varies from zero (asialoganglioside) to five or more. They are linked either directly to galactose or to a sialic acid that is linked to a galactose. The ganglioside series of sphingoglycolipids is characteristic of nervous tissue, particularly gray matter, whereas the globoside series is nonneural. Globosides consist of glucosylceramide to which galactose, galactose, and N-acetylgalactosamine are sequentially linked. Globosides are also β-glycosodically linked, except for an α-glycosidic link between the two galactose moieties. A wide variety of additional glycosylceramide derivatives is possible [10] by virtue of different glycosidic linkages, and it is not surprising that these lipids have frequently been identified as immunodeterminants. Gangliosides appear to play a role in the receptor for cholera toxin and possibly tetanus toxin [11]. The fatty acid component of ganglioside ceramide is usually 18:0. Some elongated (C_{20}) sphingosine is present in gangliosides.

Biosynthesis of sphingolipids

There is uncertainty with regard to the synthesis of sphingosine. At present, the favored synthetic pathway involves a condensation between palmitoyl-CoA and serine, followed by reduction of the resulting 3-ketodihydrosphingosine to dihydrosphingosine and then dehydrogenation to sphingosine. Following N-acylation of sphingosine to ceramide, phosphocholine is transferred from PC to form SM and DG [12]. There is also evidence for dehydrogenation of the dihydroceramide. The reaction of ceramide with CDP-choline has also been described but is thought to play a minor biosynthetic role at most. Galactocerebrosides are formed by reaction of ceramide with UDP-gal. The significance of the reaction of sphingosine with UDP-gal to form galactosylsphingosine (psychosine) is unclear. A number of sphingolipids, including sphingosine and psychosine, are potent blockers of protein kinase C [13]. Conversion of galactocerebroside to its sulfatide requires the presence of phosphoadenosine phosphosulfate (PAPS). Myelin contains a glucuronide sulfosphingolipid.

Glucocerebroside is found by reaction of ceramide with UDP-glu. Gangliosides are then formed by sequential glycosylation of glucocerebroside with UDP sugars (Fig. 9). Sialic acid is synthesized by condensation of mannosamine and pyruvate. It is transferred to gangliosides via CMP-sialic acid (Fig. 7). Degradation of sphingolipids occurs primarily via lysosomal enzymes, and deficiency in a given degradative step can lead to a number of inborn metabolic errors, most of which are associated with mental retardation (see Chap. 37).

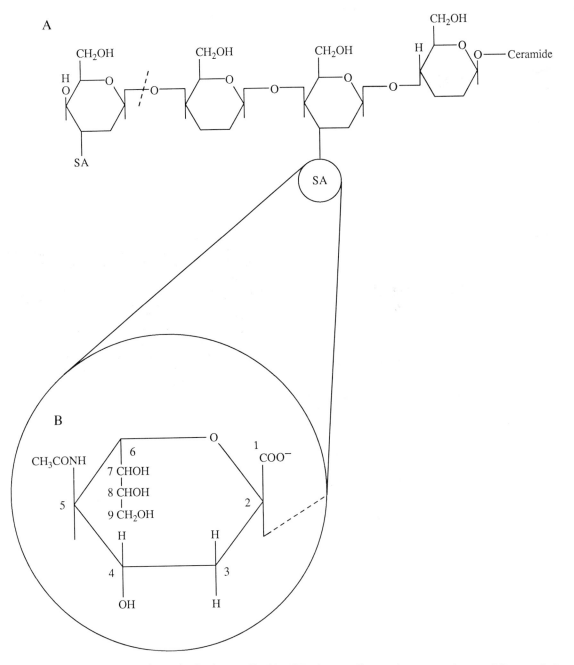

FIG. 7. **A:** The structure of a major brain ganglioside (GD$_{1a}$) according to the nomenclature of Svennerholm (Yu [9]). "G" denotes ganglioside, "D" indicates that there are two sialic acid residues, and "1" refers to the presence of the complete ganglioside tetrasaccharide. The "a" distinguishes positional isomers in terms of the location of the sialic acid residues (see Fig. 9). If the terminal galactose and sialic are removed (*dotted line*), the resulting sialylated trisaccharidyl ceramide is GM2, the Tay-Sachs ganglioside (see Chap. 37). **B:** The structure of sialic acid (SA), also called *N*-acetylneuraminic acid (NANA). Some tissues contain in addition *N*-glycolylneuraminic acid. The metabolic biosynthetic precursor for sialylation of glycoconjugates is CMP-sialic acid, in which the nucleotide is diesterified to the 9-hydroxyl position of the sugar.

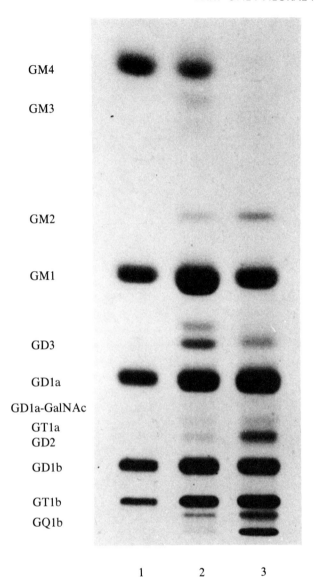

FIG. 8. Thin-layer chromatograms of gangliosides from normal human white matter (*lane 2*) and gray matter (*lane 3*). *Lane 1* contains a mixture of isolated standards. Each lane contains about 7 μg sialic acid. Merck precoated HPTLC plates (silica gel 60, 200 μm thick) were used. The plate was developed with chloroform-methanol-water, 60:40:9 (containing 0.02 percent $CaCl_2 \cdot 2\ H_2O$). The bands were visualized with resorcinol-hydrochloric acid reagent. (Courtesy of R. K. Yu, see also Leeden and Yu [8].)

FIG. 9. Known and proposed pathways for biosynthesis of gangliosides (designated as *a*, *b*, and *c*), (*solid arrows*) reactions demonstrated *in vitro*; (*dashed arrows*) proposed reactions not yet observed. (SA) sialic acid; (A, M, D, T, Q, P) 0, 1, 2, 3, 4 and 5 sialic acid residues, respectively. From Yu [9].)

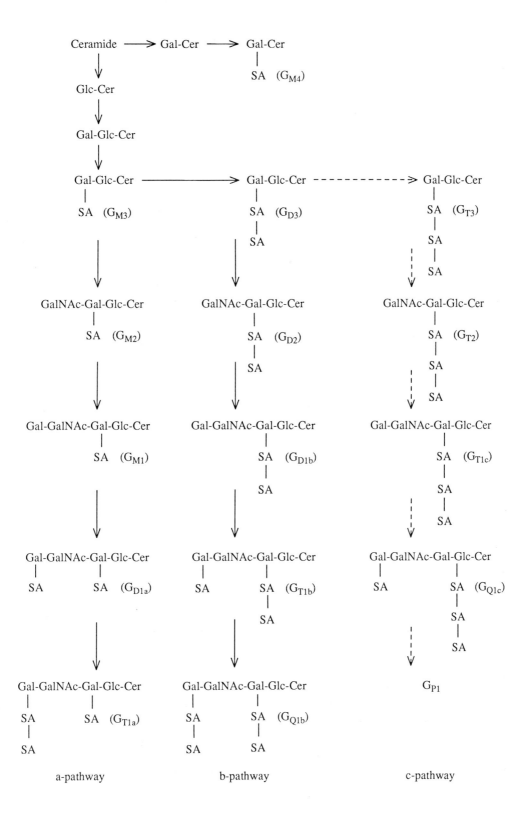

Brain lipids contain long, polyunsaturated fatty acids

Cerebroside acyl chains may be α-hydroxylated or have an odd number of carbon atoms, mainly 23 and 25. Normally, very small amounts of free fatty acids are found in the brain. Cholesterol esters accumulate in the inherited metabolic disease adrenoleukodystrophy (ALD) [14]. Fatty acids containing 24, 25, or 26 carbon atoms are predominant in these esters. Gangliosides also contain these fatty acids rather than 18:0 in this disease. The metabolic basis of ALD is not known, but a defect in fatty acid degradation cannot be excluded. It is probably a dysfunction in peroxisomal metabolism of long-chain fatty acids.

It is not yet clear how the difference in the amount of saturation between fatty acids at position C-1 and those at C-2 in phosphoglycerides originates. There is considerable evidence to indicate that newly biosynthesized phospholipids do not show great selectivity between the two positions. It appears that following biosynthesis, there is a deacylation by phospholipase A_2 to produce lysolipid, quickly followed by reacylation with an unsaturated long-chain acyl-CoA to yield the naturally occurring form of the lipid. These enzymatically catalyzed exchanges may be of importance in understanding how arachidonate is introduced into phospholipids and how it is released for synthesis of the prostanoids (see Chap. 20).

Metabolism of brain fatty acids

In addition to the classical β-oxidation of fatty acids, known to occur in all tissues, significant α-oxidation also occurs in the brain: Position 2 of a fatty acid is hydroxylated, then oxidized to form an α-keto acid, which is then decarboxylated. In this way, one carbon at a time may be removed. This minor pathway may explain the origin of both odd-carbon fatty acids and 2-hydroxy fatty acids in brain cerebrosides. Additionally, there is a known metabolic defect in humans in which α-oxidation of a dietary fatty acid cannot occur. This results in the failure to metabolize the branched-chain fatty acid phytanic acid (see Fig. 3). Such branched-chain fatty acids, the metabolism of which can only be initiated by α- and not by β-oxidation, accumulate in individuals with Refsum's disease [15], in which there is a severe neuropathy.

ANALYSIS OF BRAIN AND BRAIN FRACTIONS FOR LIPID CONTENT

There are many variations of the chloroform/methanol extraction originally reported by Folch et al. [16]. For health and economic considerations, alternative extraction mixtures have been suggested, the most successful of which is a hexane/isopropanol mixture, but it is not yet commonly used [17]. In most extraction procedures, one volume of a 1:3 to 1:10 aqueous tissue homogenate is treated with 19 volumes of a 2:1 v/v mixture of chloroform/methanol. A single liquid phase is formed, leaving behind a residue of macromolecular material, primarily protein, with lesser amounts of DNA, RNA, and polysaccharides. The subsequent addition of a small amount of water to the supernatant fraction leads to separation of the chloroform and aqueous methanol phases; the lower (chloroform) phase contains the lipids, whereas low-molecular-weight metabolites are in the upper phase. If the lower phase is evaporated to dryness and taken back up in a lipid solvent such as chloroform, proteolipid protein remains undissolved and can be removed at this point. Ganglioside can be extracted from the aqueous phase by repartitioning into an apolar solvent. The polyphosphoinositides and PA are poorly extracted at neutral pH, and it is therefore necessary to acidify the initial chloroform/methanol mixture for their recovery [18]. Unfortunately, the acidity leads to cleavage of plasmalogen, primarily alkenyl-acyl PE. There is thus no one single procedure that results in quantitative recovery of all brain lipids.

Lipid classes are separated from a lipid extract by thin-layer chromatography (TLC) or by high-performance liquid chromatography (HPLC). To analyze individual fatty acids in a given lipid class, methyl esters can be prepared directly by alkaline methanolysis of extracted bands scraped from TLC plates following visualization, usually with a fluorescent spray. The methyl esters are then separated by gas-liquid chromatography (GLC). It is possible to separate subclasses of intact phospholipids on the basis of the number of fatty acid double bonds if Ag^+ is present in the silica gel of the TLC plates. This separation is based on π-bonding between Ag^+ and the fatty acid double bonds [18]. The molecular species can also be separated by reverse-phase HPLC. The amide-bound fatty acids of the sphingolipids require more vigorous conditions, such as treatment with hot HCl-methanol.

LIPIDS AS MEMBRANE COMPONENTS

Membranes vary in their lipid and protein content

Table 2 illustrates the wide range in lipid content of different membranes. Note that the mitochondrial membrane, in addition to containing a characteristic lipid (cardiolipin), is relatively low in lipid content. By contrast, myelin membranes have a very high lipid content. They, too, contain characteristic lipids, such as galactocerebroside and galactocerebroside sulfate. The lipid enrichment in myelin accounts for the high lipid content of white matter in brain and to a great extent the high lipid content of brain itself. Most organs contain twice as much protein as lipid, whereas the brain contains approximately equal amounts. Note in Table 3 that white matter has nearly three times the lipid content of gray matter, based on fresh weight. This difference is not as great on a dry weight basis, since gray matter has a higher water content than white matter. Note that cholesterol, PE,

TABLE 2. Protein/lipid ratios in various eukaryotic membranes[a]

Membrane	Ratio
Myelin	0.23
Liver (mouse)	0.85
Retinal rods (bovine)	1.0
Erythrocyte (human)	1.1
Mitochondrial outer membrane	1.1
Ameba	1.3
Cultured cells (Hela)	1.5
Sarcoplasmic reticulum	2.0
Mitochondrial inner membrane	3.2

[a] From Singer [19].

and PC account for over 80 percent of brain lipids. In other tissues, for example, heart, PC prevails over PE as the major lipid and contains the major plasmalogen content. Bear in mind that the various phospholipid classes in both gray and white matter contain very different fatty acids (see Table 1).

Orientation of lipids within membrane leaflets

Much of our concept of membranes at the molecular level originated with surface tension studies of compressed monomolecular films of lipids, which showed that when a monolayer of fatty acids over an aqueous surface is compressed, the fatty acids become oriented with their chains perpendicular to the surface and their methyl ends out of the water. Particles made of a spherical monolayer array (micelles) can be made artificially, but in membranes, lipids form biomolecular leaflets with the polar functions of the lipid molecules back-to-back. Proteins may be embedded in the inner or outer leaflet only or may span the membrane, depending on their primary, secondary, and tertiary structures. Studies on the polarity of amino acids comprising membrane-spanning proteins such as receptors indicate that a single receptor molecule may span the membrane several times (see Chap. 4). Gangliosides are generally regarded to be enriched in plasma

TABLE 3. Lipid composition of normal adult human brain[a]

Constituent	Gray matter (%)			White matter (%)		
	Fresh wt.	Dry wt.	Lipid	Fresh wt.	Dry wt.	Lipid
Water	81.9	—	—	71.6	—	—
Chloroform-methanol—insoluble residue	9.5	52.6	—	8.7	30.6	—
Proteolipid protein	0.5	2.7	—	2.4	8.4	—
Total lipid	5.9	32.7	100	15.6	54.9	100
Upper phase solids	2.2	12.1	—	1.7	6.0	—
Cholesterol	1.3	7.2	22.0	4.3	15.1	27.5
Phospholipid, total	4.1	22.7	69.5	7.2	25.2	45.9
PE	1.7	9.2	27.1	3.7	13.2	23.9
PC	1.9	10.7	30.1	2.4	8.4	15.0
SM	0.4	2.3	6.9	1.2	4.2	7.7
Phosphoinositides (PI, PIP, PIP$_2$)	0.16	0.9	2.7	0.14	0.5	0.9
PS	0.5	2.8	8.7	1.2	4.3	7.9
Galactocerebroside	0.3	1.8	5.4	3.1	10.9	19.8
Galactocerebroside sulfate	0.1	0.6	1.7	0.9	3.0	5.4
Ganglioside, total[b]	0.3	1.7	—	0.05	0.18	—

[a] Modified from Suzuki [20].
[b] Phospholipid fractions include plasmalogen, assuming that all plasmalogen is present as PE and PC with a ratio of 4:1 in white matter and 1:1 in gray matter. In intact brain (based on microwaved rat brain), phosphoinositides are present in both white and gray matter in the ratio of 5:0.3:1 for PI, PIP, and PIP$_2$. Gangliosides are calculated on the basis of total sialic acid, assuming that sialic acid constitutes 30 percent of the weight of a typical ganglioside; G_{DIa} is the major ganglioside of both gray and white matter.

membranes, with their complex carbohydrate functions bathing in the extracellular space. Phospholipids with quaternary nitrogen functions, such as PC and SM, are enriched in the outer (extracellular) plasma membrane leaflet, whereas PE and PS are in general considered to be in the inner leaflet. Although PI, PIP, and PIP$_2$ are all considered to be in the inner leaflet, some proteins appear to be linked to PI in the outer leaflet, and they are released by a PI-specific phospholipase C (see Chap. 16).

REFERENCES

1. Inoue, T., Deshmukh, D. S., and Pieringer, R. A. The association of the galactosyl diglycerides of brain with myelination. I. Changes in the concentration of monogalactosyl diglyceride in the microsomal and myelin fractions of brain of rats during development. *J. Biol. Chem.* 246:5688–5694, 1971.

2. O'Brien, J. S., and Sampson, E. L. Lipid composition of the normal human brain: Gray matter, white matter, and myelin. *J. Lipid Res.* 6:537–544, 1965.

3. Hajra, A. K. Biosynthesis of *O*-alkylglycerol ether lipids. In H. K. Mangold and F. Paltauf (eds.), *Ether Lipids: Biochemical and Biomedical Aspects.* New York: Academic Press, 1983, pp. 85–106.

4. Datta, N. S., Wilson, G. N., and Hajra, A. K. Deficiency of enzymes catalyzing the biosynthesis of glycerol-ether lipids in Zellweger syndrome. *New England J. Med.* 311:1080–1083, 1984.

5. Kennedy, E. P. The biosynthesis of phospholipids. In J. A. F. Op den Kamp, B. Roelofsen, and K. W. A. Wirtz (eds.), *Lipids and Membranes: Past, Present and Future.* Amsterdam: Elsevier, 1986, pp. 171–206.

6. Barany, M., and Glonek, T. Identification of diseased states by phosphorus-31 NMR. In D. G. Gorenstein (ed.), *Phosphorus-31 NMR: Principles and Applications*. Orlando: Academic Press, 1984, pp. 511–545.

7. Kanfer, J. N. The base exchange enzymes and phospholipase D of rat brain microsomes. In L. A. Horrocks, G. B. Ansell, and G. Porcellati (eds.), *Phospholipids in the Nervous System, Metabolism*. New York: Raven Press, 1982, pp. 13–20.

8. Ledeen, R. W., and Yu, R. K. Gangliosides: Structure, isolation and analysis. In V. Ginsburg (ed.), *Methods in Enzymology, Vol. 83: Complex Carbohydrates, Part D*. New York: Academic Press, Inc., 1982, pp. 139–191.

9. Yu, R. K., and Ando, S. Structures of some new complex gangliosides. In L. Svennerholm, P. Mandel, H. Drefus, and P.-F. Urban (eds.), *Structure and Function of Gangliosides*. New York, Plenum Press, 1980, pp. 33–45.

10. Wiegandt, H. The gangliosides. In B. W. Agranoff and M. H. Aprison (eds.), *Advances in Neurochemistry*. New York: Plenum Press, 1982, Vol. 4, 149–223.

11. Fishman, P. H. Role of membrane gangliosides in the binding and action of bacterial toxins. *J. Membrane Biol.* 69:85–97, 1982.

12. Radin, N. S. Biosynthesis of the sphingoid bases: A provocation. *J. Lipid Res.* 25:1536–1540, 1984.

13. Hannun, Y. A., and Bell, R. M. Lysosphingolipids inhibit protein kinase C: Implications for the sphingolipidoses. *Science* 235:670–674, 1987.

14. Singh, I., Moser, A. E., Moser, H. W., and Kishimoto, Y. Andrenoleukodystrophy: Impaired oxidation of very long chain fatty acids in white blood cells, cultured skin fibroblasts and amniocytes. *Pediatric Res.* 18:286–290, 1984.

15. Steinberg, D. Phytanic acid storage disease (Refsum's disease). In J. B. Stanbury, J. B. Wyngaarden, D. S. Fredrickson, J. L. Goldstein, and M. S. Brown (eds.), *The Metabolic Basis of Inherited Disease*, 5th ed. New York: McGraw-Hill, 1983, pp. 731–747.

16. Folch, J., Lees, M., and Sloane-Stanley, G. H. A simple method for the isolation and purification of total lipids from animal tissues. *J. Biol. Chem.* 226:497–509, 1957.

17. Hara, A., and Radin, N. S. Lipid extraction of tissues with a low-toxicity solvent. *Anal. Biochem.* 90:420–426, 1978.

18. Hajra, A. K., Fisher, S. K., and Agranoff, B. W. Isolation, separation and analysis of phosphoinositides from biological sources. In A. A. Boulton, G. B. Baker, and L. A. Horrocks (eds.), *Neuromethods (Neurochemistry), Volume 8: Lipids and Related Compounds*. Clifton, NJ: Humana Press, 1987.

19. Singer, S. J. Architecture and topography of biologic membranes. In G. Weissmann and R. Claiborne (eds.), *Cell Membranes: Biochemistry, Cell Biology and Pathology*. New York: HP Publishing Co., Inc. 1975, p. 35.

20. Suzuki, K. Chemistry and metabolism of brain lipids. In G. J. Siegel, R. W. Albers, B. W. Agranoff, and R. Katzman (eds.), *Basic Neurochemistry*, 3rd ed. Little, Brown and Company: Boston, 1981, pp. 355–370.

GENERAL REFERENCES

Bradford, H. F. *Chemical Neurobiology. An Introduction to Neurochemistry*. New York: W. H. Freeman and Company, 1986, pp. 22–28.

Gurr, M. I., and James, A. T. (eds.), *Lipid Biochemistry: An Introduction*. London: Chapman and Hall, 1980.

Hucho, F., Membrane molecules. In M. Dickins (translator), *Neurochemistry: Fundamentals and Concepts*. Weinheim, FRG: VCH, 1986, pp. 25–72.

Lajtha, A. (ed.), *Handbook of Neurochemistry, 2nd ed., Vol. 7: Structural Elements of the Nervous System*. New York: Plenum Press, 1985.

Svennerholm, L., Mandel, P., Dreyfus, H., and Urban, P.-F. (eds.), *Structure and Function of Gangliosides*. New York: Plenum Press, 1980.

Vance, D. E., and Vance, J. E. (eds.), *Biochemistry of Lipids and Membranes*. Menlo Park, CA: The Benjamin/Cummings Publishing Company, Inc., 1985.

CHAPTER 6

Formation, Structure, and Biochemistry of Myelin

Pierre Morell, Richard H. Quarles, and William T. Norton

The morphological distinction between white matter and gray matter is a useful one for the neurochemist. White matter, so called for its glistening white appearance, is composed of myelinated axons, glial cells, and blood vessels. Gray matter contains, in addition, the nerve cell bodies with their extensive dendritic arborizations and very different ratios of the other ele-

Basic Neurochemistry: Molecular, Cellular, and Medical Aspects, 4th Ed., edited by G. J. Siegel et al. Raven Press, Ltd., New York, 1989. Correspondence to Pierre Morell, Biological Sciences Research Center, University of North Carolina, Chapel Hill, North Carolina 27599-7250.

ments. The predominant element of white matter is the myelin sheath, which comprises approximately 50 percent of the total dry weight. Myelin is mainly responsible for the gross chemical differences between white and gray matter.

THE MYELIN SHEATH

The myelin sheath is a greatly extended and modified plasma membrane that is wrapped around the nerve axon in a spiral fashion (for review, see Raine [1]). The myelin membranes originate from and are part of the Schwann cell in the peripheral nervous system (PNS) and the oligodendroglial cells (oligodendrocytes) in the central nervous system (CNS) (see Chap. 1). Each myelin-generating cell furnishes myelin for only one segment of any given axon. The periodic interruptions in the myelin sheath, where short portions of the axon are left uncovered by myelin, are the nodes of Ranvier, and they are critical to the functioning of myelin.

Myelin facilitates conduction

Myelin is an electrical insulator; however, its function of facilitating conduction in axons has no exact analogy in electrical circuitry. In unmyelinated fibers, impulse conduction is propagated by local circuits of ion current that flow into the active region of the axonal membrane, through the axon, and out through adjacent sections of the membrane (Fig. 1). These local circuits depolarize the adjacent region of membrane in a continuous sequential fashion. In myelinated axons, the excitable axonal membrane is exposed to the extracellular space only at the nodes of Ranvier. The remainder of the axolemma is covered by the myelin sheath. This stack of unit membranes has much higher resistance and much lower capacitance than the axonal membrane. When the membrane at the node is excited, the local circuit generated cannot flow through the high-resistance sheath; it therefore flows out through and depolarizes the membrane at the next node, which might be 1 mm or farther away (see Fig. 1). The low capacitance of the sheath means that little energy is required to depolarize the remaining membrane between the nodes, which results in increased speed of local circuit spreading. Active excitation of the axonal membrane jumps from node to node; this form of impulse propagation is therefore called saltatory conduction (Latin *saltare*, "to jump"). Such movement of the

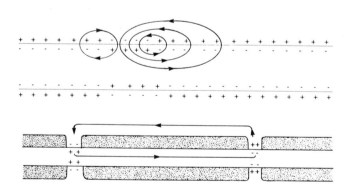

FIG. 1. Impulse conduction in unmyelinated (*top*) and myelinated (*bottom*) fibers. The *arrows* show the flow of action currents in local circuits into the active region of the membrane. In unmyelinated fibers, the circuits flow through the adjacent piece of membrane, but in myelinated fibers the circuit flow jumps to the next node.

wave of depolarization is much more rapid than is the case in unmyelinated fibers. Furthermore, because only the nodes of Ranvier are excited during conduction in myelinated fibers, sodium ion flux into the nerve is much less than in unmyelinated fibers, where the entire membrane is involved. An example of the advantage of myelination is obtained by comparison of two different nerve fibers that both conduct at 25 m/sec at 20°C. The 500-μm-diameter unmyelinated squid giant axon requires 5,000 times as much energy and occupies about 1,500 times as much space as a 12-μm-diameter myelinated axon in a frog.

Conduction velocity in myelinated fibers is proportional to the diameter, whereas in unmyelinated fibers it is proportional to the square root of the diameter. Thus, differences in energy and space requirements between the two types of fibers are exaggerated at higher conduction velocities. If nerves were not myelinated and equivalent conduction velocities were maintained, the human spinal cord would need to be as large as a good-sized tree trunk. Myelin, then, facilitates conduction while conserving space and energy.

A quantitative treatment (see Ritchie [2] for references) of the relationship between conduction velocity and myelination indicates that the optimal internodal distance and thickness of the myelin sheath for a given axon should be proportional to fiber diameter. The calculated ratio of axon diameter to overall myelinated fiber diameter is about 0.6 for optimal conduction velocity. This ratio is close to that observed in myelinated fibers in both PNS and CNS. Another factor is that as the fiber diameter approaches 0.2 μm, the core resistance of the axon becomes a limiting factor in impulse propagation. In the CNS, the observed minimum diameter of myelinated fibers is approximately 0.3 μm, close to the critical minimum size to make myelination useful. In the PNS, the observed minimum diameter of myelinated fibers is approximately 1 μm. The greater diameter is possibly a consequence of the longer internodal distance range, 0.5–1.5 mm, dictated by the morphology of the Schwann cell relative to the shorter internodes of oligodendrocyte-generated myelin in the CNS. (Literature references and a more detailed treatment of this topic may be found in Ritchie [2] and several chapters in Waxman [3].)

Myelin has a characteristic ultrastructure

Myelin, as well as many of its morphological features, such as the nodes of Ranvier and Schmidt-Lantermann clefts, can be seen readily under the light microscope (Fig. 2); however, much of our understanding of the organization of this structure is derived from studies by three physical techniques: polarized light, X-ray diffraction, and electron microscopy. Myelin, when examined by polarized light, exhibits both lipid-dependent and protein-dependent birefringence. These results suggest that myelin is built up of ordered layers; the lipid component of these layers is oriented radially to the axis of the nerve fiber, whereas the protein component is oriented tangentially to the nerve. Low-angle X-ray diffraction studies of PNS myelin have provided an electron density plot of the repeating unit that shows three peaks (each corresponding to protein plus lipid polar groups) and two troughs (lipid hydrocarbon chains), with a repeat distance of 180 Å. The results from these two techniques are thus consistent with a protein-lipid-protein-lipid-protein structure in which the lipid portion is a bimolecular leaflet, and adjacent protein layers are different in some way. Although it is useful to think of myelin in terms of alternating protein and lipid layers, this concept has been modified somewhat in recent years to be compatible with the "fluid mosaic" model of membrane structure, which includes intrinsic transmembrane proteins as well as extrinsic proteins (this is discussed in detail later).

Similar electron density plots of mammal-

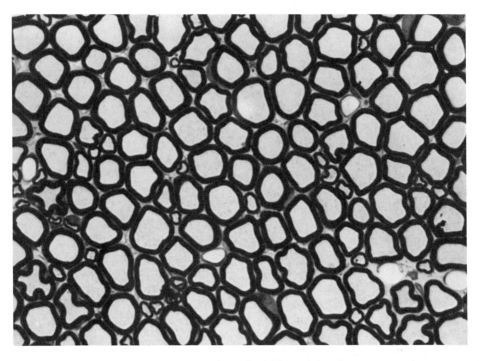

FIG. 2. Light micrograph of a 1-μm Epon section of rabbit peripheral nerve (anterior root), stained with toluidine blue. The myelin sheath appears as a thick black ring around the pale axon. ×600, before 30 percent reduction. (Courtesy of Dr. Cedric Raine.)

ian optic nerve showed a repeat distance of 80 Å (Fig. 3); that is, adjacent protein layers reacted identically to the X-ray beam. Because 80 Å can accommodate one bimolecular layer of lipid (~50 Å) and two protein layers (~15 Å each), 80 Å represents the width of one unit membrane; the main repeating unit of two fused unit membranes is twice this figure, or 160 Å. (Results obtained using this methodology, as well as high-resolution studies, are reviewed in Kirschner et al. [5].)

The conclusions noted above are fully supported by electron microscope studies. This technique visualizes myelin as a series of alternating dark and less dark lines (protein layers) separated by unstained zones (the lipid hydrocarbon chains) (Figs. 4–7). The asymmetry in the staining of the protein layers results from the way the myelin sheath is generated from the cell plasma membrane (see next section and Figs. 8–10). The less dark, or intraperiod, line represents the closely apposed outer protein coats of the original cell membrane; the dark, or major period, line is the fused, inner protein coats of the cell membrane. Confirmation of this interpretation comes from examination of myelin of the PNS that has been swollen in hypotonic solutions. Electron microscopy reveals splitting only at the intraperiod line, and the electron density plots show that broadening occurs at the wider of the three peaks in the repeating unit. This approach shows the continuity of the membrane junction of the intraperiod line with the extracellular space and proves that the wide electron density peak in plots of peripheral nerve corresponds to the intraperiod lines seen in electron micrographs.

The repeat distances observed by electron

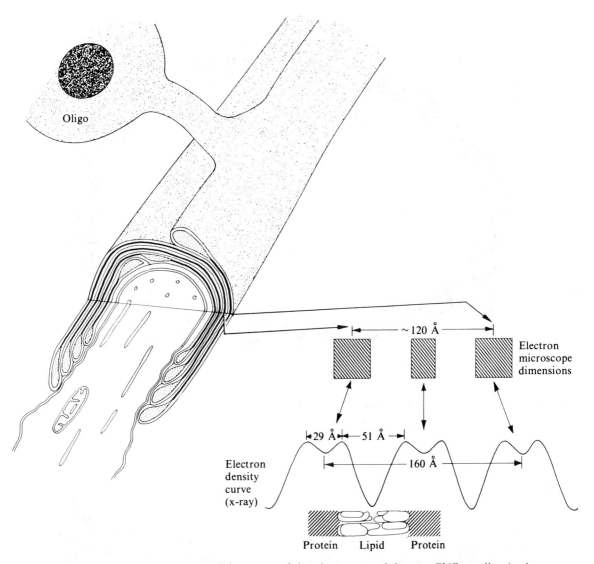

FIG. 3.   A composite diagram summarizing some of the ultrastructural data on CNS myelin. At the *top*, an oligodendroglial cell is shown connected to the sheath by a process. The cutaway view of the myelin and axon illustrates the relationship of these two structures at the nodal and paranodal regions. (Only a few myelin layers have been drawn for the sake of clarity.) At the internodal region, the cross section reveals the inner and outer mesaxons and their relationship to the inner cytoplasmic wedges and the outer loop of cytoplasm. Note that in contrast to PNS myelin (see Fig. 4), there is no full ring of cytoplasm surrounding the outside of the sheath. The *lower part* of the figure shows roughly the dimensions and appearance of one myelin repeating unit as seen with fixed and embedded preparations in the electron microscope. This is contrasted with the dimensions of the electron density curve of CNS myelin obtained by X-ray diffraction studies in fresh nerve. The components responsible for the peaks and troughs of the curve are sketched below. (From Norton [4]. Reprinted courtesy of Lea & Febiger, publishers.)

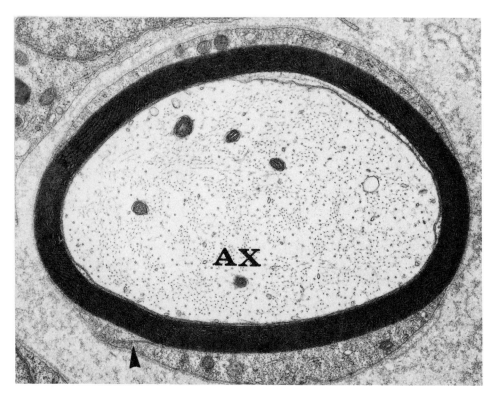

FIG. 4. Electron micrograph of a single peripheral nerve fiber from rabbit. Note that the myelin sheath has a lamellated structure and is surrounded by Schwann cell cytoplasm: (*arrow, lower left*) outer mesaxon; (AX) axon. ×18,000. (Courtesy of Dr. Cedric Raine.)

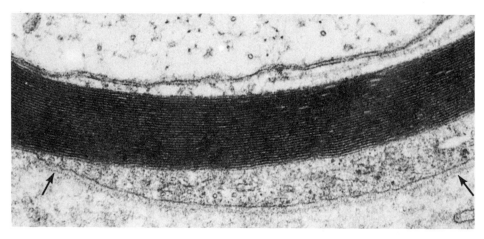

FIG. 5. Higher magnification of Fig. 4 to show the Schwann cell cytoplasm covered by basal lamina (*arrow*). ×50,000.

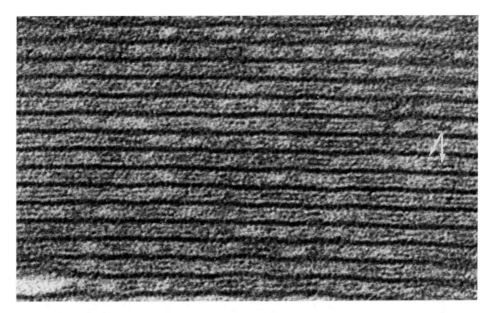

FIG. 6.   Magnification of the myelin sheath of Fig. 4. Note that the intraperiod line (*arrows*) at this high resolution is a double structure. ×350,000. (Courtesy of Dr. Cedric Raine.)

microscopy are less than those calculated from the low-angle X-ray diffraction data, a consequence of the considerable shrinkage that takes place after fixation and dehydration. However, the difference in periodicity between the PNS and CNS myelin is maintained; PNS myelin has an average repeat distance of 119 Å, that of CNS myelin, 107 Å. Also, with improved methods of perfusion fixation and tissue staining, the intraperiod line is now routinely seen as a double line rather than a single one (see Figs. 6 and 7). This ultrastructural appearance indicates that the extracellular sides of the unit membranes are closely apposed but not fused.

Nodes of Ranvier

Two adjacent segments of myelin on one axon are separated by a node of Ranvier. In this region the axon is not covered by myelin. At the paranodal region and the Schmidt-Lantermann clefts, the cytoplasmic surfaces of myelin are not compacted, and Schwann or glial cell cy-

toplasm is included within the sheath. To visualize these structures, one may refer to Figs. 8 and 9, adapted from those of Hirano and Dembitzer [6], which show that if myelin were unrolled from the axon it would be a flat, spade-shaped sheet surrounded by a tube of cytoplasm. Thus, as shown in electron micrographs of longitudinal sections of axon paranodal regions, the major dense line formed by apposition of the cytoplasmic faces opens up at the edges of the sheet, enclosing cytoplasm within a loop (see Figs. 3 and 9). These loop-shaped terminations of the sheath at the node are called lateral loops. The loops form membrane complexes with the axolemma, called transverse bands, whereas myelin in the internodal region is separated from the axon by a gap of periaxonal space. The transverse bands are helical structures that seal the myelin to the axolemma but provide, by spaces between them, a tortuous path from the extracellular space to the periaxonal space.

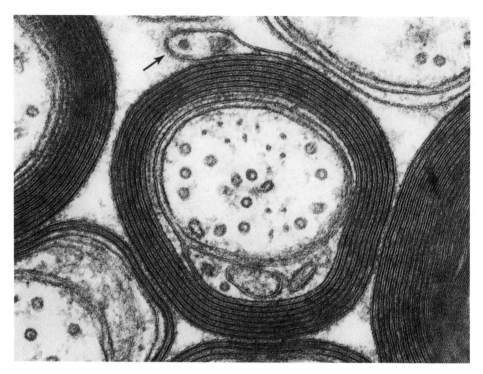

FIG. 7.   A typical CNS myelinated fiber from the spinal cord of an adult dog. Contrast this figure with the PNS fiber in Fig. 4. The course of the flattened oligodendrocytic process, beginning at the outer tongue (*arrow*), can be traced. Note that the fiber lacks investing cell cytoplasm and a basal lamina, as is the case in the PNS. The major dense line and the paler, double intraperiod line of the myelin sheath can be discerned. The axon contains neurotubules and neurofilaments. ×135,000.

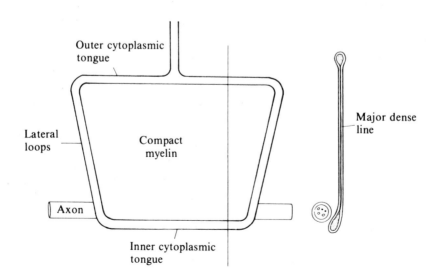

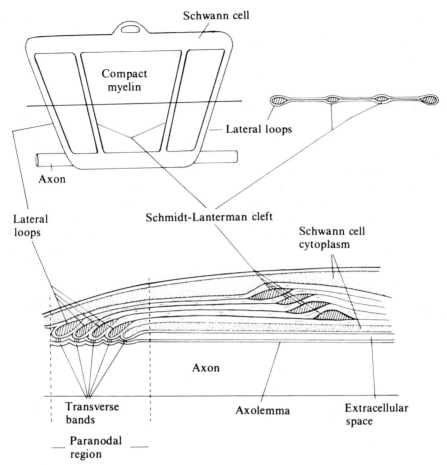

FIG. 9. A diagram similar to Fig. 8 but showing one Schwann cell and its myelin sheath unrolled from a peripheral axon. The sheet of PNS myelin (*top left*) is, like CNS myelin, surrounded by a tube of cytoplasm and has additional tubes of cytoplasm that make up the Schmidt-Lantermann clefts, running through the internodal regions. The cross section of the sheet taken horizontally (*top right*) shows that these additional tubes of cytoplasm arise from regions where the cytoplasmic membrane surfaces have not fused. Diagram at *bottom* is an enlarged longitudinal cross section through the Schwann cell and its myelin wrappings around the axon. The tube forming the lateral loop seals to the axolemma at the paranodal region, and the cytoplasmic tubes in the internodal region form the Schmidt-Lantermann clefts. (These drawings are not to scale.) (Adapted from Hirano and Dembitzer [5].)

FIG. 8. Diagram showing the appearance of CNS myelin were it unrolled from the axon. One can visualize this structure arising from Fig. 3 if the glial cell process were pulled straight up and the myelin layers separated at the intraperiod line. The whole myelin internode forms a spade-shaped sheet surrounded by a continuous tube of oligodendroglial cell cytoplasm. This diagram shows that the lateral loops and inner and outer cytoplasmic tongues are part of the same cytoplasmic tube. The drawing on the *right* shows the appearance of this sheet were it sectioned along the vertical line, indicating that the compact myelin region is formed of two unit membranes fused at the cytoplasmic surfaces. (The drawing is not necessarily to scale.) (Adapted from Hirano and Dembitzer [5].)

Schmidt-Lantermann Clefts

The Schmidt-Lantermann clefts, structures common in peripheral, but rare in central, myelinated axons are regions where the cytoplasmic surfaces of the myelin sheath have not compacted to form the major dense line and therefore contain Schwann or glial cell cytoplasm (Fig. 9). These inclusions of cytoplasm are present in each layer of myelin. The clefts can therefore be visualized in the unrolled myelin sheet as tubes of cytoplasm similar to the tubes making up the lateral loops, but in the middle regions of the sheet rather than at the edges (Fig. 9). (See Raine [1] for a more complete description of myelin morphology.)

Myelin is an extension of a cell membrane

Myelination in the PNS

Myelination in the PNS is preceded by invasion of the nerve bundle by Schwann cells, rapid multiplication of these cells, and segregation of the individual axons by Schwann cell processes. Small axons (≤ 1 μm), which will remain unmyelinated, are segregated; several may be enclosed in one cell, each within its own pocket, similar to the structure shown in Fig. 10A. Large axons (>1 μm) destined for myelination are enclosed singly, one Schwann cell per axon per internode. These cells line up along the axons with intervals between them; the intervals become the nodes of Ranvier.

Before myelination, the axon lies in an invagination of the Schwann cell (see Fig. 10A). The plasmalemma of the cell then surrounds the axons and joins to form a double-membrane structure that communicates with the cell surface [7]. This structure, called the mesaxon, then elongates around the axons in a spiral fashion (see Fig. 10). Thus, mature myelin is formed in this "jelly roll" fashion; the mesaxon winds about the axon, and the cytoplasmic surfaces

condense into a compact myelin sheath and form the major dense line. The two external surfaces form the myelin intraperiod line.

Myelination in the CNS

The structure of myelin in the CNS, formed by the oligodendroglial cell [8], has many similarities to, but also points of difference from, that in the PNS. CNS nerve fibers are not separated by connective tissue, nor are they surrounded by cell cytoplasm, and specific glial nuclei are not obviously associated with particular myelinated fibers. CNS myelin is a spiral structure similar to PNS myelin; it has an inner mesaxon and an outer mesaxon that ends in a loop, or tongue, of glial cytoplasm (Fig. 3). Unlike peripheral nerve, where the sheath is surrounded by Schwann cell cytoplasm, the cytoplasmic tongue in the CNS is restricted to a small portion of the sheath. This glial tongue is continuous with the plasma membrane of the oligodendroglial cell through slender processes. One glial cell, through extension of multiple processes, can myelinate many (40 or more) separate axons [9].

Mechanism of myelin deposition

The actual mechanism of myelin deposition is still obscure. In the PNS, a single axon may have up to 100 myelin layers, and it is therefore improbable that myelin is laid down by a simple rotation of the Schwann cell nucleus around the axon. In the CNS, such a postulate is precluded by the fact that one glial cell can myelinate several axons. During myelination, there are increases in the length of the internode, the diameter of the axon, and the number of myelin layers. Myelin therefore expands in all planes at once. Any mechanism to account for this growth must assume that the membrane system is able to expand and contract and that the layers slip over each other.

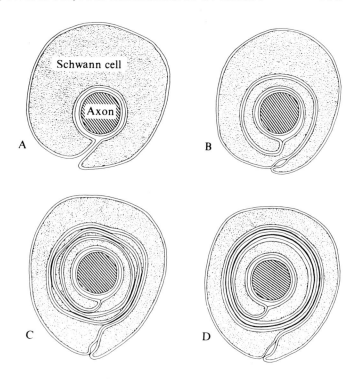

FIG. 10. Myelin formation in the PNS. **A:** The Schwann cell has surrounded the axon, but the external surfaces of the plasma membrane have not yet fused in the mesaxon. **B:** The mesaxon has fused into a five-layered structure and spiraled once around the axon. **C:** A few layers of myelin have formed but are not completely compacted. Note the cytoplasm trapped in zones where the cytoplasmic membrane surfaces have not yet fused. **D:** Compact myelin showing only a few layers for the sake of clarity. Note that Schwann cell cytoplasm forms a ring both inside and outside the sheath. (From Norton [4]. Reprinted courtesy of Lea & Febiger, publishers.)

Myelin can be isolated in high yield and purity by conventional methods of subcellular fractionation

CNS myelin isolation

If CNS tissue is homogenized in media of low ionic strength, myelin peels off the axons and reforms in vesicles of the size range of nuclei and mitochondria. Because of their high lipid content, these myelin vesicles have the lowest intrinsic density of any membrane fraction of the nervous system. Procedures for isolation of myelin take advantage of both of these properties—large vesicle size and low density.

In a widely used method, a homogenate of nervous tissue in isotonic sucrose (0.3 M) is layered directly onto 0.85 M sucrose and centrifuged at high speed. Mitochondria and synaptosomes sediment through the denser sucrose, and many of the smaller membrane fragments from other organelles remain in the 0.3-M sucrose layer. A crude myelin layer collects at the interface. The major impurities, microsomes and axoplasm, trapped in the vesicles during the homogenization procedure, are released by subjecting the myelin to osmotic shock in distilled water. The larger myelin particles can then be separated from the smaller membranous material by low-speed centrifugation or by repeating the density gradient centrifugation on continuous or discontinuous gradients, usually of sucrose. On sucrose gradients, myelin forms a band centering at approximately 0.65 M sucrose, equivalent to a density of 1.08 g/ml. For comparison, mitochondria have a density of 1.2 (equivalent to ~1.55 M sucrose). These preparations of purified myelin can be further subdivided arbitrarily into fractions of different densities and compositions by centrifugation on expanded continuous or discontinuous density gradients (described later).

Demonstration of purity for a myelin preparation includes electron microscopic appearance (the typical five-layered structure and repeat period of ~120 Å seen *in situ*); however, the difficulty of identifying small membrane vesicles of microsomes in a field of myelin membranes and the well-known sampling problems inherent in electron microscopy make this characterization unreliable after a certain purity level has been reached.

The biochemical markers that have been commonly used to assay contamination of myelin by other subcellular fractions are succinic dehydrogenase (mitochondria); Na, K-ATPase and 5'-nucleotidase (plasma membranes); NADH-cytochrome-C reductase (microsomes); DNA (nuclei); RNA (nuclei, ribosomes, microsomes); lactate dehydrogenase (cytosol); β-glucosidase (lysosomes); and acetylcholinesterase (neuronal fragments). Although all of these markers are low in purified myelin and set an upper limit for levels of contamination by other membranes, the actual contamination may be less than calculated by such methods, since low levels of many different enzymes appear to be intrinsic to myelin (discussed later).

Markers characteristic of myelin are less useful than negative markers for establishing myelin purity, both because they are minimally affected by small amounts of impurities and because they will all be expressed to varying degrees, depending on the developmental stage, by components of oligodendroglial or Schwann cells. Thus, the myelin-typical marker galactosylceramide (cerebroside); the myelin-specific enzyme 2',3'-cyclic nucleotide 3'-phosphohydrolase (CNPase); and the content of myelin-specific proteins are probably more useful in assaying myelin and oligodendroglial plasma membrane contamination in other fractions than in establishing myelin purity.

PNS myelin isolation

PNS myelin can be isolated by similar techniques, but especially vigorous homogenization conditions are required because of the large amounts of connective tissue and, sometimes, adipose tissue present in the nerve. The slightly lower density of PNS myelin requires some adjustment of gradient composition to prevent loss of myelin.

CHARACTERISTIC COMPOSITION OF MYELIN

Myelin *in situ* has a water content of approximately 40 percent. The dry mass of both CNS and PNS myelin is characterized by a high proportion of lipid (70–85 percent) and, consequently, a low proportion of protein (15–30 percent). In contrast, most biological membranes have a higher ratio of protein to lipid.

CNS myelin is enriched in certain lipids

Table 1 lists the composition of bovine, rat, and human myelin compared to bovine and human white matter, human gray matter, and rat whole brain. (The classification of brain lipids is discussed in Chap. 5.) It can be seen that all the lipids assayed in whole brain are also present in myelin; that is, there are no lipids localized exclusively in some "nonmyelin compartment" (with the exception of the mitochondrial specific lipid, diphosphatidylglycerol, not included in Table 1). We also know that the reverse is true; that is, there are no myelin lipids that are not also found in other subcellular fractions of the brain. Although, strictly speaking, there may be no completely "myelin-specific" lipids, cerebroside is the most typical of myelin. During development, the concentration of cerebroside in brain is directly proportional to the amount of myelin present.

In addition to cerebroside, the major lipids of myelin are cholesterol and ethanolamine-containing plasmalogens (glycerophospholipids containing a alkenyl ether bond; see Chap. 5). Lecithin is also a major myelin constituent and

TABLE 1. Composition of CNS myelin and brain[a]

Substance[b]	Myelin			White matter		Gray matter (human)	Whole brain (rat)
	Human	Bovine	Rat	Human	Bovine		
Protein	30.0	24.7	29.5	39.0	39.5	55.3	56.9
Lipid	70.0	75.3	70.5	54.9	55.0	32.7	37.0
Cholesterol	27.7	28.1	27.3	27.5	23.6	22.0	23.0
Cerebroside	22.7	24.0	23.7	19.8	22.5	5.4	14.6
Sulfatide	3.8	3.6	7.1	5.4	5.0	1.7	4.8
Total galactolipid	27.5	29.3	31.5	26.4	28.6	7.3	21.3
Ethanolamine phosphatides	15.6	17.4	16.7	14.9	13.6	22.7	19.8
Lecithin	11.2	10.9	11.3	12.8	12.9	26.7	22.0
Sphingomyelin	7.9	7.1	3.2	7.7	6.7	6.9	3.8
Phosphatidylserine	4.8	6.5	7.0	7.9	11.4	8.7	7.2
Phosphatidylinositol	0.6	0.8	1.2	0.9	0.9	2.7	2.4
Plasmalogens[c]	12.3	14.1	14.1	11.2	12.2	8.8	11.6
Total phospholipid	43.1	43.0	44.0	45.9	46.3	69.5	57.6

[a] From W. Norton. In G. J. Siegel, R. W. Albers, B. W. Agranoff, and R. Katzman (eds.), Basic Neurochemistry, 3rd. ed. Boston: Little, Brown, 1981, p. 77.
[b] Protein and lipid figures in percent dry weight; all others in percent total lipid weight.
[c] Plasmalogens are primarily ethanolamine phosphatides.

sphingomyelin a relatively minor one. Data for lipid compositions can be expressed in terms of molar ratios for cholesterol, phospholipid, and galactolipid; for mammalian myelin, these ratios range from 2:2:1 to 4:3:2. Thus, cholesterol constitutes the largest proportion of lipid molecules in myelin, although the galactolipids may constitute a greater proportion of the lipid weight.

The data in Table 1 indicate that myelin accounts for much of the total lipid of white matter and that the lipid composition of gray matter is very different from that of myelin. It is of interest that the composition of brain myelin from all mammalian species studied is very much the same; however, there are some obvious species differences. For example, myelin of rat has less sphingomyelin than that of bovine or human brain (Table 1). Although not shown in Table 1, there are also regional variations; for example, myelin isolated from the spinal cord has a higher lipid/protein ratio than brain myelin from the same species. Not only is the lipid class

composition of myelin highly characteristic of this membrane, the fatty acid composition of many of the individual lipids is distinctive (see Chap. 5). For example, the cerebroside fatty acids include a high proportion of primarily long chains (22–26 carbon atoms) and a high content of α-hydroxy groups.

Besides the lipids listed in Table 1, there are several others of importance. If myelin is not extracted with acid organic solvents, the polyphosphoinositides (see Chap. 16) remain tightly bound to the myelin protein and are therefore not included in lipid analysis. Phosphatidylinositol bisphosphate accounts for between 4 and 6 percent of the total myelin lipid phosphorous and phosphatidylinositol phosphate for 1 to 1.5 percent of the myelin lipid phosphorous.

In addition to cerebrosides and sulfatides, there are several minor neutral galactolipids. These include at least three fatty acid esters of cerebroside and two glycerol-based lipids, diacylglycerylgalactoside and monoalkylmonoacylglycerylgalactoside, collectively called galactosyldiglyceride. Some long-chain alkanes also appear to be present.

Also, it is now apparent that myelin from mammals contains 0.1 to 0.3 percent ganglioside (complex sialic acid-containing glycosphingolipids). This is 10 to 20 percent of ganglioside levels in cerebral gray matter. Myelin is greatly enriched in the monosialoganglioside GM_1), whereas other brain membranes are enriched in the polysialo series. Myelin from certain species (including humans) contains an additional unique ganglioside as a major component, sialosylgalactosylceramide (GM_4) (see Chap. 37).

PNS myelin lipids are similar to those of CNS myelin

Myelin from the PNS contains many of the same lipids as myelin from the CNS, although there are quantitative differences [10,12]. Analyses reveal that PNS myelin has less cerebroside and sulfatide and considerably more sphingomyelin than CNS myelin. An interesting observation is the presence of ganglioside LM_1 (sialosyl-lactoneotetraosylceramide) as a characteristic component of myelin in the PNS of some species. These differences in lipid composition between CNS and PNS myelin are not, however, as dramatic as the differences in protein composition discussed below.

CNS myelin contains unique proteins

The protein composition of CNS myelin is simpler than that of other brain membranes, with the proteolipid protein (PLP) and myelin basic protein(s) (MBP), making up 60 to 80 percent of the total in most species. Many other proteins and glycoproteins are present to a lesser extent. With the exception of the MBPs, myelin proteins are neither easily extractable nor soluble in aqueous media; however, like other membrane proteins, they are soluble in sodium dodecylsulfate (SDS) solutions and can be separated readily by electrophoresis of these solutions in polyacrylamide gels. This technique separates proteins primarily according to their molecular weight (a common notation is M_r for relative molecular mass). The presence of bound carbohydrates or unusual structural features disrupts somewhat the relationship between migration and molecular weight so that location of a protein in such a gel is taken to mean apparent molecular weight. Protein composition of human and rat brain myelin are illustrated in Fig. 11B and D, respectively. The quantitative predominance of two proteins, the positively charged MBP ($M_r = 18,500$) and PLP, in the gel pattern of human CNS myelin is clear. These proteins are major constituents of all mammalian CNS myelins, and similar proteins are present in myelins of many lower species. (The interested reader will find extensive reviews and references in Benjamins et al. [11] and Lees and Brostoff [13].)

Proteolipid protein

Myelin PLP is the major component of the organic solvent extractable lipoprotein complexes of whole brain. This protein, also known as the Folch-Lees protein (see Lees and Brostoff [13] for review), has been the subject of much study because of its unusual physical properties: It remains soluble in chloroform even after essentially all of its bound lipids have been removed. The molecular weight of PLP from sequence analysis is approximately 30,000, although it migrates anomalously (fast) on SDS gels and gives a lower apparent molecular weight. It has approximately 60 percent nonpolar amino acids and 40 percent polar amino acids. It is very hydrophobic, forms large aggregates in aqueous solution, and is relatively resistant to proteolysis. The amino acid sequence is known from work done on the isolated protein as well as through sequencing of a cDNA clone. (References to applications of recombinant DNA technology in this work are given in Lemke [14].) The protein sequence is exceedingly conserved during evolution; the bovine and rat proteins differ in only a few amino acids. PLP contains approximately 3 mol fatty acids (primarily palmitate, oleate, or stearate)/mol protein in ester linkage to hydroxy amino acids. The amino acid sequence suggests that there are three membrane-spanning domains. Presumably, the properties of this protein promote the formation and stabilization of the characteristic compact multilamellar structure of myelin (Fig. 13).

The human gene for PLP maps to the X chromosome. An unusual feature of its molecular biology is the presence of more than one functional polyadenylation site, giving rise to more than one functional mRNA coding for the same protein [15]. The isolation of DNA clones was the starting point for an explanation of the presence in myelin from many species of a protein known to have related properties in terms of organic solvent solubility. This protein, variously named IM for intermediate (between MBPs and PLPs in molecular weight) or DM-20 (since M_r = 20,000), is coded by an alternative splicing of the RNA, which gives rise to the major PLP [16]. DNA and protein sequencing data both indicate that the structure of DM-20 is related to that of PLP by a deletion of 40 amino acids.

Myelin basic proteins

The major basic protein of myelin (MBP) has long been of interest because it is the antigen that, when injected into an animal, elicits a cellular immune response that produces the CNS autoimmune disease, experimental allergic encephalomyelitis (see Chap. 36). MBP can be extracted from myelin as well as from brain with either dilute acid or salt solutions; once extracted, it is very soluble in water. The complete amino acid sequences of both bovine and human MBP are well known (see Lees and Brostoff [13] for references): Bovine MBP has 169 residues and differs from human MBP by only 11 residues. MBP shows microheterogeneity on electrophoresis in alkaline conditions. This is due

to a combination of phosphorylation, loss of the C-terminal arginine, and deamidation. There is also heterogeneity in the degree of methylation of an arginine at residue 106.

The major MBPs of all species studied are very similar. They are highly unfolded, with essentially no tertiary structure in solution. These proteins have molecular weights of approximately 18,500 and contain approximately 52 percent polar amino acids and 48 percent nonpolar amino acids.

In addition to the major MBP, most species of mammals that have been studied contain various amounts of other basic proteins related in sequence to 18.5-kilodalton (kDa) protein. As noted above, mice and rats have a second smaller MBP (M_r = 14,000). Small MBP has the same N- and C-terminal sequences as larger MBP but differs by a deletion of 40 residues. The ratio of these two basic proteins to one another changes during development: Mature rats and mice have more of the 14-kDa protein than the 18-kDa protein. Two other MBPs seen in many species include a 21.5- and a 17-kDa protein. These two proteins are related structurally to large and small MBP, respectively, by an addition near the N-terminal end of a polypeptide sequence of approximately 3 kDa. Another protein, present to some extent in humans, is the 17.2-kDa MBP [17], which is now known to be slightly different from 17-kDa protein in other species. The relationship among this group of proteins was recently clarified [18,19] with a demonstration that the various MBPs arise from alternative splicing of a common mRNA precursor.

MBP is located on the cytoplasmic face of the myelin membranes corresponding to the major dense line (Fig. 13). Whether MBP has a functional role other than structural is not known; however, the rapid turnover of the phosphate groups [20] present on about one-quarter of the MBP molecules might influence the close apposition of the cytoplasmic surfaces of the membrane.

CNPase

In addition to PLP and MBP, there are many high-molecular-weight proteins present in the gel electrophoretic pattern of myelin. These vary in amount depending on species (mouse and rat may have as much as 30 percent of total myelin protein in this category) and degree of maturity (the younger the animal, the more high-molecular-weight proteins). Although some of these high-molecular-weight proteins may be due to contaminating membranes, many are undoubtedly intrinsic myelin components. A number of these proteins have been characterized. One example that is clearly identifiable on gel electrophoretic profiles of myelin from most species is 2':3'-cyclic nucleotide 3'-phosphodiesterase (CNPase). Although there are low levels of this enzymatic activity associated with the surface membranes of many different types of cells, it is much enriched in myelin and in cells committed to the formation of myelin. This enzyme activity has been purified (see Sprinkle et al. [21] for references), and it corresponds to a double band visible in gels of myelin protein. The doublet is centered around an apparent molecular weight between 44 and 50 kDa (there is some species-specific variation with regard to apparent molecular weight). These two protein bands are often referred to as W_1 and W_2 (after F. Wolfgram). The CNP is extremely active against the substrate 2':3'-cAMP as well as the GMP, CMP, and UMP analogs, which are all hydrolyzed to the corresponding 2'-isomer. The physiological significance of this activity is obscure, since the biologically active cyclic nucleotides are those with a 3':5' structure.

Myelin-associated glycoprotein

Another component in the high-molecular-weight region of SDS gels is the 100 kDa myelin-associated glycoprotein (MAG) (see Quarles [22] for review). Its position is indicated in Fig. 6-11, although it is a quantitatively minor component that electrophoreses diffusely and does not correspond to one of the discrete Coomassie blue-stained bands seen in this figure. MAG is an integral membrane glycoprotein: about one-third of its weight consists of oligosaccharides N-linked with sialic acid, fucose, galactose, mannose, N-acetylglucosamine, and sulfate. Immunocytochemical investigations have shown that MAG is concentrated in the inner periaxonal membrane of myelin sheaths. This position is compatible with its postulated involvement in oligodendrocyte-axon interactions. Most studies indicate that it is absent from the compact multilamellar myelin. Although MAG is a very minor constituent of the isolated myelin fraction (<1 percent of total protein), it is present in substantially higher concentration in the periaxonal membrane that interacts with the axon.

Studies [23–25] have identified cDNA clones for MAG. Amino acid sequences derived from cDNA clones indicate that MAG has a single-membrane-spanning domain separating a C-terminal tail from a heavily glycosylated N-terminal region that is composed of five domains related in sequence to each other and to immunoglobulin-like molecules. Thus, MAG appears to be a member of the immunoglobulin superfamily that includes other nervous system molecules involved in cell-cell interactions, such as neural cell adhesion molecule (N-CAM). An additional relationship of MAG to N-CAM and the immune system is demonstrated by the antibody HNK-1 (anti-leu 7) that binds to a carbohydrate determinant that is on MAG, N-CAM, other adhesion molecules of the nervous system, and a subset of human lymphocytes.

Availability of the MAG/1B236 cDNA clones has led to experiments explaining the decrease in the molecular weight of MAG that occurs during CNS development. There are two MAG proteins resulting from alternative splicing of its mRNA. The mRNA switches to one for a shortened C-terminus of MAG during development.

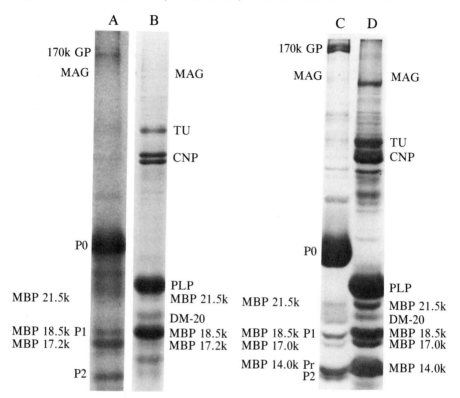

FIG. 11. Polyacrylamide gel electrophoresis of myelin proteins in the presence of SDS. The proteins of human PNS myelin (*A*), human CNS myelin (*B*), rat PNS myelin (*C*) and rat CNS myelin (*D*) were solubilized with the detergent SDS, electrophoresed, and stained with Coomassie Brilliant Blue. The electrophoretic system separates proteins primarily according to their molecular size, with the smallest proteins migrating the furthest toward the bottom of the gel: (P0, P1, P2, Pr) refer to P_0, P_1, P_2, P_r in text; (170 k GP) 170-kDa glycoprotein; (TU) tubulin. Note that in *lane D*, the location noted for MAG (which stains too faintly to be photographed on this gel) is above the discrete Coomassie-stained band (the stained band may correspond to Na, K-ATPase).

There are a large number of glycoproteins in isolated myelin that have not yet been well characterized. Small amounts of proteins characteristic of membranes in general can also be identified on gels of myelin proteins. Noted in Fig. 11 is tubulin; there is evidence suggesting that it is an authentic myelin component. Other minor protein bands can be visualized on gels of myelin with various high-resolution techniques. These may relate to the presence of numerous enzyme activities associated with the myelin sheath (discussed in a following section).

The major PNS myelin protein is P_0, a glycoprotein

PNS myelin proteins are very different from those of CNS myelin (for review, see Smith [12] and Lees and Brostoff [13]). Peripheral nerves do not have the proteolipid protein characteristic of the CNS, and the content of MBP is low. Gel electrophoretic analysis (Fig. 11A and C) shows that a single protein, P_0 (M_r = 30,000), accounts for more than half of the PNS myelin protein. The N-terminal sequence has 28 uncharged and/or nonpolar amino acids, presumably a signal sequence required for insertion of the protein into a membrane. A single, large hydrophobic region is assumed to be located within the membrane and separates an extracellular domain, which contains the glycosylation site, from a cytoplasmic (C-terminal) domain [14]. The P_0 glycoprotein is phosphorylated, sulfated, and, probably, acylated. No trace of PLP, the predominant protein of CNS myelin, is present in myelin of the PNS [26]. It is interesting to note that proteolipid protein and P_0 protein (so different in sequence, posttranslational modifications, and, possibly, structure) may have similar roles in the formation of structures as closely related as myelins of the CNS and PNS.

Myelin basic proteins

MBP content in the PNS varies from approximately 5 to 18 percent of total protein in contrast to the CNS, where it is on the order of 30 percent. As in the CNS, the 18-kDa MBP is the most prominent component in many species,

and it is often referred to as the P_1 protein in the nomenclature of peripheral myelin proteins. In rodents, the same four MBPs found in the CNS are present in the PNS with molecular weights of 21, 18.5, 17, and 14 kDa. In adult rodents, the 14-kDa MBP is the most prominent component and is termed P_r in the PNS nomenclature. Another species-specific variation occurs in humans. In human PNS, the major basic protein is not the 18.5-kDa form that is most prominent in the CNS, but the 17.2-kDa form produced by alternate splicing, as shown in Fig. 12. MBP may not play as critical a role in myelin structure in the PNS as it does in the CNS. The murine mutant, shiverer, is lesioned with respect to MBP synthesis. Whatever CNS myelin present has no dense line structure; this contrasts with the PNS, which has almost normal myelin amounts and structure but lacks MBP (see Hogan and Greenfield [27] for review).

The MBPs of PNS myelin differ further from CNS myelin [13]. They include another positively charged protein ($M_r \simeq 14,000$) that is unrelated in sequence to either P_1 or P_r and is

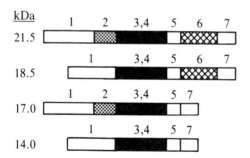
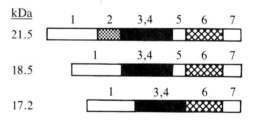

FIG. 12. Exons for mouse (*left*) and human (*right*) MBP isoforms. The amino acid sequences corresponding to the mouse MBPs are encoded in a gene containing at least seven exons (separated by *introns*, which are DNA regions whose base sequences do not code directly for protein). The precursor RNA transcribed from this gene can be spliced to give a message containing all seven exons; this message codes for the 21.5-kDa MBP. Alternative splicings result in RNA species with deletions of exons 2 and/or 6, which code for the other MBPs. The corresponding gene in humans also contains seven exons, which have minor base changes relative to the corresponding mouse sequences. The messenger for 21.5- and 18.5-kDa MBPs are formed in a manner analogous to the corresponding mouse proteins. Note, however, that the 17.2-kDa human protein contains a slightly different exon complement than does the 17-kDa mouse MBP. (Adapted from Kamholz et al. [19].)

referred to as P_2 in PNS terminology [13]. The amount of P_2 protein is variable from species to species accounting for approximately 15 percent of total protein in bovine PNS myelin, 5 percent in humans, and less than 1 percent in rodents. The P_2 protein is difficult to separate electrophoretically from the 14-kDa MBP of rodents (P_r), and this has led to some confusion about the relative amounts of P_2 and MBP. The P_2 protein is generally considered in the context of PNS myelin proteins, since it was originally identified there and is quantitatively a prominent component of PNS in some species. However, experiments utilizing sensitive immunological techniques demonstrate that P_2 is also expressed in small amounts in CNS myelin sheaths of some species. The P_2 protein is the antigen for experimental allergic neuritis (EAN), the PNS counterpart of experimental allergic encephalomyelitis (EAE) (see Chap. 36); P_2 appears to be present in the major dense line of myelin sheaths, where it may play a structural role similar to MBP, and there appears to be substantially more P_2 in large sheaths than small ones.

In addition to the MBPs, there are a number of low-molecular-weight glycoproteins in PNS myelin that migrate below P_0 on SDS gels [13]. The most prominent migrate between P_0 and the 18.5-kDa MBP, and have been referred to as the X and Y proteins or the 19- and 23-kDa proteins.

Myelin-associated glycoprotein

The content of high-molecular-weight proteins is somewhat lower in the PNS than the CNS. MAG is present, and immunocytochemical studies have shown that, as in the CNS, MAG is in the periaxonal membrane of Schwann cells, where it may be involved in Schwann cell-axon interactions [22]. In the PNS, MAG is also in Schmidt-Lantermann incisures, paranodal loops, and the outer mesaxon. All of these locations are characterized by 12- to 14-nm spaces between the extracellular surfaces of adjacent membranes and the presence of cytoplasm on the inner side of the membrane. Correlative data have been obtained suggesting that MAG is involved in maintaining this spacing of membranes. A molecular model has been proposed to explain how MAG could function to maintain this membrane spacing by interacting with binding sites on the adjacent axolemma or Schwann cell membrane and with cytoskeletal elements inside the Schwann cell [22]. Sequence information obtained about MAG from its cDNA clones is compatible with many aspects of the proposed model and give further insights into how MAG may play this structural role. Clinical interest in PNS MAG has developed from the demonstration that human IgM monoclonal antibodies in patients with neuropathy associated with paraproteinemia react with MAG (see Chap. 36).

An additional glycoprotein with a molecular mass of approximately 170 kDa that is specific for PNS myelin has been identified by Schuman et al. [28]. This glycoprotein accounts for approximately 5 percent of the total myelin protein and appears to be distributed throughout the compact myelin sheath.

Myelin contains enzymes that function in synthesis and transport

It was generally believed that myelin was an inert membrane with few if any biochemical functions. Recently, however, a large and growing number of enzymes have been discovered in myelin, which implies that myelin plays an active metabolic role in synthesis and transport. (For review and references, see Norton and Cammer [10] and Lees and Sapirstein [29].) These enzymatic activities can be divided into two classes: those believed to be fairly myelin specific (but probably also present in oligodendroglial membranes) and those known to be present in other subcellular fractions as well.

The first group presently includes only two enzymes: CNPase and, possibly, a cholesterol ester hydrolase. Isolated myelin contains approximately 60 percent of total brain CNPase activity. The enzyme increases in brain and spinal cord during development in parallel with myelination, and low levels are present in the myelin-deficient jimpy and quaking mouse mutants. CNPase is concentrated more in heavy myelin subfractions (see section on myelin subfractions) than in compact myelin and is also high in oligodendroglial cells and their plasma membranes. Curiously, it is very low in peripheral nerve and PNS myelin. Some of the characteristics of CNPase have been described in the section on proteins of CNS myelin.

A cholesterol ester hydrolase active at pH 7.2 may also be relatively myelin specific. Although the enzyme is prominent in myelin, it is unknown whether it is a different molecular species from that present in the extramyelin compartment.

In the second group, there are many enzymes that are not myelin specific but appear to be intrinsic to myelin. Neutral protease activity has been well documented. The presence in myelin of cAMP-stimulated kinase, calcium/calmodulin-dependent kinase, and protein kinase C (PK-C) activities has been reported. Phosphoprotein phosphatases are also present. The PK-C and phosphatase activities are presumed to be responsible for the rapid turnover of phosphate groups of MBP. Enzyme activity for acylation of proteolipid protein is also intrinsic to myelin.

Enzymes involved in metabolism of structural lipids (for review, see Ledeen [30]) include a cholesterol esterifying enzyme, UDP-galactose:ceramide galactosyltransferase, and many enzymes of glycerophospholipid metabolism. The latter grouping includes CDP-choline:1,2-diradyl-*sn*-glycerol choline phosphotransferase; CDP-ethanolamine:1,2-diradyl-*sn*-glycerol ethanolamine phosphotransferase; CTP:ethanol-amine phosphate cytidyltransferase; choline kinase and ethanolamine kinase. Thus, all the enzymes necessary for phosphatidyl ethanolamine synthesis from diradyl-*sn*-glycerol and ethanolamine are present; it is likely that phosphatidylcholine can also be synthesized within myelin. Perhaps even more elemental building blocks can be assembled into lipids by myelin enzymes. Acyl-CoA synthetase is present in myelin, suggesting the capacity to integrate free fatty acids into myelin lipids. The actual extent of the contribution of these enzymes in myelin (relative to enzymes within the oligodendroglial perikaryon) to metabolism of myelin lipids is not known.

Other enzymes of glycerol phospholipid synthesis present in myelin include phosphatidylinositol kinase, phosphatidylinositol phosphate kinase, and the corresponding phosphatases. These are of interest because of the high concentration of polyphosphoinositides in myelin and the rapid turnover of their phosphate groups.

Enzymes of myelin implicated in transport include carbonic anhydrase, 5'-nucleotidase, and Na, K-ATPase. Carbonic anhydrase has generally been considered a soluble enzyme and a glial marker, but myelin accounts for a large part of the membrane-bound form in brain. This enzyme may play a role in removal of carbonic acid from metabolically active axons. The enzymes 5'-nucleotidase and Na, K-ATPase have long been considered specific markers for plasma membranes. The 5'-nucleotidase activity may be related to a transport mechanism for adenosine, and Na, K-ATPase is involved in transport of monovalent cations. The presence of these enzymes suggests that myelin may have an active role in transport of material in and out of the axon. In connection with this hypothesis, it is of interest that proteolipid protein, when inserted into artificial bilayers, has proton ionophore properties.

The protein kinases and carbonic anhydrase have also been shown to be present in PNS myelin, but little else is known about PNS enzymes.

DEVELOPMENTAL BIOLOGY OF MYELIN

Myelination follows the order of phylogenetic development

As the nervous system matures, portions of the PNS myelinate first, then the spinal cord, and the brain last. In all parts of the nervous system there are many small fibers that never myelinate. Even within the brain, different areas myelinate at different rates, the intracortical association areas being the last to do so. In humans, the motor roots begin to myelinate in the fifth fetal month, and the brain is almost completely myelinated by the end of the second year of life.

It is generally true that pathways in the nervous system become myelinated before they become completely functional. A relevant observation is that the CNS of rats and other nest-building animals myelinates largely postnatally and that the animals are quite helpless at birth. Grazing animals, such as horses, cows, and sheep, have considerably more myelin in the CNS at birth and a correspondingly much higher level of complex activity immediately postnatally. Despite the attractiveness of the hypothesis that myelination is the terminal step in preparing a nervous system pathway for function, it should be noted that the period of maximum myelination also coincides with many other less-known changes in the nervous system.

Although it is easy to ascertain when myelination begins, it is difficult to determine when the process of accumulation stops. In the rat, myelin is still depositing in the brain well past 1 year of age and possibly longer. The rat, however, continues to grow in body size and brain

weight for most of its life span, and such a prolonged period of myelination may not occur in all species. Even in the human, myelination continues in the neocortex, at least through the end of the second decade.

Composition of myelin changes during development

Nervous system development is marked by several overlapping periods, each defined by one major event in brain growth and structural maturation (see Chap. 25). In the rat, in which the CNS undergoes considerable development postnatally, the maximal rate of cellular proliferation, much of this involving oligodendroglial precursor cells, occurs at 10 days. The rat brain begins to form myelin postnatally at about 10 to 12 days. Although the maximal rate of accumulation of myelin in the rat is at about 20 days of age, in this species myelin accumulation continues at a decreasing rate throughout adulthood. At 6 months of age, 60 mg myelin can be isolated from one brain. This represents an increase of approximately 1,500 percent over the brain myelin content of 15-day-old animals. During the same $5\frac{1}{2}$-month period, the brain weight increases by 50 to 60 percent [17].

Myelin that is first deposited is very different in composition from that of the adult (for review, see Norton and Cammer [10]). As the rat matures, the myelin galactolipids increase by approximately 50 percent, and lecithin decreases by a similar amount. Similar changes are seen in human myelin. The very small amount of desmosterol declines, but the other lipids remain relatively constant. In addition, the polysialogangliosides decrease, and the monosialoganglioside GM_1 increases to become the predominant ganglioside. These changes are not complete until the rat is approximately 2 months old. There is also a change in the composition of the protein portion as well as in the lipid portion. Both MBP and PLP increase in the myelin sheath during development, whereas the amount of higher molecular weight protein decreases.

Transitional forms of myelin can be isolated

The studies summarized above on the composition of myelin from immature brains are consistent with the idea that myelin first laid down by the oligodendroglial cell may represent a transitional form with properties intermediate between those of mature compact myelin and the oligodendroglial cell membrane. As mentioned earlier, in the section on isolation, myelin can be separated into subfractions of various densities. The lighter fractions are enriched in multilamellar myelin, whereas the denser fractions contain a large proportion of single-membrane vesicles that resemble microsomes or plasma membrane fragments. Generally, as one goes from light myelin fractions to heavier, the lipid/protein ratio decreases; the amount of basic protein decreases; the amount of MAG and of unidentified high-molecular-weight proteins increases; CNPase, carbonic anhydrase, and other enzymes increase; and the amount of proteolipid protein stays relatively constant. Metabolic studies described later lend support to the view that the dense fractions represent transitional forms.

Myelin metabolism varies during development

The principal features of myelin metabolism are its high rate of synthesis during the early stages of myelination and the relative metabolic stability of many of its components in the adult (for review, see Benjamins et al. [11] and Benjamins and Smith [31]). A remarkable amount of synthetic work is done by the oligodendroglial cell during the period of maximum myelination. Myelin accumulates in a 20-day-old rat brain at

a rate of approximately 3.5 mg/day. Rough calculations show that there are about 20×10^6 oligodendroglia in such a brain, with each cell body having a dry weight of approximately 50×10^{-9} mg. Thus, on average, each cell makes approximately 175×10^{-9} mg myelin/day, an amount more than three times the weight of the perikaryon. The rates of myelin accumulation increase rapidly prior to this peak and decrease rapidly afterward. These rates of accumulation depend on three potentially independent biochemical processes: synthesis of separate myelin components, their degradation, and their assembly into myelin. It is not always possible to measure these processes independently.

In vivo, the activity of UDP-galactose: ceramide galactosyltransferase (the enzyme that catalyzes the last step of cerebroside synthesis) in mouse brain microsomes increases fourfold from 10 days to a peak activity at 20 days, just preceding the age of maximal rate of myelin accumulation. It then gradually declines, paralleling the declining rate of myelination. The synthesis of glucocerebroside, which is not a myelin lipid, follows a completely different developmental pattern. Many other enzymes involved in lipid synthesis show increases during the period of rapid myelination, even though their products are not myelin specific. Most of the lipid synthesis of brain during this period is directed to formation of myelin, independently of whether the lipids are myelin specific, like the galactolipids, or nonspecific, like cholesterol and the phospholipids.

In vivo studies using radioactive precursors generally furnish results similar to those of enzyme assays *in vitro*. Incorporation of precursor into myelin-specific lipids is greatest when the injection of precursor coincides with greatest myelin accumulation (~20 days in rat) but is decreased at earlier or later ages. Similar results are obtained also when radioactive precursors, such as acetate for lipids or leucine for proteins, are presented to brain and spinal cord slices *in vitro*. Incorporation of radioactive precursors into myelin is greatest when slices are obtained from rats approximately 20 days of age.

The slice system has been used to estimate total brain effort devoted to production and maintenance of myelin. It is interesting that, although myelin lipid synthesis decreases greatly with increasing age, so does total lipid synthesis in the nervous system; thus, the proportion devoted to myelin synthesis remains about the same at 60 days. This varies in different nervous system regions according to the extent of myelination; in the cerebrum, approximately 50 percent of lipid synthesis is devoted to myelination. It should be noted that the rate of synthesis of an individual myelin lipid is related not only to the accumulation of myelin, but to the metabolic turnover of that lipid as well (see section on myelin turnover).

SYNTHESIS AND METABOLISM OF MYELIN

Some lipids and proteins must be processed and transported to the site of myelin assembly

After myelin components have been synthesized in the cell they have to be assembled to form the membrane. Following intracranial injection of a radioactive amino acid or application of a labeled precursor to tissue slices, radioactive MBP is synthesized and integrated into myelin very rapidly; there is a lag time of only a few minutes (see Benjamins and Smith [31] for references). In contrast, substantial amounts of radioactive PLP are not found in myelin until approximately 45 min later. Thus, following synthesis, PLP enters a pool that is on its way to being integrated into new myelin; in contrast, MBP is incorporated into myelin as soon as it is made. This interpretation is compatible with other data, demonstrating that PLP is synthesized on bound polysomes in the perikaryon [31]. Presumably, the pool of PLP consists of membranous vesicles on their way to the myelin being formed at the end of the oligodendroglial cell processes. In contrast, MBP is synthesized on free polysomes that are actually associated with, or in very close proximity to, the myelin sheath [31]. Another difference in the processing of the two proteins during myelin assembly is that, following a pulse of incorporation of radioactive amino acids into newly synthesized protein, radioactive MBP appears more or less simultaneously in myelin subfractions of different densities. In contrast, PLP appears first in the densest myelin fractions and later in lighter, more mature, myelin fractions in a manner that suggests a precursor-product relationship. Metabolic experiments suggest that MAG resembles PLP, whereas other high-molecular-weight proteins resemble MBP with respect to their kinetics of entry into myelin.

The kinetics of incorporation of individual lipids into myelin as a function of time after pulse labeling with a radioactive precursor has also been studied. Choline and ethanolamine phospholipids, as well as cerebroside, are found in myelin very soon after they are synthesized. In contrast the entry of sulfatide shows a delay; that is, it undergoes some period of intracellular processing, as does PLP. There is some heterogeneity among the glycerol phospholipids in terms of integration into the myelin membrane. Following a pulse label, ethanolamine phospholipids are first found in the heavier myelin fractions; then they rapidly enter the lighter, more mature, myelin. In contrast, choline phospholipids also appear rapidly and simultaneously in myelin subfractions differing in density.

Although available information is not yet sufficient to provide a detailed model of membrane assembly, a general picture emerges. Many high-molecular-weight proteins are present in a lipid-poor precursor membrane (oligodendroglial cell membrane), with all of the PLP and some MBP added during the early stages of myelin formation. More of the MBP and other high-molecular-weight proteins are added at later states of transition. The addition of PLP may be a rate-limiting step in myelin formation. The bulk of the lipids are added at later stages of myelin assembly, and their entry is directed by the proteins already present.

It is important to emphasize that synthesis and assembly are separate processes. There are examples, with respect to both CNS and PNS myelin, where the synthesis of myelin proteins occurs at a much greater rate than that at which these proteins are incorporated into myelin. For example, the quaking mouse has a defect in myelin assembly and incorporation of MBP and PLP into myelin is reduced considerably below normal. However, the synthesis of these proteins in the extramyelin pool is near normal, even though the synthesis of myelin lipids is defective in these mutants (see Hogan and Greenfield [27] for review and references). The synthesized but unincorporated myelin proteins are presumably degraded relatively rapidly.

Some but not all, myelin components turn over slowly

Experiments by Smith [12] confirmed the relative metabolic stability of myelin relative to other membranes but demonstrated that some components turn over with a half-life of weeks and thus cast doubt on the idea that myelin is metabolized as a unit. Long-term experiments showed that radioactivity is lost from individual myelin lipids at different rates.

Reutilization of lipids

The relationship between loss of radioactivity, usually referred to as apparent half-life, and the real rate of degradation of a lipid is complicated by reutilization. For example, radioactive acetate is incorporated into fatty acids, which are further processed to become part of glycerolipid molecules. At some future time when these lipids are degraded, that is, broken down to their constituent moieties, the fatty acid can to a large extent be reutilized for synthesis of new lipids. In contrast, radioactive glycerol is also incorporated into glycerolipids, but on degradation the glycerol moiety is preferentially metabolized rather than reutilized for biosynthesis. The apparent half-life, or time course of loss of radioactivity, from phosphatidylcholine might vary depending on whether the molecule was labeled with radioactive phosphate, acetate, choline, or glycerol; glycerol yields the shortest and, presumably, most accurate estimate.

Metabolic pools for lipids

Many different metabolic turnover studies suggest that at a minimum there are two metabolic pools in myelin. When young animals incorporate radioactive precursors, much of the labeled myelin is present in the more metabolically stable pool. When older animals are injected with a radioactive tracer, although much less radioactivity is incorporated into myelin, most of the label that is incorporated is in the more labile metabolic pool. One interpretation of these data is on the basis of morphology, the stabler metabolic pool consisting of deeper layers of myelin. Myelin deposited in young animals, during the period of rapid myelin accumulation, is rapidly transferred to this compartment. In adult animals, when myelin is accumulating much less rapidly, the newly formed myelin may remain in outer layers and stay accessible for whatever mechanisms are involved in catabolism for a longer time period.

Data in Table 2 illustrate several of the problems discussed above [31]. In the first experiment, rats were injected at 17 days of age with various precursors; turnover was calculated for the first 15-day period after injection (fast-turnover phase) and for the period of 15 to 80 days after injection (slow-turnover phase). The turnover times in days for three myelin phospholipids are given in Table 2.

It can be seen that with all precursors, mye-

TABLE 2. Metabolic half-lives of glycerophosphatides of myelin and microsomes of rat brain[a]

Precursor	Phosphatidylcholine		Phosphatidylethanolamine		Phosphatidylethanolamine	
	MY	MIC	MY	MIC	MY	MIC
Animals injected at 17 days of age[b]						
[³H]Glycerol	25(10)	13(4)	25(6.5)	14(3)	34(11)	20(4)
[¹⁴C]Choline	39	26	—	—	—	—
[¹⁴C]Ethanolamine	—	—	33	26	58	40
[³²P]Phosphate	30	17	30	29	44	33
[¹⁴C]Glucose	56	35 ·	108	55	Stable	54
[¹⁴C]Acetate	54	28	125	65	Stable	Stable
Animals injected at 60 days of age[c]						
[³H]Glycerol	11	6.0				
[¹⁴C]Choline	22	11				
[¹⁴C]Glucose	27	14				

[a] (MY) myelin; (MIC) microsomes; all times are in days and represent half-lives of the slow phase; numbers in parentheses are half-lives of the rapid phase and are calculated for the first 15 days following injection.
[b] Data from S. L. Miller et al., *J. Biol. Chem.* 252:4025–4037, 1977.
[c] Data from S. L. Miller and P. Morell, *J. Neurochem.* 31:771–778, 1978.

lin lipids turned over more slowly than microsomal lipids. The data in Table 2 indicate extensive reutilization of several radioactive precursors relative to turnover assayed with [³H]glycerol. The biosynthetic process for ethanolamine lipids (including plasmalogens) seems to reutilize precursors more efficiently than does phosphatidylcholine, giving the appearance of considerable metabolic stability for plasmalogens when glucose or acetate is employed as precursor. If animals are labeled at 60 days instead of at 17 days, turnover times for phosphatidylcholine remain relatively rapid for a prolonged period of time, very much like the faster phase of turnover seen in young animals. This presumably would also hold true for other glycerophospholipids (Table 2).

Metabolic turnover of proteins

Myelin proteins show the same type of biphasic turnover as myelin lipids. The major myelin-specific proteins have been extensively studied in this regard. Whereas, in the fast phase, both MBP and PLP show half-lives of the order of 2 to 3 weeks, several studies show that both proteins are metabolically stable in the slow phase, showing half-lives too long to be calculated accurately. Again, as with the lipids, myelin protein decay curves vary with the precursor used and the age of the animals injected. Shorter half-lives are seen if adult animals are labeled.

Although the previous discussion indicates a half-life of the order of days to months for most myelin components, it is now known that there are some components of myelin metabolism that have a half-life of the order of minutes. The phosphate group of MBPs is in this category. Measurements of its half-life are limited by the time taken for injected [³²P]phosphate to equilibrate with ATP, but it is clear that much of the phosphate cycles on and off the peptide backbone with a half-life that is of the order of minutes or faster [20]. It is also known that the monoesterified phosphate groups of polyphosphoinositides (those at positions 4 and 5) are labeled very quickly, even in mature animals, and also presumably have a rapid half-life. Finally, there is recent evidence that a significant portion of the phosphatidylinositol of myelin rapidly incorporates phosphate into the phosphodiester position, indicating cleavage and resynthesis of at least a pool of the phosphatidylinositol of myelin.

In summary, then, myelin lipids and proteins are more stable than similar components of other membranes. There is metabolic heterogeneity; different lipids have different turnover rates. Furthermore, turnover of a given lipid class varies as a function of age and/or the location of that fragment of myelin within the sheath. Some myelin components, such as cerebroside, sulfatide, and cholesterol, exhibit great metabolic stability. It is possible that some aspects of myelin metabolism such as phosphorylation are metabolically linked to electrical activity of the axon.

MOLECULAR ARCHITECTURE OF MYELIN

The currently accepted view of membrane structure is that of a lipid bilayer with some proteins fully or partially embedded in the bilayer and others attached to one surface or the other by weaker linkages. Both proteins and lipids are asymmetrically distributed; asymmetry of the lipids is partial. Presumably, the galactolipids in myelin, as in other membranes, are preferentially at the extracellular membrane surfaces. Diffraction studies demonstrate that cholesterol is enriched in the extracellular face of the membrane (intraperiod domain), whereas ethanolamine plasmalogen is asymmetrically localized to the cytoplasmic half of the bilayer (for review, see Kirschner et al. [5]).

The orientation of protein molecules in membrane bilayers is presumably fixed. Extrinsic proteins are attached to only one side of the bilayer, and the integral proteins have their orientations defined by how their hydrophobic domains penetrate the bilayer. Detailed discussion of the orientation of proteins in the membrane of myelin sheaths is presented by Braun [34].

A diagrammatic representation of the molecular organization of myelin protein in the CNS and PNS is shown in Fig. 13 (similar in many ways to one in Braun [34]). PLP is depicted as an integral membrane protein that passes through the bilayer several times and has domains in both the intraperiod and major dense line. This hypothesis is derived both from model building based on sequence information and surface probe studies. PLP is probably involved in stabilizing the intraperiod lines. MBP is an

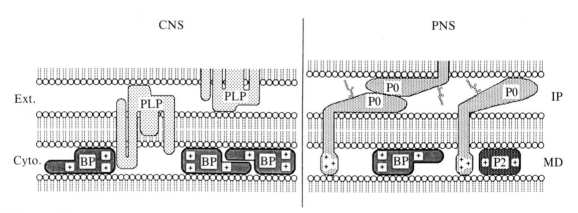

FIG. 13. Diagrammatic representation of current concepts of the molecular organization of compact CNS and PNS myelin. *Upper*: Apposition of the extracellular (Ext.) surfaces of the oligodendrocyte or Schwann cell membranes to form the intraperiod (IP) line. *Lower*: Apposition of the cytoplasmic (Cyto.) surfaces of the membranes of the myelin-forming cells to form the major dense (MD) line. See the text for a detailed description of this model; (BP) myelin basic protein.

extrinsic protein localized in the major dense lines, a conclusion based on knowledge of the amino acid sequence, inaccessibility to surface probes, and immunocytochemistry at the electron microscopic level. MBP probably stabilizes the major dense lines, as noted earlier. The positively charged MBP probably interacts with negatively charged lipids. There is evidence to suggest that MBPs are often associated in the dimer form. Figure 13 does not include MAG or the other high-molecular-weight protein components.

In the PNS, the major protein is P_0, which traverses the membrane once and has a relatively large hydrophobic domain in the intraperiod lines. It may stabilize the intraperiod line by interacting with itself [14], or it may exist as a monomer. In any case, the large extracellular domain of P_0 probably accounts for the greater separation of the extracellular surfaces in PNS myelin compared to the situation in CNS myelin. The P_0 protein also has a relatively large positively charged domain at the cytoplasmic side, which could contribute significantly to stabilization of the major dense line. The positively charged MBP and P_2 protein also are presumably localized at the cytoplasmic face and contribute to stabilization of the major dense line. However, the role of MBP in the PNS is not as important as in the CNS, as demonstrated by the normal major dense line in the PNS of the shiverer mutant.

Studies that demonstrate relatively rapid metabolism of certain myelin components suggest that there may be some dynamic aspect of myelin structure, such as occasional separation of the cytoplasmic faces of the membranes.

ACKNOWLEDGMENT

We wish to thank Dr. Cedric Raine for supplying the elegant photomicrographs that illustrate this chapter. The assistance of Jeffrey Hammer in developing and drafting the model shown in Fig. 13 on a personal computer is gratefully acknowledged.

REFERENCES

1. Raine, C. S. Morphology of myelin and myelination. In P. Morell (ed.), *Myelin*, 2nd ed. New York: Plenum, 1984, pp. 1–41.
2. Ritchie, J. M. Physiological basis of conduction in myelinated nerve fibers. In P. Morell (ed.), *Myelin*, 2nd ed., New York: Plenum, 1984, pp. 117–141.
3. Waxman, S. G. *Physiology and Pathobiology of Axons*. New York: Raven Press, 1978.
4. Norton, W. T. The myelin sheath. In: E. S. Goldensohn and S. H. Appel (eds.), Scientific Approaches to Clinical Neurology. Philadelphia: Lea & Febiger, 1977, pp. 259–298.
5. Kirschner, D. A., Ganser, A. L., and Caspar, D. L. D. Diffraction studies of molecular organization and membrane interactions in myelin. In P. Morell (ed.), *Myelin*, 2nd ed. New York: Plenum, 1984, pp. 51–91.
6. Hirano, A., and Dembitzer, H. M. A structural analysis of the myelin sheath in the central nervous system. *J. Cell Biol.* 34:555–567, 1987.
7. Geren, B. H. The formation from the Schwann cell surface of myelin in the peripheral nerves of chick embryos. *Exp. Cell Res.* 7:558–562, 1984.
8. Bunge, R. P. Glial cells and the central myelin sheath. *Physiol. Rev.* 48:197–248, 1968.
9. Davison, A. N., and Peters, A. *Myelination*. Springfield: Thomas, 1970.
10. Norton, W. T., and Cammer, W. Isolation and characterization of myelin. In P. Morell (ed.), *Myelin*, New York: Plenum, 1984, pp. 147–180.
11. Benjamins, J. A., Morell, P., Hartman, B. K., and Agrawal, H. C. CNS Myelin. In A. Lajtha (ed.), *Handbook of Neurochemistry*, Vol. 7. New York: Plenum, 1984, pp. 361–415.
12. Smith, M. E. Peripheral nervous system myelin properties and metabolism. In A. Lajtha (ed.), *Handbook of Neurochemistry*, Vol. 3, 2nd ed. New York: Plenum, 1983, pp. 201–223.
13. Lees, M. B., and Brostoff, S. W. Proteins of myelin. In P. Morell (ed.), *Myelin*, 2nd ed. New York: Plenum, 1984, pp. 197–217.
14. Lemke, G. Molecular biology of the major myelin genes. *Trends Neurosci.* 9:266–269, 1986.
15. Milner, R. J., Lai, C., Nave, K.-.A., Lenoir D., Ogata, J., and Sutcliffe, J. G. Nucleotide sequences of two mRNAs for rat brain myelin proteolipid protein. *Cell* 42:931–939, 1985.

16. Hudson, L. D., Berndt, J. A., Puckett, C., Kozak, C. A., and Lazzarini, R. A. Aberrant splicing of proteolipid protein mRNA in the dysmyelinating jimpy mouse. *Proc. Natl. Acad. Sci. USA* 84:1454–1458, 1987.

17. Deibler, G. E., Krutzsch, H. C., and Kies, M. W. A new form of myelin basic protein found in human brain. *J. Neurochem.* 47:1219–1225, 1986.

18. Takahashi, N., Roach, A., Teplow, D. B., Prusiner, S. B., and Hood, L. Cloning and characterization of the myelin basic protein gene from mouse: One gene can encode both 14 kd and 18.5 kd MBPs by alternate use of exons. *Cell* 42:139–148, 1985.

19. Kamholz, J., de Ferra, F., Puckett, C., and Lazzarini, R. Identification of three forms of human myelin basic protein by cDNA cloning. *Proc. Natl. Acad. Sci. USA*, 83:4962–4966, 1986.

20. DesJardins, K. C., and Morell, P. The phosphate groups modifying myelin basic proteins are metabolically labile; the methyl groups are stable. *J. Cell Biol.* 97:438–446, 1983.

21. Sprinkle, T. J., McMorris, F. A., Yoshino, J., and DeVries, G. H., Differential expression of 2′:3′-cyclic nucleotide 3′-phosphodiesterase in cultured central, peripheral, and extraneural cells. *Neurochem. Res.* 10:919–931, 1985.

22. Quarles, R. H. Myelin-associated glycoprotein: functional and clinical aspects. In P. J. Marangos, I. Campbell, and R. M. Cohen (eds.), *Neurobiological Research, Vol. II: Neuronal and Glial Proteins Structure, Function, and Clinical Application.* New York: Academic, 1988, pp. 295–320.

23. Arquint, M., Roder, J., Chia, L.-.S., Down, J., Wilkinson, D., Bayley, H., Braun, P., and Dunn, R. Molecular cloning and primary structure of myelin-associated glycoprotein. *Proc. Natl. Acad. Sci. USA* 83:1–5, 1986.

24. Salzer, J. L., Holmes, W. P., and Colman, D. R., The amino acid sequences of the myelin associated glycoproteins: Homology to the immunoglobulin gene superfamily. *J. Cell Biol.* 104:957–965, 1987.

25. Lai, C., Brow, M.A., Nave, K.-R., Noronha, A. B., Quarles, R. H., Bloom, F. E., Milner, R. J., and Sutcliffe, J. G. Two forms of 1B236/myelin associated glycoprotein (MAG), a cell adhesion molecule for postnatal neural development, are produced by alternative splicing. *Proc. Natl. Acad. Sci. USA* 84:4337–4341, 1987.

26. Puckett, C., Hudson, L., Ono, K., Friedrich, V., Benecke, J., Dubois-Dalcq, M., and Lazzarini, R. A. Myelin-specific proteolipid protein is expressed in myelinating Schwann cells but is not incorporated into myelin sheaths. *J. Neurosci. Res.* 18(4):511–518, 1987.

27. Hogan, E. L., and Greenfield, S. Animal models of genetic disorders of myelin. In P. Morell (ed.), *Myelin*, 2nd ed. New York: Plenum, 1984, pp. 489–535.

28. Shuman, S., Hardy, M., and Pleasure, D. Peripheral nervous system myelin and Schwann cell glycoproteins: identification by lectin binding and partial purification of a peripheral nervous system myelin-specific 170,000 molecular weight glycoprotein. *J. Neurochem.* 41:1277–1285, 1983.

29. Lees, M. B., and Sapirstein, V. S. Myelin-associated enzymes. In A. Lajtha (ed.), *Handbook of Neurochemistry, Vol. 4, 2nd ed.*, New York: Plenum, 1983, pp. 435–460.

30. Ledeen, R. W., Lipid-metabolizing enzymes of myelin and their relation to the axon. *J. Lipid Res.* 25:1548–1554, 1984.

31. Benjamins, J. A., and Smith, M. E., Metabolism of myelin. In P. Morell (ed.), *Myelin*, 2nd ed. New York: Plenum, 1984, pp. 225–249.

32. Colman, D. R., Kreibich, G., Frey, A. B., and Sabatini, D. D. Synthesis and incorporation of myelin polypeptides into CNS myelin. *J. Cell Biol.* 95:598–608, 1982.

33. Miller, S. L., Benjamins, J. A., and Morell, P. Metabolism of glycerophospholipids of myelin and microsomes in rat brain. Reutilization of precursors. *J. Biol. Chem.* 252:4025–4037, 1977.

34. Braun, P. E., Molecular organization of myelin. In P. Morell (ed.), *Myelin*, 2nd ed. New York: Plenum, 1984, pp. 97–113.

CHAPTER 7

Molecular Biology of Vision

Hitoshi Shichi

PHYSIOLOGICAL BACKGROUND

Light-absorbing pigments differentiate rod cells, for black-white vision, and three types of cone cells, for color vision

The eye, a remarkable photosensor, can detect a single photon and transmit its signal to the brain. The receptors for light in the vertebrate eye are the visual (photoreceptor) cells of the retina. Each visual cell comprises two principal parts: the outer segment, which contains light-absorbing (visual) pigments; and the inner segment, which contains the nucleus, mitochondria, and other subcellular organelles and which metabolically supports the functions of the

Basic Neurochemistry: Molecular, Cellular, and Medical Aspects, 4th Ed., edited by G. J. Siegel et al. Raven Press, Ltd., New York, 1989. Correspondence to Hitoshi Shichi, Eye Research Institute, Oakland University, Rochester, Michigan 48063.

outer segment (Fig. 1). The segments are connected by the ciliary process, or cilium. The inner segments of visual cells have terminals that synapse with horizontal cells and bipolar cells. The bipolar cells, in turn, form synapses with ganglion and amacrine cells.

Visual cells are of two types. Rod cells, which have elongated outer segments, contain rhodopsin [light wave length for maximum absorption (λ_{max}), ~500 nm], the visual pigment responsible for dim-light (black-and-white, or scotopic) vision. Cone cells, possessing cone-shaped outer segments, are the photoreceptors for daylight (color, or photopic) vision. In the human retina there are three types of cone cells, each containing one of three pigments: λ_{max} - 445, 535, and 570 nm. According to one estimate, the human eye contains 120 million rod cells in the peripheral region of the retina and 6.5 million cone cells, concentrated mainly in the central, or foveal, region.

Absorption of light causes inhibition of vertebrate photoreceptor cells, which then initiate programs of responses among retinal neurons

The plasma membrane of each rod outer segment possesses several thousand Na^+ channels through which Na^+ enters the cell at a rate of about 2.5×10^4 Na^+ per channel per second. In contrast, the plasma membrane of the rod inner segment has ATP-dependent Na^+/K^+ pumps that pump Na^+ out of the cell. The Na^+ permeability of the outer segment is higher in the dark than in the light. Thus, the plasma membrane of the vertebrate rod cell shows a membrane potential of 35 to 45 mV (inside negative) and is depolarized in the dark. Light reduces the Na^+ permeability of the outer segment and hyperpolarizes the membrane. Therefore, "visual excitation" in the vertebrate photoreceptor means hyperpolarization, or in-

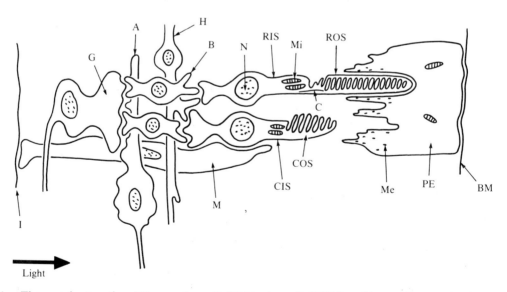

FIG. 1. The vertebrate retina: (A) amacrine cell; (B) bipolar cell; (BM) Bruch's membrane; (C) ciliary process (cilium); (CIS) cone inner segment; (COS) cone outer segment; (G) ganglion cell; (H) horizontal cell; (I) inner limiting membrane; (M) Müller cell (glial cell); (Me) melanine granule; (Mi) mitochondrion; (N) nucleus; (PE) retinal pigmented epithelium; (RIS) rod inner segment; (ROS) rod outer segment.

hibition, of the visual cell plasma membrane. The release of a chemical transmitter, such as aspartate or glutamate, at the synaptic terminal of a visual cell in the dark is also inhibited by light. The retina, which is part of the central nervous system, contains putative neurotransmitters, such as acetylcholine, dopamine, γ-aminobutyric acid (GABA), serotonin, taurine, glycine, glutamate, aspartate, and neuropeptides. Active research is under way to determine which transmitters are associated with which types of retinal neurons.

Intercellular communication among retinal neurons is very complex. In goldfish retina, for example, excitation of bipolar cells by transmitters from photoreceptors is counteracted or inhibited by horizontal cells, which release inhibitory transmitters such as GABA. Amacrine cells are diverse, and some synthesize dopamine, releasing it in light to excite horizontal cells. Other amacrine cells accumulate the inhibitory transmitter glycine; still others contain various neuropeptides. The mechanism by which retinal neurons are mutually regulated by transmitters remains largely unknown.

Retinal responses to different light frequencies are encoded in the retina and conveyed to the thalamus and visual cortex

Absorption of photons by visual cells triggers a series of events that results in a particular pattern of stimulation of retinal and, eventually, cerebral neurons. In rod cell vision (dim light), the magnitude of neural response is directly related to the perception of brightness. In cone cell (color) vision, absorption of light by at least two cone cell pigments with different absorption maxima is essential to discriminate color. The ratio of magnitudes of the induced photoresponses determines the color perceived. The arrays of visual signals generated by the photoreceptor cells and programmed by retinal neurons, principally bipolar cells, are transmitted to the lateral geniculate bodies via ganglion cell axons, which make up the optic nerves and tracts. Impulses are conveyed by the geniculolcalcarine radiations to the visual cortex of the brain, where the signals representing light intensity and wavelength are decoded separately by different neurons. The coding and decoding of visual signals, an important area of neurophysiology, is not covered here. This chapter deals primarily with the structure and function of photoreceptors and the molecular events that take place after photon absorption by the visual cells. (General reviews may be found in refs. 1–4.)

PHOTORECEPTOR MEMBRANES AND VISUAL PIGMENTS

Rod outer segment membranes are arranged in stacks of disks containing rhodopsin

The outer segment of a rod cell consists of a stack of several hundred disks encased in a sack of plasma membrane. It is presumed that the disks are formed by evagination of the plasma membrane in the proximal region of the outer segment, followed by fusion of two adjacent evaginates, and detachment from the plasma membrane. This process is probably controlled by the ciliary process. The effect of this repeated envagination and disk formation is to increase greatly the area of rod cell membrane and, thus, the amount of rhodopsin, a protein-bound membrane, that is exposed to light. As new disks are formed, older disks are pushed toward the apex of the outer segment. Disks that eventually reach the apex are shed from the tip and are phagocytized by the pigmented epithelial cells. In higher order animals, disk shedding is minimal in the dark and follows a circadian rhythm—a burst of shedding occurs soon after the onset of light [5]. The life cycle of a single disk may last from a few days to months, depending on the species [6]. Disk membrane components, such as proteins, carbohydrates, and lipids, are synthesized in the inner segment and then transported to the basal region of the ciliary process, where membrane assembly occurs. In contrast to rod disks, cone disks generally remain continuous with the plasma membrane.

Abnormalities of disk membrane turnover cause retinal degeneration, and animals known to have hereditary retinal dystrophy are studied as models for human retinal degenerations, such as retinitis pigmentosa. In rats with retinal dystrophy, rod outer segments grow abnormally long and accumulate as lamellar bundles in the extracellular space between the visual cell and the pigmented epithelium. This overproduction is the result of the failure of the pigmented epithelium to phagocytize the rod membranes. In another type of hereditary retinal dystrophy that occurs in mice, the rod outer segments fail to develop to full maturation, probably because of a genetic defect in the disk assembly mechanism.

Rod outer segment membranes (>95 percent disk membranes, <5 percent plasma membrane) consist of 60 percent protein and 40 percent phospholipid. In vertebrate photoreceptors, phosphatidylethanolamine and phosphatidylcholine account for about 80 percent of the phospholipid. The most abundant polyunsaturated fatty acid is docosahexaenoic acid (22 carbons and six unsaturated bonds), linked to the middle carbon of the glycerol moiety of phospholipids. Their high levels of polyunsaturated fatty acids make rod membranes as fluid as olive oil, at physiological tempera-

tures, allowing the integral membrane protein rhodopsin to rotate freely and diffuse within the membrane. This fluidity may be important in allowing photoactivated rhodopsin to collide quickly with so many molecules of the peripheral membrane proteins, such as guanine nucleotide-binding protein (G protein).

Rhodopsin is a transmembrane protein linked to 11-cis-retinal, which, on photoabsorption, decomposes to opsin and all-trans-retinal

Rhodopsin has a molecular weight of about 40,000. Its C-terminal is exposed on the cytoplasmic surface of the disk, and its sugar-containing N-terminal sequence is exposed on the intraluminal surface. Half of the mass is embedded in the hydrophobic region of the membrane lipid bilayer, with the remaining half distributed equally on both surfaces of the membrane. The primary structures have been determined in bovine [4,7], sheep [8], human [9], and fruitfly [10,11] rhodopsins (Fig. 2). The three mammalian rhodopsins show a high degree of sequence homology. All rhodopsins possess seven segments of hydrophobic sequences separated by segments of hydrophilic sequences. It has been hypothesized that the seven hydrophobic sequences (designated helices 1–7 in Fig. 3) are in α-helical conformation and form a bundle that spans the membrane from one side to the other. Two sugar moieties, each composed of three mannoses and three N-acetylglucosamines, are linked to asparagine-2 and asparagine-15 in bovine rhodopsin. The C-

$\longrightarrow$

FIG. 2. The primary structures of rhodopsins. The fly sequence is from drosophila. All other sequences are human. The lower three are cone cell rhodopsins deduced from cDNA sequences: (b) blue-sensitive; (r) red-sensitive; and (g) green-sensitive. The single-letter amino acid code used here is defined in the Glossary. Residues identical in all sequences are shown in *boldface*. Gaps necessary to maintain the alignment are connected by *dashed lines*. The transmembrane segments shown in Fig. 3 are indicated by the numbered *arrows* below the corresponding sequences. The lysine to which retinal is linked to form the chromophore (Fig. 4) is indicated as *K* near the center of transmembrane segment 7.

```
MESFAVAAQLGPHFAPLSNGSVVDKVTPDMAHLI___SPYWNQFPAMDPI   (fly)
MNGTEGPNFYVPFSNATGVV_____RSPFEYPQYYLAEP    (rod)
MRKMSEEQFYLFKNISSV_____GPWDGPQYHIAPV     (b)
MAQQWSLQRLAGRHPQDSYEDSTQSSIFTYTNSNSTRGPFEGPNYHIAPR   (r)
MAQQWSLQRLAGRHPQDSYEDSTQSSIFTYTNSNSTRGPFEGPNYHIAPR   (g)

W_AKILTAYMIMIGMISWCGNGVVIYIFATTKSLRTPANLLVINLAISDF   (fly)
WQFSMLAAYMFLLEVLGFPINFLTLYVTVQHKKLRTPLNYILLNLAVADL   (rod)
WAFYLQAAFMGTVFLIGFPLNAMVLVATLRYKKLRQPLNYILVNVSFGGF   (b)
WVYHLTSVWMIFVVTASVFTNGLVLAATMKFKKLRHPLNWILVNLAVADL   (r)
WVYHLTSVWMIFVVIASVFTNGLVLAATMKFKKLRHPLNWILVNLAVADL   (g)
        ←————————— 1 —————————→        ←———————— 2 ——

GIMITNTPMMGINLYFETWVLGPMMCDIYAGLGSAFGCSSIWSMCMISLD   (fly)
FMVLGGFTSTLYTSLHGYFVFGPTGCNLEGFFATLGGEIALQSLVVLAIE   (rod)
LLCIFSVFPVFVASCNGYFVFGRHVCALEGFLGTVAGLVTGWSLAFLAFE   (b)
AETVIASTISIVNEVSGWFVLGHPMCVLEGYTVSLCGITGLWSLAIISWE   (r)
AETVIASTISVVNQVYGYFVLGHPMCVLEGYTVSLCGITGLWSLAIISWE   (g)
  —— 2 —————————→           ←——————————— 3 ————————

RYQVIVKGMAGRPMTIPLALGKIAYIWFMSSIWCLAPAFGWSRYVPEGNL   (fly)
RYVVVCKPMSNFRFGENHAIMGVAFTWVMALACAAPPLAGWSRYIPEGLQ   (rod)
RYIVICKPFGNFRFSSKHALTVVLATWTIGIGVSIPPFFGWSRFIPEGLQ   (b)
RWLVVCKPFGNVRFDAKLAIVGIAFSWIWSAVWTAPPIFGWSRYWPHGLK   (r)
RWMVVCKPFGNVRFDAKLAIVGIAFSWIWAAVWTAPPIFGWSRYWPHGLK   (g)
  —3 —→       ←——————————————— 4 ———————————————→

TSCGIDYLERDWNPRSYLIFYSIFV__YYIPLFLICYSYWFIIAAVSAHE   (fly)
CSCGIDYYTLKPEVNNESFVIYMFVVHFTIPMIIIFFCYGQLVFTVKEAA   (rod)
CSCGPDWYTVGTKYRSESYTWFLFIFCFIVPLSLICFSYTQLLRALKAVA   (b)
TSCGPDVFSGSSYPGVQSYMIVLMVTCCIIPLAIIMLCYLQVWLAIRAVA   (r)
TSCGPDVFSGSSYPGVQSYMIVLMVTCCITPLSIIVLCYLQVWLAIRAVA   (g)
            ←———————————————— 5 ————————————————→

KAMREQAKKMNV_____  (fly)

KSLRSSEDAEKSAEGKLAKVALVTITLWFMAWTPYLVINCMGLFKFEG_LT (fly)
AQQQESATTQKAEKEVTRMVIIMVIAFLI_CWVPYASVAFYIFTHQGSNFG (rod)
AQQQQSQTTQKAEREVSRMVVVMVGSFCV_CYVPYAAFAMYMVNNRNHGLD (b)
KQQKESESTQKAEKEVTRMVVVMIFAYCV_CWGPYTFFACFAAANPGYAFH (r)
KQQKESESTQKAEKEVTRMVVVMVLAFCF_CWGPYAFFACFAAANPGYPFH (g)
              ←————————————— 6 —————————————→

PLNTIWGACFAKSAACYNPIVYGISHPKYRLALKEKCPCCVFGKVDDGKS  (fly)
PIFMTIPAFFAKSAAIYNPVIYIMMNKQFRNCMLTTICCGKNPLGDDEAS  (rod)
LRLVTIPSFFSKSACIYNPIIYCFMNKQFQACIMKMVCEKAMTDESDTCS  (b)
PLMAALPAYFAKSATIYNPVIYVFMNRQFRNCILQLFGKKVDDGSELSSA  (r)
PLMAALPAFFAKSATIYNPVIYVFMNRQFRNCILQLFGKKVDDGSELSSA  (g)
      ←————————— 7 —————————→

SDAQSEATASEAE___SKA   378                            (fly)
ATVSKTETS_____QVAPA   348                            (rod)
S__QKTEVSTVSSTQVGPN   348                            (b)
S___KTEVSSVSS__VSPA   364                            (r)
S___KTEVSSVSS__VSPA   364                            (g)
```

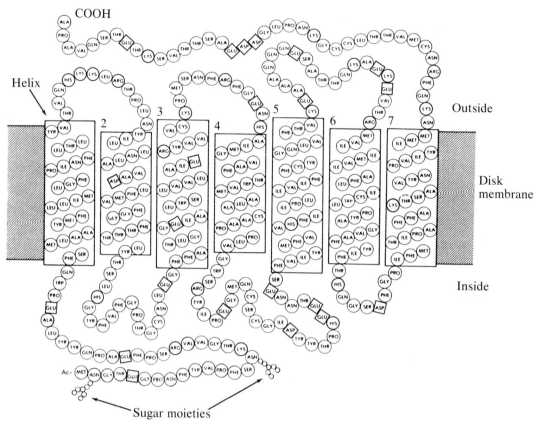

FIG. 3. Proposed transmembrane disposition of bovine rhodopsin. Acidic residues are in *squares* and basic residues in *bold-outline circles*. The N-terminal methionine is acetylated.

terminal sequence contains a cluster of serine and threonine residues that serve as phosphorylation sites.

The chromophore 11-*cis*-retinal is linked to the ε-amino group of lysine-296 by a protonated Schiff base. Protonated Schiff bases usually absorb light maximally at around 440 nm, but the λ_{max} of rhodopsin is near 500 nm. The 60-nm shift of λ_{max} toward the longer wavelength side can be explained by delocalization of the positive charge of the protonated Schiff base. According to a current model [12], the first negative charge is placed near the Schiff base nitrogen and the second negative charge about

3 Å away both from C-12 and C-14 to delocalize the positive charge (Fig. 4). These negative charges may be provided by three acidic residues (aspartic acid-83, glutamic acid-122, and glutamic acid-134) in the helical regions of the rhodopsin molecule (Fig. 3). When the helices are bundled together, two of the acidic residues may move in the vicinity of the chromophore and donate the necessary electrons. On absorption of light, rhodopsin is decomposed to the opsin protein and all-*trans*-retinal. The reaction occurs through several spectrally distinct intermediates (Fig. 5). The formation of bathorhodopsin involves photoisomerization of the 11-

cis-retinylidene chromophore to a constrained all-*trans* form and takes place within a few picoseconds after light absorption at physiological temperature. Bathorhodopsin then undergoes thermal relaxation, giving rise first to lumirhodopsin and then metarhodopsin I. Decay of metarhodopsin I (lifetime, 3×10^{-4} sec) is believed to be related to the photocurrent generation (latency, 10^{-4} sec) by the rod.

Bleached rhodopsin must be regenerated to maintain normal vision

Regeneration of rhodopsin occurs by several mechanisms. The major mechanism involves isomerization of all-*trans*-retinal to the 11-*cis* form, presumably in the pigmented epithelium, transport of 11-*cis*-retinal to the outer segment, and recombination with opsin [13]. Isomerization of all-*trans*-retinal to the 11-*cis* form in the dark is believed to occur as an enzymic reaction in the pigmented epithelium, and attempts to characterize the enzyme are being made. The shuttle of retinoids between the photoreceptor and pigmented epithelium may involve several retinoid-binding proteins. A second mechanism is photoconversion of thermal intermediates, such as metarhodopsins, to rhodopsin. For example, regeneration of squid rhodopsin occurs mainly by· photoisomerization of opsin-linked retinal at pH 10 and subsequent dark adaptation [14]. In a third mechanism, the photoisomerization of all-*trans*-retinal to the 11-*cis* form may take place within the rod outer segment. For

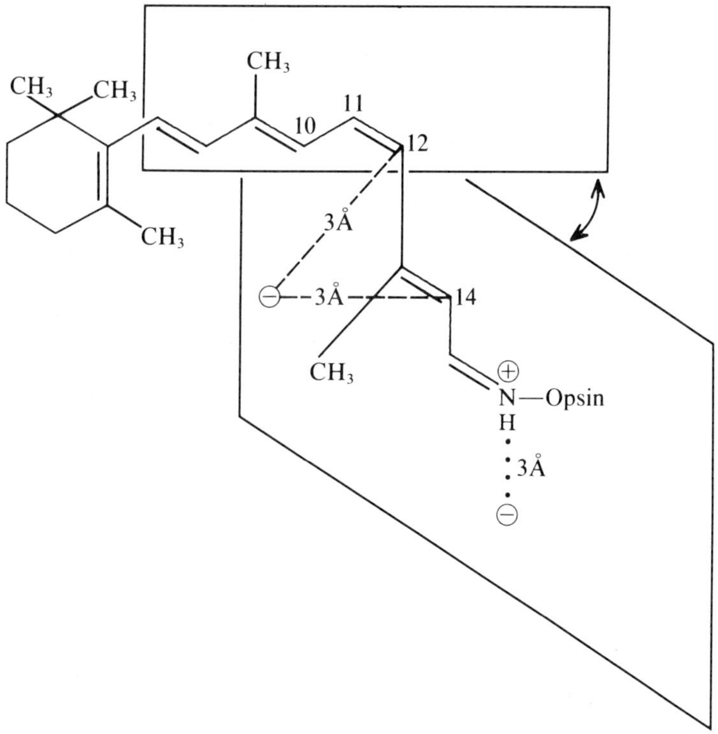

FIG. 4. External point-charge model of rhodopsin chromophore. The C-7–C-12 and C-12–C-15 conjugated systems are not in the same plane. Neither are the cyclohexene ring and the C-7–C-12 conjugated system in the same plane.

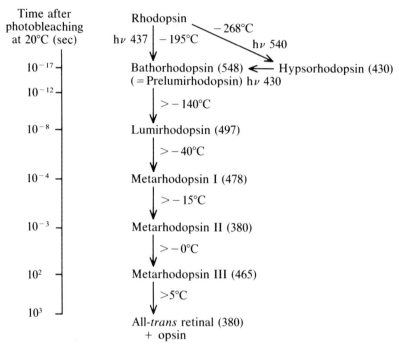

FIG. 5. Intermediates detected spectrally after photic bleaching of vertebrate rhodopsin. *Numbers in parentheses* are wavelengths of light (in nanometers) absorbed maximally by the individual intermediates. Numbers after hν indicate wavelengths of irradiating light.

example, all-*trans*-retinylidene phospholipid is photoisomerized to the 11-*cis* form within the disk membrane and reacts with opsin [15].

Cone cell pigments contain different opsins but with high sequence homology

The primary structure of the three human cone pigments was deduced from analysis of genomic and complementary DNA clones encoding them [16] (Fig. 2). The sequences of cone pigments show 41 percent identity with rhodopsin. Red and green pigments show high sequence homology: Only 15 of 364 residues are different. Genetic analysis locates the rhodopsin gene on chromosome 3 and the blue pigment gene on chromosome 7. Although none of the human cone pigments have been isolated, the chicken

cone pigment iodopsin has been partially purified and characterized. Iodopsin (λ_{max} = 475 nm) forms bathoiodopsin λ_{max} = 640 nm on light absorption at $-196°C$ [17]. This intermediate reverts back to iodopsin on warming. If iodopsin is illuminated by 600-nm light at $-183°C$, lumi-iodopsin (λ_{max} = 575 nm) is formed and thermally decays to metaiodopsin I (λ_{max} = 495 nm) and metaiodopsin II (λ_{max} = 380 nm).

PHOTOTRANSDUCTION

Light absorption by rhodopsin leads to closure of Na$^+$ conductance channels via a chemical messenger system

Light is known to close the Na$^+$ channels on outer segment plasma membrane and induce hyperpolarization of the membrane within 100 msec. The magnitude of light response reaches a maximum by absorption of several hundred photons per rod cell. Below the saturation light intensity, the relationship between the magnitude of light response (I) and energy of irradiating light (A) is given by

$$I = I_{max} A/(A + K)$$

where I_{max} is the magnitude of response at the saturation light intensity, and K is light energy required for 50 percent of the maximum response [18]. This equation has the same form as the Michaelis-Menten equation of enzyme kinetics. By analogy to enzyme kinetics, we may assume that rhodopsin reacts with light to form a complex, photoactivated rhodopsin (probably metarhodopsin II), which gives rise to an intracellular messenger X that links the photochemical reaction of rhodopsin to the plasma membrane. It is logical to postulate such a messenger because the disk membrane, where rhodopsin is localized, is not continuous with the plasma membrane that contains the Na^+ channels.

The messenger compound must satisfy at least two properties. First, its concentration in the outer segment cytoplasm must change rapidly on light irradiation and return to the original level after light is turned off. Second, when the compound is introduced in the outer segment cytoplasm in the dark, it must mimic the effect of light. The first candidate proposed for messenger X is Ca^{2+} [19]. The Ca^{2+} hypothesis assumes that a large number of Ca^{2+} ions are sequestered within the disk in the dark and are released into the cytoplasm when a single rhodopsin molecule in the disk membrane absorbs a photon. Ca^{2+} is assumed to close the Na^+ channels in the plasma membrane. In support of the hypothesis, injection of Ca^{2+} into the outer segment in the dark suppresses Na^+ permeability and induces membrane hyperpolarization; however, several findings contradict the hypothesis. Cytoplasmic Ca^{2+} concentration in the outer segment does not increase on

light illumination but decreases instead. There is no evidence that the disks can actively accumulate Ca^{2+} in the dark, and in patch-clamp experiments in which a small piece of outer segment plasma membrane is attached by suction to the tip of an electrode, exposure of the cytoplasmic surface of membrane to Ca^{2+} does not inhibit Na^{2+} conductance of the membrane fragment [20]. Thus, the Ca^{2+} hypothesis remains unresolved.

A G-protein/cGMP system in outer segments is responsive to photoactivated rhodopsin

Another candidate for messenger X is related to guanosine cyclic 3′,5′-phosphate (cGMP). According to the cGMP hypothesis, the Na^+ channel is kept open by cGMP and closes when cGMP is hydrolyzed in light. Exposure of an outer segment membrane fragment to cGMP in patch-clamp experiments increases its Na^+ conductance in the dark [20]. This effect is reversible. Concentration of cGMP in dark-adapted rod outer segments is high and decreases rapidly when the rod is irradiated at low Ca^{2+} concentrations. The decrease of cGMP is proportional to the log of light intensity. Since messenger X is expected to accumulate in light, cGMP cannot be messenger X. Rather, messenger X is assumed to be proportional to the amount of cGMP hydrolyzed. Rod cGMP concentration is restored to its original level by guanylate cyclase during dark adaptation. cGMP phosphodiesterase, the enzyme that hydrolyzes cGMP to 5′-GMP, is activated by light. This activation is mediated by a G protein ($G_{\alpha\beta\gamma}$), which is activated by photoactivated rhodopsin (R*) [21] (Fig. 6). According to the cGMP hypothesis, a single R* molecule may produce as many as 500 active G-protein molecules. The G protein consists of three subunits, α, β, and γ, and has GDP bound to the α subunit in inactive form. The R* catalyzes exchange of GTP for GDP, and the $G_\alpha \cdot$GTP thus formed dis-

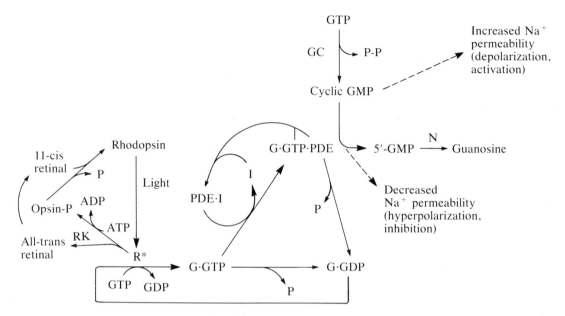

FIG. 6. Light-elicited biochemical reactions leading to cGMP hydrolysis: (G) guanine nucleotide-binding protein; (PDE) phosphodiesterase; (GC) guanyl cyclase; (N) 5′-nucleotidase; (RK) rhodopsin kinase; (R*) photoactivated rhodopsin; (I) PDE inhibitory γ subunit.

sociates from the β and γ subunits. Each $G_\alpha \cdot GTP$ molecule then activates a phosphodiesterase ($PDE_{\alpha\beta\gamma}$) molecule by dissociating the γ subunit (internal inhibitor). A family of G proteins is known as mediators of extracellular signals (e.g., hormones, neurotransmitters, or antigens) to intracellular enzymes. The G_β subunit is common to G proteins associated with various receptors, and G_α is specific to the individual receptors. Rod and cone outer segments seem to have different G_α subunits. The primary structure of rod G-protein subunits has been elucidated (references are found in Sugimoto et al. [22]).

The cGMP hypothesis is by no means complete. The rate of light-induced cGMP decrease, for instance, does not always correlate with suppression of the membrane Na^+ current. Peculiarly, light does not affect the cGMP level in invertebrate photoreceptors, and a different mechanism may exist in invertebrates. Nevertheless, the hypothesis can explain many aspects of phototransduction in vertebrate photoreceptors, including the effect of Ca^{2+}. The Ca^{2+} and cGMP concentrations in the photoreceptors are reciprocally related. Reduced Ca^{2+} concentration after irradiation is therefore expected to enhance cGMP level and open Na^+ channels. Thus, Ca^{2+} will play an important role in the regulation of light adaptation [23].

Another proposed mechanism of photosignal transduction involves light-stimulated hydrolysis of phosphatidylinositol-4,5-bis-phosphate (PIP_2). Reception of an external signal by a variety of receptors can evoke hydrolysis of PIP_2 to diacylglycerol (DG) and inositol-1,4,5-triphosphate (IP_3) by activating phospholipase C (see Chap. 16, Fig. 3) [24]. Both IP_3 and DG serve as intracellular messengers: IP_3 increases intracellular Ca^{2+}, DG stimulates protein kinase C. Injection of IP_3 into *Limulus* ventral photoreceptors in the dark mimics the light effect, evoking membrane depolarization without latency, and an increase in the intracellular Ca^{2+} level as well [25,26]. Injection of IP_3 into salamander rod outer segments induces membrane hyperpolarization in the dark.

Whatever mechanism is involved in phototransduction, the process must be regulated to reset the system. Hydrolysis of G-protein-bound GTP to GDP inactivates G protein. Thermal decay of R* (presumably metarhodopsin II) to opsin and all-*trans*-retinal terminates activation of G protein; R* is also inactivated by phosphorylation [27]. Regulation of membrane receptors by phosphorylation may be of general importance. Different membrane receptors may have structural similarities. The mammalian β-adrenergic receptor and the muscarinic acetylcholine receptor show significant amino acid sequence homology with rhodopsin [28], and a β-receptor-specific protein kinase phosphorylates rhodopsin [29]. Similarities between the photoreceptor system and these membrane receptor systems suggest that they are evolutionarily related.

REFERENCES

1. Fuortes, M. G. F. (ed.). *Handbook of Sensory Physiology. Physiology of Photoreceptor Organs.* Heidelberg: Springer-Verlag, 1972, Vol. 7/2.
2. Jung, R. (ed.). *Handbook of Sensory Physiology.* Part A, *Central Processing of Visual Information*; Part B, *Visual Centers in the Brain.* Heidelberg: Springer-Verlag, 1973, Vol. 7/3.
3. Shichi, H. *Biochemistry of Vision.* New York: Academic Press, 1983.
4. Hargrave, P. Molecular dynamics of the rod cell. In R. Adler and D. Farber (eds.), *The Retina.* New York: Academic Press, 1986, pp. 207–237.
5. LaVail, M. M. Rod outer segment disk shedding in rat retina: Relationship to cyclic lighting. *Science* 194:1071–1074, 1976.
6. Young, R. W. Visual cells and the concept of renewal. *Invest. Ophthalmol.* 15:700–725, 1976.
7. Ovchinnikov, Y. A. Rhodopsin and bacteriorhodopsin: Structure-function relationships, *FEBS Letters* 148:179–191, 1982.
8. Findlay, B. C., and Pappin, D. J. C. The opsin family of proteins. *Biochem. J.* 238:625–642, 1986.
9. Nathans, J., and Hogness, D. S. Isolation and nucleotide sequence of the gene encoding human rhodopsin. *Proc. Natl. Acad. Sci. U.S.A.* 81:4851–4855, 1984.
10. O'Tousa, J. E., Baehr, W., Martin, R. L., Hirsh, J., Pak, W. L., and Applebury, M. L. The drosophila *nina E* gene encodes an opsin. *Cell* 40:839–850, 1985.
11. Zucker, C. S., Cowman, A. F., and Rubin, G. M. Isolation and structure of a rhodopsin gene from *D. melanogaster. Cell* 40:851–858, 1985.
12. Honig, B., Dinur, U., Nakanishi, K., Balogh-Nair, V., Gawinowicz, M. A., et al. An external point-charge model for wavelength regulation in visual pigments. *J. Am. Chem. Soc.* 10:7084–7086, 1979.
13. Bridges, C. D. Vitamin A and the role of the pigment epithelium during bleaching and regeneration of rhodopsin in the frog eye. *Exp. Eye Res.* 22:435–455, 1976.
14. Suzuki, T., Sugahara, M., and Kito, Y. An intermediate in the photoregeneration of squid rhodopsin. *Biochim. Biophys. Acta* 275:260–270, 1972.
15. Shichi, H., and Somers, R. L. Possible involvement of retinylidene phospholipid in photoisomerization of all-*trans* to 11-*cis* retinal. *J. Biol. Chem.* 249:6570–6577, 1974.
16. Nathans, J., Thomas, D., and Hogness, D. S. Molecular genetics of human color vision: The genes encoding blue, green, and red pigments. *Science* 232:193–202, 1986.
17. Yoshizawa, T. The Behaviour of visual pigments at low temperatures. In Dartnall, H. J. A. (ed.), *Handbook of Sensory Physiology. Photochemistry of Vision.* Heidelberg: Springer-Verlag, 1972, vol. 7/1, pp. 146–179.
18. Korenbrot, J. I. Signal mechanisms of phototransduction in retinal rod. *CRC Critical Rev. Biochem.* 17:223–256, 1985.
19. Hagins, W. A. The visual process: Excitatory mechanisms in the primary receptor cells. *Annu. Rev. Biophys. Bioeng.* 1:131–158, 1972.

20. Fesenko, E., Kolesnikov, S. S., and Lyubarsky, A. L. Induction by cyclic GMP of cationic conductance in plasma membrane of retinal rod outer segment. *Nature* 313:310–313, 1985.

21. Stryer, L. Cyclic GMP cascade of vision. *Annu. Rev. Neurosci.* 9:87–119, 1986.

22. Sugimoto, K., Nukada, T., Tanabe, T., Takahashi, H., Noda, M., et al. Primary structure of the β-subunit of bovine transducin deduced from the cDNA sequence. *FEBS Letters* 191:235–240, 1985.

23. Torre, V., Matthews, H. R., and Lamb, T. D. Role of calcium in regulating the cyclic GMP cascade of phototransduction in retinal rods. *Proc. Natl. Acad. Sci. U.S.A.* 83:7109–7113, 1986.

24. Hokin, L. E. Receptors and phosphoinositide-generated second messengers. *Annu. Rev. Biochem.* 54:205–235, 1985.

25. Brown, J. E., Rubin, L. J., Ghalayini, A. J., Tarver, A. P., Irvine, R. F., et al. *Myo*-inositol polyphosphate may be a messenger for visual excitation in *Limulus* photoreceptors. *Nature* 311:160–163, 1984.

26. Fein, A. Excitation and adaptation of *Limulus* photoreceptors by light and inositol 1,4,5-triphosphate. *Trends Neurosci.* 9:110–114, 1986.

27. Liebman, P. A., and Pugh, E. N. ATP mediates rapid reversal of cyclic GMP phosphodiesterase activation in visual receptor membranes. *Nature* 287:734–736, 1980.

28. Kubo, T., Fukuda, K., Mikami, A., Maeda, A., Takahashi, H., et al. Cloning, sequencing and expression of complementary DNA encoding the muscarinic acetylcholine receptor. *Nature* 232:411–416, 1986.

29. Benovic, J. L., Mayor, F., Somers, R. L., Caron, M. G., and Lefkowitz, R. J. Light-dependent phosphorylation of rhodopsin by β-adrenergic receptor kinase. *Nature* 321:869–872, 1986.

PART TWO

Synaptic Function

CHAPTER 8

Chemically Mediated Synaptic Transmission: An Overview

S. D. Erulkar

Basic Neurochemistry: Molecular, Cellular, and Medical Aspects, 4th Ed., edited by G. J. Siegel et al. Raven Press, Ltd., New York, 1989.
Correspondence to S. D. Erulkar, Department of Pharmacology, University of Pennsylvania School of Medicine, Philadelphia, PA 19104-
6084.

CHARACTERISTICS OF CHEMICAL NEUROTRANSMISSION

*Neurotransmitters are substances that,
on release from nerve terminals, act
on receptor sites at postsynaptic
membranes to produce either excitation
or inhibition of the target cell*

These changes are brought about by changes in
the distribution of ions across postsynaptic
membranes of nerves, muscles, and glands.
Chemically mediated transmission is one of the
means by which an appropriate signal is transferred from one nerve cell to another, or from
nerve fibers to muscle cells or even gland cells.

Elliott in 1904 [1] first suggested the possibility that information was transferred from one
neuron to the next by the release of a chemical
substance from nerve fibers; it was Loewi [2],
however, who first showed the existence of a
chemical substance in the perfusion fluid on
stimulation of the vagus nerve. He and his col-
laborator Navratil later showed that this substance was acetylcholine.

Chemically mediated transmission involves the following processes:

1. Synthesis of the neurotransmitter at the
   presynaptic terminal.
2. Storage of the neurotransmitter or its precursor in the presynaptic terminal.
3. Release of the substance into the synaptic
   extracellular space.
4. Recognition and binding of the compound
   by postsynaptic receptors.

5. Inactivation and termination of the action of the neurotransmitter.

Some neurotransmitters such as acetylcholine (ACh), glycine, glutamate, and γ-aminobutyric acid (GABA), have an inherent biological activity such that the neurotransmitter directly causes an increase in conductance to certain ions at the postsynaptic membrane. Other neurotransmitters, such as norepinephrine, dopamine, and serotonin, have no direct activity but act through an adenylate cyclase system, or some other messenger system, to cause metabolic changes in the postsynaptic membrane, leading to changes in conductance for a specific ion or other biological effects. Transmitter-dependent changes in adenylate cyclase activity, many of which lead to changes in protein kinase activity, are discussed in Chapters 17–19. Effects of other transmitters are mediated through increases in polyphosphoinositide turnover that lead to changes in intracellular concentrations of Ca^{2+} and activation of protein kinase C (see Chap. 16).

Molecular mechanisms of synaptic transmission have been studied mainly in the vertebrate neuromuscular junction and the giant synapse of the squid, Loligo

The vertebrate neuromuscular junction, especially that of amphibia, provides convenient and available recording sites at which electrical activity resulting from transmitter release can be measured for long periods of time. The neurotransmitter is known to be ACh, and the structure is well defined. The disadvantage of this preparation is that electrodes cannot be placed within the presynaptic terminal to measure activity directly; rather, one relies on extracellular recording across a volume conductor. Studies using the squid giant synapse provide a means of circumventing this limitation. Electrodes can be placed intracellularly within the terminal as well as postsynaptically at the synaptic junction; however, the identity of the neurotransmitter is still unknown. Other preparations in which both pre- and postsynaptic nerve elements can be successfully impaled by microelectrodes have also been used and are becoming more popular. These include giant synapses in the lamprey, lobster, and cockroach; the photoreceptor of the barnacle; and the synapses of the Mauthner cells of fish.

In all these preparations, there is a close approximation of the nerve terminal and postsynaptic cell, with transmission occurring at discrete sites characterized by specializations of pre- and postsynaptic membranes. The released substance diffuses across the synaptic gap and interacts with postsynaptic receptors. The time delay from entry of action potentials into presynaptic nerve terminals to a response mediated by postsynaptic receptors includes time required for the following events to occur:

1. Activation of presynaptic mechanisms related to release.
2. Diffusion across the synaptic gap (~50 μsec at the frog neuromuscular junction).
3. Response time of the postsynaptic receptor (~150 μsec at the frog neuromuscular junction).

The total time required varies from 0.5 to 3.5 msec. Most of this time (at least 350 μsec) must therefore be occupied by processes of release at the terminal, originally termed mobilization of neurotransmitter. It has now been suggested that this time is taken by the opening of Ca^{2+} gates to allow free ions to enter the terminal (see later).

This direct effect of a chemical substance crossing a short distance to act on its target site is thought of classically as neurotransmitter action: an effect that occurs rapidly but has limited duration. Our ideas have been somewhat modified, however, since it has been learned that certain substances can be released into the circulation to travel some distance before reaching their receptors. These substances were first called neurohormones to account for the effects of substances secreted into the bloodstream by neurosecretory cells in response to nerve impulses relayed via synapses. Although classical neurotransmitters are believed to act rapidly, some hypothalamic neuron terminals release peptides that cross a synaptic gap to act on other neurons where the action is slow and long-lasting. This is true also in the spinal cord, where the release of substance P (an undecapeptide) gives rise to a long-lasting depolarizing response.

In some tissues, such as the intestine, nerve terminals are not closely associated with specific smooth muscle cells, and transmitter is released into the extracellular space, where it diffuses locally to influence a number of cells. A particular transmitter may act locally at some synapses but may be released from other cells into the bloodstream to act at different receptors. Norepinephrine neurons in the central nervous system form contacts with close association to postsynaptic cells; chromaffin cells of the adrenal medulla release norepinephrine and epinephrine into the circulation from which they are carried to smooth muscle throughout the body.

A single transmitter may have different effects at different neurons

In the abdominal ganglion of the mollusc *Aplysia californica,* ACh can elicit depolarization of the membranes of certain neurons, leading to increased frequency of action potential firing; in other neurons, the same neurotransmitter causes a hyperpolarization and depression of firing. Sometimes, both postsynaptic effects can be seen at the same neuron. The mechanisms underlying the responses involve a nonspecific increase in conductance to cations, causing membrane depolarization at some postsynaptic sites and an increase in Cl^- conductance, causing hyperpolarization, at others.

Several criteria must be satisfied before a substance can be defined as a neurotransmitter

The presynaptic neuron should be able to synthesize the substance or its precursor. The putative transmitter must be present in the terminal, usually in association with enzymes required for its synthesis; however, peptides are synthesized in the soma and transported via the axon to the terminal. The content of the terminal may be demonstrated by chemical measurement, histofluorescence, or immunological markers. The terminal should release the transmitter in a pharmacologically identifiable form. This is not to say that every substance released is necessarily a neurotransmitter. For instance, adrenal medullary cells release adenine, ATP, ADP, AMP, and dopamine-β-hydroxylase, together with catecholamines, yet the postsynaptic response is due to norepinephrine.

At the postsynaptic neuron, the putative neurotransmitter should reproduce in every way the specific events of transmission resulting from stimulating the presynaptic neuron. This includes membrane changes, ionic conductances, and reversal potential. The effects should be obtained at concentrations that are as low as those present after release by nerve stimulation. The effects of a putative transmitter should be blocked by known competitive antagonists in a dose-dependent manner similar to that seen with neuronal stimulation.

Finally, there should be some mechanism to terminate the action of the substance. This can include an enzyme capable of destroying the transmitter, such as acetylcholinesterase, which hydrolyzes acetylcholine and thus makes it inactive. Catecholamines are either transported into nerve terminals or degraded; amino acids are either taken up into the nerve terminal or into glial cells that surround the synapse (or both); peptides are probably degraded by peptidases.

Acetylcholine was the first neurotransmitter in the central nervous system to be identified

The experimental evidence that led to this conclusion fulfilled the criteria described above. Basic to these studies was a statement by Sir Henry Dale [3] to the effect that when a cholinergic or adrenergic neuron undergoes regeneration, the original transmitter is always restored and is ''unchangeable.'' A corollary of Dale's principle applies to two different endings of the same neuron, one peripheral, the other central. In this case, identification of the peripheral transmitter may yield clues to the identity of the central transmitter. Eccles extended this concept to synapses at neurons in the ventral horn of the spinal cord. Spinal motoneurons of mammals have a main axon that innervates a specific skeletal muscle. This motor axon is known to release ACh at the neuromuscular junction (or end-plate region). There is, however, a motor axon collateral that branches from the main axon back into the spinal cord and projects to interneurons that in turn synapse on the original and other motoneurons. Eccles and his colleagues [4] showed by electrophysiological techniques that the neurotransmitter released from the terminals of the motor axon collateral was ACh. Inspection of Table 1 shows that concentrations of choline acetyltransferase, the enzyme responsible for ACh synthesis, acetylcholinesterase, the enzyme responsible for ACh hydrolysis, and ACh itself are high in the ventral region of the spinal cord. Finally, it was shown that ACh was present in the perfusate at the spinal cord after stimulation of the ventral root. The criteria for neurotransmitter identification have thus been satisfied.

It should be noted, however, that although application of Dale's principle has proved helpful, in certain cases, for neurotransmitter identification, the laws underlying it can no longer be thought of as inviolate. There is convincing evidence that invertebrate neurons contain more than one neurotransmitter, although there is still no proof that all are released. In addition, there is morphological evidence that in certain mammalian neurons, peptide and nonpeptide neurotransmitters can coexist in the same terminal [5].

TABLE 1. Distribution of components of ACh systems in dog tissues[a]

	ACh content (μg/g fresh tissue)	Choline acetylase activity (mg/ACh synthesized/ g wet wt/hr)	Acetylcholinesterase[b]
Sensory cortex	2.8	—	150
Motor cortex	4.5	3	178
Caudate nucleus	2.7	13.3	3936
Thalamus	3	3.1	409
Hypothalamus	1.8	2.0	323
Pons-medulla	—	—	—
Cerebellum	0.18	0.09	1075
Dorsal roots	0.04	<0.02	—
Ventral roots	15	11	149
Sympathetic ganglion	30	—	—

[a] From Paton [32].
[b] Rate of hydrolysis of methacholine, in μl CO_2 evolved/g wet wt/10 min, as an estimate of true cholinesterase activity.

A large number of substances that may act as transmitters have been identified in nerve cells

In addition to ACh, the catecholamines, such as dopamine, norepinephrine, and epinephrine, have been shown convincingly to be neurotransmitters in both peripheral and central nervous systems. For dopamine, norepinephrine, and the indoleamine 5-hydroxytryptamine (serotonin), identification of neurons containing the transmitter has been facilitated by the development of fluorescent histochemical techniques (see Chaps. 11 and 12). Other primary amines, such as histamine, octopamine, phenylethylamine, and phenylethanolamine, and polyamines, such as putrecine, spermine, and spermidine, may also be transmitters. A number of amino acids also have well-documented effects on neurons. These include glutamic and aspartic acids, glycine, β-alanine, GABA, taurine, and, possibly, proline (Chap. 15). Evaluation of the physiological function of these substances is complicated by their ubiquitous distribution in cells. Other relatively small molecules have at times been suggested as neurotransmitters; these include Ca^{2+}, adenosine, ATP, cyclic AMP, GTP, cyclic GMP, CTP, estrogen, testosterone, corticosterone, and various prostaglandins.

A major development has been the appreciation of the role of small peptides as neurotransmitters

Substance P, an 11-amino acid peptide, was described as an active agent as early as 1931, but only with the work of Leeman and her associates [6], who determined the sequence and developed radioimmunoassay methods for identification, has this peptide become widely recognized as an important neurotransmitter. A variety of peptides are present and distributed asymmetrically in nervous tissue. These range in size from carnosine and thyrotropin-releasing hormone (TRH), 2- and 3-amino acid peptides, respectively, to neurotensin and somatostatin, 13- and 14-amino acid peptides, respectively. Other putative peptide neurotransmitters include the enkephalins and endorphins, which may be the brain's natural morphine; agents known to be hormonally active, including insulin, angiotensin I and II, vasoactive intestinal polypeptide, cholecystokinin, prolactin, vasopressin, and oxytocin; and releasing factors, such as luteinizing hormone-releasing hormone (LHRH), melanocyte-stimulating hormone–release-inhibiting hormone, and somatostatin release-inhibiting hormone. A number of other active peptides have been described in both vertebrates and invertebrates, but less is known about their structures and actions (see Chaps. 13 and 14).

The number of substances that must be considered putative neurotransmitters at present is at least 50 and is growing rapidly; however, rigorous proof of transmitter function has been obtained for only a very few of these substances. The realization that small peptides can be neurotransmitters increases the number of possible active agents, and the difficulties in chemical and physiological identification become enormous.

Fast and slow systems are involved in chemically mediated synaptic transmission

The first system involves fast, short-lived transmission resulting from relatively small molecules that bring about brief conductance changes at the postsynaptic membrane. These so-called classical neurotransmitters are synthesized in the nerve terminal and are classified by their chemical structure, e.g., ACh, catecholamines, indoleamines, and amino acids. A second system that involves neuroactive peptides may coexist in the terminals with the classical neurotransmitters; however, unlike the classical transmitters, they are synthesized in the cell bodies. The peptides can be grouped in families; each family is structurally related and contains long stretches of amino acid sequences that are homologous. Their actions are apparently long-lasting and are modulatory to those of the classical neurotransmitters.

STRUCTURAL, MOLECULAR, AND FUNCTIONAL CORRELATIONS OF TRANSMISSION

The model for studies on synaptic transmission is usually the amphibian neuromuscular junction

Certain structural features are seen universally at chemical synapses, even where the transmitter is unknown. Critical questions include: First, how does the structure of the presynaptic terminal correlate with its known function? Second, can the morphology provide clues to understanding the mechanisms of transmitter release? Several techniques have been used to study the morphology of the synapse. These include the use of transmission electron microscopy and freeze-fracture techniques. Specific receptors for neurotransmitters or peptides, especially at postsynaptic membranes, have been identified by immunocytochemical techniques that have proved to be particularly useful in the central nervous system.

The presynaptic terminal displays specific structural characteristics

Figure 1 shows an electron micrograph of longitudinal (Fig. 1A) and transverse (Fig. 1B) sections through a nerve terminal on frog sartorius muscle in the absence of nerve stimulation. The presynaptic terminal displays four characteristic features:

1. Synaptic vesicles, usually about 20 to 60 nm in diameter. At the neuromuscular junc-

tion they are spherical; in the central nervous system, they can also be ellipsoid or flattened in shape. A motor nerve terminal at a frog neuromuscular junction contains about 500,000 vesicles, and each vesicle is believed to contain a quantum of neurotransmitter that is released by exocytosis. The concept that each quantum of transmitter is contained in a vesicle is known as the vesicular hypothesis.
2. Mitochondria that are usually located at some distance away from the synaptic surface.
3. Intramembranous specializations, including an endoplasmic reticulum.
4. Presynaptic densities.

Transmitter release is quantal at chemically mediated synapses

The vesicle, in which the neurotransmitter can be packaged, provides a structural choice for the quantal nature of the release; release itself is accomplished by means of exocytosis, whereby the vesicle membrane fuses with the terminal membrane. Is there proof that this process actually occurs? Electron microscopy has been used to show the morphological events in real time by quick-freezing the synapse within a few milliseconds of eliciting release, so that the number of quanta released at a frog nerve muscle synapse could be compared to the number of exocytotic events that result from a single nerve stimulation. Over a wide range of transmitter release, augmented by K^+-blocking agents such as 4-aminopyridine, one quantum accompanies one exocytotic event (Fig. 2) [7].

Freeze-fracture technique permits visualization of synaptic vesicle openings during exocytosis

Generally, it is difficult to visualize exocytosis directly in conventional electron micrographs, perhaps because the exocytotic opening is usu-

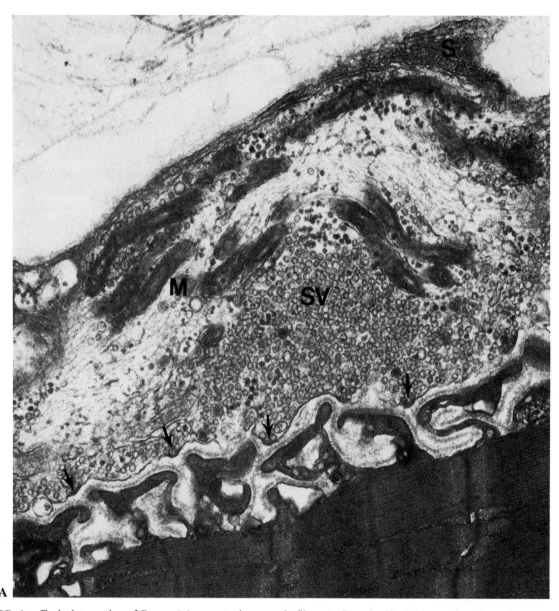

FIG. 1. End-plate region of *Rana pipiens* sartorius muscle fiber. **A:** Longitudinal thin section through a nerve terminal. *Arrows* denote active zones. Also shown are synaptic vesicles (SV), mitochondria (M), and Schwann cells (S). The postsynaptic component is represented by the thicker membrane at the top of the folds in the muscle surface (×30,400). **B:** Transverse section of a motor nerve terminal. Contents of the terminal include synaptic vesicles (SV), mitochondria (M), and cistern (C). (×36,800.) (Courtesy of A. Stieber, N. D. Gonatas, and S. D. Erulkar.)

158

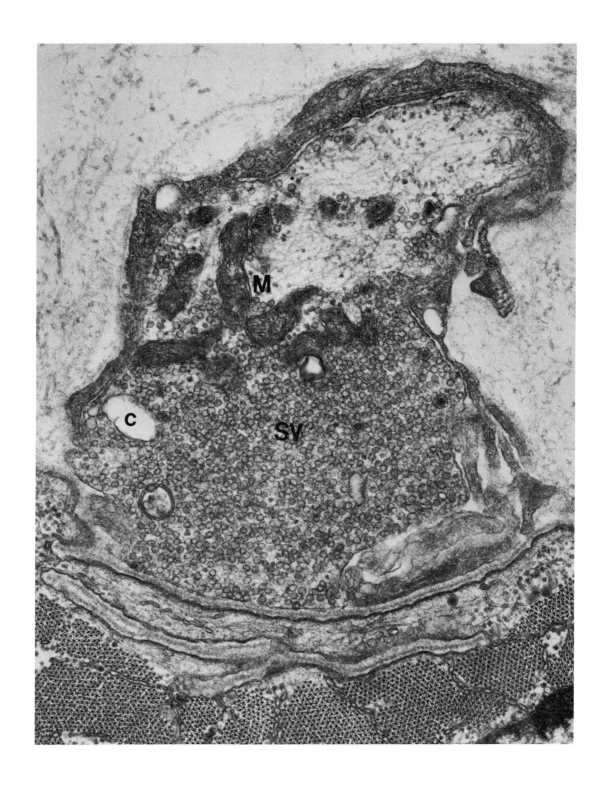

159

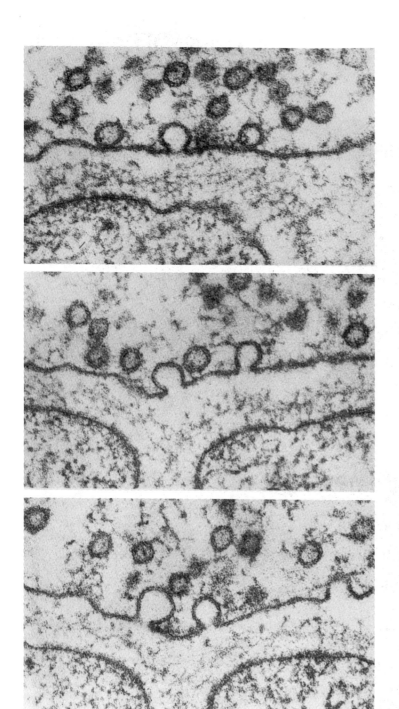

FIG. 2. Three separate high-magnification ($\times 145,000$) views of freeze-substituted neuromuscular junctions in a muscle frozen during the abnormally large burst of ACh release that is provoked by a single nerve stimulus in 2 mM 4-aminopyridine, in this case delivered 5.1 msec before the muscle was frozen. These sections were cut unusually thin (~ 200 Å) to show the fine structure of the presynaptic membrane, which displayed many examples of synaptic vesicles apparently caught in the act of exocytosis. In all cases, these open vesicles were found just above the mouths of the postsynaptic folds, hence at the site of the presynaptic active zones. (From Heuser [7].)

ally smaller than the thickness of typical sections. The freeze-fracture technique is more suitable for this purpose, because when tissue is fixed, frozen, and broken open, the fracture tends to split membranes and therefore to follow their hydrophobic interiors. While still frozen, this fractured surface can be replicated with platinum and examined with a resolution of 2 nm, which is high enough to see where intrinsic membrane proteins cross the lipid bilayer (Fig. 3) [8]. With this technique, it was possible to see the stomata of synaptic vesicles in the act of exocytosis during quantal release either during nerve stimulation or after application of a toxin such as black or brown widow spider venom. Furthermore, any agent that blocked release also blocked the exocytosis. The process of exocytosis did not depend on action potentials in the nerve because it could be elicited by neurotoxins such as spider venom acting directly on the terminal.

Synaptic vesicles cluster over regions where neighboring membranes of two neurons appear thickened

Using transmission electron microscopy, Palay suggested in 1956 [9] that these areas may represent sites of vesicle discharge, and he later named these areas "synaptic complexes." Indeed, much evidence has accumulated to support the idea that these synaptic complexes adhere to each other. Even when the neurons are disrupted, thickened portions of the postsynaptic membranes cling to the presynaptic densities of the synaptosomes and can be separated only by strong proteolytic agents.

Couteaux and Pecot-Dechavassine [10] suggested in 1970 that a nerve has "active zones" for transmitter release, and evidence from freeze-fracture suggests that exocytosis is limited to these active zones of the synaptic membrane surface. However, it is known that the majority of individual active zones fail to release a quantum of neurotransmitter after a

nerve impulse. There are approximately 500 active zones per nerve terminal at the frog nerve-muscle synapse, yet less than 250 quanta are released by action potentials after nerve stimulation.

The morphology of active zones suggests important questions for further investigation. Large intramembrane particles are present near the active zone, and consideration of their universal deployment and numbers at presynaptic active zones leads to the suggestion that they are the channels that admit Ca^{2+} that initiates transmitter release [11]. The cytoplasm of nerve terminals near active zones always contains a fuzzy material that makes contact with the releasable vesicles at the active zone. It is important to know the role of this material in inserting a new vesicle back into the active zone after it undergoes exocytosis, or for initiating the membrane interactions that lead to exocytosis. Finally, it remains to be determined whether all chemical synaptic transmission occurs at active zones [11].

Synaptic vesicles associated with presynaptic densities are in a favorable position to be discharged, and they contain an immediately available pool of transmitter

Prolonged stimulation would be expected to cause depletion of vesicles from the terminal. Experiments to show this have been frustrating, and some investigators have shown that the number of vesicles near the presynaptic densities actually increases after a few minutes of nerve stimulation. In fact, although vesicles are in some way altered in number after repetitive nerve stimulation, they are not readily depleted. Stimulation of the frog neuromuscular junction can cause the release of millions of quanta with no resultant depletion of vesicles.

It appears that the vesicle membrane is somehow conserved during repetitive stimulation. The most detailed study on this topic was

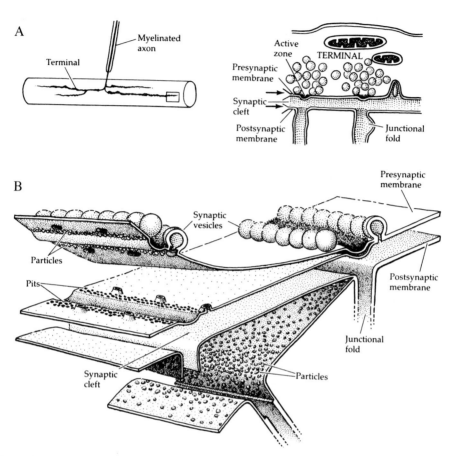

FIG. 3. Synaptic membrane structure. **A:** Entire frog neuromuscular junction (*left*) and longitudinal section through a portion of the nerve terminal (*right*). *Arrows* indicate planes of cleavage during freeze-fracture. **B:** Three-dimensional view of presynaptic and postsynaptic membranes with active zones and immediately adjacent rows of synaptic vesicles. Plasma membranes are split along planes indicated by the *arrows* in **A** to illustrate structures observed on freeze-fracturing. The cytoplasmic half of the presynaptic membrane at the active zone shows on its fracture face protruding particles whose counterparts are seen as pits on the fracture face of the outer membrane leaflet. Vesicles that fuse with the presynaptic membrane give rise to characteristic protrusions and pores in the fracture faces. The fractured postsynaptic membrane in the region of the folds shows a high concentration of particles on the fracture face of the cytoplasmic leaflet; these are probably ACh receptors. (Courtesy of U. J. McMahan; from Kuffler et al. [8].) **C, D:** Freeze-fractured active zones from frog resting and stimulated neuromuscular junction. The active zone is the region of presynaptic membrane surrounding double rows of intramembrane particles, which may be channels for Ca^{2+} entry that initiates transmitter release. Holes that appear in active zones during transmitter release (*lower picture*) are openings of synaptic vesicles engaged in exocytosis. This muscle was prepared by quick-freezing, and transmitter release was augmented with 4-aminopyridine, so that the morphological events (opening of synaptic vesicles) could be examined at the exact moment of transmitter release evoked by a single nerve shock. ($\times$120,000.) (From Heuser and Reese [34], with permission.)

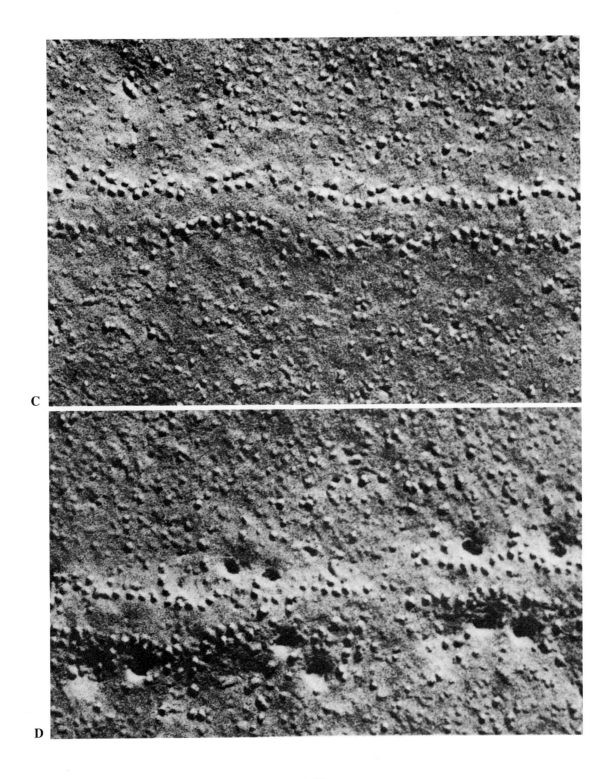

C

D

that of Heuser and Reese [12], who showed that during brief tetanic stimulation of frog motor nerve, horseradish peroxidase (HRP), which had been added to the extracellular space previously, appeared in the nerve terminal in coated vesicles and cisternae that became more evident with stimulation. When stimulation was stopped, the cisternae resolved, and HRP was then seen in vesicles (Fig. 4). The authors suggested that after fusion with the terminal membrane, synaptic vesicle membrane is retrieved by coated vesicles and cisternae and then recycled as new synaptic vesicles (Fig. 5). Whether this is the exclusive pathway for retrieval of vesicle membrane is still uncertain. Heuser and Reese themselves caution that HRP only marks the "fluid" phase, not the "adsorptive," or membrane, phase, so they have no direct proof that synaptic vesicle membrane is being recycled. Later studies with the use of

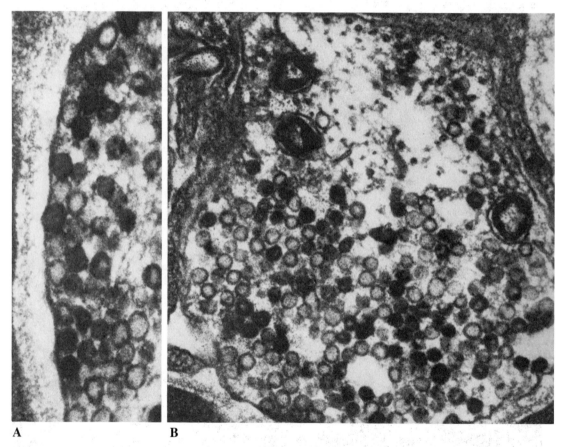

A　　　　　　　　**B**

FIG. 4. Cross sections through normal regions of loaded terminals. Nearly 50 percent of the vesicles contain HRP, which corresponds to the number that should have been depleted by the stimulation and reformed from HRP-containing cisternae. **B:** The HRP-containing vesicles appear to be distributed randomly within the nerve terminal, including the area near the presynaptic surface, shown in more detail in **A** to illustrate that HRP-containing vesicles in contact with the plasma membrane do not discharge HRP, even though the tracer has been washed out of the synaptic cleft. (**A,** ×72,250; **B,** ×28,050.) (From Heuser and Reese [12], with permission.)

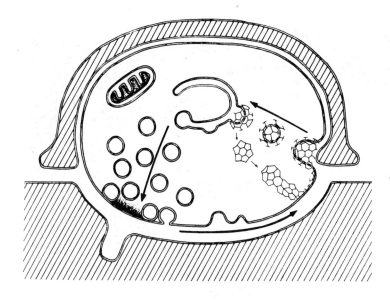

FIG. 5. Current view of synaptic vesicle recycling at the frog neuromuscular junction, supported by the new views shown here of synaptic vesicle exocytosis as it looks in quick-frozen frog neuromuscular junctions treated with 4-aminopyridine and given a single electrical shock. *Arrows* indicate the sequence of vesicle recycling. (From Heuser and Reese [12], with permission.)

membrane markers, however, have shown that membranes from the terminal are incorporated in the formation of new synaptic vesicles (Fig. 6).

Postsynaptic active zones are observed where synaptic terminals make contact with nerves or muscles

The position, but not necessarily the size, of the postsynaptic active zone matches that of the presynaptic active zone [11]. The internal membrane structure of the postsynaptic active zones varies with the type of transmitter used. At most types of postsynaptic active zones, intramembrane particles are more concentrated than over the rest of the membrane. The concentration of intramembrane particles varies up to 10,000/μm^2 in cholinergic systems (a 100-fold increase over that on the remaining membrane) and down to aggregates barely discernible from those in the rest of the membrane at certain central nervous system synapses (Fig. 7). The organization within the aggregate can also vary from linear arrays to dispersed types of spacing,

where distances between particles are relatively constant.

For cholinergic nerve-muscle synapses, there is good evidence that the intramembrane particles at the postsynaptic active zones are the sites of ion channel-receptor complexes. The heads of these particles protrude beyond the outer surface of the postsynaptic active zone into the synaptic cleft. The synaptic cleft contains a basement membrane, or a similar, fuzzy material, concentrated in the center of the cleft at nerve-nerve synapses, and side-arms periodically arise from the central skein of cleft material to make contact with the surface of the postsynaptic active zone. At nerve-muscle synapses, the cytoplasmic side of this membrane is also thickened by a coat of fuzzy material, 5 to 10 nm wide, and similar coats of material seem to be a general feature of postsynaptic active zones, regardless of the chemical nature of the synapse.

The active zones of different types of chemical synapses vary mainly in the concentration, size, and fracturing characteristics of the intramembrane components and in the extent to which this and perhaps additional components

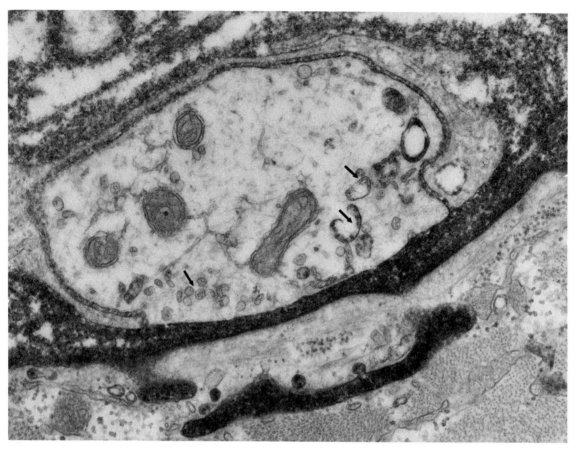

FIG. 6. Transverse section of motor nerve terminal of sartorius muscle of *Rana pipiens* double-labeled with wheat germ-ferritin and free HRP. The protocol for this experiment was as follows: The frog, *Rana pipiens,* was anesthetized with tricaine methanesulfonate and the sartorius muscle exposed. Wheat germ-ferritin was then injected at many areas in the muscle, the skin sewn together, and the animal allowed to revive over a 2-hr period. It was then decapitated and a conventional nerve-muscle preparation of the sartorius made. The nerve-muscle preparation was then allowed to soak in HRP, D-tubocurarine, and Ringer's solution for 30 min, at the end of which the nerve was stimulated at 10 Hz for 15 min. When the stimulation was stopped, the muscle was left in the solution for a period of 30 min. It was then fixed in glutaraldehyde and prepared for electron microscopy. (×50,250.) (Courtesy of A. Stieber, N. D. Gonatas, and S. D. Erulkar.)

extend into the cytoplasm. The postsynaptic active zone, therefore, is a membrane complex that involves both the cytoplasmic and external surfaces of the postsynaptic membrane [11]. Its edges are very sharp, and the sharpness persists even at the edges of large postsynaptic active zones, where groups containing several hundred receptors separate into patches. These membrane complexes are more stable than the rest of the membrane. Turnover of cholinergic receptors in the active zone has a time course of days, and active zones in general maintain

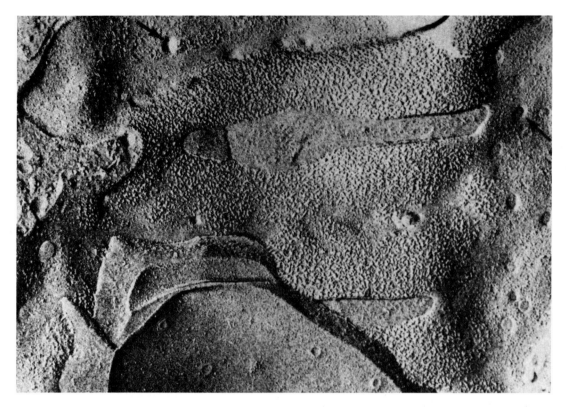

FIG. 7. In this freeze-fracture view the nerve terminal (*bottom*) has been ripped away, exposing the surface of muscle under it. The postsynaptic active zones clearly differ from the rest of the muscle membrane, which is marked by the caveolae characteristic of muscle cells (*arrow*). More important are the numerous intra-membrane particles at the active zones on the tops of the folds; these are thought to be ACh receptors. The vesicle openings on the outer leaflet of the nerve terminal (*bottom*) are formation sites of coated pits. These occur following transmitter release, but outside the active zones. (×75,000.) (From Heuser and Reese [11], with permission.)

their organization in the face of metabolic or mechanical damage that alters the rest of the surface membrane.

Development of the postsynaptic active zones requires the laying down of synaptic cleft material and deployment of receptors and submembranous components

The exact sequences of the different structural changes are not known, although it is known that the postsynaptic active zone in muscle regenerates at its former position, provided that the cleft material, a basement membrane in this instance, is left intact. Alternatively, brains of mutant mice show instances in which the postsynaptic active zone is completed in the absence of presynaptic nerve terminals or a cleft.

In cultured muscle, receptors exchange rapidly between the insides of cells and the surface membrane and are spread out over the entire muscle surface. The intramembrane components of receptors seem to enter or leave the surface membrane in small groups. This finding suggests that the transmitter-sensitive regions of the muscle fibers could be assembled from small, prefabricated arrays of receptor membrane. Studies on the development of intracellular junctions in other systems suggest that an anlage, manifested by shape changes within the membrane, may be established prior to the deployment of intramembrane components. The intramembrane components at the presynaptic active zone also seem to be assembled in patches suggestive of prefabricated arrays.

In some instances, postsynaptic active zones are deployed on special folds or protrusions of the postsynaptic cell

At many types of nerve-muscle synapses, the surface of the muscle postsynaptic membrane is a series of folds, as in vertebrates (Fig. 1B), cylindrical invaginations, as in electric organ, or cylindrical protrusions, as in insects. The postsynaptic active zones are typically found at the apices of these protrusions, although the purpose of this arrangement is not yet clear. At the frog neuromuscular junction, the folds themselves are supported by a core of intermediate-sized filaments and microtubules that run parallel to the axis of the fold. A fine network of neurofilaments, in turn, connects this core with the fuzz on the cytoplasmic side of the active zone.

In the brain, cylindrical protrusions, called dendritic spines, are also sites of postsynaptic active zones; a single cortical neuron has on the order of 50,000 such spines. Although the special detail afforded by current freezing and staining techniques is not yet available for brain, it has been shown that spines are characterized by their content of fine filamentous material. Active zones isolated from the cerebral cortex show further details of the relationship between the postsynaptic membrane and the cytoskeleton. The cytoplasmic side of the active zone shows a prominent band of fuzz, which, in turn,

is in contact with a meshwork of microfilaments. The similarity of central nervous system spines with the folds at the neuromuscular junction lies in this contact between the active zone and the cytomatrix; the difference lies in the lack of a microtubule-filament complex in the core of the spine. Cortical spines are of particular interest, because there is evidence that the size and shape of the spines may affect the input from their active zones to the cell body. Furthermore, spines change shape under certain experimental conditions. This suggests that they may act similarly in life; they are in a strategic position for these shape changes to result in changes in information processing.

THE NEUROMUSCULAR JUNCTION

The end-plate region also has been used to provide information on the nature of synaptic transmission with respect to its associated electrical activity

While the neuromuscular junction has the advantage of being a single synapse at which the neurotransmitter is known to be acetylcholine, it has the disadvantage that a microelectrode cannot penetrate the presynaptic terminal without causing damage.

Microelectrode recordings are used in two ways:

1. Intracellular recording, in which the electrode penetrates the muscle membrane close to the end-plate region and records a transmembrane potential between the interior of the muscle and the outside.

2. Focal recording, in which the microelectrode records extracellularly from the surface of the muscle fiber. In this situation, the electrode records potentials from sites of the muscle membrane of approximately only 5 μm^2 compared to 500 μm^2 with intracellular recording. Furthermore, focal

recording also allows the potential from the presynaptic nerve terminal to be recorded; while this is not as satisfactory as an electrode placed within the terminal, it does provide an indication of the time of the peak of the presynaptic current.

In the absence of motor nerve stimulation, intracellular recording at the end plate has revealed the presence of small subthreshold depolarizing potentials that appear to occur randomly

In 1952, Fatt and Katz [13] hypothesized that these events represented the release of packages or "quanta" of ACh from the nerve terminal. An interesting aspect of these potentials was their similarity in configuration, except for their amplitudes, to the end-plate potential (EPP) that is elicited when the motor nerve is stimulated. In view of the fact that the "miniature" end-plate potentials (MEPPs), as they were called, appeared to represent the basic unit of transmitter release, it was suggested that release was quantal and that the EPP itself reflected the release of many quanta of ACh. In fact, the rate of secretion of quanta is increased by the nerve impulse. Indeed, if the external Ca^{2+} concentration is reduced (see below), the evoked EPP becomes extremely small and its amplitude can become the same as those of the MEPPs. When the nerve terminal membrane is depolarized, the rate of spontaneous MEPPs is increased, provided that Ca^{2+} is present in the external medium. The amplitude of each MEPP is unchanged. Similar events have been shown to occur at synapses of central neurons.

A histogram relating the amplitude of the MEPP with its frequency of occurrence can be constructed that shows that the MEPP amplitudes fall into peaks that are multiples of the mean MEPP amplitude. This experiment requires reduction of the external Ca^{2+} concentration and an increase in the concentration of

Mg^{2+} (Fig. 8) [14]. This result allowed the formulation of a statistical model of the release process such that if there are n available release sites on nerve terminals and each has a probability p of releasing a quantum, then $m = np$, which is the mean number of quanta released per nerve impulse, called *quantal content*.

Since this concept was first proposed a large literature has appeared concerning the interpretation of both n and p and the conditions under which they are valid. In particular, if n varies with time or p varies from different sites, these parameters will no longer be valid. Nevertheless, it is possible with these parameters under certain conditions to define the probability of x quanta being released by an impulse. The probability will follow a binomial distribution such that

$$P_x = \frac{n_x}{N} = \frac{n!}{x!(n-x)!} p^x q^{(n-x)} \qquad (1)$$

where n_x is the number of trials in which x quanta are released; N is the total number of trials; p is the probability of release of a single quantum; and q is the probability that a quantum will not be released, $(1 - p)$. When p becomes small (<0.05) and n becomes large ($n > 100$), the Poisson distribution applies:

$$f(x) = \frac{n_x}{N} = \frac{e^{-m}m^x}{x!} \qquad (2)$$

This means that each event is not influenced by its previous history. Quantal content can also be measured by

$$m = \frac{\text{Mean amplitude of EPP}}{\text{Mean amplitude of MEPPs}} \qquad (3)$$

or by the number of failures of transmission (n_0) that occur in N trials. If a Poisson distribution is followed, then

$$n_0/N = e^{-m} \qquad \text{and} \qquad m = \ln(N/n_0) \qquad (4)$$

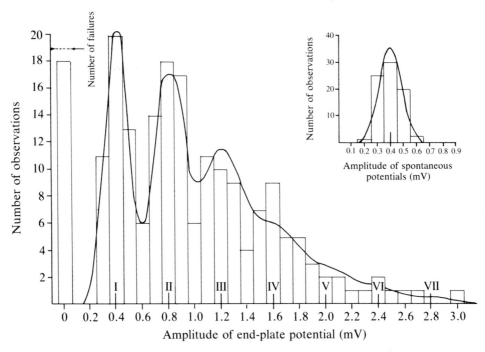

FIG. 8.   The distribution of amplitudes of evoked EPPs and of spontaneous MEPPs (inset), from a mammalian end-plate blocked with high Mg^{2+}. Peaks of the EPP amplitude histogram occur at one, two, three, and four times the mean amplitude of the spontaneous potentials. A gaussian curve is fitted to the latter and used to calculate the theoretical distribution of EPP amplitudes (*continuous curve*); *arrows* indicate expected number of failures. (From Boyd and Martin [14].)

Calcium ions are necessary for transmission at synaptic junctions

In the nervous system, at the perfused superior cervical ganglion, when Ca^{2+} is withdrawn from the perfusing medium, there is no release of ACh from the preganglionic endings, either during stimulation of the sympathetic trunk or following the addition of K^+ to the external medium, and thus causing depolarization of the membrane. Katz and Miledi [15] provided the ultimate proof of the role of Ca^{2+} in transmitter release in an elegant series of experiments with the use of a Ca^{2+} pipette. They used a frog sartorius neuromuscular junction preparation and

perfused it with a medium deficient in Ca^{2+} but with Mg^{2+} present. Stimulation of the motor nerve failed to elicit EPPs even though an action potential was conducted to the nerve terminal (Fig. 9A and D). When they used an electrode filled with 0.5 M $CaCl_2$, however, a small voltage applied to it either caused or prevented the release of Ca^{2+} from the pipette, depending on the polarity of the voltage. Release of Ca^{2+} before the stimulus caused an EPP to be elicited (Fig. 9B and C); after the stimulus, no EPP was elicited. What is clear is that for transmitter release to take place, Ca^{2+} must be present externally at the terminal when the depolarization, in the form of the nerve impulse, arrives at the terminal.

The antagonism of Ca^{2+} by Mg^{2+} suggested that two parallel reactions may occur at the nerve terminal such that

$$[Ca] + [X] = [CaX],$$

with dissociation constant K_1

$$[Mg] + [X] = [MgX],$$

with dissociation constant K_2

where [X] is the binding site. With this in mind, the law of mass action could be applied. If quantal release were simply proportional to [CaX], then the EPP should be linearly proportional to [Ca] at all values of [Ca]. If this were true, one would find that

$$CaX = \frac{W[Ca]}{1 + [Ca]/K_1 + [Mg]/K_2} \qquad (5)$$

where $W = [X_0]/K_1$ and $[X_0]$ is the concentration of unbound sites. However, the experimental data of Dodge and Rahamimoff [16] show a marked curvature of the graphs at low values (Figs. 10 and 11). Then, the EPP amplitude is

$$k = \left[\frac{W[Ca]}{1 + [Ca]/K_1 + [Mg]/K_2} \right]^4 \qquad (6)$$

A Lineweaver-Burk plot of the inverse of the fourth root of the EPP amplitude versus 1/[Ca] yielded a straight line, which suggests that competitive inhibition may indeed describe the opposite actions of Ca^{2+} and Mg^{2+} (Fig. 11). However, the fourth-power dependency also suggests that at low concentrations of Ca^{2+}, cooperativity is involved and that either four Ca^{2+} are necessary for the release of one quantum of transmitter or four Ca^{2+} sites have to be occupied for the release of one quantum of transmitter. The value of four, however, is not always found and differs according to the

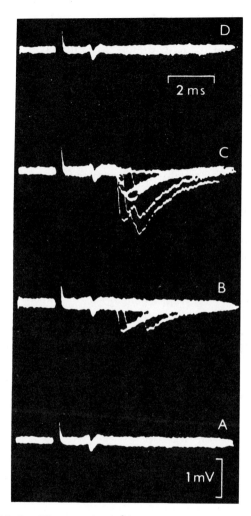

FIG. 9. The use of a Ca^{2+} pipette in exploring neuromuscular transmission. The frog sartorius was immersed in Ca^{2+}-free solution containing 0.84 mM Mg^{2+}. A pipette filled with 0.5 M $CaCl_2$ was used to record focal external potentials from a junctional spot. Efflux of Ca^{2+} was controlled electrophoretically. In the four records, *A–D,* Ca^{2+} efflux was stopped initially by applying sufficient negative voltage to the pipette; the bias was then reduced in two steps, and finally reapplied. Several superimposed traces are shown at each stage. (From Katz and Miledi [15], with permission.)

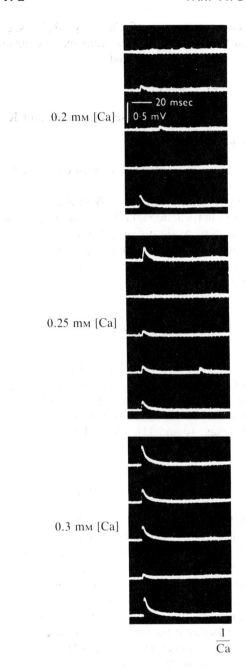

0.2 mm [Ca]

20 msec
0.5 mV

0.25 mm [Ca]

0.3 mm [Ca]

$$\frac{1}{Ca}$$

FIG. 10. The dependence of transmitter release on [Ca^{2+}]. Sample records of EPPs at three different Ca^{2+} concentrations. The same calibrations apply to all concentrations. (From Dodge and Rahamimoff [16], with permission.)

preparation; at the crayfish neuromuscular junction, for example, the relationship is linear.

The Ca^{2+} hypothesis thus suggested that with depolarization of the nerve terminal, Ca^{2+} attached to defined sites and entered the terminal, where by some unknown process it caused the release of neurotransmitter. There was, however, no direct proof of Ca^{2+} entry until Llinás and Nicholson showed, by means of the luminescent dye aequorin, that at the squid giant synapse, Ca^{2+} entered the terminal during presynaptic depolarization. In the presence of tetraethylammonium (TEA), to block K^+ currents, and tetrodotoxin (TTX), to block Na^+ currents, an inwardly directed Ca^{2+} current could be recorded presynaptically in response to the depolarization. If the excitatory postsynaptic potential (EPSP) was recorded simultaneously, a delay of several milliseconds was obtained. On repolarization, the delay for the Ca^{2+} current was less than 0.2 msec. This shows that much of the time associated with the synaptic delay is due to the activation of Ca^{2+} conductance [17,18].

Calcium, once it enters a terminal, has numerous effects, including activation of protein kinases

Greengard and his colleagues [19] reported on the isolation of a substance, synapsin I, that acts as a substrate for cyclic AMP (cAMP)-dependent protein kinase, Ca^{2+}-calmodulin–dependent protein kinase, and protein kinase C in the brain (see Chap. 19). It is interesting that synapsin I was found to be phosphorylated when nerve terminals were depolarized. Bahler and Greengard (Greengard et al. [19]) have shown an "actin-bundling" activity associated with synapsin I, such that the activity only occurs with the dephosphorylated form of synapsin I. On phosphorylation, the bundling activity disappears and the significance of this bundling activity lies in the possibility that synapsin I may

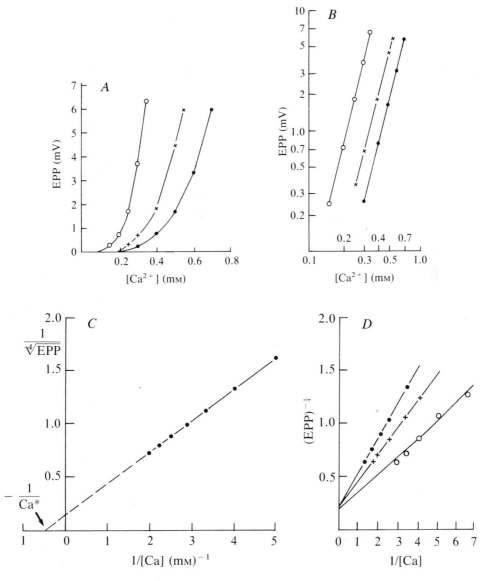

FIG. 11. **A/B:** Relation between $[Ca^{2+}]$ and the amplitude of EPP. **A:** Linear plot at three different Mg^{2+} concentrations: (○) 0.5 mM Mg^{2+}; (X) 2.0 mM Mg^{2+}; (●) 4.0 mM Mg^{2+}. Each value represents the average amplitude of 128 or 256 EPPs. **B:** Same as **A** on double logarithmic coordinates. **C/D:** Lineweaver-Burk plot for relationship between $[CaX]^4$ and response. *Ordinate*: Reciprocal of fourth root of EPP. *Abscissa*: Reciprocal of [Ca]. **C:** The intersection with the abscissa gives $-1/Ca^*$. **D:** Note that *straight lines* have approximately the same intercept. (From Dodge and Rahamimoff [16], with permission.)

be involved in a mechanism whereby synaptic vesicles are held in a protein complex in the terminal with dephosphorylated synapsin I and not allowed to coalesce with the terminal membrane. Once depolarization occurs, phosphorylation takes place and the vesicles are freed to enable them to fuse with the terminal membrane, allowing exocytosis and neurotransmitter release. Indeed Llinás and his collaborators [20] have shown that dephosphorylated synapsin I could block synaptic transmission when injected into squid synapse preterminals. This occurred even when Ca^{2+} influx was unaffected. It appears that with depolarization, Ca^{2+} enters the terminal, activates a protein kinase that phosphorylates synapsin I, which allows the debundling of actin, which in turn allows synaptic vesicles to fuse with the terminal membrane. The fusion itself probably results through the action of another protein that can promote membrane-membrane fusion, and it may be that once the vesicle is freed, Ca^{2+} in the cytoplasm activates the protein, resulting in vesicular fusion and exocytosis.

The delay between the influx of Ca^{2+} into the presynaptic terminal and the postsynaptic response to the neurotransmitter consists of the initiation of release, the diffusion of the transmitter across the cleft, and the response time of the postsynaptic receptor. The total time for this process is extremely small, yet it is clear that several reactions must take place at the terminal before release occurs. The rate constants of the reactions described must be extremely high, or the sites of Ca^{2+} entry must be very close to the location of the protein kinase that it activates, or both.

Finally, transmitter release can be elicited by some divalent cations other than Ca^{2+}; these include Sr^{2+} and Ba^{2+}. The release mechanism is most sensitive to Ca^{2+}, followed by Sr^{2+} and then Ba^{2+}, suggesting a higher affinity of Ca^{2+} for binding to the appropriate protein at the terminal.

A hypothesis has emerged suggesting that quantal transmitter release may be at least partly cytoplasmic rather than vesicular

Up to now, we have discussed quantal transmitter release as if it were entirely vesicular in nature. Indeed, there is substantial evidence that the vesicles are responsible for quantal transmitter release, as originally suggested by del Castillo and Katz [21]. Using a chemoluminescent technique to measure ACh release, Israel and Lesbats [22] found that in response to a single cycle of freezing and thawing, about 30 percent of the ACh in *Torpedo* electric organ synaptosomes is cytoplasmic. Furthermore, they reported that in response to various treatments these synaptosomes released an amount of ACh that exactly matched the depletion of cytoplasmic ACh. Synaptosomal membrane sacs filled with ACh released transmitter in response to Ca^{2+} influx [23]. Finally, proteoliposomes filled with ACh and made from purified presynaptic membranes and synthetic lecithin also released ACh in a Ca^{2+}-dependent manner. The results were interpreted to suggest that cytoplasmic, in addition to vesicular, release of ACh occurs.

EFFECTS OF TRANSMITTERS ON POSTSYNAPTIC NEURONAL EXCITABILITY

Neurotransmitters can alter the excitability of a postsynaptic cell by changing membrane potential and resistance

Although many common synaptic responses result in a change of both potential and resistance, this is not always the case. Furthermore, the effects of changing potential may either add to or oppose the effects of changing resistance.

In a typical electrically excitable neuron that has an axon projecting to some distant point, there is an integration of synaptic inputs from dendrites and soma at the axon hillock. If threshold depolarization is reached at this site, an action potential is initiated that will ultimately trigger transmitter release at the axon terminals. The level of depolarization that must be reached at the axon hillock for spike initiation is relatively constant, and thus the effect of membrane potential at the hillock is simple, in that depolarization brings the neuron closer to firing threshold, whereas hyperpolarization takes the neuron further from threshold.

Binding of a transmitter to a specific receptor causes a change in the transmembrane permeability to one or more ions

The effect on potential depends on which ionic permeabilities are changed. Because the ions in a tissue are not present in equal concentration on both sides of the cell membrane, there is a driving force, determined by the concentration gradient, for each ionic species (see Chap. 4). The asymmetrical ionic concentrations are maintained by the relative membrane impermeability to some ions and the activity of the Na^+-K^+ pump (see Chap. 3). By the Nernst equation

(see Chap. 4), we can define an equilibrium potential (E) for any ion. The equilibrium potential is the one at which the electrical gradient is exactly equal to the chemical concentration gradient for that ion.

Figure 12 shows in diagrammatic form the equilibrium potentials for the major ionic species involved in determining potential shifts in neurons. To a first approximation, resting membrane potential (RMP) can be described by the Goldman-Hodgkin-Katz equation [24], which considers the contributions of Na^+, K^+, and Cl^- (see Chap. 4). Since the interior of cells is high in K^+ and low in Na^+ and Cl^-, RMP is determined by the balance of the electrical and chemical driving forces on all of these ions. Under resting conditions, K^+ permeability predominates and RMP is relatively near to E_{K^+}. The degree to which RMP deviates from E_{K^+} reflects active transport and the relative permeabilities to and the concentration gradients of the other ions. Ca^{2+} is not in electrochemical equilibrium, but its resting permeability is low enough so that the Ca^{2+} gradient does not contribute significantly to RMP.

Increased permeability to any ion can easily be detected by measuring transmembrane resistance. Permeability has an inverse relation to resistance, so the resistance falls during a response associated with an increased permea-

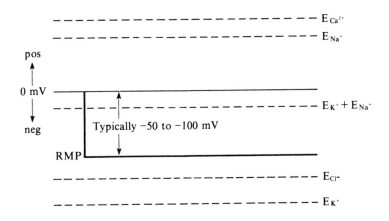

FIG. 12. Typical ionic equilibrium potentials in excitable tissues. The resting membrane potential (RMP) is usually between -50 and -100 mV. The equilibrium potentials (E) for various ions are indicated. At the equilibrium potential, the electrical gradient for that ion is exactly equal to the concentration gradient, so that as many ions enter as leave the cell.

bility to any ion. Resistance is usually measured by passing small pulses of current across the membrane and measuring the resulting voltage deflection. If the current is kept constant, the voltage produced will reflect changes in resistance according to Ohm's law.

When a transmitter increases permeability to a single ion, the membrane potential will move in the direction of the equilibrium potential for that ion

If a transmitter causes a specific decrease in the permeability to one ionic species, the membrane potential will move away from the equilibrium potential for that ion and toward that of the ion with the dominant permeability. Acetylcholine and glutamate regulate receptors that open ion channels, allowing cations to flow through nonspecifically so that the equilibrium potentials will, under the right conditions, be at 0 mV. GABA and glycine increase Cl^- conductances, so that neuronal membranes become hyperpolarized as they strive to achieve the Cl^- equilibrium potential. The voltage-activated conductances for Na^{2+} (I_{Na}) and Ca^{2+} (I_{Ca}), which carry inward currents that depolarize the membrane, do not appear to be affected by neurotransmitters. On the other hand, K^+ and some Ca^{2+} conductances are regulated by some transmitters. Table 2 lists the established transmitter-regulated ion channels in the vertebrate central nervous system. The best studied responses are the result of increased permeabilities to one or two ionic species.

Because E_{K^+} is more negative than RMP, an increase in K^+ permeability will hyperpolarize the cell whereas an increase in Na^+ permeability will depolarize the cell. In most neurons E_{Cl^-} is more negative than RMP, and, consequently, most specific Cl^- permeability increases are hyperpolarizing. In some neurons,

such as dorsal root ganglion cells, however, E_{Cl^-} is less negative than RMP, and an increase in Cl^- permeability results in depolarization. At the vertebrate neuromuscular junction, and perhaps at most receptors mediating fast excitation in vertebrates, the transmitter acts to open a channel that allows nonspecific movement of cations. This is a different channel from those specific for cations such as Na^+ and K^+, which are turned on sequentially to generate and repolarize action potentials. In invertebrates, several transmitters have been found that activate a slower pharmacologically distinguishable increase in permeability to Na^+ and Ca^{2+}. Because Ca^{2+} has so many regulatory influences on a variety of neuronal functions, transmitter control of permeability to Ca^{2+} may have significant influences beyond the immediate voltage changes (see Chaps. 15 and 19).

Some responses to neurotransmitters are not associated with a decrease in resistance

These responses may be either hyperpolarizing, presumably the result of a specific decrease in Na^+ permeability [25], or depolarizing, a decreased K^+ permeability [25], and they tend to have a slower time course than those with increased permeability. The mechanisms that generate the potentials are unknown, but they are probably energy-requiring, in contrast to those where the permeability increases (which require no energy beyond that necessary to maintain concentration gradients), and may involve a second messenger. Although it has been suggested that cAMP and cyclic GMP (cGMP) are involved in several of these slow responses and although synthesis of both substances may be stimulated by neurotransmitters, it is not yet possible to correlate rigorously these biochemical changes with electrical changes. Some responses not accompanied by clear changes in

TABLE 2. Transmitter-regulated ion channels in the vertebrate central nervous system[a]

Conductance	Transmitter	Receptor	Change	Cell effect
K$^+$ conductances				
I_A	Norepinephrine	α_1	Closes	Speeds
	Acetylcholine	M	Closes	Speeds
I_{AHP}	Acetylcholine	M_1	Reduces	Prolongs excitability
	Norepinephrine	β	Reduces	Decreases accommodation
	Norepinephrine	α_1	Reduces	Prolongs bursts
	Corticotropin-releasing factor		Reduces	Decreases accommodation
	Glutamate	KA	Reduces	Increases excitability
	Histamine	H_2	Reduces	Increases excitability
	Serotonin	1A	Reduces	Decreases accommodation
	Adenosine		Increases	Increases accommodation
	Bradykinin		Increases	Hyperpolarizes
I_{IR}	Glutamate	KA	Closes	Depolarizes
	Substance P		Closes	Depolarizes
	Dopamine	D2	Closes	Depolarizes
	Adenosine		Opens	Hyperpolarizes
	Norepinephrine	α_2?	Opens	Hyperpolarizes
	Opioids	μ, δ	Opens	Hyperpolarizes
	Dopamine	D1	Opens	Hyperpolarizes
	5-Hydroxytryptamine	1a	Opens	Hyperpolarizes
	GABA	B	Opens	Hyperpolarizes
I_M	Acetylcholine	M_1	Closes	Depolarizes
	Serotonin	1a	Closes	Depolarizes
	Substance P		Closes	Depolarizes
	Bradykinin		Closes	Depolarizes
	Somatostatin		Opens	Hyperpolarizes
Ca^{2+} conductances	Opioids	κ	Closes	Shortens action potential
	Opioids	?δ	Closes	Shortens action potential
	GABA	B	Closes	Shortens action potential
	Norepinephrine	?α_1	Closes	Shortens action potential
	Dopamine		Closes	Shortens action potential
	Acetylcholine	M	Closes	Shortens action potential

(I_A) Fast transient, rapidly inactivating outward current; (I_{AHP}) Ca^{2+}-activated outward K$^+$ current responsible for hyperpolarization that follows a burst of action potentials; (I_{IR}) inward rectifier current whose K$^+$ channel conductance decreases with membrane depolarization and increases with membrane hyperpolarization; (I_M) current due to K$^+$ channels that are closed by ACh through its muscarinic receptor.
[a] This table offers a beginning formulation of transmitter-regulated ionic conductances based on recent articles and on the emerging criteria for characterizing specific forms of ion- and voltage-regulated channels and for assessing the specific receptor subtypes involved. Because most reports before 1985 could not utilize the full range of evaluative procedures now available, it is likely that these initial designations will require modification. (From Bloom [33].)

conductance have been ascribed to activation of an electrogenic Na$^+$-K$^+$ pump, but this conclusion is controversial (see also Chap. 3). An elucidation of the mechanisms involved in responses not caused by permeability increases is one of the obvious challenges in neurobiology today.

In presynaptic inhibition, the effects of neurotransmitters on membrane resistance are of greater importance than is potential change

In some neurons, E_{Cl^-} is very near to RMP. If a transmitter increases permeability to Cl$^-$, and

E_{Cl^-} is equal to RMP, there would be no change in potential. Even so, any other input would be reduced in effectiveness. This is most easily understood by viewing the action of the second input as a current which, by Ohm's law, will produce less voltage when resistance has fallen. Since E_{Cl^-} is never very far from RMP, the short-circuiting effect of increasing Cl^- permeability may be very significant. An example is presynaptic inhibition, a process that has best been studied in the spinal cord, where it results from a synaptic ending on the presynaptic terminal of primary afferent fibers. The effect of activating this pathway onto the presynaptic terminal is to release GABA, which causes increased Cl^- permeability and a Cl^--dependent depolarization in the presynaptic terminal; in these fibers, E_{Cl^-} is less negative than RMP. In a manner not totally understood, there is a reduction in the amount of transmitter released from the presynaptic terminal when the afferent fiber discharges. The mechanism may be a short-circuiting of the terminal, due to increased Cl^- permeability, with blockade of impulse invasion into the terminal branches where transmitter release occurs. In a second type of transmitter action, the effects of neurotransmitters associated with a decrease, rather than increase, in permeability may increase the responsiveness of neurons to other synaptic inputs. Also, in this type of synapse, the permeability decreases are often associated with only modest voltage shifts, and the alteration of membrane resistance may be the most significant result.

The patch-clamp technique allows measurement of currents resulting from ion transfer through single channels of the membrane

The principle of this technique is to establish a very high resistance seal between the rim of the micropipette and the membrane of the cell [26,27]. This large recording resistance (in the gigaohm range), plus special input amplifiers, allows measurement of currents of less than 1 pA.

Four configurations of the patch-clamp have been described (Fig. 13). In one configuration, currents from the whole cell can be conveniently obtained, provided that the cell is not too large and does not have many processes. In the other three configurations, single-channel recordings are obtained. Unitary current values, conductance values for neurotransmitter-activated channels, and single-channel kinetics for durations of channel open and closed times can all be obtained using this technique.

Studies using the patch-clamp technique have measured the kinetics for opening and closing of ion channels in response to ACh. These studies were initiated by measurement of the end-plate current elicited in response to stimulation of the motor nerve. There occurs an initial delay, a rise of the end-plate current, and finally a decay, whose time course follows a single exponential with a rate constant α. This decay is voltage-dependent, being much faster at depolarizing voltages.

The decay is also temperature-dependent, with a Q_{10} of 2.8. Magleby and Stevens [28], therefore, applied a kinetic model for the binding of the agonist A to the receptor R, leading to opening of the channel. This was the model originally suggested by del Castillo and Katz [29] for the kinetics of agonist binding to the ACh receptor:

$$A + R \underset{k_{-1}}{\overset{k_{+1}}{\rightleftharpoons}} AR \underset{\alpha}{\overset{\beta}{\rightleftharpoons}} AR^* \qquad (7)$$

If the rate constants k_{+1} and k_{-1} are such that this reaction is very fast, AR is in equilibrium with A + R. If free ACh can no longer be detected in a short time period, the decay of the end-plate current can be thought of as the exponential closing of open channels AR^* with rate constant α. The AR complex could then dissociate quickly to free receptor, and the agonist would be removed by hydrolysis, as in the case

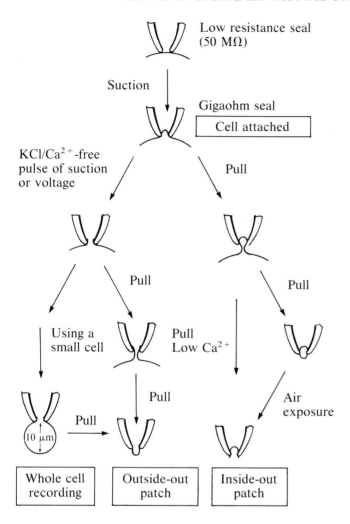

FIG. 13. Configurations of the patch-clamp technique. (From Hamill et al. [27].)

for ACh, or by uptake into the nerve terminals or glial cells. The voltage dependence of α could be explained by a gating process.

Studies on single-channel current kinetics show that the ACh receptor has several identifiable states whose transitions have known rate constants

Originally characterized electrophysiologically by Anderson and Stevens [30], these states were measured for current fluctuation and power spectra from resting and ACh-activated channels. The resulting curves showed a Lorentzian distribution such that:

$$S(f) = \frac{s(0)}{1 + (f/f_c)^2} = \frac{s(0)}{1 + (2\pi f\tau)^2} \quad (8)$$

where f is frequency; $s(0)$ is the low-frequency intercept; f_c is the corner frequency; and $\tau = \frac{1}{2}f_c$ is the relaxation time constant. The relaxation time measured by these means lengthens with cooling and hyperpolarization as shown for the end-plate current. Experiments using different agonists have shown that the open-channel lifetime is much longer with suberyldicholine and much shorter with carbamylcholine than with ACh. It is interesting that this sequence is also true at snail neurons, where suberyldicholine acts as a hyperpolarizing agent.

The early studies on single-channel currents by patch-clamp techniques showed distributions for open times with a single exponential with time and a time constant that shortened with depolarization; however, it became clear that so-called single-channel openings were interrupted by extremely short closures, and this suggests a deviation from the

kinetic scheme shown in Eq. 7. There had been some question with regard to the applicability of Eq. 7, for it was known that two molecules of ACh must combine with the receptor to cause the channel to open.

Once the two molecules are bound, the channel must be able to isomerize from the closed to the open state. The following scheme may then apply:

$$A + R \underset{k_{-1}}{\overset{k_{+1}}{\rightleftharpoons}} AR \underset{k_{-2}}{\overset{k_{+2}}{\rightleftharpoons}} A_2R \underset{\alpha}{\overset{\beta}{\rightleftharpoons}} A_2R^* \quad (9)$$

If, however, the binding reactions are much faster than the open-shut isomerization reaction, there may be many brief events resulting in this fast opening and closing. This would sug-

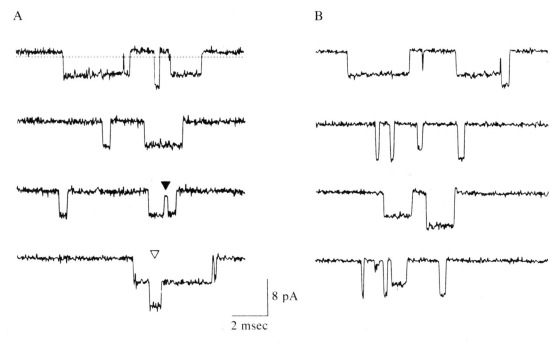

FIG. 14. ACh receptor channel currents elicited by 0.2 μM ACh from "cell-attached" patches of (**A**) 1-day- and (**B**) 6-day-cultured myotomal muscle. In the top trace (**A**) the threshold for event discrimination is indicated by a *dashed line,* computed to be 2.5 times the standard deviation of base-line fluctuations. The data were digitized at 50-μsec intervals and redisplayed in analog fashion on a Hewlett-Packard monitor. The pipette potential was +40 mV, and the intracellular potential was approximately −85 mV in both recordings. This results in an estimated patch potential of −125 mV. (▲) An example of an opening to a subconductance state; (△) coincident opening by two low-conductance channels. (From Brehm et al. [31].)

gest that there are multiple openings and closings during a single occupancy by an agonist. With high concentrations of agonist, desensitization occurs, and the pattern of channel openings becomes typically one that progresses from bursts to clusters of bursts. The clusters are separated by long silent intervals.

At the present time, single-channel responses to ACh, glutamate, GABA, and serotonin have been obtained at various sites. Table 2 shows the changes in permeability to, and postsynaptic effects of, known transmitters. Although results of early studies showed that ACh-activated channels were permeable to Na^+ and K^+, it is now clear that these channels are permeant virtually nonselectively to cations. Hille [26] states that "every monovalent or divalent cation that can fit through a 6.5 Å × 6.5 Å hole is permeant." The same appears to be also true insofar as selectivity is concerned for glutamate-activated channels, although GABA channels are selectively permeant to Cl^-.

The use of the patch-clamp technique has resulted in the finding that there are at least two populations of ACh receptor channels in muscle cells of many vertebrate species [31]: One type located at the synapse of innervated adult muscle fibers has a high (25 pS) single-channel conductance and fast kinetics; the other, found in nonsynaptic membrane of both embryonic and adult denervated muscle fibers has a lower conductance (45 pS) and slower kinetics (Fig. 14). The separation into different channel populations is not confined to neurotransmitter-activated channels but has been described also for voltage-dependent channels.

ACKNOWLEDGMENTS

I am grateful to Drs. David O. Carpenter and Thomas S. Reese for allowing me to use much of the chapter that was prepared for the earlier edition of this book. Support was provided by USPHS grant NS12211.

REFERENCES

1. Elliott, T. R. The action of adrenalin. *J. Physiol. (Lond.)* 32:401–467, 1905.
2. Loewi, O. Über humorole Übertragbarkeit der Herznervenwirkung. I. Mitteilung. *Pflugers Arch.* 189:239–242, 1921.
3. Dale, H. H. Pharmacology and nerve endings. *Proc. R. Soc. Med.* 28:319–332, 1935.
4. Eccles, J. C., Fatt, P., and Koketsu, K. Cholinergic and inhibitory synapses in a pathway from motor-axon collaterals to motoneurones. *J. Physiol. (Lond.)* 126:524–562, 1954.
5. Chan-Palay, V., and Palay, S. L. (eds). *Co-existence of Neuroactive Substances in Neurons.* New York: Wiley, 1984.
6. Leeman, S. E., and Mroz, E. A. Substance P. *Life Sci.* 15:2033–2044, 1975.
7. Heuser, J. E. Synaptic vesicle exocytosis revealed in quick-frozen frog neuromuscular junctions treated with 4-aminopyridine and given a single electrical shock. In: W. M. Cowan and J. Ferrendelli (eds.), *Approaches to the Cell Biology of Neurons.* Bethesda: Society for Neuroscience, 1976, pp. 215–239.
8. Kuffler, S. W., Nicholls, J. G., and Martin, A. R. *From Neuron to Brain.* Sunderland, MA: Sinauer, 1984.
9. Palay, S. L. Synapses in the central nervous system. *J. Biophys. Biochem. Cytol.* 2(Suppl.):193–202, 1956.
10. Couteaux, R., and Pecot-Dechavassine, M. Vesicules synaptiques et poches au niveau des "zones actives" de la junction neuromusculaire. *C. R. Acad. Sci. Ser. C. Sci. Chem.* 271:2346–2349, 1970.
11. Heuser, J. E., and Reese, T. S. Structure of the synapse. In E. R. Kandel (ed.), *Handbook of Physiology, The Nervous System I.* Bethesda: American Physiological Society, 1977, pp. 261–294.
12. Heuser, J. E., and Reese, T. S. Evidence for recycling of synaptic vesicle membrane during transmitter release at the frog neuromuscular junction. *J. Cell Biol.* 57:315–344, 1973.
13. Fatt, P., and Katz, B. Spontaneous subthreshold activity at motor nerve endings. *J. Physiol. (Lond.)* 117:109–128, 1952.

14. Boyd, I. A., and Martin, A. R. The end-plate potential in mammalian muscle. *J. Physiol. (Lond.)* 132:74–91, 1956.

15. Katz, B., and Miledi, R. The effect of calcium on acetylcholine release from motor nerve terminals. *Proc. R. Soc. Lond. (Biol.)* 161:496–503, 1965.

16. Dodge, F. A., and Rahamimoff, R. Cooperative action of calcium ions in transmitter release at the neuromuscular junction. *J. Physiol. (Lond.)* 193:419–432, 1967.

17. Llinás, R., Steinberg, I. Z., and Walton, K. Presynaptic calcium currents in squid giant synapse. *Biophys. J.* 33:289–322, 1981.

18. Llinás, R., Steinberg, I. Z., and Walton, K. Relationship between presynaptic calcium current and postsynaptic potential in squid giant synapse. *Biophys. J.* 33:323–351, 1981.

19. Browning, M. D., Huganir, R., and Greengard, P. Protein phosphorylation and neuronal function. *J. Neurochem.* 45:11–23, 1985.

20. Llinás, R., McGuinness, T. L., Leonard, C. S., Sugimori, M., and Greengard, P. Intraterminal injection of synapsin I or calcium/calmodulin-dependent protein kinase II alters neurotransmitter release at the squid giant synapse. *Proc. Natl. Acad. Sci. U.S.A.* 82:3035–3039, 1985.

21. del Castillo, J., and Katz, B. Quantal components of the end-plate potential. *J. Physiol. (Lond.)* 124:560–573, 1954.

22. Israel, M., and Lesbats, B. Continuous determination by a chemoluminescent method of acetylcholine release and compartmentation in *Torpedo* electric organ synaptosomes. *J. Neurochem.* 37:1475–1483, 1981.

23. Israel, M., Lesbats, B., and Manarande, R. ACh release from osmotically shocked synaptosomes refilled with transmitter. *Nature* 294:474–475, 1981.

24. Hodgkin, A. L., and Katz, B. The effect of sodium ions on the electrical activity of the giant axon of the squid. *J. Physiol. (Lond.)* 108:37–77, 1949.

25. Weight, F. F., and Padjen, A. Acetylcholine and slow synaptic inhibition in frog sympathetic ganglion. *Brain Res.* 55:225–228, 1973.

26. Hille, B. *Ionic Channels of Excitable Membranes.* Sunderland, MA: Sinauer, 1984.

27. Hamill, O. P., Marty, A., Neher, E., Sakmann, B., and Sigworth, F. J. Improved patch-clamp techniques for high-resolution current recording from cells and cell-free membrane patches. *Pflugers Arch.* 391:85–100, 1981.

28. Magleby, K. L., and Stevens, C. F. A quantitative description of end-plate currents. *J. Physiol. (Lond.)* 223:173–197, 1972.

29. del Castillo, J., and Katz, B. Interaction at end-plate receptors between different choline derivatives. *Proc. R. Soc. Lond. (Biol.)* 146:369–381, 1957.

30. Anderson, C. R., and Stevens, C. F. Voltage clamp analysis of acetylcholine produced end-plate current fluctuations at frog neuromuscular junction. *J. Physiol. (Lond.)* 235:655–691, 1973.

31. Brehm, P., Kidokoro, Y., and Moody-Corbett, F. Acetylcholine receptor channel properties during development of *Xenopus* muscle cells in culture. *J. Physiol. (Lond.)* 357:203–217, 1984.

32. Paton, W. D. M. Central and synaptic transmission in the nervous system (pharmacological aspects). *Annu. Rev. Physiol.* 20:431–470, 1958.

33. Bloom, F. E. Neurotransmitters: Past, present and future directions. *FASEB J.* 2:32–41, 1988.

34. Heuser, J. E., and Reese, T. S. Synaptic vesicle exocytosis captured by quick freezing. In F. O. Schmitt and F. G. Worden (eds.), *The Neurosciences Fourth Intensive Study Program.* Cambridge, MA: M.I.T. Press, 1979, pp. 573–600.

CHAPTER 9

Quantitative Aspects of Drug-Receptor Interactions

Paul McGonigle and Perry B. Molinoff

Basic Neurochemistry: Molecular, Cellular, and Medical Aspects, 4th Ed., edited by G. J. Siegel et al. Raven Press, Ltd., New York, 1989. Correspondence to Paul McGonigle, Department of Pharmacology, School of Medicine, University of Pennsylvania, Philadelphia, Pennsylvania 19104-6084.

BINDING ASSAYS WITH RADIOLIGANDS TO STUDY RECEPTORS FOR NEUROTRANSMITTERS, HORMONES, AND DRUGS

In 1971, the first successful binding assays with radioligands made it possible to study nicotinic cholinergic receptors in the electric organs of fish and eels. In 1973, the stereospecific binding of radiolabeled opiates to binding sites in mammalian brain was described. Over the next ten years, quantitative radioligand binding assays were developed for receptors for a variety of drugs and transmitters, and ligands radiolabeled with ^{3}H or ^{125}I are now available for the study of many classes of receptors. This widespread availability of suitable ligands has led to a rapid expansion in the use of binding assays with radioligands to characterize receptors and receptor subtypes [1].

Before the widespread use of *in vitro* binding assays, the properties of receptors were inferred from the measurement of biological responses. This approach proved to be productive in the classification of receptors and even led to the identification of subtypes of receptors; however, measuring a biological response either *in vivo* or *in situ* can raise several questions. For example, the tissue distribution of a drug administered *in vivo* may vary depending on its ability to cross diffusion barriers, such as the blood-brain barrier, or on the extent to which the drug binds to plasma proteins. The lipophilic or hydrophilic nature of a compound can determine whether or not it has equal access to all of the receptors in a given tissue. Drugs can also be metabolized before they have an opportunity to interact with a receptor. These metabolic transformations can yield compounds that are either more or less active than the parent drug and thus can markedly alter the observed pharmacological specificity. Drugs not subject to structural alterations are often removed from the extracellular environment by

neuronal and extraneuronal uptake mechanisms. Furthermore, *in vivo* the response to a drug is frequently attenuated by compensatory feedback mechanisms. Interpretation of a measured biological response can also be difficult if the drug has multiple sites of action—a phenomenon that can also occur *in vitro* with tissues that contain multiple classes of receptor subtypes. In some cases, the receptor subtypes mediate the same physiological response, and they may exert these effects through the same effector system. The observed pharmacological response will then be affected by the degree of selectivity of the drug and by the relative densities of the subtypes present in the tissue. In general, the most reliable characterization of receptors results from studies carried out with simple, isolated tissue preparations that exhibit reproducible, graded dose-response curves. Even with such preparations, it is often impossible to define accurately the kinetic characteristics of drug-receptor interactions.

Radioligand binding techniques supplement and overcome many limitations of studies of biological responses

Radioligands provide precise probes that permit specific examination of the initial interaction between a drug and its binding site. For example, the kinetics of association and dissociation of a receptor-radioligand complex can be accurately determined by using simple tissue homogenates. A pharmacological profile that is based on the equilibrium dissociation constants of a series of unlabeled ligands can be defined by measuring the inhibition of the binding of a radioligand by these unlabeled compounds. The use of radioligands also permits characterization of receptors in the absence of a measurable biological response. This may be important, for example, in the study of central nervous system receptors, where the effects of neurotransmitters are complex and isolated tissue preparations difficult to obtain. The use of binding assays with radioligands can result in meaningful estimates of the number or density of receptors in a particular tissue. Consequently, changes in the density of receptors resulting from pathological conditions or pharmacological interventions can be monitored. Binding assays can also be used to discriminate multiple classes of receptors in a single tissue and to estimate their relative proportions. Moreover, binding assays with radioligands provide the only means by which receptors can be measured during solubilization, purification, and reconstitution—steps necessary for the complete understanding of receptor function.

Two basic types of assays utilize radioligands. The first, direct binding assays, measure the direct interaction of a radioligand with a receptor. Direct binding assays permit determination of both kinetic and equilibrium properties and provide estimates of the receptor density. They are also used to choose appropriate conditions and radioligands to determine the pharmacological properties of receptors. The second, indirect binding assays, measure the inhibition of the binding of a radioligand by an unlabeled ligand to deduce indirectly the affinity of receptors for the unlabeled ligand. This approach is particularly useful in the pharmacological characterization of receptors because studies can be carried out with compounds that would not be suitable radioligands, either because they are too lipophilic or because the receptor affinity for these compounds is too low.

DIRECT BINDING ASSAYS MEASURE BINDING OF A RADIOLIGAND TO A RECEPTOR

Equilibrium analysis

Analysis of untransformed data

The simplest model describing the interaction of a receptor, R, with a radioligand, L, to form a complex, RL, is the bimolecular reaction

$$[L] + [R] \underset{k_{-1}}{\overset{k_{+1}}{\rightleftharpoons}} [RL] \qquad (1)$$

(see Table 1). The concentration of the receptor-radioligand complex [RL] is frequently referred to as the amount bound [B]. According to the laws of mass action, at equilibrium,

$$K_d = \frac{[R][L]}{[B]} \qquad (2)$$

where K_d is the equilibrium dissociation constant. When studying receptors, it is important to distinguish between the total concentration

TABLE 1. Symbols used in this chapter

[L]	Concentration of radioligand
[R]	Concentration of receptor
[RL] = [B]	Concentration of receptor-radioligand complex
k_{+1}	Rate constant for association
k_{-1}	Rate constant for dissociation
K_d, K_{d1}, K_{d2}	Equilibrium dissociation constant, k_{-1}/k_{+1}
B_{max}, B_{max1}, B_{max2}	Total concentration of receptors
F	Free ligand concentration
t	Time
$[L_t]$	Total concentration of radioligand
$[B_e]$	Concentration of receptor-radioligand complex at equilibrium
[I]	Concentration of competitive inhibitor
$[B_i]$	Concentration of receptor-inhibitor complex
K_i, K_{i1}, K_{i2}	Equilibrium dissociation constant for a competitive inhibitor
IC$_{50}$, IC$_1$, IC$_2$	Concentration of competitive inhibitor that inhibits 50 percent of the binding of a radioligand to a receptor
B, B_0, B_1, B_2	Concentration of receptor-radioligand complex in the absence of a competitive inhibitor
n_H	Hill coefficient

of ligand [L] in an assay and the free concentration of ligand in solution at equilibrium ([L] − [B]). The kinetic rate constants, k_{+1} and k_{-1}, and the equilibrium dissociation constant, K_d, are related such that

$$K_d = k_{-1}/k_{+1} \qquad (3)$$

Since the total number of receptors B_{max} = [R] + [B], substitution for [R] in Eq. 2 yields

$$K_d = \frac{(B_{max} - [B])[L]}{[B]} \qquad (4)$$

which can be rearranged to form

$$[B] = \frac{B_{max}[L]}{[L] + K_d} \qquad (5)$$

In a typical "saturation" experiment, increasing amounts of a radioligand are added to a fixed concentration of receptors, and the amount of radioligand bound to the receptor, [B], is measured as a function of the concentration of radioligand. The concentration of radioligand is increased until virtually all the receptors are occupied by the ligand (Fig. 1). Nonlinear regression analysis can be used to fit Eq. 5 to the data to provide estimates of both K_d and B_{max}.

In practice, the radioligand binds not only to the receptor, but also to other components of the assay system, including the wall of glass test tubes, filter paper, and constituents of the tissue. Although the exact nature of this nonspecific binding is unknown, it usually occurs instantaneously. Nonspecific binding is generally nonsaturable and is proportional to the concentration of radioligand (Fig. 1). An incorrect definition of this nonspecific component is a common source of error in the analysis of radioligand binding data (see p. 200), resulting in an overestimate of the density of receptors and in some cases to the incorrect conclusion that multiple classes of receptors coexist in a given tissue [2]. Nonspecific binding can be quantified

by adding high concentrations of an unlabeled competing ligand that is specific for the receptor of interest. The amount of radioligand that remains bound in the presence of the unlabeled ligand is defined as nonspecific binding. In a saturation experiment, the nonspecific component of binding at each concentration of radioligand is subtracted from the total amount of radioligand bound to yield the amount of radioligand specifically bound to the receptor (Fig. 1). The amount of nonspecific binding should be the same in experiments carried out with a variety of unlabeled ligands, including both agonists and antagonists. In general, the best results are obtained when the drug used to define specific binding is of a different chemical class from that of the radioligand and when the concentration of the competing ligand is approximately 100 times its K_d value. Higher concentrations of a competing ligand can inhibit nonspecific as well as specific binding.

Scatchard analysis

A useful method for analyzing binding data is to construct a Scatchard plot [3]. Rearrangement of Eq. 4 for equilibrium binding yields the following relationship:

$$\frac{[B]}{[L]} = \frac{B_{max}}{K_d} - \frac{[B]}{K_d} \qquad (6)$$

A plot of the ratio of bound [B] to free [L] ligand against the concentration of bound ligand is a straight line that has a slope equal to the negative reciprocal of the dissociation constant, $(-1/K_d)$, and an intercept on the abscissa equal to the total concentration of receptors (B_{max}) (Fig. 1).

An advantage of using Scatchard analysis is that it provides an estimate of the total concentration of receptors without requiring saturating concentrations of radioligand. The concentration of receptors can be estimated by extrapolating a straight line to the abscissa;

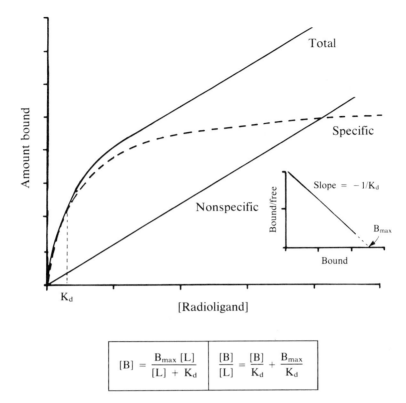

$$[B] = \frac{B_{max}\,[L]}{[L] + K_d} \qquad \frac{[B]}{[L]} = \frac{[B]}{K_d} + \frac{B_{max}}{K_d}$$

FIG. 1. Analysis of saturation data. The amount of radioligand specifically bound to the receptor is determined by subtracting the amount of radioligand bound nonspecifically from the total amount bound. The left-hand equation describes the relationship between specific binding $[B]$ and the concentration of radioligand $[L]$ in terms of the total number of receptors B_{max} and the equilibrium dissociation constant K_d. **Inset:** Transformation of the saturation equation by the Scatchard method results in the right-hand equation, which describes the linear relationship between bound/free and bound. The slope of this line is $-1/K_d$ and the intercept on the abscissa is B_{max}.

however, estimates of B_{max} made by nonlinear regression analysis or Scatchard analysis are subject to significant error if the highest concentration of radioligand does not at least exceed the K_d value. This is particularly important in systems with high levels of nonspecific binding. Another advantage of the Scatchard plot is that visual inspection provides insight into whether or not a simple bimolecular reaction adequately describes the interaction between ligand and receptor. Curvature of a Scatchard plot implies that this interaction is complex. A Scatchard plot that is concave upward can re-

sult from a heterogeneous population of receptors, a multistep/multicomponent binding reaction, or negative cooperativity between the binding sites. These possibilities can be discriminated by detailed kinetic analysis [4]. A Scatchard plot that is concave downward can result from positive cooperativity between the binding sites or from failure of the reaction to reach equilibrium at low concentrations of the ligand, since the time to reach equilibrium is a function of the concentration of ligand. These possibilities can also be discriminated by kinetic analysis.

Curvilinear Scatchard plots can also be produced artifactually by a variety of factors (see below). Some of the more common factors include an incorrect definition of nonspecific binding, incomplete separation of bound and free ligand, and dissociation of the receptor-ligand complex during the separation of bound and free ligand. If too high a concentration of competing ligand is used to define nonspecific binding (see above), a Scatchard plot that is concave upward will result. These factors are discussed in detail by Boeynaems and Dumont [5] and Weiland and Molinoff [6].)

Kinetic analysis

Rate of association

The rate of association of a radioligand with a receptor is determined by measuring the amount of bound ligand $[B]$ as a function of time. At time $t = 0$, a specific concentration of radioligand $[L]$ is added, and the amount of bound ligand $[B]$ is measured at various times until equilibrium is reached. The amount of radioligand bound at a given time depends on the simultaneously occurring processes of association and dissociation. In the simple bimolecular reaction described in Eq. 1, the rate of association of ligand receptor complex is $k_{+1}[L][R]$, and the rate of dissociation of this complex is $k_{-1}[B]$. Thus, the measured rate of formation of $[B]$ is

$$\frac{d[B]}{dt} = k_{+1}[L][R] - k_{-1}[B] \qquad (7)$$

At equilibrium, $d[B]/dt = 0$, and

$$k_{+1}[L][R] = k_{-1}[B] \qquad (8)$$

The values $[L]$ and $[R]$ can be expressed in terms of equilibrium measurements as follows:

$$[L] = [L_t] - [B_e]; \qquad [R] = B_{max} - [B_e]$$

Substitution into Eq. 8 yields

$$k_{+1}([L_t] - [B_e])(B_{max} - [B_e])$$
$$= k_{-1}[B_e] \qquad (9)$$

which can be rearranged to form

$$k_{-1} = k_{+1} \frac{([L_t] - [B_e])(B_{max} - [B_e])}{[B_e]} \qquad (10)$$

Substitution for k_{-1} in Eq. 7 yields

$$\frac{d[B]}{dt} = k_{+1}([L_t] - [B_e])(B_{max} - [B_e])$$
$$- k_{+1}[B] \frac{[L_t] - [B_e](B_{max} - [B_e])}{[B_e]} \qquad (11)$$

which describes the formation of receptor-ligand complex in terms of the association rate constant k_{+1}. The second-order rate equation (Eq. 11) can be integrated to give

$$\ln \frac{[B_e]([L_t] - [B][B_e])/B_{max}}{[L_t]([B_e] - [B])}$$
$$= \left[k_{+1}t \frac{[L_t](B_{max} - [B_e])}{[B_e]} \right] \qquad (12)$$

The rate constant of association can be determined from the slope of a plot of the expression on the left-hand side of Eq. 12 against time (Fig. 2). If the reaction obeys simple bimolecular kinetics, this plot will result in a straight line. The only parameter in Eq. 12 that varies as a function of time is $[B]$. $[L_t]$ is the total amount of radioligand added at the start of the reaction; $[B_e]$ is the amount of radioligand bound at equilibrium; and B_{max} is the number of receptors determined by Scatchard analysis of a saturation experiment performed with the same tissue. One disadvantage of this analysis is that the association rate constant is not independent of the equilibrium dissociation constant K_d be-

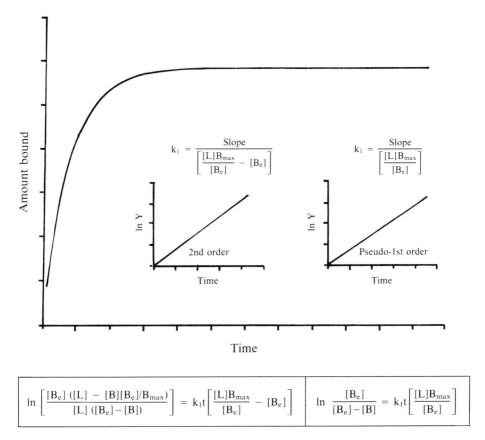

FIG. 2. Determination of association rate. The amount of radioligand bound is measured at various times. **Left inset:** Association is plotted according to the integrated form of the second-order rate equation, where $[B_e]$ is the amount of radioligand bound at equilibrium; k_{+1} is the association rate constant; and $Y = [B_e]([L] - [B] \cdot [B_e])/B_{max}/[L]([B_e] - [B])$. This plot is linear, and k_{+1} is directly related to the slope. **Right inset:** Association is plotted according to the integrated form of the pseudo-first-order rate equation, where $Y = [B_e]/([B_e] - [B])$. This equation assumes that the concentration of radioligand $[L]$ is much greater than the total concentration of receptors B_{max}. This plot is linear, and k_{+1} is directly related to the slope.

cause the term B_{max} appears in Eq. 12; however, the advantage of using the full second-order equation is that no assumptions are made about the relative concentrations of radioligand or receptor.

In many studies of the binding of radioligands, the total concentration of radioligand $[L_t]$ is much greater than the total concentration of receptors $[B_{max}]$. Under these conditions there is little or no change in the concentration of free ligand $[L]$ as the reaction proceeds to equilibrium. Even at equilibrium, only a small fraction of the total concentration of ligand $[L_t]$ is bound to the receptor. For all practical purposes, $[L]$ is a constant, and the reaction can be considered a "pseudo-first-order" reaction. Thus, Eq. 12 can be simplified to [6]:

$$\ln \frac{[B_e]}{[B_e] + [B]} = k_{+1}t \frac{[L_t]B_{max}}{[B_e]} \quad (13)$$

A plot of the term on the left-hand side of Eq. 13 versus time is called a pseudo-first-order plot (Fig. 2). The association rate constant, k_{+1}, is related to the slope of the pseudo-first-order plot, as follows:

$$k_{+1} = \frac{\text{Slope}}{[L_t]B_{max}/[B_e]} \qquad (14)$$

where $[L_t]$, B_{max}, and $[B_e]$ are constants. In addition to the assumption that $[L_t] \gg [B_e]$, the determination of k_{+1} again depends on the equilibrium measurement of B_{max}.

One method of analyzing the pseudo-first-order time course eliminates the need for an in-

dependent determination of B_{max}. This method requires measurement of the slopes of pseudo-first-order plots over a range of ligand concentrations. The slope of the pseudo-first-order plot is called k_{obs}. It can be shown that k_{obs} is related to the ligand concentration [L] as follows:

$$k_{obs} = k_{+1}[L] + k_{-1} \qquad (15)$$

A plot of k_{obs} versus ligand concentration results in a straight line with a slope equal to k_{+1} and an intercept on the ordinate equal to k_{-1} (Fig. 3).

The association and dissociation rate constants determined by this method can be com-

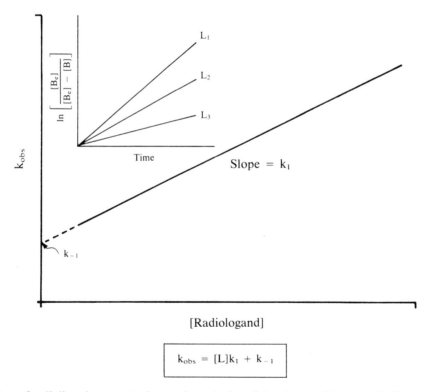

FIG. 3. Effect of radioligand concentration on k_{obs}. A plot of the slopes of the pseudo-first-order rate plots (k_{obs}) versus the concentrations of radioligand at which the association rates were measured is linear. The equation describing the relationship of k_{obs} to the rates of association (k_{+1}) and dissociation (k_{-1}) is shown. Use of this method to determine the association rate constant k_{+1} does not require independent determination of the total number of receptors. **Inset:** Pseudo-first-order rate plots measured at different concentrations of radioligand.

pared to the rate constants determined at a single concentration of ligand to confirm their accuracy. Curvilinear second-order plots and pseudo-first-order plots imply that a simple bimolecular reaction is not adequate to describe the interaction between the ligand and the receptor. More complex kinetics may result from the same factors that yield curvilinear Scatchard plots [2,6–8]. Moreover, under certain conditions, the use of radioligands that are racemic mixtures will result in multiple rate constants for association and dissociation [6]. Even when second-order or pseudo-first-order plots are linear, a more complex interaction is implied if the relationship between k_{obs} and concentration of the ligand is nonlinear. A ligand-induced conformational change in the receptor would cause such a relationship; however, detailed kinetics and equilibrium analysis are required to verify this model [6].

Rate of dissociation

The rate of dissociation is determined by stopping the association of the ligand and receptor and measuring the amount of radioligand that remains bound as a function of time. In practice, the reaction between receptor and ligand is allowed to reach equilibrium, and the forward reaction is stopped by "infinite dilution" or by the addition of a high concentration of an unlabeled competing ligand. The rate of change of the concentration of the receptor-ligand complex is defined by

$$d[B]/dt = -k_{-1}[B] \tag{16}$$

Integration of Eq. 16 yields

$$\ln[B]/[B_0] = -k_{-1}t \tag{17}$$

where $[B_0]$ is the concentration of receptor-ligand complex just prior to dilution or the addition of a competing ligand. The dissociation rate constant, k_{-1}, a simple first-order rate constant, is the negative of the slope of a plot of

$\ln[B]/[B_0]$ versus time (Fig. 4). A simple bimolecular reaction should be completely reversible; therefore, if the experiment is carried out for a sufficiently long time, the ligand should completely dissociate from the receptor.

Determining the dissociation rate constant has important methodological implications for the study of receptors. The most common technique used to study the binding of radioligands utilizes vacuum filtration to separate bound from free ligand. This process usually involves a 15-sec exposure to buffer during dilution, filtration, and rinsing of the filter. If the dissociation rate is too rapid, as indicated by a high rate constant, there will be a measurable loss of bound ligand during the filtration. This can sometimes be prevented by stopping the reaction and measuring bound ligand at a low temperature.

Nonlinear first-order dissociation plots may result from the same factors that can account for curvilinear second-order and pseudo-first-order association plots. In addition, if k_{-1} is dependent on the method of displacement, then cooperativity in binding should be suspected [9]. A more rapid dissociation by dilution than by competitive displacement implies positive cooperativity, whereas a more rapid dissociation by displacement than by dilution implies negative cooperativity. A two-step binding reaction that involves a third component can also cause the dissociation rate to vary with the method of displacement [7,8]. When using competitive displacement, it is sometimes useful to examine effects of both agonists and antagonists.

Once the association and dissociation rate constants have been determined, their ratio can be calculated to provide a kinetically determined estimate of the dissociation constant ($K_d = k_{-1}/k_{+1}$). This value can be compared to the dissociation constant derived from saturation experiments carried out under equilibrium conditions to verify its accuracy and to validate the assumptions made during the analysis. A sig-

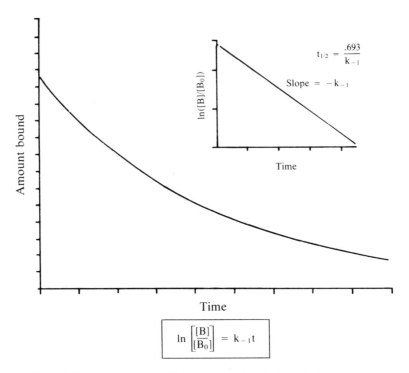

$$\ln\left[\frac{[B]}{[B_0]}\right] = k_{-1}t$$

FIG. 4. Determination of dissociation rate. The amount of radioligand that remains bound following the termination of association is measured at various times. **Inset:** Dissociation is plotted according to the integrated form of the first-order rate equation, where $[B]/[B_0]$ is the ratio of the amount of ligand bound at a given time to the amount of radioligand bound just prior to the termination of association. The slope of this linear plot is equal to the negative of the dissociation rate constant k_{-1}.

nificant discrepancy between the K_d value determined kinetically and at equilibrium implies that a simple bimolecular reaction is an inadequate model for the system and a more detailed kinetic analysis is required.

INDIRECT BINDING ASSAYS MEASURE INHIBITION OF RADIOLIGAND BINDING TO A RECEPTOR

Equilibrium analysis

The interactions of unlabeled ligands with a receptor can be characterized by studying their ability to inhibit the binding of a radioligand. Since unlabeled ligands are far more numerous than radioligands, indirect binding assays are essential to characterize a population of receptors completely. Traditionally, receptors have been classified in terms of the order of potency of various compounds that either cause or antagonize a functional response. Indirect binding assays make it possible to define the pharmacological specificity of a receptor based on the dissociation constants for a variety of compounds determined from inhibition of the binding of a radioligand. Another important use of indirect binding assays is to define the level of nonspecific binding. An accurate definition of nonspecific binding is required for the analysis of both direct and indirect binding data and should be established prior to determining the kinetic and equilibrium properties of the radioligand.

Analysis of untransformed data

The simplest model describing the interaction of a radioligand [L] and a competitive inhibitor [I] with a receptor is

$$[L] + [R] \underset{k_{-1}}{\overset{k_{+1}}{\rightleftharpoons}} [B] \tag{18}$$

$$[I] + [R] \underset{k_{-1i}}{\overset{k_{+1i}}{\rightleftharpoons}} [B_i] \tag{19}$$

According to the laws of mass action, the rates of formation of $[B]$ and $[B_i]$ are

$$\frac{d[B]}{dt} = k_{+1}[L](B_{max} - [B] - [B_i]) - k_{-1}[B] \tag{20}$$

$$\frac{d[B_i]}{dt} = k_{+1i}[I](B_{max} - [B] - [B_i]) - k_{-1i}[B_i] \tag{21}$$

At equilibrium, $d[B]/dt = d[B_i]/dt = 0$, and the following equation for $[B_i]$ can be derived from Eqs. 20 and 21:

$$[B_i] = \frac{B_{max}[I]}{[I] + K_i(1 + [L]/K_d)} \tag{22}$$

In this equation, K_i is the equilibrium dissociation constant of the competitive inhibitor. If K_d is much greater than the concentration of receptors in the assay, Eq. 22 may be simplified to

$$[B_i] = \frac{B_{max}[I]}{[I] + IC_{50}} \tag{23}$$

where IC_{50} is the concentration of inhibitor that blocks 50 percent of the binding measured in the absence of inhibitor.

In a typical competition experiment, the binding of a fixed concentration of radioligand is inhibited by increasing concentrations of an unlabeled ligand. The amount of radioligand that is bound to the receptor, $[B]$, is

$$[B] = [B_0] - \frac{[B_0] - [I]}{[I] + IC_{50}} \tag{24}$$

Equation 24 can be rearranged to a simpler form:

$$[B] = \frac{[B_0]}{1 + [I]/IC_{50}} \tag{25}$$

Nonlinear regression analysis can be used to fit Eq. 25 to experimental data to provide an estimate of the IC_{50} value (Fig. 5).

Cheng and Prusoff correction

The equilibrium dissociation constant K_i of an unlabeled competing ligand, [I], is related to the IC_{50} value, as described by Cheng and Prusoff [10]:

$$K_i = \frac{IC_{50}}{1 + [L]/K_d} \tag{26}$$

Since the concentration of free unlabeled ligand is difficult to determine experimentally, it is approximated by the total concentration of unlabeled ligand in the assay. This calculation is valid if the concentration of receptors is much lower than the dissociation constant of the unlabeled ligand. Furthermore, the amount of radioligand bound should be much less than the total concentration of radioligand; otherwise, a significant change in the concentration of free radioligand will occur in the presence of high concentrations of unlabeled competing ligand. If assay conditions are such that $[L]/K_d \ll 1$, then $K_i \approx IC_{50}$.

Hill plot

Another useful method for analyzing indirect binding data is the construction of an indirect

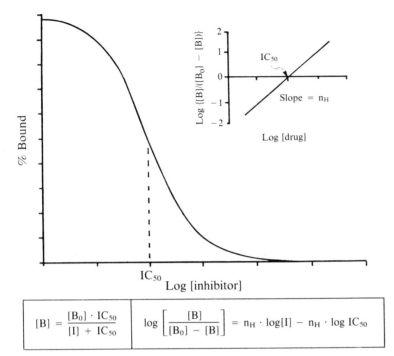

FIG. 5. Analysis of competition data. The amount of radioligand bound in the presence of increasing concentrations of an unlabeled competing ligand is measured. The left–hand equation describes the relationship between the amount of radioligand bound $[B]$ and the concentration of inhibitor $[I]$ in terms of the amount of radioligand bound in the absence of inhibitor $[B_0]$ and the concentration of inhibitor that inhibits 50 percent of the binding of the radioligand (IC_{50}). **Inset.** A Hill plot is constructed according to the transformation described by the right-hand equation. The slope of this linear plot is equal to the Hill coefficient (n_H) and the intercept is log IC_{50}. The Hill plot deviates from linearity when the amount bound is greater than 90 percent or less than 10 percent of $[B_0]$.

$$[B] = \frac{[B_0] \cdot IC_{50}}{[I] + IC_{50}} \qquad \log\left[\frac{[B]}{[B_0] - [B]}\right] = n_H \cdot \log[I] - n_H \cdot \log IC_{50}$$

Hill plot [11] from the following equation:

$$\log \frac{[B]}{[B_0] - [B]} = n_H \cdot \log[I] - n_H \cdot \log IC_{50}$$

$$(27)$$

A plot of log $([B]/([B_0] - [B]))$ versus log[I] has a slope value of n_H, which is the apparent Hill coefficient, and an intercept on the abscissa of log IC_{50}. Only those concentrations of unlabeled ligand that inhibit between 10 and 90 percent of specific binding are included, since the Hill plot deviates from linearity at the extremes [12]. If the reaction follows mass action principles at equilibrium, the apparent Hill coefficient will be equal to 1. A Hill coefficient significantly different from 1 indicates a more complex interaction between ligand and receptor. This may result from a heterogeneous population of binding sites, a two-step/three-component binding system, negative or positive cooperativity between sites or an incorrect definition of nonspecific binding [12].

It is important to note that addition of a competing ligand increases the time required for a binding reaction to reach equilibrium. Thus the incubation time of a binding assay carried out in the presence of a competing ligand should be greater than the time required for the binding of a radioligand to reach equilibrium in a direct binding assay. Under pseudo-first-order conditions, the time to equilibrium will be increased at most by a factor of $1 + [L]/K_d$ in the presence of a competing ligand [6].

Kinetic analysis

The rates of association and dissociation of an unlabeled competing ligand with a receptor can be determined by measuring the time course of the binding of a radioligand in the presence of a competing ligand. The concentration of receptors that can interact with a radioligand at any given time in the presence of a competing ligand will be reduced by an amount dependent on the rate of approach to equilibrium and the concentration of the competitor. Thus, the presence of competing ligand alters the time course of binding of radioligand. One of two approaches may be taken to determine the rates of association and dissociation of the unlabeled ligand. The kinetic rate constants for the radioligand may be determined in a separate experiment and substituted in the equation for the time course of the binding of the radioligand in the presence of a competing ligand [14]. Nonlinear regression analysis of data obtained in the presence of a competing ligand is used to derive estimates of the kinetic rate constant for the competing ligand. Alternatively, the time course for the binding of the radioligand can be measured in the absence and presence of the competing ligand. Simultaneous nonlinear regression analysis of both sets of data will provide estimates of the kinetic rate constants for both the radioligand and the competing ligand. The validity of this indirect method of determination of kinetic rate constants has been verified for several ligands that bind to β-adrenergic receptors [15].

There are two important limitations to the application of this method. Derivation of the equations assumes that pseudo-first-order conditions prevail, and violation of this assumption will invalidate the results of the analysis [14]. Thus assays should be carried out under conditions where less than 5 percent of the radioligand is bound to receptor at equilibrium. In addition, if binding of the competing ligand reaches equilibrium before the radioligand is bound to an appreciable extent, the kinetic rate constants cannot be resolved statistically [15].

RECEPTOR SUBTYPES

Subtypes of receptors for a variety of neurotransmitters exist in the central nervous system and peripheral tissues

Radioligand binding assays are routinely used to characterize the kinetic properties of receptor subtypes in a wide variety of tissues. This characterization is independent of the functional responses elicited by the receptors. The ligand-binding properties are particularly important in the study of the central nervous system because the effects mediated by neurotransmitter receptors are often complex behaviors that are not easily quantified. Under these circumstances, it is difficult to use classical pharmacological techniques to characterize the relevant receptors. Studies of the binding of radioligands, used extensively in the central nervous system, make it possible to discriminate subtypes of receptors that coexist in the same tissue. For example, β_1- and β_2-adrenergic receptors have been shown to coexist in a variety of mammalian tissues. Both subtypes stimulate the enzyme adenylate cyclase and both contribute to the chronotropic effects of catecholamines on the heart [16]. Characterization of β-adrenergic receptor subtypes based on studies of the chronotropic effects of various drugs would be likely to yield ambiguous results, whereas radioligand binding studies can provide a pharmacological profile for each subtype in a tissue and a measure of the relative proportion of each. Two approaches, based on direct and indirect assays, have been developed to study receptors in tissues that contain multiple receptor subtypes.

Direct binding assays utilize a radioligand selective for one subtype

If a radioligand is completely selective, the density of a single receptor subtype can be determined from a saturation experiment, and the pharmacological profile for this receptor subtype can be determined from studies of the inhibition of the binding of this radioligand by various competing ligands. Many radioligands have been shown to be highly selective. These include prazosin at the α_1, clonidine at the α_2, and receptor, α-bungarotoxin at the nicotinic cholinergic receptors and iodobenzamide and SCH 23390 at D_2 and D_1 receptors. If, as is more common, multiple classes of receptors bind a given radioligand with different affinities, nonlinear regression analysis of the saturation data provides estimates of the relative densities of the subtypes and their affinities for the radioligand.

Nonlinear regression analysis

In addition to the existence of receptor subtypes, it is possible for a radioligand to have a high affinity for receptors for multiple neurotransmitters. For example, both dopamine and serotonin receptors in mammalian brain have a high affinity for [^{3}H]spiroperidol. Multiple populations of receptors or receptor subtypes can be detected in a saturation experiment if the radioligand is selective in that it has a significantly lower dissociation constant for its interaction with one class of receptors than for its interaction with the other. The interaction of a radioligand with two types of receptors is modeled as the sum of two independent bimolecular reactions. At equilibrium, the total amount of radioligand bound [B] is

$$[B] = \frac{[L]B_{max1}}{[L] + K_{d1}} + \frac{[L]B_{max2}}{[L] + K_{d2}} \quad (28)$$

Nonlinear least-squares regression analysis can be used to fit Eq. 28 to saturation data (Fig. 6) to provide estimates of the dissociation constants and the densities of each population of receptors. Results from this analysis must be interpreted with caution, since all of the factors identified above that lead to curvilinear Scatchard plots also cause complex saturation curves. The statistical validity of the two-site model is tested by comparing the goodness of fit of the one-site (Eq. 5) and two-site (Eq. 28) models. The improvement of fit is estimated from an F-test on the sum of squares of the residuals [19].

Scatchard transformation

Scatchard transformation of saturation data for the interaction of a selective radioligand with multiple subtypes of receptor will result in a curvilinear plot (Fig. 6, inset). The degree of curvature will be determined by the selectivity of the radioligand and the relative proportions of binding sites with high and low affinities for the radioligand. The greater the selectivity of the radioligand, the more marked will be the curvature observed in the Scatchard plot. It is difficult to use transformed data of this kind to obtain estimates of the parameters of the two subtypes. The dependent variable, amount of ligand bound, appears on both the abscissa and the ordinate; therefore, individual Scatchard equations cannot be simply added together. Moreover, any error in the measurement of the amount of radioligand bound is propagated from the abscissa to the ordinate. The ratio of bound to free ligand also demonstrates nonuniformity of variance, thus violating a basic assumption of regression analysis [4]. In the presence of multiple classes of receptors, the Scatchard plot is most effectively used to provide visual confirmation of the existence of a heterogeneous population of binding sites.

Indirect binding assays utilize a selective competing unlabeled ligand

Since selective radioligands are not available for most subtypes of receptor, an approach has been developed to take advantage of the availability of numerous selective unlabeled ligands. This method involves studies of the inhibition of the binding of a nonselective radioligand by unlabeled competing selective ligands. The relative proportions of the subtypes and their affinities for each ligand can be determined by nonlinear regression analysis of inhibition curves. Regardless of the ligand used for the determination, the number and relative proportions of the subtypes in a specific tissue should always be the same. In practice, it is usually impossible to discriminate more than two or at most three receptor subtypes on the basis of nonlinear regression analysis. The limits of resolution of

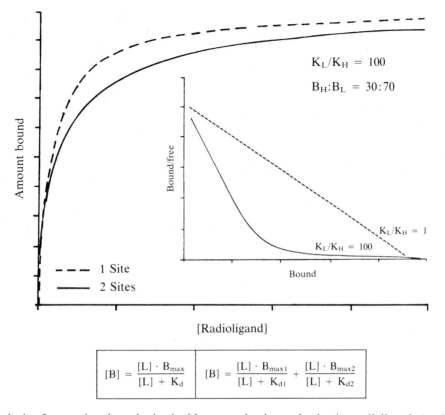

$$[B] = \frac{[L] \cdot B_{max}}{[L] + K_d} \qquad [B] = \frac{[L] \cdot B_{max1}}{[L] + K_{d1}} + \frac{[L] \cdot B_{max2}}{[L] + K_{d2}}$$

FIG. 6. Analysis of saturation data obtained with a nonselective and selective radioligand: (- - -) binding of a nonselective ligand according to the one-site equation (*left*), (—) binding of a 100-fold selective (K_L/K_H = 100) radioligand according to the two-site equation (*right*), assuming that 30 percent of the receptors have a high affinity for the radioligand. **Inset:** Scatchard transformation of the saturation data results in a linear plot for the nonselective radioligand and a markedly curvilinear plot for the selective ligand.

nonlinear regression analysis depend on the relative proportions of the subtypes present and on the selectivity of the ligands. These limits have been experimentally evaluated in studies of β-adrenergic receptors by combining various proportions of previously characterized preparations of β_1- and β_2-adrenergic receptors [17]. A mixture of receptor subtypes present in a ratio of 9:1 or 1:9 required ligands that were at least 70-fold selective to resolve the properties of each subtype. Alternatively, a competing ligand that was only sixfold selective discriminated a 50:50 mixture of receptor subtypes [17].

It is also important to verify that all the ligands are interacting with the receptors according to the principles of mass action. This is accomplished by performing indirect binding assays in tissues that contain only one subtype of receptor. Analysis of inhibition data from these tissues should yield Hill coefficients equal to 1. This has been demonstrated for subtypes of the β-adrenergic receptor in studies of the binding of [125I]iodohydroxypindolol in rat cortex, rat liver, and guinea pig ventricle. The rat cortex contains both β_1- and β_2-adrenergic receptors and studies carried out with selective unlabeled antagonists resulted in markedly biphasic inhibition curves. In contrast, in the guinea pig ventricle, which contains only β_1 receptors, and the rat liver, which contains only β_2 receptors, each antagonist produced monophasic inhibition curves and Hill coefficients of 1 [18].

If the concept of a receptor is to have any meaning, the properties of the receptor should be conserved in different tissues. Thus, the pharmacological profile of a receptor subtype should be the same, regardless of whether it is derived from tissues that contain a single subtype or tissues that contain multiple subtypes. This has been demonstrated in the β-adrenergic system where the dissociation constants for seven selective drugs measured in heterogeneous and homogeneous tissues were compared. The correlation coefficient for both β_1 and β_2 receptors for heterogeneous, compared to homogeneous, tissues was found to be 0.99 [18].

Nonlinear regression analysis

A Hill coefficient less than 1 often results from the presence of multiple classes of receptors. If an unlabeled competing ligand is selective for one of the subtypes—if it has a measurably lower dissociation constant for one population of sites than for the other—then inhibition curves will be shallow and Hill coefficients will be less than 1. Inhibition of the binding of a nonselective radioligand by a selective competing ligand is described by

$$[B] = \frac{[B_1]}{1 + [I]/IC_1} + \frac{[B_2]}{1 + [I]/IC_2} \quad (29)$$

Nonlinear regression analysis is used to provide estimates for each of the parameters. This analysis assumes that the interaction of both the radioligand and the competing ligand with each receptor subtype follows the principles of mass action. The improvement in fit with the two-site model (Eq. 29) compared to the one-site model (Eq. 25) is determined from the F value calculated from the residual sum of squares [20] (Fig. 7).

Accurate estimates of the density of each

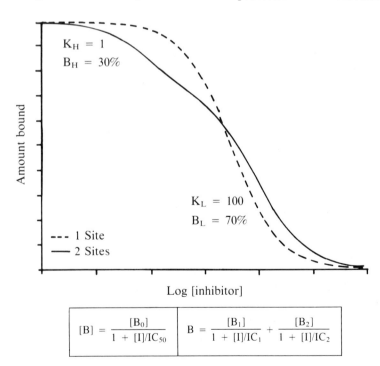

$K_H = 1$
$B_H = 30\%$

$K_L = 100$
$B_L = 70\%$

--- 1 Site
— 2 Sites

Amount bound

Log [inhibitor]

$$[B] = \frac{[B_0]}{1 + [I]/IC_{50}} \qquad B = \frac{[B_1]}{1 + [I]/IC_1} + \frac{[B_2]}{1 + [I]/IC_2}$$

FIG. 7. Analysis of untransformed competition data. The inhibition of the binding of a nonselective radioligand by a selective and a nonselective competing ligand is illustrated: (- - -) inhibition resulting from a nonselective ligand (*left-hand equation*); (—) inhibition by a 100-fold selective (K_L/K_H) competing ligand, assuming that 30 percent of the receptors have a high affinity for the competing ligand.

class of receptors and the affinity of each class of site for a selective competing ligand will only be obtained if the radioligand is entirely non-selective. Selectivity of only two- to threefold can markedly influence the results of subtype analysis [21]. The conclusion that a radioligand is nonselective is usually based on analysis of a saturation binding curve as discussed above; however, the ability of these analytical methods to determine the selectivity of a radioligand is limited. Even under ideal conditions, selectivity is unlikely to be detected reliably unless the two classes of binding sites differ in their affinity for the radioligand by at least five- to sevenfold. Such slight selectivity can be detected by the analysis of multiple inhibition curves. The interaction of a selective radioligand and a selective competing ligand with two classes of receptors is described by Eq. 30:

$$[B] = \frac{B_{max1}[I]}{1 + K_{i1}(1 + [L]/K_{d1})}$$
$$+ \frac{B_{max2}[I]}{1 + K_{i2}(1 + [L]/K_{d2})} \quad (30)$$

This approach requires that a series of inhibition curves with a highly selective competing ligand be generated in the presence of increasing concentrations of radioligand. Simultaneous non-linear regression analysis of these multiple inhibition curves provides accurate estimates of the density of each class of binding sites and the affinity of each class of sites for the labeled and unlabeled ligand. This method has been used to detect a threefold selectivity of [^{125}I]iodopindolol for β_2-adrenergic receptors [21].

Interpretations of curvilinear Scatchard or Hofstee plots alternative to receptor heterogeneity

Ternary complex formation

A Hill coefficient less than 1 for the interaction of an agonist with a receptor can result from a two-step reaction that involves three components and leads to the formation of a ternary complex [8,22]. According to this reaction scheme, an agonist [H] binds to the receptor [R]:

$$[H] + [R] \rightleftharpoons [HR] \quad (31)$$

The agonist occupies the receptor according to the principles of mass action as described above. The low-affinity receptor-agonist complex [HR] then interacts with a third component in the membrane, [N], to form a high-affinity ternary complex [HRN]:

$$[HR] + [N] \rightleftharpoons [HRN] \quad (32)$$

Only one class of receptors is required in this two-step model. The receptors can exist in two different states, however, with distinct affinities for agonists. The extent of formation of ternary complex is limited by the concentration of [N] in the membrane relative to that of [R] and by the affinity of [HR] for [N]. These factors also affect the apparent affinity of the receptor for the agonist and the shape of the agonist competition curve.

This ternary complex model appears to describe accurately interactions of agonists with receptors in a number of systems in which receptors are linked to the stimulation or inhibition of adenylate cyclase activity (see Chap. 18) or to the turnover of phosphoinositides (Chap. 16). For example, the interaction of agonists with β-adrenergic receptors results in the formation of a high-affinity ternary complex composed of agonist, β receptor, and guanine nucleotide binding protein [13]. The formation of this ternary complex appears to be a required step in the stimulation of adenylate cyclase activity. Addition of a guanine nucleotide like GTP or $G_{pp}NH_p$ appears to destabilize the ternary complex so that only the initial interaction of the agonist with the receptor can be detected. In the presence of GTP, the affinity of the receptor for the agonist is decreased, and the slope of the inhibition curve is increased. Such effects of guanine nucleotides on the interactions of agonists with receptors have been reported for β-adrenergic receptors, dopamine receptors, and α-adrenergic receptors. Thus, in systems coupled to the enzyme adenylate cyclase, addition of GTP in radioligand binding assays appears to prevent the accumulation of ternary complex and permits characterization of the initial reaction between agonist and receptor.

Incorrect definition of nonspecific binding

One of the most common errors in the interpretation of binding data is an incorrect definition of nonspecific binding. In general, nonspecific binding is defined with a concentration of competing ligand that is 100 times its K_d value. This concentration will displace up to 99 percent of the specifically bound radioligand. If the concentration of competing ligand is higher than 100 times that of the radioligand, nonspecific binding as well as specific binding may be displaced. Depending on the percentage of nonspecific binding, this may result in a markedly curvilinear Scatchard plot. In a similar manner, displacement of nonspecific binding by a competing ligand can produce a markedly biphasic inhibition curve. Such curves are easily misinterpreted as providing evidence for the existence of multiple subtypes of receptor with significantly different affinities for the radioligand or competing drug. Such errors can be avoided by careful examination of the displacement curve of the competing ligand used to define nonspecific binding. The binding of the radioligand should decrease to a plateau at high concentrations of competing ligand, and this plateau should be the same for several different agonists and antagonists. Moreover, the competing ligand used to define nonspecific binding should be structurally different from the radioligand. This frequently means using agonists to define the nonspecific binding of antagonists and antagonists to define the nonspecific binding of agonists. A correct definition of nonspecific binding is an absolute requirement for the quantitative measurement of receptor subtypes.

ACKNOWLEDGMENTS

During the preparation of this manuscript, the authors were supported by USPHS grants NS 18591, NS 18479, and GM 34781.

REFERENCES

1. Snyder, S. Drug and neurotransmitter receptors in the brain. *Science* 224:22–31, 1984.
2. Molinoff, P. B., Wolfe, B. B., and Weiland, G. A. Quantitative analysis of drug-receptor interactions. II. Determination of the properties of receptor subtypes. *Life Sci.* 29:427–443, 1981.
3. Scatchard, G. The attractions of proteins for small molecules and ions. *Ann. N.Y. Acad. Sci.* 51:660–672, 1949.
4. Munson, P. J., and Rodbard, D. LIGAND: A versatile computerized approach for characterization of ligand-binding systems. *Anal. Biochem.* 107:220–239, 1980.
5. Boeynaems, J. M., and Dumont, J. E. Quantitative analysis of the binding of ligands to their receptors. *J. Cyclic Nucleotide Res.* 1:123–142, 1976.
6. Weiland, G. A., and Molinoff, P. B. Quantitative analysis of drug-receptor interactions. I. Determination of kinetic and equilibrium properties. *Life Sci.* 29:313–330, 1981.
7. Boeynaems, J. M., and Dumont, J. E. The two step model of ligand-receptor interaction. *Mol. Cell. Endocrinol.* 7:33–47, 1977.
8. Jacobs, S., and Cuatrecasas, P. The mobile receptor hypothesis and "cooperativity" of hormone binding. Application to insulin. *Biochem. Biophys. Acta.* 433:482–495, 1976.
9. DeLean, A., and Rodbard, D. Kinetics of cooperative binding. In R. D. O'Brien (ed.), *The*

Receptors, A Comprehensive Treatise. New York: Plenum Press, 1979, pp. 143–192.

10. Cheng, Y. C., and Prusoff, W. H. Relationship between the inhibition constant (K_i) and the concentration of inhibitor which causes 50% inhibition (I_{50}) of an enzymatic reaction. *Biochem. Pharmacol.* 22:3099–3108, 1973.

11. Hill, A. V. The possible effects of the aggregation of the molecules of haemoglobin on its dissociation curves. *J. Physiol.* (London). 40:iv–vii, 1910.

12. Cornish-Bowden, A., and Koshland, D. E. Diagnostic uses of the Hill (Logit and Nernst) plots. *J. Mol. Biol.* 95:201–212, 1975.

13. Limbird, L. E. *Cell Surface Receptors: A Short Course on Theory and Methods.* Boston: Martinus Nijhoff, 1985, pp. 51–96.

14. Motulsky, H. J., and Mahan, L. C. The kinetics of competitive radioligand binding predicted by the laws of mass action. *Mol. Pharmacol.* 25:1–9, 1984.

15. Contreras, M. L., Wolfe, B. B., and Molinoff, P. B. Kinetic analysis of the interactions of agonists and antagonists with *beta* adrenergic receptors. *J. Pharmacol. Exp. Ther.* 239:136–143, 1986.

16. Liang, B. T., Frame, L. H., and Molinoff, P. B. β_2-Adrenergic receptors contribute to catechola-mine-stimulated shortening of action potential duration in dog atrial muscle. *Proc. Natl. Acad. Sci. U.S.A.* 82:4521–4525, 1985.

17. DeLean, A., Hancock, A. A., and Lefkowitz, R. J. Validation and statistical analysis of a computer modelling method for quantitative analysis of radioligand binding data for mixtures of pharmacological receptor subtypes. *Mol. Pharmacol.* 21:5–16, 1982.

18. Minneman, K. P., Hedberg, A., and Molinoff, P. B. Comparison of *beta* adrenergic receptor subtypes in mammalian tissues. *J. Pharmacol. Exp. Ther.* 211:502–508, 1979.

19. McGonigle, P., Huff, R. M., and Molinoff, P. B. A comprehensive method for the quantitative determination of dopamine receptor subtypes. *Ann. N.Y. Acad. Sci.* 430:77–90, 1984.

20. Snedecor, G. W., and Cochran, W. G. *Statistical Methods.* Ames, Iowa, Iowa State University, University Press, 1967.

21. McGonigle, P., Neve, K. A., and Molinoff, P. B. A quantitative method of analyzing the interaction of slightly selective radioligands with multiple receptor subtypes. *Mol. Pharmacol.* 30:329–337, 1986.

22. De Haën, C. The non-stoichiometric floating receptor model for hormone sensitive adenylyl cyclase. *J. Theoret. Biol.* 58:383–400, 1976.

CHAPTER 10

Acetylcholine

Palmer Taylor and Joan Heller Brown

Basic Neurochemistry: Molecular, Cellular, and Medical Aspects, 4th Ed., edited by G. J. Siegel et al. Raven Press, Ltd., New York, 1989.
Correspondence to Palmer Taylor, Department of Pharmacology, University of California, San Diego, La Jolla, California 92093.

There is considerable evidence that acetylcholine arrived within the evolutionary scheme long before the design of the nervous system and functional synapses. Bacteria, fungi, protozoa, and plants store acetylcholine and possess biosynthetic and degradative capacities for turnover of the molecule. Even in higher systems, acetylcholine distribution is far wider than the nervous system. For example, acetylcholine is found in the cornea, certain ciliated epithelia, the spleen of ungulates, and in the human placenta [1]. Although definitive evidence is lacking, acetylcholine has been proposed to play a role in development and tissue differentiation.

Acetylcholine was first identified as a possible mediator of cellular function by Hunt in 1907, and in 1914 Dale [2] pointed out that its action closely mimicked the response of parasympathetic nerve stimulation (see also Chap. 8). Loewi, in 1921, provided clear evidence for acetylcholine release by nerve stimulation. Separate receptors that explained the variety of actions of acetylcholine became apparent in Dale's early experiments [2]. The nicotinic acetylcholine receptor was the first transmitter receptor to be purified and to have its primary structure determined [3,4]. Over the past decade the primary structures of several subtypes of both nicotinic and muscarinic receptors have been ascertained as have the structures of the various cholinesterases and of choline acetyltransferase.

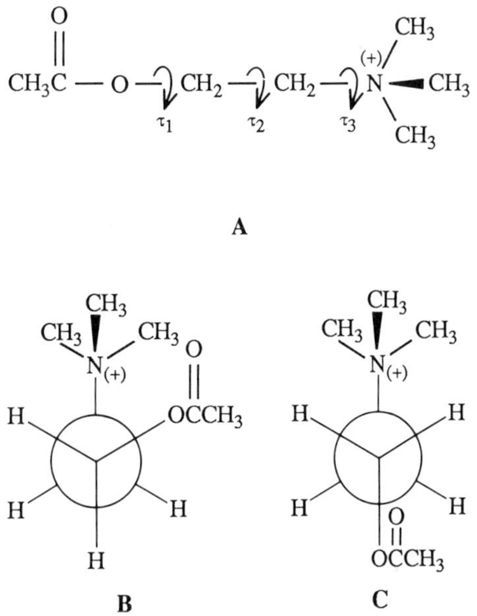

FIG. 1. Structure of acetylcholine. **A:** The three torsion angles τ_1, τ_2, τ_3. **B:** Newman projection of the *gauche* conformation. **C:** Newman projection of *trans* conformation. The molecule is viewed in the plane of the paper from the left side and the bond angles around τ_2 compared.

CHEMISTRY OF ACETYLCHOLINE

Free rotation in the acetylcholine molecule can occur around bonds τ_1, τ_2, and τ_3 (Fig. 1). Since the methyl groups are symmetrically disposed around τ_3, and constraints may be placed on τ_1 by the planar acetoxy group, the most important torsion angle determining acetylcholine conformation in solution is τ_2. A view from the side of the molecule (Fig. 1) shows the lowest energy configurations around τ_2. Nuclear magnetic resonance (NMR) studies indicate that the *gauche* conformation is predominant in solution [5]. Studies on the activity of rigid analogues of acetylcholine suggest that the *trans* conformation may be the active conformation at muscarinic receptors [6], while recent results of studies with NMR show that the acetoxy and quaternary nitrogens in the bound state of acetylcholine are too close together for this conformation to exist when acetylcholine is bound to the nicotinic receptor. Hence the bound conformations of this flexible molecule appear to differ substantially with receptor subtype. This finding may not emerge as a great surprise, since it

has been known for years that the structural modifications that enhance or diminish activity on muscarinic receptors are very different from those modifications that influence activity on nicotinic receptors [7].

ORGANIZATION OF THE CHOLINERGIC NERVOUS SYSTEM

Chemical specificity of acetylcholine receptors

The subtyping of the receptors in the cholinergic nervous system was initially based on the pharmacologic activity of two alkaloids: nicotine and muscarine (Fig. 2). This classification occurred long before the structures of these naturally occurring agonists were determined. The

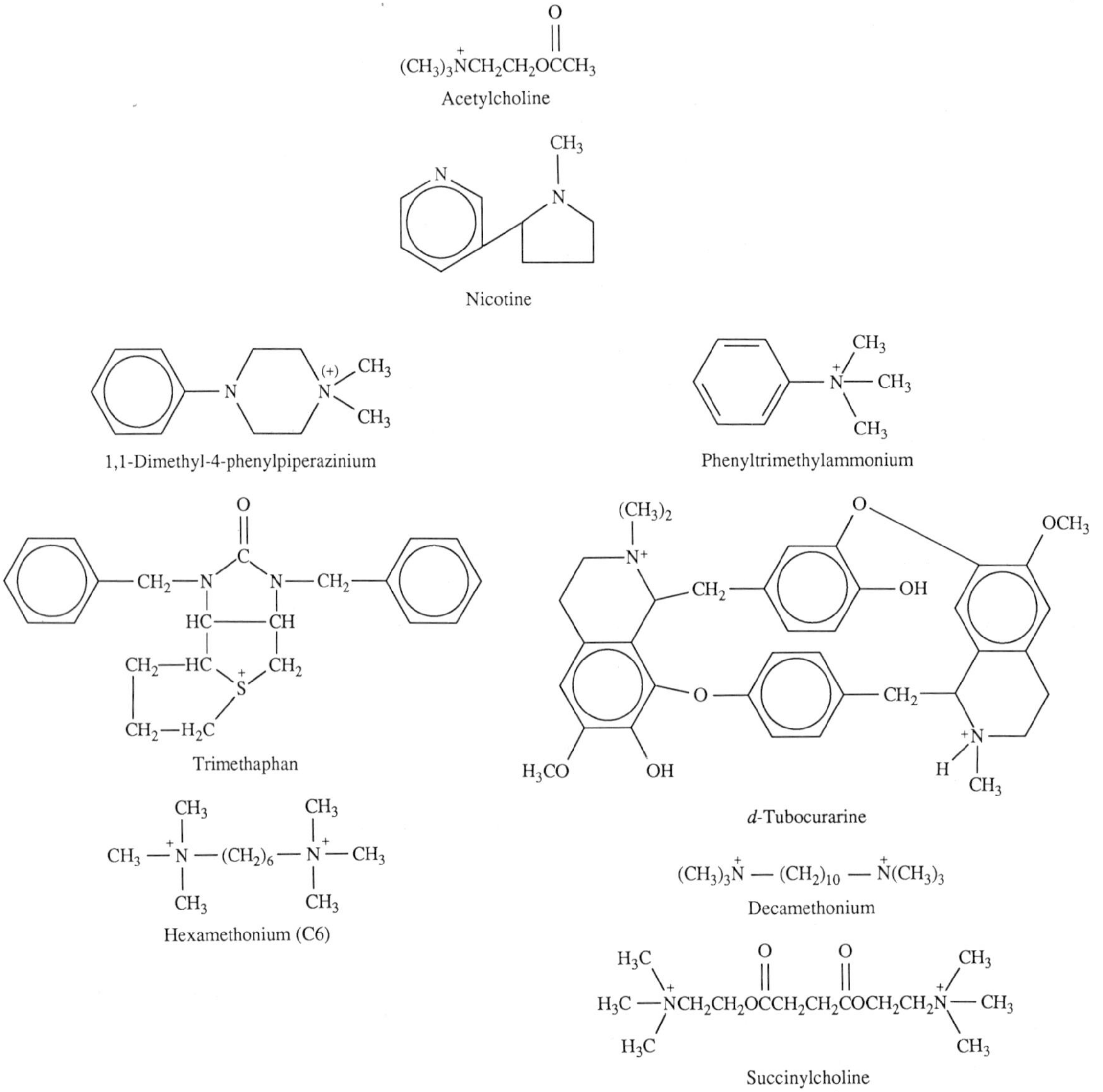

$$(CH_3)_3\overset{+}{N}CH_2CH_2OCCH_3$$

Acetylcholine

Nicotine

1,1-Dimethyl-4-phenylpiperazinium

Phenyltrimethylammonium

Trimethaphan

d-Tubocurarine

$$CH_3 - \overset{\overset{\displaystyle CH_3}{|}}{\overset{+}{N}} - (CH_2)_6 - \overset{\overset{\displaystyle CH_3}{|}}{\overset{+}{N}} - CH_3$$

Hexamethonium (C6)

$$(CH_3)_3\overset{+}{N} - (CH_2)_{10} - \overset{+}{N}(CH_3)_3$$

Decamethonium

Succinylcholine

FIG. 2. Structure of compounds important to the classification of receptor subtypes at cholinergic synapses. Compounds are subdivided as nicotinic and muscarinic. The compounds interacting with nicotinic receptors are further subdivided according to whether they are neuromuscular (N_1) in the right column or ganglionic selective (N_2) in the left column. The receptor agonists and antagonists with general specificity are listed above those that are subtype selective.

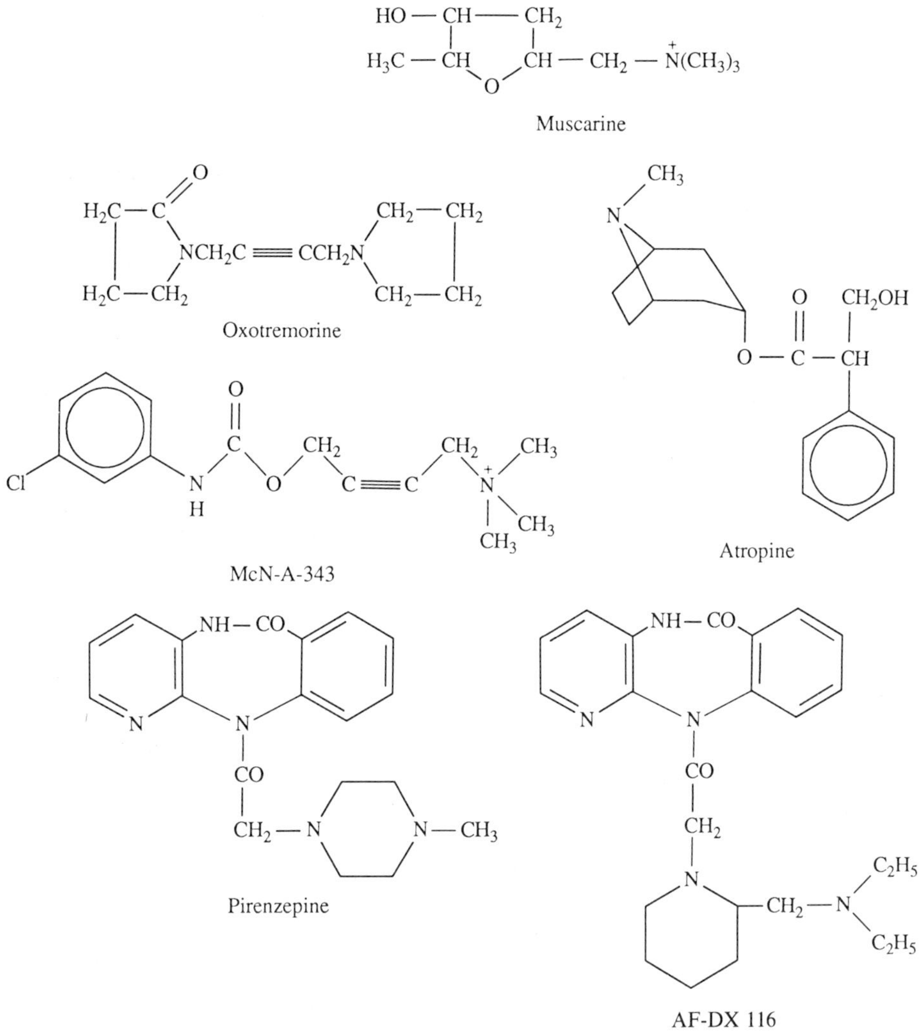

Muscarine

Oxotremorine

Atropine

McN-A-343

Pirenzepine

AF-DX 116

FIG. 2. *continued*

greatly different activities of the antagonists, atropine activity on muscarinic receptors and *d*-tubocurarine on nicotinic receptors, further supported the argument that multiple classes of receptors exist for acetylcholine. It was subsequently found that all nicotinic receptors are not identical. Those nicotinic receptors found in the neuromuscular junction, sometimes denoted as N_1 receptors, show selectivity toward phenyltrimethylammonium as an agonist; elicit a membrane depolarization in the presence of bisquaternary agents, with decamethonium being the most potent; are preferentially blocked by the competitive antagonist *d*-tubocurarine; and are irreversibly blocked by the snake α toxins. Nicotinic receptors in ganglia, N_2 receptors, are preferentially stimulated by tetramethylammonium; competitively blocked by trimethaphan; blocked by bisquaternary agents, with hexamethonium being most potent; and are resistant to the snake α toxins [8].

Muscarinic receptors also exhibit distinct subtypes, although the differences in ligand specificity are not as apparent. The drug pirenzepine (PZ) appears to have higher affinity for some subtypes of muscarinic receptors compared to others. Using this pharmacologic agent as a standard, it has been suggested that receptors with high affinity for PZ be termed M_1, whereas receptors with low affinity be termed M_2. Another agent, AF-DX 116, is selective for certain M_2 receptors. Molecular biological experiments discussed below indicate even greater complexity.

Developments in subtyping of receptors emerged from their molecular cloning

Not only do the ganglionic and neuromuscular types of the nicotinic receptors differ in primary structure, but each of these receptors also presents several subtypes. In the case of the extrajunctional neuromuscular receptor, an additional subunit may substitute for one of the subunits found in junctional receptors. Ligand selectivity and the potential dependence for channel opening differ only slightly between junctional and extrajunctional receptors. These properties alone may not be sufficient to warrant a separate classification; however, a difference in subunit composition may have important implications with respect to receptor regulation and turnover. In the central nervous system, at least four different sequences of α subunits of the nicotinic receptor have been identified [9]. Expression of the cloned genes encoding the individual α subunits shows a different sensitivity toward various toxins and agonists. Hence multiple subtypes of neuronal nicotinic receptors are in evidence. *In situ* hybridization studies also reveal discrete and different regional locations of the mRNAs encoding the α subunits in brain.

At least four distinct muscarinic receptor

genes have been cloned and sequenced. The genes are called m_1, m_2, m_3, and m_4 to distinguish them from M_1 and M_2 receptors identified pharmacologically. The pharmacologically defined M_1 and M_2 classes appear to include m_1 and m_2, respectively, but the relationships of the other gene products remain to be deduced. It is possible that subtypes differ in their ability to couple to different G proteins. The muscarinic receptor subtypes also exhibit distinct regional locations in the brain based on hybridization with mRNA. (The subtypes of receptors and genes are discussed later in this chapter.)

Taxonomy of receptor subtypes is based on ligand specificity and on the primary structures of the molecules

The individual subtypes of receptors often show discrete anatomic locations, and this has further facilitated their classification and study. Nicotinic receptors are found in peripheral ganglia and skeletal muscle. On innervation of skeletal muscle, receptors congregate in the junctional or postsynaptic end-plate area. On denervation or in noninnervated embryonic muscle, the receptors appear to be distributed across the surface of the muscle, and these extrajunctional receptors are synthesized and degraded rapidly. Junctional receptors exhibit far slower rates of turnover. Small differences in the binding of *d*-tubocurarine have been distinguished in studies of junctional and extrajunctional receptors. The basis for this difference may be a different subunit composition, but it could also occur through post-translational modifications of the expressed genes.

Ganglionic nicotinic receptors are found on postsynaptic neurons in both parasympathetic and sympathetic ganglia and in the adrenal gland. Ganglionic nicotinic receptors appear in tissues of neural crest embryonic origin and exhibit identical properties in sympathetic and parasympathetic ganglia.

Muscarinic receptors are the mediator of postganglionic parasympathetic neurotransmission. Some sympathetic responses, such as sweating and piloerection, are also mediated through muscarinic receptors. Subtypes of muscarinic receptors have been distinguished on the basis of their affinity for PZ, although the precise localization of the subtypes has yet to be determined. Receptors with a high affinity for PZ predominate in ganglia and in neurons, whereas receptors with a low affinity for PZ are found in smooth muscle cells, secretory glands, and the myocardium.

FUNCTIONAL ASPECTS OF CHOLINERGIC NEUROTRANSMISSION

Cholinergic neurotransmission is primarily nicotinic in the spinal cord, whereas both muscarinic and nicotinic responses are found in cortical and subcortical areas of the brain

Some specific cholinergic pathways have been studied. For example, Renshaw cells in the spinal cord play a role in modulating motoneuron activity by a feedback mechanism. Stimulation of Renshaw cells occurs through branches of the motoneuron, and the transmitter is acetylcholine acting on nicotinic receptors. If analyzed on the basis of excitability of individual cells, muscarinic responses dominate in higher centers; however, some areas of the brain such as the optic tectum rely on nicotinic responses. Muscarinic receptors with a high affinity for PZ appear to predominate in corpus striatum, hippocampus, and cerebral cortex, whereas receptors with a low affinity for PZ, although in low abundance, predominate in the cerebellum. The mapping of cholinergic pathways in the brain continues to be actively studied and relies on several techniques [10]. Histochemical studies that employ antibodies selective for acetylcholinesterase and choline acetyltransferase and receptor autoradiography with labeled ligands have produced detailed maps of the central nervous system. The wide distribution of some of these markers in pre- and postsynaptic cells and even nonneuronal cells limits the usefulness of these techniques. Studies involving iontophoretic application of transmitter, local stimulation, and intracellular or cell surface measurements of responses establish appropriate functional correlates.

Neurotransmission in autonomic ganglia is more complex than a simple depolarization event mediated by a single transmitter

The primary electrophysiologic event following preganglionic nerve stimulation is the rapid depolarization of postsynaptic sites by released acetylcholine acting on nicotinic receptors. Their activation gives rise to an initial excitatory postsynaptic potential (EPSP), which is due to an inward current through a cation channel (see Chaps. 4 and 8). This mechanism is virtually identical to that in the neuromuscular junction with an immediate onset of the depolarization and decay over a few milliseconds. Nicotinic antagonists such as trimethaphan competitively block ganglionic transmission, whereas agents such as hexamethonium produce blockade by occluding the channel. An action potential is generated in the postganglionic nerve when the initial EPSP attains a critical amplitude.

Several secondary events amplify or suppress this signal. These include the slow EPSP; the late, slow EPSP; and an inhibitory postsynaptic potential (IPSP). The slow EPSP is generated by acetylcholine acting on muscarinic receptors and is blocked by atropine or the selective antagonist PZ. It has a latency of approximately 1 sec and a duration of 30 to 60 sec. The late, slow EPSP can last for several minutes and is mediated by peptides found in ganglia, including substance P, angiotensin, leutinizing hormone-releasing hormone (LHRH), and the enkephalins. The slow EPSP and late, slow EPSP result from decreased K^+ conductance and are believed to regulate the sensitivity of the postsynaptic neuron to repetitive depolarization [11]. The IPSP seems to be mediated by the catecholamines, dopamine and/or norepinephrine. The IPSP is blocked by α-adrenergic antagonists and atropine. Acetylcholine released from presynaptic terminals may act on a catecholamine-containing interneuron to stimulate the release of norepinephrine or dopamine. As in the case of the slow EPSP, the IPSP has a longer latency and duration of action than the fast EPSP. These secondary events vary with the individual ganglia and are believed to modulate the sensitivity to the primary event. Hence drugs that selectively block the slow EPSP, such as atropine, will diminish the efficiency of ganglionic transmission rather than completely ablating it. Similarly, drugs such as muscarine and the ganglion-selective muscarinic agonist McN-A–343 are not thought of as primary ganglionic stimulants. Rather, they enhance the initial EPSP under conditions of repetitive stimulation.

Since parasympathetic and sympathetic ganglia exhibit comparable sensitivities to nicotine and acetylcholine in producing the initial EPSP, the pharmacologic action of ganglionic stimulants depends on the profile of innervation to particular organs or tissues (Table 1). For example, blood vessels are only innervated by the sympathetic nervous system; thus, ganglionic stimulation should only produce vasoconstriction. Similarly, the pharmacologic effects of ganglionic blockade will depend on which component of the autonomic nervous system is exerting predominant tone at the organ.

Administration of acetylcholine to an intact animal elicits a response characteristic of stimulation of postganglionic effector sites rather than of the ganglia

Only when muscarinic receptors are blocked with atropine or an M_2 antagonist are the effects of stimulation of the ganglia by administered acetylcholine observed. This is a consequence of the greater abundance of muscarinic receptors at effector sites in innervated tissues and the relatively poor plasma perfusion of ganglia.

In addition to their presence in the central nervous system, ganglia, and assorted peripheral nerve plexuses, muscarinic receptors are widely distributed in the body. They are found in visceral smooth muscle, in secretory glands, and in the endothelial cells of the vasculature. Aside from endothelial cells, each of these sites receives a cholinergic innervation. Responses can be excitatory or inhibitory depending on the tissue. Even within a single tissue the responses may vary. For example, muscarinic stimulation

TABLE 1. Predominance of sympathetic or parasympathetic tone at effector sites; effects of autonomic ganglionic blockade

Site	Predominant tone	Effect of ganglionic blockade
Arterioles	Sympathetic (adrenergic)	Vasodilatation; increased peripheral blood flow; hypotension
Veins	Sympathetic (adrenergic)	Dilatation; pooling of blood; decreased venous return; decreased cardiac output
Heart	Parasympathetic (cholinergic)	Tachycardia
Iris	Parasympathetic (cholinergic)	Mydriasis
Ciliary muscle	Parasympathetic (cholinergic)	Cycloplegia
Gastrointestinal tract	Parasympathetic (cholinergic)	Reduced tone and motility of smooth muscle; constipation, decreased gastric and pancreatic secretion
Urinary bladder	Parasympathetic (cholinergic)	Urinary retention
Salivary glands	Parasympathetic (cholinergic)	Xerostomia
Sweat glands	Sympathetic (cholinergic)	Anhidrosis

causes gastrointestinal smooth muscle to depolarize and contract, except at sphincters, where hyperpolarization and relaxation is seen (Table 2). Many tissues that are innervated by the cholinergic nervous system exhibit intrinsic electrical and/or mechanical activity. This activity is modified rather than initiated by cholinergic nerve activity. Cardiac muscle and smooth muscle exhibit spikes of electrical activity that are propagated between cells. These spikes are initiated by rhythmic fluctuations in resting membrane potential. In intestinal smooth muscle, cholinergic stimulation will cause a partial depolarization and increase the frequency by spike production. By contrast, cholinergic stimulation of atria will decrease the rate of depolarization of the spikes, and this appears to be a consequence of hyperpolarization of the membrane.

Membrane depolarization appears to be a consequence of an increase in Na^+ and, perhaps, Ca^{2+} conductances

In addition, Ca^{2+} fluxes across the cell membrane and the mobilization of intracellular Ca^{2+} from the endoplasmic or sarcoplasmic reticulum appear to be elicited by acetylcholine acting on muscarinic receptors (see Chap. 16). The increase in intracellular free Ca^{2+} is involved in activation of contractile, metabolic, and secretory events. Stimulation of muscarinic receptors has also been linked to changes in cyclic nucleotide concentrations. Reductions in cyclic AMP (cAMP) levels and increases in cyclic GMP (cGMP) levels are typical responses (see Chap. 17). The cyclic nucleotides may facilitate contraction or relaxation, depending on the particular tissue. The inhibitory responses appear to be associated with hyperpolarization and this is a consequence of an increased K^+ conductance. Increases in K^+ conductance may be mediated by a direct receptor linkage to a K^+ channel or by increases in intracellular Ca^{2+}, which in turn activate K^+ channels. The mechanisms through which muscarinic receptors might couple to multiple events are considered later.

Stimulation of the motorneuron for skeletal muscle results in the release of acetylcholine and contraction of the skeletal muscle fibers

Contraction and associated electrical events can be produced by the intra-arterial injection of acetylcholine close to the muscle. Since skeletal muscle does not possess inherent myogenic tone, the tone of apparently resting muscle is maintained by spontaneous and basal release of acetylcholine. The consequences of sponta-

TABLE 2. Effects of ACh stimulation on peripheral tissues

Tissue	Effect of ACh
Vasculature (endothelial cells)	Release of EDRF (nitric oxide) and vasodilatation
Eye iris (pupillae sphincter muscle)	Contraction and miosis
Ciliary muscle	Contraction and accommodation of lens to near vision
Salivary glands and lacrimal glands	Secretion—thin and watery
Bronchi	Constriction; increased secretions
Heart	Bradycardia, decreased conduction (A–V block at high doses)—small negative inotropic action
Gastrointestinal tract	Increased tone; increased GI secretions; relaxation at sphincters
Urinary bladder	Contraction of detrusor muscle; relaxation of the sphincter
Sweat glands	Diaphoresis
Reproductive tract, male	Erection
Uterus	Variable, dependent on hormone influence

neous release at the motor end-plate of skeletal muscle are small spontaneous depolarizations from the quantized release of acetylcholine—miniature end-plate potentials (MEPPs) (see Chaps. 8 and 32). Decay times for the MEPPs range between 1 and 2 msec, a value of about the same magnitude as the mean channel open time seen with acetylcholine stimulation of the receptor. Stimulation of the motorneuron results in the release of several hundred quanta of acetylcholine. The summation of MEPPs gives rise to a postsynaptic excitatory potential (PSEP), also termed motor end-plate potential. A sufficiently large and abrupt potential change at the end-plate will elicit an action potential by activating voltage-sensitive Na^+ channels. The action potential propagates in two-dimensional space across the surface of the muscle to release Ca^{2+} and elicit contraction. The PSEP may therefore be thought of as a generator potential. It is found only in junctional regions and arises from the opening of the receptor channel. Normal resting potentials in end-plates are about -70 mV. The postsynaptic excitatory potential causes the end-plate to depolarize partially to about -55 mV. It is the transition from -70 to -55 mV in localized areas of the end-plate that triggers action potential generation [12].

Competitive blocking agents such as d-tubocurarine cause muscle paralysis by preventing access of acetylcholine to its binding site on the receptor

The end-plate potential with competitive blockade is maintained at -70 mV. Without frequent PSEPs, action potentials are not triggered, and there is flaccid paralysis of the muscle. Depolarizing neuromuscular blocking agents, such as decamethonium or succinylcholine, produce depolarization of the end-plate such that the end-plate potential is found to reside at -55 mV. The high concentrations of depolarizing agent that are present do not allow the end-plate to repolarize, as would occur with a labile trans-

mitter such as acetylcholine. Since it is the transition between -70 and -55 mV that triggers the action potential, flaccid paralysis will also occur with a depolarizing block [8]. As might be expected if depolarization occurs in a non-uniform manner in microscopic areas within individual end-plates and in individual motor units, the onset of depolarization blockade is characterized by muscle twitching and fasciculations that are not evident in competitive block. Once paralysis is evident, the overall pharmacologic actions of competitive and depolarizing blocking agents are similar, yet an intracellular measurement of end-plate potential would distinguish these two classes of agents.

SYNTHESIS, STORAGE, AND RELEASE OF ACETYLCHOLINE

Acetylcholine is synthesized from its two immediate precursors, choline and acetyl coenzyme A

This reaction is a single step catalyzed by the enzyme choline acetyltransferase (ChAT) (EC 2.3.1.6):

Choline + Acetyl coenzyme A

$\rightleftharpoons$ Acetylcholine + coenzyme A

This enzymatic activity was first assayed in a cell-free preparation by Nachmansohn and Machado in 1943. ChAT has subsequently been purified from several sources and cloned in *Drosophila* [13]. The purification of ChAT has allowed production of specific antibodies, and it is now possible to carry out immunohistochemical mapping of cholinergic pathways using this enzyme as a specific marker. Whereas acetylcholinesterase, the enzyme responsible for degradation of ACh is produced by cells containing cholinoceptive sites as well as in cholinergic neurons, ChAT is found in the nervous system specifically at sites where ACh synthesis takes place. For example, the enzyme is found in relatively high concentration in the caudate nucleus but in relatively low amounts in the cerebellum. Within cholinergic neurons, ChAT is concentrated in nerve terminals, although it is also present in axons, where it is transported from its site of synthesis in the soma. When subcellular fractionation studies are carried out, ChAT is recovered in the synaptosomal fraction, and within synaptosomes it is primarily cytoplasmic. It has been suggested that ChAT is also bound to the outside of the storage vesicle under physiological conditions and that ACh synthesized in that location may be favorably situated to enter the vesicle.

The purified enzyme is a protein of 66 to 70 kilodaltons (kDa). There may be several isozymes with different isoelectric points; possibly, these differ in their association with the vesicles. The brain enzyme has a K_D for choline of approximately 1 mM and a K_D for acetyl CoA of approximately 10 μM. The activity of the isolated enzyme, assayed in the presence of optimal concentrations of cofactors and substrates, appears far greater than that reflected by the rate at which choline is converted to ACh *in vivo*. This suggests that the full activity of ChAT is not expressed *in vivo*. Inhibitors of ChAT do not decrease ACh synthesis when used *in vivo;* this may reflect a failure to achieve a sufficient local concentration of inhibitor but also suggests that this step is not rate limiting in the synthesis of acetylcholine.

What limits ACh formation in vivo *could be the intracellular concentrations of its precursors*

The acetyl coenzyme (CoA) used for ACh synthesis in mammalian brain comes from pyruvate formed from glucose. It is uncertain how the acetyl CoA, generally thought to be formed at the inner membrane of the mitochondria, ac-

cesses the cytoplasmic ChAT, and it is possible that this is a rate-limiting step. It appears more likely, however, that ACh formation is limited by the intracellular concentration of choline, which is determined by uptake of choline into the nerve ending.

Choline is present in the plasma at a concentration of about 10 μM. A "low-affinity" choline uptake system with a K_m of 10 to 100 μM is present in all tissues, but cholinergic neurons also have an Na$^+$-dependent "high-affinity" choline uptake system with a K_m for choline of 1 to 5 μM [14]. This high-affinity choline uptake system appears linked, in a still undefined way, to both ACh synthesis and release. The high-affinity uptake mechanisms would be saturated at 10 μM choline so the plasma choline concentration is probably adequate for sustained ACh synthesis even under conditions of high demand, as observed in ganglia. Furthermore, since the plasma concentration of choline is above the K_m of the high-affinity choline transport system, one would not expect to increase choline in the nerve ending by increasing the plasma concentration of choline or by changing the K_m of the uptake system. One might, however, change neuronal choline content by altering the capacity of the high-affinity choline uptake mechanism, i.e., changing the V_{max} for transport, and this has been reported to occur in some brain regions in response to increased or decreased neuronal activity. There is some dispute about whether the capacity of the uptake system is increased or whether choline influx is regulated by changes in the intraterminal concentration of choline; but it is agreed that some event associated with neuronal activity serves to enhance choline entry into neurons [14]. If the K_m of ChAT for choline *in vivo* is as high as that seen with the purified enzyme, one would expect ACh synthesis to increase in proportion to the greater availability of choline. Conversely, ACh synthesis should be diminished when high-affinity choline uptake is blocked. Hemicholinium-3 is a potent inhibitor of the high-affinity choline uptake system (Fig. 3). Treatment with this drug decreases ACh synthesis and leads to a reduction in ACh release during prolonged stimulation; these findings lend support to the notion that choline uptake is the major rate-limiting factor in the biosynthesis of ACh.

Neurons cannot synthesize choline de novo, and it must therefore be supplied either from plasma or by metabolism of choline-containing compounds

Approximately half of the choline used in ACh synthesis is thought to come directly from recycling of released ACh, hydrolyzed to choline by cholinesterase. Presumably, the uptake of this metabolically derived choline occurs rapidly, before the choline diffuses away from the synaptic cleft. Another source of choline is from the breakdown of phosphatidylcholine, which may be increased in response to locally released ACh. Choline derived from these two sources becomes available in the extracellular space and is then subject to high-affinity uptake into the nerve ending. In the central nervous system these metabolic sources of choline may be particularly important, because choline in the plasma cannot pass the blood-brain barrier. Thus, in the central nervous system the high-affinity uptake of choline into cholinergic neurons might not be saturated, and ACh synthesis could be limited by the supply of choline during sustained activity. This would be consistent with the finding that ACh stores in the brain are subject to variation, whereas ACh stores in ganglia and muscles remain relatively constant.

The slow release of ACh from neurons at rest probably occurs at all cholinergic synapses

This was first described by Fatt and Katz who recorded small spontaneous depolarizations at frog neuromuscular junctions that were sub-threshold for triggering action potentials. These MEPPs were shown to be due to the release of ACh. When the nerve was then stimulated and end-plate potentials recorded and analyzed, the magnitude of these potentials was always found to be some multiple of the magnitude of the MEPPs. It was suggested that each MEPP resulted from a finite quantity or quantum of released ACh and that the end-plate potentials resulted from release of greater numbers of quanta during nerve stimulation (see also Chap. 8).

A possible structural basis for these discrete units of transmitter was discovered shortly thereafter when independent electron microscopic and subcellular fractionation studies by de Robertis and Whittaker revealed the presence of vesicles in cholinergic nerve endings. Subcellular fractionation of mammalian brain and *Torpedo* electric organs yields re-sealed nerve endings, or synaptosomes, that can be lysed to release a fraction enriched in vesicles. More than half of the ACh in the synaptosome is found associated with particles that look like the vesicles seen by electron microscopy. It is therefore clear that ACh is associated

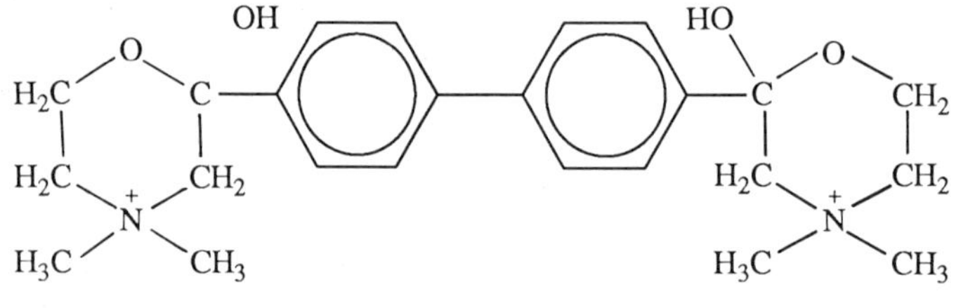

FIG. 3. Structure of hemicholinium (HC-3).

with a vesicle fraction, and it is likely that it is contained within the vesicle. The origin of the ACh that is free within the synaptosome is less clear. It may be ACh that is normally in the cytosol of the nerve ending, or it may be an artifact of release from the vesicles during their preparation (see Chap. 8).

The relationship between the amount of ACh in a vesicle and the quanta of ACh released can only be estimated

Estimates of the amount of ACh contained within cholinergic vesicles vary, and there is obviously some subjectivity in correcting the values obtained, e.g., for the percent of vesicles that are cholinergic or how much ACh would be lost during their preparation. Whittaker has estimated that there are about 2,000 molecules of ACh in a cholinergic vesicle from the central nervous system. A similar estimate was made using sympathetic ganglia; there are about 1,600 molecules of ACh per vesicle. The most abundant source of cholinergic synaptic vesicles is the electric organ of *Torpedo*. Vesicles from *Torpedo* are far larger than those from mammalian species and are estimated to contain up to 100 times more ACh, i.e., 200,000 molecules per vesicle. The *Torpedo* vesicle has also been shown to contain ATP and, in its core, a proteoglycan of the heparin sulfate type. Both of these constituents may serve as counter-ions for ACh, which would otherwise be at a hyperosmotic concentration.

The amount of ACh in a quantum has been estimated by comparing the potential changes associated with MEPPs to those obtained by iontophoresis of known quantities of ACh. Based on such analysis, the amount of ACh per quantum at the snake neuromuscular junction was estimated to be something less than 10,000 molecules [16]. Given the possible error in these calculations, this would be within the range of that estimated to be contained in a vesicle. It is therefore likely that quanta are defined by the amount of releasable ACh in the vesicle. An alternative favored by some investigators is that ACh is released directly from the cytoplasm. In this model definable quanta occur because some channel in the membrane is open for finite periods of time when Ca^{2+} is elevated. A presynaptic membrane protein suggested to mediate Ca^{2+}-dependent translocation of ACh has recently been isolated by Israel and colleagues. Although there are some compelling arguments in support of this model, most investigators favor the more conventional notion that the vesicle serves not only as a unit of storage but as a unit of release. (The vesicle hypothesis is discussed also in Chapter 8.)

Depolarization of the nerve terminal by an action potential increases the number of quanta released per unit time

Release of ACh requires the presence of extracellular Ca^{2+}, which enters the neuron when it is depolarized. Most investigators feel that a voltage-dependent Ca^{2+} current is the initial event responsible for transmitter release, which occurs about 200 μsec later. The mechanism through which elevated Ca^{2+} increases the probability of ACh release is not yet known; phosphorylation or activation of proteins that cause the vesicle to fuse with the neuronal membrane are among the possibilities. Dependence on Ca^{2+} is a common feature of all exocytotic release mechanisms, and it is likely that exocytosis is a conserved mechanism for transmitter release. There is good evidence that adrenergic vesicles empty their contents into the synaptic cleft because norepinephrine and epinephrine are released along with other contents of the storage vesicle. Although less rigorous data are available for cholinergic systems, cholinergic vesicles contain ATP, and release of ATP has been shown to accompany ACh secretion from these vesicles. Furthermore, as discussed in Chap. 8, Heuser and Reese demonstrated in electron microscopic studies at frog nerve terminals that vesicles fuse with the nerve membrane and that vesicular contents appear to be released by exocytosis; it has been difficult to ascertain, however, whether the fusions are sufficiently frequent to account for release on stimulation. The nerve ending also appears to endocytose the outer vesicle membrane to form vesicles that are subsequently refilled with ACh [16].

Torpedo synaptic vesicles have also been used to study the mechanisms through which ACh, formed in the cytoplasm by ChAT, is concentrated in storage vesicles [15]. The purified *Torpedo* vesicle does not incorporate much ACh compared to the amount seen *in vivo*, but this preparation has nonetheless provided valuable information that presumably reflects the *in vivo* situation. It appears that there is a specific ACh transporter and that ACh uptake is driven by an ATPase that pumps protons so that the inside of the vesicle becomes acidified and positively charged. There must also be a coupled mechanism for the movement of ions such that the vesicle remains isoosmotic and electroneutral, but this activity has not yet been directly demonstrated. An inhibitor of ACh transport into the vesicle has been studied in detail by Parsons and colleagues [15]. The inhibitor vesamicol (Fig. 4), formerly AH5183, inhibits ACh uptake with an IC_{50} of about 40 nM. The inhibition is noncompetitive, suggesting that the drug does not act at the ACh binding site on the transporter although it may act at another site on the same protein. Significantly, vesamicol blocks the evoked release of newly synthesized ACh from a number of preparations without significantly affecting high-affinity choline uptake, ACh synthesis, or Ca^{2+} influx. That ACh release is lost secondary to blockade of its uptake by the vesicle is powerful evidence that the vesicle is the site of ACh release.

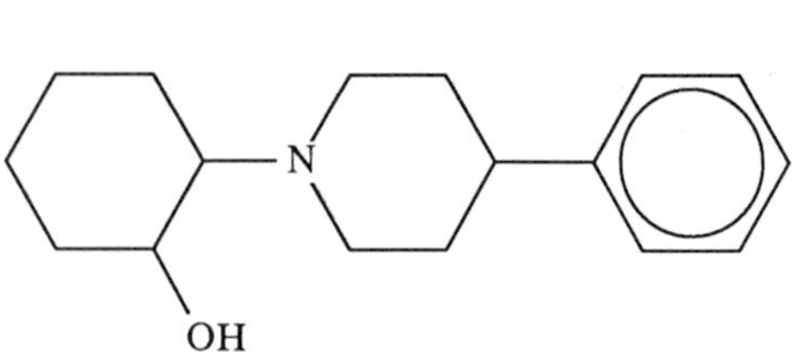

All of the ACh contained within the cholinergic neuron does not behave as if in a single compartment

Results of a variety of neurophysiological and biochemical experiments suggest that there are at least two distinguishable pools of ACh, only one of which is readily available for release. These have been referred to as the "readily available" or "depot" pool and as the "reserve" or "stationary" pool. The reserve pool serves to refill the readily available pool as it is utilized. Unless the rate of mobilization of ACh into the readily available pool is adequate, the amount of ACh that can be released may be limited. It must also be the case that newly synthesized ACh is used to fill the readily available pool of ACh because it is the newly synthesized ACh that is preferentially released during nerve stimulation. The relationship between these functionally defined pools and ACh storage vesicles is not known with certainty. It is possible that the readily available pool resides in vesicles poised for release near the nerve ending membrane, whereas the reserve pool is in more distant vesicles. Although cholinergic vesicles appear to be homogeneous, there may be subpopulations of vesicles. Density gradient separation of cholinergic vesicles from *Torpedo* reveals two populations of vesicles that differ in size and density. There is some evidence that the smaller and denser vesicles (VP_2) are vesicles that are used and recycled by refilling with ACh and that VP_1 vesicles form the reserve pool. VP_2 vesicles also differ from VP_1 vesicles in terms of their relative capacities for ACh transport and vesamicol binding. Evidence for distinct populations of vesicles provides a morphological basis for the concept of pools.

FIG. 4. Structure of vesamicol (AH5183).

ACETYLCHOLINESTERASE AND THE TERMINATION OF ACETYLCHOLINE ACTION

Cholinesterases are widely distributed throughout the body in both neuronal and nonneuronal tissues

Wide distribution of the cholinesterases in fact limits their use in identifying cholinergic nerve tracks. Based largely on substrate specificity, the cholinesterases are subdivided into the acetylcholinesterases (EC 3.1.1.7) and the butyryl or pseudocholinesterases (EC 3.1.1.8) [17]. Acylcholines with an acyl group of the size of butyric acid or larger are very slowly hydrolyzed by the former enzyme; organophosphates that are selective inhibitors for each enzyme have been identified. Substantial amounts of butyrylcholinesterase are made in the liver and appear in plasma; however, it is highly unlikely that appreciable concentrations of ACh would diffuse away from a synapse and elicit a systemic response. Thus, the function of butyrylcholinesterase remains obscure. In general, acetylcholinesterase levels correlate most directly with innervation and development. The acetylcholinesterases are also most apt to exhibit synaptic localization.

Acetylcholinesterase exists in several molecular forms that differ in their solubility and mode of membrane attachment rather than in catalytic activity

One class of molecular forms exists as a homologous assembly of catalytic subunits that appear as monomers, dimers, or tetramers (Fig. 5). These forms also differ in their degree of hydrophobicity, and the hydrophobic character arises from a post-translational addition of a glycophospholipid on the C-terminal carboxyl group. The glycophospholipid allows the enzyme to be tethered on the external surface of the cell membrane. The hydrophobic form of the enzyme is widely distributed in both excitable and nonexcitable tissues. Soluble globular forms of the enzyme have been identified in brain. In certain dopamine-containing neurons, acetylcholinesterase is co-released in a soluble form with dopamine on nerve stimulation; however, the function of the released enzyme is unknown.

The second class of acetylcholinesterase forms exists as assemblies of heterologous subunits. One form consists of catalytic subunits (up to 12) linked by a disulfide bond to filamentous, collagen-containing structural subunits. These forms are often termed asymmetric, since the tail unit imparts substantial dimensional asymmetry to the molecule. Studies in avian muscle show that both acetyl- and butyrylcholinesterases are linked to tail units, and it is possible that a single molecular assembly is a hybrid containing both acetyl- and butyrylcholinesterases. The asymmetric species appear on synapse formation and are localized to synaptic areas. The collagenous tail unit is responsible for this molecular form being associated with the basal lamina of the synapse rather than the plasma membrane. Asymmetric forms are particularly abundant in the neuromuscular junction. Recently, a second type of structural subunit, to which catalytic subunits are linked by disulfide bonds, has been identified in brain. This subunit contains covalently attached lipid. The different subunit assemblies and post-translational modifications lead to distinct localizations of acetylcholinesterase on the cell surface but appear not to affect their intrinsic catalytic activity.

The primary structures of several cholinesterases are now known

Cholinesterase genes encode a leader peptide, but the cholinesterases do not have obvious membrane-spanning regions in their primary structure [18]. Hence they are designed for secretion from the cell. It is interesting that the

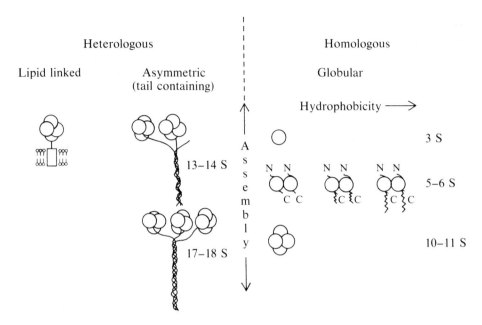

FIG. 5. Molecular species of acetylcholinesterase. Two classes of enzyme species may be defined. The homologous class consists of associations of identical catalytic subunits. The individual species differ in the degree of association (monomer, dimer, and tetramer) and in their hydrophobicity. The latter appears to be a consequence of addition of a glycophospholipid on the C-terminal carboxyl group. This modification serves to localize the enzyme on the extracellular surface of the membrane. The second class is a heterologous association of disulfide-linked catalytic and structural subunits. One form exists as an association of up to 12 catalytic subunits with a collagen-like, filamentous unit and has been termed the asymmetric form. A second form appears to be a tetramer of catalytic subunits associated with a lipid-linked tail unit.

cholinesterases do not show homology or structural similarity to the chymotrypsin family of serine hydrolases despite having virtually identical catalytic mechanisms. Rather, the cholinesterases have defined a new family of secreted proteins. Within this growing family are several nonneuronal esterases, thyroglobulin, and an inducible protein from *Dictyostelium* of unknown function.

tains two splicing alternatives that give rise to distinct C-terminal sequences for the two classes (heterologous and homologous) of acetylcholinesterase forms. The unique sequences encoded by exon 3 apparently provide the signal for the different subunit assemblies and posttranslational modifications inherent to the different molecular species of acetylcholinesterase.

The diversity of molecular species of acetylcholinesterase arises from alternative mRNA processing of a single gene

Within the open reading frame of the gene, exons 1 and 2 are identical for the two classes of acetylcholinesterase species. Exon 3 con-

The catalytic mechanism for ACh hydrolysis involves formation of an acyl enzyme, followed by deacylation and formation of the parent enzyme

The acylation step proceeds through the formation of a tetrahedral transition state. Alkylphosphates are tetrahedral in configuration, and this geometric resemblance to the transition state, in part, accounts for their effectiveness as inhibitors of acetylcholinesterase. Acylation occurs on the active-site serine, which is rendered nucleophilic by a charge-relay system involving a histidine. The acetyl enzyme that is formed is short-lived, which accounts for the high catalytic efficiency of the enzyme (Fig. 6).

Inhibition of acetylcholinesterase occurs by several distinct mechanisms

Some acetylcholinesterase inhibitors are useful therapeutically, whereas others have proven useful as insecticides. Still others have been manufactured for a more insidious use in chemical warfare. Reversible inhibitors such as edrophonium bind reversibly to the active site of the enzyme and prevent access of the substrate. Other reversible inhibitors, such as gallamine and propidium, bind to a peripheral site on the enzyme. The carbamoylating agents, such as neostigmine and physostigmine, form a carbamoyl enzyme by reacting with the active-site serine. The carbamoyl enzymes are more stable than the acetyl enzyme; their deacylation occurs over several minutes. Since the carbamoyl enzyme will not hydrolyze ACh, the carbamoy-

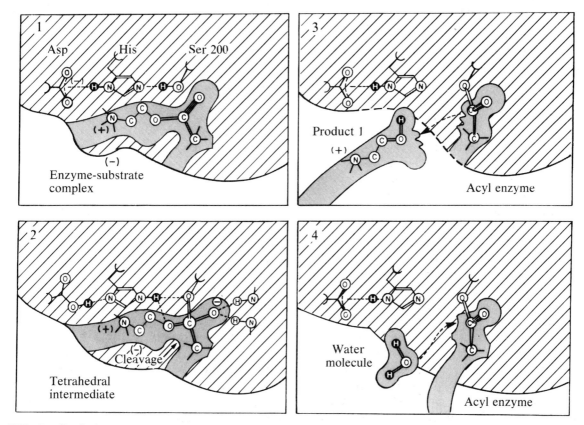

FIG. 6. Catalytic sequence in ACh hydrolysis. The active-site serine (position 200 in the *Torpedo* sequence) is rendered nucleophilic by a charge-relay system involving a dicarboxylic amino acid (ASP) serving as a proton sink and an imidazole group of histidine. The serine attacks the carbonyl carbon (*panel 1*) forming a tetrahedral intermediate (*panel 2*). The carbonyl oxygen is likely stabilized through hydrogen bonding. Removal of the choline-leaving group forms an acyl enzyme (*panel 3*). Attack by water is rapid and generates the free enzyme (*panel 4*).

lating agents are alternative substrates that are effective inhibitors of ACh hydrolysis. The alkylphosphates, such as di-isopropylfluorophosphate or echothiophate, act in a similar manner; however, the alkylphosphates and alkylphosphonates form extremely stable bonds with the active-site serine on the enzyme. The time required for their hydrolysis exceeds that for biosynthesis and turnover of the enzyme. Accordingly, inhibition with the alkylphosphates is often irreversible.

The consequences of acetylcholinesterase inhibition differ from synapse to synapse

At postganglionic parasympathetic effector sites, acetylcholinesterase inhibition enhances or potentiates the action of administered ACh or ACh released by nerve stimulation. This, in part, is a consequence of stimulation of receptors extending over a larger area from the point of transmitter release. Similarly, ganglionic transmission is enhanced by cholinesterase inhibitors. Although the behavioral and physiologic action of cholinesterase inhibition in the central nervous system has been well studied, its precise action on individual cholinergic pathways is not understood; however, since atropine and other muscarinic antagonists are effective antidotes of the toxicity of inhibitors of acetylcholinesterase [8], we assume that the central nervous system manifestations result largely from excessive muscarinic stimulation.

By prolonging the residence time of ACh in the synapse, acetylcholinesterase inhibition in the neuromuscular junction promotes a persistent depolarization of the motor end-plate. The decay of end-plate currents or potentials resulting from spontaneous release of ACh are prolonged from 1 to 2 msec to 5 to 10 msec. This indicates that the transmitter activates multiple receptors before diffusing from the synapse. Excessive depolarization of the end-plate and a diminished capacity to initiate coordinated ac-

tion potentials follow. In a fashion similar to depolarizing blocking agents, fasciculations and muscle twitching are initially observed with acetylcholinesterase inhibition, followed by flaccid paralysis.

NICOTINIC RECEPTORS

The nicotinic ACh receptor is the best characterized neurotransmitter receptor

Investigators were able to purify the nicotinic receptor about a decade before purification of other receptor types was possible. Electric organs of the *Torpedo* species are a rich source of nicotinic receptors and consist of stacks of electrocytes that have emerged from an embryologic tissue similar to skeletal muscle. On differentiation, the electrogenic bud in the electrocyte proliferates, but the contractile elements atrophy. The excitable membrane encompasses the entire ventral surface of the electrocyte rather than being localized to junctional areas, as occurs in skeletal muscle. The electrical discharge in *Torpedo* relies solely on a postsynaptic excitatory potential resulting from depolarization of the postsynaptic membrane. Depolarization arises directly from the opening of receptor channels; in skeletal muscle and in the fresh water electric eel, *Electrophorus electricus*, depolarization at the end-plate activates a voltage-sensitive Na^+ channel that, in turn, causes the depolarization to spread across the surface of the muscle or electric organ. The density of receptors in *Torpedo* electric organs approaches 100 pmol/mg protein, which may be compared with 0.1 pmol/mg protein in skeletal muscle.

Studies of C. Y. Lee and his colleagues in the early 1960s established that several snake α toxins, including α-bungarotoxin, irreversibly inactivated receptor function in intact skeletal muscle, and this finding led directly to the identification and subsequent isolation of the nicotinic ACh receptor from *Torpedo* [3]. By virtue of their high affinity and slow rate of dissociation, labeled α toxins serve as markers of the receptor during solubilization and purification.

Purification of the nicotinic ACh receptor facilitated examination of its overall structure

Antibodies were raised to the purified protein, and sufficient amino acid sequence of the receptor itself became available to enable the cloning and sequencing of the genes encoding the individual subunits of the receptor [4]. Recently, cDNAs encoding the four subunits have been stably integrated into the genome of mouse fibroblasts and expression of active receptor obtained [19]. Owing to the high density of nicotinic ACh receptors in the postsynaptic membranes of *Torpedo*, sufficient order of the receptor is achieved in isolated membrane fragments that image reconstructions from electron micrographs have allowed a more detailed analysis of structure [20]. Finally, labeling of functional sites and determination of subunit composition contributed to the development of our understanding of the structure of nicotinic receptors.

The nicotinic ACh receptor consists of five subunits arranged around a pseudoaxis of symmetry

The subunits display partially homologous amino acid sequence, 30 to 40 percent identity of amino acid residues [20]. One of the subunits, designated α, is expressed in two copies; the other three, β, γ, and δ, are present as single copies (Fig. 7). Thus, the receptor is a pentamer of molecular mass near 280 kDa. Structural studies show the subunits to be arranged around a central cavity, with the largest portion of the protein exposed toward the extracellular surface. The central cavity is believed to be the ion channel, which in the resting state is imperme-

able to ions; on activation, however, it opens to a diameter of 6.5 Å. The open channel is selective for cations; permeation of the channel by particular cations appears to be limited primarily by the diameter of the open channel. The α subunits form the site for binding of agonists and competitive antagonists and the primary surface with which the larger snake α toxins associate. A site for ligand binding exists on each of the α subunits; occupation of both sites is necessary for receptor activation. Electrophysiologic and ligand binding measurements, together with analysis of the functional states of the receptor, indicate positive cooperativity in the association of agonists; Hill coefficients greater than unity have been described for agonist-elicited channel opening, agonist binding, and agonist-induced desensitization of the receptor [21].

The sequence of the individual subunits is shown in Fig. 8; sequence identity among the subunits appears to be greatest in the hydrophobic regions. Various models for the disposition of the peptide chains have been proposed on the basis of hydropathy and reactivity of various residues to modifying agents and antibodies. Five candidate membrane-spanning regions have been proposed. Four of these are hydrophobic (M_1-M_4), whereas one (A) can be constructed as an α helix containing negative charges aligned to one surface. All of these potential membrane-spanning domains appear after residue 200, with the N-terminal portion of the molecule on the extracellular surface. The homology among the four subunits strongly suggests that the same pattern is found in all subunits. The validity of such models remains to be ascertained as they are subjected to more rigorous structural studies, since it has not been established that M_1 to M_4 and A do in fact span the membrane. Further details about the structure of the receptor are likely to emerge from analysis of disulfide linkages, reactivity of particular residues, and high-resolution structural methods.

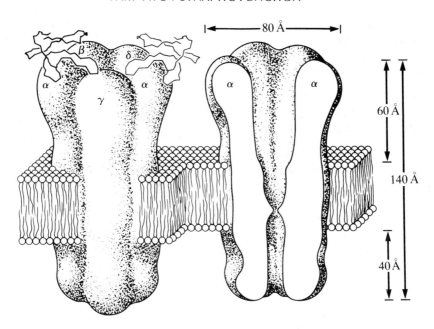

FIG. 7. Structure of the nicotinic ACh receptor. The structure is from image reconstruction analyses of Brisson and Unwin [20], employing electron microscopy on isolated membrane tubes enriched in receptor. The receptor is a pentamer of five distinct subunits; α_1, α_2, β, γ, δ ($M_r \cong 55,000$), and shown is one proposal for the subunit arrangement. Recent findings indicate that the γ subunit may reside between the two α subunits. The internal channel surrounded by the five subunits appears funnel-shaped, with the primary constriction at the membrane surface. Most of the membrane protein extends toward the outer, or extracellular, surface. A nonintegral peptide, often termed ν or 43K, is associated with the cytoplasmic surface of the receptor. Although not essential to the function of the receptor, it appears to play a role in immobilization and aggregation of receptors in junctional regions. This peptide may contribute to the cytoplasmic density seen in the proposed structure. Two α-toxin molecules (peptides of 7,500 Da) bind to each receptor. Their binding surface primarily resides on the α subunit, and these sites seem to be located near the outer perimeter of the molecule. The α subunits also contain recognition sites for agonists, reversible antagonists, and coral lophotoxin. The stoichiometry of these agents is identical to that of α toxins.

Asp 141 in the α subunit is at least partially glycosylated and hence is on the outside surface. After reduction of the receptor by dithiothreitol to convert disulfide bonds to free thiols, bromoacetylcholine and *N*-maleimidobenzyltrimethyl ammonium react with cysteine 192 or 193. Since the adjacent cysteines at residues 192 to 193 are unique to the α subunit, this region is believed to play a role in the binding of agonists and α toxins. Cysteine 192 and 193 appear to be linked by a disulfide bond, as are cysteines 128 and 145. Residues in the β and δ chain (serine 254 and 262) in the M_2 domain have been labeled with the noncompetitive inhibitors chlorpromazine and tetraphenylphosphonium. These residues may define a sequence lining the channel. Conformational changes in this region could prove critical to channel opening. The cobra α toxins and α-bungarotoxin have a flat, leaflike structure and bind to an extended surface area that is mainly encompassed by the α subunit. Fluorescence energy-transfer measurements and electron microscopic imaging indicate that the α toxin and agonist binding sites are closer to the outer perimeter of the receptor than a central pseudo axis of symmetry.

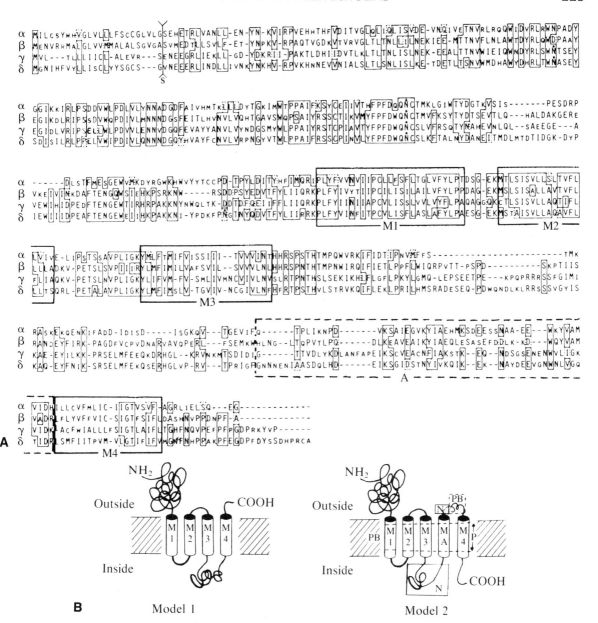

FIG. 8. A: Amino acid sequence homology among the four subunits (α, β, γ, δ) of the *Torpedo californica* ACh receptor [3,4]. Amino acid positions identical in at least three of the four subunits are enclosed in *solid boxes*. In cases where the fourth residue is replaced with an amino acid of equivalent hydrophilic/hydrophobic character, it is denoted by a *dotted line*. The four hydrophobic, helical domains and one amphipathic α helix, which are candidates for spanning the membrane, are denoted by M_1–M_4 and A, respectively. The *arrow* denoted by S represents the cleavage point of the signal peptide. Cysteines 192 and 193 are noted by the *asterisk*. **B:** Two possible arrangements of the polypeptide chain of the subunits of the ACh receptor with respect to the membrane surface. (From Guy and Hucho, *Trends Neurosci.* 10:318–321, 1987.)

*The events associated with ligand
binding and activation of the receptor
have been studied by the analysis of
opening and closing events of individual
channels*

Current electrophysiological studies use high-resistance patch electrodes that form tight seals on the membrane surface over a diameter of 1 to 2 μm and have the capacity to record conductance changes of individual channels within the lumen of the electrode (see Chap. 4). The patch of membrane affixed to the electrode may be excised, inverted, or studied on the intact cell. The individual opening events for ACh achieve a conductance of 25 pS across the membrane and have an opening duration that is exponentially distributed around a value of about 1 msec. The duration of channel opening is dependent on the particular agonist, whereas the conductance of the open-channel state appears to be agonist-independent. Analyses of the frequencies of opening events have permitted an estimation of the kinetic constants for channel opening and ligand binding, and these numbers are in reasonable agreement with estimates of ligand binding and activation from fast kinetic, or stopped-flow, studies. Overall, activation events can be described by Scheme 1. Two ligands (L) associate with the receptor (R) prior to the isomerization step to form the open-channel state L_2R^*. For ACh, the forward rate constant for binding, k_{+1}, is $1 - 2 \times 10^8 \, M^{-1} \, sec^{-1}$; k_{+2} and k_{-2}, forward and reverse rate constants for isomerization, yield rates of isomerization consistent with opening events in the millisecond time frame. Since k_{+2} and k_{-2} are greater than k_{-1}, the rate constant for ligand dissociation, several opening and closing events with the fully liganded receptor occur prior to the

dissociation of the first ligand. Binding of the first and second ligands appears not to be identical, even allowing for the statistical differences arising from the two sites. Such a conclusion is consistent with receptor structure, since different subunits are adjacent to the α subunits in the pentamer.

Desensitization of receptors

Continued exposure of nicotinic receptors to agonist leads to a diminution of the response, even though the concentration of agonist available to the receptor has not changed. The loss of response from prior agonist exposure is called desensitization. Katz and Thesleff examined the kinetics of desensitization with microelectrodes and found that a cyclic scheme in which the receptor existed in two states, R and R', prior to exposure to the ligand best described the process.

To achieve receptor desensitization and activation by a single ligand, multiple conformational states of the receptor must be proposed. The binding steps represented in horizontal equilibria are rapid; vertical steps reflect the slow, unimolecular isomerizations involved in desensitization (Scheme 2). Rapid isomerization for channel opening should be added. To accommodate the additional complexities of the observed fast and slow steps of desensitization, additional states would have to be included.

A simplified scheme, in which only one desensitized and one open-channel state of the receptor exist, is represented in Scheme 2, where R is the resting (activatible), R* the active (open channel), R' the desensitized state of the receptor; M is an allosteric constant defined by R'/R, and K and K' are equilibrium constants

$$2L + R \underset{k_{-1}}{\overset{2k_{+1}}{\rightleftharpoons}} LR \underset{2k_{-1}}{\overset{k_{+1}}{\rightleftharpoons}} L_2R \underset{k_{-2}}{\overset{k_{+2}}{\rightleftharpoons}} L_2R^*$$

(Closed)   (Closed)   (Closed)   (Open)

Scheme 1

$$
\begin{array}{ccccc}
2L + R & \xrightarrow{K/2} & LR & \xrightarrow{2K} & L_2R \longrightarrow L_2R^* \\
M \downarrow & & \downarrow & & \downarrow \\
2L + R' & \xrightarrow{K'/2} & LR' & \xrightarrow{2K'} & L_2R'
\end{array}
$$

Scheme 2

for the indicated reactions. In this scheme, $M < 1$ and $K' < K$. Addition of ligand will eventually result in an increased fraction of R' species due to the way the equilibrium constants are set. Direct binding experiments have confirmed the generality of this scheme for nicotinic receptors. Thus, distinct conformational states dictate the different temporal responses that ensue on addition of a ligand to the nicotinic receptor.

The ganglionic and neuromuscular subtypes of nicotinic receptors differ in their ligand selectivity

Several agonists and antagonists show partial selectivity for subtypes of nicotinic receptors. The most striking difference in specificity is seen with α-bungarotoxin and cobra α toxin (elapid α toxins). These peptides have dissociation constants $\leq 10^{-10}$ M for the neuromuscular receptor and are virtually inactive at ganglia or other nicotinic receptors derived from the embryonic neural crest. Other toxins that block neuromuscular nicotinic receptors, e.g., κ toxins from snake venoms, lophotoxin from coral, and conotoxin from snails, block at autonomic ganglia.

Nevertheless, the absence of an enriched source of nicotinic receptors from ganglia or brain has meant that progress in isolating these receptor subtypes has lagged behind that for receptors in the neuromuscular junction. However, the cDNAs encoding the neuromuscular receptor subunits appear to have provided the necessary key to obtaining detailed structural information about neuronal nicotinic receptors. Since considerable sequence homology exists among nicotinic receptor subtypes, cross-species hybridization using cDNA clones in neuronal libraries has yielded several candidate cDNAs encoding nicotinic receptors from the central nervous system and tissues of neural crest origin. Localization of mRNAs, which hybridize with particular cDNA clones, to selective regional areas in the central nervous system documents the central origin and regional distributions of other types of nicotinic receptors. More difficult will be the assignment of particular cDNAs to receptor subtypes that are actually isolated from discrete brain areas.

At least four genes encode α subunits and two encode β subunits of subtypes of nicotinic receptors

Additional nicotinic receptor subunits may be uncovered, but early evidence suggests that brain nicotinic receptors may in fact be tetramers or pentamers of only two distinct subunits, α and β. Results of molecular cloning have also suggested that junctional and extrajunctional receptors in muscle are different. Although small biophysical differences have been detected between junctional and extrajunctional receptors and the multiple classes of brain receptors, a rigorous receptor subtyping solely on this basis would have been difficult.

Both the nicotinic receptor and acetylcholinesterase are tightly regulated during synapse formation

The different distributions of the nicotinic receptor in innervated and noninnervated muscle were alluded to earlier. Acetylcholinesterase expression is under similar control. Peptides, such as calcitonin gene-related peptide which colocalizes in motorneurons, influence the synthesis of receptors. Moreover, specific molecules within the basal lamina of the synapse, such as agrin, play an important role in establishing nerve-muscle contacts on reinnervation and localizing the receptor and acetylcholinesterase at these sites. Proteins on the cytoplasmic surface of the end-plate appear to immobilize the receptor in the junctional region. One of these proteins is a 43-kDa protein (*ν* protein) that is tightly associated with junctional receptors. The 43-kDa protein may also be involved in receptor aggregation at the end-plate and diminishing the rate of receptor turnover.

MUSCARINIC RECEPTORS

Muscarinic and nicotinic receptors are structurally and functionally closer to other receptors in their respective families than to one another

The nicotinic receptor is much more like other ligand-gated ion channels such as the γ-aminobutyric acid receptor, which are rapidly activated on ligand binding, than the muscarinic receptor. The muscarinic receptor is in turn closer to other cell surface proteins such as adrenergic receptors [22], which transduce their signals across membranes by interacting with GTP binding proteins (G proteins). (The G proteins are described in Chap. 17.) The involvement of several macromolecular interactions in muscarinic receptor activation contributes to the observation that muscarinic responses are slow (100–250 msec latency) compared to those mediated by nicotinic receptors.

The final cellular responses to muscarinic receptor stimulation include inhibition of adenylate cyclase, stimulation of phospholipase C, and activation of K^+ channels

A variety of effector cell types in brain and periphery receive cholinergic innervation, and they respond in different ways to muscarinic receptor stimulation. Muscarinic receptors are also located on presynaptic neurons, where they regulate transmitter release. Despite this obvious functional diversity, the initial event that follows ligand binding to the muscarinic receptor may be in all cases the interaction of the receptor with a G protein. Depending on the nature of the G protein, the receptor-G protein interaction initiates one of several early bio-

chemical events seen with muscarinic receptor occupation: inhibition of adenylate cyclase, stimulation of phosphoinositide hydrolysis, or activation of a K^+ (or other ion) channel (Fig. 9) [23].

Inhibition of adenylate cyclase

Muscarinic inhibition of cAMP formation is most apparent when adenylate cyclase is stimulated, for example by activation of adrenergic receptors with catecholamines. Simultaneous addition of cholinergic agonists decreases the amount of cAMP formed in response to the catecholamine, in some tissues almost completely. The result would be diminished activation of cAMP-dependent protein kinase and decreased substrate phosphorylation catalyzed by this kinase. The mechanism by which the muscarinic receptor inhibits adenylate cyclase is through activation of an inhibitory GTP-binding protein, G_i. This molecule competes with the G protein activated by stimulatory agonists (G_s) for regulation of adenylate cyclase (see also Chaps. 17 and 19).

Stimulation of phospholipase C

Muscarinic agonists stimulate phosphoinositide hydrolysis by activating a phosphoinositide-specific phospholipase C. Activation of this enzyme also requires GTP, implying the involvement of a GTP-binding protein. The hydrolysis of phosphatidylinositol bisphosphate yields two potential second messengers, inositol trisphosphate ($InsP_3$) and diacylglycerol (see Chap. 16). Diacylglycerol increases the activity of the Ca^{2+} and phospholipid-dependent protein kinase (protein kinase C). Inositol trisphosphate can mobilize Ca^{2+} from intracellular stores in the endoplasmic reticulum and thereby elevate cytosolic free Ca^{2+}. Subsequent responses are triggered by direct effects of Ca^{2+} on Ca^{2+}-regulated proteins and by phosphorylation mediated through Ca^{2+}-dependent kinases and protein kinase C.

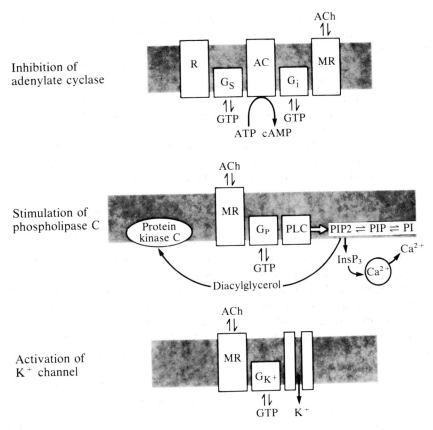

FIG. 9. Primary biochemical responses mediated by muscarinic ACh receptor. ACh interacts with a muscarinic receptor (MR), which may differ for the three responses. The MR interacts with a GTP-binding protein, G_i, known to inhibit adenylate cyclase (AC), or the putative GTP-binding proteins G_p and G_{K+}, to activate phospholipase C (PLC) and K^+ channels, respectively. Mediators formed within the cell are cAMP, inositol trisphosphate (IP_3), and diacylglycerol (DAG).

Activation of K^+ channels

Muscarinic agonists also increase specific K^+ conductance and thereby hyperpolarize cardiac and other cell membranes. This muscarinic effect can be mimicked by GTP analogs in whole-cell clamp experiments, and the response is sensitive to pertussis toxin, which ribosylates and inactivates G_i and a related protein, G_o (see Chap. 7). The likelihood that a G protein links the muscarinic receptor to the K^+ channel is supported by recent data showing that purified G-protein subunits regulate K^+ conductance

and by evidence that other receptor-activated channels are likewise coupled to their receptors in a GTP-dependent fashion [23].

Intracellular mediators of muscarinic receptor action

The three events described above—inhibition of adenylate cyclase, stimulation of phosphoinositide hydrolysis, and activation of K^+ channels—all occur within the plasma membrane. They are triggered directly by muscarinic receptor occupation and are apparently independent of changes in cytosolic mediators. These primary events lead to changes in cell Ca^{2+}, cAMP, and protein phosphorylation, which generate other metabolic sequelae. For example, an increase in cytosolic free Ca^{2+} probably contributes to activation of phospholipase A_2, generating arachidonic acid, prostaglandins, and related eicosanoids (see Chap. 20). These products in turn can stimulate cGMP formation and can regulate ion channel activity. Increased Ca^{2+} can also activate Ca^{2+}-dependent ion channels (K^+, Cl^-) and regulate cAMP phosphodiesterase. Protein kinase C has effects on ion-channel activity and appears necessary for cholinergic secretory and contractile responses. Given the obviously complex set of possible interactions between the intracellular mediators, it is easy to explain how diverse cellular responses can be mediated through a single receptor activating relatively few primary responses (see Chap. 19).

Radiolabeled antagonists, such as quinuclidinylbenzilate, N-methylscopolamine, and propylbenzilylcholine, have been used to characterize muscarinic receptors

In membranes or homogenates from heart, brain, and other tissues, muscarinic agonists compete for these antagonist binding sites with Hill slopes of less than unity, i.e., agonists appear to interact with more than a single population of muscarinic receptors [24]. Direct binding experiments with agonists also show multiple binding sites for agonists. The competition curves are best fit by a model in which there are sites with low, high, and, in some cases, superhigh affinity for agonists. The addition of GTP to the binding assay can have a dramatic effect on the agonist competition curve or on direct agonist binding. The effect is to "convert" high-affinity binding sites to low

affinity or to decrease the apparent affinity of the receptor for agonists.

One mechanism underlying the apparent heterogeneity in agonist binding, as suggested by the effects of GTP and by analogy with adrenergic receptors, is that the receptor interacts with the GTP-binding protein that transduces its effects. This interaction increases the affinity of the receptor for agonist. In the heart, most receptor heterogeneity for agonists can be explained on the basis that a portion of receptors interact with the G protein. In brain this cannot be the only explanation for heterogeneity, since the effects of GTP are often minimal, and guanine nucleotides never fully convert the receptor to a state in which the sites reveal a single dissociation constant [23,24].

Not all agonists show the same amount of heterogeneity in their binding. Some, like ACh, carbamylcholine, and methacholine, bind with high affinity to a large percentage of the total sites or show a large difference in affinity for the low- and high-affinity sites (K_L/K_H). Others, like oxotremorine and pilocarpine, bind more homogeneously and show relatively little high-affinity binding. The capacity of an agonist to induce high-affinity binding correlates with the efficacy of that agonist for eliciting contractile responses or for stimulating phosphoinositide breakdown. It therefore appears that interaction of the receptor and G protein is critical to production of the cellular response.

Unlike agonists, most muscarinic antagonists bind to the receptor with Hill slopes of unity, as expected for a mass action interaction with a single receptor type. There is little difference in affinity for atropine or scopolamine in various tissues. Similar findings with other antagonists suggest that all muscarinic receptors are the same. There are, however, a number of functional studies suggesting that muscarinic receptors are heterogeneous, and several atypical antagonists have been described throughout the years. Results of molecular biology studies of muscarinic receptors suggest that there are at least four distinct subtypes of receptor.

The selectivity of the antagonist pirenzepine forms the cornerstone for the classification of muscarinic receptors into M_1 and M_2 subtypes

Pirenzepine binds to muscarinic receptors in cortex, hippocampus, and ganglia with relatively high affinity, and these sites have been termed M_1, as mentioned earlier. Heart, gland, and smooth muscle muscarinic receptors, as well as those in cerebellum, show 30- to 50-fold lower affinity, and these receptors have been termed M_2 [25]. The affinity for classical antagonists like *N*-methylscopolamine is the same in all of these regions, emphasizing the unique selectivity of pirenzepine (PZ). Direct binding studies using [^{3}H]PZ confirm that only certain tissues and brain regions have receptors with high affinity for this antagonist. Results of pharmacological studies also indicate that PZ blocks muscarinic responses in ganglia better than responses in heart. Another agent described more recently is AF-DX 116. This antagonist discriminates between cardiac and glandular M_2 receptors, suggesting that the M_2 receptor subtype can be further subdivided.

The question of whether the M_1 and M_2 receptors are specifically linked to particular functional responses, such as adenylate cyclase inhibition and phosphoinositide hydrolysis, has been addressed but not yet resolved. Thus, in some tissues the receptor-mediated phosphoinositide responses can be blocked by low concentrations of PZ, suggesting that the M_1 receptor couples to this effector. On the other hand, phosphoinositide hydrolysis in a number of tissues is blocked only at higher concentrations of PZ, consistent with an M_2 receptor-mediated response. The relationship between receptor subtypes and functional responses will likely be resolved in studies carried out on cloned receptors (see below).

Muscarinic receptors from porcine brain and atria have been purified to homogeneity

The receptor consists of a single subunit of about 70 kDa and is a glycoprotein. In general, the characteristics of the purified receptors from heart and brain exhibit similar physical properties. Oligonucleotide probes based on amino acid sequences from these proteins were used to screen porcine brain and heart cDNA libraries. The screening yielded cDNAs encoding the entire open reading frame. The cDNAs code for proteins predicted to have seven transmembrane-spanning regions, similar to what is seen for the β-adrenergic receptor and other receptors that couple to G proteins (Fig. 10). There is only 38 percent homology between the proteins cloned from porcine brain and heart, and most of this is in the transmembrane region [22]. The long cytoplasmic loop between the sixth and seventh transmembrane domain is markedly different for the two receptors. In addition, when the cloned cDNAs are expressed, that from brain binds PZ with high affinity, whereas that from heart binds with low affinity. Thus, the cDNA encoding the receptor initially cloned from the brain has been termed m_1 and is clearly included in the pharmacologically defined class of M_1 receptors, whereas that cloned from the heart has been termed m_2 and appears to be included in the M_2 class of receptors.

Clones encoding muscarinic receptors that differ from the M_1 and M_2 receptors have been isolated from human and rat tissues

Thus, there appear to be at least two additional subtypes of receptor. It remains to be seen whether all of these putative subtypes of muscarinic receptors are normally expressed in mammalian cells and what their function might be. When the cDNA for the receptor from pig

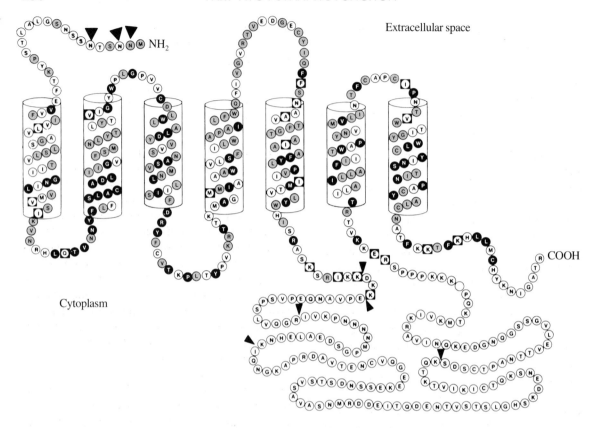

FIG. 10. Predicted transmembrane domain structure of the myocardial muscarinic receptor. Amino acids are indicated by the single-letter code in the *circles*. *Shaded circles* indicate identities between the sequences of the myocardial receptor shown here and the cerebral muscarinic receptor cloned from porcine brain. *Solid circles* indicate additional homology between muscarinic receptors and β-adrenergic receptors. (See Peralta et al., *Science* 236:600, 1987, for additional information.)

heart is expressed in Chinese hamster ovary cells it can couple to and regulate either adenylate cyclase or phospholipase C [22]. Thus, although there are likely to be multiple receptor subtypes, a single subtype may be able to interact with various G proteins and turn on multiple effectors present in the cell. Whether or not there is a preferred and therefore most efficient coupling between a receptor subtype and a particular G protein or effector remains to be determined.

REFERENCES

1. Rama-Sastry, B. V., and Sadavongvivad, C. Non-neuronal acetylcholine. *Pharmacol. Rev.* 30:65–132, 1979.
2. Dale, H. H. The action of certain esters and ethers of choline and their relation to muscarine. *J. Pharmacol.* 6:147–190, 1914.
3. Changeux, J. -P., Devilers-Thierry, A., and Chemuivilli, P. Acetylcholine receptor: An allosteric protein. *Science* 25:1335–1345, 1984.
4. Numa, S., Noda, M., Takahashi, H., Tanabe, T.,

Toyosoto, M., et al. Molecular structure of the acetylcholine receptor. *Cold Spring Harbor Symp. Quant. Biol.* 48:57–69, 1983.

5. Partington, P., Feeney, J., and Burgen, A. S. V. The conformation of acetylcholine and related compounds in aqueous solution as studied by nuclear magnetic resonance spectroscopy. *Mol. Pharmacol.* 8:269–277, 1972.

6. Portoghese, P. S. Relationships between stereostructure and pharmacological activity. *Annu. Rev. Pharmacol.* 10:51–76, 1970.

7. Baker, R. W., Pauling, P., and Petcher, T. J. Structure and activity of muscarinic stimulants. *Nature* 230:439–445, 1971.

8. Weiner, N., and Taylor, P. Drugs acting at synaptic and neuroeffector junctional sites. In Goodman & Gilman's *Pharmacological Basis of Therapeutics.* Gilman, A. G., Goodman, L. S., Rall, T. W. and Murad, F. (eds.). New York: MacMillan, 1985, pp. 66–235.

9. Bolter, J., Evans, K., Goldman, D., Martin, G., Treco, D., et al. Isolation of a cDNA clone coding for a possible neural nicotinic acetylcholine receptor subunit. *Nature* 319:368–373, 1986.

10. Kasa, P. The cholinergic systems in brain and spinal cord. *Prog. Neurobiol.* 26:211–272, 1986.

11. Adams, P. R., Brown, D. A., and Constitini, A. Pharmacological inhibition of the M-current. *J. Physiol. (Lond.)* 332:223–262, 1982.

12. Llinas, R., and Precht, W. (eds.). *Neurobiology of the Frog.* Berlin: Springer-Verlag, 1976.

13. Itoh, N., Slemmon, R., Hawke, D., Williamson, R., Morita, E., et al. Cloning of *Drosophila* choline acetyltransferase cDNA. *Proc. Natl. Acad. Sci. U.S.A.* 83:4081–4085, 1986.

14. Jope, R. High affinity choline uptake and acetylcholine production in brain. Role in regulation of ACh synthesis. *Brain Res. Rev.* 1:313–344, 1979.

15. Parsons, S. M., Bahv, B. A., Graez, M., Kaufman, R., Kornreich, W. D., et al. Acetylcholine transport: Fundamental properties and effects of pharmacological agents. *Ann. N.Y. Acad. Sci.* 493:220–233, 1987.

16. Kuffler, S. W., Nicholls, J., and Martin, R. A. *From Neuron to Brain: A Cellular Approach to the Function of the Nervous System.* Sunderland, MA: Sinauer Associates Inc., 1984.

17. Massoulie, J., and Bon, S. Acetylcholinesterase. *Ann. Rev. Neurosci.* 5:57–106, 1982.

18. Schumacher, M., Camp, S., Maulet, Y., Newton, M. MacPhee-Quigley, K., et al. Primary structure of *Torpedo californica* acetylcholinesterase deduced from its cDNA sequence. *Nature* 319:407–409, 1986.

19. Claudio, T., Green, W. N., Hartman, D. S., Mayden, D., Paulson, H. L., et al. Genetic reconstitution of functional acetylcholine receptor channels in mouse fibroblasts. *Science* 238:1688–1694, 1987.

20. Brisson, A., and Unwin, P. N. T. Quaternary studies of the acetylcholine receptor. *Nature* 315:414–417, 1985.

21. Maelicke, A. (ed.) *Nicotinic Acetylcholine Receptor Structure and Function.* Berlin: Springer-Verlag, 1986. [NATO ASI Series, Vol. H-3]

22. Peralta, E., Winslow, J., Ashkenazi, A., Smith, D., Ramachandran, J., and Capon, D. Structural basis of muscarinic acetylcholine receptor subtype diversity. *Trends Pharmacol. Sci.* (Suppl.) III 6-11, 1988.

23. Nathanson, N. Molecular properties of the muscarinic acetylcholine receptor. *Annu. Rev. Neurosci.* 10:195–236, 1987.

24. Birdsall, N. J. M., Burgen, A. S. V., and Hulme, E. The binding of agonists to brain muscarinic receptor. *Mol. Pharmacol.* 14:723–736, 1978.

25. Hammer, R., Berrie, C. P., Birdsall, N. M. J., Burgen, A. S. V., and Hulme, E. C. Pirenzepine distinguishes between different subclasses of muscarinic receptors. *Nature* 283:90–92, 1980.

CHAPTER **11**

Catecholamines

Norman Weiner and Perry B. Molinoff

Basic Neurochemistry: Molecular, Cellular, and Medical Aspects, 4th Ed., edited by G. J. Siegel et al. Raven Press, Ltd., New York, 1989.
Correspondence to Perry B. Molinoff, Department of Pharmacology, University of Pennsylvania School of Medicine, Philadelphia, PA 19104-6084.

The catecholamines dopamine, norepinephrine, and epinephrine are neurotransmitters and/or hormones in peripheral tissues and central nervous system. Norepinephrine is the principal postganglionic, sympathetic neurotransmitter in both peripheral and central nervous systems. Dopamine, the precursor of norepinephrine, has biological activity in peripheral tissues, most particularly in the kidney, and serves as a neurotransmitter in several important pathways in the central nervous system. Epinephrine, formed by the N-methylation of norepinephrine, is a hormone released from the adrenal gland, and it stimulates catecholamine receptors in a variety of organs. Small amounts of epinephrine are also found in the central nervous system, particularly in the brain stem. (For reviews, see Axelrod and Molinoff [1] and Trendelenburg and Weiner [2].)

BIOSYNTHESIS OF CATECHOLAMINES

The enzymatic processes involved in the formation of catecholamines have been more completely characterized than those for any other neurotransmitter

The component enzymes in the pathway have been purified to homogeneity, which has allowed for detailed analysis of their kinetics, substrate specificity, and cofactor requirements and for the development of inhibitors (Fig. 1). Furthermore, the use of specific antibodies raised against the purified enzymes has permitted precise localization of the enzymes through immunocytochemical techniques.

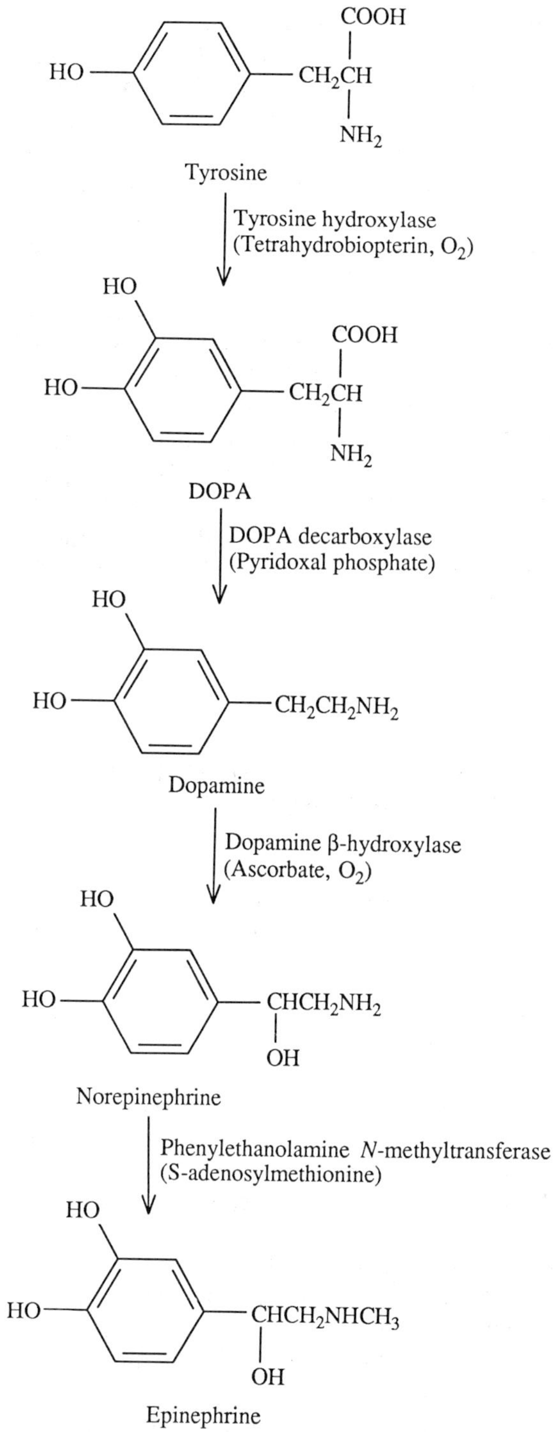

Tyrosine

Tyrosine hydroxylase
(Tetrahydrobiopterin, O_2)

DOPA

DOPA decarboxylase
(Pyridoxal phosphate)

Dopamine

Dopamine β-hydroxylase
(Ascorbate, O_2)

Norepinephrine

Phenylethanolamine *N*-methyltransferase
(S-adenosylmethionine)

Epinephrine

Tyrosine hydroxylase is found in all cells that synthesize catecholamines and is the rate-limiting enzyme in their biosynthetic pathway

Tyrosine hydroxylase (TH) is a mixed-function oxidase that uses molecular oxygen and tyrosine as its substrates and biopterin as its cofactor [3]. It catalyzes the addition of a hydroxyl group to the meta position of tyrosine, thus forming 3,4-dihydroxy-L-phenylalanine (L-dopa). Tyrosine hydroxylase can also hydroxylate phenylalanine to tyrosine, which is then converted to L-dopa; this alternative synthetic route may be of significance in patients affected with phenylketonuria, in which phenylalanine hydroxylase activity is depressed (see Chap. 38). Tyrosine hydroxylase has a K_m value for tyrosine in the micromolar range. As a result, it is virtually saturated by the high tissue concentrations of endogenous tyrosine. Although tyrosine does not ordinarily limit the rate of amine synthesis, recent evidence indicates that the cofactor, biopterin, is at subsaturating concentrations within catecholamine-containing neurons and thus may play an important role in regulating norepinephrine biosynthesis. Tyrosine hydroxylase is primarily a soluble enzyme, localized in the cytosol of catecholamine-containing neuronal processes; however, interactions with membrane constituents, such as phosphatidylserine, or with polyanions, such as heparin sulfate, have been shown to alter its kinetic characteristics. Analogues of tyrosine, such as α-methyl-*p*-tyrosine, are competitive inhibitors of tyrosine hydroxylase.

Dopa decarboxylase is a pyridoxine-dependent enzyme that catalyzes the removal of the carboxyl group from dopa to form dopamine

Dopa decarboxylase (DDC) has a low K_m and high V_m with respect to L-dopa; thus, endogenous L-dopa is efficiently converted to dopa-

FIG. 1. Biosynthetic pathway for catecholamines.

mine, and negligible amounts of L-dopa occur in catecholamine-containing tissues [4]. DDC also decarboxylates 5-hydroxytryptophan, the precursor of serotonin, as well as other aromatic amino acids; accordingly, it has also been called aromatic amino acid decarboxylase. DDC is widely distributed throughout the body, where it is found both in catecholamine- and serotonin-containing neurons and in nonneuronal tissues, such as kidney and vascular pericytes. For dopamine-containing neurons, this is the final step in the pathway. α-Methyldopa inhibits DDC *in vitro* and leads to a reduction in blood pressure after being converted to the false transmitter α-methylnorepinephrine (see also Chap. 42).

For neurons that synthesize epinephrine or norepinephrine, dopamine-β-hydroxylase is the next step in the biosynthetic pathway

Like tyrosine hydroxylase, dopamine-β-hydroxylase (DBH) is a mixed-function oxidase that uses molecular oxygen to form the hydroxyl group added to the β-carbon on the side chain of dopamine [5]. Ascorbate, reduced to dihydroascorbate during the reaction, provides a source of electrons. DBH contains Cu^{2+}, which is involved in electron transfer in the reaction; accordingly, copper chelators, such as diethyldithiocarbamate, are potent inhibitors of DBH. The enzyme is concentrated within the vesicles that store catecholamines; most of the DBH is bound to the inner vesicular membrane, but some is free within the vesicles. DBH is released along with catecholamines from nerves and from the adrenal gland and is found in plasma.

For cells that produce epinephrine, the final step in the pathway is catalyzed by the enzyme phenylethanolamine N-methyltransferase

These cells include a small group of neurons in the brain stem that utilize epinephrine as their neurotransmitter and the adrenal medullary cells for which epinephrine is the primary neurohormone. Phenylethanolamine N-methyltransferase (PNMT) transfers a methyl group from S-adenosylmethionine to the nitrogen of norepinephrine, forming a secondary amine [6]. PNMT activity is regulated by corticosteroids. The high activity of PNMT in the adrenal medulla reflects the high concentrations of corticosteroids released into the venous sinuses that drain the adrenal cortex. Hypophysectomy, which causes a decrease in corticosteroid levels, results in marked reductions in the amount of this enzyme in adrenergic tissues; conversely, administration of large amounts of corticosteroids, particularly during the neonatal period, results in the synthesis of PNMT in sympathetic neurons that do not ordinarily contain the enzyme.

STORAGE AND RELEASE OF CATECHOLAMINES

Catecholamines are concentrated in storage vesicles that are present in high density within nerve terminals

Ordinarily, low concentrations of catecholamines are free in the cytosol, where they may be metabolized by enzymes including monoamine oxidase (MAO). Thus, conversion of tyrosine to L-dopa and L-dopa to dopamine occurs in the cytosol; dopamine then is taken up into the storage vesicles. In norepinephrine-containing neurons, the final β-hydroxylation occurs within the vesicles. In the adrenal gland, norepinephrine is N-methylated by PNMT in the cytoplasm. Epinephrine is then transported back into the chromaffin granules for storage. The mechanism that concentrates catecholamines within the vesicles is an ATP-dependent process linked to a proton pump [7]. The intravesicular concentration of catecholamines is approximately 0.5 M, and they exist in a complex with adenosine triphosphate (ATP) and acidic proteins known as chromogranins. The vesicular uptake process has broad substrate specificity and can transport a variety of biogenic amines, including tryptamine, tyramine, and amphetamines; these amines compete with endogenous catecholamines for vesicular storage sites. Reserpine is a specific, irreversible inhibitor of the vesicular amine pump that terminates the ability of the vesicles to concentrate the amines. Treatment with reserpine causes a profound depletion of endogenous catecholamines in neurons. The effect of reserpine is to inhibit the uptake of dopamine and other catecholamines into vesicles.

The vesicles play a dual role: they maintain a ready supply of catecholamines at the terminal available for release, and they mediate the process of release. When an action potential reaches the nerve terminal, Ca^{2+} channels open, allowing an influx of the cation into the terminal; increased intracellular Ca^{2+} promotes the fusion of vesicles with the neuronal membrane (see Chap. 8). The vesicles then discharge their soluble contents, including norepinephrine, ATP, and DBH, into the extraneuronal space [8]. The demonstration that DBH is released concurrently and proportionately with norepinephrine established that release occurs by the process of exocytosis, since proteins would not be expected to diffuse across cell membranes. Exocytotic release from sympathetic neurons may be the source of some of the DBH found in the plasma and cerebrospinal fluid (CSF) of animals and humans. Indirectly acting sympathomimetics, like tyramine and amphetamine, release catecholamines by a mechanism that is neither dependent on Ca^{2+} nor associated with release of DBH. These drugs displace catecholamines from storage vesicles, resulting in leakage of neurotransmitter from the nerve terminals.

Despite marked fluctuations in the activity of catecholamine-containing neurons, the level of catecholamines within nerve terminals remains relatively constant

Efficient regulatory mechanisms must operate to modulate the rate of synthesis of catecholamines, depending on need [9]. A long-term process affecting catecholamine synthesis involves alterations in the amounts of TH and DBH present in nerve terminals [1]. When the level of neuronal activity of sympathetic neurons is increased for a prolonged period of time, the amounts of mRNA coding for TH and DBH are increased in the neuronal perikarya. DDC does not appear to be modulated by this process. The newly synthesized enzyme molecules are then transported down the axon to the nerve terminals.

Whereas alteration in the rate of synthesis of biosynthetic enzymes provides a gradual and delayed method of control, two mechanisms operative at the level of the nerve terminal play an important role in the short-term modulation of catecholamine synthesis and are responsive to momentary changes in neuronal activity. First, TH, the rate-limiting enzyme in the synthesis pathway, is modulated by end-product inhibition [9]. Thus, free intraneuronal catecholamine inhibits the further activity of TH by competing at the site that binds the pterin cofactor; conversely, neuronal activity results in the release of catecholamines, a decrease in cytoplasmic levels and disinhibition of the enzyme. An additional and probably more important effect of depolarization of catecholaminergic terminals is activation of TH. The kinetic characteristics of the enzyme change so that it has a higher affinity for the pterin cofactor, and the enzyme becomes less sensitive to end-product inhibition. The results of recent experiments suggest that this transient modification of the enzyme occurs as a result of reversible phosphorylation following the influx of Ca^{2+}. Protein kinase C appears to be the kinase responsible for the phosphorylation of TH *in vivo* (see Chap. 19). Thus, through such mechanisms as end-product inhibition, transient activation by phosphorylation, and enzyme induction, the neuron can respond to alterations in utilization of catecholamine neurotransmitters [10].

Two enzymes are primarily responsible for the catabolic inactivation of catecholamines: MAO and catechol-O-methyltransferase

MAO and catechol-*O*-methyltransferase (COMT) are widely distributed throughout the body (Fig. 2). MAO is a flavin-containing enzyme located on the outer membrane of the mi-

tochondria [11]. This enzyme oxidatively deaminates catecholamines to their corresponding aldehydes; in turn, these can be converted by aldehyde dehydrogenase to corresponding acids or by aldehyde reductase to form glycols. Because of its intracellular localization, MAO plays a strategic role in inactivating catecholamines that are free within the nerve terminal and not protected by storage vesicles. Accordingly, drugs that interfere with vesicular storage, such as reserpine, or indirectly acting sympathomimetics, such as amphetamine, which displaces catecholamines from vesicles, cause a marked increase in deaminated metabolites. Isozymes of MAO with differential substrate specificities have been identified. MAO-A preferentially deaminates norepinephrine and serotonin, and

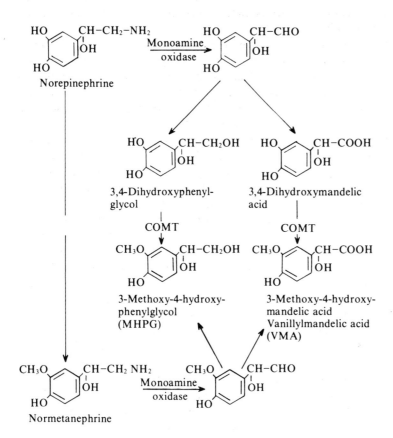

FIG. 2. Pathways of norepinephrine degradation.

it is selectively inhibited by clorgyline, whereas MAO-B acts on a broad spectrum of phenylethylamines, including β-phenylethylamine. MAO-B is selectively inhibited by deprenyl. MAO plays an important protective role in the gastrointestinal tract and liver by preventing access to the general circulation of ingested, indirectly acting amines, such as tyramine and phenylethylamine, that are contained in food; however, patients being treated for depression or hypertension with MAO inhibitors are not afforded this protection and can suffer severe hypertensive crises after ingesting foods that contain large amounts of tyramine. Such foods include port wine, Stilton cheese, and herring. A methyl substituent on the α-carbon of the phenylethylamine side chain protects against deamination by MAO; the prolonged action of amphetamine and related indirectly acting stimulants is one consequence of the presence of an α-methyl group, which prevents their inactivation by MAO.

COMT is found in nearly all cells, including erythrocytes [12]; thus, COMT acts on extraneuronal catecholamines. Most studies of COMT are carried out with enzyme purified from homogenates of liver. The enzyme, which requires Mg^{2+}, transfers a methyl group from the cosubstrate, S-adenosylmethionine, to the 3-hydroxy group on the catecholamine ring. COMT has broad substrate specificity, methylating virtually any catechol regardless of the side-chain constituents; for this reason, competitive inhibitors of the enzyme that are of pharmacological significance have not been developed.

Measurement of catecholamine metabolites can provide insight into the rate of release or turnover of catecholamines in the brain. In clinical studies, metabolites of catecholamines are generally assayed in the CSF, because the large quantities derived from the peripheral sympathomedullary system obscure the small contribution from the brain to urinary levels. However, acid metabolites are actively excreted from the CSF; more reliable estimates of turnover in the brain are obtained when this transport process is blocked by pretreatment with the drug probenecid.

4-Hydroxy-3-methoxy-phenylacetic acid, more commonly known as homovanillic acid (HVA), is a major metabolite of brain dopamine. Spinal fluid levels of HVA provide insight into the turnover of dopamine in the striatum. Levels of HVA are decreased, for example, in CSF of patients with Parkinson's disease (see Chap. 42). A metabolite of norepinephrine formed relatively selectively in the brain is 3-methoxy-4-hydroxyphenylglycol (MHPG). Because this is a minor metabolite of the much larger amounts of norepinephrine metabolized in the periphery, it is estimated that between 30 and 50 percent of the MHPG excreted in urine is derived from brain. Levels of MHPG have been measured in CSF and in urine to provide an index of norepinephrine turnover in the brain, and levels have been shown to be decreased in certain forms of depression (see Chap. 46).

The action of catecholamines released at the synapse is terminated by reuptake into presynaptic nerve terminals

Catecholamines that have not been effectively removed from the synaptic cleft by the transport process diffuse into the extracellular space, where they may be catabolized by MAO and COMT in the liver and kidney. The catecholamine reuptake process was originally described by Axelrod [13]. He observed that when radioactive norepinephrine was injected intravenously, it accumulated in tissues in direct proportion to the density of the sympathetic innervation in the tissue. The amine taken up into the tissues was protected from catabolic degradation, and studies of the subcellular distribution of catecholamines showed that they are localized in synaptic vesicles. Ablation of the sympathetic input to organs abolished the ability of vesicles to accumulate and store radioactive norepinephrine. Subsequent studies demonstrated that this Na^+-dependent uptake process is a characteristic feature of catecholamine-containing neurons in both the periphery and the brain; the transport process has been extensively studied in sheared-off nerve terminals or synaptosomes isolated from brain.

The uptake process is mediated by a carrier located on the outer membrane of the catecholaminergic neurons. It is saturable and obeys Michaelis-Menten kinetics. A transport process selective for norepinephrine is found only in noradrenergic neurons, whereas a carrier with different specificity is found on dopamine-containing neurons [14]. The uptake process is energy-dependent, since it can be inhibited by incubation at a low temperature or by a metabolic inhibitor. The energy requirements reflect a coupling of the uptake process with the Na^+ gradient across the neuronal membrane; drugs such as ouabain, which inhibits Na^+, K^+-ATPase, or drugs like veratridine, which opens Na^+ channels, inhibit the uptake process. The linkage of uptake to the Na^+ gradient may be of physiological significance, since transport temporarily ceases at the time of depolarization-induced release of catecholamines. Because of the differential specificity of the transport processes for dopamine and norepinephrine, uptake of catecholamines can be inhibited selectively by drugs including tricyclic antidepressants and cocaine. In addition, a variety of phenylethylamines, such as amphetamine, bind to the carrier; thus, they can be concentrated within catecholamine-containing neurons and can compete with the catecholamines for transport.

Once an amine has been taken up across the neuronal membrane, it may be sequestered within adrenergic storage vesicles. Neuronal uptake is Na^+-dependent and is not affected by drugs like reserpine; uptake across the vesicle membrane requires Mg^{2+} and is inhibited by reserpine. Once a compound is taken up into the vesicles, it can be released in place of norepinephrine. Such substances are called false transmitters. Active uptake is also the mechanism whereby the neurotoxin 6-hydroxydopamine is accumulated in catecholamine-containing neurons, destroying them through the auto-oxidative liberation of hydrogen peroxide or through formation of a quinone.

ANATOMY OF CATECHOLAMINERGIC SYSTEMS

Our understanding of the function of catecholamine-containing neurons has been aided by neuroanatomical methods of visualizing these neurons

Nearly two decades ago, Falck and Hillarp took advantage of the fact that in the presence of formaldehyde, catecholamines cyclize to form intensely fluorescent products [15]. With a fluorescence microscope, neurons containing catecholamines could be visualized in thin sections obtained from tissue previously exposed to formaldehyde vapor. Numerous investigators have used this technique to map the distribution of catecholamine-containing cell bodies and axonal pathways in the brain. A modification of the method uses glyoxylic acid and has resulted in enhanced sensitivity and a more stable fluorophor for even better visualization of the fine axons and terminals.

Once the enzymes that synthesize catecholamines were purified, it was possible to elicit antiserum against each enzyme. Thin sections of tissue can be incubated with antibody against a particular enzyme, e.g., rabbit anti-DBH. The section is then incubated with a second antibody linked to a marker, such as fluorescein (fluorescein-labeled goat anti-rabbit IgG) or horseradish peroxidase. The neurons containing these enzymes are thus stained specifically. By using this technique, the PNMT-containing neurons that synthesize epinephrine can be distinguished from noradrenergic neurons that are devoid of PNMT; similarly, noradrenergic neurons that contain DBH can be separated from the dopamine-containing neurons that do not possess this enzyme. Cloning the genes that encode for catecholaminergic biosynthetic enzymes makes it possible to use *in situ* hybridization to localize mRNAs within particular neurons (see Chaps. 21 and 22).

Finally, experimental advantage has been taken of the highly selective uptake process for catecholamines. Thus, after incubation with radioactive norepinephrine, noradrenergic axons can be demonstrated at the ultrastructural level by autoradiographic techniques. Alternatively, after administration of the congener 5-hydroxydopamine, which is taken up actively and stored within the vesicles, catecholamine-containing terminals can be distinguished by the presence of dense precipitates of 5-hydroxydopamine within their vesicles.

Cell bodies of noradrenergic neurons are clustered in the medulla oblongata, pons, and midbrain and are considered to be anatomically part of the reticular formation

On the basis of their major axonal projections, noradrenergic fibers can be divided into two major pathways: the dorsal and ventral bundles (Fig. 3). The cell bodies of origin for the dorsal bundle are contained in a dense nucleus known as the locus coeruleus, located on the lateral aspect of the fourth ventricle. Axons of neurons in the locus coeruleus have endings in the spinal cord and cerebellum and course anteriorly through the medial forebrain bundle to innervate the entire cerebral cortex and hippocampus. The ventrally located cell bodies send fibers that innervate the brain stem and hypothalamus. As demonstrated by immunocytochemical techniques, in the ventral portion of the pons and medulla there are a small num-

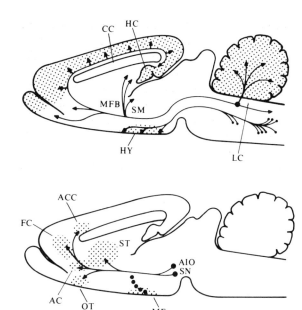

FIG. 3. Catecholaminergic neuronal pathways in the rat brain. **Upper:** Noradrenergic neuronal pathways. **Lower:** Dopaminergic neuronal pathways. (AC) nucleus accumbens; (ACC) anterior cingulate cortex; (CC) corpus callosum; (FC) frontal cortex; (HC) hippocampus; (HY) hypothalamus; (LC) locus coeruleus; (ME) median eminence; (MFB) median forebrain bundle; (OT) olfactory tubercle; (SM) stria medullaris; (SN) substantia nigra; (ST) striatum. (Courtesy of J. T. Coyle and S. H. Snyder).

ber of neurons that contain PNMT; the axons of these epinephrine-containing neurons terminate primarily in the brain stem and hypothalamus.

Cell bodies of dopamine-containing neurons are located primarily in the midbrain

Dopamine-containing neurons can be divided into three main groups: nigrostriatal, mesocortical, and tuberohypophysial. The major dopaminergic tract in brain originates in the zona compacta of the substantia nigra and sends axons that provide a dense innervation to the caudate nucleus and putamen of the corpus striatum; nearly 80 percent of all the dopamine in the brain is found in the corpus striatum. In Parkinson's disease, the nigrostriatal tract degenerates. This accounts for a profound depletion of dopamine from the striatum and for the symptoms of this disorder. The compound MPTP may be formed as a side product in the synthesis of an analogue of the synthetic opiate meperidine. Ingestion or administration of small amounts of MPTP causes biochemical and clinical changes identical to those seen in Parkinson's disease (see also Chap. 42).

Dopamine-containing cell bodies that lie medial to the substantia nigra provide a diffuse, but modest, innervation to the forebrain, including the frontal and cingulate cortex, septum, nucleus accumbens, and olfactory tubercle. It has been hypothesized that antipsychotic neuroleptic drugs exert their therapeutic action though blockade of the effects of dopamine released by this system (see Chap. 45).

Dopamine-containing cell bodies in the arcuate and periventricular nuclei of the hypothalamus send axons that innervate the intermediate lobe of the pituitary and the median eminence. These neurons play an important role in regulating the release of pituitary hormones, especially prolactin (see Chaps. 14 and 47). In addition to these major pathways, dopamine-containing interneurons have been found in the olfactory bulb and in the neural retina.

The brain contains at least six classes of receptors for catecholamines

The six classes are D_1, D_2, α_1, α_2, β_1, and β_2. Postsynaptic receptors for dopamine and norepinephrine are distinct (Table 1). It is not yet known whether receptors for epinephrine-containing neurons differ in their properties from receptors postsynaptic to norepinephrine-containing neurons, because the limited distribution of epinephrine-containing neurons in the brain

TABLE 1. Distinguishing features of multiple classes of catecholamine receptors

DOPAMINE RECEPTORS

Dopamine-1 (D_1) receptors
  Linked to stimulation of adenylate cyclase
  Ergot alkaloids (e.g., bromocryptine) are antagonists
  SKF-38393 is a specific agonist
  Butyrophenone neuroleptics are weak antagonists
  Largely absent in pituitary, but present in parathyroid gland
  Present in corpus striatum on intrinsic neurons sensitive to kainic acid
  Studied with [^{3}H]SCH-23390 or [^{125}I]SCH-23982

Dopamine-2 (D_2) receptors
  Linked to inhibition of adenylate cyclase
  Ergot alkaloids are agonists
  N-propylnorapomorphine is a specific agonist
  Butyrophenone neuroleptics are potent antagonists
  Present in pituitary
  Present in corpus striatum on axons and terminals of corticostriate neurons
  Studied with [^{3}H]spiroperidol or [^{125}I]iodobenzamide

NOREPINEPHRINE AND EPINEPHRINE RECEPTORS

β_1 Receptors
  Linked to stimulation of adenylate cyclase
  Found in high density in the heart and cerebral cortex
  Epinephrine and norepinephrine are equally potent agonists
  Practolol and ICI 89,406 are selective antagonists
  Marked regional variations in brain
  No selective radioligands. Studied with [^{125}I]iodopindolol, [^{3}H]dihydroalprenolol, or [^{3}H]CGP-12177 (hydrophilic)

β_2 Receptors
  Linked to stimulation of adenylate cyclase
  Found in high density in the lung and cerebellum
  Epinephrine is more potent than norepinephrine
  Terbutaline and salbutamol are selective agonists
  ICI 118,551 is a selective antagonist
  No selective radioligands. Studied with [^{125}I]iodopindolol, [^{3}H]dihydroalprenolol, or [^{3}H]CGP-12177 (hydrophilic)

α_1 Receptors[a]
  Located postsynaptically on blood vessels and in the spleen and peripheral tissues
  Prazosin, indoramin, and WB-4101 are selective antagonists of receptors localized in heart and vas deferens
  Studied with [^{3}H]WB-4101, [^{3}H]prazosin, or [^{125}I]BE-2254

continued

TABLE 1. (*continued*)

α_2 Receptors[a]

Located on presynaptic nerve terminals in the periphery

Piperoxan and yohimbine are relatively selective antagonists

Clonidine and other imidazolines are selective agonists

Localized in pancreas and rabbit duodenum

Effects mediated through stimulation of phospholipase α_2 activity and mobilization of intracellular Ca^{2+}

Clonidine, epinephrine, and norepinephrine are selective ligands

Studied with [^{3}H]clonidine, [^{3}H]yohimbine, or [^{3}H]idazoxan

[a] α_1 and α_2 receptors are blocked to a similar extent by ergot alkaloids and by phentolamine. Both classes of receptors are present throughout the brain, although regional variations in rat are greater for α_2 receptors.

has precluded a detailed characterization of their receptors.

Autoreceptors

The postsynaptic receptors on any given neuron receive information from transmitters released by another neuron. Typically, the postsynaptic receptor is located on the dendrite or cell body of the neuron, but it also may occur on axons or nerve terminals; in the latter case, an axoaxonic synaptic relationship causes presynaptic inhibition or excitation (see Chap 8). In contrast, autoreceptors are situated on a given neuron and respond to transmitter molecules released by the same neuron. Autoreceptors may be distributed over the entire surface of the neuron. At the nerve terminal, they respond to transmitter molecules released into the synaptic cleft; on the cell body, they may respond to transmitter molecules released by dendrites. Functionally, autoreceptors appear to regulate transmitter release in such a way that the released transmitter, acting on the autoreceptors, inhibits further release. Autoreceptors have

been identified for norepinephrine-, dopamine-, serotonin-, and GABA-containing neurons; however, the most detailed information is available from studies of norepinephrine-containing neurons. The major type of autoreceptor described in both the peripheral sympathetic nervous system and the brain has pharmacological properties resembling those of the α_2-adrenergic receptor, [16–18]. In general, the drug specificity of dopamine autoreceptors appears to be similar to that of the postsynaptic dopamine receptors.

In the peripheral sympathetic nervous system, autoreceptors of the β-adrenergic type have also been described. These differ markedly from most other autoreceptors, since norepinephrine acting on these receptors facilitates transmitter release and thus amplifies the effects of neuronal firing. This effect contrasts with the inhibitory action of α-adrenergic and dopamine autoreceptors, which exert negative feedback control on transmitter release.

The most extensive biochemical data about catecholamine receptors deal with the postsynaptic receptors that can be labeled readily in binding studies. In contrast, autoreceptors have not been directly labeled. One can study a neurotransmitter receptor biochemically either indirectly by measuring a related biochemical response, such as stimulation or inhibition of adenylate cyclase activity, or directly by studying the binding of a radioligand.

DOPAMINE RECEPTORS

There is general agreement that there are multiple subtypes of dopamine receptors

Kebabian and Calne [19] classified dopamine receptor subtypes in terms of whether or not they were linked to activation of the enzyme adenylate cyclase. It is now believed that D_1 receptors are linked to stimulation of adenylate cyclase activity, whereas D_2 receptors inhibit the activity of this enzyme. Although many neuroleptics interact with several different classes of receptors, the strongest correlation between clinical dose of antipsychotic drug and *in vitro* potency at a receptor has been observed for D_2 receptors. Spiroperidol, a butyrophenone, and sulpiride, a benzamide, are relatively selective antagonists of D_2 receptors. Furthermore, ergot derivatives used in the treatment of Parkinson's disease, including bromocriptine, lisuride, and pergolide, are potent agonists at D_2 receptors but weak antagonists or partial agonists at D_1 receptors.

The recent availability of a D_1-selective antagonist, SCH-23390, as well as a D_1-selective agonist, SKF-38393, has made it possible to carry out functional studies designed to determine the role of the D_1 receptor in the CNS. The results of these studies suggest complex interactions of D_1 and D_2 receptors in controlling behaviors formerly thought to be mediated solely by D_2 receptors. For example, catalepsy, a behavior previously thought to be mediated by inhibition of D_2 receptors, was induced when rats were given SCH-23390. Moreover, catalepsy induced by this D_1-selective antagonist could be inhibited in a dose-dependent manner by D_2-selective agonists. SCH-23390 also blocked amphetamine-induced hyperlocomotion and apomorphine-induced stereotypy, behaviors thought to be mediated by D_2 receptors.

A number of different approaches have been developed that can distinguish the different subclasses of receptor for a given transmitter

One approach is to use a radioligand that binds with approximately the same affinity to multiple subtypes of receptors. Inhibition of the binding of $[^3H]\alpha$-flupenthixol by ligands including domperidone and spiroperidol made it possible to determine the densities of D_1 and D_2 receptors in tissues that contain both major subtypes of dopamine receptors. A second approach to characterization of receptor subtypes employs radioligands that show selectivity for one or the other subclass of receptors. If the radioligand has a measurable affinity for both of the putative subtypes, curvilinear Scatchard plots will result (see Chap. 9). Computer-assisted analysis of such data can provide estimates of the densities and properties of the putative subtypes present in a given tissue. Alternatively, it is sometimes possible to use a radioligand that is highly selective for a given subtype of receptor. This approach is appropriate for the study of subtypes of dopamine receptors. In particular, SCH-23390 labeled with tritium or its iodinated analog $[^{125}I]$SCH-23982 is highly selective for D_1 receptors. In autoradiographic studies [20], only a small percentage of the binding of $[^3H]$SKF-83566, a brominated analog of SCH-23390, was nonspecific. $[^3H]$Spiroperidol ($[^3H]$SPD) is a useful ligand for the study of D_2 receptors. It is not as specific as the ligands available for D_1 receptors, since $[^3H]$SPD also labels 5-HT$_2$ receptors and the so-called spirodecanone sites. The use of $[^3H]$SPD to study D_2 receptors is facilitated by the use of a highly D_2-selective ligand such as sulpiride to define specific binding. An iodinated derivative of raclopride (^{125}I-iodobenzamide) has recently become available. This ligand has a high affinity for D_2 receptors, and it does not appear to label 5-HT$_2$ receptors (see Chap. 12) or spirodecanone sites. These properties, together with its high specific activity, suggest that it will be a useful ligand for the study of D_2 receptors in homogenates and after detergent solubilization. It is worth noting that no ligand is entirely selective for a single receptor or receptor subtype. Thus, SCH-23390, initially thought to label only D_1 receptors, also binds with high affinity to 5-HT$_{1c}$ receptors in the choroid plexus and elsewhere throughout the brain.

Injection of kainic acid into the corpus striatum selectively destroys intrinsic neurons and essentially abolishes dopamine-stimulated adenylate cyclase activity, but it reduces binding of antagonists to dopamine receptors by only about 50 percent. The remaining dopamine receptors labeled by tritiated antagonists are removed by lesions of the major neuronal projection from the cerebral cortex to the corpus striatum. This suggests that receptors labeled by antagonists include those dopamine receptors localized on intrinsic neurons in the corpus striatum that are linked to stimulation of adenylate cyclase activity and dopamine receptors situated on axons and nerve terminals of the corticostriate projection that are not associated with stimulation of adenylate cyclase activity (Fig. 4).

Two experimental approaches have been used for solubilization of membrane-associated D₂ receptors

The first approach has been to solubilize the receptor using the detergent digitonin. A second approach for solubilization of D₂ receptors has been to extract tissue with a low concentration of a synthetic detergent in the presence of a high concentration of salt. A potential advantage of the second approach is that synthetic detergents often have a higher critical micelle concentration than does digitonin, and they can therefore be removed by dialysis. However, membrane fragments rather than soluble proteins may result when using the low-detergent/high-salt extraction protocol [21].

Results of recent studies indicate that preparations of caudate tissue solubilized with digitonin are sources of D₁, as well as D₂, receptors. Studies of the binding of [³H]SCH-23390 to receptors in solubilized preparations have been carried out. The same rank order of po-

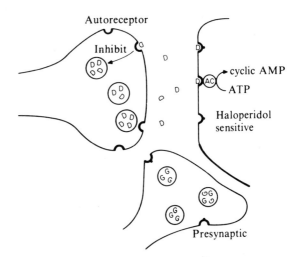

FIG. 4. Dopamine receptor heterogeneity. A postsynaptic receptor (D_1) is linked to adenylate cyclase (AC). A second dopamine receptor (D_2), which exhibits high affinity for butyrophenones such as haloperidol, is found on postsynaptic neurons as well as on the terminals of striatal glutaminergic (G) afferents. The third dopamine receptor (autoreceptor) is localized on dopaminergic terminals (D) and regulates the release of dopamine. (Courtesy of J. T. Coyle and S. H. Snyder).

tency for the binding of agonists and antagonists exists as with D_1 receptors associated with membranes [22]. The observation of different elution profiles for the binding sites labeled with [³H]SPD and [³H]SCH-23390 strongly suggests that D_1 and D_2 receptors are distinct proteins.

α- AND β-ADRENERGIC RECEPTORS

The pharmacological responses to catecholamines were ascribed to effects of α-adrenergic and β-adrenergic receptors in the late 1940s

Norepinephrine and epinephrine act at both α and β receptors, but isoproterenol, a synthetic agonist, acts only at β receptors. Numerous antagonists also differentiate between α and β receptors. The prototypic β-adrenergic receptor antagonist propranolol is essentially inactive at α receptors; the α-adrenergic receptor antagonist phentolamine is very weak at β receptors.

Physically distinct subtypes of β-adrenergic receptors exist and have important pharmacological consequences

Of the β receptors, those known as β_1-adrenergic receptors predominate in the heart and in the cerebral cortex whereas β_2-adrenergic receptors predominate in the lung and cerebellum. However, in many cases, β_1- and β_2-adrenergic receptors coexist in the same tissue, sometimes mediating the same physiological effect. A major side effect of β_2-selective agonists like metaproterenol, used to treat asthma, is cardiac acceleration. This is due to the coexistence of β_1- and β_2-adrenergic receptors in the heart. Both classes of receptors are coupled to the electrophysiologic effects of catecholamines in the heart.

The brain contains both β_1 and β_2 receptors, which cannot, however, be differentiated in terms of their physiological functions. Moreover, radioactive drugs that bind exclusively to one or the other type of β receptor are not yet available. However, one can label all of the β-adrenergic receptors in a given tissue with a nonselective radioligand and then selectively inhibit the binding to one of the subtypes of β receptors with increasing concentrations of β_1- or β_2-selective agents. ICI 89,406 and ICI 118,551 are highly selective antagonists at β_1- and β_2-adrenergic receptors, respectively. A similar approach can be used to define the anatomical localization of β_1- and β_2-adrenergic receptors using the technique of quantitative autoradiography. The density of β_1 receptors varies more markedly in different brain areas than does that of β_2 receptors [23]. It has been suggested that this is due to the presence of β_2-adrenergic receptors on glia or blood vessels.

Using the tools of molecular biology, the amino acid sequences of β-adrenergic receptors in brain and various tissues have been determined

A striking structural feature of all β-adrenergic receptors that have been cloned and sequenced (from turkey erythrocytes, hamster lung, and human placenta and brain) is their topographical orientation with respect to the membrane [24]. Analysis of hydropathicity profiles suggests that there are seven hydrophobic regions, each of 20 to 25 amino acids. These are potentially membrane-spanning. Other structural features include a long C-terminal hydrophilic sequence thought to be extracellular, a somewhat shorter N-terminal hydrophilic sequence thought to be intracellular, and a long cytoplasmic loop between presumptive transmembrane segments V and VI (Fig. 5). Specific functions associated with different portions of the receptor have not yet been established. Sites for N-linked glycosylation are found in the N-terminal extracellular portion of the molecule, whereas numerous sites that may be phosphorylated are found in the C-terminal portion of the molecule and on the third intracellular loop. Evidence from studies involving limited proteolysis and site-directed mutagenesis have led to the conclusion that the hydrophobic transmembrane helices are involved in the formation of the binding site for catecholamines, and the third intracellular loop may play a role in the interaction of the receptor with a GTP-binding protein (see Chap. 17).

The multiple serine and threonine residues and consensus sites for cyclic AMP (cAMP)-dependent phosphorylation may be important in explaining processes including agonist-induced receptor sequestration and desensitization. cAMP- and non-cAMP-dependent phosphorylation of β-adrenergic receptors has been im-

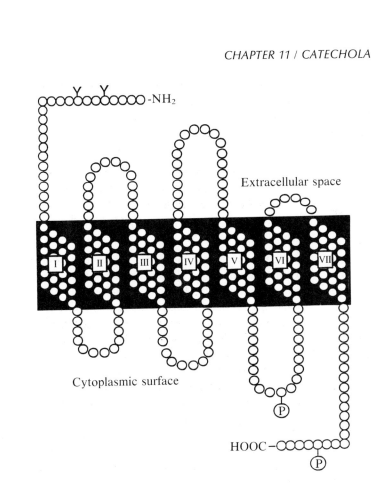

FIG. 5. Schematic diagram of the generic structure of G-protein-related receptors. The seven membrane-spanning regions are indicated with Roman numerals: (Y) sites of glycosylation; (P) positions at which phosphorylation may occur.

plicated in the process known as desensitization. In particular, occupancy of β-adrenergic receptors by agonists results in the activation of β-adrenergic receptor kinase, which catalyzes phosphorylation of the receptor. Although the specific residues phosphorylated by β-adrenergic receptor kinase have not been identified, this reaction appears to contribute to a decrease in the ability of the receptor to activate G_s and thus adenylate cyclase. (Desensitization is presented in Chap. 18.)

The proposed structure of the β-adrenergic receptor is strikingly similar in sequence and topography to that of bacterial rhodopsin (see Chap. 7) and the muscarinic acetylcholine receptor, whose cDNA has recently been cloned from porcine brain and heart (see Chap. 10). Although these proteins mediate widely dispar-

ate biological effects, they show a high degree of homology. This is almost certainly related to the fact that in each case, the immediate consequence of receptor activation is to promote an interaction between the receptor and a GTP-binding protein. The homologies between the members of this extended family of proteins are most evident within the presumed membrane-spanning helices.

Distinct subtypes of postsynaptic α-adrenergic receptors have also been described

Radiolabeled agonists and antagonists have been used to label α receptors in both the brain and the peripheral tissues. As with β receptors, the binding properties of α receptors are essentially the same in the brain and the periphery. Some tissues possess only postsynaptic α_1, others postsynaptic α_2, and some organs have a mixture of both. Results of pharmacological and physiological studies have led to the suggestion that there are multiple types of both α_1 and α_2 receptors. Of particular clinical importance are differences in the properties of junctional and extrajunctional α receptors. The proportions of α_1 and α_2 receptors also vary in different brain regions. Some areas possess exclusively α_1, others exclusively α_2, and a third area has mixtures of the two [25]. The physiological consequences of the two types of α receptors in the brain are unclear at the present time. It is striking that the drug specificity of postsynaptic α_2 receptors closely resembles that of adrenergic autoreceptors, which are therefore also referred to as α_2 receptors. In peripheral tissues, the pharmacological effects of drugs in contracting smooth muscle of various organs differ, and these differences in relative potencies parallel differences in binding properties of α receptors in the various organs.

Studies involving the binding of radioligands are also consistent with the suggestion that there are subtypes of both α_1- and α_2-adrenergic receptors. The suggestion that there are subtypes of α_1-adrenergic receptors was based on a comparison of the properties of [3H]prazosin and [3H]WB-4101 binding to α_1-adrenergic receptors in rat brain and uterus. Heterogeneity of α_2-adrenergic receptors was based on a comparison between the binding of [3H]guanidine and [3H]yohimbine in a variety of tissues and species [26]. The observation that prazosin is more potent in neonatal rat lung [25] and cerebral cortex than in the human platelet, the prototypic tissue for the study of α_2 receptors, was interpreted as indicating a heterogeneity in the pharmacological characteristics of α_2-adrenergic receptors. α_2-Adrenergic receptors have been purified to homogeneity from human platelets and porcine brain. In both

cases, the receptor migrates as a single band on sodium dodecylsulfate (SDS)-polyacrylamide gels at approximately 65,000 daltons.

The purified α_2-adrenergic receptor has been functionally reconstituted with various guanine nucleotide-binding regulatory proteins in phospholipid vesicles

In the presence of epinephrine, reconstituted receptor stimulated the GTPase activity of several guanine nucleotide-binding proteins (G proteins). Maximal stimulation was observed when α_2-adrenergic receptors were coupled with G_i and G_o [27]. Much lower levels of stimulation were obtained with G_s or transducin, a GTP-binding protein found in the retina. This order of efficacy is not surprising, since G_i is thought to be involved in biochemical events normally mediated by α_2-adrenergic receptors, including inhibition of adenylate cyclase activity. Although the function of G_s is unknown at present, one may speculate that its function is more similar to that of G_i than that of G_s (see Chap. 17).

Recently, a gene coding for the α_2-adrenergic receptor has been cloned and sequenced [28]. The protein sequence deduced from the DNA shows significant homology to that of the β_2-adrenergic receptor and shows the now typical seven membrane-spanning regions of high hydrophobicity. On the other hand, the third intracellular loop of the α_2-adrenergic receptor is much longer than the corresponding region of the β_2-adrenergic receptor. This feature of a long, third intracellular loop is shared with the several muscarinic receptors that have been cloned and sequenced. As observed with other G-protein-coupled receptors, the α_2-adrenergic receptor has asparagine residues (positions 10 and 14) that are likely to be sites of N-linked glycosylation. Using somatic cell hybridization analysis, it was shown that the gene coding for the human α_2-adrenergic receptor resides on chromosome 10.

DYNAMICS OF CATECHOLAMINE RECEPTORS

Neurotransmitter receptors are not static entities; changes in the number of receptors appear to be associated with altered synaptic activity

In both the peripheral sympathetic nervous system and the brain, destruction of catecholamine-containing nerves is associated with functional supersensitivity of postsynaptic sites [29]. Conversely, administration of tricyclic antidepressants or inhibitors of MAO leads to functional subsensitivity. These changes appear to be a compensatory response to altered levels of sympathetic stimulation. Destruction of the dopamine-containing nigrostriatal pathway has well-observed behavioral consequences. Because this pathway is uncrossed, a unilateral nigrostriatal lesion causes asymmetry in dopamine innervation between the two cerebral hemispheres. Behavioral studies demonstrate that the dopamine receptors in the denervated corpus striatum are supersensitive. Apomorphine, a dopamine agonist that stimulates dopamine receptors selectively, causes rotational behavior in rats with unilateral lesions. The extent of receptor supersensitivity can be quantified by measuring the amount of rotational behavior.

After selective nigrostriatal lesions have been produced in rats by injections of 6-hydroxydopamine in the substantia nigra, the number of dopamine receptors in the ipsilateral corpus striatum increases markedly, and the increase in the number of receptors may correlate with the extent of behavioral supersensitivity as monitored by rotational behavior [30]. Thus, the increase in receptor density appears to play a role in the behavioral supersensitivity of these animals.

Changes in the number of dopamine receptors may also be involved in pharmacological actions of neuroleptic drugs

One of the most serious side effects of the neuroleptic drugs is tardive dyskinesia, a disfiguring, excessive motor activity of the tongue, face, arms, and legs in patients treated chronically with large doses of the drugs (see Chap. 42). Paradoxically, reduction of the dosage worsens the symptoms, whereas increasing the dosage alleviates the symptoms, so clinicians have speculated that tardive dyskinesia reflects supersensitivity of dopamine receptors that have been chronically blocked. This hypothesis gains support from direct demonstration that chronic treatment with neuroleptics leads to an increase in the number of dopamine receptors in the corpus striatum [30]. Moreover, the ability of neuroleptics to elicit this increase correlates with their ability to block dopamine receptors.

α-Adrenergic and β-adrenergic receptors also demonstrate supersensitivity in binding studies

The number of α_1 and α_2 receptors increases after the noradrenergic neurons in the brain have been destroyed by injections of 6-hydroxydopamine. It is interesting that after this induced destruction of norepinephrine-containing neurons, the number of β_1 receptors increases markedly, but no change occurs in the number of β_2 receptors [23]. This may be a consequence of the fact that β_2 receptors have a low affinity for norepinephrine and that the concentration of epinephrine in the brain is relatively low. Similarly, the chronic administration of tricyclic antidepressants leads to a selective decrease in the density of β_1-adrenergic receptors in the cerebral cortex. This suggests that the β_1-adrenergic receptors in the cortex are functionally innervated. On the other hand, studies using quantitative autoradiography have revealed increases in the density of β_2-adrenergic receptors in particular thalamic nuclei following administration of 6-hydroxydopamine.

ACKNOWLEDGMENTS

We are indebted to Drs. Joseph T. Coyle and Solomon H. Snyder for allowing us to use much of the chapter they prepared for the 3rd edition of this book. Support was provided by NIH grants NS 18479 and NS 18591.

REFERENCES

1. Molinoff, P. B., and Axelrod, J. Biochemistry of catecholamines. *Annu. Rev. Biochem.* 40:465–500, 1971.
2. Trendelenburg, U., and Weiner, N. (eds.). *Catecholamines.* Berlin: Springer-Verlag, 1988, Vol. II (*in press*).
3. Shiman, R., Akino, M., and Kaufman, S. Solubilization and partial purification of tyrosine hydroxylase from bovine adrenal medulla. *J. Biol. Chem.* 246:1330–1340, 1971.
4. Christenson, J. G., Dairman, W., and Udenfriend, S. Preparation and properties of homogeneous aromatic L-amino acid decarboxylase from hog kidney. *Arch. Biochem. Biophys.* 141:356–367, 1970.
5. Craine, J. E., Daniels, G., and Kaufman, S. Dopamine-β-hydroxylase: The subunit structure and anion activation of the bovine adrenal enzyme. *J. Biol. Chem.* 248:7838–7844, 1973.
6. Connett, R. J., and Kirshner, N. Purification and properties of bovine phenylethanolamine-*N*-methyltransferase. *J. Biol. Chem.* 245:329–334, 1970.
7. Holz, R. W. Evidence that catecholamine transport into chromaffin vesicles is coupled to vesicle membrane potential. *Proc. Natl. Acad. Sci. U.S.A.* 75:5190–5194, 1978.
8. Weinshilboum, R. M., Thoa, N. B., Johnson, D. G., Kopin, I. J., and Axelrod, J. Proportional release of norepinephrine and dopamine-β-hydroxylase from sympathetic nerves. *Science* 174:1349–1351, 1971.
9. Masserano, J. M., Vulliet, P. R., Tank, A. W., and Weiner, N. The role of tyrosine hydroxylase in the regulation of catecholamine synthesis. Berlin: Springer-Verlag, 1988, Vol. II (*in press*).
10. Joh, T. H., Park, D. H., and Reis, D. J. Direct phosphorylation of brain tyrosine hydroxylase by cyclic AMP-dependent protein kinase: Mechanism of enzyme activation. *Proc. Natl. Acad. Sci. U.S.A.* 75:4744–4748, 1978.
11. Costa, E., and Sandler, M. *Monoamine Oxidase: New Vistas.* New York: Raven, 1972.
12. Nikodejevic, B., Sinoh, S., Daly, J. W., and Creveling, C. R. Catechol-*O*-methyltransferase II: A new class of inhibitors of catechol-*O*-methyltransferase; 3,5-dihydroxy-4-methoxybenzoic acid and related compounds. *J. Pharmacol. Exp. Ther.* 174:83–93, 1970.
13. Axelrod, J. Noradrenaline: Fate and control of its biosynthesis. *Science* 173:598–606, 1971.
14. Coyle, J. T., and Snyder, S. H. Catecholamine uptake by synaptosomes in homogenates of rat brain: Stereospecificity of different areas. *J. Pharmacol. Exp. Ther.* 170:221–231, 1969.
15. Lindvall, O., and Bjorklund, A. Organization of catecholamine neurons in the rat central nervous system. In L. L. Iversen, S. D. Iversen, and S. H. Snyder (eds.), *Handbook of Psychopharmacology.* New York: Plenum, 1978, Vol. 9, pp. 139–231.
16. Langer, S. Z. Presynaptic regulation of catecholamine release. *Biochem. Pharmacol.* 23:1793–1800, 1974.
17. Starke, K. Regulation of noradrenaline release by presynaptic receptor systems. *Rev. Physiol. Biochem. Pharmacol.* 77:1–124, 1977.
18. Stjarne, L. Basic mechanisms and local feedback control of secretion of adrenergic and cholinergic neurotransmitters. In L. L. Iversen, S. D. Iversen, and S. H. Snyder (eds.), *Handbook of Psychopharmacology.* New York: Plenum, 1975, Vol. 6, pp. 179–233.
19. Kebabian, J. W., and Calne, D. B. Multiple receptors for dopamine. *Nature* 277:93–96, 1979.
20. Boyson, S. J., McGonigle, P., and Molinoff, P.

B. Quantitative autoradiographic localization of the D_1 and D_2 subtypes of dopamine receptors in rat brain. *J. Neurosci.* 6:3177–3188, 1986.

21. Luedtke, R., and Molinoff, P. B. Characterization of binding sites for ^{3}H-spiroperidol. *Biochem. Pharmacol.* 36:3255–3264, 1987.

22. Niznik, H. B., Otsuka, N. Y., Dumbrille-Ross, A., Grigoriadis, D., Tirpak, A., and Seeman, P. Dopamine D_1 receptors characterized with [^{3}H]SCH 23390: Solubilization of a guanine nucleotide-sensitive form of the receptor. *J. Biol. Chem.* 261:8397–8406, 1986.

23. Minneman, K. P., Dibner, M. D., Wolfe, B. B., and Molinoff, P. B. β_1- and β_2-adrenergic receptors in rat cerebral cortex are independently regulated. *Science* 204:866–868, 1979.

24. Dohlman, H. G., Caron, M. G., and Lefkowitz, R. J. A family of receptors coupled to guanine nucleotide regulatory proteins. *Biochemistry* 26:2657–2664, 1987.

25. U'Prichard, D. C., and Snyder, S. H. Distinct α-noradrenergic receptors differentiated by binding and physiological relationships. *Life Sci.* 24:79–88, 1979.

26. Latifpour, J., Jones, S. B., and Bylund, D. B. Characterization of [^{3}H]yohimbine binding to putative *alpha*-2 adrenergic receptors in neonatal rat lung. *J. Pharmacol. Exp. Ther.* 223:606–611, 1982.

27. Cerione, R. A., Regan, J. W., Nakata, H., Codina, J., Benovic, J. L., et al. Functional reconstitution of the α_2-adrenergic receptor with guanine nucleotide regulatory proteins in phospholipid vesicles. *J. Biol. Chem.* 261:3901–3909, 1986.

28. Kobilka, B. K., Dixon, R. A. F., Frielle, T., Dohlman, H. G., Bolanowki, M. A., et al. cDNA for the human β_2-adrenergic receptor: A protein with multiple membrane-spanning domains and encoded by a gene whose chromosomal location is shared with that of the receptor for platelet-derived growth factor. *Proc. Natl. Acad. Sci. U.S.A.* 84:46–50, 1987.

29. Snyder, S. H. Receptors, neurotransmitters, and drug responses. *N. Engl. J. Med.* 300:465–472, 1979.

30. Creese, I., Burt, D. R., and Snyder, S. H. Biochemical actions of neuroleptic drugs: Focus on the dopamine receptor. In L. L. Iversen, S. D. Iversen, and S. H. Snyder (eds.), *Handbook of Psychopharmacology.* New York: Plenum, 1978, Vol. 10, pp. 37–90.

CHAPTER 12

Histamine and Serotonin

Jack Peter Green

Basic Neurochemistry: Molecular, Cellular, and Medical Aspects, 4th Ed., edited by G. J. Siegel et al. Raven Press, Ltd., New York, 1989. Correspondence to Jack Peter Green, Department of Pharmacology, Mount Sinai School of Medicine, New York, New York 10029.

HISTAMINE

Over 20 years ago, there was evidence to suggest that histamine functions in brain as a neuroregulator; however, only in the past few years has enough evidence accumulated to provide convincing support for this assertion [1–5]. The lag in recognizing histamine as a neuroregulator is due to the low concentration of histamine in the brain, which made it difficult to use histochemical methods to detect a histaminergic system *in situ*. The recent development of immunocytochemical methods represents an important advance in the study of histamine-containing neurons.

The pharmacological effects of histamine are similar to those of the anaphylactic reaction: Hypotension and bronchoconstriction

Dale [6] emphasized these similarities soon after the discovery of histamine in ergot, before it was shown to be present in nearly all animal tissues. Later work focused on the role of histamine in acid secretion and peptic ulcer disease. The concern "with this mainly pathological aspect of its significance" [6] contrasts with the histories of other biogenic amines, which, from the start, or soon after, were postulated to function in the nervous system. Yet, despite the relatively limited emphasis on the study of histamine in the brain, such studies led to the development of psychotropic drugs [7]. The phenothiazines were synthesized as antihistamines, and one of them, chlorpromazine, was observed to produce an unusual effect on mood, which led to its use in treating schizophrenia. Chemical modification produced another drug, imipramine, that proved disappointing in treating schizophrenia. Clinical observation revealed, however, that this drug was effective in treating depression. Curiously, until about ten years ago, no attention was given to histamine receptors as sites of action for these drugs. Now it is clear that many of these and other psychotropic drugs such as lysergic acid diethylamide (LSD) react with histamine receptors [7]. Which of the numerous pharmacological effects of these drugs may be attributable to interactions with histamine receptors remains to be determined.

Histamine, found in food and formed by intestinal bacteria, is taken up from blood by many peripheral tissues but not readily by the brain

Histamine in brain [1,3–5,8] is formed from L-histidine (Fig. 1), which is taken up by an active process. Histidine is decarboxylated by a specific histidine decarboxylase (E.C.4.1.1.22), which has no other naturally occurring substrate, and by aromatic L-amino acid decarboxylase (E.C.4.1.1.28). Both enzymes require pyridoxal-5′-phosphate. The enzymes differ in their pH optima, K_m for histidine, response to inhibitors, and in their distribution in brain. (*S*)-α-Fluoromethylhistidine irreversibly inactivates histidine decarboxylase and lowers brain levels of histamine without influencing the activity of aromatic L-amino acid decarboxylase [3]. Administration of L-histidine raises brain histamine levels, reflective of the high K_m of histidine decarboxylase for histidine and the comparably low concentrations of histidine normally present in brain and blood; this circumstance differs in some invertebrate neural tissue where the concentration of histidine saturates the enzyme. Since both mammalian decarboxylases can form histamine, it is not known whether raising histamine levels by injection of histidine influences only histaminergic activity, since histamine could rise at sites containing aromatic L-amino acid decarboxylase; histidine may also compete with other amino acids for the uptake system.

Since the activity of histidine decarboxylase in brain is very low, the enzyme was purified from fetal rat liver [9], which has high histidine decarboxylase activity with properties not different from those of the enzyme in the brain. The purified native enzyme has a molecular weight of 110,000 and is a dimer. Antibody to the purified enzyme from fetal liver cross-reacted with the enzyme from brain [9]. Histidine decarboxylase from the bacterium *Morganella morganii*, a tetramer with subunits of M_r 43,000, has many of the same properties as the mammalian enzyme, including a requirement for pyridoxal phosphate and sensitivity to α-fluoromethylhistidine [10]. α-Fluoromethylhistidine, which competes with histidine for binding at the active site, requires pyridoxal phosphate to inactivate the enzyme. Catalytic action of the holoenzyme produces a compound that covalently reacts with a specific serine residue in each subunit and with pyridoxal phosphate [10]. The nucleotide sequence of the gene that encodes the enzyme from *M. morganii* and the derived amino acid sequence are known [10].

A portion of the histamine in brain is stored in particulate fractions containing synaptosomes

In addition to the synaptosomal portions, about 20 percent of the histamine is found in the denser P_1 fraction that contains relatively few synaptosomes [1,3–5]. Because of this it has been suggested that there are at least two pools of histamine in brain; this is supported by other observations. Acute treatment with α-fluoromethylhistidine about halves the content of histamine; chronic treatment is needed to eliminate most of the histamine from brain. One of these pools, the pool of histamine that turns over slowly, may be nonneuronal, since lesioning histaminergic fibers reduces histamine content in the fraction containing nerve endings without influencing the content in the P_1 fraction [3]. This nonneuronal pool may be in mast cells or in vascular cells or both. Histamine turns over slowly in both mast cells and microvessels. The prevalence and regional distribution of mast cells in brain differ among species, but they are not abundant and probably make slight contribution to histamine in brain [4]; however, pe-

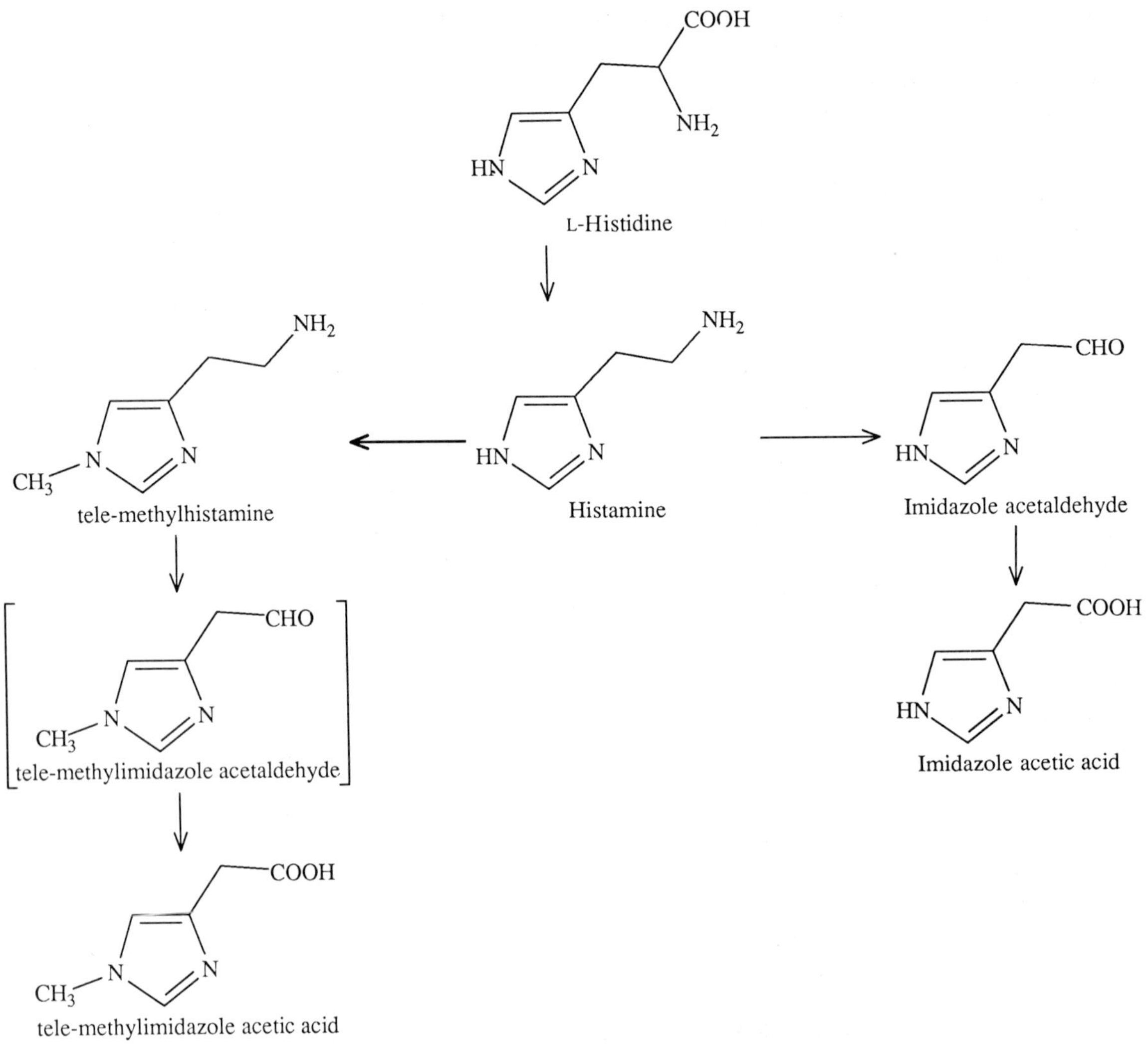

FIG. 1. Formation of histamine and its main metabolic pathways.

ripheral neural structures are rich in mast cells [1].

Histaminergic cell bodies and nerve endings have been visualized with antibodies to histidine decarboxylase and to histamine coupled to proteins

These two approaches yield similar results that are consonant with those that support conclu-sions based on the effects of lesions [2–5,11]. The large bipolar or multipolar cell bodies (20–30 μm in diameter) are found only in the ventral part of the posterior hypothalamus. These cells are mainly in the tuberal and caudal nuclei and, most prominently, in the caudal magnocellular nucleus. The fibers project predominantly ipsi-laterally to almost all regions of the brain and to the spinal cord (Fig. 2). Fibers and nerve terminals are numerous in the posterior hypo-

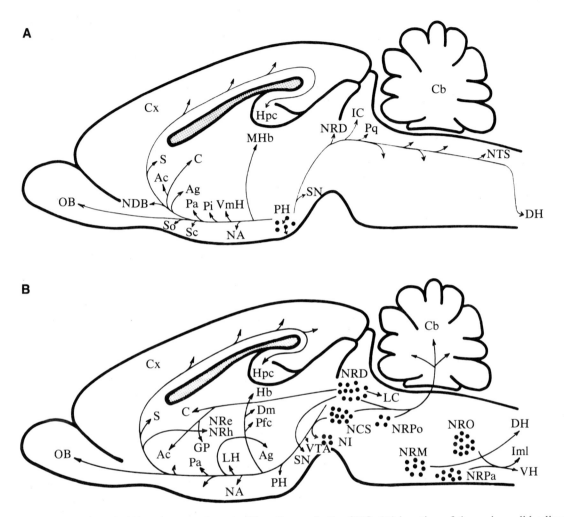

FIG. 2. Histaminergic (**A**) and serotoninergic (**B**) pathways in the CNS: (●) location of the major cell bodies; (Ac) nucleus accumbens; (Ag) amygdala; (C) caudate nucleus; (Cb) cerebellum; (Cx) cerebral cortex; (DH) dorsal horn of spinal cord; (Dm) dorsomedial thalamic nucleus; (GP) globus pallidus; (Hb) habenula; (Hpc) hippocampus; (IC) inferior colliculus; (Iml) intermediolateral nucleus; (LC) locus coeruleus; (LH) lateral hypothalamus; (MHb) medial habenular nucleus; (NA) arcuate nucleus; (NCS) nucleus centralis superior (B8 group); (NDB) diagonal band nucleus; (NI) nucleus interpeduncularis; (NRD) nucleus raphe dorsalis (B7); (NRe) nucleus reuniens; (NRh) nucleus rhomboideus; (NRM) nucleus raphe magnus (B3); (NRO) nucleus raphe obscurus (B2); (NRPa) nucleus raphe pallidus (B1); (NRPo) nucleus raphe pontis; (NTS) nucleus tractus solitarius; (OB) olfactory bulb; (Pa) paraventricular nucleus; (Pfc) parafascicular nucleus; (PH) posterior hypothalamus; (Pi) periventricular nucleus; (Pq) periaqueductal grey; (S) septum; (Sc) suprachiasmatic nucleus; (SN) substantia nigra; (VH) ventral horn of spinal cord; (VmH) ventromedial hypothalamus; (VTA) ventral tegmental area.

thalamus. The tuberal, caudal, and caudal magnocellular nuclei also contain glutamate decarboxylase and adenosine deaminase, a coexistence that could imply a functional relationship among histamine, γ-aminobutyrate, and adenosine [12]. Cells in this area also contain 5-hydroxytryptophan and its decarboxylase and thyrotropin-releasing hormone. In addition, the caudal magnocellular nucleus contains substance P, the peptide galanin, and an enkephalin-containing peptide [12]. Immunocytochemistry also revealed histidine decarboxylase-containing enterochromaffin-like cells in the stomach and histidine decarboxylase in neuronal elements in the stomach, intestine (notably the myenteric ganglia), and adrenal medulla [5]. Histamine-containing cells are present in the superior cervical ganglion in mast cells and other cells.

Many studies on the release of histamine from brain slices have been carried out on slices preincubated with exogenous histamine

The release of exogenous histamine by either K^+ or electrical stimulation is Ca^{2+} dependent and temperature sensitive, as has been shown for other biogenic amines believed to be neuroregulators; however, the meaning of the experiments on the release of exogenous histamine is not clear. In experiments on slices of rat cerebral cortex in which the release of radioactive exogenous histamine was compared with the release of endogenous histamine, clear differences were observed [3]. Both the spontaneous release and the K^+-induced release of exogenous histamine were much greater than the release of endogenous histamine. Addition of histamine did not influence the K^+-induced release of exogenous histamine but reduced the release of endogenous histamine. These observations imply that exogenously administered histamine does not equilibrate with the pool of endogenous histamine [8].

The effect of histamine in reducing the release of endogenous histamine from depolarized brain slices and from synaptosomes is due to action on a presynaptic histamine autoreceptor [3]. The release process is influenced by Ca^{2+} and Mg^{2+} as is the release of other biogenic amines by their autoreceptors. A K^+-induced increase in histamine synthesis is also inhibited by histamine, and evidence suggests that the histamine autoreceptor, i.e., the H_3 receptor (see below), is linked to both effects [3].

Histamine is metabolized by histamine methyltransferase and monoamine oxidase

Studies in many laboratories have failed, however, to demonstrate a high-affinity uptake system. Some invertebrate nerves may contain a high-affinity uptake system [1,4]. It is highly probable that unlike some other biogenic amines, histamine released from mammalian nerve endings is inactivated solely by metabolism [1,3–5,8].

Histamine methyltransferase

Histamine is metabolized mainly by methylation of the *tele*-nitrogen, or N^τ-nitrogen, by histamine methyltransferase (E.C.2.1.1.8). The methyl group is transferred from *S*-adenosyl-L-methionine to form *tele*-methylhistamine (Fig. 1) and *S*-adenosyl-L-homocysteine. Both products inhibit the activity of the enzyme. Since histamine is tautomeric, the other nitrogen in the ring, the *pros*-nitrogen (or N^π-nitrogen), could theoretically be methylated. Efforts to show methylation of the *pros*-nitrogen by histamine methyltransferase have failed, and *pros*-methylhistamine cannot be found in brain by a gas chromatographic-mass spectrometric method that easily quantifies *tele*-methylhistamine [8].

Histamine methyltransferase is found in glia and in postsynaptic sites in neurons. The enzyme was purified to homogeneity from both guinea pig brain and rat kidney. The enzymes are very similar in their amino acid composition and in their catalytic properties [13], supporting the suggestion that the enzymes from the two sources may be identical. The enzyme is highly selective for histamine, acting on no other known endogenous substance with the possible exception of N^α-methylhistamine, which has not been unequivocally shown to exist in the nervous system.

Tele-Methylhistamine is oxidatively deaminated by both monoamine oxidase and diamine oxidase (Fig. 1). Diamine oxidase activity is lacking in brain, where the oxidation is carried out by monoamine oxidase B. The intermediate aldehyde, which has not been isolated, is oxidized to *tele*-methylimidazoleacetic acid, or, conceivably, reduced to *tele*-methylimidazole ethanol, in analogy with the metabolism of serotonin (see below), which, in this regard, has been more extensively studied. If there are alternative pathways for histamine metabolism by mammalian brain, they are minor ones [1,3–5,8]. The concentrations of histamine, *tele*-methylhistamine, and *tele*-methylimidazoleacetic acid in regions of brain are highly correlated with the highest concentrations found in the hypothalamus. The turnover rate of histamine is also highest in hypothalamus, but the rate constants are highest in the caudate nucleus and cortex [1,14]. The relatively low rate constant in hypothalamus implies that only a portion of the histamine there is turning over; the presence of histamine-containing cell bodies, as well as nerve terminals, in the hypothalamus can account for the low rate constant. Although the steady-state levels of histamine in brain are low, its turnover rate is similar to that of other biogenic amines; the half-life of histamine in rat cortex and striatum is, in fact, shorter than that of dopamine [14].

Diamine oxidase

The other major route of histamine metabolism is direct oxidative deamination by diamine oxidase to form imidazoleacetaldehyde and then imidazoleacetic acid (Fig. 1). That the aldehyde is an intermediate was shown by the formation of imidazole ethanol after inhibition of aldehyde dehydrogenase. This route of metabolism to form imidazoleacetic acid is important in mammalian peripheral tissues, but it has not been unequivocally demonstrated in mammalian brain. However, the nervous systems of several invertebrates have been shown to form imidazoleacetic acid from histamine.

Other pathways

Some invertebrates lack both the methylating and the oxidative pathways [1,4]; at least in *Aplysia*, the only histamine metabolite is γ-glutamylhistamine, which may be a minor metabolite in mammalian brain. In mast cells, γ-glutamylhistamine is formed and incorporated into proteins. There is evidence that the hypothalamus may form other peptides containing histamine [1].

Histamine metabolites have slight or no activity on histamine receptors, but they are active on other systems

Imidazoleacetic acid has activity like γ-aminobutyrate on both vertebrate and invertebrate neurons, showing similar potency and similar sensitivity to blockade by bicuculline [8]. Imidazoleacetic acid also blocks the uptake of γ-aminobutyrate; and imidazoleacetic acid, formed in mammalian peripheral tissues, enters mammalian brain [1,4]. Imidazoleacetic acid acts like γ-aminobutyrate on the γ-aminobutyrate-benzodiazepine-chloride receptor complex, increasing the affinity of the receptor for benzodiazepines. In contrast, *tele*-methylimidazoleacetic acid decreases the affinity of the receptor for benzodiazepines. In this system, *tele*-methylimidazoleacetic acid acts at a distinct site, since bicuculline blocks the effects of both γ-aminobutyrate and imidazoleacetic acid but not the effect of *tele*-methylimidazoleacetic acid.

RECEPTORS AND SECOND MESSENGERS

H_1 receptors exist in the brain

Most work on the H_1 receptor in brain [1,3–5,7] has been based on the high-affinity binding of the labeled antagonist pyrilamine (i.e., mepyramine) or of labeled doxepin, an antidepressant drug with very high affinity for the H_1 receptor. The density of H_1 receptors in regions of the brain shows surprising variation among species. Autoradiography shows that the CA3 region of the hippocampus has a high density of H_1 receptors in rat and a low density in guinea pig. In the rat at least, there is no similarity between the regional distribution of the H_1 receptor and the regional distribution of histamine, its metabolites, the enzymes that synthesize and metabolize histamine, or histaminergic nerve endings.

Binding of H_1 agonists to the H_1 receptor is modulated by Na^+ and GTP, which decrease the affinity of the receptor for histamine. Affinities of receptors for agonists are enhanced by Mn^{2+} and Mg^{2+} but not by Ca^{2+}. None of these effects is seen in studies with antagonists.

Stimulation of the H_1 receptor in various tissues is associated with increased formation of cAMP and cGMP, increased phosphoinositide turnover, and ion shifts

In addition, stimulation of H_1 receptors in vascular tissues releases a relaxing factor from the endothelium. Stimulation of H_1 receptors in conventionally prepared homogenates does not increase cAMP formation, but in slices or a cell-free preparation containing large vesicular sacs or synaptoneurosomes, stimulation of the H_1 receptor increases cAMP formation. The increased cAMP formation on stimulation of the H_1 receptor is indirect, dependent on stimulation of H_2 receptors and the presence of adenosine. The effect of adenosine is especially interesting since, as noted above, immunocytochemistry suggests that histamine and adenosine may coexist in the same neurons.

Histamine increases the cGMP content of cerebral cortical slices and of other mammalian neural tissues. Histamine-stimulated cGMP formation in mouse neuroblastoma cells is linked to the H_1 receptor. This effect of histamine requires Ca^{2+}. Increased glycogenolysis after stimulation of H_1 receptors in brain slices is also mediated by increased cytosolic Ca^{2+}, which could depend on H_1 stimulation of the turnover of the phosphoinositides. Increased turnover of phosphoinositides in brain and in many other cells results from stimulation of H_1 receptors. Hydrolysis of the phosphoinositides produces both inositol phosphates and a 1,2-diacylglycerol, mainly 1-stearoyl-2-arachidonyl-sn-glycerol (see Chap. 16). In many cells, inositol-1-4,5-trisphosphate has been shown to elevate cytosolic Ca^{2+}; Ca^{2+} and diacylglycerol are required for maximal activation of protein kinase C. (This is discussed fully in Chap. 16.)

The association of H_1 receptors with more than one second messenger may be attributed to interaction among the second-messenger systems

Products of the phosphoinositides influence other second messengers. In neuroblastoma cells, stimulation of H_1 receptors increases phosphoinositide turnover, thereby releasing arachidonate. Increases in cGMP formation are also observed. Both effects are blocked not only by H_1 antagonists but by inhibitors of the lipoxygenase pathway of arachidonate metabolism (see Chap. 20). Thus, a lipoxygenase product(s) of arachidonate, for example, hydroxyeicosatetraenoic acids and leukotrienes, influences the cGMP response, acting like a tertiary messenger(s) [4].

Labeling of the H_2 receptor is difficult because of the high nonspecific binding of H_2 antagonists

Specific labeling of the H_2 receptor has not been observed in brain regions where results of electrophysiologic studies and measurements of adenylate cyclase activity suggest that H_2 receptors are present. H_2 receptors are directly linked to adenylate cyclase in many tissues including brain [4,7]. Activity is highest in homogenates of the hippocampus and neocortex; however, other regions of brain show small or nondetectable responses of adenylate cyclase activity, even where results of electrophysiological studies show the H_2 receptor to be present. The receptor is found in neurons and in glial cells. In the myenteric plexus of the guinea pig ileum, stimulation of H_2 receptors results in contractions that are associated with released acetylcholine, 5-HT, a peptide(s), and cyclooxygenase product(s) of arachidonate metabolism.

Postulated mechanism of H_2 receptor activation

Application of quantum chemical calculations led to a hypothesis on the mechanism of activation of H_2 receptors by histamine and other H_2 agonists [15]. The proton relay mechanism that was proposed is based on tautomerism of the imidazole ring. It is known from both experimental and theoretical studies that the tautomeric preference of histamine changes with ionization of the side–chain amino group. As the free base, where the side-chain amino group is uncharged, i.e., $-NH_2$, the more stable tautomer has the proton on the *pros*-nitrogen of the ring; as the monocation, where the side-chain amino group is protonated, i.e., $-NH_3$, the more stable tautomer has the proton on the *tele*-nitrogen. It is proposed that the cationic amino group of histamine interacts with an anionic site of the receptor, while the *tele*-NH and *pros*-N interact

with additional sites of the receptor. The effect of the interaction of the cationic amino group with an anionic site is to confer on the ring the properties of the free base of histamine: The *pros*-N becomes more nucleophilic and becomes protonated by the receptor; and the *tele*-NH releases its proton to the receptor. It is proposed that this charge relay triggers the biological response.

Stimulating the H_3 presynaptic receptor reduces histamine release

The H_3 autoreceptor is prominent in brain areas rich in histaminergic nerve endings [3]. Treatment with an antagonist of the H_3 receptor results in reduced brain levels of histamine by increasing histamine release. The receptor is also found in lung, perhaps in mast cells. Vascular smooth muscle also contains this receptor, probably at presynaptic sites on autonomic nerves; its stimulation may produce vasodilation by inhibiting sympathetic tone. These findings may explain older observations showing that histamine, released after sympathetic activity, mediates active vasodilation [1].

In vivo *and* in vitro *studies of the electrophysiological effects of histamine on mammalian neurons have yielded paradoxical results*

Local application, e.g., iontophoresis, of histamine agonists on almost all neurons in the brain, with the notable exception of hypothalamus, and spinal cord produces inhibitory responses. These are defined as decreased firing rates, hyperpolarization, decreased excitatory postsynaptic potentials, and reduction of both glutamate-evoked and electrically evoked excitation. The inhibitory responses appear to be mediated by the H_2 receptor. On perfusion of histamine *in vitro*, most neurons in culture or in brain slices exhibit excitatory responses.

These are characterized by increased firing rates and reductions in the magnitude and duration of the late hyperpolarization, due to a reduction of a Ca^{2+}-dependent K^+ conductance. Excitatory responses are also mediated by H_2 receptors. To account for the inhibitory responses observed on local application of histamine and the excitatory responses on perfusion of histamine, it was proposed that the inhibitory responses are overcome by excitatory actions when a larger population of H_2 receptors on neurons is stimulated [2].

The effects of histamine on neurons are slow in onset and of long duration, like the effects of norepinephrine and 5-hydroxytryptamine, and different from the rapid and brief effects of amino acid transmitters

Like norepinephrine and 5-hydroxytryptamine, histamine potentiates the effects of amino acids on many mammalian neurons. In *Aplysia* there is evidence that histamine functions as a modulator. The C2 cells, rich in histamine, project to cells that potentiate feeding behavior by releasing 5-hydroxytryptamine. C2 cells fire when stimuli are applied to the perioral area of *Aplysia*, and they continue to fire as long as rhythmic mouth movements persist. Since mechanical stimuli to the mouth generate spikes, C2 is probably a primary mechanosensory afferent neuron. The C2 cell requires a high rate of axon input to pass proprioceptive information to the follower cell; in its normal state it does not convey information. Its role in feeding, then, is modulatory rather than obligatory [4].

Among the roles attributed to histamine in brain are arousal, regulation of biological rhythms, thermoregulation, and various vegetative and neuroendocrine functions

The rapid turnover of histamine in the hypothalamus may be consonant with some of these functions. Most of the observations supporting these and other postulated functions derive from observations on the effects of injected histamine [3,5]. In some cases, the effects of histamine and its antagonists depend on which parts of the brain they are injected into, e.g., in the effects on response to painful stimuli [5]. There is physiological evidence that histamine in the hypothalamus contributes to the control of blood pressure: Histamine release is increased when the posterior caudal hypothalamus is electrically stimulated, a procedure that increases blood pressure; the release of histamine from the posterior hypothalamus of spontaneously hypertensive rats is higher than that of controls. Hypothalamic neurons, in contrast to other neurons in other areas of the brain, respond to iontophoretically applied histamine with excitation, which appears to be mediated by H_1 receptors [2]. Among these neurons are the vasopressin-secreting and oxytocin-secreting neurons in the supraoptic nucleus. Injections of histamine into this nucleus produce antidiuresis and a release of vasopressin, effects that are sensitive to H_1 antagonists [2]. Of special interest are observations showing state dependence: Some osmosensitive neurons in the supraoptic nucleus that failed to respond to iontophoretically applied histamine did respond after injection of hypertonic NaCl. This may be another example of histamine's functioning as a neuromodulator [2].

SEROTONIN

Serotonin (5-hydroxytryptamine) derives its name from the observation in 1868 that after blood clots, the resultant serum increases vascular tone

It is now known that the active substance is serotonin and that it is released from aggregating platelets. Its crystalization from blood and proof of structure in 1949 [16] coincided with heightened interest in neurochemistry. It is widely distributed in nature, including neural structures of many vertebrates and invertebrates.

Serotonin, which does not readily enter the brain, originates from dietary L-tryptophan

L-tryptophan [17] is acted on by tryptophan-5-monooxygenase (E.C.1.14.16.4), also known as tryptophan-5-hydroxylase, to form 5-hydroxytryptophan (Fig. 3). Molecular oxygen and L-erythro-tetrahydrobiopterin are required. One atom of oxygen is used to form 5-hydroxytryptophan, and the other atom is reduced to water. On donation of electrons, the tetrahydrobiopterin becomes quininoid, and it is regenerated by NADPH-linked quininoid dehydropteridine reductase (see also Chap. 38). Other reduced pterins can serve as cofactors, but the affinity of the enzyme for tryptophan and oxygen is highest with L-erythro-tetrahydrobiopterin. The K_m of the enzyme for tryptophan is 50 to 120 μM. The concentration of tryptophan in the brain is about 30 μM; therefore, increasing levels of tryptophan result in increases in the level of serotonin. Transport of tryptophan into brain competes with transport of some other amino acids (see Chap. 30). It has also been suggested that since plasma tryptophan is largely bound to plasma albumin, substances like fatty acids that compete for the albumin binding sites can raise the levels of free tryptophan and hence its levels in brain. Tryptophan-5-hydroxylase is found only in cells that synthesize serotonin, and its distribution in the brain parallels that of serotonin. The hydroxylation of tryptophan is the rate-limiting step in the formation of serotonin. Among numerous inhibitors of this enzyme, the one most commonly used is *p*-chlorophenylalanine, which, though only a weak competitive inhibitor of the enzyme *in vitro*, produces an inhibition of the

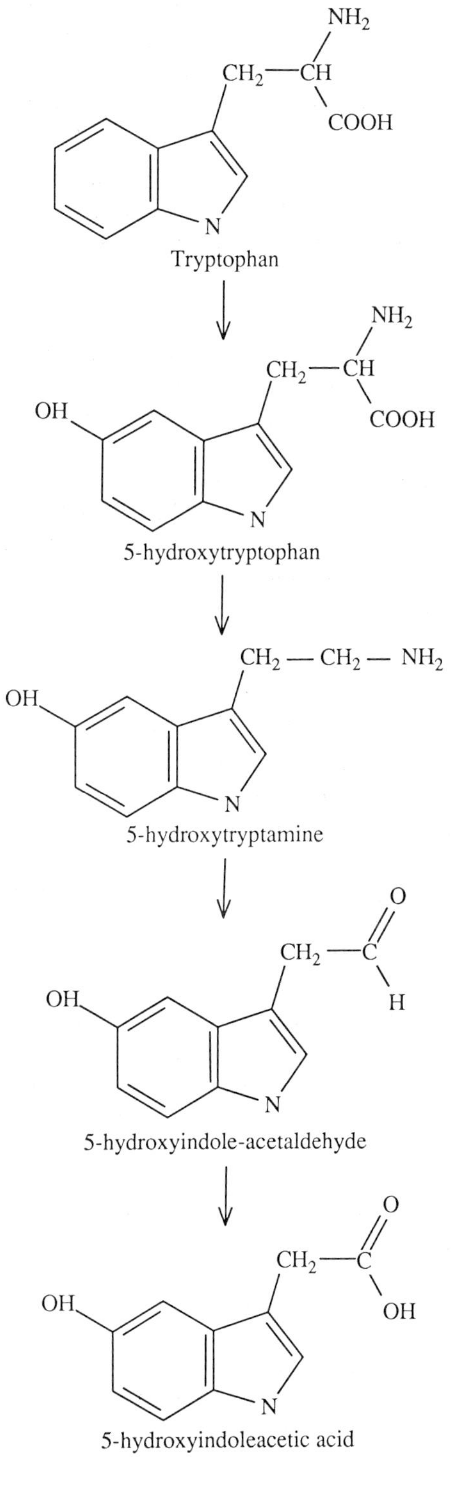

FIG. 3. Formation of serotonin and its main metabolic pathway.

enzyme *in vivo* of long duration. *p*-Chlorophenylalanine reduces transport into brain of other amino acids, e.g., tyrosine, and can thereby lower brain levels of other biogenic amines.

Electrical stimulation of serotonin-containing cell bodies increases the synthesis of 5-hydroxytryptophan from tryptophan in a frequency-dependent manner

The stimulation of synthesis is dependent on Ca^{2+} and is accompanied by an increase in the V_{max} of the enzyme for tryptophan, but additional factors contribute to the persistent increase in serotonin synthesis. It has been suggested that Ca^{2+}-dependent phosphorylation is involved in the activation of tryptophan hydroxylase by depolarization [18].

Endogenous 5-hydroxytryptophan in brain is decarboxylated by aromatic L-amino acid decarboxylase

This reaction is dependent on pyridoxal-5'-phosphate. The serotonin that is formed is stored in synaptosomes, at least some of it bound to a specific protein [17]. Under usual conditions, little or no 5-hydroxytryptophan is detectable in cells because of the relatively high activity of the decarboxylase. The decarboxylase is nonspecific, acting on 3,4-dihydroxyphenylalanine as well as 5-hydroxytryptophan. The enzyme is not saturated under physiological conditions, and administration of 5-hydroxytryptophan increases serotonin levels in tissues. Because of the nonspecific nature of the decarboxylase, administration of 5-hydroxytryptophan increases the levels of serotonin in cells that normally lack serotonin, e.g., in cells that contain catecholamines. The enzyme also decarboxylates exogenously administered aromatic amino acids, e.g., α-methyldopa, which competes with endogenous substrates and is itself decarboxylated to form a false transmitter. An irreversible inhibitor of the decarboxylase,

α-fluoromethyldopa, greatly reduces levels of serotonin and dopamine.

The cell bodies of serotonin-containing neurons are localized primarily in the raphe nuclei of the brain stem, from where they project to almost all levels of the central nervous system

The serotoninergic projections depicted in Fig. 2 are based mainly on findings from histofluorescence and immunohistochemistry [19], with additional information derived from anterograde and retrograde mapping, studies of serotonin uptake, studies of the effects of lesions, and electrophysiological investigations. The nuclei raphe dorsalis (the B7 group) project to the neocortex, pyriform cortex, olfactory bulb, neostriatum, thalamus, amygdala, hippocampus, substantia nigra, and locus coeruleus. The nucleus centralis superior (B8) projects to the cerebral cortex, hippocampus, suprachiasmatic nucleus, anterior hypothalamic area, medial preoptic area, arcuate nucleus, and to the nuclei raphe dorsalis. The nucleus raphe magnus (B3) projects to the medulla and the dorsal horn of the spinal cord. The nucleus raphe obscurus (B2) and the nucleus raphe pallidus (B1), which contain substance P, project to the intermediolateral cell column and ventral horn of the spinal cord. Many of the raphe nuclei project to the ependyma lining the ventricles of the brain, the pia and the arachnoid sheath. In nonmammalian vertebrates and mammals, the terminal arborizations of the serotoninergic systems in brain are structurally similar, suggesting that the systems are phylogenetically old and that they may serve similar functions in all vertebrates.

Depolarization causes release of serotonin by a Ca^{2+}-dependent exocytotic mechanism

Serotonin is released by stimulation of its cell bodies in the raphe nuclei [17]. These cells contain serotonin autoreceptors (see below) that receive input from serotonin-containing axon collaterals. In some neurons, serotonin may coexist with other neuroregulators. Cells in the medullary raphe nuclei contain both serotonin and substance P, and some serotonin-containing cells contain leucine-enkephalin, whereas others contain thyrotropin-releasing hormone. These peptides may function to modulate the release of serotonin. Numerous other neuroregulators have been implicated in the release of serotonin, including dopamine, norepinephrine, acetylcholine, and prostaglandins. Many drugs and experimental compounds cause release of serotonin, including reserpine and *p*-chloroamphetamine.

Effects of serotonin are terminated by reuptake into presynaptic terminals

The uptake system for serotonin in nerve terminals, like the uptake systems for some other biogenic amines, has high affinity, low capacity, and high specificity. It is saturable, following Michaelis-Menten kinetics; it is Na^+ and temperature dependent and inhibited by metabolic inhibitors; it is reduced or eliminated by destruction of the serotoninergic cell bodies or the nerve endings; its regional distribution in brain is similar to that of serotonin. A similar or identical uptake mechanism is present in the pineal gland, retina, the myenteric plexus of the guinea pig ileum, and platelets. The serotonin uptake site can be blocked relatively selectively by citalopram and fluoxetine. The selectivity of the uptake sites for serotonin offers a means of changing serotonin levels without concomitantly changing the levels of dopamine and norepinephrine. Highly selective uptake blockers have also been used to reveal serotoninergic nerve terminals.

The primary metabolite of serotonin is 5-hydroxyindoleacetaldehyde

This reaction (Fig. 3) is catalyzed by the flavoprotein monoamine oxidase (E.C.1.4.3.4),

preferentially by monoamine oxidase A [20]. 5-Hydroxyindoleacetaldehyde is oxidized by NAD^+-dependent aldehyde dehydrogenase (E.C.1.2.1.3) to 5-hydroxyindoleacetic acid. 5-Hydroxyindoleacetaldehyde is also reduced by NADPH-dependent aldehyde reductase (E.C.1.1.1.2) to the alcohol 5-hydroxytryptophol. The same aldehyde dehydrogenase oxidizes the acetaldehyde that results from oxidation of ethanol and of other biogenic amines, including histamine. The levels of 5-hydroxytryptophol increase in ethanol intoxication [20].

The regional distribution of 5-hydroxyindoleacetic acid is similar to that of serotonin. Measurements of 5-hydroxyindoleacetic acid in brain and other tissues provide an index of serotoninergic activity. At least in brain, efflux of 5-hydroxyindoleacetic acid is energy dependent and inhibited by probenecid. Administration of both a monoamine oxidase inhibitor and an inhibitor of serotonin uptake results in increased serotoninergic activity, showing that both monoamine oxidase and uptake are included in termination of the action of serotonin. Effects resulting from these treatments may not rest exclusively on increased serotoninergic activity, since monoamine oxidase A also oxidizes dopamine and norepinephrine.

Other pathways for metabolism of serotonin have been suggested [20]. The sulfate ester is formed by peripheral tissues. Enzymatic methylation of the side-chain amino group can occur in brain to form N^α-methylserotonin and then bufotenine, i.e., N^α,N^α-dimethylserotonin. Serotonin can be converted to a tetrahydro-β-carboline by condensation of an aldehyde, e.g., formaldehyde or acetaldehyde, with the side-chain amino group and carbon-2 (adjacent to the ring nitrogen) of serotonin. This reaction occurs nonenzymatically. Other biogenic amines, including histamine, can form analogous derivatives with aldehydes. The carboline that is formed from serotonin has been found in brain and platelets, and it has numerous pharmacological effects, but it is not certain that the compound is present in sufficient concentration *in vivo* to exert biologically meaningful effects.

The pineal gland synthesizes serotonin and converts it to melatonin, i.e., 5-methoxy-N^α-acetylserotonin; the initial step is catalyzed by serotonin-N-acetyltransferase in the presence of acetylcoenzyme A to form N-acetylserotonin, which is then O-methylated by hydroxyindole-O-methyltransferase in the presence of S-adenosylmethionine [21]. The synthesis and release of melatonin by the pineal gland depends on adrenergic input. Melatonin has negligible serotonin-like activity but has an array of distinct biological effects including influences on gonadal maturation [21]. The hypothalamus and the pineal body also methylate serotonin to form 5-methoxytryptamine, a compound whose potency is similar to that of serotonin on many serotonin receptors.

Many classes of high-affinity binding sites for serotonin have been described, and almost all have been shown to be receptors

Occupation of the binding sites by serotonin elicits a response, and the relative potencies of agonists and/or antagonists for the receptor accord with the affinities for the binding site [22]. The 5-HT$_{1A}$ receptor, in the hippocampus, is linked to control of adenylate cyclase activity. If cyclase activity is first stimulated with forskolin, serotonin inhibits enzyme activity. Results of electrophysiological studies also imply that in whole cells, the 5-HT$_{1A}$ receptor is linked to inhibition of cyclase activity. Hippocampal membranes contain a second serotonin receptor associated with stimulation of cyclase activity. It is characterized by much lower affinity than the 5-HT$_{1A}$ receptor for serotonin. This receptor, unnamed and lacking a ligand for binding studies, may be the same as one described in infant rat brain colliculi. The 5-HT$_{1B}$ receptor, found in high density in the striatum, functions as a serotonin autoreceptor. The 5-HT$_{1C}$ receptor is linked to stimulation of phosphoinositide

turnover, and it is found in highest concentration in the choroid plexus. The 5-HT$_2$ receptors are present in high density in neocortex, hippocampus, and platelets and in cardiac and many smooth muscles. These receptors are also linked to stimulation of phosphoinositide turnover. There are as many as three serotonin receptors, collectively called 5-HT$_3$ or 5-HT$_M$ receptors, that have been defined exclusively by functional studies, since ligands are not available to perform binding assays. These receptors are present on peripheral neuronal structures: sympathetic neurons, vagal afferent fibers, and sensory fibers. Evidence also indicates that still other undefined serotonin receptors exist in brain and in other organs.

Discharge of raphe neurons is normally regular, and the rate correlates with the state of arousal: Activity is highest on active waking and lowest during REM sleep

This pattern of activity is due to pacemaker potentials of long duration that are followed by hyperpolarizing afterpotentials; the afterhyperpolarization may be due to an increase in Ca^{2+}-dependent K^+ conductance [23,24]. Other intrinsic control mechanisms in the raphe are inhibitory interactions among serotoninergic neurons under control of autoreceptors. Serotonin suppresses the pacemaker potentials. The neurons in the mesencephalic raphe nuclei, e.g., nucleus raphe dorsalis, are more sensitive to serotonin than are the neurons in the medullary raphe nuclei, e.g., nucleus raphe magnus. Inhibition of the firing of raphe cells by serotonin may be mediated by the 5-HT$_{1A}$ receptor.

Unlike the effects of histamine, discussed in the previous section, the effects of serotonin are similar whether applied by iontophoresis or by perfusion. On most neurons, the postsynaptic effect of serotonin is inhibitory, but on some neurons serotonin is excitatory and on others it facilitates excitatory actions. In the hippocampus, the effects of serotonin are particularly complex. The complexity is probably due to the multiplicity of serotonin receptors, their relative distribution and densities within the region, the different and possibly interacting second messengers, and the varying efficiencies of coupling to second messengers. A further source of complexity may be a heterogeneous distribution of heterologous presynaptic receptors. For example, at some sites, serotonin influences the release of dopamine, norepinephrine, and other substances.

Serotonin decreases the firing rate of hippocampal neurons through an increase in K^+ conductance

Evidence has been presented that this effect is Ca^{2+} independent and mediated by the 5-HT$_{1A}$ receptors directly coupled to a G-protein. In addition to activating K^+ conductances, serotonin suppresses a Ca^{2+}-dependent K^+ conductance that leads to increased firing in response to depolarization; this action may be linked to the 5-HT$_{1B}$ receptor [25]. The latter effect may explain the facilitation of excitatory actions produced by serotonin: On facial motoneurons, serotonin itself does not excite but greatly facilitates the excitatory actions produced either by electrical stimulation of afferent nerves or by application of glutamate [23]. These experiments are consistent with a modulatory role of serotonin, a role analogous to that of histamine and norepinephrine. In gastropods, serotonin also has modulatory functions [17].

In the mammalian CNS, serotonin modulates body temperature, blood pressure, endocrine secretion, appetite, sexual behavior, movement, emesis, and pain

The modulatory role for these various functions serves to coordinate activities [23,24]. For example, in the spinal cord, a serotoninergic dorsal horn projection inhibits somatosensory input, whereas the ventral horn projection facilitates discharge of motoneurons. Serotonin thus simultaneously inhibits algesia and facilitates motor activity [26]. It has been emphasized that the firing of the nucleus raphe dorsalis or of the nucleus centralis superior in response to changes in body temperature, blood pressure, or pain is indistinguishable from the response to behavioral activation that these specific changes produce [24]; however, the serotoninergic system, in responding to behavioral activation, may modulate and coordinate these responses. The diffuse projection of serotoninergic neurons and the arborizations of the terminals that permit action at many postsynaptic sites provide the means for coordinating and modulating functions. It has been postulated [27] that the serotoninergic system may be important in modulating human behavior, reduced serotoninergic transmission producing a facilitation or disinhibition of some behaviors. This effect could be manifested as impulsivity (and/or aggression). Supporting these ideas are results showing low levels of 5-hydroxyindoleacetic acid in the cerebrospinal fluid of people with histories of aggression, suicidal behavior, or criminality [27].

ACKNOWLEDGMENTS

The author is grateful to the authors of papers that could not be cited and to Dennis Healy and William Clarke who helped with the anatomy and electrophysiology, respectively. The author's original work cited here was supported by grants from the National Institute of Mental Health (MH 31805) and the National Institute on Drug Abuse (DA 01875).

REFERENCES

1. Hough, L. B., and Green, J. P. Histamine and its receptors in the nervous system. In A. Lajtha

(ed.), *Handbook of Neurochemistry*, 2nd ed. New York: Plenum, 1984, Vol. 6, pp. 145–211.

2. Haas, H. L. Histamine. In M. A. Rogawski and J. L. Barker (eds.), *Neurotransmitter Actions in the Vertebrate Nervous System.* New York: Plenum, 1985, pp. 321–337.

3. Schwartz, J.-C., Garbarg, M., and Pollard, H. Histaminergic transmission in brain. In V. B. Mountcastle, F. E. Bloom, and S. R. Geiger (eds.), *Handbook of Physiology, Volume 4, Section 1, Neurophysiology.* Bethesda: American Physiological Society, 1986, pp. 257–316.

4. Prell, G. D., and Green, J. P. Histamine as a neuroregulator. *Annu. Rev. Neurosci.* 9:209–254, 1986.

5. Hough, L. B. Cellular localization and possible functions for brain histamine: Recent progress. *Prog. Neurobiol.* 30:469–505, 1987.

6. Dale, H. H. Foreword. *Handb. Exp. Pharmacol.* 18/I:XXVI–XXXV, 1966.

7. Green, J. P. Histamine receptors. In H. Y. Meltzer, W. E. Bunny, J. T. Coyle, K. L. Davis, I. J. Kopin, et al. (eds.), *Psychopharmacology, The Third Generation of Progress.* New York: Raven Press, 1987, pp. 273–279.

8. Green, J. P., Prell, G. D., Khandelwal, J. K., and Blandina, P. Aspects of histamine metabolism. *Agents Actions* 22:1–15, 1987.

9. Taguchi, Y., Watanabe, T., Kubota, H., Hayashi, H., and Wada, H. Purification of histidine decarboxylase from the liver of fetal rats and its immunochemical and immunohistochemical characterization. *J. Biol. Chem.* 259:5214–5221, 1984.

10. Vaaler, G. L., Brasch, M. A., and Snell, E. E. Pyridoxal 5'-phosphate-dependent histidine decarboxylase. Nucleotide sequence of the *hdc* gene and the corresponding amino acid sequence. *J. Biol. Chem.* 261:11010–11014, 1986.

11. Steinbusch, H. W. M., and Mulder, A. H. Immunohistochemical localization of histamine in neurons and mast cells in brain. In A. Bjorklund, T. Hokfelt, and M. J. Kuhar (eds.), *Handbook of Chemical Neuroanatomy, Volume 3, Part II: Classical Transmitters and Transmitter Receptors in the CNS.* Amsterdam: Elsevier, 1984, pp. 126–140.

12. Köhler, C., Ericson, H., Watanabe, T., Polak, J., Palay, S. L., Palay, V., and Chan-Palay, V. Galanin immunoreactivity in hypothalamic histamine neurons: Further evidence for multiple chemical messengers in the tuberomammillary nucleus. *J. Comp. Neurol.* 250:58–64, 1986.

13. Borcharat, R. T., and Matuszewska, B. S-Adenosylmethionine-dependent transmethylation of histamine: Purification and partial characterization of guinea pig brain and rat kidney histamine *N*-methyltransferase. *Adv. Biosci.* 51:163–172, 1985.

14. Green, J. P., and Khandelwal, J. K. Histamine turnover in regions of rat brain. *Adv. Biosci.* 51:185–194, 1985.

15. Green, J. P., Johnson, C. L., and Weinstein, H. Histamine as a neurotransmitter. In M. A. Lipton, A. DiMascio, and K. F. Killam (eds.), *Psychopharmacology, A Generation of Progress.* New York: Raven Press, 1978, pp. 319–332.

16. Page, I. H. The discovery of serotonin. *Perspect. Biol. Med.* 20:1–8, 1976.

17. Osborne, N. N. (ed.), *Biology of Serotonergic Transmission.* New York: Wiley, 1982, pp. 1–522.

18. Hamon, M., Bourgoin, S., Artaud, F., and El Mestikawy, S. The respective roles of tryptophan uptake and tryptophan hydroxylase in the regulation of serotonin synthesis in the central nervous system. *J. Physiol. Paris* 77:269–279, 1981.

19. Steinbusch, H. W. M. Serotonin-immunoreactive neurons and their projections in the CNS. In A. Bjorklund, T. Hokfelt, and M. J. Kuhar (eds.), *Handbook of Chemical Neuroanatomy, Volume 3, Part II: Classical Transmitters and Transmitter Receptors in the CNS.* Amsterdam: Elsevier, 1984, pp. 68–125.

20. Beck, O., Lundman, A., and Jonsson, G. 5-Hydroxytryptophol and 5-hydroxyindoleacetic acid levels in rat brain: Effects of various drugs affecting serotonergic transmitter mechanisms. *J. Neural Transm.* 69:287–298, 1987.

21. Wurtman, R. J. Introduction: Melatonin in humans. *J. Neural Transm. (Suppl.)* 21:1–8, 1986.

22. Green, J. P., and Maayani, S. Nomenclature, classification and notation of receptors: 5-hydroxytryptamine receptors and binding sites as examples. In J. W. Black, D. H. Jenkinson, and V. P. Gerskowitch (eds.), *Perspectives on Receptor Classification, Receptor Biochemistry*

and Methodology. New York: Alan R. Liss, 1987. Vol. 6, pp. 237–267.

23. Aghajanian, G. K., and Vandermaelen, C. P. Specific systems of the reticular core: Serotonin. In V. B. Mountcastle, F. E. Bloom, and S. R. Geiger (eds.), *Handbook of Physiology, Volume 4, Section 1: Neurophysiology.* Bethesda: American Physiological Society, 1986, pp. 237–256.

24. Fornal, C. A., and Jacobs, B. L. Physiological and behavioral correlates of serotonergic single-unit activity. In N. N. Osborne and C. A. Fornal (eds.), *Neuronal Serotonin.* Chichester: Wiley, 1987, pp. 305–345.

25. Colino, A., and Halliwell, J. V. Differential modulation of three separate K-conductances in hippocampal CA1 neurons by serotonin. *Nature* 328:73–77, 1987.

26. Anderson, E. G. The serotonin system of the spinal cord. In R. A. Davidoff (ed.), *Handbook of the Spinal Cord, Volume 1, Pharmacology.* New York: Marcel Dekker, 1983, pp. 241–274.

27. Soubrié, P. Reconciling the role of serotonin neurons in human and animal behavior. *Behav. Brain Sci.* 9:319–363, 1986.

CHAPTER 13

Opioid Peptides and Opioid Receptors

Eric J. Simon and Jacob M. Hiller

Basic Neurochemistry: Molecular, Cellular, and Medical Aspects, 4th Ed., edited by G. J. Siegel et al. Raven Press, Ltd., New York, 1989. Correspondence to Eric J. Simon, Departments of Psychiatry and Pharmacology, New York University Medical Center, 550 First Avenue, New York, New York 10016.

Opium is one of the oldest medications known to humans. Its efficacy in relieving pain and diarrhea has been known for thousands of years. During the nineteenth century, morphine was recognized as the principal alkaloid responsible for most of the beneficial effects of opium. It is also responsible for its undesirable side effects, the most important of which is the development of addiction on chronic use.

This chapter discusses developments in the neurochemical and neuropharmacological aspects of opiate research, most of which have occurred during the past two decades. The field is a very active and rapidly moving one, and the reader will find in the reference list a number of books and reviews that provide detailed information and complete literature citations [1–7].

HISTORICAL SUMMARY

Discovering stereospecificity of opiate actions was a most significant advance

The hypothesis that specific receptors for opiate drugs exist in the central nervous system of animals and humans arose from pharmacological studies of narcotic analgesics and from the large-scale efforts mounted in many industrial, governmental, and university laboratories to attempt synthesis of a nonaddictive analgesic. Many very useful compounds were synthesized, and some of these are in clinical use; however, synthesis of the perfect nonaddictive analgesic has not yet been achieved. A large body of important information about the structural requirements for pharmacological action has resulted from this work. It was recognized that many of the actions of opiates, such as analgesia and addiction liability, are stereospecific; that is, these activities reside in only one of the enantiomers of a racemic mixture. It was also shown that relatively small alterations in parts of the morphine molecule result in drastic changes in its pharmacology. The most interesting and important such change is the substitution of the methyl on the tertiary amino group by an allyl or cyclopropylmethyl group, which endows the resulting molecule with potent and specific antagonistic activity against many of the pharmacological actions of morphine and related opiates. Some antagonists, such as nalorphine and cyclazocine, retain some of their analgesic or agonist potency (agonist/antagonist drugs); others, such as naloxone and naltrexone, become pure antagonists, devoid of detectable agonist properties.

Stereospecificity was explained by postulating specific receptors for opiates

The remarkable stereospecificity and structural constraints placed on these drugs for many of their actions were most readily explained by the existence of highly specific binding sites to which these drugs must attach to exert their effects. Binding to these sites, or receptors, is presumed to trigger a series of reactions that result in the observed response. Antagonists are thought to act by binding to the receptors with high affinity but without the ability to trigger the subsequent events (see Chap. 9).

Although the receptor postulate for the actions of opiates had existed for several decades, the biochemical demonstration of its validity did not occur until 1973, when several laboratories simultaneously and independently reported the existence of stereospecific opiate binding, which represented the major portion of total binding to animal brain homogenates [8–10]. Stereospecific binding is represented by that portion of bound, labeled opiate that is replaceable by an excess of unlabeled opiate but not by its inactive enantiomer. There is now much evidence that these binding sites are pharmacological opiate receptors; some of this evidence is summarized in the next section.

Why do animal tissues contain receptors for plant opiate alkaloids?

The existence of opiate receptors is now firmly established for all vertebrates examined, from hagfish to humans, as well as for some invertebrates. This gave rise to the questions: Why are so many species endowed with highly specific receptors for alkaloids produced by opium poppies, and why have such receptors survived the eons of evolution? A physiological function that confers a selective advantage on the organism that carries them seemed probable. Such a function required the existence of endogenous ligands, the binding of which was the real reason for the existence of the receptors. The possibility that an endogenous analgesic system exists was also supported by the finding, which dates back to 1969, that electrical stimulation of the central gray region of the brain could produce powerful, long-lasting analgesia [11].

Opiate-like activity is found in the brain and pituitary gland

When none of the known neurotransmitters or hormones were found to be bound to opiate receptors with high affinity or to be active in bioassays specific for opiates, the search for novel endogenous substances with opiate-like (opioid) activity began. First reports of the existence of such substances came simultaneously from John Hughes in Hans Kosterlitz's laboratory and from Terenius and Wahlström. The presence of opioid activity in extracts of the pituitary was first reported by Goldstein and his group.

The identification of the first endogenous opioids was accomplished by Hughes and Kosterlitz and their collaborators [12], who found that the opioid activity present in aqueous extracts of pig brain resided in two pentapeptides, Tyr-Gly-Gly-Phe-Met and Tyr-Gly-Gly-Phe-

Leu, which they named methionine (met) enkephalin and leucine (leu) enkephalin, respectively (enkephalin, Greek, "in the head").

The finding of opioid activity in the pituitary and the observation by Hughes et al. that the met-enkephalin sequence is present in the pituitary hormone β-lipotropin (β-LPH) as residues 61–65 led to the discovery of three longer peptides with opioid activity, all representing sequences present in β-LPH. These peptides were named α-, β-, and τ-endorphin, following a suggestion by Simon that the term endorphin, a contraction of endogenous and morphine, might be an appropriate and useful term for endogenous substances with opioid activity. More recently, Goldstein and co-workers [13] discovered another potent endogenous opioid peptide, not derived from β-LPH, which they named dynorphin. The number of peptides with opioid activity currently known is approximately 12. Since it is now evident that the primary function of opiate receptors is to bind endogenous opioids, they have been renamed opioid receptors and are so referred to henceforth in this chapter.

OPIOID RECEPTORS

Properties and distribution of opioid receptors provide important leads in the elucidation of function

Opioid binding sites are found in the CNS and in a number of peripheral tissues; isolated guinea pig ileum and vasa deferentia from several species are peripheral tissues extremely useful as *in vitro* bioassay systems for opioids and their receptors. Opioid binding sites are tightly attached to cell membranes, and cell fractionation experiments suggest that they exist predominantly in the synaptic region. Stereospecific binding is saturable and of high affinity, ranging from 10^{-11} to 10^{-7} M for substances with strong to moderate opioid activity. The pH optimum for binding is in the physiological range (pH 7–8).

Biochemical properties of opioid receptors

Biochemical studies have indicated that opioid binding is highly sensitive to various proteolytic enzymes and to a large number of reagents capable of reacting with amino acids and functional groups present in proteins. Thus, opioid binding is inhibited by sulfhydryl-reactive reagents, such as *N*-ethylmaleimide (NEM) and iodoacetate. These studies suggest that one or more proteins play an essential role in specific opioid binding. Recent studies, using immobilized plant lectins able to bind specific sugars, have shown the existence of sugar moieties in opioid receptors, indicating that these integral membrane proteins are glycoproteins. The role of lipids in opioid binding is less clear. Binding is highly sensitive to some preparations of phospholipase A but not to others, nor to phospholipases C and D. Phospholipids may have a role in holding receptors in their proper conformation in the membrane lipid bilayer.

The evidence that opioid receptors can exist in different conformational states is of considerable interest. In brief, results from the laboratories of Simon and Hiller and of Snyder showed that Na^+ in the incubation medium increases the affinity of antagonist binding while decreasing that of agonist binding. The suggestion that this is due to a conformational change was supported by the finding of Simon and Hiller that Na^+ decreases the rate of inactivation of receptor sulfhydryl groups by reagents such as NEM. Both effects are highly specific for Na^+; only Li^+ has been found to have a similar, albeit weaker, effect. The knowledge that opioid binding sites have this kind of plasticity may prove important in understanding the steps subsequent to opioid binding that lead to the observed nervous system responses.

Distribution of opioid receptors

Detailed studies of the distribution of opioid binding sites within the CNS have been carried out in a number of species including humans, monkeys, cows, guinea pigs, and rats. The early experiments were done by dissecting and homogenizing discrete regions of the brain and spinal cord and binding labeled opiates to the homogenates. More recent studies have used autoradiography of brain and spinal cord slices to achieve detailed mapping of receptors, even in subnuclei of various regions. Two methods have been used successfully: injection of animals with labeled opioids and isolation of tissue slices at various times; and the incubation of tissue slices from various CNS regions with labeled opioids *in vitro*. The results from many different laboratories can be summarized by stating that large differences exist in the levels of opioid binding sites between different CNS regions. Moreover, the areas rich in opioid receptors tend to be in, or associated with, the limbic system and in all areas that have been implicated in pain perception and modulation and some of the other actions of opioid drugs. Table 1 summarizes the regions containing high receptor levels and the putative opiate, or opioid, responses mediated by these regions.

The question of pre- or postsynaptic localization of opioid receptors has been investigated in numerous ways. Suffice it to say that there is evidence for both. As discussed in the next section, there are multiple types of opioid receptors. It is not yet known whether some types of receptors are pre- and some postsynaptic, or whether a given type can have either location.

Multiple types of opioid receptors have been found to exist

The existence of many opioid peptides and the knowledge that receptors for classical neurotransmitters often exist in multiple forms led scientists to search for multiple classes of opioid

TABLE 1. Location of opioid receptors proposed to mediate specific opioid effects[a]

Opioid effect	Location of opioid receptors
ANALGESIA	
Spinal (body)	Laminae I and II of dorsal horn
Trigeminal (face)	Substantia gelatinosa of trigeminal nerve
Supraspinal	Periaqueductal grey matter, medial thalamic nuclei, intralaminar thalamic nuclei, striatum (?)
AUTONOMIC REFLEXES	
Suppression of cough, orthostatic hypotension, inhibition of gastric secretion	Nucleus tractus solitarius, commissuralis, ambiguous, and locus coeruleus
Respiratory depression	Nucleus tractus solitarius, parabrachial nuclei
Nausea and vomiting	Area postrema
Meiosis	Superior colliculus, pretectal nuclei
ENDOCRINE EFFECTS	
Inhibition of vasopressin secretion	Posterior pituitary
Hormonal effects	Hypothalamic infundibulum, hypothalamic nuclei, accessory optic system, amygdala (?)
BEHAVIORAL AND MOOD EFFECTS	Amygdala, nucleus stria terminalis, hippocampus, cortex, medial thalamic nuclei, nucleus accumbens, basal ganglia (?)
MOTOR RIGIDITY	Striatum

[a] From Atweh and Kuhar [1].

receptors. The first evidence for multiple opioid receptors came from experiments of Martin and co-workers [14] in chronic spinal dogs. Striking differences in pharmacological responses to different narcotic analgesics and their inability to substitute for one another in suppressing withdrawal symptoms in addicted dogs led them to postulate the existence of at least three types of receptors. These were named for the prototype drugs used: μ for morphine, κ for ketocyclazocine, and σ for SKF 10047 (*N*-allylnormetazocine).

Following the discovery of the enkephalins, Kosterlitz's group provided evidence for yet another receptor type [15]. They found that the electrically evoked contractions of the isolated guinea pig ileum were much more sensitive to inhibition by morphine and related opiate alkaloids than by enkephalins, whereas the opposite was observed with the mouse vas deferens. They suggested that the two bioassay systems contain different populations of receptors. The major receptors present in the guinea pig myenteric plexus seem to prefer opiates and resemble Martin's μ receptors, whereas the vas deferens seems to contain a preponderance of receptors that exhibit higher affinity for enkephalins and their analogues. These new receptors were named δ (deferens) receptors. *In vitro* binding competition studies in guinea pig brain homogenates supported the existence of these two receptor types.

The existence of κ-type binding sites has also been confirmed by *in vitro* binding studies, although this proved more difficult because of the low level of such sites present in the rat, the animal used in the early experiments. More important, all κ opiates known at that time also exhibited high affinity for μ and δ sites. Only when μ and δ sites were saturated with ligands selective for them could κ sites be demonstrated.

The existence of σ sites has also been established, but the fact that actions mediated by these receptors are not reversed by naloxone, and the finding that there appears to be an overlap of σ sites with binding sites for the nonopiate drug of abuse, phencyclidine (angel dust), has led to the suggestion that σ receptors should not be defined as opioid receptors.

A large amount of evidence from many laboratories supports the existence of μ, δ, and κ opioid receptors, and a number of other receptor types have been postulated, for example, ε and ι, as well as receptor subtypes, such as μ_1, μ_2, κ_1, κ_2. The reader is referred to the review articles listed at the end of this chapter for details on these topics.

The existence of multiple types of opioid receptors appears to be well established. It is further supported by the finding that the three major types of opioid receptors vary significantly in their distribution within the CNS. The question that is more difficult to answer is whether different types represent different conformations of a single receptor molecule or whether some or all of the different types of receptors are separate molecular entities. Some experiments bearing on this subject are summarized in a subsequent section.

What are the functions and endogenous ligands of the different receptor types?

The current notion as to which are the endogenous ligands for the three major types of receptors is that δ receptors mediate the effects of enkephalins, whereas κ receptors seem to bind and mediate the actions of the peptides derived from the precursor, prodynorphin (see below). These assignments should be regarded as preliminary, but there is even more uncertainty about the endogenous ligands of the μ receptor. It has been suggested as the receptor for β-endorphin or for the recently found endogenous morphine alkaloids or as an isoreceptor for the enkephalins.

A word is in order about the current state of our knowledge of the steps triggered by the binding of opioids to their receptors. There is evidence that the major types of opioid receptors use cyclic AMP (cAMP) as their second messenger. Experiments mainly with NG108-15 cells, but also with brain homogenates, indicate that opioid receptors are coupled to adenylate cyclase in a negative way; that is, opioids inhibit the enzyme via the G_i protein, the GTP-binding protein used for inhibition of the cyclase (see Chap. 17). There has also been progress by the

electrophysiologists in delineating the ionic channels involved in the effects mediated by the three major opioid receptor types. Briefly, the evidence suggests that binding to μ and δ receptors leads to the opening of synaptic K^+ channels, whereas binding to κ sites results in the closing of Ca^{2+} channels (16).

Presently, it appears as though all three major receptor types are involved in pain modulation (analgesia), δ receptors have been implicated in cardiovascular effects of opioid peptides and κ receptors seem to play a role in salt and water balance. The functions of the various types of opioid receptors are not yet clearly established. With the recent availability of highly selective ligands, the elucidation of physiological function should become easier.

Further knowledge of receptor structure and function requires isolation and purification. This is also the only way to determine molecular differences or similarities among various receptor types. There are two ways to accomplish this: (a) by linking receptors covalently to a labeled ligand—affinity labeling or cross-linking—and isolating the labeled complex; and (b) by isolating and purifying active receptor molecules. These two approaches are discussed in the next two sections.

Isolation and purification of opioid receptors can be monitored by covalent attachment of labeled ligand

The earliest attempt to isolate prelabeled opioid binding sites did not involve covalent binding but the use of a very high-affinity ligand, etorphine, which dissociates sufficiently slowly to survive the extraction and assay procedures. In 1975, a [^{3}H]etorphine-labeled macromolecular complex was solubilized with a nonionic detergent and found to have properties consistent with its being an etorphine-opioid receptor complex [17]. The complex was useful for some characterization but was not sufficiently stable to permit extensive purification.

Isolation of δ receptors

Since that time a large number of potentially useful affinity and photoaffinity ligands for opioid binding sites have been prepared. The only one that has been successfully used to achieve purification is fentanylisothiocyanate (FIT) and a more potent analogue, known as "superFIT." Klee and associates [18] have purified to homogeneity a [^{3}H]superFIT-receptor complex isolated from the neuroblastoma-glioma hybrid cell line NG108-15. Since these cells are known to contain only δ receptors, the isolated glycoprotein must be a binding unit of the δ receptor. It was found to have a molecular weight of 58,000 on sodium dodecylsulfate (SDS)-PAGE.

Separation of μ and δ receptors

More recently, affinity-cross-linking has been used to isolate binding proteins from both μ and δ receptors [19]. Iodination of the tyrosine in the 1 position of β-endorphin destroys its ability to bind to receptors; however, a second tyrosine is present in human β-endorphin (β-end$_h$), and advantage has been taken of this fact to prepare ^{125}I-labeled human β-endorphin with the label in tyrosine-27. This material was found to have high affinity for both μ and δ binding sites, but very low affinity for κ sites. The binding and cross-linking of ^{125}I-β-end$_h$ to tissues containing either μ or δ sites or both were now possible. Membranes cross-linked in this manner were solubilized in SDS, run on SDS-PAGE, and the gels submitted to autoradiography. A number of labeled bands were seen, all of which were opioid-binding-site related, since labeling could be prevented by the presence of excess unlabeled opioids during the binding.

For this discussion, two bands are of importance: a band of 65 kilodaltons (kDa), present in all tissues containing μ sites, including rat thalamus with a large preponderance of μ sites, and a 53-kDa band, present in all tissues containing δ sites, including the NG108-15 cells, which contain only δ sites. Further support for the idea that the 65-kDa protein is the major μ binding protein was obtained by showing that it fails to be cross-linked when binding of ^{125}I-β-end$_h$ is carried out in the presence of the highly selective μ ligand, D-Ala^2-MePhe^4-Gly-ol-enkephalin (DAGO). Similarly, the putative major δ binding protein (53 kDa) is not labeled when binding is done in the presence of the highly specific δ ligand, D-Pen^2-D-Pen^5-enkephalin (DPDPE).

This work represents the first evidence indicating that μ and δ binding sites may be distinct molecules. The results do not, however, distinguish between differences in the polypeptides (primary gene products) or in post-translational modifications. This information will only be available once the total amino acid sequences of the various opioid receptor types are known.

Active opioid binding sites can be extracted from membranes and purified

The first step in the isolation of opioid binding sites involves their solubilization from the cell membranes with which they are tightly associated, a step that proved more difficult than anticipated; however, several laboratories have now developed methods that extract soluble active binding sites from membranes derived from a variety of tissues. Digitonin, CHAPS, and Triton X-100 have been the detergents most frequently used.

The first receptor type to be separated in its active form was the κ receptor. This was accomplished by sucrose density gradient centrifugation of a digitonin extract of guinea pig brain [20]. Two peaks of opioid binding were obtained. The first was found to be virtually pure κ sites, and the second peak contained a mixture of μ and δ sites. A similar separation was achieved by Chow and Zukin using molecular exclusion chromatography of CHAPS extracts of rat brain membranes.

The purification of active opioid binding sites has been accomplished for the μ opioid receptor in several laboratories. In the first such achievement digitonin extracts of bovine striatal membranes were purified by two major chromatographic steps: ligand affinity chromatography on immobilized naltrexyl-6-ethylenediamine, and lectin affinity chromatography on a column of wheat germ agglutinin-agarose [21]. The total purification obtained was 60,000 to 70,000 times, with a specific activity of opioid binding of approximately 12,000 to 14,000 pmol/mg protein. These values are in excellent agreement with the theoretical values for a 65-kDa protein containing a single binding site. The purified receptor exhibits a single band of 65 kDa on SDS-PAGE.

Active δ sites have not yet been purified. There has been some progress toward purification of κ sites from frog brain, though homogeneity has not yet been achieved.

Investigating the structure of opioid receptors

The next important step in this research is the elucidation of the complete amino acid sequence of opioid-binding proteins. This is most readily accomplished by cloning and sequencing the cDNA corresponding to receptor mRNA. Two methods are used to screen suitable cDNA libraries. One involves the synthesis of oligonucleotide probes based on a partial amino acid sequence derived from the purified receptor protein. The other involves the use of antibodies against the receptor protein to detect expression of the protein in a phage (λgt11) system (see Chaps. 21 and 22).

Still another approach involves the technique of expression cloning. The gene for the opioid receptor in question is transferred to a cell line that does not normally express it. Receptor expression is monitored either by a sensitive binding assay or by the use of receptor antibodies. The DNA present in transformed cells, but not in the parental line, is isolated and

cloned. Evidence must then be obtained to prove that this DNA is the gene coding for the receptor polypeptide. This method is currently being applied to the δ opioid receptor from NG108-15 cells.

OPIOID PEPTIDES

Progress has been rapid in our knowledge of the biosynthesis and molecular genetics of the opioid peptides

The relatively large number of opioid peptides, whose sequence includes either met- or leu-enkephalin, isolated in recent years is a reflection of the complexity of the endogenous opioid system. Investigators have used various approaches to study the biosynthesis of opioid peptides. These include the classical technique of incorporation of radiolabeled amino acids into cultures of cells known to synthesize the peptide in question, and the use of antibodies to demonstrate the presence of peptides in putative precursor proteins. Recombinant DNA technology has been used to determine the amino acid sequence of polypeptide precursors from the nucleotide sequence of mRNA isolated from cells that produce the precursor and to study the structure of the genes that code for the precursor proteins.

The major opioid peptides are cleavage products of three distinct protein precursors

These proteins, in turn, are coded for by three separate genes. The precursor proteins are proopiomelanocortin (POMC), which contains β-lipotropin (β-LPH) and gives rise to β-, α-, and τ-endorphin; proenkephalin, whose cleavage products are met-enkephalin, leu-enkephalin, met-enkephalin-arg[6]-phe[7], met-enkephalin-arg[6]-gly[7]-leu[8], and peptide E; and prodynorphin, the precursor protein of α-neodynorphin, β-neoendorphin, dynorphin A-(1-8), dynorphin A-(1-17), and dynorphin B (rimorphin). The amino acid sequences of these opioid peptides are listed under their respective precursor proteins in Table 2.

Proopiomelanocortin

Proopiomelanocortin (POMC) is also the precursor of the nonopioid hormones adrenocorticotropin (ACTH) and α-, β-, and τ-melanocyte-stimulating hormones (MSH) (see Chap. 47). Its discovery [22,23] is of considerable importance, since it was the first time that a precursor was found to give rise to several different biologically active peptides. It was also the first of the three opioid peptide precursors to be sequenced [24]. The intermediate lobe of the pituitary gland is the major source of POMC. β-Endorphin, the 31-amino acid C-terminal peptide of β-LPH, is the predominant active opioid peptide product (Table 2). The gene coding for POMC contains two introns (areas within the gene not present in mature mRNA) and three

exons (areas transcribed into mRNA). Post-translational processing of precursor proteins is tissue specific. Pairs of basic amino acid residues border each of the peptides in the precursor molecule and are the presumed targets of proteolytic cleavage. Processing of POMC in the arcuate nucleus of the brain appears to be similar to that in the intermediate lobe of the pituitary. Post-translational modification may also lead to inactivation of opioid peptides. Thus, the N-acetylation of the N-terminal tyrosine of β-endorphin produces a peptide devoid of activity at the opioid receptor.

Proenkephalin

Proenkephalin was first discovered in bovine adrenal cortex where enkephalin biosynthesis was elucidated [25]. It contains one copy of leu-enkephalin, four copies of met-enkephalin, and one copy each of a met-enkephalin C-terminal-extended heptapeptide and octapeptide, all separated by basic dipeptides (Table 2). Human proenkephalin (267 amino acids) is coded for by

TABLE 2. Opioid precursors and major active opioid peptide products

Precursor	No. of amino acids	Peptide	Structure[a]
POMC Human	267	β-Endorphin	YGGFLTSEKSQTPLVTLFKNAIIKNAYKKGE
		γ-Endorphin	YGGFLTSEKSQTPLVTL
		α-Endorphin	YGGFLTSEKSQTPLVT
Proenkephalin A Human	269	Met-enkephalin	YGGFM
		Leu-enkephalin	YGGFL
		Heptapeptide	YGGFMRF
		Octapeptide	YGGFMRGL
		Peptide E	YGGFMRRVGRPEWWMDYQKRYGGFL
Prodynorphin (Proenkephalin B) Porcine	256	α-Neoendorphin	YGGFLRKYPK
		β-Neoendorphin	YGGFLRKYP
		Dynorphin A (1–17)	YGGFLRRIRPKLKWDNQ
		Dynorphin A –(1–8)	YGGFLRRI
		Leumorphin [Dynorphin B (1–29)]	YGGFLRRQFKVVTRSQQDPNAYYEELFDV
		Dynorphin B (Rimorphin)	YGGFLRRQFKVVT

[a] (A) Ala; (D) Asp; (E) Glu; (F) Phe; (G) Gly; (H) His; (I) Ile; (K) Lys; (L) Leu; (M) Met; (N) Asn; (P) Pro; (Q) Gln; (R) Arg; (T) Thr; (S) Ser; (V) Val; (W) Trp; (Y) Tyr.

a gene containing four exons and five introns. An N-terminal signal peptide, 24 amino acids in length, is present in the precursor protein. A body of evidence exists supporting the finding that proenkephalin of the bovine adrenal medulla is identical to that of the brain. The processing in the brain of this precursor appears to be more complete in that free enkephalins are the principal cleavage products, whereas high-molecular-weight enkephalin-containing peptides predominate in the adrenal medulla.

Prodynorphin

Prodynorphin, the latest of the opioid peptide precursors to be characterized, has been isolated from mammalian tissues, such as brain, anterior pituitary, adrenal gland, spinal cord, and reproductive organs. Sequencing of the human prodynorphin gene revealed four exons and three introns. The amino acid sequence of leu-enkephalin is repeated three times in the precursor. All active opioid peptides processed from prodynorphin are C-terminal extensions of leu-enkephalin (Table 2). They are α- and β-neoendorphin, dynorphin A (1-17), dynorphin A (1-8), and dynorphin B (1-29), also called leumorphin, processed at double basic amino acids that serve as processing signals. However, it is likely that enzymes able to cleave at single arginine sites exist, as demonstrated by the formation of dynorphin A (1-8) and rimorphin by the cleavage between isoleucine-8 and arginine-9 of dynorphin A and between threonine-13 and arginine-14 of leumorphin, respectively.

The distribution of proteolytic enzymes responsible for particular types of cleavage, leading to the production of various opioid peptides, is not uniform. Therefore, the species of product derived from post-translational processing of the same precursor molecule is dependent on the type of enzyme a neuronal cell body or its proximal dendrites is programmed to manufacture. Thus, for example, dynorphin A (1-8) may be the principal product of prodynorphin in one area of the brain, whereas longer forms of dynorphin are abundant in other brain areas.

Similarities among precursors of opioid peptides

It is of great interest to note that POMC, proenkephalin, and prodynorphin possess many shared characteristics. The three precursor proteins contain almost the same number of amino acids. All possess multiple sequences of opioid peptides contained in the C-terminal half of the molecule, and these peptides are almost always framed by pairs of basic amino acids. In addition, all contain a cysteine-rich N-terminal sequence preceded by very similarly sized signal peptides. The position of six separate cysteine residues in the N-terminal regions of proenkephalin and prodynorphin have almost equivalent placement. Finally, amino acid sequence homology between proenkephalin and prodynorphin exceeds 50 percent.

The structural organization of the genes encoding for the three precursors also possesses impressive similarities in the placement and size of their respective introns and exons. Thus, it has been suggested that these genes have developed by evolution from a common gene.

Distribution and tissue levels of opioid peptides can be measured by several techniques

In order to study the anatomical distribution and tissue levels of opioid peptides, highly specific and sensitive methods for their identification and quantitation are needed. Assays making use of highly specific polyclonal antibodies, generated against opioid peptides or opioid peptide-protein conjugates in rabbits and other animals, and monoclonal antibodies, raised by hybridoma technology, have been developed. Radioimmunoassays (RIAs) have been developed for all members of the three opioid peptide families. They measure the amount of peptide present in a tissue or plasma extract by competition with radiolabeled peptide for binding to the specific antibody. RIAs with sensitivities enabling them to detect femtomoles of a given peptide have been developed. Since a number of the antibodies employed in these assays demonstrate some degree of immunological cross-reactivity, in such cases a preparatory step using high-pressure liquid chromatography has been employed to separate the peptide of interest from other cross-reacting peptides.

Immunohistochemial techniques have proven extremely useful in mapping the distribution of opioid peptides. These methods consist of incubating an opioid peptide antibody with freeze-dried sections of tissue. The antigen-antibody complex is then visualized by the use of a second antibody (against the first) conjugated with a fluorescent marker or radioactive label or by the peroxidase-antiperoxidase method of Sternberger.

Peptidergic axons are widely distributed from central nuclei

RIAs and immunohistochemical techniques have been used for the detailed mapping of β-endorphin, enkephalin, and dynorphin in the CNS. Results of these studies are summarized below. It has been well established that areas of the brain that contain nerve fibers and terminals that transport and release opioid peptides exceed the number of areas in the brain containing cell bodies that produce opioid peptides.

β-Endorphin

Major concentrations of β-endorphin are found in the arcuate nucleus of the medial basal hypothalamus and the nucleus of the solitary tract, which lies within the medulla oblongata; however, nerve fibers containing β-endorphin have been found to project from these two centers to many areas of the brain. From the arcuate nucleus, β-endorphin-containing tracts are seen

projecting forward through the preoptic area, around the anterior commissure, and into the periaqueductal region of the diencephalon. Midline structures containing β-endorphin include the anterior paraventricular nucleus and the locus coeruleus. Neurons containing β-endorphin project laterally from the nucleus of the solitary tract to many pontine reticular sites and from there continue into the medulla to innervate the nuclei raphe magnus, reticularis gigantocellularis, paragigantocellularis, and reticularis lateralis.

Enkephalins

The most widely distributed opioid peptides are the enkephalins, which are found in many neuronal systems from the telencephalon to the spinal cord. The enkephalins have been shown to form local circuits or to be transplanted via lengthy neuronal projections to areas distant from the cell bodies in which they were synthesized. The distribution of leu-enkephalin and met-enkephalin has so far proved to be identical. In all areas, the level of leu-enkephalin is lower than that of met-enkephalin. This finding is in accord with the ratio of copies of these two pentapeptides in the proenkephalin precursor molecule. The enkephalins have their highest concentration in the globus pallidus, followed by, in descending order of concentration, the remainder of the telencephalon (except for low concentrations in the hippocampus and cortical areas), the diencephalon, pons, mesencephalon, and cerebellum.

Prodynorphin peptides

In general, the anatomical localization of peptides derived from the prodynorphin precursor follows the distribution map established for the enkephalin peptides. Dynorphins have their highest concentrations in the posterior pituitary and the hypothalamus. RIAs have also shown high concentrations to be present in the amygdala, septum, spinal cord, midbrain, and striatum. Somewhat lower levels have been detected in the hippocampus, thalamus, and pons, and very low concentrations in the cortex and cerebellum.

There is a problem in matching peptidergic fibers and opioid peptide receptors

Finally, it should be noted that there is poor correlation between the anatomical distribution of opioid peptide-containing nerve fibers and terminals and the distribution of the major types of opioid binding sites. The following are a few examples of these incongruous distribution patterns. The caudate and various cortical areas possess high concentrations of opioid binding sites but low concentrations of opioid peptides. This is in contrast to the situation seen in the globus pallidus, which has a very high concentration of enkephalin but only low levels of δ-opioid binding sites. The same is true for the substantia nigra and the hippocampus, which receive dense innervation from the dynorphin system but have sparse populations of κ-type opioid binding sites. On the other hand, areas of dense κ binding have been identified autoradiographically in the hypothalamus, an area possessing the highest concentration of dynorphin.

The reasons for the discrepancies between peptide and receptor localization are at present unknown. The discrepancies may be due to the use of ligands that have less than optimal specificity for *in situ* receptor labeling or to the conditions employed for *in vitro* labeling studies. Either of these procedures could lead to labeling of only high-affinity receptors when it may be that the low-affinity receptors are more closely aligned with the release sites of the peptides.

How is the expression of opioid peptides and precursors regulated?

The methods described above for the localization of opioid peptides leave open the question whether the genes coding for their precursors are expressed in the same cells. The possibility that the peptides may be synthesized at some distance and transported to their site of storage or action is especially relevant to the CNS. Another important question is whether changes in peptide levels resulting from physiological, pharmacological, or pathological alterations are due to changes in gene expression or to other events, such as altered transport, precursor processing, breakdown, or release. Answers are now possible by the use of modern methods of molecular biology. Gene expression, i.e., the level of mRNA, can be measured by hybridization with suitable labeled oligonucleotide probes prepared from the known nucleotide sequence of the cDNA (or mRNA) coding for the peptide precursor. The amount of labeled hybrid can be measured by dot blots on nitrocellulose. The size of the message can be determined by Northern blot analysis. The technique of *in situ* hybridization permits the cellular localization of a specific mRNA (see Chaps. 21 and 22).

These techniques have already been widely applied to opioid peptides, especially to proenkephalin. For example, it has long been known that enkephalin levels are very low in rat adrenals but that they increase ten- to 15-fold following surgical denervation. This increase was shown by Udenfriend and co-workers to be due to increased gene expression, since a comparable increase in the level of proenkephalin mRNA was observed. This provides evidence for transcriptional and/or translational control of enkephalin biosynthesis. This technique also led to the unexpected finding of high levels of proenkephalin message in rat testis, ovary, and heart. All of these tissues have barely measurable levels of enkephalin. The significance of the presence of untranslated mRNA is not understood.

In situ hybridization has been used to obtain the cellular distribution of proenkephalin mRNA in the caudate putamen and cerebellar cortex of the rat. The subpopulations of cells that express the message were delineated. The potential of this technique for the quantitation of mRNA on a cellular level is just beginning to be exploited.

Many physiological functions have been suggested for the endogenous opioid system

The putative functions of opioid peptides have been deduced from their observed pharmacological effects; their anatomical distribution in regions known to control various physiological and behavioral functions; as well as from the effects of the administration of the opiate antagonist, naloxone. One should be aware that pharmacological activity is only indicative of physiological function. Our understanding of how and under what conditions a given peptide activates a physiological mechanism is still sparse and much remains to be learned.

Physiological and behavioral systems

The properties of opioid peptides can best be summarized by stating that their pharmacological effects are remarkably similar to those of the plant-derived and synthetic opiate alkaloids. The physiological areas in which the endogenous opioid system seems to have a role include pain perception, stress mechanisms, respiratory regulation, temperature control, tolerance development, and physical dependence, as well as modulation of diuretic and cardiovascular functions. Behavioral patterns that seem to be under some influence of opioid peptides include sexual behavior, feeding and drinking, grooming, locomotor activity, and operant behavior. Opioid peptides may also serve a role in memory storage and recall (see Chap. 48). Like opiates, opioid peptides interact with the endocrine system, producing increases in the release of growth hormone, ACTH, prolactin, and antidiuretic hormone, and decreases in the circulating levels of thyrotropin, luteinizing hor-

mone and follicle-stimulating hormone (see Chaps. 14 and 47).

Role in disease

The participation of opioid peptides and their receptors in a number of pathological conditions has been investigated. The finding that in rats naloxone can rapidly reverse the hypotensive effects of bacterial endotoxin, which is commonly used as a model of human septic shock, led to the hypothesis that the profound hypotension produced during shock may be mediated via the endogenous opioid peptides. The psychopathological states of schizophrenia and depression have also been investigated. Based on the finding that the major behavioral response after intraventricular injection of β-endorphin in rats was the induction of catatonia, two essentially opposite hypotheses have been developed for the role of opioid peptides in schizophrenia (see also Chap. 45). One holds that catatonic symptoms may be the result of excess opioid peptides; the second argues that a deficiency in opioid peptide content could account for this behavior. The first hypothesis justified the administration of opiate antagonists to schizophrenic patients; the second was the rationale for administering opioid peptides and their analogues. Variable results have been reported with both regimens. The administration of naloxone to patients with endogenous depression has given promising results in the hands of some investigators.

Possible roles in neuromodulation and neurotransmission

The ability of opioid peptides to inhibit the release of various neurotransmitters, such as epinephrine, dopamine, acetylcholine, and substance P, supports their possible function as neuromodulators. In those instances in which opioid receptors are located postsynaptically, the peptides may function as neurotransmitters. Additional evidence supporting their role in synaptic transmission comes from the finding that they are largely located in nerve terminals and that they can be released from nervous tissue in response to depolarization in a Ca^{2+}-dependent manner.

ACKNOWLEDGMENTS

The research carried out in the authors' laboratory was supported by Grant DA-00017 from the National Institute on Drug Abuse.

REFERENCES

1. Hughes, J. (ed.), Opioid Peptides. *Br. Med. Bull.* 39, 1983.
2. Simon, E. J. Opiate receptors. In A. Lajtha (ed.), *Handbook of Neurochemistry.* New York: Plenum Press, 1984, Vol. 6, pp. 331–352.
3. Hughes, J., Collier, H. O. J., Rance, M. J., and Tyers, M. B. (eds.), *Opioids Past, Present and Future.* London: Taylor and Francis, 1984.
4. Höllt, V. Opioid peptide processing and receptor selectivity. *Annu. Rev. Pharmacol. Toxicol.* 26:59–77, 1986.
5. Gubler, U. Enkephalin genes. In J. F. Habener (ed.), *Molecular Cloning of Hormone Genes.* Clifton, NJ: Humana Press, 1986, pp. 229–276.
6. Uhl, G. R. *In Situ Hybridization in Brain.* New York: Plenum Publ. Corp., 1986.
7. Simon, E. J., and Hiller, J. M. Solubilization and purification of opioid binding sites. In G. W. Pasternak (ed.), *The Opiate Receptors.* Clifton, NJ: Humana Press 1988, pp. 165–194.
8. Simon, E. J., Hiller, J. M., and Edelman, I. Stereospecific binding of the potent narcotic analgesic ^{3}H-etorphine to rat brain homogenate. *Proc. Natl. Acad. Sci. U.S.A.* 70:1947–1949, 1973.
9. Terenius, L. Stereospecific interaction between narcotic analgesics and a synaptic plasma membrane fraction of rat cerebral cortex. *Acta Pharmacol. Toxicol.* (Copenhagen) 32:317–320, 1973.
10. Pert, C. B., and Snyder, S. H. Opiate receptor: Demonstration in nervous tissue. *Science* 179:1011–1014, 1973.
11. Liebeskind, J. C., Mayer, D. J., and Akil, H. Central mechanisms of pain inhibition: Studies of analgesia from focal brain stimulation. *Advan. Neurol.* 4:261–268, 1974.
12. Hughes, J., Smith, T. W., Kosterlitz, H. W., Fothergill, L. A., Morgan, B. A., and Morris, H. R. Identification of two related pentapeptides from the brain with potent opiate agonist activity. *Nature* 258:577–579, 1975.
13. Goldstein, A., Tachibana, S., Lowney, L. I., Hunkapiller, M., and Hood, L. Dynorphin (1-13), an extraordinarily potent opioid peptide. *Proc. Natl. Acad. Sci. U.S.A.* 76:6666–6670, 1979.
14. Martin, W. R., Eades, C. G., Thompson, J. A., Huppler, R. E., and Gilbert, P. E. The effects of morphine- and nalorphine-like drugs in the nondependent and morphine-dependent chronic spinal dog. *J. Pharmacol. Exp. Ther.* 197:517–532, 1976.
15. Lord, J. A. H., Waterfield, A. A., Hughes, J., and Kosterlitz, H. W. Endogenous opioid peptides: Multiple agonists and receptors. *Nature* 267:495–499, 1977.
16. North, R. A. Opioid receptor types and membrane ion channels. *Trends Neurosci.* 9:114–117, 1986.
17. Simon, E. J., Hiller, J. M., and Edelman, I. Solubilization of a stereospecific opiate-macromolecular complex from rat brain. *Science* 190:389–390, 1975.
18. Simonds, W. F., Burke, T. R., Jr., Rice, K. C., Jacobson, A. E., and Klee, W. A. Purification of the opiate receptor of NG 108-15 neuroblastoma-glioma hybrid cells. *Proc. Natl. Acad. Sci. U.S.A.* 82:4974–4978, 1985.
19. Howard, A. D., de la Baume, S., Gioannini, T. L., Hiller, J. H., and Simon, E. J. Covalent labeling of opioid receptors with radioiodinated human β-endorphin. *J. Biol. Chem.* 260:10833–10839, 1985.
20. Itzhak, Y., Hiller, J. M., and Simon, E. J. Solubilization and characterization of μ, δ and κ opioid binding sites from guinea pig brain: Physical separation of κ receptors. *Proc. Natl. Acad. Sci. U.S.A.* 81:4217–4221, 1984.
21. Gioannini, T. L., Howard, A. D., Hiller, J. M., and Simon, E. J. Purification of an active opioid-binding protein from bovine striatum. *J. Biol. Chem.* 260:15117–15121, 1985.

22. Mains, R. E., Eipper, B. A., and Ling, N. Common precursor to corticotropins and endorphins. *Proc. Natl. Acad. Sci. U.S.A.* 74:3014–3018, 1977.

23. Roberts, J. L., and Herbert, E. Characterization of a common precursor to corticotropin and β-lipotropin: Cell-free synthesis of the precursor and identification of corticotropin peptides in the molecule. *Proc. Natl. Acad. Sci. U.S.A.* 74:4826–4830, 1977.

24. Nakanishi, S., Inoue, A., Kita, T., Nakamura, M., Chang, A. C. Y., Cohen, S. N., and Numa, S. Nucleotide sequence of cloned cDNA for bovine corticotropin-β-lipotropin precursor. *Nature* 278:423–427, 1979.

25. Lewis, R. V., Stern, A. S., Kimura, S., Rossier, J., Stein, S. and Udenfriend, S. An about 50,000-dalton protein in adrenal medulla: A common precursor of [Met]- and [Leu]enkephalin. *Science* 208:1459–1461, 1980.

CHAPTER **14**

Neuropeptides

Michael J. Brownstein

Basic Neurochemistry: Molecular, Cellular, and Medical Aspects, 4th Ed., edited by G. J. Siegel et al. Raven Press, Ltd., New York, 1989.
Correspondence to Michael J. Brownstein, National Institute of Mental Health, National Institutes of Health, Bldg. 36, Rm. 3A17, Bethesda,
Maryland 20892.

287

PEPTIDERGIC NEURONS

Several independent avenues of work have led to the recognition that peptides are involved in nervous system function. The discovery of the peptidergic neurosecretory cell in vertebrates by Ernst Scharrer led to the proposal of the "peptidergic neuron" concept and its subsequent amplification [1]. Initially, the term peptidergic neuron referred to those neurosecretory cells in the hypothalamus that release oxytocin and vasopressin directly into the circulation from their nerve terminals in the posterior pituitary; however, two major lines of investigation have been largely responsible for the subsequent broadening of this concept. The first relates to the development of the "releasing-factor" concept by G. W. Harris and co-workers (for historical development, see Fink [2]) and the culmination of this conceptual revolution in the isolation and characterization of a tripeptide-releasing factor, that is, thyrotropin-releasing factor [3]. The latter effort represented a landmark event in the field of neuroendocrinology and provided the impetus for the discovery of other peptide-releasing factors [3]. The second major development was the detection of substance P by von Euler and Gaddum in 1931 [4] and its isolation and characterization by Leeman and Mroz [5]. The significance of the finding was that this peptide was clearly concentrated in specific extrahypothalamic areas (such as the sensory ganglia); hence, physiologists were alerted to the possibility that peptides might act as neurotransmitters [5].

Peptidergic neurons commonly occur throughout the animal kingdom [6]. In fact, in lower invertebrates, such as annelids, at least one-half of the cerebral ganglion consists of such neurons [1]. Amino acid sequences are known for several of the invertebrate neuropeptides: the red chromatotropin of crustaceans; the adipokinetic hormone and proctolin [6] of insects; the egg-laying hormone and peptides A and B of *Aplysia*; and the head activator of *Hydra*.

Many peptide structures appear to be phylogenetically conserved, since vertebrate peptides have been detected in invertebrates, and vice versa. In addition, there appear to be significant redundancies of peptide structure in different tissues of a single species [7].

Ever since the discovery of the endogenous opioid peptides (see Chap. 13), neuropeptide research has become one of the most rapidly expanding areas in neurobiology. Several books providing both background and current information on the subject have been published [7–10]. This chapter will give an overview of the field, which should provide the reader with a basis for further study. Much of our understanding of the functional organization of peptidergic neuronal systems comes from studies of the hypothalamus and pituitary, and therefore, we begin with an exposition of this area.

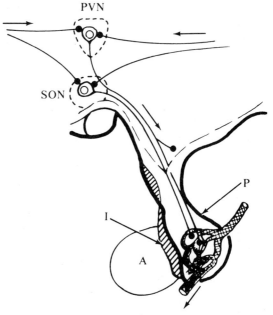

Vasopressin/oxytocin/neurophysins

FIG. 1. The hypothalamoneurohypophysial system. Magnocellular neurons in the supraoptic nucleus (SON) and paraventricular nucleus (PVN) of the hypothalamus project via the median eminence to the posterior pituitary (P). There they release their hormones into capillaries. The magnocellular neurons are influenced both by ascending and descending afferents. Note that the axons of some neurons in the PVN terminate in the zona externa of the median eminence and release their contents into the portal capillary plexus. (A) anterior lobe; (I) intermediate lobe.

PEPTIDES INVOLVED IN HYPOTHALAMIC AND PITUITARY FUNCTION

The pituitary is composed of anterior or distal, intermediate, and posterior or neural lobes

The posterior lobe is of neuronal origin and comes from the floor of the hypothalamus. It is connected to the median eminence of the hypothalamus by a stalk (Fig. 1). The anterior and intermediate parts of the pituitary arise from epithelial cells that migrate up from the roof of the embryonal mouth cavity (Rathke's pouch). The three parts of the pituitary eventually join one another and take up residence beneath the diencephalon, those derived from Rathke's pouch becoming most rostral.

Axons of large neurons in the supraoptic and paraventricular hypothalamic nuclei travel through the median eminence and stalk to the posterior pituitary, where they terminate near blood vessels

These axons discharge the peptide hormones vasopressin and oxytocin into these vessels (Fig. 1). Separate populations of neurons manufacture the two peptide hormones along with their so-called carrier proteins, the neurophysins. The posterior pituitary is best thought of as the part of the brain that secretes into the peripheral circulation.

Vasopressin, or antidiuretic hormone, inhibits water diuresis. Without this hormone, animals have to consume large amounts of water each day in order to replace their fluid losses. If water is not freely available, depletion of body fluids and cardiovascular collapse rapidly ensue. Vasopressin also increases arterial blood pressure; the physiological importance of this effect is beginning to be appreciated [11].

Moderate to severe dehydration is associated with an outpouring of vasopressin. Theoretically, this outpouring could be triggered either by the decrease in plasma volume that is associated with dehydration or the increase in osmolarity; the latter seems to be the more important factor. Osmoreceptor cells in the central nervous system are concerned with regulating vasopressin release. Cells elsewhere in the body that are sensitive to changes in osmolarity or blood pressure also influence vasopressin secretion.

A number of pharmacological agents alter the firing patterns of vasopressin-producing neurons and affect the release rate of the hormone. Acetylcholine and histamine are especially potent in releasing vasopressin; norepinephrine has the opposite action. Many other neurotransmitters present in a variety of ascending and descending central pathways probably participate in controlling vasopressin secretion, mediating changes in its release in response to pain, stress, hemorrhage, transfusion, orthostasis, and anoxia.

Oxytocin, the second neurohypophysial hormone to be characterized, plays an important role in reproduction and lactation. The word oxytocin ("quick birth") was coined because the hormone stimulates uterine contractions. There is no doubt that oxytocin is secreted during parturition, but its precise role in promoting the ordered evacuation of the fetus from the uterus is still debated.

The part played by oxytocin in milk ejection is clearer. When suckling commences, afferent stimuli from the teats cause reflex release of oxytocin from the posterior pituitary. The oxytocin activates a contractile mechanism, and alveolar milk is expressed through the lactiferous ducts into the sinuses or cisterns connecting to the teat ducts. In the absence of oxytocin, only the milk stored in the cisterns is available to the infant.

It has been suggested that oxytocin influences sperm transport in the female genital tract, milk secretion, male reproductive function, the estrous cycle of certain animals, and maternal behavior, but these suggestions are not yet universally accepted.

The anterior pituitary contains several types of cells that manufacture and secrete hormones

Growth hormone and prolactin have similar primary structures and, to an important degree, similar functions. Growth hormone probably affects metabolic processes in all tissues of the body. Its most obvious action is to cause growth of the immature animal by stimulating elongation of long bones and by stimulating protein biosynthesis at the expense of sugar and fat stores. Some of the actions of growth hormone are mediated by another group of peptides, the somatomedins, which are made in the liver. The effects of prolactin, on the other hand, seem to result from the direct influence of this hormone on target cells. Although prolactin can stimulate protein biosynthesis just as growth hormone does, its only certain physiological function is to stimulate lactation in the breast that has been primed with estrogen, progesterone, glucocorticoids, insulin, and thyroxine.

Thyroid-stimulating hormone (TSH), luteinizing hormone (LH), and follicle-stimulating hormone (FSH), as well as human chorionic gonadotropin (CG), are glycoproteins formed from two peptide subunits called α and β chains. Fifteen to 30 percent of the total weight of the molecules is contributed by their sugar moieties (polymers of fucose, mannose, galactose, *N*-acetylglucosamine, *N*-acetylgalactosamine, and sialic acid) and the rest by the peptide chains. The amino acid sequence of the α chain, which is not biologically active, seems to be the same in TSH, LH, FSH, and CG. The biologically active β chains differ in primary structure.

TSH increases the volume and vascularization of the thyroid gland and stimulates the synthesis and release of thyroid hormones. It also promotes lypolysis in adipose tissue, but the physiological importance of this extrathyroid effect is not understood.

In women, FSH causes growth and development of the ovarian follicle. Subsequently, LH acts on the follicle, causing it to mature and secrete estrogens. LH then induces ovulation and participates in transforming the follicle into the progesterone-secreting corpus luteum. In men, FSH promotes spermatogenesis, and LH stimulates androgen production by the testis (Leydig cells).

Adrenocorticotropic hormone (corticotropin or ACTH), α-melanocyte-stimulating hormone (α-MSH), β-MSH, β-lipotropic hormone (β-LPH), and β-endorphin comprise a family of peptides that are synthesized as parts of a common precursor molecule, pro-opiocortin [11], which has a molecular weight of about 31,000 Da. This glycoprotein has β-LPH (β-endorphin and β-MSH) on its C-terminal end, ACTH(α-MSH) in the middle, and γ-MSH near the N-terminal end.

In all species studied, ACTH has 39 amino acid residues. Its first 24 amino acids are constant from species to species. The first 13 amino acids of ACTH are required for the only significant physiological action of the hormone, adrenocorticotropic activity. Adding the next seven amino acids one at a time progressively enhances the molecule's potency. The remaining 19 amino acids are not required for optimum biological activity.

Melanotropic and small nonsecretory cells comprise the intermediate lobe of the pituitary gland. α-MSH contains the first 13 amino acids of ACTH. It is *N*-acetylated and C-amidated, and, consequently, resistant to most peptidases.

β-MSH, β-LPH, α-MSH, and ACTH secreted from the anterior and/or intermediate lobes of the pituitary have seven amino acids in common (ACTH residues 4 to 10). These residues are the minimum required for melanotropic activity in amphibians and reptiles. The role of MSH in mammals is still unknown. In fact, humans have a vestigial intermediate pituitary and have little or no circulating α-MSH.

The anterior pituitary is an organ that is separate from, but regulated by, the brain

The anterior pituitary is connected to the hypothalamus by a special portal vascular system [12] (Fig. 2). This system consists of two connected capillary beds, one in the external zone of the median eminence, the other in the pituitary. Axons of a variety of neurons terminate adjacent to portal capillaries in the median eminence. Some of the nerve endings in the median eminence release hypothalamic hormones that enter the portal vessels and travel to the anterior pituitary (undiluted by blood from the general circulation). Others release neurotransmitters that probably influence by presynaptic mechanisms the secretion of the hypothalamic hormones.

On reaching the anterior pituitary, hypothalamic hormones stimulate or inhibit the synthesis and secretion of tropic hormones made in the pituitary

A number of releasing hormones and release-inhibiting hormones are present in the hypothalamus. Four releasing hormones—thyrotro-

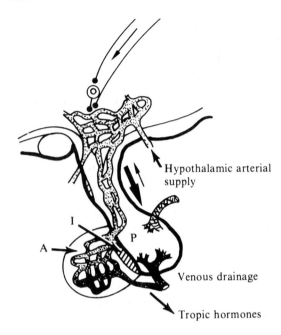

Hypothalamic arterial
supply

I

P

A

Venous drainage

Tropic hormones

FIG. 2. Control of anterior pituitary function. Releasing hormones and release-inhibiting hormones are secreted into portal capillaries in the zona externa of the median eminence. The hormones travel to the anterior pituitary; there they act on tropic hormone-producing cells. These cells secrete into the general circulation; tropic hormones may also travel back to the brain through the portal vessels. Cells that make releasing or release-inhibiting hormones are excited or inhibited by other neurons. Furthermore, release of hypothalamic hormones may be modulated at the median eminence level by a presynaptic mechanism.

pin-releasing hormone (TRH); gonadotropin-releasing hormone (GnRH); corticotropin-releasing hormone (CRH), and growth hormone-releasing hormone (GHRH)—and one release-inhibiting hormone (growth hormone release-inhibiting hormone, or somatostatin) have been isolated and characterized (see Table 1 for the amino acid sequences of these and other peptides). A number of other peptides—vasopressin, vasoactive intestinal polypeptide, and cholecystokinin, to name a few—may be involved in regulating anterior pituitary function as well.

The general properties of the hypothalamic hormones are defined in Table 2. It is noteworthy that the properties of a releasing factor (or release-inhibiting factor) are quite similar to those of a neurotransmitter. Indeed, the releasing factors are best thought of as a special class of neurotransmitters that act on a variety of cells among which are cells in the anterior pituitary.

TRH stimulates the secretion of thyrotropin and prolactin; GnRH stimulates the secretion of LH and FSH; CRH stimulates ACTH and β-endorphin release; and GHRH stimulates growth hormone secretion. Somatostatin inhibits the secretion of growth hormone, thyrotropin, and prolactin *in vitro*, but it seems unlikely that somatostatin participates in regulating prolactin *in vivo*. Dopamine, on the other hand, is a potent inhibitor of prolactin secretion and is found in high concentrations in the median eminence. Hence, it has been suggested that dopamine is a prolactin release-inhibiting hormone.

In addition to controlling anterior pituitary function, the hypothalamic hormones may act in the central nervous system and the periphery

GnRH, for example, induces mating behavior in female rats. This orchestration of reproductive phenomena—mating and ovulation—by a single peptide may represent a special case. Peptides may also mediate diverse and unrelated events.

In addition to acting within the central nervous system, hypothalamic hormones function in the periphery. Thus, somatostatin has been shown to play an important role outside the brain in the pancreas and gastrointestinal tract. It inhibits the secretion of insulin, glucagon, and gastrin and decreases gastric acidity. Conversely, a number of peptides first isolated from gut extracts and thought of as gastrointestinal hormones are now known to operate in the brain.

TABLE 1. Amino acid sequences of representative mammalian biologically active peptides

Adrenocorticotropic hormone
H-Ser-Tyr-Ser-Met-Glu-His-Phe-Arg-Trp-Gly-Lys-Pro-Val-Gly-Lys-Lys-Arg-Arg-Pro-Val-Lys-Val-Tyr-Pro-Asn-Gly-Ala-Glu-Asp-Glu-Leu-Ala-Glu-Ala-Phe-Pro-Leu-Glu-Phe-OH

Angiotensin II
H-Asp-Arg-Val-Tyr-Ile-His-Pro-Phe-OH

Arginine vasopressin
H-Cys-Tyr-Phe-Glu-Asn-Cys-Pro-Arg-Gly-NH$_2$

Arginine vasotocin
H-Cys-Tyr-Ile-Glu-Asn-Cys-Pro-Arg-Gly-NH$_2$

Atrial natriuretic polypeptide
Ser-Leu-Arg-Arg-Ser-Ser-Cys-Phe-Gly-Gly-Arg-Met-Asp-Arg-Ile-Gly-Ala-Gln-Ser-Gly-Leu-Gly-Cys-Asn-Ser-Phe-Arg-Tyr

Bradykinin
H-Arg-Pro-Pro-Gly-Phe-Ser-Pro-Phe-Arg-OH

Calcitonin
Cys-Gly-Asn-Leu-Ser-Thr-Cys-Met-Leu-Gly-Thr-Tyr-Thr-Gln-Asp-Phe-Asn-Lys-Phe-His-Thr-Phe-Pro-Gln-Thr-Ala-Ile-Gly-Val-Gly-Ala-Pro-NH$_2$

Calcitonin gene-related peptide
Ala-Cys-Asp-Thr-Ala-Thr-Cys-Val-Thr-His-Arg-Leu-Ala-Gly-Leu-Leu-Ser-Arg-Ser-Gly-Gly-Val-Val-Lys-Asn-Asn-Phe-Val-Pro-Thr-Asn-Val-Gly-Ser-Lys-Ala-Phe-NH$_2$

L-Carnosine
N-β-alanyl-L-histidine

Cholecystokinin octapeptide
Asp-Tyr(SO$_3$)-Met-Gly-Trp-Met-Asp-Phe-NH$_2$

Corticotropin-releasing hormone
Ser-Glu-Glu-Pro-Pro-Ile-Ser-Leu-Asp-Leu-Thr-Phe-His-Leu-Leu-Arg-Glu-Val-Leu-Glu-Met-Ala-Arg-Ala-Glu-Gln-Leu-Ala-Gln-Gln-Ala-His-Ser-Asn-Arg-Lys-Leu-Met-Glu-Ile-Ile-NH$_2$

Dynorphin A
Tyr-Gly-Gly-Phe-Leu-Arg-Arg-Ile-Arg-Pro-Lys-Leu-Lys-Trp-Asp-Asn-Gln

β-Endorphin
H-Tyr-Gly-Gly-Phe-Met-Thr-Ser-Glu-Lys-Ser-Gln-Thr-Pro-Leu-Val-Thr-Leu-Phe-Lys-Asn-Ala-Ile-Ile-Lys-Asn-Ala-Tyr-Lys-Lys-Gly-Glu-OH

Gonadotropin-releasing hormone (also called luteinizing hormone-releasing hormone (LHRH))
pGlu-His-Trp-Ser-Tyr-Gly-Leu-Arg-Pro-Gly-NH$_2$

Growth hormone-releasing hormone
Tyr-Ala-Asp-Ala-Ile-Phe-Thr-Asn-Ser-Tyr-Arg-Lys-Val-Leu-Gly-Gln-Leu-Ser-Ala-Arg-Lys-Leu-Leu-Gln-Asp-Ile-Met-Ser-Arg-Gln-Gln-Gly-Glu-Ser-Asn-Gln-Glu-Arg-Gly-Ala-Arg-Ala-Arg-Leu-NH$_2$

Leu-enkephalin
H-Tyr-Gly-Gly-Phe-Leu-OH

α-Melanocyte-stimulating hormone
Acetyl-Ser-Tyr-Ser-Met-Glu-His-Phe-Arg-Trp-Gly-Lys-Pro-Val-NH$_2$

Met-enkephalin
H-Tyr-Gly-Gly-Phe-Met-OH

TABLE 1. (*continued*)

Neurotensin
  pGlu-Leu-Tyr-Glu-Asn-Lys-Pro-Arg-Arg-Pro-Tyr-Ile-Leu-OH

Oxytocin
  H-Cys-Tyr-Ile-Glu-Asn-Cys-Pro-Leu-Gly-NH$_2$

Somatostatin
  H-Ala-Gly-Cys-Lys-Asn-Phe-Phe-Trp-Lys-Thr-Phe-Thr-Ser-Cys-OH

Substance P
  H-Arg-Pro-Lys-Pro-Glu-Glu-Phe-Phe-Gly-Leu-Met-NH$_2$

Thyrotropin-releasing hormone
  pGlu-His-Pro-NH$_2$

Vasoactive intestinal peptide
  H-His-Ser-Asp-Ala-Val-Phe-Thr-Asp-Asn-Tyr-Thr-Arg-Leu-Arg-Lys-Glu-Met-Ala-Val-Lys-Lys-Tyr-Leu-Asn-Ser-Ile-Leu-
  Asn-NH$_2$

The neuroendocrine system is a hierarchy with higher centers regulating lower ones

This hierarchical control of secretory activity involves feedback loops (Fig. 3). That is, some

TABLE 2. Criteria for assessing the physiological role of any proposed substance as a releasing factor*

1. The putative releasing factor must be extractable from hypothalamic or stalk-median eminence tissue
2. It must be present in hypophysial portal blood in greater amounts than in systemic blood (i.e., it is released into the portal capillaries)
3. Varying concentrations of the substance in portal vessel blood should be related to varying secretion rates of one of the anterior pituitary hormones under a number of different experimental and environmental conditions
4. The factor should stimulate (or inhibit) secretion of one or more anterior pituitary hormones when administered *in vivo* or *in vitro*. Inhibitors, if available, should antagonize the actions of the endogenous peptide and block (or stimulate) anterior pituitary hormone secretion
5. Target cells should have receptors for the candidate peptides; e.g., corticotropes should, and indeed do, have CRH binding sites

* After Harris, G. W. *J. Endocrinol.* 53:ii–xii, 1972.

change related to secretory activity is detected by a control center, and the information is used to adjust the output of the control mechanism in an appropriate way. Consequently, Fig. 3 could be redrawn with many extra arrows pointing upward to indicate feedback.

Negative, or inhibitory, feedback is the usual means of maintaining a particular level of output in the face of uncontrolled or unpredictable disturbances. For example, an increase in the blood level of adrenocorticosteroids causes a decrease in the release of ACTH from the anterior pituitary. This, in turn, results in a decrease in the secretion rate of corticosteroids, and they return toward their original level. Gonadal steroids and thyroxine also exert negative feedback control over their respective tropic hormones.

There is evidence for positive, or stimulatory, feedback as well as negative feedback. Implantation of estrogen in the rat pituitary during a critical period of the estrous cycle causes advancement of ovulation, which is probably due to an increase in the plasma level of LH. By acting on the developing ovarian follicle, the LH causes a further increase in estrogen level. Unlike negative feedback systems, positive feed-

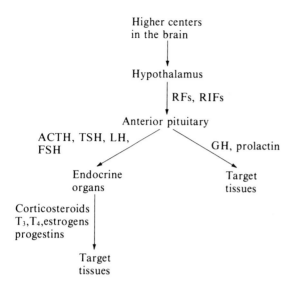

FIG. 3. Neuronal control of anterior pituitary function: (RF) releasing factor; (RIF) release-inhibiting factor.

back controls are inherently unstable. Once set in motion, they rapidly produce a high level of activity. For example, estrogen stimulation of LH secretion seems responsible for the peak of LH output that triggers ovulation when the follicle is mature. Inhibitory mechanisms are required for turning off positive feedback control loops. Inhibition by LH of its own secretion may provide such a mechanism in the example cited above.

In general, the higher a regulatory center is in the neuroendocrine hierarchy, the more opportunities it has to be fed back on, positively or negatively. Theoretically, the feedback control of a center can be mediated by the secretory product of the center itself (this sort of feedback—releasing hormones onto the very cells that make them—is termed ultrashort feedback), by the secretory products of lower centers, or by reflexes triggered by these secretory products. Cells in the anterior pituitary and in

the hypothalamus are sensitive to peripheral hormone levels. These hormone-brain and hormone-pituitary interactions are responsible for so-called long-feedback effects. For example, repeated injection of exogenous thyroxine into an animal with an isolated pituitary will cause atrophy of its thyroid gland, just as in the intact animal. This is taken to indicate that the isolated pituitary gland, in addition to maintaining a low rate of TSH secretion, is sensitive to the level of thyroxine in the general circulation. Increasing the thyroxine level inhibits the TSH release and produces atrophy of the target organ. There is also evidence that thyroxine affects the synthesis and secretion of TRH (Fig. 4).

After stalk section, the thyroid is unresponsive to many of the stimuli that would have increased its secretory activity in the intact animal, such as environmental stress. The input to the pituitary-thyroid axis from these stimuli must be mediated via TRH secretion into the hypophysial portal system. Similar observations have been made for ACTH and the gonadotropic hormones.

Feedback control of brain centers by adenohypophysial tropic hormones is referred to as internal or short feedback. There is evidence that each of the tropic hormones except prolactin may act on the hypothalamus in such an inhibitory short loop. Since the pressure in pituitary portal vessels is low, blood flow in this vascular system is probably bidirectional, although predominantly toward the pituitary (Fig. 2). Therefore, pituitary secretions can return to the median eminence, to the cerebrospinal fluid, and finally, to the rest of the brain either directly by this route or indirectly (and much diluted) through systemic circulation. Peripheral hormones must be carried to the brain through the general circulation. Once there, these peripheral hormones act, along with pituitary tropic hormones, on a variety of neurons that are involved in neuroendocrine regulation (for more detail, see Lightman and Everitt [13]).

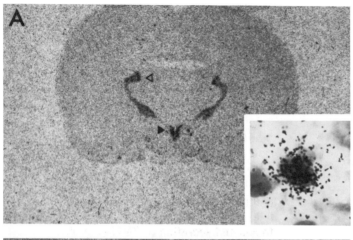

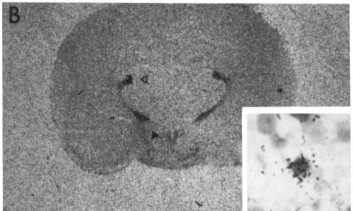

FIG. 4. *In situ* hybridization histochemistry of TRH mRNA-containing cells in the paraventricular nucleus (PVN) of the hypothalamus and the reticular nucleus of the thalamus. The autoradiographic hybridization signal on X-ray film appears as an area of darkening over the PVN (*solid arrowhead*) and reticular nucleus (*open arrowhead*) of a rat treated with propylthiouracil (PTU) (**A**) and of a PTU-treated rat injected with T₃ (**B**). The hybridization appears as dense clusters of grains over individual cell bodies within the PVN of a PTU-treated rat (*inset* **A**) and of a PTU-treated rat injected with T₃ (*inset* **B**). Each inset shows the most intensely labeled cells within the respective PVN [34].

EXPERIMENTAL APPROACHES TO THE STUDY OF NEUROPEPTIDES

There is no single best approach to the detection and isolation of biologically active neuropeptides

One general paradigm that has been used with success [14] is presented in Table 3. In this approach, the biochemist is directed by the biological phenomenon of interest, that is, the bioactivity of the peptide. The biological assay may be either a physiologically relevant one, as was the case for the hypothalamic releasing factors (see above), or a reproducible response to

the peptide in a neuronal or nonneuronal tissue that may have no apparent relationship to its actual physiological role in the nervous system, as was the case for substance P and the sialogogic bioassay [14]. In some cases, if it is feasible, even a complex behavioral response can be used as the basis for a bioassay.

Development of a quantitative bioassay depends on effective extraction of the peptide

The extraction should be done under conditions that protect the peptide from degradative processes (e.g., proteolytic enzymes), and a sol-

TABLE 3. Steps in the analysis of a neuropeptide[a]

1. Development of a quantitative bioassay
2. Evidence that the biologically active material is peptidic in nature
3. Development of extraction and separation procedures for maximum yields of the purified peptide
4. Chemical and physical characterization of the pure peptide (e.g., molecular weight determination and amino acid composition)
5. Obtain amino acid sequence of the peptide
6. Chemical synthesis of the peptide (which is then tested for bioactivity using quantitative bioassay)
7. Produce antibodies to peptide
8. Characterization of antibodies using synthetic analogs of the peptide (purification of antibodies)
9. Development of immunologic assays and procedures for use on neural tissues (e.g., radioimmunoassay and immunocytochemistry)
10. Isolation of cDNA that encodes the peptide's precursor. Characterization and chromosomal localization of the gene that gives rise to the precursor. Development of methods for detecting and measuring the precursor's mRNA (Northern blotting, *in situ* hybridization histochemistry)

[a] Although it is highly desirable to have at the outset a biological activity of the peptide that can be monitored by a quantitative bioassay, not all studies on peptides begin with this step; however, the value of a bioassay is emphasized by its role in the establishment of purity criteria for the isolated and the synthetic peptides.

vent should be used in which the peptide is highly soluble. Methods for preventing degradation of the peptide during extraction include microwave treatment or freezing of the tissue with liquid nitrogen, adding protease inhibitors to the extraction solvent, and boiling the tissue in dilute acid. In addition to the problems of degradation, one must also attend to the problem of recovery. Peptides tend to bind to glass surfaces, may be associated with binding proteins, and may be destroyed by such processes as oxidation and esterification of sensitive amino acid residues during extraction. Obviously, the initial extraction step is critical and often must be tailored to the specific peptide being extracted and to the specific tissue from which it is to be extracted [14].

Even with a good extraction procedure, one may find that the biological activity in the extract is altered or masked by other substances that are coextracted. Only by sequential separation steps and bioassay at each step can one determine if this is indeed the case. Herein lies the major value of the quantitative bioassay. The bioassay provides a major criterion for purity of the peptide as it is being fractionated. The aim is to subject the extract to a variety of sequential separation procedures until the isolated peptide is at maximum and constant specific activity (i.e., where the units of biological activity per amount of peptide are maximal and constant). In addition, the bioassay can be used early to determine whether the bioactive substance is a peptide. Preliminary evidence of its peptidic nature can be obtained by evaluating its size by molecular filtration chromatography, by determining whether it maintains activity after boiling at neutral pH (most, but not all, peptides do), and by determining whether the bioactivity is destroyed by incubation of the material with proteolytic enzymes (e.g., pronase, trypsin) or by acid hydrolysis.

A variety of separation procedures can be used to isolate a purified peptide

These include molecular filtration chromatography (which also provides information about the size of the peptide), selective extractions in diverse solvents, ion-exchange chromatography, thin-layer chromatography, high-voltage electrophoresis, and, where possible, specific affinity chromatography. The latter procedure is particularly efficacious, as it provides a large purification in a single step because of a specific property of the peptide (i.e., it may bind specifically to a protein and will be eluted from a column on which this protein is attached only in the presence of an excess of a competing ligand). High-performance liquid chromatography (HPLC) has proven especially useful for peptide separation. The point of using these separation procedures is to generate a pure peptide. One criterion of purity has already been discussed; that is, the peptide is at maximum and constant specific biological activity. Several other criteria should also be fulfilled: N-terminal and C-terminal analyses of the peptide show that there is only one N-terminal and one C-terminal amino acid, and analysis of the amino acid composition of the peptide demonstrates that the molar ratios of its constituent amino acids remain constant integrals throughout sequential fractionation procedures.

After a peptide has been isolated in sufficient quantity (50 pmol to 1 nmol, depending on whether or not it is N-terminally derivatized), its amino acid sequence can be determined by automated Edman degradation and/or fast atom bombardment mass spectroscopy [15]. Alternatively, a partial sequence for the peptide can be used to generate oligonucleotide probes for screening a cDNA library. The amino acid sequence of the peptide can be inferred from the sequence of its precursor protein. Ultimately, the peptide can be synthesized chemically in large quantities, and the purified molecule can be compared to the natural product and bioassayed.

Tatemoto and Mutt [16] have devised another strategy for identifying and purifying biologically active peptides. They recognized the fact that many such peptides are C-terminally amidated and developed a method for detecting amidated amino acids liberated when peptides are hydrolyzed. Using this method they have found a number of novel species that subsequently proved to be quite active *in vivo* and *in vitro*, e.g., peptide histidine-isoleucine (PHI) related to vasoactive intestinal peptide (VIP), neuropeptide Y (NPY), and galanin. Care must be taken not to jump too quickly to the conclusion that a new "biologically active" peptide is a chemical messenger [17].

Characterization of peptide precursors by molecular biological techniques has also led to the discovery of novel peptides. It is not uncommon for a precursor to contain more than one active agent. In addition, differential splicing of peptide genes can give rise to mRNAs encoding different products; witness the case of calcitonin and the calcitonin gene-related peptide [18] (see also Chap. 21).

Immunological techniques are the methods of choice for studying neuropeptide distribution and cellular compartmentation

Radioimmunoassay (RIA) techniques can detect extremely low levels of peptides (femtomoles). Immunological reactions are relatively specific, and RIAs require little technical investment [19]. Similarly, the techniques of immunocytochemistry provide a unique morphological approach to the cellular and subcellular localization of peptides even in a tissue as heterogeneous as the brain.

The production of antibodies to a peptide involves the immunization of rabbits, goats, mice, or guinea pigs with a peptide that has been emulsified in Freund's adjuvant. Relatively impure peptides can be used for immunization, and slight denaturation of the antigens may actually improve their immunogenicity. Small peptides that may not be antigenic can be made so by coupling them to larger proteins, such as bovine serum albumin or thyroglobulin. Antibody concentration tends to increase with repeated immunization, reaching a maximum after about three to five immunizations. The presence and characteristics of the antibody are usually tested, using RIA methods [19], after each reimmunization.

Despite the obvious power of RIA for the analysis of peptides, there are many potential pitfalls and sources of artifacts that may confront the naive user. It must be remembered that, even in the best of cases, the unique value of RIA is its extraordinary sensitivity and simplicity. Its specificity, however, is based on immunological reactions with antigenic determinants that may be shared by diverse molecules (e.g., prohormones versus peptide hormones). Hence, in a strict sense, peptides cannot be shown to exist in a tissue by means of immunological procedures. What is measured is specific peptide-like immunoreactivity, and definitive proof of a specific peptide's presence in the tissue still requires a biochemical approach.

The principle of immunocytochemistry is to detect the antigen in tissue by light and electron microscopy using a labeled antibody

The various markers for antibodies include covalently bound fluorescent molecules, ferritin, enzymes (peroxidase), and radioactive substances. The recent uses of enzymatic [5] and radioactive markers in antigen-antibody complexes have greatly enhanced the sensitivity of this method and have reduced some of the problems inherent in covalent labeling of the antibodies. Although immunocytochemical techniques are extremely useful and provide a unique approach to the cellular localization of peptides, proof of specificity of the immunoreaction is very difficult to obtain. It is generally agreed that the specificity manifested by antiserum in an RIA does not guarantee specificity in an immunocytochemical procedure that uses the same antiserum, partly because of the much higher antisera dilutions used in RIA [14]. One approach used to deal with this problem is to purify the antibodies by means of affinity chromatography, that is, to produce so-called monospecific antibodies. In this approach, purified antigen is covalently coupled to Sepharose beads. Specific antibody will attach to the beads and after removing nonspecific antibodies by washing, the specific antibodies can be selectively eluted and used. Another approach is to adsorb out the specific antibody in the immunocytochemical procedure by the addition of excess antigen as a control for nonspecific labeling [20]. In any case, evidence for the detection of a "specific" peptide by immunocytochemistry is usually regarded as less compelling than evidence obtained by RIA methods. As with RIA, the peptide visualized immunocytochemically is referred to as "specific-peptide-like immunoreactivity."

PEPTIDE DISTRIBUTION IN THE NERVOUS SYSTEM

One reason for studying the distribution of peptides in the central nervous system is to determine whether they are present in neurons

The peptide's presence in neurons must be shown first if it is to be considered a neurotransmitter candidate. By examining the neuroanatomy of peptidergic systems, one does much more than satisfy this criterion, however. If one function of a peptide is known, its distribution can hint at the role of brain areas where it is found. For example, the presence of LHRH in the septum and preoptic areas suggested (but certainly did not guarantee) that these regions might be involved somehow in reproduction. Indeed, these regions may provide the anatomical substrate for LHRH-induced lordotic behavior (see Chap. 47).

If the central role of a peptide is a mystery, as was the case with substance P, looking at its distribution may provide clues about its actions. The presence of large amounts of substance P in the dorsal part of the spinal cord hinted that it might mediate pain sensation. In addition to providing a starting point for physiological and behavioral studies, neuroanatomical studies are necessary as first steps for biochemical and cell biological investigations. Conversely, the demonstration that specific cells in which a peptide has been visualized are capable of manufacturing the peptide provides a final vindication of the anatomical data.

Many peptides have unique distributions reflecting the location of neuronal perikarya that produce them and the processes that store and release them

Peptides that are produced as parts of the same precursor typically have very similar distributions, but need not be identically distributed; variations in post-translational processing of a precursor in the different cells that make it can give rise to variations in the products formed.

Axons and nerve endings are especially rich in peptides

The cell bodies seem to manufacture peptide precursors and send them down the axons rather rapidly, so that peptide levels in perikarya are normally not very high. For this reason, peptidergic cell bodies have proven difficult to visualize immunocytochemically. Agents such as colchicine that block axonal transport have been used by immunohistochemists to promote the build-up of peptides in cell bodies. After colchicine treatment, peptide-containing perikarya that are impossible to see otherwise can sometimes be visualized.

Anatomists interested in neuropeptides have introduced a nonimmunological technique, in situ *hybridization histochemistry*

This method is based on the ability of radiolabeled DNA that is complementary to a specific mRNA to bind to specific mRNA in tissue sections. The technique is relatively sensitive and because mRNA is confined mainly to the cell body, it is useful for mapping peptidergic perikarya. In addition, it can be used to detect changes in mRNA levels that follow pharmacological, physiological, or surgical manipulations (see Siegel [21] and Fig. 3).

There is nothing about the anatomy of central peptidergic neurons that distinguishes them from other classes of neurons: some are large,

some small; some are local-circuit neurons, others project to distant regions. Consequently, in the absence of immunological staining techniques, peptide-producing neurons cannot be separated from their nonpeptide-producing neighbors. In fact, it has been shown that peptides can coexist with one another or with nonpeptide transmitters in many neurons [22]. Whether these neurons can release different transmitters at different times or under different circumstances is unknown, but not unlikely (see Chap. 8).

Many peptides have been found in unexpected places

Pituitary tropic hormones, such as prolactin and growth hormone, have been shown to be present in the brain and seem to be there in specific populations of neurons. Insulin has also been detected in brain extracts. Hormones present in the blood or in structures that are in close proximity to the brain, such as the pituitary or pineal gland, may not be made by central neurons; they may be taken up and stored by them. Alternatively, part of the hormone in the brain may be made endogenously, and part may be provided by an outside source.

In addition to demonstrating that numerous gut and pituitary hormones are widely distributed in the central nervous system, workers in this field have shown that hypothalamic hormones are not as narrowly distributed as they were at first thought to be. Somatostatin, for example, is found both inside the hypothalamus and outside it. In fact, only about one-quarter of the somatostatin in the brain is in the hypothalamus. Therefore, it has been suggested that somatostatin may act as a neurotransmitter at sites other than the median eminence. Similarly, based on their widespread distributions, it has been said that TRH and CRH may be central neurotransmitters. (For specific information on neuroanatomical studies of peptidergic pathways, the reader should consult detailed reviews of this topic, e.g., Björklund and Hökfelt [8].)

BIOSYNTHESIS OF NEUROPEPTIDES

Much of our understanding of peptide biosynthesis comes from studies on tissues other than brain

To date, the mechanisms for the biosynthesis of neuronal peptides appear to be similar to those mechanisms found in other eukaryotic tissues. Two major alternatives exist: (a) the synthesis of oligopeptides by enzymatic mechanisms, that is, synthetases; and (b) synthesis by conventional ribosomal protein synthesis mechanisms, usually as a prohormone that is degraded by limited proteolysis to specific peptide products in the cell before release. Mechanism (a) is used for small peptides, such as carnosine (β-alanyl-L-histidine) and glutathione (γ-L-glutamyl-L-cysteinylglycine), which are found in various eukaryotic tissues (including brain) and are synthesized by such enzymes as carnosine synthetase and γ-glutamyl-L-cysteine (plus tripeptide) synthetase, respectively. Larger peptides, such as insulin, nerve growth factor, ACTH, endorphin, vasopressin, and oxytocin, appear to be synthesized as prohormones.

If protein synthesis inhibitors block peptide synthesis, there is presumptive evidence for the prohormone mode of synthesis

If protein synthesis inhibitors like cycloheximide or puromycin do not block the synthesis of a peptide, a search for a specific enzymatic mechanism is in order. Another approach is to employ RIAs for the peptide to see whether on biochemical separation (e.g., gel filtration), higher molecular weight, heterogeneous immunoreactive forms of the peptide can be detected. This also represents presumptive evidence, but not proof, of a prohormone (''big''

forms of insulin, ACTH, growth hormone, calcitonin, and other peptides have been detected by this method).

Biosynthesis of a peptide from a prohormone can be studied by means of pulse-chase labeling

A tissue known to contain substantial quantities of the peptide of interest is exposed to radioactive amino acids for a short time (pulse). Immediately after this pulse, a larger form of the peptide should be detected. The tissue, having been pulsed in this manner, is then exposed to a large excess of nonradioactive amino acids to dilute out the radioactive ones (chase) or, alternatively, to protein synthesis inhibitors to block further *de novo* protein synthesis, and is incubated for various periods. The minimum requirement in these experiments is to show that radioactivity associated with the higher molecular weight precursor (or prohormone) decreases with time after the chase or addition of inhibitor. Concurrently, there is an increase in the radioactivity of the peptide product. To demonstrate this, it is necessary in many cases (particularly with heterogeneous tissue such as brain) to use an antibody to the peptide that also reacts with the precursor in a quantitative immunoprecipitation procedure to resolve the relevant labeled molecules. Labeled presumptive precursors can be purified from the immunoprecipitates and evaluated for the presence of the peptide sequence by limited proteolysis mapping *in vitro* and by analysis of amino acid sequences.

The use of cell-free protein-synthesizing systems (e.g., wheat germ and reticulocyte in vitro *systems) and polyribosomes from the tissue of interest can lead to the synthesis of the prohormone*

This approach has the advantage of also identifying the preprohormone, that is, the prohormone with a characteristic peptide still attached to its N-terminal that is used as a signal to direct the prohormone into the cisternae of the endoplasmic reticulum.

Isolation of DNA complementary to mRNAs that encode peptide precursors is used to characterize propeptides

The various methods described above have in large measure been superceded by paradigms involving the use of recombinant DNA. The sequences of almost all of the neuropeptide precursors are now known [7,9,22].

The cDNAs that encode precursors can be put to many uses:

1. They can be used to probe genomic libraries for their respective genes. Regulatory domains of these genes can be studied.
2. cDNA probes can be used for Northern blotting to measure mRNA levels.
3. cRNA and cDNA probes can be generated for *in situ* hybridization histochemistry.
4. cDNAs can be expressed, intact or mutated, to examine intracellular sorting or to make substrates for studies of processing enzymes.

Development of the prohormone concept began with proinsulin

The discovery in 1967 by Steiner and Dyer [23] that insulin is synthesized in a large precursor form as proinsulin provided the impetus for further studies, which have shown that this is a common mode of biosynthesis of eukaryotic peptides destined for secretion. The studies on proinsulin offer a useful intellectual and experimental paradigm. Proinsulin is a single polypeptide chain ordered as follows: NH_2-(B-chain)-Arg-Arg-(C-peptide)-Lys-Arg-(A-chain)-COOH. The presumed function of the C peptide is to ensure the correct folding and sulfhydryl oxidation between the A and B chains in proinsulin.

The higher rate (15 times) of mutation in the C peptide compared to the insulin moiety suggests that the C peptide may not have a physiological function; however, immunoassay of C peptide may be a useful differential diagnostic procedure for hypoglycemia.

The transformation of proinsulin to insulin in the β cells begins in the Golgi apparatus, where new secretory granules are formed, and continues in the granules thereafter. The half-time of conversion is about 1 hr. Two major processing enzymes have been identified in the granules: a trypsin-like endopeptidase and a carboxypeptidase B-like exopeptidase. The insulin is maintained in the granule in a crystalline form (in combination with zinc). This system leads to several important generalizations: (a) peptide hormones can be synthesized in larger precursor forms (i.e., as prohormones); (b) post-translational processing of the prohormone occurs in the secretory granule; and (c) peptides other than the known biologically active one(s) will emerge from this biosynthetic mechanism, and, if processing occurs intragranularly, all will be released simultaneously by the cell.

The intracellular compartmentation [24] following synthesis of the protein on the rough endoplasmic reticulum (RER) is determined, in part, by the translocational process itself. The initial N-terminal amino acid sequence of the protein serves as a signal for the protein to traverse the RER membrane and enter the cisternae, where the signal sequence is immediately cleaved off. Similar signal sequences exist for secreted proteins and intrinsic membrane proteins (Chap. 21). The prohormone, plus its transient N-terminal sequence, which usually contains 20 to 30 amino acids, is referred to as a preprohormone.

Peptide biosynthesis in neurons also involves propeptide precursors

The first hypothesis for the existence of a prohormone derived from studies on the nervous system. In 1964, Sacks and Takabatake hypothesized that vasopressin, a nonapeptide, and neurophysin, a protein of about 10,000 M_r, were formed by post-translational processing of a common precursor protein. Two precursors of neurophysin ($\sim$ 20,000 M_r each), one associated with vasopressin synthesis and the other with oxytocin synthesis, were identified in pulse-chase and immunoprecipitation experiments on the rat hypothalamoneurohypophysial system [25], and, subsequently, DNAs complementary to the RNAs that encode the precursors were isolated [26].

Neuropeptide precursors appear to be processed in much the same way as insulin. Sulfhydryl oxidation and proximal glycosylation take place in the RER cisternum. In the Golgi apparatus, they are further glycosylated and sorted into secretory granules. In the granule, the precursors come in contact with a variety of peptidases and with enzymes that add functional groups to specific amino acids.

A general peptide precursor is depicted in Fig. 5. This propeptide has already had its signal sequence removed. It has two pairs of basic residues: lysine (K) and arginine (R). The first step in processing such a protein is cleavage at the paired basic amino acids by an endopeptidase. The cleavage can occur between the two amino acids or on the C-terminal side of the pair (arrows). In the former case, basic residues are left attached to both the N-terminal and the C-terminal of the peptide P. Trimming enzymes are required to remove these appendages—a basic-residue-specific aminopeptidase and a basic-residue-specific carboxypeptidase, referred to as carboxypeptidase H.

Note that the precursor in Fig. 5 has a single arginine (R) residue. Some precursors (e.g., that of vasopressin) are cleaved at single basic residues. The enzyme(s) responsible for this are thought to be different from the paired-base-specific endopeptidase.

The glycine (G) just N-terminal to the second KR pair in the precursor is required for peptide P to be amidated. The amidating enzyme requires molecular oxygen, ascorbic acid, and Ca^{2+}. The glycine will donate its amino group to the amino acid that precedes it.

A number of other enzymes may act to modify peptides. α-MSH and β-endorphin both undergo N-acetylation; cholecystokinin and gastrin are tyrosine sulfated. In theory, peptides can also be carboxymethylated or phosphorylated.

Since precursor processing appears to take place in the secretory granules during axonal transport, one would expect that all of the products generated from a precursor protein would be released during stimulus-induced exocytosis. A hypothetical model of the peptidergic neuron is illustrated in Fig. 6.

SECRETION OF NEUROPEPTIDES

The neuropeptide secretion mechanism appears to be similar to that of conventional neurotransmitter secretion [27]. The principal events in the release of neuropeptides occur as follows: The propagated action potential depolarizes the nerve terminal and induces an influx of Ca^{2+}, which produces exocytosis and extrusion of secretory granule (or vesicle) contents into the extracellular space. The dependence of the stimulus-secretion coupling on extracellular Ca^{2+} is

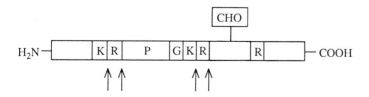

FIG. 5. A general peptide precursor.

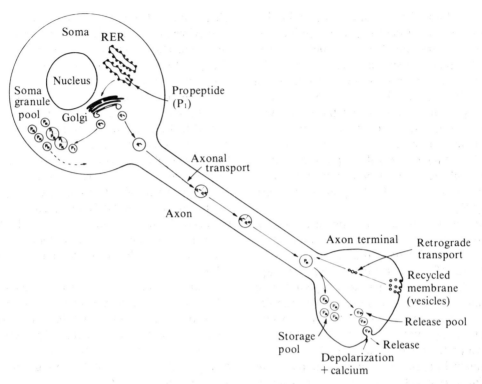

FIG. 6. Hypothetical model of biosynthesis, translocation, processing, and release of peptides in a peptidergic neuron: (RER) rough endoplasmic reticulum; (P_1) propeptide or precursor molecule; ($P_1 \cdots P_n$) intermediates between P_1 and P_n; (P_n) final peptide product of processing. (From Gainer, H., Sarne, Y., and Brownstein, M. J., *J. Cell Biol.* 73:366–381, 1977.)

well established [28], and various morphological features of the exocytotic process have been visualized in freeze-fracture studies. Retrieval of the granule membranes after exocytosis is in large vacuoles [29], but in contrast to cholinergic terminals, where recycling of vesicle membrane occurs (Chap. 10), little is known at present about the fates of the retrieved peptidergic granule membranes.

Peptide secretion from nerve terminals depends on Ca²⁺ entry during depolarization

This feature of the basic mechanism has been used as a criterion for the physiological rele-

vance of stimulation-induced release of peptides from a variety of experimental preparations. The release experiments are usually performed on either thin tissue slices, or blocks, or on synaptosomes, isolated nerve endings, prepared from a specific brain area incubated in a well-oxygenated physiological medium. After an initial washing of the tissue by repeated changes of medium, a stimulus is applied. The stimulus may be field electrical stimulation, depolarization by an excess of K^+, or the addition of veratridine (Na^+ channel activation) to the medium. In all cases, removal of Ca^{2+} from the medium should prevent secretion of the peptides. In some cases, the membrane depolarization step is bypassed by direct application of a Ca^{2+} ionophore (e.g., A23187), which causes an increase in intracellular Ca^{2+} and thus induces exocytosis. In some cases, release experiments can be done in the intact animal either by using push-pull cannulas in specific brain regions [30] or by monitoring the cerebrospinal fluid for peptide release after specific brain areas have been stimulated.

Peptidergic neurosecretory cells tend to fire in bursts, each burst followed by inactivity

This temporal pattern of release *in vivo*, although poorly understood, is significant; it suggests that periodicity is important for sustained secretory activity in these cells. Periodicity may also be important to the target organ; this has been elegantly demonstrated in a study in which monkeys with hypothalamic lesions that abolish LH and FSH release by the pituitary were infused with GnRH. Constant infusion of GnRH failed to restore LH and FSH secretion, whereas once-hourly infusion of GnRH reestablished normal hormone release. Thus, the cyclic pattern of GnRH delivery to the target organ was more important than the amount delivered. The intermittent delivery may avoid down-regulation or desensitization of the GnRH receptors in the target tissue.

INACTIVATION MECHANISMS

The time course and extent of neurotransmitter action are determined, in part, by the mechanisms involved in the reduction of the neurotransmitter concentration around the receptor. This can occur either by diffusion of the substance away from the receptor; by reuptake by the presynaptic terminals or surrounding glia, or both; or by enzymatic degradation of the substance (see Chap. 8). So far there have been no convincing data to indicate that reuptake of neuropeptides takes place, and enzymatic degra-

dation appears to be the principal mechanism for inactivation of neuropeptides.

In general, proteolytic enzymes are described as either exopeptidases or endopeptidases (proteinases). Exopeptidases hydrolyze peptides from either their C- or N-terminal regions by removal of single amino acids (or dipeptides). Endopeptidases cleave internal bonds of proteins and peptides. They often show specificity with regard to the nature of the peptide bond [for example, trypsin hydrolyzes exclusively at basic amino acid (lysine and arginine) residues] but rarely are specific to only one substrate. The probable reason is that the specificity of limited proteolysis is determined by the three-dimensional structure (conformation) of the peptide substrate and of the protease [31]. The substrate region containing the susceptible peptide bond must match the active site of the enzyme for hydrolysis to occur. Thus, proteases may degrade diverse substrates with conformational homologies.

Keeping the above caveats about protease specificity in mind, it is worth noting that enzymes that show selective degradation of biologically active peptides have been found in various tissues, including brain. Many neuropeptides have groups blocked by N-terminal acetylation, C-terminal amidation, or by addition of N-terminal pyroglutamate. These prevent the action of exopeptidases. Therefore, relatively specific endopeptidases are involved in their degradation.

PEPTIDE RECEPTORS

Biological effects are correlated with binding measurements

A great deal can be learned about the affinity and specificity of a biological receptor for its natural ligand by means of dose-response measurements either in the whole animal or in isolated organs *in vitro*. Alternatively, binding of radiolabeled agonists or antagonists to whole cells, suspension of plasma membranes, or solubilized membrane components can be studied. The latter is fast, relatively simple to perform, and serves as a first step in receptor purification. It must be undertaken cautiously, however, because not all binding is to biologically relevant sites (i.e., receptors). Several criteria must be satisfied to establish that the interaction of a ligand with any given preparation represents binding to a receptor (Table 4) (see also Chap. 9 for detailed discussions of receptor quantification).

Whenever possible, quantitative comparisons between binding and biological effects should be made. The activation of a ligand-dependent, membrane-localized enzyme, such as adenylate cyclase or phosphatidylethanolamine *N*-methyltransferase, might be measured at the same time that binding is determined. Similar sets of parallel measurements can sometimes be made on isolated membrane preparations, but there is no guarantee that ligand-induced modulation of enzyme activity will be the same in the intact cell as it is in an isolated membrane.

Intact homogeneous populations of cells

TABLE 4.   Characteristics of ligand-receptor interactions

BIOLOGICAL ACTIVITY
The labeled ligand should have the same biological potency as its unlabeled parent compound

HIGH AFFINITY
Concentrations of ligand as low as those that are biologically effective should specifically bind to receptors

REVERSIBILITY
Agonists with rapidly reversible biological actions should dissociate rapidly from their binding sites

STRUCTURAL OR STERIC SPECIFICITY
Binding of a labeled ligand and displacement of this ligand by other agonists or antagonists should quantitatively reflect the biological potencies of the agonists and antagonists treated

SATURABILITY
A biologically relevant concentration of ligand should saturate specific binding sites

cannot easily be obtained from the brain for direct comparisons of binding and biological activity. Nevertheless, it is possible to compare binding of a variety of agonists and antagonists and, in this way, to determine the structural specificity of binding sites in the central nervous system. Thus, most of the criteria listed in Table 4 can be met. To the extent that cells or membranes harvested from the central nervous system are heterogeneous, though, little can be learned by comparing the properties of receptors of various brain regions. Meaningful comparisons of this sort can be made only by isolating purified populations of plasma membranes from cells and measuring the number of receptors per milligram of membrane (see Chap. 9).

Biologically active peptides can be labeled and used in binding studies

Common problems encountered in studies of peptide receptors have included (a) difficulties in labeling the peptide; iodinated peptides may be inactive; tritiation may prove difficult or may yield a product with too low a specific activity; and (b) enzymatic degradation of the labeled peptide.

Insulin, for example, can be iodinated without losing its biological activity, and its degradation by peptidases in membrane preparations can be inhibited by bacitracin [32]. Although the density of insulin receptors on cells is low, specific binding of insulin to cells and membranes can be detected by using radioiodinated insulin (1,000 Ci/mmol). It would be difficult, if not impossible, to study insulin binding by using a tritiated ligand; but tritiated ligands have been used successfully to study other classes of receptors, among them the receptors for the opioid peptides (Chap. 13). The latter are unique in that they can be occupied by members of a large group of well-characterized nonpeptide agonists and antagonists. Labeled antagonists with high affinities for the opiate receptor and with conveniently long receptor-antagonist half-lives have been used in lieu of the peptides to study binding sites in the brain and elsewhere.

Agonists and antagonists have been synthesized that are resistant to peptidase action. These should prove to be useful ligands for binding studies of the receptors and receptor purification by affinity chromatography.

PEPTIDES AND NEURONAL FUNCTION

Hypothalamic peptides are physiologically important messages in the regulation of the anterior pituitary by brain, but the situation for the rest of the brain is less clear. Extensive pharmacological evidence suggests that there are a variety of peptide receptors in extrahypothalamic areas. In addition, exposure of the nervous system to specific peptides often produces profound changes in the biochemistry and physiology of the nervous system as well as specific modifications of behavior (Table 5). Immunocytochemical procedures can demonstrate that neurons containing biologically active peptides are distributed throughout the brain. Nevertheless, it is still not possible to state whether peptides play a unique role in neuronal function.

Can neuropeptides act as neurotransmitters?

The work on invertebrate peptides proves that they can. Although the criteria for the identification of a neurotransmitter are well established (Chap. 8), it is often difficult to satisfy them in any specific case. Thus, although substance P fulfilled many of the desiderata of a candidate for primary afferent transmitter [5], its time course of action was too slow in comparison to natural afferent activity, and hence, its candidacy as the primary afferent transmitter was not credible. However, substance P might be associated specifically with slow-conducting

TABLE 5. Potential sites and mechanisms of neuropeptide action

Acts as a conventional neurotransmitter in a synaptic pathway
Influences a synaptic pathway by its presynaptic action
  Affects amount and time course of transmitter release
  Affects transmitter reuptake at synapse
  Alters "releasable" and "nonreleasable" transmitter pools
  Affects transmitter biosynthesis
Influences a synaptic pathway by its postsynaptic action on receptor
  Alters receptor sensitivity
  Affects receptor-ionophore coupling
    Kinetics
    Specific ionic conductances
Influences a synaptic pathway by its effects on electrogenesis
  Change in electrically excitable membrane properties
    Resting conductance
    Spike threshold
    Intracellular electrical resistance (length constant)
    Current-voltage relations of membrane
    Coupling resistance at electrotonic junctions
    Alters electrogenic pump activity
  Excitation-coupled phenomena
    Muscle contraction
    Metabolic processes

fibers in pain pathways [33]. The point is that unless the neuronal circuit in which the peptide may be involved is understood and amenable to experimental analysis, it is extremely difficult to evaluate the status of any putative transmitter. Because of this difficulty, and because the morphology of peptidergic synapses is poorly understood, the term *neuromodulatory* is often ascribed to a peptide's action. It should be apparent that the criteria for identification of *neuromodulators* are identical to those of neurotransmitters and that the use of this term does not obviate the necessity for rigorous analysis of the mechanisms of action of the substance in question.

Neurochemists are as excited about neuropeptides as they were about monoamines in the early 1960s. This is in part because the peptides are so potent biologically and in part because they are present in discrete systems of neurons. Undoubtedly many peptides remain to be discovered and characterized. In fact, the number of peptides two to ten amino acids long that might theoretically exist is astronomical ($>10^{13}$). There are 10^{10} neurons in the human brain, so it is possible, although unlikely, that each neuron makes its own unique peptide.

REFERENCES

1. Scharrer, B. Peptidergic neurons: Facts and trends. *Gen. Comp. Endocrinol.* 34:50–62, 1978.
2. Fink, G. The development of the releasing factor concept. *Clin. Endocrinol.* 5(Suppl.):245s–260s, 1976.
3. Guillemin, R. Peptides in the brain: The new endocrinology of the neuron. *Science* 202:390–402, 1978.
4. von Euler, U. S., and Gaddum, J. H. An unidentified depressor substance in certain tissue extracts. *J. Physiol.* (*Lond.*) 72:74–87, 1931.
5. Leeman, S., and Mroz, E. A. Substance P. *Life Sci.* 15:2033–2044, 1974.
6. Frontali, N., and Gainer, H. Peptides in invertebrate nervous systems. In H. Gainer (ed.), *Peptides in Neurobiology.* New York: Plenum, 1977, pp. 259–294.
7. Martin, J. B., Brownstein, M. J., and Krieger, D. T. (eds.), *Brain Peptides Update.* New York: Wiley, 1987.
8. Björklund, A., and Hökfelt, T. (eds.), *Handbook of Chemical Neuroanatomy.* New York: Elsevier, 1985, Vol. 4.
9. Iverson, L. L., Iverson, S. D., and Snyder, S. H. (eds.), *Handbook of Psychopharmacology. Neuropeptides.* New York: Plenum, 1983, Vol. 16.
10. Martin, J. B., and Barchas, J. D. (eds.), *Neuropeptides in Neurologic and Psychiatric Disease.* New York: Raven Press, 1986.
11. Mains, R. E., Eipper, B. A., and Ling, N. Common precursor to corticotropins and endorphins. *Proc. Natl. Acad. Sci. U.S.A.* 74:3014–3018, 1977.
12. Green, J. D., and Harris, G. W. The neurovascular link between the neurohypophysis and adenohypophysis. *J. Endocrinol.* 5:136–146, 1947.
13. Lightman, S. L., and Everitt, B. J. (eds.), *Neuroendocrinology.* Boston: Blackwell, 1986.
14. Leeman, S. E., Mroz, E. A., and Carraway, R. Substance P and neurotensin. In H. Gainer (ed.), *Peptides in Neurobiology.* New York: Plenum, 1977, pp. 99–144.
15. Marshak, D. R., and Fraser, B. A. Structural analysis of brain peptides. In J. B. Martin, M. J. Brownstein, and D. T. Krieger (eds.), *Brain Peptides Update.* New York: Wiley, 1987, pp. 9–36.
16. Tatemoto, K., and Mutt, V. Isolation of two novel candidate hormones using a chemical method for finding naturally occurring polypeptides. *Nature* 285:417–418, 1980.
17. Koller, K. J., and Brownstein, M. J. Use of a cDNA clone to identify a supposed precursor protein containing valocin. *Nature* 325:542–545, 1987.
18. Rosenfeld, M. G., Mermod, J.-J., Amara, S. G., Swanson, L. W., Sawchenko, P. E., et al. Production of a novel neuropeptide encoded by the calcitonin gene via tissue-specific RNA processing. *Nature* 304:129–135, 1983.
19. Yalow, R. S. Radioimmunoassay: A probe for the fine structure of biological systems. *Science* 200:1236–1242, 1978.
20. Swaab, D. F., Pool, C. W., and Van Leeuwen, F. W. Can specificity ever be proved in immunocytochemical staining? *J. Histochem. Cytochem.* 25:388–389, 1977.
21. Siegel, R. E. *In situ* hybridization histochemistry. In J. B. Martin, M. J. Brownstein, and D. T. Krieger (eds.), *Brain Peptides Update.* New York: Wiley, 1987, pp. 81–100.
22. Hökfelt, T., Fuxe, K., and Pernow, B. *Coexistence of Neuronal Messengers: A New Principle in Chemical Transmission.* (Progress in Brain Research, Vol. 68.) New York: Elsevier, 1986.
23. Steiner, D. F., and Dyer, P. E. The biosynthesis of insulin and a probable precursor of insulin by a human islet cell adenoma. *Proc. Natl. Acad. Sci. U.S.A.* 57:473–480, 1967.
24. Palade, G. Intracellular aspects of the process of protein synthesis. *Science* 189:347–358, 1975.
25. Russell, J. T., Brownstein, M. J., and Gainer, H. Biosynthesis of vasopressin, oxytocin, and neurophysins: Isolation and characterization of two common precursors (propressophysin and prooxyphysin). *Endocrinology* 107:1880–1891, 1980.

26. Richter, D., and Ivell, R. Gene organization, biosynthesis, and chemistry of neurohypophysial hormones. In H. Imura (ed.), *The Pituitary Gland. Comprehensive Endocrinology.* New York: Raven Press, 1985, pp. 127–148.

27. Douglas, W. W. How do neurones secrete peptides? Exocytosis and its consequences, including "synaptic" vesicle formation, in the hypothalamo-neurohypophysial system. *Prog. Brain Res.* 39:21–39, 1973.

28. Thorn, N. A., Russell, J. T., Torp-Pedersen, C., and Treiman, M. Calcium and neurosecretion. *Ann. N.Y. Acad. Sci.* 307:618–639, 1978.

29. Nordman, J. J., and Morris, J. F. Membrane retrieval at neurosecretory axon endings. *Nature* 261:723–725, 1976.

30. Gaddum, J. H. Push-pull cannulae. *J. Physiol. (Lond)* 155:1–2, 1961.

31. Neurath, H., and Walsh, K. A. Role of proteolytic enzymes in biological regulation (a review). *Proc. Natl. Acad. Sci. U.S.A.* 73:3825–3832, 1976.

32. Cuatrecasas, P. Insulin receptor of liver and fat cell membranes. *Fed. Proc.* 32:1838–1846, 1973.

33. Collu, R., et al. (eds.), *Central Nervous System Effects of Hypothalamic Hormones and Other Peptides.* New York: Raven Press, 1979.

34. Koller, K. J., Wolff, R. S., Warden, M. K., and Zoeller, R. T. Thyroid hormones regulate levels of thyrotropin-releasing-hormone mRNA in the paraventricular nucleus. *Proc. Natl. Acad. Sci. U.S.A.* 84:7329–7333, 1987.

CHAPTER 15

Amino Acid Neurotransmitters

P. L. McGeer and E. G. McGeer

Basic Neurochemistry: Molecular, Cellular, and Medical Aspects, 4th Ed., edited by G. J. Siegel et al. Raven Press, Ltd., New York, 1989.
Correspondence to P. L. McGeer and E. G. McGeer, Kinsmen Laboratory of Neurological Research, Department of Psychiatry, University
of British Columbia, Vancouver, British Columbia, Canada V6T 1W5.

There are several amino acids for which neurotransmitter roles have either been proven or considered possible. Physiological and anatomical evidence suggest that amino acid transmitters carry the major "yes/no" (excitatory/inhibitory) commands in the central nervous system (CNS) and that other types of CNS transmitters play more diffuse modulatory roles. Of the aliphatic amino acids with 2 to 6 carbons, those with one acidic and one amine function are inhibitory, and those with two acidic functions and only one α-amino group are excitatory. γ-Aminobutyric acid and glycine are the principal inhibitory transmitters, whereas glutamate and, to a lesser extent, aspartate are presumed to be the excitatory transmitters. Most of the neurons in the brain probably use one of these amino acids as a transmitter. They are described as ionotropic because they usually interact with receptors to open ionic channels. Most evidence suggests that taurine, proline, and serine do not function as transmitters in the CNS. (For detail and further references, the interested reader is referred to McGeer et al. [1].)

γ-AMINOBUTYRIC ACID

γ-Aminobutyric acid (GABA) is one of the most thoroughly documented neurotransmitters. It has been the object of intensive study, and many elegant chemical and physiological techniques have been applied to elucidation of its role.

Roberts and Awapara independently discovered the presence of GABA in brain tissue in 1950. In 1953, Florey discovered in mammalian brain a mysterious "factor I" that inhibited the crayfish stretch-receptor neuron. Bazemore, Elliott, and Florey identified this as GABA the year before Kuffler and Edwards showed that it duplicated transmitter action at certain crayfish cord synapses. Obata and Takeda first showed its release in mammalian systems, demonstrating its presence in the fourth ventricle after stimulation of Purkinje cells.

Fonnum and co-workers then demonstrated that cutting Purkinje cell axons resulted in the disappearance of glutamic acid decarboxylase (GAD), the synthesizing enzyme, from the terminals. Elegant final proof of GABA's role in Purkinje cells was developed by the Roberts team. They purified GAD, developed antibodies against it, and showed by the immunohistochemical method that it was localized to specific neuronal elements [2]. Many GABAergic neurons and pathways have since been established through immunohistochemical studies of GAD and of GABA itself and through histochemical studies of GABA α-oxoglutarate transaminase (GABA-T) (Table 2).

Glucose, the main energy source in brain, is the principal precursor of GABA

Although glucose is probably the main source *in vivo*, pyruvate and several other amino acids can also serve as GABA precursors, since they feed into the GABA shunt (Fig. 1). The shunt is a closed loop that acts to conserve the supply of GABA. The first step is the transamination of α-ketoglutarate, an intermediate in the Krebs cycle, to glutamic acid. Glutamic acid is then decarboxylated by GAD to form GABA. GABA is transaminated by GABA-T to form succinic semialdehyde, but the transamination can only take place if α-ketoglutarate is the acceptor of the amine group. This transforms α-ketoglutarate into the GABA precursor glutamate; thus, a molecule of GABA can be destroyed metabolically only if a molecule of precursor is formed to take its place. The succinic semialdehyde formed from GABA is rapidly oxidized by succinic semialdehyde dehydrogenase (SSADH) to succinic acid, which reenters the Krebs cycle (see Chap. 28). Ancillary to the GABA shunt is a glutamine loop: Released GABA is taken up by glial cells, where a similar transamination by GABA-T can take place. The glutamate formed cannot, however, be converted to GABA in the glia, since they lack

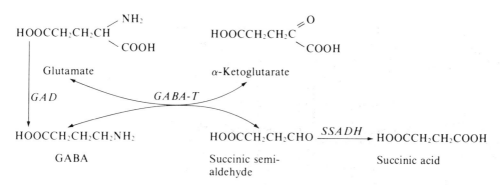

FIG. 1. Reactions of the GABA shunt.

GAD. Instead, it is transformed by glutamine synthetase (Glu Synth) into glutamine, which is returned to the nerve ending. In the nerve ending, the enzyme glutaminase converts glutamine back to glutamate, thus completing the loop and conserving the supply of GABA precursor.

Enzymes of the GABA shunt and glutamine loop are located in neuronal and glial components of the synapse

As shown in Fig. 2, GABA-T and SSADH are attached to mitochondria. Glutaminase, GAD, and Glu Synth are cytoplasmic enzymes, with GAD occurring only in neurons, Glu Synth only in glia, and glutaminase in both. An internal segment of the shunt operates entirely within the nerve ending, but the glutaminase loop comes into play when GABA is released from the nerve ending. The released GABA can be taken back into the nerve ending or picked up by glial cells by high-affinity transport systems; in either location, transamination by mitochondrial GABA-T can take place. The final enzyme in the GABA shunt, SSADH, is closely coupled to GABA-T and is similarly distributed in brain. The high tissue content of substrate required to saturate the enzyme relative to that required for GABA-T saturation probably explains why succinic semialdehyde has never been detected as an endogenous metabolite in neuronal tissue.

That which is formed from GABA is very rapidly converted to succinic acid.

Other routes have been described for GABA in brain. It can be formed from putrescine or from γ-hydroxybutyrate. It may be a precursor of other significant brain metabolites, such as homocarnosine (the dipeptide derivative of GABA and histidine), γ-hydroxybutyrate, γ-aminobutyrylcholine, γ-butyrylbetaine, γ-guanidinobutyric acid, and several others (see also Chap. 38). None of these alternate routes, however, has been established as being of major importance either metabolically or physiologically.

Characteristics of GABA metabolic routes and enzymes

GAD, the key enzyme in the formation of GABA, has been purified. It has a molecular weight of 85,000 and requires pyridoxal phosphate as a cofactor (see Chap. 34). The K_m is 0.7 mM for glutamate and 0.05 mM for pyridoxal phosphate — in each case well below the *in vivo* tissue level. Consequently, the enzyme should normally be fully saturated with its substrate and its cofactor.

The complementary DNA corresponding to GAD messenger RNA (mRNA) has been cloned from brain and pheochromocytoma cell

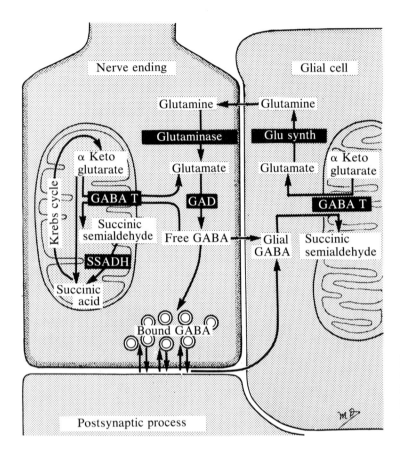

FIG. 2. Schematic diagram showing relationship of GABA nerve ending, a postsynaptic process, and a glial cell: (*black rectangles*) enzymes; (*white rectangles*) endogenous intermediates.

lines. The mRNA is approximately 3.7 kilobases in size.

GABA-T has also been purified to homogeneity, and antibodies to it have been prepared. It has a molecular weight of 109,000 and, like GAD, requires pyridoxal phosphate as cofactor. The K_m for GABA is 1.1 mM. The availability of α-ketoglutarate may play an important role in the destruction of GABA. This is particularly true when respiration ceases: Since the Krebs cycle depends on aerobic metabolism, the level of α-ketoglutarate rapidly declines during anoxia. GABA cannot then be destroyed, although it can still be formed from glutamate because GAD is an anaerobic enzyme. There is therefore a rapid increase in brain GABA levels postmortem, accompanied by a rapid decline in glutamate content.

Physiology and pharmacology of GABA and its receptors

The physiological actions of GABA as an inhibitory neurotransmitter of mammalian synapses can be summarized by considering the following classical evidence obtained for its action in the cerebellar Purkinje cell:

1. Stimulation of Purkinje cells results in hyperpolarization of postsynaptic cells in the deep cerebellar nuclei and Deiters' nucleus. This hyperpolarization becomes a

depolarization when the resting membrane potential of the postsynaptic cell is artificially increased beyond the equilibrium potential for the inhibitory postsynaptic potential (IPSP).

2. The postsynaptic membrane is permeable to chloride and other anions of comparably small size during transmitter action.
3. Picrotoxin and bicuculline, which are classical GABA antagonists, block the effects of stimulation; strychnine, which is not a GABA blocker, is ineffective.
4. Stimulation of Purkinje cells results in the release of detectable amounts of GABA into the perfusion fluid of the fourth ventricle or into the output field of a push-pull cannula inserted into the area of the deep cerebellar nuclei.

The action of GABA at its postsynaptic receptor (GABA$_A$ site) can be described as ionotropic because it results in a brief (~ 1 msec) opening of a Cl$^-$ channel. The influx of Cl$^-$ from the extracellular fluid hyperpolarizes the membrane of the postsynaptic cell, thus inhibiting its ability to fire. However, both physiological and binding studies indicate at least one other action of GABA based on the existence of a second receptor (GABA$_B$). The properties of these two receptors are as follows. GABA$_A$ is sensitive to bicuculline (antagonist), muscimol (agonist), 3-aminopropanesulfonic acid (agonist), and isoguvacine (agonist). It is insensitive to baclofen. Binding to GABA$_B$ sites is insensitive to ions but enhanced by Triton X-100 treatment. GABA$_B$ is insensitive to bicuculline, 3-aminopropanesulfonic acid, and isoguvacine. It is only weakly sensitive to muscimol, but stereospecifically sensitive to baclofen (agonist). Binding to GABA$_B$ sites is inhibited by guanyl nucleotides, dependent on Ca^{2+} or Mg^{2+}, and reduced by Triton X-100 treatment. GABA$_A$ sites are thought to be largely postsynaptic and concentrated on central neurons and

peripheral sympathetic neurons, whereas GABA$_B$ sites are on presynaptic autonomic and central nerve terminals [3].

Activation of GABA$_A$ receptors is responsible for the classic postsynaptic inhibitory action. At the GABA$_B$ receptor, GABA (or baclofen) acts to reduce the outflow of other neurotransmitters, such as norepinephrine, glutamate, dopamine, or serotonin. The GABA$_B$ receptor may work by decreasing the inward flux of Ca^{2+} into the presynaptic nerve terminal.

Much remains to be learned about GABA receptors. Some, but not all, appear to be coupled to modulatory sites. At these modulatory sites, drugs, such as the benzodiazepines and picrotoxinin (the active form of picrotoxin), can act to modify the effect of GABA on the Cl$^-$ channel. The picrotoxinin site is believed to be distinct from the benzodiazepine site (Fig. 3). The benzodiazepines affect GABA binding, whereas picrotoxin does not. Instead, picrotoxinin inhibits the increase in Cl$^-$ flux triggered by the binding of GABA to its receptor. The GABA/benzodiazepine (GABA$_A$) receptor has been purified and consists of two α- and two β-subunits. On sequencing, these two peptides and a peptide from a glycine receptor have shown strong homologies with each other and with the nicotinic receptor. This provides the first strong evidence that membrane proteins mediating transmission of information in the brain probably fall into genetically related families [4].

Endogenous ligands for the benzodiazepine and picrotoxinin sites have not been identified, but several peptides and low-molecular-weight compounds have been suggested: for example, the 104-amino-acid peptide called the diazepam binding inhibitor (DBI), has been proposed as a ligand or ligand precursor for some benzodiazepine sites.

Pharmacological agents exist that are capable of interacting with GABA in all the classic

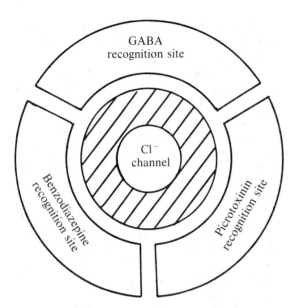

FIG. 3. Theoretical model of the GABA receptor-ionophore complex, including recognition sites for convulsant and anticonvulsant drugs as viewed from outside the postsynaptic membrane looking down the Cl⁻ channel. The complex contains three binding sites: the GABA recognition site, the picrotoxinin recognition site, and the benzodiazepine recognition site. The ion channel may be a separate component or part of one of the ligand binding proteins. The model proposes that GABA function (opening of the Cl⁻ channel) can be modulated by endogenous ligands or drugs that bind to the picrotoxinin or benzodiazepine recognition sites, or both. The effect can be either positive (i.e., enhancement of GABA inhibition) or negative (i.e., reduction of GABA inhibition) at the GABA-Cl⁻ ionophore. (Modified from Olsen and Leeb-Lundberg [17].)

areas for manipulation of neurotransmitter systems. These are the sites of synthesis, storage, extraneuronal release, presynaptic reuptake, postsynaptic destruction, and postsynaptic activation. In particular, many drugs appear to modulate GABA binding to its receptor or the coupling of the GABA receptor to the Cl⁻ channel. It is these modulators that comprise the most clinically effective drugs.

The better known agents affecting GABA action are listed in Table 1. Some interact prominently with other systems, so that their specificity is limited. Although inconsistencies appear in a number of cases between the presumed mechanism of action and their overall physiological effects, drugs that diminish GABA activity generally cause excitation leading to convulsions, whereas those that enhance its activity cause depression, leading to anticonvulsant activity or sedation. Such global effects would be anticipated for a general inhibitory neurotransmitter.

The benzodiazepines, of which diazepam represents the prototype compound, are among the most widely used drugs in clinical practice. They are extremely effective in alleviating anxiety and certain of them are also used as anticonvulsants and muscle relaxants. Considerable evidence now indicates that the benzodiazepines exert many of their effects by action at a site coupled to a postsynaptic GABA receptor in such a way as to increase GABA binding, thus augmenting GABA's physiological action. However, not all benzodiazepine and GABA sites are coupled to each other. Two major types of benzodiazepine receptors are found in brain: Type I is defined as a GABA-independent site at which the benzodiazepines have their anxiolytic effect; type II is defined as a GABA-dependent site at which the benzodiazepines have their anticonvulsive and sedative hypnotic effects (4). Another benzodiazepine binding site found to a limited extent in brain is called a peripheral type because of its greater occurrence in peripheral organs such as kidney. Peripheral-type binding is insensitive to GABA and of unknown function, although it may be related to purine uptake.

There have been suggestions that barbiturates act either at a benzodiazepine site to facilitate GABA binding or at the same site as picrotoxinin. One action of the anticonvulsant valproate (sodium dipropylacetate) is believed to be at the picrotoxinin binding site to facilitate the coupling of the GABA site with the Cl⁻ channel.

TABLE 1. Some drugs that affect GABA action

Drug	Presumed action mechanism	Physiological effect
Receptor site modulators		
Diazepam (benzodiazepines)	Facilitate GABA binding	Anticonvulsants, tranquilizers
Barbiturates	Facilitate GABA binding	Anticonvulsants
Valproate	Facilitates GABA binding	Anticonvulsant
Picrotoxinin	Uncouples GABA site from Cl^-	Convulsant
Synthesis		
Allylglycine	GAD inhibitor	Convulsant
β-N-γ-Glutamyldiamino-propionic acid	GAD inhibitor	Convulsant and neuritic
3-Mercaptopropionic acid	GAD inhibitor	Convulsant
High-pressure oxygen	GAD inhibitor	Convulsant
Isonicotinylhydrazide	B_6 antagonist	Convulsant at high doses
Thiosemicarbazide	B_6 antagonist	Convulsant at high doses
Methionine sulfoximine	Glutamine synthetase inhibitor	Convulsant
Release		
Tetanus toxin	Inhibitor of GABA and glycine release	Convulsant
Pump		
cis-3-Aminocyclohexane-carboxylic acid	GABA neuronal pump inhibitor	—
Nipecotic acid	GABA neuronal pump inhibitor	—
β-Alanine	GABA glial pump inhibitor	—
Destruction		
n-Dipropylacetate	GABA-T inhibitor	Anticonvulsant
Hydrazinopropionic acid	GABA-T inhibitor	Sedative
Gabaculine	GABA-T inhibitor	Anticonvulsant
γ-AcetylenicGABA	GABA-T inhibitor	—
Ethanolamine-O-sulfate	GABA-T inhibitor	—
Antagonist		
Bicuculline	$GABA_A$ antagonist	Convulsant
Agonist		
Muscimol	$GABA_A$ agonist	Psychotomimetic
Progabide	Metabolized to GABA agonist	Anticonvulsant
Baclofen	$GABA_B$ agonist	Muscle relaxant
γ-Hydroxybutyric acid	Possible GABA agonist	Sedative

So far, no way is known for increasing GABA levels in brain by administering either the substance itself or its precursors. Neither glutamate nor GABA crosses the blood-brain-barrier (BBB) with ease except in neonates, and administration of either glutamine or pyridoxal phosphate, both of which do cross the BBB, is ineffective (see Chap. 30). As expected from the K_m data, normal tissue levels of both precursor and cofactor appear to be sufficient to saturate the enzyme.

On the other hand, GABA levels can be lowered by a variety of agents that inhibit GABA synthesis. The so-called carbonyl trapping agents, which act against the cofactor pyridoxal phosphate, form the largest family (see Chap. 34). Classic members are such hydrazides as isoniazid, semicarbazide, and thiosemicarbazide, which will inhibit GAD in the concentration range of 10^{-4} to 10^{-3} M *in vitro* and *in vivo*. Since GABA-T also requires pyridoxal phosphate, these cofactor antagonists may have variable effects on GABA levels, depending on dose and time.

3-Mercaptopropionic acid, at a concentration of 10^{-3} M, inhibits GAD almost totally and markedly inhibits K^+-induced release of GABA. Following administration of this agent to rats, convulsions occur in approximately 7 min. At that time, GABA levels are reduced by about one-third. Allylglycine and high-pressure oxygen, which also inhibit GAD activity and reduce GABA levels, produce the same effect.

The importance of glutamine as a precursor of GABA is suggested by the convulsant activity of methionine sulfoximine, an irreversible inhibitor of glutamine synthetase.

Tetanus toxin, a convulsant protein, acts on the CNS apparently by reducing the synaptic release of the inhibitory neurotransmitters GABA and glycine. In studies *in vitro*, tetanus toxin has been shown to affect GABA release from slices of the hippocampus, substantia nigra, and striatum.

Uptake inhibitors enhance and prolong the inhibitory action of GABA, but the physiological effects of the compounds investigated so far vary according to their actions on other systems.

A GABA pump exists in glia as well as in synaptosomes. The two uptake processes are not identical because they are affected by different inhibitors. β-Alanine and proline, for example, inhibit glial uptake of GABA hundreds of times more powerfully than they do neuronal uptake, whereas *cis*-3-aminocyclohexane-carboxylic acid is a selective neuronal uptake inhibitor.

Levels of GABA in brain can be increased by inhibiting the metabolizing enzyme, GABA-T. In animals, the inhibitors tend to produce sedation; however, many are of limited clinical usefulness because they are relatively nonspecific, highly toxic, or do not cross the BBB. The most useful GABA-T inhibitor developed so far is sodium *n*-dipropylacetate (valproate), which, however, may owe its anticonvulsant activity primarily to an interaction with the GABA receptor-ionophore complex. Valproate may also have some interaction with excitatory amino acid systems. Clinically, this drug has proven to be effective in treating certain forms of epilepsy.

Some other GABA-T inhibitors, such as ethanolamine-*O*-sulfate and gabaculine (5-amino-1,3-cyclohexadienecarboxylic acid), have long-lasting action because they irreversibly destroy the GABA-T present at the time of administration; hence, metabolism is slowed until new enzyme can be synthesized. They have use in a pharmacohistochemical method for GABA-T.

Picrotoxin and bicuculline have been regarded as potent and specific blockers of GABA. Both cause convulsions. As previously mentioned, picrotoxin probably does not act directly at the GABA recognition site but modifies the effect of GABA at that site. Bicuculline, however, appears to block the GABA$_A$ receptor and is thus a true antagonist.

It has been proposed that anticonvulsants might be made by synthesizing "prodrugs" that are capable of crossing the BBB and being metabolized within the brain to GABA-like molecules. The agent of this type that has so far been the most widely studied is Progabide (SL 76002) {4-[2′-hydroxy-4′-fluoro-α-(4-chlorophenyl)-benzenemethanimino]butyramide}, which readily enters the brain following peripheral administration and is metabolized to a GABA agonist.

Muscimol, a psychotomimetic isoxazole isolated from the mushroom *Amanita muscaria*, is a potent agonist at GABA$_A$ receptors. The reason for its seemingly unrelated psychotomimetic pharmacological action is unknown. β-(*p*-Chlorophenyl)GABA, also termed baclofen, has become the drug of choice in treatment of spasticity and is reported effective in some forms of chorea. It is believed to have its clinical effects because it acts on GABA_B receptors. γ-Hydroxybutyric acid (γ-OH) is another GABA-like agent in clinical use in some countries as a basal anesthetic or, at lower doses, as a mild sedative. It readily crosses the BBB, but its mechanism of action is unknown.

Anatomical distribution of GABA pathways in brain

The concentration of GABA in the brain (Table 4) is 200 to 1,000 times greater than that of such neurotransmitters as dopamine, norepinephrine, acetylcholine, and serotonin. GABA is widely distributed, as might be anticipated for

a transmitter believed to serve the inhibitory neurons of almost all areas of brain.

A great deal of information is now available on the distribution of GABA cells and pathways in brain (Table 2), largely as a result of immunohistochemistry for GAD (Fig. 4A), immunohistochemistry for GABA (Fig. 4B), and pharmacohistochemistry of GABA-T (Fig. 4C), supplemented by lesion, axoplasmic flow, and [3H]GABA-uptake studies.

Complete brain mapping has been performed only with the pharmacohistochemical GABA-T method [5]. Although GABA-T is present in glia, pretreating animals with an irreversible inhibitor of GABA-T several hours before sacrifice permits only newly synthesized enzyme to be visualized. The new enzyme ap-

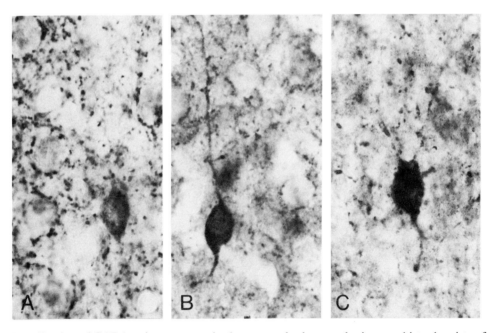

FIG. 4. Localization of GABAergic structures in the rat cerebral cortex by immunohistochemistry for GAD (**A**) and GABA (**B**) and by pharmacohistochemistry for GABA-T (**C**). **A:** GAD immunohistochemical stain is of moderate intensity in a round neuron but of greater intensity in the surrounding punctate nerve endings, some of which are outlining clear neurons. **B:** GABA immunohistochemical stain is of stronger intensity in a cell of similar morphology to that in **A** and also shows prominent staining of fibers. **C:** GABA-T positive cerebral cortical neuron, of morphology similar to the cells in **A** and **B**, stained by the pharmacohistochemical method. (Photomicrographs courtesy of H. Tago and H. Kimura, University of British Columbia, Vancouver, Canada, and Shiga University, Kyoto, Japan.)

TABLE 2. Some proposed neuronal pathways involving GABA

Anatomical system	Evidence[a]
Cortex to substantia nigra	P, L
Corticorubral	P
Hippocampal commissural	P, D
Hippocampus to septal area	D
Diagonal band to medial habenula	L
Diagonal band to olfactory bulb	D
Septum to habenula	L
Septum to interpeduncular nucleus	L
Septal area to hippocampus	L
Amygdala to bed nucleus of the stria terminalis	L
Nucleus accumbens to globus pallidus	P
Nucleus accumbens to substantia innominata (ventral pallidum)	P, L
Nucleus accumbens to entopeduncular nucleus	P
Nucleus accumbens to hypothalamus	L
Nucleus accumbens to substantia nigra	(P), (L)
Nucleus accumbens to A10	P, (L)
Striatopallidal and striatoentopeduncular	P, L
Striatonigral neurons	P, R, (L), A
Pallidosubthalamic	P, (L)
Pallidonigral neurons	R, (L), A, D
Entopeduncular to lateral habenula	P, L, D
Entopedunculothalamic	L
Hypothalamus to cortex	D
Hypothalamus to lateral habenula	D
Hypothalamus to central gray matter	L
Nigrothalamic and nigrotectal	P, R, L, A, D
Nigrotegmental	P, (L), A
Subthalamus to entopeduncular nucleus	P
Zona incerta to superior colliculus and basilar pons	D
Purkinje cells	P, L, A, R
Lateral cerebellum to basilar pons	D

[a] (P) inhibitory action; (R) GABA release; (L) lesion effect; (A) axoplasmic flow; (D) dual labeling; parentheses signify that the literature is controversial. Similar types of evidence have been used to support the existence of GABA interneurons in the cortex, olfactory bulb, olfactory tubercle, hippocampus, septal area, amygdala, nucleus accumbens, neostriatum, thalamus, hypothalamus, inferior colliculus, lateral geniculate, raphe, cerebellum, cochlear nucleus, rostral ventrolateral medulla, spinal cord, ventral pallidum, and retina. Neurons staining for GABA-T by the pharmacohistochemical method have been found in all these and other regions, and many have also been shown to stain immunohistochemically for GAD or GABA. GABA neurons are also found in some peripheral regions, notably the gastrointestinal tract [1].

pears first in neurons presumed to be of the GABA type, since they would be the ones requiring high concentrations of the enzyme. Glial cells regenerate GABA-T much more slowly.

Figure 4 compares staining of presumed GABA cells in rat cortex by the three techniques. They show a highly concordant pattern of staining, providing convincing evidence of the nature and distribution of cerebral cortical GABA cells. The GAD method shows (Fig. 4A) relatively light staining of cells but intense staining of fibers and nerve endings. The GABA method (Fig. 4B) shows staining of both cells and fibers, and the GABA-T method (Fig. 4C) shows more intense staining of cells. The latter result would be anticipated, since, in the pharmacohistochemical technique, newly synthesized GABA-T must reach the fibers and nerve endings by axoplasmic transport. GABA cells are observed in all layers of the cortex; they show round or fusiform morphology. Comparable results are available for many other areas of brain [1].

GABAergic projections are defined by several means: decreases in GAD or GABA after various lesions; axoplasmic flow of radioactive GABA or of a marking agent, such as a lectin or dye; release of GABA on electrical stimulation of the pathway; or physiological demonstration that the tract exerts an inhibitory effect on target cells and that the effect can be blocked by GABA antagonists (Table 2).

GLYCINE

Glycine has the anatomical distribution and physiological effect of an inhibitory neurotransmitter in the spinal cord

Glycine is the simplest of the amino acids in structure and is involved in a multitude of metabolic pathways. As a consequence, it was not seriously considered as a neurotransmitter candidate at the time its inhibitory neurophysiological properties were first noted by Purpura and co-workers and by Curtis and co-workers, who considered it only a weakly active agent. A study of its distribution in spinal cord by Werman et al. [7], however, showed that glycine had the predicted distribution of the postsynaptic inhibitory transmitter. This study was quickly followed by one which showed that, after temporary aortic occlusion, there was a significant loss of glycine and aspartate, but not of GABA or glutamate, in the gray matter of the spinal cord. Moreover, the loss of glycine and aspartate correlated with the amount of interneuronal disruption seen in histological sections.

A rigorous neurophysiological comparison showed that glycine iontophoresed onto motoneurons duplicated the action of the inhibitory transmitter released on stimulation of these spinal interneurons [6].

Further confirmatory chemical evidence came when it was shown that there was a high-affinity uptake system for glycine in slices and homogenates of cat or rat spinal cord and that glycine was preferentially localized to synaptosomes following subcellular fractionation. On the basis of these findings in spinal cord, it can be said that glycine is a proven neurotransmitter.

Glycine participates in many biochemical pathways

In mammals, glycine is a nonessential amino acid that makes up 1 to 5 percent of typical dietary proteins. It is incorporated into peptides, proteins, nucleotides, and nucleic acids, and its fragments participate in other metabolic sequences. Thus, it is one of the more versatile compounds in brain. It can be synthesized from glucose and other substrates. The immediate precursor of glycine is serine. Studies using radioactive precursors suggest that much of the glycine in brain is derived from *de novo* synthesis from glucose through serine (Fig. 5) and not from transport from the blood. The enzyme serine hydroxymethyltransferase (SHMT) is responsible for converting serine to glycine. It requires tetrahydrofolic acid, pyridoxal phos-

phate, and manganese ions and is strongly inhibited by such antipyridoxal compounds as aminooxyacetic acid (see also Chaps. 34 and 38). Unfortunately, the activity of SHMT cannot be used as an index of the presence of glycinergic neurons. The rate of formation from serine appears constant from area to area, and there is no distinct correlation with the presumed presence of glycinergic cell bodies or nerve endings.

The metabolic disposal of glycine is unclear. It has been shown *in vitro* that glycine can be converted to glutathione, guanidinoacetic acid, glyoxylate, or even back to serine through a cleavage mechanism (Fig. 5). Again, however, there is no correspondence between the activity of this cleavage system or other disposal mechanisms and the probable occurrence of glycine neurons.

Sodium-ion-dependent synaptosomal high-affinity uptake of radioactive glycine has been demonstrated in the spinal cord and in certain areas of the brain

This system is easily distinguished from the low-affinity-uptake system; the latter is shared by other small amino acids, is present in all CNS areas, and is presumably concerned with other aspects of glycine metabolism (see Chaps. 28 and 30).

Glycine and strychnine bind to synaptosomal membrane fragments by a high-affinity Na^+-independent system characteristic of specific receptor sites. The parallelism between regional [3H]strychnine binding and glycine uptake and the correlation between the neurophysiological actions of glycine-like amino acids and their ability to inhibit [3H]strychnine binding have been taken to mean that such binding involves synaptic receptor sites for glycine. Action of glycine at a second, strychnine-insensitive glycine receptor has been reported to modulate some excitatory amino acid recep-

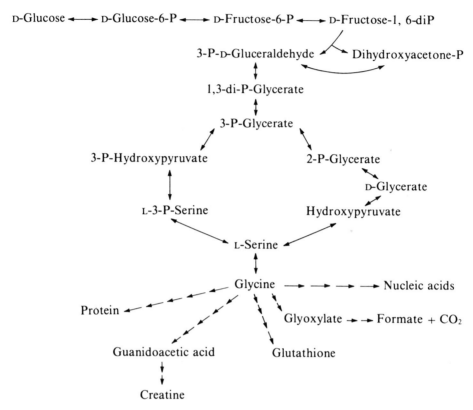

FIG. 5.   Probable synthetic pathway and possible metabolic routes for glycine in nervous tissue.

tors. Cloning and sequencing of the cDNAs of the strychnine-binding subunit of the rat brain glycine receptor indicates a significant structural homology with components of the nicotinic receptor and the GABA$_A$ receptor complex [7].

Much remains to be discovered about the chemical reactions important for glycine synthesis and disposal, the control of glycine levels, and the chemistry of the glycinergic receptor.

Physiology and pharmacology of glycine and its receptor

Glycine fulfills the physiological criteria expected of the transmitter released by inhibitory interneurons in the spinal cord. Its iontophoretic action hyperpolarizes the membrane, brings about a large fall in membrane resistance, and increases Cl^- permeability, all of which duplicates the effects of synaptic activation. Although these actions are also produced by GABA, those of glycine are blocked by strychnine and those of GABA by bicuculline. The action of spinal inhibitory interneurons is prevented by strychnine but not by bicuculline, confirming that glycine is the true transmitter.

There are several other substances besides strychnine that block the action of glycine but not of GABA on spinal neurons. Examples are brucine, thebaine, 4-phenyl-4-formyl-*N*-methylpiperidine, and *N,N*-dimethylmuscimol.

TABLE 3. Some suggested pathways using glycine[a]

Spinal cord interneurons
Spinal afferents from the raphe and reticular formation
Cortical projection to the hypothalamus
Brain stem afferents to the substantia nigra
Cerebellar Golgi cells
Glossopharyngeal nerve
Retinal amacrine cells
Ventral cochlear nucleus to contralateral cochlear nucleus

[a] In most cases, the only evidence is physiological [1], although the last has been suggested by retrograde transport combined with immunohistochemistry for glycine.

Anatomical distribution of glycine

As a dietary amino acid, glycine is found in all tissues. The discovery of unusually high levels in the spinal cord was fundamental in indicating a neurotransmitter role. Similarly, high glycine levels and specific uptake in particular regions of the retina suggest a neurotransmitter function in some retinal interplexiform and amacrine cells. The demonstration in retina of K^+-stimulated, Ca^{2+}-dependent release of glycine and of lesion-induced decreases in synaptosomal glycine uptake provides supporting evidence. Immunohistochemical studies using antibodies to a glycine conjugate have indicated glycine-positive neurons in the retina, cerebellum, brain stem, and spinal cord. Regional distribution data suggest the presence of glycine nerve endings in the pons, medulla, midbrain, and, possibly, diencephalon. Evidence has been accumulated for a few glycine pathways and neuronal groups, as indicated in Table 3.

GLUTAMATE AND ASPARTATE

Glutamate and aspartate meet many of the criteria for neurotransmitter status

Glutamate and aspartate are present in appropriate concentrations in brain and are released in a Ca^{2+}-dependent fashion on electrical stimulation *in vitro*. Both have powerful excitatory effects on neurons when iontophoresed *in vivo*. They have high-affinity uptake systems in nerve endings of a number of neuronal pathways. They have selective binding sites that can be demonstrated radiochemically *in vitro* and selective receptor sites that can be identified pharmacologically *in vivo*.

Although the evidence for neurotransmitter status is not as thorough as it is for some other neurotransmitters, glutamate and aspartate (Glu/Asp) are probably the ionotropic transmitters for most excitatory neurons in brain and therefore could belong to some of the most populous neuronal types. One problem with defining their role as neurotransmitters is that they obviously have other roles in the CNS. For example, glutamate is incorporated into proteins and peptides, is involved in fatty acid synthesis, contributes (along with glutamine) to the regulation of ammonia levels and the control of osmotic or anionic balance, serves as precursor for GABA and for various Krebs cycle intermediates, and is a constituent of at least two important cofactors (glutathione and folic acid). It is not surprising that glutamate should be the most plentiful amino acid in the adult CNS, its concentration being three to four times as high as the concentration of taurine, glutamine, or aspartate, the three amino acids that are next most abundant (Table 4).

TABLE 4. Content of some amino acids in whole rat brain (in μmol/g wet wt)

Glutamate	13.6 ± 0.4
Taurine	4.8 ± 0.3
Glutamine	4.4 ± 0.2
Aspartate	3.7 ± 0.2
GABA	2.3 ± 0.1
Glycine	1.7 ± 0.1
Serine	1.4 ± 0.1
Alanine	1.1 ± 0.1
Lysine	0.4 ± 0.0

Chemistry and metabolism of glutamate and aspartate

Glutamate and aspartate are nonessential amino acids that do not cross the BBB; therefore, they are not supplied to the brain by the blood. Instead, they are synthesized from glucose and other precursors by several biochemical routes within brain. Glutamate may be produced from α-ketoglutarate by transamination (Fig. 6), from glutamine by glutaminase action (Eq. 1), from α-ketoglutarate by reversal of the glutamic acid dehydrogenase action (Eq. 2), and from ornithine by ornithine aminotransferase (Orn-T) via Δ^1-pyrroline-5-carboxylic acid (P5C) and glutamate semialdehyde (Eq. 3). P5C can also be formed from proline by proline oxidase (not shown). The precise role of glutamate formed by each of these routes is unknown.

Metabolic studies have revealed the existence of several different pools or compartments for both glutamate and aspartate [8]. Unfortunately, it has not yet been possible to associate definitively any of these metabolic pools with anatomical structures, such as neurons or glia, or with distinct glutamate or aspartate neuronal systems.

No definite single source of neurotransmitter glutamate has been identified, although formation from glutaminase (Eq. 1) seems most probable in some, but not all, brain regions. It has been suggested that a combination of routes may exist, with the critical factor being the existence of specialized synaptic vesicles that could concentrate the available glutamate.

As far as the aspartate transmitter pool is concerned, oxaloacetate, glutamate, glutamine, and asparagine have all been suggested as precursor sources. Lesioning Glu/Asp afferents to the hippocampus did not cause a decrease in aspartate transaminase (Asp-T), which argues against oxaloacetate being an exclusive or even primary source for the transmitter pool of aspartate. Evidence for synthesis from glutamine or asparagine is equally slim.

Physiology and pharmacology of glutamate and aspartate and their receptors

Highly convincing evidence that L-glutamate and L-aspartate should be neurotransmitters comes from their iontophoretic actions. Both these dicarboxylic amino acids powerfully ex-

$$H_2NOCCH_2CH_2\overset{\overset{\displaystyle NH_2}{|}}{C}HCOOH + H_2O \xrightarrow{\text{Glutaminase}} HOOCCH_2CH_2\overset{\overset{\displaystyle NH_2}{|}}{C}HCOOH + NH_3 \qquad (1)$$

Glutamine Glutamic acid

$$HOOCCH_2CH_2COCOOH + NH_4^+ + NADH \xrightarrow{\substack{\text{Glutamic acid} \\ \text{dehydrogenase}}} HOOCCH_2CH_2\overset{\overset{\displaystyle NH_2}{|}}{C}HCOOH + NAD^+ + H_2O \qquad (2)$$

α-Ketoglutaric acid Glutamic acid

$$H_2N CH_2CH_2CH_2\overset{\overset{\displaystyle NH_2}{|}}{C}HCOOH \xrightarrow{\text{Orn-T}} \underset{\substack{\Delta^1\text{-Pyrroline-} \\ 5\text{-carboxylic acid}}}{\begin{array}{c} H_2C\text{---}CH_2 \\ HC\diagdown_N\diagup CHCOOH \end{array}} \xrightarrow{\substack{\text{P5C} \\ \text{dehydrogenase}}} \underset{\substack{\text{Glutamic} \\ \text{semialdehyde}}}{\begin{array}{c} H_2C\text{---}CH_2 \\ | \quad\quad | \\ OHC \quad CHCOOH \\ | \\ H_2N \end{array}} \qquad (3)$$

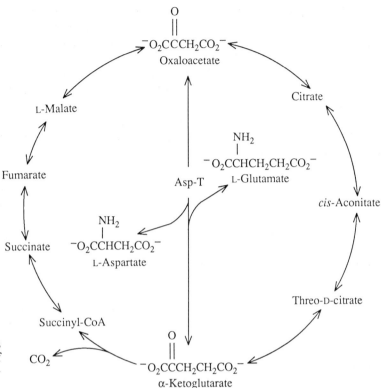

FIG. 6. Intermediates of the Krebs cycle, showing the formation of L-glutamate and L-aspartate by transamination reactions.

cite virtually all neurons with which they come in contact. Under optimal conditions, cells can be excited with as little as 10^{-14} mol. Effects of glutamate are instantaneous in onset, and are rapidly terminated. Glutamate iontophoresis is accompanied by a marked fall in membrane resistance and an increase in Na^+ and other ion permeability comparable to that observed when acetylcholine is applied near the muscle end-plate. The action is not blocked by tetrodotoxin, so that a specific excitation of receptor sites and not a stimulation of the Na^+ channels is responsible for the propagated action potential. In most respects, L-aspartate has an iontophoretic action comparable to that of glutamate, although it is generally less potent. Glutamate has been well established as the transmitter at the locust neuromuscular junction and the squid giant ganglion synapse [9].

Glutamate and aspartate excite a multiplicity of receptors in brain when applied iontophoretically, but it has so far not been possible to associate these receptors with any particular glutamate or aspartate pathway. A variety of agonists and antagonists for these iontophoretically defined receptors have been found [10]. Autoradiography of specific ligand binding is being used to demonstrate the anatomical distribution of these receptor systems.

Some of the many excitatory and blocking agents that have been discovered are shown in Table 5. They reveal four main receptor subtypes: N-methyl-D-aspartate (NMDA), quisqualic acid (QA), kainic acid (KA), and L-aminophosphonobutyric acid (AP4) receptors [10].

The NMDA receptor is functionally different from the other types. It is blocked in a voltage-dependent manner by physiological concentrations of Mg^{2+} at rest and only becomes operative when the membrane is depolarized due to an influx of Na^+ presumably from excitation of other types of glutamate receptors. Thus, the NMDA-induced current is regenerative, as is the action potential (see Chap. 4). Activation of the NMDA receptor permits not only Na^+ but Ca^{2+} ions to flow into the cell, which activates a Ca^{2+}-calmodulin-dependent kinase in the postsynaptic membrane. The NMDA receptor in the hippocampus has been strongly implicated in the phenomenon of long-term potentiation (LTP), which many believe may be a mechanism for short-term memory [1,10]. It might also be involved in epilepsy (see Chap. 41). The NMDA receptor seems to be modulated not only by Mg^{2+} in a voltage-de-pendent manner, but also by glycine and by a receptor that accepts anesthetics, such as phencyclidine or ketamine, and sigma opioids. Blockers of the NMDA receptor (Table 5) have shown some promise as anticonvulsants and as neuroprotective agents in animal models of ischemia and stroke [11].

Other receptors

The QA receptor is activated by QA and has a high affinity for L-glutamate and α-amino-3-hydroxy-5-methyl-4-isoxazolepropionic acid (AMPA). It may be modulated in similar fashion to the NMDA receptor and is supposedly concerned in the long-term depression that may play a role in motor learning in the cerebellum [12].

TABLE 5.   Acidic amino acid receptor classes

	Receptor class[a]			
	NMDA	*QA*	*KA*	*L-AP4*
Agonists	NMDA	QA	KA	L-AP4[b]
	Aspartate	AMPA	Domoate	(L-Glutamate)?[b]
	Glutamate	L-Glutamate		
Antagonists	MK-801	GDEE		
	D-AP5	GAMS		
	CPP			
	Glu-Amp			
Presumed *in vitro* binding site [13]	A₁	A₂	A₃	(A₄)
Radioligands	D-AP5	AMPA	KA	(D)L-AP4
	L-Glutamate	L-Glutamate		L-Glutamate
	CPP			
Binding characteristics	Independent of Cl⁻ and Na⁺	Enhanced by freeze-thawing	Not affected by freeze-thawing	Dependent on Cl⁻
	Enhanced by freeze-thawing	Displaced by μM QA	Displaced by nM– μM domoate, QA, or glutamate	Stimulated by Ca²⁺
	Moderately sensitive to NMLA			Inhibited by Na⁺
	Less sensitive to AP4, QA, and KA			Abolished by freeze-thawing
				Displaced by nM QA; less by KA or NMDA

[a] (AMPA) α-amino-3-hydroxy-5-methyl-4-isoxazolepropionic acid; (AP4) 2-amino-4-phosphonobutyric acid; (AP5) 2-amino-5-phosphonovaleric acid; (CPP) 3-[(±)-2-carboxypiperazin-4-yl]-propyl-1-phosphoric acid; (GAMS) γ-D-glutamylaminoethyl sulfonate; (GDEE) diethyl glutamate; (Glu-Amp) γ-D-glutamylaminomethylphosphonic acid; (KA) kainate; (MK-801) (+)-5-methyl-10,11-dihydro-5H-dibenzo[a,d]cyclohepten-5,10-imine maleate; (NMDA) N-methyl-D-aspartic acid; (NMLA) N-methyl-L-aspartic acid; (QA) quisqualate. Brackets indicate that identification is questionable.
[b] Not known if compound is agonist or antagonist at this receptor.

The KA receptor is activated by KA and seems to be particularly important for excitotoxicity, which is discussed later. Only limited studies have been conducted to determine the nature of AP4-sensitive receptors; however, L-AP4 is a potent antagonist of excitatory synaptic responses at such sites as the spinal cord and hippocampal perforant path synapses, which presumably use Glu/Asp as their neurotransmitter agent.

In addition to the multiple receptor sites for Glu/Asp that have been discovered *in vivo* through iontophoretic studies multiple binding sites have been identified *in vitro*. Foster and Fagg [13] adopted A_1-A_4 as the binding site nomenclature and attempted to correlate these with physiologically defined receptors (Table 5). Some recent evidence indicates, however, that the Cl^--dependent site A_4 is a glutamate sequestration site rather than a receptor.

In addition to the four binding sites discussed in Table 5, there is also an Na^+-dependent, high-affinity-uptake site that exists presumably for the purpose of removing the amino acids from the synapse and concentrating them in nerve endings and glia. At this site, cysteinesulfinate and D-aspartate are effective competitors of L-glutamate and L-aspartate.

Excitotoxic effects

A physiological consequence of the fact that glutamate, aspartate, and a number of structurally related amino acids powerfully excite neurons in the CNS is that they will bring about neuronal destruction if administered in sufficient excess. This neurotoxic consequence of excitatory activity, unnoticed for many years, is being exploited by neuroscientists as a means of providing much new information about the operation of neuronal systems.

Systemically administered L-glutamate or L-aspartate, as well as any one of several excitatory analogs, produces degeneration of cells in the retina and the hypothalamus in immature animals when given at sufficiently high doses. Seizures may also occur, and the same result is produced in mature animals with intraventricular administration. Microinjections of many excitatory amino acids into various brain areas can produce an acute reaction that selectively destroys certain neurons in the area [1,10,14]. Examples of such excitotoxic amino acids include kainic acid, ibotenic acid, quinolinic acid, cysteinesulfinic acid, homocysteic acid, and folic acid (Fig. 7). They all have two acidic groups and can be thought of as analogs of glutamate and aspartate.

Three factors seem to play a role in the extent of neuronal damage produced by various excitotoxins: (1) the nature and concentration of amino acid receptors affected by that excitotoxin; (2) the synergistic effect of endogenous Glu/Asp input to the injected area; and (3) trans-synaptic spread of damage due to induced epileptiform activity. Excessive activity of endogenous excitatory amino acids has been postulated to play a role in a variety of neurodegenerative diseases including ischemia, Huntington's disease, Alzheimer's disease, and epilepsy [11,15]. β-*N*-Oxalylamino-L-alanine (ODAP) and β-*N*-methylamino-L-alanine (L-BMAA) are two chemically related amino acids isolated, respectively, from the seeds of the chickling pea and *Cycas* palm flour; it has been suggested that consumption of these materials is linked to the occurrence of lathyrism in India and an amyotrophic lateral sclerosis/Parkinsonism/dementia syndrome occurring in Guam and some other Pacific rim regions. There is considerable evidence that ODAP is an excitotoxin [14,15]. An excitotoxic role for L-BMAA has also been proposed since, on chronic oral administration, it produces symptoms in monkeys suggesting neuronal damage. The dibasic amino acid structure of L-BMAA, however, makes it unlikely to be an excitotoxin in itself, but it could be metabolized to such a material.

It might be anticipated that high doses of

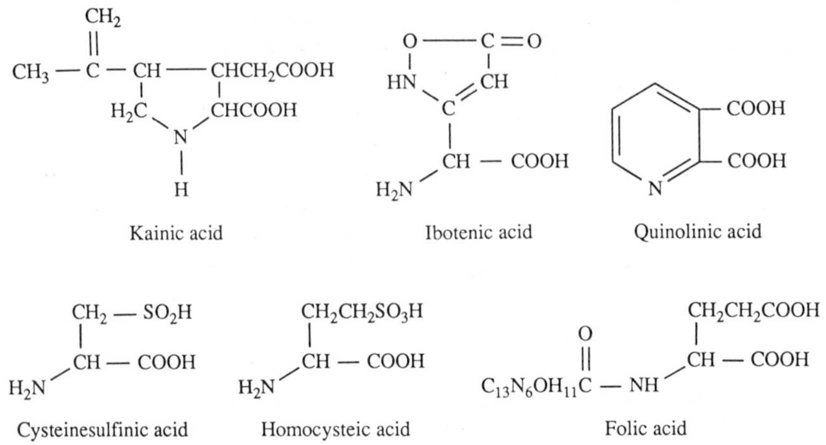

FIG. 7. Structures of some excitatory and neurotoxic amino acids.

glutamate and aspartate would be toxic in humans, but there are no firm data to support this supposition. A few anecdotal reports of symptoms in individuals consuming large amounts of the structurally related artificial sweetener Aspartame have appeared, and some people experience strange sensations after eating in Chinese restaurants. This "Chinese restaurant syndrome" involves the production of burning sensations, facial pressure, and chest pains in sensitive individuals. The effects are probably at least partially peripheral. Caution should be exercised with infants, however, in whom the BBB might not be fully developed.

Anatomy of pathways containing glutamate and aspartate

Some proposed Glu/Asp pathways are shown in Fig. 8. Most are tentative, but they serve as a base on which future data may be built.

Immunohistochemistry for glutamate itself is perhaps the most promising approach for definitive localization of glutamate neurons and pathways. It depends on developing antibodies to a chemically coupled glutamate-protein complex. Several investigators have obtained excellent staining of rat cortical pyramidal neurons. Both the distribution and morphology of the cells are different from that of the cortical GABA cells (see Fig. 4).

The most firmly based assignments for glutamate are descending pathways from cortical and hippocampal pyramidal cells. These tracts include the corticostriatal, entorhinal-hippocampal, and hippocampal and cortical pathways to various hypothalamic, thalamic, and brain stem nuclei. For aspartate, the hippocampal commissural path has been suggested. Granule cells of the cerebellum also appear to be largely Glu/Asp in nature. It must be iterated that the present techniques for identifying and distinguishing between glutamate and/or aspartate paths have major weaknesses. Physiological methods are technically difficult and suffer from lack of selective antagonists. Biochemical approaches involve measuring changes in release, uptake, or levels of the amino acid in a given area after various lesions. Release measurements have technical difficulties, uptake measurements do not distinguish between aspartate and glutamate, and levels tend to be an insensitive index of the neuronal pools.

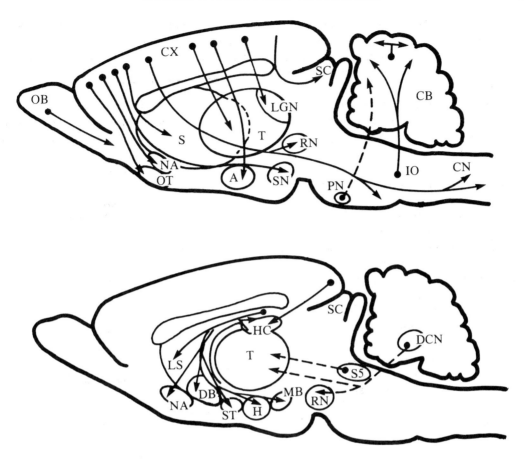

FIG. 8. Some pathways proposed to use acidic amino acid transmitters in the mammalian brain: (A) amygdala; (CB) cerebellum; (CN) cuneate nucleus; (CX) cerebral cortex; (DB) nucleus of the diagonal band; (DCN) deep cerebellar nuclei; (H) hypothalamus; (HC) hippocampus; (IO) inferior olive; (LGN) lateral geniculate nucleus; (LS) lateral septum; (MB) mammillary body; (NA) nucleus accumbens; (OB) olfactory bulb; (OT) olfactory tubercle; (PN) pontine nuclei; (RN) red nucleus; (S) striatum; (SC) superior colliculus; (SN) substantia nigra; (ST) bed nucleus of the stria terminalis; (S5) spinal nucleus of nerve 5; (T) thalamus.

OTHER AMINO ACIDS

A number of other amino acids occur in brain and possess some physiological activity. These include taurine, serine, proline, pipecolic acid, *N*-acetylaspartic acid, α- and β-alanine, and L-cysteinesulfinic acid. Of these, only the first three deserve further mention as neurotransmitter candidates.

Taurine

A decade after the discovery of high concentrations of taurine in brain by Awapara and Roberts, Curtis and Watkins demonstrated that it had a strong inhibitory action on spinal neurons. Jasper and Koyama added further interest by demonstrating its increased release from the cerebral cortex of cats during arousal. Since these initial reports, there has been continuing controversy as to whether taurine might play a neurotransmitter role in brain. It is now believed that taurine modulates membrane excitability by decreasing the concentration of intracellular free Ca^{2+}.

Taurine is believed to be formed in brain by a route starting from cysteine. This is converted to cysteinesulfinic acid, hypotaurine, and, finally, taurine (Fig. 9). The key enzyme is believed to be the decarboxylase that converts cysteinesulfinic acid to hypotaurine. Some taurine may also be taken up from the periphery, particularly in newborn animals. Alternative routes through cysteic acid or cysteamine are generally considered less probable. (Metabolic diseases related to taurine, and these metabolites are discussed in Chap. 38.)

Most taurine is excreted unchanged or is conjugated with bile acids. Turnover of total brain taurine is far slower than that of the established neurotransmitters (9–16 hr for fast decay; 40–238 hr for slow decay). In view of this, as well as the postnatal decrease in total taurine levels and the rather even regional distribution, it is generally accepted that much of the taurine in brain is present in nonneurotransmitter pools.

Higher than average levels are found in the pituitary and pineal glands, the retina, cerebellum, olfactory bulb, and striatum. Particular taurine systems proposed therefore include cerebellar stellate cells, retinotectal neurons, and interneurons of the retina, olfactory bulb, and striatum.

Although a neurotransmitter role has not been proven for taurine, it seems to be clearly involved in maintaining the structural integrity of the retina, and a defect in taurine transport or storage, or both, may be related to retinitis pigmentosa, a degenerative disease in humans. An association of taurine deficiency with epilepsy has also been suggested, and mild anticonvulsant activity of taurine has been reported in humans and in some, but not all, experimental models of epilepsy.

Serine

The chief interest in serine is that it is interconvertible with glycine in the CNS. It also has a weak glycine-like action in iontophoretic studies. Serine does not influence the high-affinity-uptake system of glycine, and thus far it has been associated only with low-affinity uptake in brain tissue from adult animals. Thus, evidence for neurotransmitter action is very weak.

Proline

Although proline is present at relatively low concentrations in mammalian brain, very high

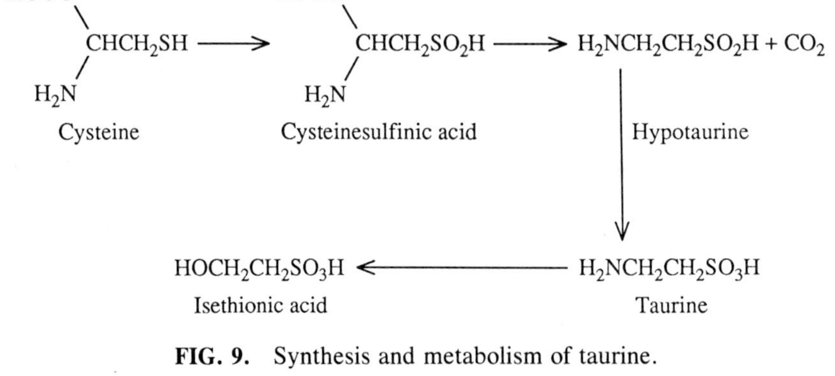

FIG. 9. Synthesis and metabolism of taurine.

concentrations have been reported in the nervous systems of both crabs and lobsters. Significantly higher concentrations occur in dorsal than in ventral roots in the spinal cord. It has a weak glycine-like action on cat spinal neurons and appears to be taken up into synaptosomes by a high-affinity Na^+-dependent system. Some believe, however, that it may be taken up nonspecifically by many neurons or as a precursor for thyrotropin releasing hormone (TRH). Again, evidence for neurotransmitter action is weak. Inborn errors of metabolism in which high levels of proline or pipecolic acid occur are generally characterized by mental retardation, suggesting a role in brain development.

SUMMARY

There is excellent evidence that four amino acids are the major ionotropic neurotransmitters in brain, with GABA and, to a lesser extent, glycine being inhibitory and glutamate and aspartate excitatory. There is little convincing evidence that any other amino acid serves as a neurotransmitter in mammalian brain. GABAergic and glycinergic systems can be distinguished both chemically and physiologically, but good methods are not yet available for a clear distinction between aspartate and glutamate neurons. Both physiological and binding studies suggest that more than one type of receptor exists for each amino acid neurotransmitter. Considerable attention is being given to defining the characteristics and functions of these various types of receptors and, particularly, the NMDA receptor for excitatory amino acids and that type of GABA receptor which is coupled with a benzodiazepine recognition site into a unit that allows interaction between GABA and the benzodiazepines.

REFERENCES

1. McGeer, P. L., Eccles, J. C., and McGeer, E. G. *Molecular Neurobiology of the Mammalian Brain*, 2nd ed. New York: Plenum Press, 1987, pp. 149–224; 553–594.

2. Roberts, E., Chase, T. N., and Tower, D. B. (eds.) *GABA in Nervous System Function*. New York: Raven Press, 1976.

3. Hill, D. R., and Bowery, N. G. ³H-Baclofen and ³H-GABA bind to bicuculline-insensitive $GABA_B$ sites in rat brain. *Nature* 290:119–152, 1981.

4. Stevens, C. F. Channel families in the brain. *Nature* 328:198–199, 1987.

5. Hirsch, J. D., Garrett, K. M., and Beer, B. Heterogeneity of benzodiazepine binding: A review of recent research. *Pharmacol. Biochem. Behav.* 23:681–685, 1985.

6. Nagai, T., McGeer, P. L., Araki, M., and McGeer, E. G. GABA-T intensive neurons in the rat brain. In A. Björklund, T. Hökfelt, and M. J. Kuhar (eds.), *Classical Transmitters and Transmitter Receptors in the CNS, Part II* (*Handbook of Chemical Neuroanatomy, Vol. 3*). Amsterdam: Elsevier, 1984, pp. 247–272.

7. Werman, R., Davidoff, R. A., and Aprison, M. H. Inhibitory effect of glycine in spinal neurons of the cat. *J. Neurophysiol.* 31:81–95, 1968.

8. Fonnum, F. Glutamate: A neurotransmitter in mammalian brain. *J. Neurochem.* 42:1–11, 1984.

9. Kawai, N., Yamagishi, S., Saito, M., and Furuya, K. Blockade of synaptic transmission in the squid giant synapse by a spider toxin (JSTX). *Brain Res.* 278:346–349, 1983.

10. Cotman, C. W., Iversen, L. L., Watkins, J. C., et al. Special Issue: Excitatory amino acids in the brain—focus on NMDA receptors. *Trends Neurosci.* 10:263–301, 1987.

11. Lodge, D. Modulating glutamate pharmacology. *Trends Pharmacol. Sci.* 8:243–244, 1987.

12. Knao, M., and Kato, M. Quisqualate receptors are specifically involved in cerebellar synaptic plasticity. *Nature* 325:276–279, 1987.

13. Foster, A. C., and Fagg, G. E. Acidic amino acid binding sites in mammalian neuronal membranes: Their characteristics and relationship to synaptic receptors. *Brain Res. Rev.* 7:103–164, 1984.

14. McGeer, E. G., Olney, J. W., and McGeer, P. L. *Kainic Acid as a Tool in Neurobiology*. New York: Raven Press, 1978.

15. McGeer, E. G., and McGeer, P. L., Neurotoxin-

induced animal models of human disease. In K. Blum and L. Manzo (eds.), *Neurotoxicology.* New York and Basel: Marcel Dekker, 1985, pp. 515–533.

16. Spencer, P. S., Nunn, P. B., Hugon, J., et al. BMAA and BOAA: Chemically related primate motor neuron toxins isolated respectively from Guamanian *Cycas circinalis* and Indian *Lathyrus sativus. Neurology* 36(Suppl. 1):135–136, 1986.

17. Olsen, R. W., and Leeb-Lundberg, F. Convulsant and anticonvulsant drug binding sites related to GABA-regulated chloride ion channels. *Adv. Biochem. Psychopharmacol.* 26:93–102, 1981.

CHAPTER 16

Phosphoinositides

Bernard W. Agranoff

Basic Neurochemistry: Molecular, Cellular, and Medical Aspects, 4th Ed., edited by G. J. Siegel et al. Raven Press, Ltd., New York, 1989.
Correspondence to Bernard W. Agranoff, Neuroscience Laboratory, University of Michigan, 1103 East Huron, Ann Arbor, MI 48104-1687.

333

HISTORICAL REVIEW

A growing list of ligands, including neurotransmitters, neuromodulators, and hormones, have been shown to exert their physiological action via an intracellular second-messenger system in which the activated receptor ligand complex stimulates the turnover of inositol-containing phospholipids. In this chapter, the chemistry, enzymology, and physiology of this ubiquitous pathway are examined in the context of the nervous system. A brief historical review will prove useful to present the logical sequence of events leading to our current view and to provide an understanding of the technological and conceptual obstacles that were overcome in the process.

Stimulation of secretion is accompanied by incorporation of inorganic phosphate into phospholipids

In 1953, Hokin and Hokin [1] reported that slices of pancreas incubated with labeled inorganic phosphate ($^{32}P_i$) exhibited increased phospholipid labeling under conditions of stimulation by muscarinic agents, such as carbamylcholine (carbachol). Although unphysiologically high concentrations of carbachol were required to produce maximal stimulation, both the lipid labeling and secretion of amylase into the medium were blocked when the alkaloid atropine, a known muscarinic blocker, was also present. They had thus discovered a biochemical "handle" to our understanding of receptor action. The observed labeling was confined to two quantitatively minor phospholipid components: phosphatidate (PA) and phosphatidylinositol (PI). This demonstration of receptor-stimulated lipid labeling was quickly extended and generalized to a number of other ligands, each in the presence of an appropriate tissue (e.g., thyrotropin in the presence of thyroid tissue). The avian salt gland, which secretes NaCl nonexocytotically in the presence of carbachol,

also supported a muscarinic stimulation of PA and PI labeling under these conditions.

In each tissue, it was necessary to use whole cells, in the form of slices and minces, or dissociated cells to elicit the effect. An apparent exception was found in studies with brain homogenates, which support muscarinic stimulation of lipid labeling even though they are broken-cell preparations. It was eventually shown that the stimulated lipid labeling is mediated by a nerve-ending fraction of the homogenate. These pinched-off organelles may be regarded as resealed anucleate neurons, in which the vectorial inside-outside relationship of cells has been preserved. Hence, the generalization that whole cells are required for demonstration of ligand-stimulated lipid labeling was upheld. More recently, there have been claims of successful demonstration of ligand-stimulated breakdown of prelabeled phospholipids in membrane preparations (see "G-proteins" below).

Inorganic phosphate incorporation involves a cycle of glycerolipid utilization

A few years after the initial reports of receptor-mediated labeling of lipids, a unique metabolic relationship between PA and PI was elucidated via the liponucleotide intermediate cytidine diphosphate diacylglycerol (CDP·DG; see Chap. 5). CDP·DG is formed from cytidine triphosphate (CTP) and PA and serves as the biosynthetic precursor of PI (see Chap. 5); however, under conditions of ligand-stimulated labeling of PA and PI, there is no enhancement of incorporation of labeled glycerol into either of these lipids. This result indicates that the observed stimulated incorporation of $^{32}P_i$ into PA and PI very likely involves a cycle in which there is degradation and reutilization of the glycerolipid backbone. It was proposed that PI breakdown is stimulated as a result of receptor activation, with the release and reutilization of diacylglycerol (DG). It now appears likely that in most if not all instances of stimulated inositol lipid turnover, the initiating step is the breakdown of a phosphorylated derivative of PI rather than of PI itself, as discussed below.

Although the presence of highly phosphorylated inositol lipids, particularly in brain, had been known, there are no techniques for their convenient extraction from tissue incubations or for their separation using thin-layer chromatographic (TLC) systems. It was partly for this reason that their role in transmembrane signaling was not recognized earlier. Acidification of lipid extraction solvents such as chloroform-methanol assures complete extraction of all of the inositol lipids, and TLC systems incorporating oxalate salts in the silica gel matrix have been developed to facilitate their separation [2].

Following the initial demonstration of stimulated PI and PA labeling, the broad distribution of this effect became evident, and in a review of the field in 1975, Michell [3] tabulated over 60 examples. He noted a common pattern: elevation of intracellular Ca^{2+} in the activated cells was either demonstrated or inferred. It was less clear at the time whether or not the elevated intracellular Ca^{2+} was the cause or the result of the stimulated labeling of lipids.

Phospholipids, when cleaved, give rise to a dual second-messenger system

The dual system involves, on the one hand, inositol phosphates, which elevate intracellular Ca^{2+}, and on the other, DG, which activates Ca^{2+}-dependent protein phosphorylation. Although it is evident that the signal transduction process that follows receptor activation is enormously complex, this dual system is the dominant theme that has emerged. The reader should be cautioned in advance that our knowledge of this elaborate pathway continues to evolve rapidly. There are many indications that cell receptors may differ in the details of their response and may utilize to a greater or lesser extent one or both of the dual messenger systems detailed in this chapter.

CHEMISTRY OF THE INOSITOL LIPIDS AND PHOSPHATES

The three known phosphoinositides are structurally and metabolically related

The three known phosphoinositides consist of PI and the two polyphosphoinositides, phosphatidylinositol 4-phosphate (PIP) and phosphatidylinositol 4,5-bisphosphate (PIP₂) (Fig. 1A). PI consists of a DG moiety, which is phosphodiesterified to *myo*-inositol, a polycyclic alcohol. It is phosphorylated to PIP within a reaction requiring ATP and catalyzed by PI kinase; PIP is further phosphorylated via PIP kinase to PIP_2 (see Fig. 1A).

There exists an unusual uniformity in the fatty acid composition of the inositol lipids. All three phosphoinositides in brain are enriched in the 1-stearoyl, 2-arachidonoyl (ST/AR) *sn*-glycerol species (~80 percent in brain). The polyphosphoinositides are present in much lower amounts than PI and are believed to be localized to the inner leaflet of plasma membranes. Brain tissue is the best known source of the polyphosphoinositides. A recent estimate of the total amount of the three phosphoinositides was made in brains that had been extracted following microwave treatment to minimize postmortem degradation. 78, 4, and 14 nmol of PI, PIP, and PIP_2, respectively, were found per milligram of neostriatal protein (Von Dongen et al., quoted in Hajra et al. [2]). Although postmortem breakdown is rapid, a considerable fraction of brain phosphoinositide appears to be in a slowly degraded pool.

The phosphoinositides differ from other phospholipids, such as phosphatidylethanolamine, phosphatidylcholine, and phosphatidylserine, in that they contain no nitrogen. They share this property with the phosphatidylglycerol se-

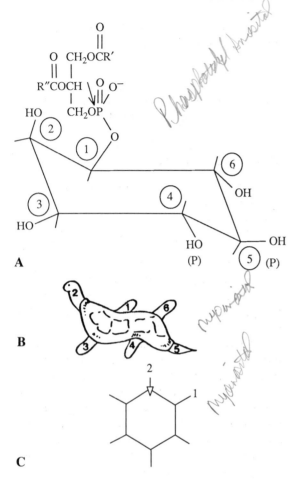

A

B

C

FIG. 1. The chemical structure of the inositol lipids. **A:** PI and the polyphosphoinositides. In the D numbering system, the 2 position is axial, and the phosphatidyl group is phosphodiesterified to the vicinal hydroxyl in the D-1 position. In PIP, there is an additional phosphate monoesterified in the D-4 position, and in PIP$_2$, a third phosphate is present on the D-5 position. The site of cleavage via phosphoinositide phosphodiesterase is shown by the *arrow.* **B:** *Myo*-inositol may be visualized as a turtle in which the 2 position is the head and the five equatorial hydroxyls constitute the four legs and tail. In the inositol lipids, the phosphatidyl group is always at the right foreleg (D-1). **C:** A convenient representation of *myo*-inositol. The *open triangle* at the D-2 position represents the axial hydroxyl (the turtle's head) projecting out of the plane of the paper toward the reader. Numbering continues in a counterclockwise direction.

ries with which they also share a common biosynthetic intermediate: CDP·DG (see Chap. 5). The cyclic polyalcohol *myo*-inositol is one of nine possible isomers of hexahydroxycyclohexane. It has one axial and five equatorial hydroxyls and is by far the most prevalent isomer in nature. Its geometry can be easily understood by regarding the cyclohexane chair configuration as a "turtle" in which the axial hydroxyl is the head, while the four limbs and tail serve as the five equatorial positions (Fig. 1B). In all of the phosphoinositides, DG is affixed to the D-1 hydroxyl, the right front leg, via a phosphodiester linkage with the *sn*-3 position of glycerol. Using the D (for dextro isomer) numbering convention, and looking down at the turtle from above (Fig. 1C), the head is then at position D-2, while the left front leg is D-3, etc. (see also Fig. 2).

At present, there are no known natural phosphoinositides containing cyclitols other than *myo*-inositol, nor are there examples in which the inositol is diesterified to DG at a position other than D-1. Monophosphate esters of the lipids have been found only at the D-4 (in PIP) or at both the D-4 and D-5 (in PIP$_2$) positions. A glycosidic link to PI appears to occur in instances in which proteins are anchored to the membrane via PI, as indicated below.

The phosphoinositides are cleaved by phosphoinositide-specific phospholipase C into two moieties

The two moieties that result are DG and either inositol 1-phosphate (IP$_1$) or inositol 1,4-bisphosphate (IP$_2$) or inositol 1,4,5-trisphosphate (IP$_3$), from PI, PIP, and PIP$_2$, respectively. Multiple forms of phospholipase C have been purified from a number of sources, and a low concentration of Ca^{2+} is generally required for activity. The enzyme has been studied most extensively with PI as substrate. Two inositol monophosphates are released in relatively equal amounts: D-*myo*-inositol 1-phosphate (1-IP$_1$)

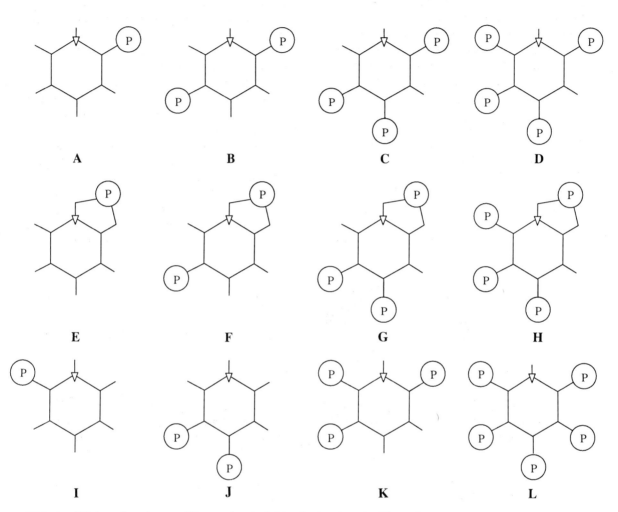

FIG. 2. Higher phosphates of D-*myo*-inositol. Numbering is as in Fig. 1. Structures (**A**), (**B**), and (**C**) depict 1-IP$_1$, 1,4-IP$_2$, and 1,4,5-IP$_3$, respectively. These are the cleavage products of PI, PIP, and PIP$_2$. Structure (**D**) is 1,3,4,5-IP$_4$, produced by phosphorylation of C at the D-3 position via IP$_3$ kinase. Structures (**E**)–(**H**) represent 1,2 cyclic derivatives of compounds (**A**)–(**D**), respectively. c1:2-IP$_1$ is the best characterized, and there is increasing evidence for the occurrence in tissues of c1:2,4-IP$_2$ and c1:2,4,5-IP$_3$. There is at present no evidence for the existence of c1:2,3,4,5-IP$_4$. Structure (**I**) is D-*myo*-inositol 3-phosphate (3-IP$_1$), also known as L-1-IP$_1$. This ester is formed from cyclization of glucose-6-phosphate. Structure (**J**) is 4,5-IP$_2$. Structure (**K**) is 1,3,4-IP$_3$, an inactive isomer of IP$_3$ (see text). Structure (**L**) is D-*myo*-inositol 1,3,4,5,6-pentakisphosphate. This isomer is present in avian erythrocytes in relatively high amounts and may be present in other tissues as well. (From Fisher and Agranoff [4].)

and D-*myo*-inositol 1:2 cyclic phosphate (c1:2-IP$_1$; see Fig. 2). The inositol lipid-specific phospholipase is of particular interest, since a membrane-bound form of the enzyme initiates stimulated phosphoinositide labeling via coupling to an activated cell-surface receptor. When PIP or PIP$_2$ is cleaved, analogous cyclic phosphates may be formed (see Fig. 2).

Cleavage of PIP$_2$ initiates two cycles: one in which the DG backbone is conserved and recycled, and one in which inositol is reutilized

As indicated above, it can be inferred that a cycle operates in which the DG is conserved, and to this end, the enzyme DG kinase was sought and found. It converts the DG released

on phosphoinositide cleavage to PA, which can then be converted to PI via CDP·DG (Figs. 3–5; also see Chap. 5). Although the latter steps are those seen in the *de novo* biosynthesis of inositol lipids, it is likely that net synthesis and stimulated lipid turnover occur in separate and distinct metabolic compartments: The receptor-stimulated cycle is likely to be confined to the plasma membrane, whereas the various steps in the *de novo* pathway occur in the mitochondrial and/or endoplasmic reticular fractions. The co-released inositol phosphates (IP$_1$, IP$_2$, or IP$_3$) are eventually cleaved via phosphatases to regenerate free inositol, which may then combine with CDP·DG to form PI. Sequential phosphorylation of PI to PIP$_2$ via PIP closes both loops of this double cycle, as is seen in Fig. 4.

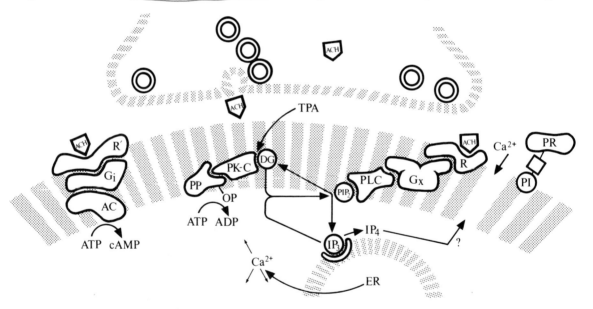

FIG. 3. Summary of signal transduction in a CNS muscarinic receptor coupled to stimulated phosphoinositide turnover. ACh released presynaptically interacts with a muscarinic receptor (R), which in turn activates a phosphoinositide-specific phospholipase C (PLC) via a G-protein (G$_x$). PIP$_2$ is cleaved to give rise to 1,4,5-inositol trisphosphate (IP$_3$) and diacylglycerol (DG). IP$_3$ interacts with the endoplasmic reticulum (ER) membrane to release Ca^{2+}. IP$_3$ can alternatively be phosphorylated to IP$_4$, which may activate a Ca^{2+} channel in the plasma membrane, shown to the right of R. To the right of the channel is a PI-linked protein (PR), as described in the text. DG released from PIP$_2$ breakdown activates protein kinase C (PK-C), which then stimulates phosphorylation of an apophosphoprotein (PP). The DG site may be deactivated by externally added tetradecanoylphorbol acetate (TPA) (a phorbol ester). To the left of PK-C is shown an inhibitory adenylate cyclase (AC)-linked muscarinic receptor (R'); R' and AC are linked via G$_i$.

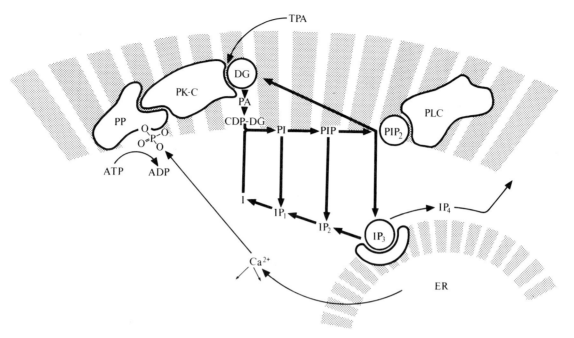

FIG. 4. Detail from Fig. 3 to show additionally the regenerative steps in the phosphoinositide cycle. DG is converted to PA via DG kinase. PA reacts with CTP to form CDP·DG. CDP·DG reacts with inositol to form PI, which in turn is converted by sequential phosphorylations to PIP and finally to PIP_2, completing a cycle. Note that PLC may also react with PIP to form DG and IP_2, or with PI to form DG and IP_1.

THE INOSITOL PHOSPHATES

D-myo-inositol 1,4,5-trisphosphate (1,4,5-IP₃) is an intracellular messenger in permeabilized cells and has been demonstrated to liberate Ca^{2+} from the endoplasmic reticulum

The cleavage products of PIP_2 and of PI, that is, inositol 1,4,-bisphosphate and inositol 1-phosphate, respectively, do not share this property. Since $1,4,5\text{-}IP_3$ uniquely liberates Ca^{2+}, this observation is one of the key arguments that it is PIP_2 cleavage, rather than breakdown of PIP or PI, that initiates the cellular response to receptor activation. The action of a 5′-phosphatase on $1,4,5\text{-}IP_3$ serves as an off-signal, since the resulting $1,4\text{-}IP_2$ does not mobilize Ca^{2+}. The latter product is identical to the IP_2 species produced on phosphodiesteratic cleavage of PIP. Thus, the presence of $1,4\text{-}IP_2$ in tissues can reflect either breakdown of PIP_2 or of $1,4,5\text{-}IP_3$ released from PIP_2. There may also be specific phosphatases that remove either the 1 or 4 phosphate from $1,4\text{-}IP_2$ (Fig. 5).

Brain contains, in addition, two other inositol monophosphates, D-2 IP_1 and D-3 IP_1. D-3 IP_1 is a stereoisomer of D-1 IP_1 and is also referred to as L-1 IP_1. It is the product of cyclization of glucose-6-phosphate and thus constitutes a biosynthetic precursor of *myo*-inositol. It is also an intermediate in the degradation of $1,3,4\text{-}IP_3$, described below. D-1 IP_1, D-3 IP_1, and D-4 IP_1 are cleaved by the same phosphatase, which is inhibited by Li^+ [4]. The action of Li^+ has facilitated the use of [³H]inositol in the study of stimulated phosphoinositide labeling [5]. In the presence of both Li^+ and a phos-

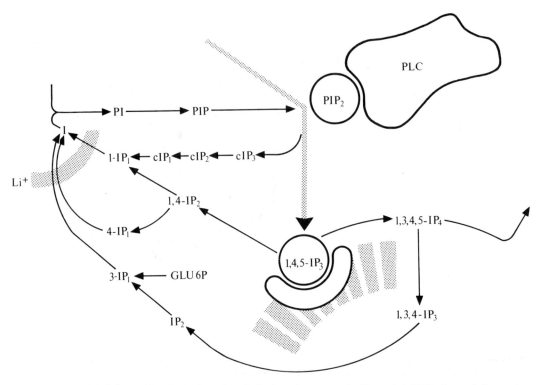

FIG. 5. Further detail from Fig. 3 to show inositol phosphate metabolism. $1,4,5\text{-IP}_3$ formed from cleavage of PIP_2 is degraded via $5'$-phosphatase to $1,4\text{-IP}_2$ and then via specific phosphatases to 1-IP_1 or 4-IP_1. 1-IP_1 is cleaved by a phosphatase, which also cleaves 3-IP_1. Formation of free inositol from 1-IP_1, 3-IP_1, or 4-IP_1 is blocked by Li^+. There is evidence that the cyclic derivative $c1{:}2,4,5\text{-IP}_3$ is formed as a product of PIP_2 cleavage, along with $1,4,5\text{-IP}_3$. While the degradation of the cyclic compound has not been described in detail, it has been proposed that the phosphomonoesters are degraded, and the resultant $c1{:}2\text{-IP}_1$ is acted on by a phosphodiesterase to yield 1-IP_1. $1,4,5\text{-IP}_3$ may be either degraded to $1,4\text{-IP}_2$ by the action of a $5'$-phosphatase, or alternatively, may be phosphorylated by IP_3 kinase to form $1,3,4,5\text{-IP}_4$. IP_4 is degraded via the $5'$-phosphatase to yield $1,3,4\text{-IP}_3$, which is eventually further degraded via phosphatases to inositol. Recently an inositol polyphosphate 1-phosphatase that degrades $1,4\text{-IP}_2$ and $1,3,4\text{-IP}_3$ has been found and reported to be Li^+-sensitive (not shown).

phoinositide-linked ligand, the amount of tritiated intracellular IP_1 that accumulates following a preincubation with $[^3H]$inositol can be stimulated as much as 50-fold, whereas the presence of either Li^+ or ligand alone has very little effect on $[^3H]IP_1$ accumulation. Thus, although ligand-activated turnover is initiated by PIP_2 breakdown with the generation of $1,4,5\text{-IP}_3$, this product is quickly degraded, so that it is far more convenient to measure the accumulation of labeled IP_1 in the presence of Li^+ than to attempt to measure the transient appearance of

labeled $1,4,5\text{-IP}_3$ a few seconds after ligand addition.

Using ^3H-labeled inositol and Li^+ is an indirect approach because IP_1 rather than IP_3 formation is measured; yet, it constitutes a more sensitive measure of stimulated phosphoinositide turnover than does the ^{32}P-labeling technique. The reason for this is that the $4'$ and $5'$ positions of the polyphosphoinositides quickly equilibrate with the $\gamma^{32}P$ in intracellular ATP via the specific lipid phosphatases and kinases, such that labeling reflects the specific radioactivity of ATP and the chemical amounts of the polyphosphoinositides rather than their turnover. This, in addition to the aforementioned technical problems in polyphosphoinositide extraction and separation, undoubtedly contributed to the delay in elucidating their role in stimulated phosphoinositide turnover.

1,3,4-IP$_3$ and 1,3,4,5,-IP$_4$

1,3,4-IP$_3$, isolated from stimulated tissues, has little Ca^{2+}-mobilizing activity. It originates from the 3' phosphorylation of 1,4,5-IP$_3$ via an IP$_3$ kinase to yield 1,3,4,5-IP$_4$, followed by dephosphorylation at the 5' position. IP$_4$ is not active in mobilizing intracellular Ca^{2+}, so that IP$_3$ kinase, like the 5'-phosphatase, can be considered to be an "off" enzyme, which terminates 1,4,5-IP$_3$ Ca^{2+}-mobilizing activity. 1,3,4,5-IP$_4$, like 1,4,5-IP$_3$ can also be cleaved by the 5'-phosphatase, to yield 1,3,4-IP$_3$, which is eventually further degraded by phosphatases. Does, then, the IP$_4$ pathway exist only for 1,4,5-IP$_3$ inactivation? This is not an appealing idea, since the 5'-phosphatase can degrade 1,4,5-IP$_3$ as readily as 1,3,4,5-IP$_4$. It has been suggested that IP$_4$ provides an alternative source of increased intracellular Ca^{2+} by opening channels to the extracellular environment. Evidence for this has been provided in studies in microinjected sea urchin eggs. It remains to be seen whether the action of IP$_4$ also holds true for other tissues, including brain [6].

Other inositol phosphates

Inositol 1,3,4,5,6-pentakisphosphate (IP$_5$) has long been known to be a component of avian erythrocytes, in which it binds to an allosteric site of hemoglobin, as does 2,3-diphosphoglycerate in mammalian erythrocytes. Inositol hexaphosphate (phytate; IP$_6$) is a well-known component of plant seeds. Labeling studies in cultured tumor cells indicate the presence of both IP$_5$ and IP$_6$, but their possible function is unclear. A small amount of 2-IP$_1$ found in brain

may be derived from degradation of intracellularly synthesized phytate.

Cyclic inositol phosphates

Just as c1:2-IP$_1$ is formed in the breakdown of PI, there is considerable evidence that c1:2,4,5-IP$_3$ may be formed, presumably along with 1,4,5-IP$_3$, on cleavage of PIP$_2$. Although a specific function for the cyclic inositol phosphates is not known, it has been suggested that c1:2,4,5-IP$_3$ has physiological actions that approximate the effects of light on the *Limulus* photoreceptor more closely than do those of 1,4,5-IP$_3$ [7]. (The metabolism of inositol phosphates has been summarized in a recent review [8].)

DIACYLGLYCEROL

Protein kinase C, a widely distributed protein kinase requiring the presence of phosphatidylserine and Ca^{2+}, is activated by DG

Protein kinase C (PK-C) consists of a catalytic as well as a regulatory subunit. The latter appears to be the site of DG, phosphatidylserine, and Ca^{2+} binding, and it may serve the enzyme as an attachment site to membranes. PK-C is particularly enriched in brain and is proposed as a regulator of critical steps in neuronal signaling [9]. It has also been suggested that PK-C plays a role in brain plasticity (see Chap. 48). It is possible that PK-C-mediated phosphorylation of receptors, G-proteins, or the phosphoinositide phospholipase affects the receptor-mediated breakdown of PIP$_2$ and could thus exert feedback control on signal transduction. It has recently been shown that four subtypes of PK-C exist and are coded by separate but interrelated genes. One form of PK-C, designated βII, is brain specific [10].

Since 1,4,5-IP$_3$ production leads to increased intracellular Ca^{2+}, which in turn stimulates PK-C action, it is also evident that the two messenger systems (i.e., DG and 1,4,5-IP$_3$) are interactive. DG could arise in cells from a number of sources other than the phosphoinositides. For example, it could be generated from the action of a phosphatidylcholine (PC)-specific phospholipase C or from the transfer of phosphorylcholine from PC to ceramide in the synthesis of sphingomyelin (see Chap. 5). If it is specifically the population of DG that is released from stimulated phosphoinositide turnover that activates cellular PK-C, one might expect that ST/AR DG would be a particularly effective activator of the enzyme. It turns out to be only marginally better than other long-chain fatty acyl DGs; however, chemical analysis indicates that brain DG is enriched in the ST/AR species. It would therefore seem that ST/AR DG is indeed the principal activator of PK-C *in vivo*, even though the enzyme shows little specificity for it. There exist in fact superior artificial DG analogs for experimental purposes, such as the relatively soluble DG species, 1-oleoyl, 2-acetyl *sn*-glycerol (OAG).

Of particular value in studying the function of PK-C are the phorbol esters. These tumor-promoting plant products and their synthetic derivatives are able to penetrate whole cells and can thus be added to tissue incubations. Many of our inferences regarding the intracellular actions of PK-C are based on studies with the phorbol esters and whole cells. Since these substances, like DG, may produce feedback-inhibition of signal transduction at a number of metabolic levels, results of experiments using phorbol esters in whole cells are often complex and must be interpreted cautiously.

Protein kinase C regulates the activity of a large number of proteins, the phosphorylation of which can result in increases or decreases in their catalytic activity

Of particular interest are the actions of PK-C on ion channels, since in this way PK-C may

directly affect the transduction process. In platelets, PK-C activity is associated with the phosphorylation of a 40-kilodalton (kDa) protein. For assay purposes, histone is a convenient substrate for phosphorylation. PK-C itself has homology with DNA binding proteins, and it has been postulated that PK-C may also play a role in the regulation of macromolecular synthesis.

If DG is considered to be an intracellular messenger that activates PK-C, what then is the "off" signal that terminates its action? Phosphorylation to PA in the lipid labeling cycle could serve this purpose, but there are several additional possibilities. For example, DG lipase can cleave DG to fatty acid and monoglyceride (MG). Although this hydrolytic activity can be demonstrated, it should be noted that for the labeling cycle to remain truly regenerative, it would be necessary to reacylate the MG to DG. Such deacylation-reacylation reactions could be of importance in the generation of arachidonate for prostanoid synthesis from inositide intermediates (see Chap. 20).

FUNCTIONAL CORRELATES OF PHOSPHOINOSITIDE-LINKED RECEPTORS IN THE NERVOUS SYSTEM

Given the complexity of the brain, it is not surprising that this tissue is a rich source of diverse receptors coupled to stimulated phosphoinositide turnover

By the same token, the nervous system is not ideal for examining in detail the interaction of a single ligand with the second-messenger system, since there is likely to be convergence of several receptors on the phosphoinositide messenger system in any given brain cell type. Table 1 summarizes the presently known extent of this diversity. It should be noted that there are neurotransmitters that have been demonstrated *not* to be coupled to phosphoinositides, and these are in general either positively or negatively coupled to adenylate cyclase. They include H_2-histaminergic, $5\text{-}HT_1$-serotonergic, β-adrenergic, $α_2$-adrenergic, nicotinic cholinergic, and GABAergic receptor systems [4].

What is the physiological significance of stimulated phosphoinositide turnover in the nervous system?

A consequence of the heterogeneity of receptors in brain is that the best understood models of signal transduction via stimulated phosphoinositide turnover are outside the nervous system—secretion by the salivary or pancreatic glands, activation of platelets by thrombin or leukocytes by chemotactic peptides, etc. At present it seems that there are diverse roles for the phosphoinositide-associated messengers in the nervous system, ranging from mediating the primary signal of neurotransmission to modulation of neuronal signals, secretion, and perhaps even contraction. In the case of one neurotransmitter in one locus studied experimentally (the muscarinic receptor in the hippocampus), the stimulated phosphoinositide turnover was shown to be postsynaptic (see Fisher and Agranoff [4]).

Does the sharing of a single system by multiple cell-surface receptors lead to degeneracy of the signal?

Given the brain's necessity for a wide variety of extracellular messengers, such as neurotransmitters and hormones, it would seem that sharing intracellular messengers would lead to degradation of signal and loss of information. In the case of the nervous system, it may be that there are anatomically discrete second-messenger domains within a single cell. The use of video-enhanced microscopic methods for studying Ca^{2+} signaling [11] may offer an experimental approach to answer this question. It is also possible that the sharing of second-mes-

senger systems has useful physiological value; for example, in heterologous desensitization. That is, the loss of response to a given receptor can lead to loss of response to another receptor, presumably by the sharing of one or more steps in the transduction process. This could be part of a physiological process whereby various neuronal inputs are integrated.

Are G-proteins involved?

By analogy to the inhibitory (G_i) and stimulatory (G_s) (also termed N_i and N_s) G-proteins that couple receptors with the cyclic AMP (cAMP) second-messenger system (see Chap. 18), one can predict the existence of a coupling G-protein between the receptors in Table 1 and the phosphoinositide-specific phosphodiesterase. There is little direct evidence for this in the nervous system, but studies in other tissues with GTP and GTPγs suggest the participation of a G-protein α-subunit in the signal transduction associated with phosphoinositide turnover [4].

Does the action of Li^+ on the phosphoinositide labeling cycle explain the therapeutic action of Li^+ in manic depressive psychosis?

It has been suggested that Li^+ will differentially block phosphoinositide turnover *in vivo*, affecting most intensively those cells in which phosphoinositide-linked receptors are being stimulated [12]. Therapeutic doses of Li^+ do in fact lead to sufficiently high concentrations of Li^+ in the brain that one might expect the inositol 1-phosphate phosphatase to be inhibited *in vivo*. Such an effect would then lower the level of brain inositol and raise the level of intracellular inositol monophosphates, and this has been seen in Li^+-fed rats. However, although the biochemical effects of Li^+ occur rapidly, the clinical action of Li^+ in human patients requires weeks. This suggests that the therapeutic action of Li^+ may involve a slower

TABLE 1. Pharmacological profile of receptor-activated phosphoinositide turnover in CNS and neural-related tissues[a]

Receptor	Subtype	Tissue	Reference
RECEPTORS DEMONSTRATED TO BE COUPLED TO PHOSPHOINOSITIDE TURNOVER			
Muscarinic cholinergic	M_1 and M_2	Brain slices	Berridge et al., *Biochem. J.* 206:587, 1982; Brown et al., *J. Neurochem.* 42:1379, 1984; Fisher et al., *J. Neurochem.* 43:1171, 1984; Gonzales and Crews, *J. Neurosci.* 4:3120, 1984; Fisher and Bartus, *J. Neurochem.* 45:1085, 1985; Gil and Wolfe, *J. Pharmacol. Exp. Ther.* 232:608, 1985; Jacobson et al., *J. Neurochem.* 44:465, 1985; Lazareno et al., *Neuropharmacology* 24:593, 1985; Eva and Costa, *J. Neurochem.* 46:1429, 1986; Heacock et al., *J. Neurochem.* 48:1904, 1987
		Primary neuronal cultures	Gonzales and Crews, *Biochem. J.* 232:799, 1985
		Primary glial cultures	Pearce et al., *J. Neurochem.* 45:1534, 1985
		Synaptoneurosomes	Gusovsky et al., *Proc. Natl. Acad. Sci. U.S.A.* 83:3003, 1986
		Astrocytoma 1321N1	Masters et al., *Mol. Pharmacol.* 26:149, 1984; Evans et al., *Biochem J.* 232:751, 1985
		Neuroblastoma N1E-115	Cohen et al., *J. Neurochem.* 40:547, 1983; Kanba et al., *Eur. J. Pharmacol.* 125:155, 1986
		Neuroblastoma-glioma NG108-15	Siman and Klein, *J. Neurochem.* 37:1099, 1981
		Superior cervical ganglion	Bone et al., *Biochem. J.* 221:803, 1984; Horwitz et al., *J. Pharmacol. Exp. Ther.* 233:235, 1984
		Pheochromocytoma	Vicentini et al., *J. Cell Biol.* 100:1330, 1985
		Adrenal medulla	Fisher et al., *J. Neurochem.* 37:491, 1981; Mohd. Adnan and Hawthorne, *J. Neurochem.* 36:1858, 1981; Ohsako and Deguchi, *FEBS Lett.* 152:62, 1983
		Pituitary	Young et al., *J. Endocrinol.* 80:203, 1979; Hauser and Parks, *J. Neurosci. Res.* 10:295, 1983
		Pituitary tumor cells	Akiyama et al., *J. Pharmacol. Exp. Ther.* 236:653, 1986
Adrenergic	α_1	Brain slices	Berridge et al., *Biochem. J.* 206:587, 1982; Minneman and Johnson, *J. Pharmacol. Exp. Ther.* 230:317, 1984; Schoepp et al., *J. Neurochem.* 43:1758, 1984; Johnson and Minneman, *Brain Res.* 341:7, 1985; Kendall et al., *Eur. J. Pharmacol.* 114:41, 1985; Fowler et al., *Eur. J. Pharmacol.* 123:401, 1986; Kemp and Downes, *Brain Res.* 371:314, 1986
		Synaptoneurosomes	Gusovsky et al., *Proc. Natl. Acad. Sci. U.S.A.* 83:3003, 1986
Histaminergic	H_1	Brain slices	Daum et al., *Eur. J. Pharmacol.* 87:497, 1983; Daum et al., *J. Neurochem.* 43:25, 1984; Carswell and Young, *Br. J. Pharmacol.* 89:809, 1986; Claro et al., *Eur. J. Pharmacol.* 123:187, 1986; Donaldson and Hill, *Eur. J. Pharmacol.* 124:255, 1986

TABLE 1. *(continued)*

Receptor	Subtype	Tissue	Reference
		Neuroblastoma N1E-115	Cohen et al., *J. Neurochem.* 40:547, 1983; Snider et al., *Soc. Neurosci. Abstr.* 10:276, 1984
		Astrocytoma 1321N1	Nakahata et al., *Mol. Pharmacol.* 29:188, 1986
Serotonergic	5-HT$_2$ and 5-HT$_{1c}$	Brain slices (cerebral cortex)	Conn and Sanders-Bush, *Neuropharmacology* 23:993, 1984; Conn and Sanders-Bush, *J. Pharmacol. Exp. Ther.* 234:195, 1985; Conn and Sanders-Bush, *Life Sci.* 38:663, 1986; Kendall and Nahorski, *J. Pharmacol. Exp. Ther.* 233:473, 1985
		Choroid plexus	Conn et al., *Proc. Natl. Acad. Sci. U.S.A.* 83:4086, 1986
Glutamatergic	?	Brain slices	Nicoletti et al., *Fed. Proc.* 44:480(Abstr.), 1985; Nicoletti et al., *J. Neurochem.* 46:40, 1986; Nicoletti et al., *Proc. Natl. Acad. Sci. U.S.A.* 83:1931, 1986
		Primary cultures	
		Cerebellum	Nicoletti et al., *J. Neurosci.* 6:1905, 1986
		Striatum	Sladeczek et al., *Nature* 317:717, 1985

RECEPTORS PURPORTED TO BE COUPLED TO PHOSPHOINOSITIDE TURNOVER[b]

Receptor	Subtype	Tissue	Reference
Substance K	—	Brain slices	Hunter et al., *Biochem. Biophys. Res. Commun.* 127:616, 1985
Neurotensin	—	Brain slices	Goedert et al., *Brain Res.* 323:193, 1984
		Neuroblastoma N1E-115	Snider et al., *J. Neurochem.* 47:1214, 1986
Cholecystokinin	—	Brain slices	Downes, *Trends Neurosci.* 6:313, 1983
Substance P	P	Brain slices	Watson and Downes, *Eur. J. Pharmacol.* 93:245, 1983; Mantyh et al., *Nature* 309:795, 1984
Vasopressin	V$_1$	Brain slices (hippocampus)	Downes, *Trends Neurosci.* 6:313, 1983; Stephens and Logan, *J. Neurochem.* 46:649, 1986
		Superior cervical ganglion	Bone et al., *Biochem. J.* 221:803, 1984
Bradykinin	—	Neuroblastoma-glioma	Yano et al., *J. Biol. Chem.* 259:10201, 1984; Osugi et al., *Brain Res.* 379:84, 1986
Thyrotropin releasing hormone (TRH)	—	GH$_3$ pituitary cells	Martin, *J. Biol. Chem.* 258:14816, 1983; Drummond and Raeburn, *Biochem. J.* 224:129, 1984; Gershengorn and Paul, *Endocrinology* 119:833, 1986
		Anterior pituitary	Simmonds and Strange, *Neurosci. Lett.* 60:267, 1985
Nerve growth factor (NGF)	—	Superior cervical ganglion	Lakshamanan, *FEBS Lett.* 92:159, 1978; Lakshamanan, *J. Neurochem.* 32:1599, 1979
		Pheochromocytoma	Traynor et al., *J. Neurochem.* 39:1677, 1982
Vasoactive intestinal peptide (VIP)	—	Superior cervical ganglion	Audigier et al., *Brain Res.* 376:363, 1986
Angiotensin	—	Anterior pituitary	Enjalbert et al., *J. Biol. Chem.* 261:4071, 1986

[a] From Fisher and Agranoff [4].
[b] Receptors in this category elicit a minimal increase in phosphoinositide turnover in tissue preparations from the CNS, even though much larger stimulations of inositol lipid turnover are on occasion observed in neurotumor cells or in other neural-related tissues.

process, such as up- or down-regulation of receptors or perhaps of enzymes of the phosphoinositide cycle.

What is the role of PI-anchored proteins?

A growing number of proteins have been shown to be linked to membranes via a glycosidic linkage to PI [13]. These include myelin basic protein, acetylcholinesterase, and Thy-1. In some PI-linked proteins, the diacylglycerol moiety contains not the ST/AR configuration, but dimyristoyl DG. An inositol glycan having messenger properties in insulin action may be derived from a PI-protein anchor [14].

REFERENCES

1. Hokin, L. E., and Hokin, M. R. Effects of acetylcholine on the turnover of phosphoryl units in individual phospholipids of pancreas slices and brain cortex slices. *Biochim. Biophys. Acta* 18:102–110, 1955.
2. Hajra, A. K., Fisher, S. K., and Agranoff, B. W. Isolation, separation and analysis of phosphoinositides from biological sources. In A. A. Boulton, G. B. Baker, and L. A. Horrocks (eds.), *Neuromethods (Neurochemistry), Vol. 8: Lipids and Related Compounds*. Clifton, New Jersey: Humana Press, 1987, *in press*.
3. Michell, R. H. Inositol phospholipids and cell surface receptor function. *Biochim. Biophys. Acta* 415:81–147, 1975.
4. Fisher, S. K., and Agranoff, B. W. Receptor activation and inositol lipid hydrolysis in neural tissues. *J. Neurochem.* 48:999–1017, 1987.
5. Berridge, M. J., Downes, C. P., and Hanley, M. R. Lithium amplifies agonist-dependent phosphatidylinositol responses in brain and salivary glands. *Biochem. J.* 206:587–595, 1982.
6. Irvine, R. F., Letcher, A. J., Heslop, J. P., and Berridge, M. J. The inositol tris/tetrakis phosphate pathway—Demonstration of inositol (1,4,5)-trisphosphate-3-kinase activity in animal tissues. *Nature* 320:631–634, 1986.
7. Wilson, D. B., Connolly, T. M., Bross, T. E., Majerus, P. W., Sherman, W. R., et al. Isolation and characterization of the inositol cyclic phosphate products of polyphosphoinositide cleavage by phospholipase C. Physiological effects in permeabilized platelets and *Limulus* photoreceptor cells. *J. Biol. Chem.* 260:13496–13501, 1985.
8. Sherman, W. R., Ackermann, K. E., Gish, B. G., and Honchar, M. P. The effects of lithium on the inositol phosphate metabolites of phosphoinositide metabolism. In N. G. Bazan, L. A. Horrocks, and G. Toffano (eds.), *Phospholipids in the Nervous System. Biochemical and Molecular Pathology*. New York: Springer-Verlag, in press.
9. Nishizuka, Y. Studies and perspectives of protein kinase C. *Science* 233:305–312, 1986.
10. Ono, Y., Kikkawa, U., Ogita, K., Fujii, T., Kurokawa, T., et al. Expression and properties of two types of protein kinase C: Alternative splicing from a single gene. *Science* 236:1116–1119, 1987.
11. Tsien, R. Y., and Poenie, M. Fluorescence ratio imaging: A new window into intracellular ionic signaling. *Trends Biochem. Sci.* 11:450–455, 1986.
12. Sherman, W. R., Gish, B. G., Honchar, M. P., and Munsell, L. Y. Effects of lithium on phosphoinositide metabolism in vivo. *Fed. Proc.* 45:2639–2646, 1986.
13. Low, M. G., Ferguson, M. A. J., Futerman, A. H., and Silman, I. Covalently attached phosphoinositol as a hydrophobic anchor for membrane proteins. *Trends Biochem. Sci.* 11:212–214, 1986.
14. Saltiel, A. R., Fox, J. A., Sherline, P., and Cuatrecasas, P. Insulin-stimulated hydrolysis of a novel glycolipid generates modulators of cAMP phosphodiesterase. *Science* 233:967–972, 1986.

ADDITIONAL REFERENCES

Inositol Phosphate Chemistry

Cosgrove, D. J. *Inositol Phosphates: Their Chemistry, Biochemistry and Physiology*. Amsterdam: Elsevier, 1980.

Posternak, T. *The Cyclitols*. San Francisco: Holden-Day, Inc., 1965.

General References

Berridge, M. J. Inositol trisphosphate and diacylglycerol: Two interacting second messengers. *Annu. Rev. Biochem.* 56:159–193, 1987.

Bleasdale, J. E., Eichberg, J., and Hauser, G. (eds.). *Inositol and Phosphoinositides. Metabolism and Regulation*. Clifton, NJ: Humana Press, 1985.

Downes, C. P. Agonist-stimulated phosphatidylinositol 4,5-bisphosphate metabolism in the nervous system. *Neurochem. Int.* 2:211–230, 1986.

Putney, J. W., Jr. (ed). *Phosphoinositides and Receptor Mechanisms (Receptor Biochemistry and Methodology*, Vol. 7). New York: Alan R. Liss, 1986.

CHAPTER 17

Regulation of Cyclic Nucleotides in the Nervous System

John K. Northup

Basic Neurochemistry: Molecular, Cellular, and Medical Aspects, 4th Ed., edited by G. J. Siegel et al. Raven Press, Ltd., New York, 1989.
Correspondence to John K. Northup, Department of Pharmacology, Yale University School of Medicine, New Haven, Connecticut 06508.

FUNCTIONS OF CYCLIC NUCLEOTIDES

Cyclic nucleotides are intracellular second messengers

In a number of different cell types, the cellular responses to circulating hormones are mediated by the intracellular second messenger, adenosine-3',5'-monophosphate [cyclic AMP (cAMP)]. In the nervous system, hormones, neurotransmitters, and autacoids have all been demonstrated to affect cellular content of cAMP. It is postulated that cAMP is the cellular mediator of the effects for many of these compounds. The system for receptor regulation of cAMP represents a prototype for the biochemical mechanisms by which intracellular processes are initiated by extracellular ligands. The transduction of the specific receptor-ligand interaction into the regulation of intracellular levels of cAMP is the initial step in a complex pathway of regulation that results in a cellular response. The single molecule, cAMP, can exert diverse actions because of the variation in expression of one or more of the components of the pathway in different cell types. Like cAMP, cyclic guanosine monophosphate (cGMP) has also been implicated as a mediator of extracellular signals. This chapter focuses on the molecular elements involved in the regulation of intracellular levels of cAMP and cGMP, second messengers that account for many of the actions of neurotransmitters, hormones, and autacoids in the nervous system.

In previous editions of *Basic Neurochemistry*, the diverse actions of cyclic nucleotides in neural systems have been described. The emphasis was on probable mediation of physiological processes by these second messengers. It is now firmly established in invertebrate model systems that the cyclic nucleotides mediate neurotransmission and neuromodulation by biogenic amines (see references in Kaczmarek and Levitan [1]). In the mammalian central nervous system, the evidence is less complete, but it is clear that the actions of catecholamines are mediated by cAMP. cAMP and cGMP play important roles in the regulation of vascular contractility and, thus, blood supply to the brain. Also, cAMP mediates the regulation of a number of nonexcitable, metabolic functions of neurons and other cell types. Most of the actions of cyclic nucleotides are mediated by the actions of cyclic nucleotide-dependent protein kinases and thus are more appropriately discussed with the function of protein kinases in brain and their regulation of ion channels (see Chap. 19).

SIX CRITERIA FOR ESTABLISHING SECOND-MESSENGER MEDIATION

Cyclic nucleoside monophosphates (NMP) and pyrophosphate (PPi) are generated from nucleoside triphosphates (NTPs), e.g., ATP and GTP, by the action of specific adenylate and guanylate cyclase enzymes:

$$NTP \xrightarrow[Mg^{2+}]{} 3',5'NMP + PP_i \qquad (1)$$

1. The existence of specific enzymes catalyzing this reaction for cAMP and cGMP is the first criterion for the participation of the cyclic nucleotides in neuronal regulation. A large amount of adenylate cyclase activity is found in the brain compared to that in other tissues. The cyclic nucleotides, once generated, are rapidly degraded by the action of one or more of the cyclic nucleotide phosphodiesterase enzymes:

$$3',5'NMP \xrightarrow[Mg^{2+}]{} 5'NMP \qquad (2)$$

The hydrolysis of the phosphodiester linkage to a 5-monophosphate terminates the biological activity of the cyclic nucleotide.

2. The existence of a pathway for the spe-

cific degradation of a cyclic nucleotide is the second criterion for the participation of these second messengers in cell regulation. Again, the activity of cyclic nucleotide phosphodiesterase is exceptionally high in the nervous system.

3. Hydrolysis-resistant analogues of cyclic nucleotide mimic the hormone or neurotransmitter action.

4. The cellular content of the cyclic nucleotide is altered in response to the neurotransmitter or hormone.

5. Potentiation of the action of hormones or neurotransmitters is produced by agents inhibiting the phosphodiesterase(s) responsible for terminating the action of the cyclic nucleotide.

6. Except for the cGMP regulation of Na^{2+} conductance in vertebrate photoreceptors, all other known actions of cyclic nucleotides are mediated by the activation of specific cyclic nucleotide-dependent protein kinases. The cyclic nucleotide-dependent protein kinases are members of a family of second-messenger-regulated protein kinases that appear to explain the general mechanism through which intracellular second messengers exert their activities. The existence of a specific cyclic nucleotide-activated protein kinase, then, is the sixth criterion for establishing mediation by a cyclic nucleotide.

By these criteria, cAMP is clearly established as the mediator of neurotransmitter regulation of ion currents in gastropod molluscan nervous systems [2]. In these cells, sophisticated reconstruction of the pathway for cAMP regulation has been performed by microinjection of many of the known regulatory ligands for this system as well as the enzymes participating in the pathway, including phosphodiesterase and cAMP-dependent protein kinase. Compelling data have also been obtained for the cAMP mediation of β-adrenergic receptor-activated, voltage-dependent Ca^{2+} channels in myocytes. Finally, data for long-term hyperpolarizing responses to catecholamines in superior cervical ganglion and hippocampus are strongly suggestive of mediation by cAMP (see references in Kaczmarek and Levitan [1]). The only established function for cGMP in neuronal tissue is its mediation of the photoreceptor response to light stimulation, which is discussed in Chap. 7.

What controls the intracellular levels of cAMP?

Intracellular levels of cAMP are determined by the rates of cAMP synthesis from ATP by hormone-sensitive adenylate cyclase and metabolism to 5′-AMP by any of several cyclic nucleotide phosphodiesterases. The activities of adenylate cyclase and cAMP phosphodiesterase are regulated by neurotransmitters and hormones in intact cells; however, only adenylate cyclase can be regulated by these agents in cell-free systems. Regulation of cAMP phosphodiesterase(s) is dependent on the generation of intracellular second messengers, such as cAMP, cGMP, and Ca^{2+}, and the activation of protein kinase(s). There is more information available on the regulation of adenylate cyclase than on regulation of the phosphodiesterases. In the central nervous system, a wide variety of neurotransmitters, autacoids, and hormones regulate cAMP levels by acting as activators and/or inhibitors of the synthesis of cAMP. Table 1 lists the categories of agents known to regulate adenylate cyclase in brain. It should be noted that such representative ligands as 5-hydroxytryptamine (5-HT), adenosine, and vasopressin are known to activate as well as inhibit adenylate cyclase. This occurs through independent, specific receptor subtypes, each recognizing the same ligand. Table 1 is not intended to be a complete list of regulators of neuronal adenylate cyclase; rather, it underscores the importance of these classes of substances as neuroregulators.

TABLE 1. Agents affecting adenylate cyclase in nervous tissue

	Activators	*Inhibitors*
Biogenic amines	Epinephrine	Norepinephrine
	Histamine	Histamine
	Serotonin	Serotonin
	Dopamine	Acetylcholine
Amino acids	—	γ-Aminobutyric acid
Prostanoids	PGE$_1$	—
	PGE$_2$	
Purines	Adenosine	Adenosine
Peptides	Glucagon	Angiotensin II
	Vasoactive intestinal peptide	Somatostatin
	Corticotropin releasing hormone	Opioid peptides
	Adrenocorticotropin hormone	
	Melanocyte stimulating hormone	

ADENYLATE CYCLASE AND REGULATION OF cAMP

Multiple independent proteins are required for regulation of adenylate cyclase

Five independent biochemical activities are involved in hormonal regulation of cAMP synthesis. Figure 1 depicts the molecular entities that carry out these functions within a patch of plasma membrane; however, it is not intended as a representation of the actual topology and distribution of the molecular components of this system. In fact, most of these components are so scarce, on the order of 1/10,000 of the membrane protein, that such a patch of membrane would be relatively rare were the individual components distributed randomly within the cell membrane. Because all of the components must be present to achieve the regulatory properties identified in plasma membranes from brain, it is hypothesized that the cytoskeleton and other factors operate to constrain the components from migrating diffusely over the cell.

Each of the molecular components necessary for the regulation of adenylate cyclase has been isolated. All have been purified to homogeneity, and the entire system reconstituted in artificial lipid bilayers. The mRNAs encoding

prototypical hormone receptors regulating the synthesis of cAMP (β-adrenergic and muscarinic cholinergic receptors) have been identified, as have those for the GTP-binding regulatory proteins, G$_s$ and G$_i$, mediating hormonal regulation of adenylate cyclase (see later).

Adenylate cyclase-linked receptors are a class of homologous proteins

Two classes of neurotransmitter and hormone receptors link to adenylate cyclase either to activate it, e.g., R$_s$, typified by the β-adrenergic receptor (see Chaps. 11 and 18), or inhibit it, e.g., R$_i$, typified by the α$_2$-adrenergic receptor. Since Chapter 18 deals with these proteins in detail, we present here only those features salient to an understanding of hormonal regulation of adenylate cyclase. The receptors are single-subunit transmembrane glycoproteins oriented to recognize neurotransmitters or hormones in the extracellular domain and transmit this information to the cytoplasmic domain. Structures for the β-adrenergic and muscarinic cholinergic receptors deduced from sequences encoded by cloned cDNA predict that these receptors share a structure similar to that of the visual pigment rhodopsin [3] (see Chap. 7). The molecules are characterized by seven hydro-

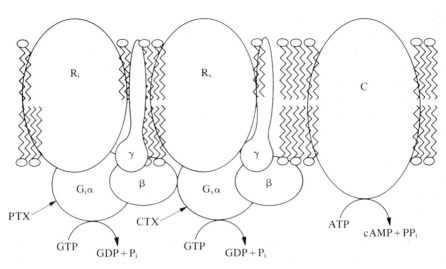

FIG. 1. Molecular components of hormone-sensitive adenylate cyclase. The identified molecular components and their hypothetical organization within the plasma membrane are depicted. The classes of hormone- and neurotransmitter-specific receptors are R_s (stimulatory) and R_i (inhibitory). The G-proteins are G_s (stimulatory) and G_i (inhibitory). Each G-protein is an oligomer of unique α (α_s, α_i) with identical β- and γ-subunits. The adenylate cyclase catalytic subunit is depicted as C. Enzymatic reactions shown are the GTPase of each G-protein and cyclization of ATP to cAMP. Sites for covalent modification by ADP-ribosylating bacterial toxins are depicted as CTX (cholera toxin) and PTX (pertussisen fraction of *Bordetella pertussis* toxin).

phobic, membrane-spanning α-helices separated by hydrophilic stretches of sequence. Indeed, a number of species of independent receptors share this same structure. Such a homology was in fact anticipated from the commonality of function for unique receptors recognizing diverse substances, all of which regulate adenylate cyclase. Further, the structural homology with the visual pigment rhodopsin, which is the primary receptor in photoreceptor neurons, also derives from a commonality of mechanism, in this case, the mediation of the receptor action by G-proteins.

Receptors of the R_s and R_i classes exhibit a characteristic guanine nucleotide-mediated alteration in affinity for agonist ligands. The K_d for activating ligands is increased (affinity is decreased) in the presence of GTP or synthetic analogues of GTP resistant to hydrolysis. Isolated receptors do not display this property, but it is restored when the receptors are reconstituted with the appropriate GTP-binding protein

(G-proteins; see below). The G_s protein produces the GTP-binding shift when added to isolated β-adrenergic receptors, whereas G_i produces this effect when added to α_2-adrenergic receptors. This characteristic is a hallmark of receptors whose function is mediated by one of the G-proteins.

Guanine nucleotide-binding proteins mediate receptor actions on adenylate cyclase

Linking the various neurotransmitter receptors to the regulation of adenylate cyclase are two species of G-proteins termed G_s (adenylate cyclase stimulatory) and G_i (adenylate cyclase inhibitory) [4]. Unlike the receptor glycoproteins, the G-proteins are oligomers of three nonidentical subunits. The GTP-binding subunits are termed the α-subunits. For the G_s protein, the α-subunit has two molecular forms of 47,000 and 44,000 daltons (Da). These represent the protein products of two species of mRNA that are alternative splicing products of a single gene [5]. The G_i protein has a 41,000-Da α-subunit. The GTP-binding α-subunits of G_s and G_i share a region of near identity in their primary structures. This portion of the G-proteins is thought to be the GTP-binding domain, and it has a high degree of homology in primary sequence to the known GTP-binding domain of the bacterial protein synthesis elongation factor EF-Tu. This sequence is also shared by a number of cDNA clones for putative G-proteins [6].

Both G_s and G_i are the cellular targets for mono-ADP ribosylation by the enterotoxins elaborated by *Vibrio cholera* and *Bordetella pertussis*, respectively. These two bacterial toxins have proved invaluable in elucidation of the molecular mechanisms of G-protein function. The α-subunits of G_s and G_i also display low intrinsic GTPase activity, which is stimulated by agonists of the receptors coupled to the G-proteins. This activity and receptor stimulation are blocked by ADP ribosylation. Cholera toxin modification of G_s leads to an irreversible activation of adenylate cyclase, whereas pertussis toxin modification of G_i abolishes hormonal inhibition.

Two other subunits, β and γ, are shared in common by the G_s and G_i proteins. There are two forms of the β-subunit, derived from two independent genes; they are 36,000 and 35,000 Da. The two forms are closely related structures, with an overall homology of greater than 90 percent of deduced amino acid sequence based on cDNA clones [7]. In the isolated G-protein oligomers, the two forms of β-polypeptides appear as a doublet on denaturing polyacrylamide gel electrophoresis. The γ-peptide associated with the G_s and G_i proteins has a mass of approximately 10,000 Da. This subunit is highly hydrophobic and it is thought to provide the membrane insertion for anchoring the G-protein oligomer within the membrane [8]. Subunit interaction then produces an oligomer of αβγ-subunits bound to the cytoplasmic face of the plasma membrane. The proteins are thus situated with access to cytoplasmic cofactors, including GTP and Mg^{2+}, and can interact with transmembrane receptors and adenylate cyclase.

The adenylate cyclase catalyst is a transmembrane glycoprotein

The catalytic component of adenylate cyclase has been purified to homogeneity [9], and an understanding of its structure is emerging. Two important findings have derived from biochemical studies of adenylate cyclase. First, adenylate cyclase appears to be a glycoprotein and may therefore be a transmembrane protein. The significance of this in terms of enzyme regulation is not yet known, but it may facilitate direct communication between extracellular signaling events and catalytic adenylate cyclase. Second, there are two species of this enzyme, as revealed by studies with monoclonal antibodies [10]. One species, found predominantly in brain, is a glycoprotein of approximately 125,000 Da. The second form has been isolated from heart; it is thought to be the predominant form outside the nervous system, and it has a molecular mass of about 150,000 Da. Adenylate cyclase in brain is distinct from that in heart in that it can be activated by Ca^{2+}-calmodulin. Stimulation by the G_s protein is much more pronounced with heart adenylate cyclase. These findings provide a molecular explanation for unique activation of adenylate cyclase in brain by Ca^{2+}-calmodulin.

Much of our understanding of the catalytic component has come from the study of a mutant of a murine lymphoma cell line S49. The cyc^- mutation in S49 lymphoma, misnamed because it was originally thought not to contain adenylate cyclase, does not synthesize the α-subunits of G_s [10]. Membranes derived from cyc^- S49 cells thus contain adenylate cyclase, which cannot be activated by agonists at β-adrenergic receptors because they lack the coupling protein. Neither can the enzyme be activated by nonhydrolyzable guanine nucleotide analogues or fluoride because these act via G_s [11]. The diterpenoid product of the roots of *Coleus forskoli*, forskolin, will directly activate cyc^- adenylate cyclase, and in the presence of Mn^{2+} rather than Mg^{2+} this activation can be as great as that with G_s and guanine nucleotide or fluoride. Forskolin will also activate a biochemically resolved adenylate cyclase catalyst, providing a powerful probe for the activity of adenylate cyclase in the absence of G_s. Affinity chromatography using a forskolin derivative was found to provide the means of isolating adenylate cyclase.

HORMONAL REGULATION AND GUANINE NUCLEOTIDE-BINDING PROTEINS

What is the molecular basis for hormonal regulation of adenylate cyclase?

The studies leading to our current understanding of the molecular mechanisms of hormonal regulation of adenylate cyclase derive from three distinct approaches. First, the biochemical properties of this system have been extensively characterized in intact cells and membrane preparations derived therefrom. The results of these types of studies have provided a basic phenomenology for molecular dissection using the approaches of biochemical resolution and reconstitution. The second approach has been the isolation and purification of identified biochemical activities associated with the membrane-bound adenylate cyclase system. Using the purified components, researchers have been able to identify a number of partial reactions in the overall process of hormonal regulation. Recently, these experiments have culminated in the reconstitution of the entire system from purified components [12]. In the third approach,

biochemical and molecular genetics are currently being applied. Biochemical genetic experiments have identified three different mutations of the G_s protein in the murine lymphoma S49, leading to a phenotype unresponsive to β-adrenergic and prostaglandin E (PGE) stimulation of adenylate cyclase [13].

The G_s protein mediates hormonal activation of adenylate cyclase

The fundamental discovery in the hormonal activation of adenylate cyclase was made in a pioneering set of experiments by Rodbell and his colleagues on the glucagon-stimulated adenylate cyclase systems in hepatocytes and adipocytes [6]. In isolated plasma membranes, the stimulation of adenylate cyclase by glucagon was not observed without the addition of micromolar concentrations of GTP. Concomitantly, addition of GTP was found to enhance dissociation of radiolabeled glucagon from its specific receptor in these membrane preparations. This work defined the existence of the three separate functional activities of R_s, G_s, and C. It required another decade to achieve the isolation of β-adrenergic receptors and the G_s protein. Even though the catalyst has only recently been isolated, the purifications of an R_s and G_s were sufficient to formulate a description of the molecular mechanism of activation of adenylate cyclase. This was possible because of the existence of the cyc^- mutant of S49 lymphoma cells.

The mechanism of activation of adenylate cyclase can be broken down into two partial reactions: (a) receptor-dependent activation of the G_s protein, and (b) activation of adenylate cyclase by G_s. To clarify what is meant by the activation of G_s protein, we now introduce empirical findings from studies of the reconstitution of adenylate cyclase activity in cyc^- membranes. First, although G_s protein has only GTPase activity as an intrinsic enzymatic activity, it is required for the physiological activation of adenylate cyclase. Activation of adenylate cyclase by nonhydrolyzable guanine nucleotide analogues or by aluminum fluoride also requires the G_s protein. Thus, G_s activation is used to describe the state of the G_s protein that confers activation on adenylate cyclase. This state of the G_s protein can be demonstrated by incubating purified G_s with aluminum fluoride or guanine nucleotide analogues in the presence of Mg^{2+}. The aluminum fluoride or guanine nucleotide can be removed, and on addition to cyc^- membranes, adenylate cyclase shows the characteristics of exposure to the activating ligands; G_s has therefore been activated prior to addition to the adenylate cyclase-containing cyc^- membranes. Using nonhydrolyzable guanine nucleotide analogues, this activated state can be maintained for hours after removal of the unbound ligand.

The ability to assess this activated state of the G_s protein allowed detailed investigation of the in vitro regulation of G_s activity by guanine nucleotides and aluminum fluoride [13]. Incorporation of radiolabeled guanine nucleotide analogues can also be assessed and correlated with the activation process. The findings reveal that the activation reaction and the formation of a slowly dissociating G_s/guanine nucleotide complex are highly correlated. The kinetics of this process are not described by a simple bimolecular binding reaction; rather, the overall activation reaction for G_s protein includes a rate-limiting dissociation of a tightly bound GDP prior to binding of guanine nucleotide and the dissociation of the guanine nucleotide-bound α-subunit from the $\beta\gamma$-complex [14]. The latter step may also become rate limiting. In vitro, the guanine nucleotide-bound $\alpha\beta\gamma$-complex can be stabilized and identified by sedimentation. Also, preparations of the G_s α-subunit free of GDP can be isolated, and these show more nearly the expected pseudo-first-order kinetics for binding guanine nucleotide. The kinetics of the activation of G_s in native membranes, measured by assaying detergent extracts of those membranes with cyc^-, more closely resemble that of the G_s $\alpha\beta\gamma$-GDP.

Activation of G_s coincides with dissociation of α- and $\beta\gamma$-subunits

On formation of the slowly dissociating bound state of G_s with nonhydrolyzable guanine nucleotide analogues, the α- and $\beta\gamma$-subunits can be resolved [15]. The guanine nucleotide-bound α-subunit is then found to activate adenylate cyclase in the absence of the $\beta\gamma$-subunit. This is true for cyc^- adenylate cyclase as well as preparations of pure catalyst. Thus, we believe that the activator of adenylate cyclase is the guanine nucleotide-bound G_s α-subunit. In vitro, the $\beta\gamma$-complex acts as an inhibitor of the activation reaction, much as would be predicted from mass action and an equilibrium between basal G_s $\alpha\beta\gamma$ and activated G_s $\alpha + \beta\gamma$ [16]. Whether such dissociation and mass-action behavior pertains to the membrane-bound G_s and hormonal activation of adenylate cyclase remains to be determined.

Stimulatory hormone receptors act as catalysts activating G_s

The above formulation for the activation of G_s and adenylate cyclase suggest that the focus of stimulatory regulation is the generation of a GTP-bound G_s α-subunit from GDP-bound G_s $\alpha\beta\gamma$. Studies with purified β-adrenergic receptors and G_s confirm this [17]. Unlike the characterization of the behavior of G_s in vitro, interaction of G_s with β-adrenergic receptors requires the proper insertion of the receptor and G_s proteins within a suitable phospholipid bilayer. Receptor regulation of the activation of G_s is characterized by an enhanced rate of guanine nucleotide binding and an increased rate of GTP hydrolysis. These are found to be concomitant with an increased rate of G_s activation on addition of β-adrenergic agonists. Under appropriate conditions, one β-adrenergic receptor can activate as many as 30 G_s molecules. The receptor, then, acts catalytically in the activation process. In addition to validating the data obtained using isolated G_s in detergent solutions, studies of reconstituted systems of β-adrenergic receptor and G_s have revealed an additional function for the βγ-complex. Receptor recognition of G_s requires both α- and βγ-subunits. The interacting species are thus thought to be agonist-occupied receptor and GDP-bound G_s αβγ. As a result of this interaction, the bound GDP is released from G_s, facilitating occupancy by GTP and subsequent dissociation of the G_s α-subunit from βγ-subunits.

The reversal from activated to basal adenylate cyclase is dependent on the hydrolysis of GTP by the G_s α-subunit and the reformation of GDP-G_s αβγ on rebinding of the βγ-complex. The G_s molecule is then in its basal state, capable of interacting with another R_s and initiating another cycle of activation. The hydrolysis of GTP has the essential role of driving the cycle of dissociation-activation. Further, it is the energy of GTP hydrolysis that is released in the activation cycle, not the energy of hormone binding to receptor. Thus, receptors are energetically allowed to act as catalysts for the activation cycle.

Using artificial liposomes containing purified β-adrenergic receptor, G_s, and adenylate cyclase, GTP-dependent epinephrine stimulation of adenylate cyclase is reconstituted [12]. Thus, it is believed that stimulation of adenylate cyclase requires only these three components. Data from several cell types, however, suggest that other, yet unidentified, cellular components can be important to the stimulation of adenylate cyclase by receptors. In C6-2B glioma cells, β-adrenergic agonists stimulate intracellular cAMP accumulation nearly 200-fold by activation of adenylate cyclase; in membrane preparations derived from these cells, stimulation is reduced to two- to threefold. If the cells are rendered permeable to substrate ATP and cofactor GTP, adenylate cyclase stimulation remains at the level of intact cells. These and other data using microtubule assembly inhibitors suggest that the cytoskeleton, and perhaps other cellular components, plays a role in the regulation of adenylate cyclase in intact cells. The molecular mechanism described above is a minimal explanation for the stimulatory regulation of adenylate cyclase.

The G_i protein mediates hormonal inhibition of adenylate cyclase

Like the stimulation of adenylate cyclase, receptor-mediated inhibition of adenylate cyclase requires the cofactors GTP and Mg^{2+}. Inhibition by hormones also requires a monovalent cation (Na^+ or Li^+) at concentrations comparable to that of extracellular Na^+. The participation of a G-protein in hormonal inhibition of adenylate cyclase is also demonstrated by the effects of ADP ribosylation of G_i by the fraction of pertussis toxin called islet activating protein (IAP). In contrast to the irreversible activation of adenylate cyclase by cholera toxin, IAP causes an irreversible blockade of the inhibition of adenylate cyclase. The ADP ribosylation of the distinct 41,000-Da G_i α-subunit by IAP identified this as the G-protein mediating the hormonal inhibition of adenylate cyclase [4]. Data obtained from studies of the biochemical properties of the isolated G_i protein, however, conflict with data obtained for hormonal inhibition of adenylate cyclase in some membrane systems. Thus, in contrast to adenylate cyclase stimulation, there is no single molecular mechanism that describes hormonal inhibition of adenylate cyclase. We shall present a model that best describes the data obtained by studies reconstituting adenylate cyclase inhibition with isolated components of the system [18], and then we will address the experimental data that are not described by this model [19].

Two mechanisms apply to the inhibition of adenylate cyclase

Figure 2 is a schematic representation of the molecular mechanisms for hormonal stimulation and inhibition of adenylate cyclase. Like the stimulatory pathway, the inhibitory receptors function catalytically to stimulate the exchange of GTP for bound GDP on the G_i protein. This process leads to the formation of GTP-G_i α and $\beta\gamma$. These reactions can be demonstrated for the isolated G_i protein and in systems of G_i reconstituted with α_2-adrenergic or muscarinic cholinergic receptors. The $\beta\gamma$-subunit released from the G_i oligomer, according to the hypothesis, acts as an inhibitory constraint on the formation of GTP-G_s α.

The data that support the $\beta\gamma$ model for hormonal inhibition of adenylate cyclase come from studies reconstituting α_2-adrenergic inhibition of adenylate cyclase in IAP-treated human platelet membranes [18]. Treatment of platelet membranes with IAP and NAD to ADP-ribosylate the endogenous substrate for IAP, substantially diminishes α_2-adrenergic inhibition of adenylate cyclase. Addition of purified G_i to IAP-treated membranes restores the epinephrine and GTP-dependent inhibition. Like the G_s protein, isolated G_i can be activated in detergent solutions with the addition of Mg^{2+} and guanine nucleotide analogues. The addition of such an activated G_i sample to the platelet membranes produces inhibition independent of GTP or epinephrine. On resolution of the G_i α- and $\beta\gamma$-subunits, the inhibitory activity frac-

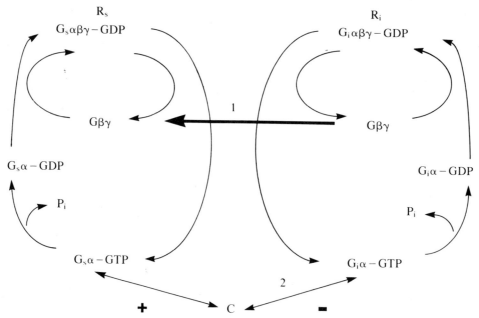

FIG. 2. Mechanisms of regulation of adenylate cyclase. The molecular mechanisms for stimulation and inhibition of adenylate cyclase discussed in the text are schematized here. Components and subunits are labeled as described in the legend for Fig. 1. The catalytic activation of G-proteins by hormone receptors is depicted by their position driving GTP-GDP exchange and subunit dissociation cycle. The potential mechanisms for G_i-mediated inhibition are given as the alternative direct interaction of G_i α-GTP with adenylate cyclase (mechanism 2) or the G_i $\beta\gamma$-subunit interaction with G_s α-GDP (mechanism 1).

tionates with the βγ-complex. The βγ-complex does not restore α_2-adrenergic inhibition to IAP-treated membranes. This requires the α-subunit or oligomer G_i.

Data obtained with pure adenylate cyclase prepared from bovine brain support the model of a βγ-mediated inhibition. In this case, no effect is observed on adding G_i α- or βγ-subunits unless adenylate cyclase is stimulated with the G_s α-subunit and GTP. When the G_s α-subunit and GTP are added to adenylate cyclase the βγ-complex is found to be inhibitory, whereas the G_i α-subunit is without effect. For both platelet membrane and purified adenylate cyclase, G_i α-GDP is found to reverse inhibition by βγ. Finally, in the system of reconstituted β-adrenergic receptor with G_s, addition of βγ inhibits the receptor activation of G_s.

Two experiments provide a discrepant view of the mechanism of hormonal inhibition of adenylate cyclase. Both use the S49 *cyc⁻* membrane as the source of adenylate cyclase. If the activity of G_i subunits is assayed with *cyc⁻* membranes rather than with platelet membranes, the α-subunit is found to inhibit, and the βγ to activate, adenylate cyclase. Second, *cyc⁻* membranes contain somatostatin receptors that are functionally coupled to a GTP-dependent inhibition of adenylate cyclase [19]. Thus, hormonal inhibition is possible in a membrane system that does not contain the G_s α-subunit; however, the activities observed in this membrane system are opposite those found for human platelet membranes, wild-type S49 membranes, or *cyc⁻* membranes reconstituted with G_s. Nevertheless, it is difficult to argue that the βγ complex could mediate inhibition in *cyc⁻* by any G_s-dependent mechanism. There is some evidence that the G_i α-subunit can directly inhibit adenylate cyclase by competing at the G_s α-subunit site on the enzyme. Direct inhibition of adenylate cyclase by βγ has also been reported. Discrepancies between test systems have yet to be resolved.

Stimulatory receptors activate G_i

Using the same procedures that efficiently reconstitute β-adrenergic receptor regulation of the G_s protein, purified turkey erythrocyte β-adrenergic receptors have been found to stimulate GTPase activity and the binding of guanine nucleotide to the isolated G_i protein. Although this is not as efficient as the stimulation of G_s (~30 percent), it is nevertheless a substantial effect. The apparent relative abundance of G_i compared to G_s, suggests that R_s can functionally interact with G_i in a native membrane structure. This could profoundly alter our understanding of the regulation of adenylate cyclase. Current speculation centers on the possibility that sequential generation of activated G_s and then G_i by β-adrenergic receptors occurs. This would provide an immediate attenuation of the stimulatory signal dependent on the degree of saturation of the β-adrenergic receptor.

Phosphorylation of G_i modifies the inhibitory response

In human platelets [20] and other cell types, exposure to tumorigenic phorbol esters that stimulate protein kinase C leads to increased responsiveness to stimulatory agonists and decreased inhibition by inhibitory hormones. Treatment of human platelet membranes with isolated protein kinase C mimics the effects of phorbol esters. Incubation with radiolabeled ATP and protein kinase C identifies an approximately 41,000-Da phosphoprotein that migrates identically with the α-subunit of G_i on sodium dodecylsulfate (SDS) gels. Finally, *in vitro*, the resolved α-subunit of rabbit liver G_i can be shown to be a substrate for phosphorylation by protein kinase C [21]. The data are preliminary, and they have not been replicated *in vivo*. Further, not all cell types in which hormonal inhibition of adenylate cyclase and protein kinase C activity are present show this effect of phor-

TABLE 2.   Identified G-protein α-subunit clones

G-protein type	kDa	Function
G_s "long" (2 types)	46	Couple receptors to activate adenylate cyclase
G_s "short" (2 types)	44.5	Couple receptors to activate adenylate cyclase
G_i (3 types)	40.5	Couple receptors to inhibit adenylate cyclase; other pertussis toxin-blocked processes
G_o	39.9	Pertussis toxin-blocked processes
G_t (2 types)	40	Couple rhodopsin to activate cyclic GMP phosphodiesterase in vertebrate photoreceptors

bol esters. Nevertheless, these data suggest that G_i may be a substrate for modification by protein kinase C and that this phosphorylation leads to diminished activity of the G_i protein. These data constitute the only evidence to date for a cellularly directed covalent modification leading to altered responsiveness of adenylate cyclase.

The βγ-subunit inhibits calmodulin-activated adenylate cyclase

Recent evidence obtained in studies of rat brain adenylate cyclase indicate that the isolated βγ-subunit from G_i is more effective at inhibiting Ca^{2+}-calmodulin-stimulated adenylate cyclase activity than forskolin- or hormone-stimulated activity [22]. This appears to be due to a direct interaction of the βγ-protein with activated calmodulin. Calmodulin and βγ are thus found to be competitive for adenylate cyclase. In addition, isolated βγ is retained by calmodulin-affinity chromatography only in the presence of Ca^{2+}, indicating a specific protein-protein interaction between activated calmodulin and the βγ-protein. The importance of this finding for the regulation of brain adenylate cyclase by hormones is still not known.

A FAMILY OF HOMOLOGOUS SIGNAL-TRANSDUCING G-PROTEINS

In addition to the G_s and G_i proteins described above for the hormone-sensitive adenylate cy-clase system, a number of structurally homologous G-proteins have been identified. A protein designated G_o (for "other") is particularly enriched in brain. Isolation of the cDNA for mRNA encoding G-protein α-subunits has revealed three distinct G_i α-subunit types as well as the G_o α-subunit, which are all pertussis toxin substrates. Table 2 presents the currently identified G-protein α-subunits. The wide variety of receptors in brain that display the hallmark GTP shift in ligand binding suggests that a number of important neural processes other than adenylate cyclase regulation may also be mediated by members of this family of signal-transducing proteins.

HYDROLYSIS OF cAMP IS ACCOMPLISHED BY MULTIPLE PHOSPHODIESTERASES

Hydrolysis of cAMP to 5'-AMP by cyclic nucleotide phosphodiesterases is also under hormonal control

Control of cAMP phosphodiesterase occurs secondarily to the regulation of intracellular second messengers [23]. Such regulation can be determined by measurement of the turnover of cellular cAMP using metabolically labeled ATP in intact cells. Using this technique, muscarinic agonists can be shown to increase the rate of hydrolysis of cAMP in astrocytoma cells. Data from a number of different experiments suggest that this regulation is due to a muscarinic receptor-mediated increase in cellular Ca^{2+} and the subsequent activation of a Ca^{2+}-calmodulin-activated phosphodiesterase. Because control of intracellular Ca^{2+} cannot be replicated in broken-cell systems, an understanding of the mechanics of this kind of regulation depends largely on extrapolation of the *in vitro* properties of the isolated phosphodiesterase.

Also, in contrast to adenylate cyclase, biochemical studies of the cyclic nucleotide phosphodiesterases show marked heterogeneity in physicochemical and regulatory properties of these enzymes [23]. Thus, the phosphodiesterases are characterized as high K_m or low K_m enzymes. Additionally, phosphodiesterase activity is found to be distributed both in cytosolic and membrane fractions. In the brain, cAMP phosphodiesterase activity is distributed approximately equally between soluble and membrane-associated forms. In the absence of purification to homogeneity, it is difficult to assess whether differences in the activities of these enzymes are due to inherent differences in the molecules or whether one or more of the activities might be derived by proteolysis or some other modification of a parent molecule. Therefore, a clear understanding of the significance of the heterogeneity of the phosphodiesterases is dependent on the biochemical characterization of the purified molecules. This has been achieved for the soluble forms of phosphodiesterase from a variety of tissues, including brain. The membrane-associated enzymes have been intransigent to biochemical resolution and purification.

Four basic types of soluble cyclic nucleotide phosphodiesterases have been described

The four basic types are (a) high-K_m Ca^{2+}-calmodulin-stimulated activity, (b) cGMP-stimulated activity, (c) low-K_m cGMP-inhibited activity, and (d) cGMP-specific activity. The first activity is the abundant soluble form of phosphodiesterase in brain. Two isozymes of calmodulin-stimulated phosphodiesterase are found in brain, with molecular masses of 61,000 and 63,000 Da. Structural studies of the isozymes of calmodulin-activated phosphodiesterase have revealed a domain of about 300 amino acid residues highly conserved among these different enzymes. This domain represents a region of the enzyme that can be released by limited tryptic digestion as an unregulated activity. It seems probable that the diverse regulatory properties of the phosphodiesterases result from the addition of specific sequences unique to each of the types of enzyme. For the Ca^{2+}-calmodulin-regulated phosphodiesterases, the N-terminal protein sequence defines the calmodulin-binding domain. Synthetic peptides based on this sequence competitively inhibit activation of the enzyme by calmodulin. The difference in calmodulin sensitivity between the two isozymes may be explained by differences in a limited number of residues in the N-terminus.

Calmodulin-stimulated phosphodiesterase is regulated by cAMP-dependent protein kinase

In addition to regulation by Ca^{2+}-calmodulin, the 61,000-Da isozyme is regulated *in vitro* by cAMP-dependent protein kinase. Phosphorylation of this isozyme decreased its affinity for activation by calmodulin. This would predict a decreased hydrolysis of cAMP during the peak rise in cellular content, with an increased hydrolysis on interruption of the hormonal activation of adenylate cyclase.

GUANYLATE CYCLASE AND REGULATION OF cGMP

Guanylate cyclase is regulated by oxidation

Intracellular levels of cGMP in nervous tissue are regulated by many of the same neurotransmitters that increase Ca^{2+}. Hydrolysis of cGMP is effected by the same family of cyclic nucleotide phosphodiesterases described above for cAMP. At least two distinct types of guanylate cyclase synthesize cGMP from GTP [24]. The soluble form, best described for liver and lung, is a dimer of 82- and 70-kDa polypeptides. This enzyme contains a copper-bound heme group, and it is principally regulated by oxidation and reduction. This regulation appears to account for the vasodilatory actions of nitric oxide-forming nitrates, such as nitroglycerin, which elevate cGMP in vascular smooth muscle. The metabolism of arachidonic acid derivatives, e.g., prostaglandins and thromboxanes, results in the generation of hydroxy and endoperoxides, and this may be the link to hormonal regulation of the soluble guanylate cyclase. Thus, the cGMP message is generated in response to extracellular signals controlling the production of prostaglandins. This may underlie the correlation between the elevation of intracellular Ca^{2+} and cGMP.

Membrane-associated guanylate cyclase is activated by atrial natriuretic peptide

An additional form of guanylate cyclase, bound to the plasma membrane, has recently been isolated as a homogeneous protein. This membrane-bound activity is also a single polypeptide chain of molecular mass 135,000 Da [24]. The protein is highly glycosylated and reduced to 72,000 Da following digestion with endoglycosidase H. This form of guanylate cyclase appears to be directly activated by the atrial natriuretic peptide (ANP) [25]. Thus, the membrane-bound guanylate cyclase appears to contain both the enzymatic activity and the cell-surface recognition site for the atrial natriuretic peptide. At present, this is the only humoral factor known to stimulate the synthesis of cGMP directly, although an active search is currently under way to identify other peptides with similar activity.

REFERENCES

1. Kaczmarek, L. K., and Levitan, I. B. *Neuromodulation. The Biochemical Control of Neuronal Excitability.* Oxford: Oxford University Press, 1987.
2. Gerschenfeld, C. M., Hammond, C., and Paupardin-Tritsch, D. Modulation of the calcium current of molluscan neurones by neurotransmitters. In P. Evans and I. Levitan (eds.), *Ion Channels and Receptors.* Cambridge: The Company of Biologists Limited, 1986.
3. Dohlman, H. G., Caron, M. G., and Lefkowitz, R. J. A family of receptors coupled to guanine nucleotide regulatory proteins. *Biochemistry* 26:2657–2664, 1987.
4. Gilman, A. G. G proteins and dual control of adenylate cyclase. *Cell* 36:577–579, 1984.
5. Harris, B. A., Robishaw, J. D., Mumby, S. M., and Gilman, A. G. Molecular cloning of complementary DNA for the alpha subunit of the G protein that stimulates adenylate cyclase. *Science* 229:1274–1277, 1985.
6. Gilman, A. G. G proteins: Transducers of receptor-generated signals. *Annu. Rev. Biochem.* 56:615–650, 1987.
7. Fong, H. K. W., Amatruda, T. T., Birren, B. W., and Simon, M. I. Distinct forms of the β subunit of GTP-binding regulatory proteins identified by molecular cloning. *Proc. Natl. Acad. Sci. U.S.A.* 84:3792–3796, 1987.
8. Sternweis, P. C. The purified α subunits of G_o and G_i from bovine brain require βγ for association with phospholipid vesicles. *J. Biol. Chem.* 261:631–637, 1986.
9. Smigel, M. D. Purification of the catalyst of adenylate cyclase. *J. Biol. Chem.* 261:1976–1982, 1986.
10. Rosenberg, G. B., and Storm, D. R. Immunological distinction between calmodulin-sensitive and calmodulin-insensitive adenylate cyclases. *J. Biol. Chem.* 262:7623–7628, 1987.
11. Bourne, H. R., Coffino, P., and Tomkins, G. M. Selection of a variant lymphoma cell deficient in adenylate cyclase. *Science* 187:750–752, 1975.
12. May, D. C., Ross, E. M., Gilman, A. G., and Smigel, M. D. Reconstitution of catecholamine-stimulated adenylate cyclase activity using three

purified proteins. *J. Biol. Chem.* 260:15829–15833, 1985.

13. Bourne, H. R., Beiderman, B., Steinberg, F., and Brothers, V. M. Three adenylate cyclase phenotypes in S49 lymphoma cells produced by mutations of one gene. *Mol. Pharmacol.* 22:204–210, 1982.

14. Northup, J. K., Smigel, M. D., and Gilman, A. G. The guanine nucleotide activating site of the regulatory component of adenylate cyclase. Identification by ligand binding. *J. Biol. Chem.* 257:11416–11423, 1982.

15. Ferguson, K. M., Higashijima, T., Smigel, M. D., and Gilman, A. G. The influence of bound GDP on the kinetics of guanine nucleotide binding to G proteins. *J. Biol. Chem.* 261:7393–7399, 1986.

16. Northup, J. K., Smigel, M. D., Sternweis, P. C., and Gilman, A. G. The subunits of the regulatory component of adenylate cyclase. Resolution of the activated 45,000-dalton (alpha) subunit. *J. Biol. Chem.* 258:11369–11376, 1983.

17. Pedersen, S. E., and Ross, E. M. Functional reconstitution of β-adrenergic receptors and the stimulatory GTP-binding protein of adenylate cyclase. *Proc. Natl. Acad. Sci. U.S.A.* 79:7228–7232, 1982.

18. Smigel, M. D., Katada, T., Northup, J. K., Bokoch, G. M., Ui, M., and Gilman, A. G. Mechanisms of guanine nucleotide-mediated regulation of adenylate cyclase activity. In P. Greengard, G. A. Robison, R. Paoletti, and S. Nicosia (eds.), *Adv. Cyclic Nucleotide Protein Phosphorylation Res.* 17:1–18, 1984.

19. Hildebrandt, J. D., Sekura, R. D., Codina, J., Iyengar, R., Manclark, C. R., and Birnbaumer, L. Stimulation and inhibition of adenylyl cyclases is mediated by distinct regulatory proteins. *Nature (Lond.)* 203:706–709, 1983.

20. Jakobs, K. H., Bauer, S., and Watanabe, Y. Modulation of adenylate cyclase of human platelets by phorbol ester. Impairment of hormone-sensitive inhibitory pathway. *Eur. J. Biochem.* 151:425–430, 1985.

21. Katada, T., Gilman, A. G., Watanabe, Y., Bauer, S., and Jakobs, K. H. Protein kinase C phosphorylates the inhibitory guanine-nucleotide-binding regulatory component and apparently suppresses its function in hormonal inhibition of adenylate cyclase. *Eur. J. Biochem.* 151:431–437, 1985.

22. Katada, T., Kusakabe, K., Oinuma, M., and Ui, M. A novel mechanism for the inhibition of adenylate cyclase via inhibitory GTP-binding proteins. Calmodulin-dependent inhibition of the cyclase catalyst by the βγ-subunits of GTP-binding proteins. *J. Biol. Chem.* 262:11897–11900, 1987.

23. Beavo, J. A. Multiple isozymes of cyclic nucleotide phosphodiesterase. In P. Greengard and G. A. Robison (eds.), *Advances in Second Messenger and Phosphoprotein Research*, Vol. 22. New York: Raven Press, 1989.

24. Waldman, S. A., and Murad, F. Cyclic GMP synthesis and function. *Pharmacol. Rev.* 39:163–196, 1987.

25. Kuno, T., Andressen, J. W., Kamisaki, Y., Waldman, S. A., Chang, L. Y., et al. Co-purification of an atrial natriuretic factor receptor and particulate guanylate cyclase from rat lung. *J. Biol. Chem.* 261:5817–5823, 1986.

CHAPTER 18

Regulation of the Responsiveness of Adenylate Cyclase to Extracellular Signals

John P. Perkins

Basic Neurochemistry: Molecular, Cellular, and Medical Aspects, 4th Ed., edited by G. J. Siegel et al. Raven Press, Ltd., New York, 1989.
Correspondence to John P. Perkins, Department of Pharmacology, Yale University School of Medicine, New Haven, Connecticut 06510.

ADAPTIVE CHANGES IN TARGET CELLS

Target cell response is a direct function of the extracellular concentration of a signal molecule under given conditions

Activation of cellular functions by catecholamines thus exhibits dose-response relationships characteristic of the affinity of α- or β-adrenergic receptors for norepinephrine or epinephrine; however, the fact that cells can exhibit states of either refractoriness or supersensitivity to normal physiological concentrations of such neurotransmitters indicates that variations in the response to a given concentration of a particular agonist are possible under different conditions. It follows that the capacity of cells to respond to extracellular signals is actively regulated. Although such regulation of responsiveness seems to occur in general for neurotransmitter-activated adenylate cyclases, evidence with regard to the specific mechanism(s) involved has come primarily from studies of the β-adrenergic receptor-linked adenylate cyclase system. It is known that changes in adenylate cyclase activity are responsible for some of the effects of neurally released norepinephrine on postsynaptic cells [1]. It is also known that when noradrenergic neuronal activity is chronically increased or decreased, the sensitivity to cate-

cholamines of the β-adrenergic receptor-linked adenylate cyclase system of postsynaptic cells is decreased or increased, respectively [2,3]. It has been proposed that adaptive changes in the capacity to make cyclic AMP (cAMP) mediate the associated adaptive changes in the function of postsynaptic cells [2,3].

REGULATION OF THE β-ADRENERGIC RECEPTOR-LINKED ADENYLATE CYCLASE SYSTEM

Adaptive changes are observed in the intact nervous system and in nonneuronal cells in culture

Clonal lines of cultured cells have been used as tools to explore the molecular basis of catecholamine-induced alterations in the β-adrenergic receptor-linked adenylate cyclase system. Thus, catecholamine-induced pathways of desensitization have been described that (a) uncouple receptors from guanine nucleotide binding (G) proteins; (b) reduce receptor number; (c) reduce G-protein activity; (d) reduce adenylate cyclase activity; and (e) increase cAMP degradation. Pathways a and b lead to receptor-specific, or homologous, desensitization. Pathways c, d, and e lead to a generalized decrease in responsiveness of receptors, or heterologous

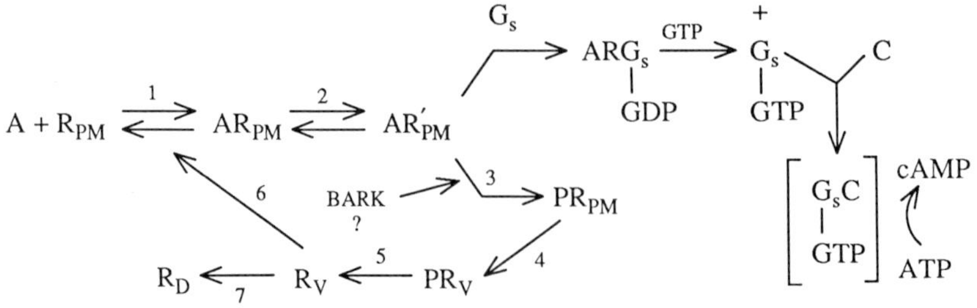

FIG. 1. Model of agonist-induced β-adrenergic receptor desensitization, internalization, and down-regulation: (A) agonist; (R) β-adrenergic receptor; (G_s) guanine nucleotide binding protein; (PM) plasma membrane; (V) cytosolic vesicle; (D) degraded; (P) phosphate; (BARK) β-adrenergic receptor kinase; (C), adenylate cyclase; numerals are reaction numbers (see text).

desensitization. Reactions leading to selective modifications of receptor function have been studied most extensively, and such studies have focused on the β-adrenergic receptor. (The interested reader is referred to more detailed reviews on this topic [2–5].)

Homologous desensitization could be accomplished by selective alteration in the quantity or functional status of the receptor for the inducing agonist

Such a mechanism would keep intact the functional state of all other receptors that influence adenylate cyclase as well as the common components of the system: the G-proteins involved in the activation (G_s) and inhibition (G_i) of adenylate cyclase, and C, the catalytic protein of adenylate cyclase. Whereas cAMP can exert a negative feedback on its own synthesis [3,4], it is possible to define mechanisms for regulation of the β-adrenergic receptor that do not require participation of either cAMP or G-proteins. The observation that the G_s-deficient (cyc^-) and cAMP-dependent protein kinase-deficient (kin^-) lines of S49 lymphoma cells undergo homologous desensitization [6,7] precludes a requirement for cAMP in this process and identifies the β-adrenergic receptor as the site of alteration.

The scheme shown in Fig. 1 has evolved as a plausible model for agonist-induced homologous desensitization. The key feature of the model is the selective phosphorylation of the agonist-occupied form of the receptor (reaction 3, Fig. 1) by a β-adrenergic receptor kinase [8] (this is discussed later). Reactions 1 and 2 in Fig. 1 generate an activated agonist-receptor complex (AR'_{PM}), which is formed in direct proportion to the efficacy of the agonist. AR'_{PM} is shown as the precursor for two pathways, one leading to activation of adenylate cyclase and the other (reaction 3) leading to inactivation of the β-adrenergic receptor. Individual agonists, partial agonists, and antagonists exhibit similar efficacies for activation of adenylate cyclase

and for inactivation of β-adrenergic receptor–mediated responses [9,10]. This relationship supports the idea that efficacy is determined in common for both pathways. The placement of the common intermediate at a location in the sequence prior to the step where β-adrenergic receptor and G_s interact is based on the observation that catecholamines induce the reactions shown in Fig. 1 [1–7] in cyc^- S49 lymphoma cells, which do not express the α subunit of G_s.

Phosphorylation of the β-adrenergic receptor is presumed to convert it to a state that does not cause activation of G_s

Since phosphorylated receptors are thought to retain the capacity to bind ligands, they can be described as being functionally uncoupled. Reaction 4 (Fig. 1) involves endocytosis of PR_{PM} to form PR_V. Reaction 5 (Fig. 1) indicates that dephosphorylation of the receptor occurs to produce R_V, which is physically uncoupled. The fate of such internalized receptors is either to recycle to the cell surface (reaction 6, Fig. 1) or to be degraded after translocation from endosomes to lysosomes (reaction 7, Fig. 1). The scheme is largely speculative but is supported by the following evidence.

Agonist-induced uncoupling of the β-adrenergic receptor-linked adenylate cyclase system may involve phosphorylation of β-adrenergic receptor

Even though it can readily be demonstrated that the β-adrenergic receptor is phosphorylated on exposure of cells to catecholamines, the functional consequences of this reaction remain unclear. It has been difficult to establish unambiguously that phosphorylation of the β-adrenergic receptor, as it occurs in the intact cell, results in either altered function or translocation of the receptor. It has been shown that exposure of frog erythrocytes to isoproterenol results in phosphorylation of the β-adrenergic receptor that was temporally correlated with loss of β-adrenergic receptor-linked adenylate cyclase activity [18]. Receptors solubilized from a crude membrane fraction of desensitized erythrocytes and purified by affinity chromatography exhibited decreased capacity in a reconstitution assay for isoproterenol-stimulated adenylate cyclase activity, relative to β-adrenergic receptors purified from control cells. Furthermore, phosphorylated receptors were associated with the plasma membrane and not with the cytosolic vesicle fraction. It was therefore concluded that β-adrenergic receptor phosphorylation is rapidly reversed on receptor internalization. This observation is consistent with results of previous work showing that internalized β-adrenergic receptors from frog erythrocytes retain functional capacity [4,19], whereas β-adrenergic receptors that accumulate in the plasma membrane of desensitized C6 rat glioma cells exhibit reduced capacity to reconstitute catecholamine-stimulated adenylate cyclase activity [14].

Although the results of studies with whole cells are consistent with the model (Fig. 1), there is no direct evidence that phosphorylation causes altered β-adrenergic receptor function; however, recent studies by Benovic et al. [8,20] could provide a basis for such direct experimentation. These investigators have isolated a seemingly unique protein kinase (β-adrenergic receptor kinase) that phosphorylates only the agonist-bound form of the β-adrenergic receptor. This kinase is a ubiquitous cytosolic enzyme that is translocated to the plasma membrane when cells are exposed to catecholamines or prostaglandins [21]. Still to be established is the effect on β-adrenergic receptor function of its phosphorylation by β-adrenergic receptor kinase. Initial observations indicated that as β-adrenergic receptor kinase is increasingly purified as measured by its phosphorylating activity, its capacity to alter β-adrenergic receptor function is markedly reduced. Additional factors may be required to translate β-adrenergic

receptor phosphorylation into functional modification. In this regard it should be pointed out that whereas phosphorylation of purified β-adrenergic receptor with purified β-adrenergic receptor kinase can achieve levels of 8 mol/mol receptor [20], *in vivo* levels of phosphorylation seldom exceed 2 mol/mol receptor [18]. Possible effects of excess phosphorylation have not been determined. No evidence is available comparing the actual sites phosphorylated *in vitro* and *in vivo*.

At present, β-adrenergic receptor phosphorylation by a kinase selective for the agonist-occupied receptor remains an appealing hypothesis as a generally applicable mechanism for homologous desensitization. Key questions remain, but the tools would appear to be at hand for addressing these concerns.

Is endocytosis of the β-adrenergic receptor involved in agonist-induced desensitization and down-regulation?

An agonist-induced change in the physical state of the β-adrenergic receptor has been described in a number of cells [11–14]. This change of state is observed as an agonist-induced translocation of β-adrenergic receptor from the plasma membrane to a vesicular form ($PR_V + R_V$) that does not sediment in association with plasma membrane markers on sucrose gradient centrifugation. This procedure for isolation of a cytosolic vesicular fraction provides a direct measure of β-adrenergic receptor internalization [12,13]. The appearance of intracellular receptors correlates well with the loss of cell surface receptors as detected by using the hydrophilic radioligand [³H]CGP-12177 [15]. The receptors in preparations such as isolated vesicles are not accessible to hydrophilic agonists or antagonists, which do not readily pass cell membranes, but can be detected with lipophilic radioligands, such as ^{125}I-iodopindolol. Treatment of such vesicles with the pore-forming antibiotic alimethacin markedly increases accessibility of β-adrenergic receptors to hydrophilic ligands. Thus, the properties of β-adrenergic receptors in this physically altered environment are most simply explained if such receptors exist in cytosolic vesicles with the ligand binding site oriented toward the inside of the vesicle; however, there is some controversy over the exact nature of the physical location of these receptors [4].

The agonist-induced translocation reaction is highly specific for the β-adrenergic receptor per se. Neither other receptors linked to adenylate cyclase nor components of the adenylate cyclase system (G_s, G_i, or C) are internalized on exposure of cells to catecholamines [13,16]. Vesicular β-adrenergic receptor exhibits only low-affinity agonist binding [9] that is unaffected by GTP, consistent with the absence of G_s from the vesicles.

The kinetics of β-adrenergic receptor internalization ($t_{1/2}$ = 2–3 min) and recycling ($t_{1/2}$ = 4–6 min) [5,16] are consistent with the kinetics of these same processes for the transferrin receptor, a receptor known to be internalized via clathrin-coated pits [17]. Internalization of the β-adrenergic receptor has been compared in the same cell line with internalization of epidermal growth factor (EGF), which also is known to undergo clathrin-coated pit-mediated endocytosis. In these studies the two processes could not be distinguished [5].

The evidence cited above supports the idea that the β-adrenergic receptor undergoes endocytosis by the clathrin-coated pit mechanism utilized for receptor-mediated endocytosis of polypeptides. No morphological evidence has been presented to confirm this specific internalization mechanism.

Functional uncoupling of the β-adrenergic receptor-linked adenylate cyclase system appears to precede receptor internalization

If β-adrenergic receptors are selectively internalized, without G_s, G_i, or C, they would exist in a physically uncoupled state. Thus, receptor internalization is sufficient to account for agonist-induced uncoupling; but is it the sole mechanism, or is it even necessary? It has been shown in studies with astrocytoma cells that functional uncoupling slightly precedes the formation of internalized β-adrenergic receptors [5,16]. Corroborating evidence for the existence of reaction 3 (Fig. 1) came from experiments in which it was possible to block agonist-induced formation of internalized β-adrenergic receptor completely without blocking agonist-induced uncoupling [5,14,16]. A plausible hypothesis would involve first a chemical modification of the β-adrenergic receptor, resulting in functional uncoupling, followed by receptor internalization, which would maintain the uncoupled state of the system even if the initial chemical modification of the β-adrenergic receptor were to be reversed, for example, by dephosphorylation, within the vesicle.

Agonist-induced down-regulation of the β-adrenergic receptor appears to be mediated by receptor degradation in lysosomes

The model (Fig. 1) indicates that R_V serves as substrate for two reactions, one leading to the return of the β-adrenergic receptor to a functional state in the plasma membrane (reaction 6) and the other leading to receptor degradation (reaction 7). The existence of a pathway for agonist-induced loss of β-adrenergic receptors is a general observation with most cell types and in various tissues. One pathway of β-adrenergic receptor loss may involve ligand-induced receptor degradation, occurring when endosomes containing the receptor fuse with lysosomes. Chuang [11] has reported the agonist-induced appearance of β-adrenergic receptors in lysosomal fractions of bullfrog erythrocytes, and other investigators have reported that exposure of cells to isoproterenol results in degradation of the β-adrenergic receptor [3,5]. *In vivo* it is probable that circumstances leading to long-term changes in the concentration of catecholamines in equilibrium with β-adrenergic receptor will result in changes in the density of receptors [2–4]. The potential physiological significance of this type of β-adrenergic receptor down-regulation should encourage continued assessment of the mechanisms involved.

Although the steps involved in catecholamine-induced desensitization and down-regulation of β-adrenergic receptor function have been elucidated to a significant extent over the past 10 years, the generality of the proposed mechanisms has not been established. For instance, very little is known about ligand-induced down-regulation of receptors for other biogenic amines, such as dopamine, histamine, and serotonin, that stimulate adenylate cyclase activity. Application of the techniques of molecular biology and immunology to studies of receptor processing should help generate the remaining details of the structural determinants of β-adrenergic receptor desensitization and down-regulation. The translation of such information to other receptors may be straightforward if all receptors that stimulate or inhibit adenylate cyclase activity are, as now seems likely, members of a closely related family of proteins [22].

cAMP and protein kinase A appear to be involved in heterologous desensitization of the adenylate cyclase system

Exposure of cells to catecholamines can result in cAMP-independent modification(s) of the β-adrenergic receptor sufficient to lead to its functional uncoupling, physical translocation, and, ultimately, its degradation. Whereas cAMP is not required for these specific changes in the β-adrenergic receptor, it may play a role in the overall cellular response to catecholamines, even to the extent of mediating receptor phosphorylation and desensitization.

Studies carried out with turkey erythrocytes have shown a clear correlation between desensitization and β-adrenergic receptor phosphorylation by a cAMP-requiring pathway [23]; however, the reactions shown in Fig. 1 do not appear to occur in avian erythrocytes. Nevertheless, cAMP-dependent phosphorylation of β-adrenergic receptor may play an important role in desensitization in mammalian cells. The mammalian β-adrenergic receptor is known to contain two consensus substrate sites for protein kinase A [22], and phosphorylation of purified mammalian β-adrenergic receptor by the catalytic subunit of protein kinase A has been reported [24]. Phosphorylation reduced the capacity of the β-adrenergic receptor to mediate isoproterenol-stimulated GTPase activity of G_s in a reconstitution assay. Thus, in the agonist-challenged cell, a rise in cAMP could induce receptor phosphorylation via protein kinase A. In fact, results of numerous studies have implicated cAMP as a component of one or more pathways for heterologous desensitization [4,5]. It will be important to determine if β-adrenergic receptors are phosphorylated at both protein kinase A and β-adrenergic receptor kinase sites during exposure of intact cells to agonists. It remains possible that these two pathways could interact, but more studies aimed at this question are required.

Phosphorylation of β-adrenergic receptor can also be catalyzed by protein kinase C with the use of purified components [24] or by activation of endogenous protein kinase C following exposure of intact cells to phorbol esters [25]. These observations suggest an additional pathway for regulation of β-adrenergic receptor function via phosphorylation; namely, via neurotransmitter-mediated activation of phospholipase C and the intracellular accumulation of diacylglycerol and Ca^{2+}.

REFERENCES

1. Nestler, E. J., and Greengard, P. Protein phosphorylation in the nervous system. New York: Wiley-Interscience, 1984.

2. Perkins, J. P., Harden, T. K., and Harper, J. F. Acute and chronic modulation of the responsiveness of receptor-associated adenylate cyclases. In: J. A. Nathanson and J. W. Kebabian (eds.), *Handbook of Experimental Pharmacology.* New York: Springer-Verlag, 1982, Vol. 58, pp. 185–224.

3. Harden, T. K. Agonist-induced desensitization of the β-adrenergic receptor-linked adenylate cyclase. *Pharmacol. Rev.* 35:5–32, 1983.

4. Sibley, D. R., and Lefkowitz, R. J. Molecular mechanisms of receptor desensitization using the β-adrenergic receptor-coupled adenylate cyclase system as a model. *Nature* 317:124–129, 1985.

5. Hertel, C., and Perkins, J. P. Receptor-specific mechanisms of desensitization of β-adrenergic receptor function. *Mol. Cell. Endocrinol.* 37:245–256, 1984.

6. Shear, M., Insel, P. A., Melmon, K. L., and Cofino, P. Agonist-specific refractoriness induced by isoproterenol. *J. Biol. Chem.* 251:7572–7578, 1976.

7. Green, D. A., and Clark, R. B. Adenylate cyclase coupling proteins are not essential for agonist-specific desensitization of lymphoma cells. *J. Biol. Chem.* 256:2105–2108, 1981.

8. Benovic, J. L., Strasser, R. H., Caron, M. G., and Lefkowitz, R. J. β-Adrenergic receptor kinase: Identification of a novel protein kinase that phosphorylates the agonist-occupied form of the receptor. *Proc. Natl. Acad. Sci. U.S.A.* 83:2797–2801, 1986.

9. Su, Y. F., Harden, T. K., and Perkins, J. P. Catecholamine-specific desensitization of adenylate cyclase: Evidence for a multistep process. *J. Biol. Chem.* 255:7410–7419, 1980.

10. Pittman, R. N., Reynolds, E. E., and Molinoff, P. B. Relationship between intrinsic activities of agonists in normal and desensitized tissue and agonist-induced loss of *beta* adrenergic receptors. *J. Pharmacol. Exp. Ther.* 230:614–618, 1984.

11. Chuang, D. M. Internalization of β-adrenergic receptor binding sites: Involvement of lysosomal enzymes. *Biochem. Biophys. Res. Commun.* 105:1466–1472, 1982.

12. Harden, T. K., Cotton, C. Y., Waldo, G. L., Lutton, J. K., and Perkins, J. P. Catecholamine-induced alteration in the sedimentation behavior of membrane-bound β-adrenergic receptors. *Science* 210:441–443, 1980.

13. Stadel, J. M., Strulovici, B., Nambi, P., Lavin, T. N., Briggs, M. M., Caron, M. G., and Lefkowitz, R. J. Desensitization of the β-adrenergic receptor of frog erythrocytes: Recovery and characterization of the down-regulated receptors in sequestered vesicles. *J. Biol. Chem.* 258:3032–3038, 1983.

14. Kassis, S., Olasmaa, M., Sullivan, M., and Fishman, P. H. Desensitization of the β-adrenergic receptor-coupled adenylate cyclase in cultured cells: Receptor sequestration versus receptor function. *J. Biol. Chem.* 261:12233–12237, 1986.

15. Staehelin, M., and Simons, P. Rapid and reversible disappearance of β-adrenergic cell surface receptors. *EMBO J.* 1:187–190, 1982.

16. Waldo, G., Northup, J. K., Perkins, J. P., and Harden, T. K. Characterization of an altered membrane form of the β-adrenergic receptor produced during agonist-induced desensitization. *J. Biol. Chem.* 258:13900–13908, 1983.

17. Bergeron, J. J. M., Cruz, J., Kahn, M. N., and Posner, B. I. Uptake of insulin and other ligands into receptor-rich endocytic components of target cells: The endosomal apparatus. *Annu. Rev. Physiol.* 47:383–403, 1985.

18. Sibley, D. R., Strasser, R. H., Benovic, J. L., Daniel, K., and Lefkowitz, R. J. Phosphorylation/dephosphorylation of the β-adrenergic receptor regulates its functional coupling to adenylate cyclase and subcellular distribution. *Proc. Natl. Acad. Sci. U.S.A.* 83:9408–9412, 1986.

19. Strulovici, B., Stadel, J. M., and Lefkowitz, R. J. Functional integrity of desensitized β-adrenergic receptors: Internalized receptors reconstitute catecholamine-stimulated adenylate cyclase. *J. Biol. Chem.* 258:6410–6414, 1983.

20. Benovic, J. L., Mayor, F., Jr., Staniszewski, C., Lefkowitz, R. J. and Caron, M. G. Purification and characterization of the β-adrenergic receptor kinase. *J. Biol. Chem.* 262:9026–9032, 1987.

21. Strasser, R. H., Benovic, J. L., Caron, M. G., and Lefkowitz, R. J. β-Agonist and prostaglandin E₁-induced translocation of the β-adrenergic receptor kinase: Evidence that the kinase may act on multiple cyclase-coupled receptors. *Proc. Natl. Acad. Sci. U.S.A.* 83:6362–6366, 1986.

22. Dohlman, H. G., Caron, M. G., and Lefkowitz, R. J. A family of receptors coupled to guanine nucleotide regulatory proteins. *Biochemistry* 26:2657–2664, 1987.

23. Sibley, D. R., Peters, J. R., Nambi, P., Caron, M. G., and Lefkowitz, R. J. Desensitization of turkey erythrocyte adenylate cyclase. *J. Biol. Chem.* 259:9742–9749, 1984.

24. Sibley, D. R., Benovic, J. L., Caron, M. G., and Lefkowitz, R. J. Regulation of transmembrane signaling by receptor phosphorylation. *Cell* 48:913–922, 1987.

25. Kelleher, D. J., Pessin, J. E., Ruoho, A. E., and Johnson, G. L. Phorbol ester induces desensitization of adenylate cyclase and phosphorylation of the β-adrenergic receptor in turkey erythrocytes. *Proc. Natl. Acad. Sci. U.S.A.* 81:4316–4320, 1984.

CHAPTER 19

Protein Phosphorylation and the Regulation of Neuronal Function

Eric J. Nestler and Paul Greengard

Basic Neurochemistry: Molecular, Cellular, and Medical Aspects, 4th Ed., edited by G. J. Siegel et al. Raven Press, Ltd., New York, 1989. Correspondence to Eric J. Nestler, Departments of Psychiatry and Pharmacology, Yale University School of Medicine, New Haven, CT 06508; Paul Greengard, Ph.D., Laboratory of Molecular and Cellular Neuroscience, The Rockefeller University, 1230 York Avenue, New York, NY 10021.

373

PROTEIN PHOSPHORYLATION IS A FINAL COMMON PATHWAY

There is now convincing evidence that protein phosphorylation is a final common pathway of fundamental importance in biological regulation. Numerous extracellular signals, both inside and outside the nervous system, are known to produce many of their diverse physiological effects by regulating the state of phosphorylation of specific phosphoproteins in their target cells [1–3]. The large number of molecular pathways involving protein phosphorylation that have been revealed over the past decade are shown schematically in Fig. 1. In this chapter, we present an overview of the vital role played by protein phosphorylation in the regulation of neuronal function.

All protein phosphorylation systems consist of a protein kinase, a protein phosphatase, and a substrate protein

These components interact according to the scheme shown in the box in Fig. 1. A substrate protein is converted from the dephospho form to the phospho form by a protein kinase, and the phospho form is converted back to the dephospho form by a protein phosphatase.

Most classes of protein kinase phosphorylate substrate proteins on serine or threonine residues, but one class, referred to as protein tyrosine kinases, phosphorylates substrate proteins solely on tyrosine residues. In all cases, the kinases catalyze the transfer of the terminal (γ) phosphate group of ATP to the hydroxyl moiety in the respective amino acid residue; Mg^{2+} is required for this reaction. Protein phosphatases catalyze the cleavage of this phosphoester bond through hydrolysis.

A change in the state of phosphorylation of a substrate protein, and thereby in its functional activity, can be achieved physiologically through increases or decreases in the activity of either a protein kinase or a protein phosphatase. Examples of each of these mechanisms are known to occur in the nervous system; however, activation of specific protein kinases appears to be the most prominent mechanism in nervous tissue by which extracellular signals regulate protein phosphorylation.

Individual steps in the molecular pathways through which extracellular signals regulate neuronal function through protein phosphorylation are shown in Fig. 2. Extracellular signals, or first messengers, in the nervous system include a variety of neurotransmitters and hor-

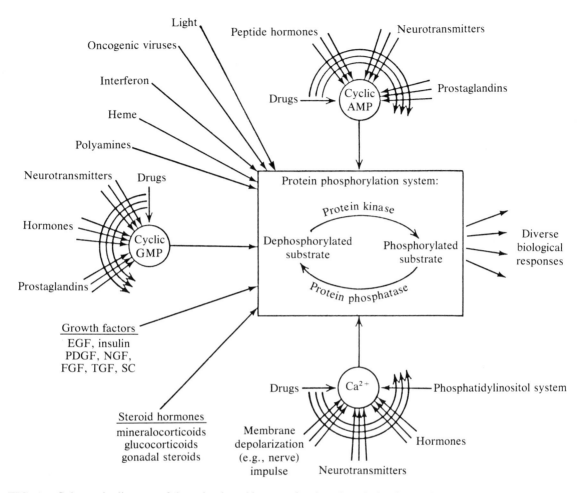

FIG. 1. Schematic diagram of the role played by protein phosphorylation in mediating some of the biological effects of a variety of regulatory agents. Many of these agents regulate protein phosphorylation through altering intracellular levels of a second messenger, cAMP, cGMP, or Ca^{2+}. Other agents appear to regulate protein phosphorylation through mechanisms that do not involve these second messengers. Most drugs regulate protein phosphorylation by affecting the ability of first messengers to alter second-messenger levels (*curved arrows*). A small number of drugs (e.g., phosphodiesterase inhibitors, Ca^{2+} channel blockers) regulate protein phosphorylation by directly altering second-messenger levels (*straight arrows*): (EGF) epidermal growth factor; (PDGF) platelet-derived growth factor; (NGF) nerve growth factor; (FGF) fibroblast growth factor; (TGF) transforming growth factor; (SC) somatomedin C. (From Nestler and Greengard [1].)

mones, as well as light and nerve impulses themselves. In most cases, these first messengers activate protein kinases indirectly by increasing the intracellular level of a second messenger in target neurons. Prominent second messengers in the nervous system include cyclic AMP (cAMP), cyclic GMP (cGMP), Ca^{2+}, and diacylglycerol. The next steps in these pathways are the activation of specific classes of protein kinase by these second messengers and the subsequent phosphorylation of specific substrate proteins, leading, through one

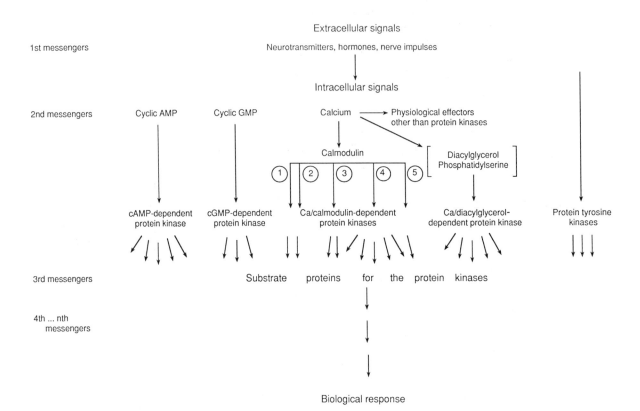

FIG. 2. Signals in the brain. Extracellular signals (first messengers) produce specific biological responses in target neurons via a series of intracellular signals (second, third, etc., messengers). Second messengers in the brain include cAMP, cGMP, Ca^{2+}, and diacylglycerol. cAMP and cGMP produce most of their second-messenger actions through the activation of virtually one type of cAMP-dependent protein kinase and one type of cGMP-dependent protein kinase, respectively. The former enzyme exhibits a broad substrate specificity and the latter a more restricted specificity. Ca^{2+} exerts many of its second-messenger actions through the activation of Ca^{2+}-dependent protein kinases, as well as through a variety of physiological effectors other than protein kinases. Ca^{2+} activates protein kinases in conjunction with calmodulin or diacylglycerol. There are at least five types of Ca^{2+}/calmodulin-dependent protein kinases in brain: (1) phosphorylase kinase, which phosphorylates only phosphorylase (and possibly glycogen synthase); (2) myosin light-chain kinase, which phosphorylates only myosin light chain; (3) Ca^{2+}/calmodulin-dependent protein kinase I; (4) Ca^{2+}/calmodulin-dependent protein kinase II; and (5) Ca^{2+}/calmodulin-dependent protein kinase III. The substrate specificities of the latter three enzymes have not been established with certainty; Ca^{2+}/calmodulin-dependent protein kinase II appears to have a broad substrate specificity, whereas Ca^{2+}/calmodulin-dependent protein kinases I and III appear to phosphorylate only a small number of substrates. Brain also contains a high level of protein tyrosine kinase activity and numerous substrates for this activity; however, the exact number of such kinases and the nature of the cellular messengers that regulate them have not been established. In some cases, the phosphorylation of substrate proteins, or third messengers, appears to result directly in the biological response. In other cases, it seems to produce the biological response indirectly through fourth, fifth, sixth, etc., messengers. (Modified from Nestler and Greengard [20].)

or more steps, to the production of specific biological responses.

The brain has extraordinarily active protein phosphorylation systems compared to nonnervous tissue

In Fig. 3, it can be seen that cAMP-dependent and Ca^{2+}-dependent protein phosphorylation are much more prominent in extracts of cerebral cortex and cerebellum than in various nonneuronal tissues, namely, liver, kidney, heart, and lung. The more prominent protein phosphorylation observed in neuronal tissue probably reflects higher concentrations of various protein kinases as well as higher concentrations and larger numbers of substrate proteins. Neuronal tissue, because it contains a myriad of distinct cell types, might be expected to contain a larger variety of substrate proteins than nonneural tissue.

PROTEIN KINASES

Protein kinases differ in their cellular and subcellular distribution, substrate specificity, and regulation by cellular messengers

Among the most prominent protein kinases in the brain are those activated by the second messengers cAMP, cGMP, Ca^{2+}, and diacylglycerol [1,2,4–6]. These protein kinases, whose characteristics are summarized in Table 1, are named for the second messengers that activate them.

The brain contains two subtypes of cAMP-dependent protein kinase

Referred to as types I and II, these subtypes contain identical catalytic subunits but distinct regulatory subunits, designated R-I and R-II, respectively. In both cases the holoenzyme,

which consists of a tetramer of two catalytic and two regulatory subunits, is inactive; cAMP activates the holoenzyme by binding to the regulatory subunits, thereby causing dissociation of the holoenzyme into free regulatory and free (active) catalytic subunits. Both types of cAMP-dependent protein kinase show a wide cellular and subcellular distribution in the brain. Both types also exhibit a broad substrate specificity; i.e., they phosphorylate a large number of physiological substrate proteins.

One type of cGMP-dependent protein kinase is known to exist

The holoenzyme is a dimer of two identical subunits, each containing a regulatory (cGMP binding) domain and a catalytic domain. As with the cAMP-dependent enzyme, cGMP activates the inactive holoenzyme by binding to the regulatory domain of the molecule; however, unlike the cAMP-dependent enzyme, activation of the cGMP-dependent holoenzyme is not accompanied by dissociation of the subunits. cGMP-dependent protein kinase shows a much more limited cellular distribution and substrate specificity than cAMP-dependent protein kinase. This probably reflects the smaller number of second-messenger actions of cGMP in the regulation of cell function.

Multiple forms of Ca^{2+}-dependent protein kinase are known to exist, and all have been found in the nervous system

The Ca^{2+}-dependent protein kinases are divided into two subclasses. One is activated by Ca^{2+} in conjunction with the Ca^{2+}-binding protein calmodulin and is referred to as Ca^{2+}/calmodulin-dependent protein kinase. The other is activated by Ca^{2+} in conjunction with phosphatidylserine and diacylglycerol and is referred to as Ca^{2+}/diacylglycerol-dependent protein kinase, Ca^{2+}/phosphatidylserine-de-

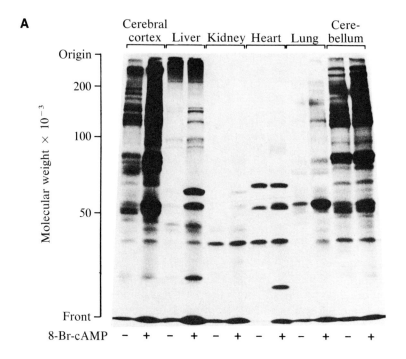

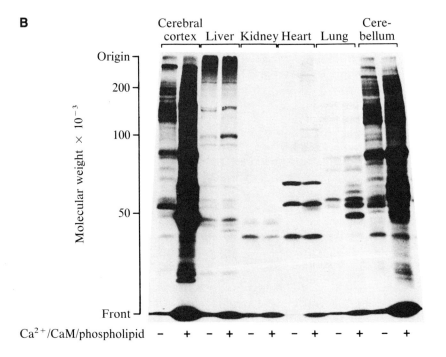

pendent protein kinase, Ca^{2+}/phospholipid-dependent protein kinase, or protein kinase C. The brain contains at least five types of Ca^{2+}/calmodulin-dependent protein kinase, each with very different properties. Multiple forms of Ca^{2+}/diacylglycerol-dependent protein kinase have been reported to exist in brain [7], but they appear to have very similar properties and may represent isozymes of this kinase. Ca^{2+}/calmodulin-dependent protein kinase II and Ca^{2+}/diacylglycerol-dependent protein kinase, like the cAMP-dependent enzyme, exhibit broad cellular distribution and substrate specificity, and each probably mediates many of the second-messenger actions of Ca^{2+} in many types of neurons. The other four types of Ca^{2+}/calmodulin-dependent protein kinase appear to phosphorylate only a few substrate proteins under physiological conditions, and each probably mediates relatively few second-messenger actions of Ca^{2+} in the nervous system [1,2,8,9].

There is evidence that second-messenger-dependent protein kinases mediate a number of physiological actions of extracellular signals

The intracellular injection of cAMP-dependent protein kinase, cGMP-dependent protein kinase, Ca^{2+}/calmodulin-dependent protein kinase II, or Ca^{2+}/diacylglycerol-dependent protein kinase into particular types of neurons has been shown to mimic specific physiological responses to known neurotransmitters in those neurons [1,10–15]. Where specific inhibitors of the kinases are available, their injection has been shown to block the ability of the neurotransmitters to elicit those responses. Taken together, these findings demonstrate that activation of protein kinases is both a necessary and sufficient step in the sequence of events by which certain first messengers produce some of their physiological effects. Most of the earlier injection studies were performed with invertebrate neurons because of their relatively large size and the ease with which they can be identified. In later years, as electrophysiological techniques have become increasingly sophisticated, it has been possible to obtain similar results in vertebrate nervous systems, including, in some cases, mammalian neurons.

The brain contains several types of protein kinase that are not regulated by the second messengers cAMP, cGMP, Ca^{2+}, and diacylglycerol

Listed in Table 2 are enzymes referred to as second-messenger-independent protein kinases [1]. Prominent among these are protein kinases that phosphorylate substrate proteins at tyrosine residues and are known as protein tyrosine kinases. The brain contains a high level of protein tyrosine kinase activity compared to most nonneuronal tissues, although it is not known how many distinct types of enzyme are involved. The brain also contains a number of endogenous substrates for this protein tyrosine

---

←

FIG. 3. Autoradiographs showing (**A**) cAMP-dependent and (**B**) Ca^{2+}-dependent endogenous protein phosphorylation in extracts of rat tissues. Various tissues were removed from rats shortly after decapitation and were homogenized and then centrifuged at low speed (700 × g) for 10 min to remove nuclei and large cellular debris. Aliquots (each containing 150 μg protein) were incubated with [γ-^{32}P]ATP for 1 min at 30°C in the presence (+) or absence (−) of 10 μM 8-bromo (8-Br)-cAMP (**A**) or 0.5 mM free Ca^{2+} plus 10 μg/ml calmodulin (CaM) plus 50 μg/ml phosphatidylserine (**B**). The reaction was terminated by the addition of sodium dodecyl sulfate (SDS), and the samples were heated at 100°C for 2 min. The entire sample was then subjected to SDS-polyacrylamide gel electrophoresis and autoradiography. Cerebral cortex and cerebellum exhibit much more prominent cAMP-dependent and Ca^{2+}-dependent protein phosphorylation than do the nonneuronal tissues liver, kidney, heart, and lung. (S. I. Walaas and P. Greengard, *unpublished observations*.) (From Nestler and Greengard [1].)

TABLE 1. Some properties of second-messenger-dependent protein kinases

Property	cAMP-dependent protein kinase	cGMP-dependent protein kinase	Phosphorylase kinase	Myosin light-chain kinase	Ca²⁺/calmodulin-dependent protein kinase I	Ca²⁺/calmodulin-dependent protein kinase II	Ca²⁺/calmodulin-dependent protein kinase III	Ca²⁺/diacylglycerol-dependent protein kinase
Holoenzyme composition	R_2C_2	Homodimer	$(\alpha, \beta, \gamma, \delta)_4$	Monomer	Monomer[a]	Unknown[b]	Monomer[a]	Monomer
Holoenzyme molecular weight[c]	Type I 170 Type II 190	150	~1,300	124	49	~600	140	87
Ratio of subunits[c]	R:C = 1:1		$\alpha:\beta:\gamma:\delta =$ 1:1:1:1			Unknown[b]		
Subunit molecular weight[d]	C = 41 R-I = 47 R-II = 54	75	α = 145 β = 128 γ = 45 δ = 17[e]	130[f]	α = 42 β = 39 γ = 37	α = 50 β = 60	α = 90 β = 85	82[g]
Catalytic subunit	C		γ		α, β, γ	α and β	α and β	
Activators	cAMP	cGMP	Ca²⁺/ calmodulin	Ca²⁺/ calmodulin	Ca²⁺/ calmodulin	Ca²⁺/ calmodulin	Ca²⁺/ calmodulin	Ca²⁺/phospha-tidylserine diacylglycerol phorbol esters
Inhibitors	PKI[h] H7, H8	H7, H8	TFP[i] W7	TFP[i] W7	TFP[i] W7	TFP[i] W7	TFP[i] W7	TFP[i] W7 H7 ? Calmodulin
Autophospho-rylation	Yes (R-II only)	Yes	Yes	Yes	Yes	Yes	Yes	Yes
Effect of autophospho-rylation	Stimulates activity by preventing reassociation	Unknown	Stimulates activity	Unknown	Unknown	Activity becomes independent of Ca²⁺/ calmodulin	Unknown	Unknown

Substrate specificity	Broad	Narrow	Narrow	Narrow	Narrow	Broad	Narrow	Broad
Known neuronal substrates[j]	Synapsin I TH AChR DARPP-32 MAP-2 Protein III Many others	G-substrate	Phosphorylase	Myosin LC	Synapsin I Protein III	Synapsin I MAP-2 Glycogen synthase Myosin LC TH Trypt. Hyd.	100 kDa	TH MAP-2 Myelin basic protein 87 kDa B-50 Many others
Regional distribution	Broad	Less broad	Broad	Broad	Broad	Broad	Broad	Broad
Subcellular distribution	Particulate and cytosolic	Predominantly cytosolic	Cytosolic	Cytosolic	Cytosolic	Particulate and cytosolic	Cytosolic	Particulate and cytosolic

[a] It is not known whether the lower molecular weight subunits represent proteolytic fragments or whether they represent distinct isozymes.

[b] Possibly a dodecamer, the ratio of α to β subunits is roughly 3:1 in whole brain, but varies significantly among different brain regions. It is not known whether the enzyme is a heteromer (α and β subunits occurring together within the same holoenzyme), in which case different brain regions would contain holoenzyme composed of different subunit ratios, or a homomer (with individual molecules containing all α or all β subunits), in which case different brain regions would contain different amounts of each isozyme.

[c] Molecular weight determined by gel filtration, and expressed as kilodaltons (kDa).

[d] Molecular weight determined by SDS-polyacrylamide gel electrophoresis, and expressed as kilodaltons (kDa).

[e] The δ subunit is calmodulin.

[f] Molecular weight varies due to proteolysis and species differences.

[g] Multiple types of this enzyme have been distinguished.

[h] (PKI) protein kinase inhibitor protein.

[i] (TFP) (trifluoperazine) and W7 are two of a large number of hydrophobic compounds that inhibit, at relatively high concentrations, all calcium/calmodulin-dependent protein kinases, as well as other calcium/calmodulin-dependent enzymes and calcium/diacylglycerol-dependent protein kinase.

[j] (TH) tyrosine hydroxylase; (MAP-2) microtubule-associated protein-2; (AChR) nicotinic acetylcholine receptor; (Myosin LC) myosin light chain; (Trypt. Hyd.) tryptophan hydroxylase.

TABLE 2.   Second-messenger-independent
protein kinases found in brain[a]

Protein tyrosine kinases
Rhodopsin kinase
β-Adrenergic receptor kinase
Casein (or phosvitin) kinase
Double-stranded RNA-dependent protein kinase
Coated-vesicle kinase
Neurofilament kinase

---

[a] Table 2 does not include the large number of second-messenger-independent protein kinases that play a role in generalized cellular processes, such as intermediary metabolism, protein synthesis, and cell growth. Although most of these have not been specifically identified in brain, it is likely that they exist in that organ, since the physiological functions that they subserve are probably common to all animal cells.

kinase activity. In nonneuronal tissue, this class of enzyme has in some cases been shown to be associated with receptors for one or another growth factor, such as insulin and epidermal growth factor [3]. In those cases for which the mechanism has been determined, the growth factor activates the kinase directly without an intervening second messenger. In such cases, the protein kinase activity resides within the growth factor receptor molecule and becomes activated when the growth factor binds to its receptor. Insulin-dependent protein kinase activity has been observed in brain, but much of the protein tyrosine kinase activity in the nervous system remains unaccounted for with respect to the extracellular messengers that regulate it. Protein tyrosine kinases have also been shown to represent the transforming agents of a number of oncogenic viruses and the normal cellular homologues of these gene products [2,3]. There is a high level of protein tyrosine kinase activity and a low level of growth and differentiation in the adult mammalian nervous system. Therefore, it seems likely that some of the protein tyrosine kinase activity of the mature, differentiated mammalian nervous system is involved in the regulation of adult neuronal function rather than in the regulation of growth and differentiation of neurons.

Virtually every known type of protein kinase undergoes autophosphorylation, a reaction in which the activated protein kinase molecule phosphorylates itself [1,2,4,5]. In most cases, autophosphorylation is known to be an intramolecular reaction; it is not known whether intermolecular reactions are also involved under physiological conditions. The autophosphorylation of a number of protein kinases is associated with an increase in kinase activity. In some instances, such as with certain protein tyrosine kinases, autophosphorylation may represent an obligatory step in the sequence of molecular events through which those kinases are activated. In other instances, such as with type II cAMP-dependent protein kinase, autophosphorylation may represent a positive feedback mechanism through which the kinases are activated to a greater extent. In the case of Ca^{2+}/calmodulin-dependent protein kinase II, autophosphorylation causes the enzyme activity to become independent of Ca^{2+} and calmodulin.

PROTEIN PHOSPHATASES

Much less is known about protein phosphatases than about protein kinases. This reflects the general inclination in biological research to concentrate on "turn-on" processes as opposed to "turn-off" processes. It also reflects the greater technical difficulties associated with the study of protein phosphatases. To study kinases, the investigator simply requires radioactively labeled ATP and purified substrate proteins. To study phosphatases, the investigator requires radioactively labeled ATP, purified substrate proteins, and purified protein kinases. Substrate proteins are phosphorylated, and then the phosphorylated substrates are purified for use in assaying phosphatase activity. Despite these difficulties, a number of investigators in recent years have begun a systematic characterization of protein phosphatases in the nervous system [16].

TABLE 3. Classification of protein phosphatases[a,b]

Type	Protein phosphatase	Inhibited by I_1 and I_2	Specificity for phosphorylase kinase (subunit)	Substrate specificity	Regulators
1	Protein phosphatase-1	Yes	β	Broad	I_1, I_2, DARPP-32
2	Protein phosphatase-2A	No	α	Broad	Unknown
2	Protein phosphatase-2B	No	α	Narrow?	Ca^{2+}/calmodulin
2	Protein phosphatase-2C	No	α	Broad	Mg^{2+}

[a] Protein phosphatases-2B and -2C are completely dependent on Ca^{2+} and Mg^{2+}, respectively, whereas protein phosphatases-1 and -2A are active in the absence of divalent cations. Protein phosphatases-1 and -2A have similar substrate specificities. Protein phosphatase-2B, also referred to as calcineurin, has been reported [16] to have very restricted specificity, since of many phosphoproteins examined in early studies, only phosphorylase kinase (α subunit), inhibitor-1, and myosin light chain were found to serve as substrates; however, several additional substrates have been found in brain for this phosphatase [18]. (Modified from Cohen [16].)
[b] (I_1) phosphatase inhibitor 1; (I_2) phosphatase inhibitor 2.

The brain contains at least four types of protein phosphatases that differ in their physicochemical properties, substrate specificity, and regulation by cellular messengers

Some characteristics of these four enzymes are summarized in Table 3 [17]. Two mechanisms for the physiological regulation of protein phosphatase activity have been described [1,16]. A phosphatase may be activated directly on binding a second messenger. This is analogous to the regulation of second-messenger-dependent protein kinases. Protein phosphatase 2B (calcineurin), which is activated by Ca^{2+} in conjunction with calmodulin, displays this type of regulation. Alternatively, a phosphatase may be regulated indirectly by second messengers via a class of proteins referred to as protein phosphatase inhibitors. In this case, second messengers activate protein kinases, which then phosphorylate phosphatase inhibitors. Phosphorylation of the inhibitor proteins then regulates their phosphatase inhibitory activity, leading to changes in the state of phosphorylation of other cellular proteins. Protein phosphatase 1, which is inhibited by three known types of inhibitor proteins (see below and Table 4), displays this type of regulation. It is likely, therefore, that many first messengers elicit physiological responses through the regulation of protein phosphatases as well as protein kinases.

There are four known species of protein phosphatase inhibitor proteins

Inhibitor 1, inhibitor 2, and DARPP-32[1] all inhibit protein phosphatase 1, while G-substrate inhibits protein phosphatase activity in cerebellar extracts [1,5,16,18]. Inhibitor 1 and DARPP-32 are substrates for cAMP-dependent protein kinase; G-substrate is a substrate for cGMP-dependent protein kinase; and inhibitor 2 is a substrate for glycogen synthase kinase 3. The phosphorylation of inhibitor 1, DARPP-32, and G-substrate leads to activation of their phosphatase inhibitory activity, and the phosphorylation of inhibitor 2 leads to inactivation of its inhibitory activity. All four inhibitors are low-molecular-weight, acid-soluble, heat-stable proteins with an elongated tertiary structure,

___
[1] Dopamine- and cAMP-regulated phosphoprotein of M_r 32, 000.

TABLE 4.   Neuronal proteins regulated by phosphorylation[a]

Enzymes involved in neurotransmitter biosynthesis
  Tyrosine hydroxylase
  Tryptophan hydroxylase
Enzymes involved in cyclic nucleotide metabolism
  Adenylate cyclase
  Guanylate cyclase
  Phosphodiesterase
Autophosphorylated protein kinases
  cAMP-dependent protein kinase
  cGMP-dependent protein kinase
  Ca^{2+}/calmodulin-dependent protein kinases
  Ca^{2+}/diacylglycerol-dependent protein kinase (protein kinase C)
  Casein kinases
  Protein tyrosine kinases
  Double-stranded RNA-dependent protein kinase
  Rhodopsin kinase
Phosphatase inhibitors
  Inhibitor 1
  Inhibitor 2
  DARPP-32
  G substrate
Proteins involved in transcription and translation regulation
  RNA polymerase
  Histones
  Nonhistone nuclear proteins
  Ribosomal protein S6
  Other ribosomal proteins
Cytoskeletal proteins
  MAP-2
  Tau
  Other microtubule-associated proteins
  Neurofilaments
  Calspectin
  Myosin light chain
  Actin
  Tubulin
Synaptic vesicle-associated proteins
  Synapsin I
  Protein III
  Clathrin
  Synaptophysin

TABLE 4.   *Continued.*

Neurotransmitter receptors
  Nicotinic acetylcholine receptor
  Muscarinic acetylcholine receptor
  β-adrenergic receptor
  α-adrenergic receptor
  GABA/benzodiazepine receptor
Ion channels[b]
  Voltage dependent
    Na^+ channel
    K^+ channel
    Ca^{2+} channel
    Ca^{2+}-dependent K^+ channel
  Neurotransmitter dependent
    Nicotinic acetylcholine receptor
    Serotonin-regulated K^+ channel in *Aplysia* sensory neurons
    Serotonin-regulated (anomalously rectifying) K^+ channel in *Aplysia* neuron R15
    Na^+ channel in rod outer segments
Miscellaneous
  B-50
  Rhodopsin
  Myelin basic protein
  87 kDa protein
  100 kDa protein
  G-proteins

[a] Some of the proteins included are specific to neurons. The others are present in many cell types in addition to neurons and are included because among their multiple functions in the nervous system is the regulation of neuron-specific phenomena. Not included are the many phosphoproteins present in diverse tissues (including brain) that play a role in generalized cellular processes, such as intermediary metabolism, and that do not appear to play a role in neuron-specific phenomena. (Modified from Nestler [24].)
[b] Several of the ion channels listed have been shown to be physiologically regulated by protein phosphorylation reactions, although it is not yet known whether such regulation is achieved directly through the phosphorylation of the ion channel or indirectly through the phosphorylation of a modulatory protein that is not a constituent of the ion channel molecule.

are phosphorylated on threonine residues, and exhibit some homology in their amino acid composition. These considerable similarities suggest that the proteins were derived, in the course of evolution, from some common precursor.

Distribution of protein phosphatase inhibitors

Inhibitors 1 and 2 appear to be widely distributed in various tissues, including brain, whereas DARPP-32 and G-substrate are neuron-specific proteins that show a restricted distribution in brain. DARPP-32 (discussed below under Neuronal Phosphoproteins) is localized to neurons that express D_1-dopamine receptors, and G-substrate is localized to cerebellar Purkinje cells. Thus, some neuronal cell types contain unique species of phosphatase inhibitor proteins. This raises the possibility that the brain contains additional species of inhibitor proteins that occur uniquely in specific neuronal cell types.

NEURONAL PHOSPHOPROTEINS

Protein phosphorylation is involved in carrying out or regulating diverse processes in the nervous system

Protein phosphorylation affects neurotransmitter biosynthesis, axoplasmic transport, neurotransmitter release, generation of postsynaptic potentials, ion channel conductance, neuronal shape and motility, elaboration of dendritic and axonal processes, and development and maintenance of differentiated characteristics of neurons. Some of the effects of protein phosphorylation on neuronal function may include biochemical events that underlie short-term and long-term memory [11,19]. The biochemical basis of short-term memory may involve the phosphorylation of presynaptic or postsynaptic proteins in response to synaptic activity, which would result in transient facilitation or inhibition of synaptic transmission. The biochemical basis of long-term memory may involve the phosphorylation of proteins that play a part in the regulation of gene expression, which would result in more permanent modifications of synaptic transmission.

Identification of the specific phosphoprotein(s) involved in each of these diverse neuronal processes is crucial to the elucidation of the molecular pathways through which those processes are achieved and regulated. Indeed, a very large number of neuronal proteins have been shown to be regulated by phosphorylation. Those neuronal phosphoproteins that have been studied most extensively fall into certain categories (Table 4) and include enzymes involved in neurotransmitter biosynthesis, enzymes involved in cyclic nucleotide metabolism, autophosphorylated protein kinases, protein phosphatase inhibitors, proteins involved in the regulation of transcription and translation, cytoskeletal proteins, synaptic vesicle-associated proteins, neurotransmitter receptors, and ion channels. In a number of cases, the functional roles of the phosphorylation reactions have already been established. (Regulation of these neuronal proteins by phosphorylation has been reviewed in detail [1,20,21].)

Neuronal phosphoproteins exhibit great diversity in the number and types of amino acid residues phosphorylated

Most neuronal phosphoproteins are phosphorylated on serine residues; some are phosphorylated on threonine residues; and a few are phosphorylated on tyrosine residues. In addition, some of the proteins are phosphorylated on only a single amino acid residue, but most are phosphorylated on multiple residues. In the latter cases, the residues phosphorylated can be the same or different types of amino acids. Some of the proteins appear to be phosphorylated by only one protein kinase, whereas others are phosphorylated by more than one protein kinase. Microtubule-associated protein-2 (MAP-2) has been reported to be phosphorylated by four distinct protein kinases. Some proteins, such as rhodopsin and synapsin I, are phosphorylated at more than one site by a single protein kinase; some, such as protein III and synapsin I, are phosphorylated on the same site by more than one protein kinase; and some, such as MAP-2, tyrosine hydroxylase, the nicotinic acetylcholine receptor, and synapsin I are phosphorylated on distinct sites by different protein kinases.

Neuronal phosphoproteins also differ in their regional, cellular, and subcellular distribution

Some of the proteins seem to be present in virtually every neuron, for example, synapsin I. Others are present in only certain neuronal cell types [22,23]. For example, DARPP-32 and ARPP-21 are highly enriched in dopaminoceptive neurons that possess D_1-dopamine receptors. G-substrate, a specific substrate for cGMP-dependent protein kinase, is present in only a single type of neuron, the cerebellar Purkinje cell. Such region-specific phosphoproteins are presumably involved in the manifestation or regulation of highly differentiated properties unique to specific neuronal cell types. Characterization of the functional roles of region-specific phosphoproteins should help provide an understanding of the diversity of neuronal cell types at the molecular level. The specific localization of phosphoproteins to certain neuronal cell types has also made it possible to use antisera against these proteins to study various anatomical, developmental, and pathophysiological aspects of the neurons in which the proteins occur [1,24]. An example of this is discussed in more detail below (see DARPP-32).

There is wide diversity of functional activities of neuronal phosphoproteins

The phosphorylation of some of the proteins appears to result directly in the physiological response being regulated, whereas the phosphorylation of other proteins appears to affect physiological responses indirectly (Table 4). Moreover, the effects of substrate protein phosphorylation can be either mediatory or modulatory with respect to the neuronal process being regulated. This point is illustrated by consideration of ion channels. Phosphorylation of certain ion channel complexes, such as the se-

rotonin-regulated K^+ channel in *Aplysia* sensory neurons, appears to play a mediatory role by being an obligatory step in the sequence of events through which those channels open or close in response to a first messenger. In contrast, phosphorylation of other channels, for example, the nicotinic acetylcholine receptor, appears to play a modulatory role by altering the sensitivity of the channels to open or close in response to the appropriate first messenger.

To illustrate some of the roles played by protein phosphorylation in the regulation of nervous system function, five of the best characterized neuronal phosphoproteins are discussed in detail. Some of the characteristics of these proteins are summarized in Table 5.

Tyrosine hydroxylase is the rate-limiting enzyme in the biosynthesis of the catecholamine neurotransmitters dopamine, norepinephrine, and epinephrine

A number of extracellular signals have been shown to stimulate catecholamine biosynthesis *in vivo*, and this effect appears to be mediated through increases in the catalytic activity of tyrosine hydroxylase (see also Chap. 11). It now appears that such changes in the catalytic activity of tyrosine hydroxylase are achieved through cAMP-dependent and Ca^{2+}-dependent phosphorylation of the enzyme.

Tyrosine hydroxylase appears to be a tetramer of identical 60-kilodalton (kDa) subunits. The enzyme is an effective substrate for three distinct protein kinases: cAMP-dependent protein kinase, Ca^{2+}/calmodulin-dependent protein kinase II, and Ca^{2+}/diacylglycerol-dependent protein kinase [1]. One serine residue (site 1) of the molecule is phosphorylated by all three kinases, whereas a second serine residue (site 2) is phosphorylated only by Ca^{2+}/calmodulin-dependent protein kinase II. Phosphorylation of

TABLE 5. Some properties of five well-characterized neuronal phosphoproteins[a]

| Phosphoprotein | Subunit M_r (kDa) | Distribution | | First-messenger regulating phosphorylation | Protein kinase(s)[b] | Phosphorylation site(s) | Effect of phosphorylation on protein[c] |
		Regional	Subcellular				
Tyrosine hydroxylase	60	Catecholaminergic neurons	Predominantly cytosol	Nerve impulses Acetylcholine	cAMP (site 1) Ca^{2+}/diacylglycerol (site 1) Ca^{2+}/calmodulin II (sites 1 and 2)	Two serine residues (sites 1 and 2) Probably additional sites on other serine residues	Increases catalytic activity (cAMP or Ca^{2+})
Rhodopsin	38	Photoreceptors	Rod outer segment membranes	Light	Rhodopsin	Approximately nine sites	Decreases ability to activate phosphodiesterase (rhodopsin)
Nicotinic acetylcholine receptor	α40 β50 γ60 δ65	Nicotinic cholinoceptive cells	Plasma membrane	CGRP	cAMP (γ, δ subunits) Ca^{2+}/diacylglycerol (α, δ subunits) Tyrosine (β, γ, δ subunits)	α: One serine residue β: One tyrosine residue γ: One serine and one tyrosine residue δ: Two serine residues and one tyrosine residue	Increases rate of desensitization to acetylcholine (cAMP, Ca^{2+}/diacylglycerol, tyrosine)
Synapsin I	Ia, 86 Ib, 80	All neurons	Synaptic vesicles	Nerve impulses (sites 1, 2, 3) Serotonin, dopamine, norepinephrine (site 1)	cAMP (site 1) Ca^{2+}/calmodulin I (site 1) Ca^{2+}/calmodulin II (sites 2 and 3)	Three serine residues (sites 1, 2, 3)	Facilitates neurotransmitter release (Ca^{2+}/calmodulin II)
DARPP-32	32	Dopaminoceptive neurons that possess D$_1$ receptors	Cytosol	Dopamine	cAMP	One threonine residue	Increases potency as phosphatase inhibitor (cAMP)

[a] First messengers regulate not only the state of phosphorylation, but also the total amount of substrate proteins. The total amount of tyrosine hydroxylase is increased by nerve impulses, acetylcholine, and glucocorticoids. The total amount of the nicotinic acetylcholine receptor is regulated by nerve impulses. The total amount of synapsin I is regulated by noradrenaline, corticosterone, and morphine.
[b] cAMP, cAMP-dependent protein kinase; Ca^{2+}/diacylglycerol, Ca^{2+}/diacylglycerol-dependent protein kinase; rhodopsin, rhodopsin kinase; Ca^{2+}/calmodulin I and Ca^{2+}/calmodulin II, Ca^{2+}/calmodulin-dependent protein kinases I and II, respectively; tyrosine, protein tyrosine kinase. Rhodopsin kinase is a substrate-activated protein kinase; cellular messengers that activate it *in vivo* have not been identified.
[c] Parentheses indicate the protein kinase that produces this effect on the substrate protein.

either site by Ca^{2+}/calmodulin-dependent protein kinase II appears to require the presence of an "activator" protein, still unidentified. It is likely that tyrosine hydroxylase also contains additional serine residues that are phosphorylated by one or more of these three kinases, but these additional sites have been less well characterized [25]. It has also been reported that other protein kinases may phosphorylate this enzyme.

Tyrosine hydroxylase is present in those neurons in the central and peripheral nervous systems that synthesize catecholamines. The enzyme is also present at high levels in cells that are developmentally related to catecholaminergic neurons, such as adrenal chromaffin cells and pheochromocytoma cells. Tyrosine hydroxylase is predominantly a cytosolic protein and is present in high levels in nerve terminals where much catecholamine biosynthesis is carried out.

Regulation of phosphorylation

The state of phosphorylation of tyrosine hydroxylase is regulated by nerve impulse conduction, by the neurotransmitter acetylcholine, and by depolarizing agents in well-defined regions of the nervous system, in the adrenal medulla, and in cultured pheochromocytoma cells.

These changes in the phosphorylation of tyrosine hydroxylase have been shown to correlate with changes in the catalytic activity of the enzyme and in the rate of catecholamine biosynthesis [1,25]. Phosphorylation appears to increase catalytic activity by increasing the V_{max} of the enzyme and the affinity of the enzyme for its pterin cofactor and by decreasing the affinity of the enzyme for its end-product inhibitor.

Several key questions remain with regard to the regulation of tyrosine hydroxylase by phosphorylation. What is the exact number of serine residues in the enzyme that undergo phosphorylation, and what is the nature of the protein kinases that phosphorylate them? What is the precise effect of the phosphorylation of each of these serine residues on the catalytic activity of the enzyme? How does the phosphorylation of multiple residues affect enzyme activity? Which protein kinase(s) mediates the actions of the various first messengers known to regulate the phosphorylation and activity of tyrosine hydroxylase?

Rhodopsin mediates the effects of light on retinal rod cells

Rhodopsin represents 90 percent of the integral protein of rod outer segment membranes. It has a molecular weight of approximately 40,000 Da and is composed of the protein opsin and the prosthetic group 11-*cis*-retinal. Light induces the isomerization of 11-*cis*-retinal to all-*trans*-retinal, which in turn leads to a conformational change in rhodopsin. This change then initiates a biochemical cascade (see below) that leads to a transient hyperpolarization of rod outer segments. (This light-sensitive process is discussed in detail in Chap. 7.) Over the past decade, it has become apparent that rhodopsin is phosphorylated by an endogenous rhodopsin kinase and that the phosphorylation of rhodopsin plays an integral role in the process by which rod outer segments become adapted, or desensitized, to light [26].

The rhodopsin kinase present in rod outer segments is a second-messenger-independent protein kinase and appears to be predominantly a cytosolic enzyme of 68 kDa. Rhodopsin kinase phosphorylates light-adapted, but not dark-adapted, rhodopsin. It appears that the conformational change induced in rhodopsin by light renders it an effective substrate for the kinase. Neither form of rhodopsin is known to be phosphorylated by second-messenger-dependent protein kinases. Rhodopsin kinase catalyzes the incorporation of up to 9 mol of phosphate into serine and threonine residues of rhodopsin, but the precise number of each type of site remains unknown. The phosphorylation sites appear to be localized in a small region of the C-terminal portion, apparently the part of the rhodopsin molecule that is exposed to the cytosol of rod outer segments. The state of phosphorylation of rhodopsin has been shown to be regulated by changes in environmental lighting *in vivo*.

To understand the role of rhodopsin phosphorylation in the regulation of rod outer segment function, it is necessary to review the role of rhodopsin itself [26]. Light leads to hyperpolarization of rod outer segment membranes via a molecular cascade (see also Chap. 7). Light induces a conformational change in rhodopsin such that light-adapted rhodopsin, referred to as R*, binds to a complex consisting of transducin (a GTP-binding membrane protein) and GDP. This binding leads to an exchange of GTP for GDP, which in turn causes the dissociation of R* and the β and γ subunits of transducin from the complex. The resulting complex of GTP and the α subunit of transducin then activate the enzyme phosphodiesterase, which leads to decreases in cGMP levels and consequently to hyperpolarization of rod outer segments. R* acts catalytically in this cascade: Once released from the R*:transducin:GTP complex, it is able to activate many additional transducin:GDP complexes. However, it is known that rod outer segments become adapted to light after very brief periods of time. This means that mechanisms exist to reverse rapidly the ability of R* to activate transducin:GDP complexes. The phosphorylation of rhodopsin represents such a mechanism [26].

Phospho-R*, like dephospho-R*, is able to activate the transducin/phosphodiesterase cascade. It appears that an additional protein, rejferred to as arrestin, a 48-kDa protein present jat high levels in rod outer segment cytosol, plays a necessary role in quenching phospho-R*. Arrestin binds with high affinity to phospho-R* but not to dephospho-R* or to dark-adapted rhodopsin, and the formation of arrestin:phospho-R* complexes makes phospho-R* unavailable for any further activation of the transducin/phosphodiesterase system. The kinetics of the various steps in this pathway are such that R* activates numerous molecules of transducin before undergoing phosphorylation by rhodopsin kinase and sequestration by arrestin.

Activation and desensitization of β-adrenergic receptor-stimulated adenylate cyclase are analogous to the regulation of rod outer segment phosphodiesterase by rhodopsin. Thus, the binding of a β-adrenergic agonist (analogous to light) to its receptor (analogous to rhodopsin) leads, through the interaction with a GTP-binding protein designated G_s (analogous to transducin), to the activation of adenylate cyclase (analogous to phosphodiesterase). Occupation of the β-adrenergic receptor by agonist also leads to desensitization of the receptor: binding of the agonist to the receptor induces a conformational change in the receptor that renders it an effective substrate for β-adrenergic receptor kinase, a second-messenger-independent protein kinase (analogous to rhodopsin kinase) [27] (see also Chap. 18). Phosphorylation of the receptor prevents its association with G_s and consequently leads to decreased activation of adenylate cyclase. An additional protein, analogous to arrestin in rod outer segments, may be involved in this uncoupling process.

In addition to the functional similarities between the rhodopsin and β-adrenergic receptor systems, there are also structural homologies. Rhodopsin and the β-adrenergic receptor show a number of similarities in their primary and tertiary structures. Transducin and G_s, which belong to a family of GTP-binding proteins with virtually identical β and γ subunits, have similar α subunits and can substitute for each other in the activation of phosphodiesterase and adenylate cyclase [26,28]. Finally, β-adrenergic receptor kinase is able to phosphorylate light-adapted rhodopsin, and rhodopsin kinase is able to phosphorylate the β-adrenergic receptor when it is bound to a β-adrenergic receptor agonist, indicating that these two kinases may be related [27]. The structural and functional similarities of these two systems raise the possibility that analogous systems may be widespread in the nervous system. It is known that the binding of many types of neurotransmitters to specific receptors elicits physiological responses through interactions with GTP-binding proteins [28]. It is possible that those receptors, in their activated states, are also phosphorylated by specific receptor-associated protein kinases and that such phosphorylation mediates desensitization of the receptors.

The nicotinic acetylcholine receptor mediates synaptic transmission at nicotinic cholinergic synapses

It has been known for many years that prolonged exposure of the nicotinic receptor to acetylcholine leads to a decrease in the sensitivity of the receptor to acetylcholine, a process referred to as desensitization (see Chap. 10). Phosphorylation of the receptor by cAMP-dependent protein kinase, and probably by Ca^{2+}/diacylglycerol-dependent protein kinase, enhances the rate at which desensitization of the receptor develops in response to acetylcholine [29]. The receptor is also phosphorylated by a protein tyrosine kinase, and that reaction enhances the rate of desensitization as well.

The nicotinic acetylcholine receptor is a 250-kDa protein that consists of four types of subunits $(\alpha,\beta,\gamma,\delta)$, with a stoichiometry of $\alpha_2\beta\gamma\delta$ (see Chap. 10). The various subunits of the receptor are effective substrates for three distinct protein kinases [29]: (a) cAMP-dependent protein kinase phosphorylates single serine residues in the γ and δ subunits; (b) Ca^{2+}/diacylglycerol-dependent protein kinase phosphorylates single serine residues in the α and δ subunits; and (c) protein tyrosine kinase phosphorylates single tyrosine residues in the β, γ, and δ subunits. The serine residues phosphorylated by the cAMP-dependent and Ca^{2+}-dependent enzymes on the δ subunit appear to represent distinct sites.

Desensitization mediated by cAMP-dependent protein kinase

Studies involving reconstitution of purified acetylcholine receptor into phospholipid vesicles have provided direct evidence for a functional role of receptor phosphorylation [29]. Purified receptor phosphorylated by cAMP-dependent protein kinase prior to reconstitution was shown to desensitize in the presence of acetylcholine at a rate seven to eight times faster than that of dephosphorylated receptor, as measured by quench-flow kinetic techniques. Other properties of the receptor, namely, the affinity of the receptor for acetylcholine, the rate of ion transport through activated receptor channels, and the mean time that activated receptor channels remain open, were found to be unaffected by receptor phosphorylation. Consistent with these observations *in vitro* is the demonstration that forskolin, which increases cellular cAMP levels by activating the enzyme adenylate cyclase, dramatically increases the rate of desensitization of the nicotinic receptor in intact muscle preparations [30].

Desensitization mediated by protein kinase C

Phorbol esters, agents that specifically activate Ca^{2+}/diacylglycerol-dependent protein kinases, also increase the rate of desensitization of the nicotinic receptor in intact cultured myotubes. These results suggest that phosphorylation of the receptor by this Ca^{2+}-dependent kinase has an effect on receptor function similar to that of phosphorylation by cAMP-dependent protein kinase. This is interesting in light of the fact that the serine residues in the δ subunit that are phosphorylated by the two kinases appear to be located 16 amino acid residues from each other. Furthermore, the tyrosine residue that appears to be phosphorylated in this subunit is located between these two sites, consistent with the fact that phosphorylation of the receptor by protein tyrosine kinase also regulates receptor desensitization. Further work is needed to elucidate the precise molecular mechanisms through which phosphorylation of the receptor by cAMP-dependent protein kinase, Ca^{2+}/diacylglycerol-dependent protein kinase, and protein tyrosine kinase results in alterations in the kinetics of receptor desensitization. It will also be important to ascertain whether phosphorylation of the receptor by one kinase alters the ability of the other kinases to phosphorylate and regulate its properties.

In vivo significance

Results of experiments using forskolin and phorbol esters indicate that phosphorylation of the receptor and the consequent regulation of its rate of desensitization can occur *in vivo*. One central question that needs to be answered is: What are the first messengers that regulate this rate of desensitization through the activation of cAMP-dependent, Ca^{2+}/diacylglycerol-dependent, and, possibly, protein tyrosine kinases? It is not known whether the state of phosphorylation of the nicotinic acetylcholine receptor is regulated by acetylcholine itself. In any case, phosphorylation of the receptor by various kinases and the resultant modulation of nicotinic cholinergic neurotransmission appear to be mediated at least in part by other first messengers.

Synapsin I, originally discovered as a phosphoprotein in particulate synaptic fractions of brain, regulates the release of neurotransmitters from nerve endings

Synapsin I has been purified to homogeneity from bovine and rat brain and extensively characterized [1,31]. It now seems probable that synapsin I plays a role in the regulation of neurotransmitter release.

Synapsin I consists of two very similar proteins, synapsin Ia and synapsin Ib, with M_r 86,000 and 80,000, respectively. Synapsin I is an effective substrate protein for at least three distinct protein kinases in brain and undergoes multi–site phosphorylation. One serine residue (site 1) of the molecule is phosphorylated both by cAMP-dependent protein kinase and by Ca^{2+}/calmodulin-dependent protein kinase I. Two other serine residues (sites 2 and 3), located in different regions of the molecule, are phosphorylated by Ca^{2+}/calmodulin-dependent protein kinase II. For each of these three protein kinases, synapsin I is one of the most effective substrates known.

Synapsin I is present solely in neurons and appears to be associated with virtually all small synaptic vesicles in all nerve terminals throughout the central and peripheral nervous systems. Synapsin I represents approximately 6 percent of the total protein present in highly purified preparations of synaptic vesicles. It is an extrinsic protein of synaptic vesicle membranes and is located on their outer or cytoplasmic surface. Synaptic vesicles contain a specific, saturable, and high-affinity (K_d = 10 nM) binding site for synapsin I. The domain of synapsin I containing phosphorylation sites 2 and 3 appears to regulate the binding of the molecule to

synaptic vesicles. It is possible that another domain of synapsin I binds to some component of the cytoskeleton, in which case synapsin I would form a bridge between synaptic vesicles and the cytoskeletal element.

Neuronal regulation of synapsin I phosphorylation

The state of phosphorylation of synapsin I has been shown to be specifically regulated by brief periods of nerve impulse conduction at physiological frequencies and by the neurotransmitters serotonin, dopamine, norepinephrine, and adenosine in a number of well-defined relatively homogeneous regions of the central and peripheral nervous systems. Impulse conduction increases phosphorylation of synapsin I in nerve terminals through an influx of Ca^{2+} into the terminals and the subsequent activation of Ca^{2+}-dependent protein kinases. In contrast, the neurotransmitters increase synapsin I phosphorylation in nerve terminals via an increase in cAMP levels and the subsequent activation of cAMP-dependent protein kinase. Since brief periods of impulse conduction, acting through Ca^{2+}, and certain neurotransmitters, acting through cAMP, are known to facilitate release of neurotransmitter from many types of nerve terminals, it seems possible that the phosphorylation of synapsin I may represent a common molecular pathway through which these different first- and second-messenger systems regulate release of neurotransmitter at the synapse (Fig. 4). Since synapsin I is ubiquitous to neurons but absent from nonneuronal tissues, including even those with secretory functions, it seems more likely that synapsin I plays a part in a neuron-specific regulation of release than in the release process itself.

Synapsin I regulation of neurotransmitter release

Direct evidence has been obtained to support a role of synapsin I in the regulation of neu-

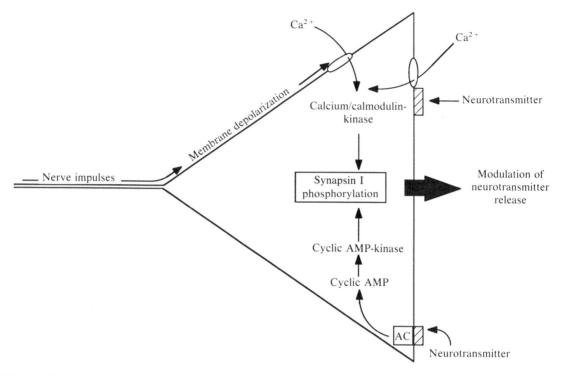

FIG. 4. Schematic diagram of the regulation of synapsin I phosphorylation in nerve terminals. Nerve impulse conduction stimulates synapsin I phosphorylation through the depolarization of the nerve terminal plasma membrane, an increase in free Ca^{2+} levels, and the activation of Ca^{2+}-dependent protein kinases. Such phosphorylation of synapsin I may be involved in various Ca^{2+}-dependent mechanisms of regulation of neurotransmitter release, including the phenomenon of post-tetanic potentiation. Some neurotransmitters stimulate (or inhibit) synapsin I phosphorylation by binding to presynaptic receptors and thereby altering Ca^{2+} levels and Ca^{2+}-dependent protein kinase activity. Such phosphorylation (or dephosphorylation) of synapsin I may be involved in Ca^{2+}-dependent mechanisms by which certain neurotransmitters acting on presynaptic receptors of axon terminals regulate neurotransmitter release. Other neurotransmitters stimulate (or inhibit) synapsin I phosphorylation by binding to other presynaptic receptors and thereby altering adenylate cyclase (AC) activity, leading to changes in cAMP levels and cAMP-dependent protein kinase activity. Such phosphorylation (or dephosphorylation) of synapsin I may be involved in cAMP-dependent mechanisms by which certain neurotransmitters acting on presynaptic receptors of axon terminals regulate neurotransmitter release. Nerve impulse conduction would be expected to stimulate synapsin I phosphorylation in all nerve terminals throughout the nervous system. In contrast, most neurotransmitters would be expected to stimulate synapsin I phosphorylation only in certain nerve terminals. (Modified from Nestler and Greengard, *Prog. Brain Res.* 69:323–340, 1986.)

rotransmitter release [13]. The injection of de-phospho-synapsin I into terminal digits at the squid giant synapse inhibited neurotransmitter release from terminals in response to membrane depolarization. The injection of synapsin I that had been phosphorylated on sites 2 and 3 by Ca^{2+}/calmodulin-dependent protein kinase II failed to produce this effect. Moreover, injection of this protein kinase itself into the terminals greatly facilitated neurotransmitter release. These results suggest that in the resting state, dephospho-synapsin I inhibits neurotransmitter release and that in the stimulated state, the phosphorylation of synapsin I at sites 2 and 3 by Ca^{2+}/calmodulin-dependent protein kinase II facilitates release by "deinhibiting" the release process. Further studies, analogous to those described here, are needed to determine whether the phosphorylation of synapsin I on site 1, by cAMP-dependent protein kinase or Ca^{2+}/calmodulin-dependent protein kinase I, also regulates neurotransmitter release.

The precise molecular mechanism through which the phosphorylation of synapsin I regulates neurotransmitter release remains unknown. Possible mechanisms include regulation of the translocation of synaptic vesicles toward, and/or their prefusion with, the nerve terminal plasma membrane [1,13,31]. In either case, phosphorylation of synapsin I might make more vesicles available for subsequent release events.

DARPP-32, originally discovered as a phosphoprotein in soluble fractions of brain, is a protein phosphatase inhibitor localized to dopaminoceptive neurons

DARPP-32 was discovered during a study of the regional distribution of neuronal phosphoproteins in rat brain. It is one of several substrates for cAMP-dependent protein kinase that are highly concentrated in the basal ganglia [18,23]. It has been purified to homogeneity and extensively characterized [18]. DARPP-32 has an apparent M_r of 32,000 by sodium dodecyl sulfate (SDS)-polyacrylamide gel electrophoresis, but its actual molecular mass based on sequencing data (202 amino acids) is 22,614 Da. It is phosphorylated at a single threonine residue by cAMP-dependent protein kinase, which converts it into a potent phosphatase inhibitor. Phospho-DARPP-32 noncompetitively inhibits protein phosphatase 1 with a K_i of about 1 nM. In contrast, it is not an effective inhibitor of protein phosphatases 2A, 2B, or 2C. Dephos-

pho-DARPP-32 possesses no detectable protein phosphatase inhibitory activity [18].

DARPP-32 is localized to the subclass of neurons in the brain that possess D_1-dopamine receptors, and it appears to be present in all such neurons (see Chaps. 11 and 42). However, it is not an integral part of the D_1-dopamine receptor per se, because the receptor molecule is a membrane-associated protein and DARPP-32 is cytosolic. Some, but not all, DARPP-32-containing neurons are GABAergic, but most GABAergic neurons do not contain DARPP-32. Thus, it would appear that DARPP-32 is not specifically associated with any one neurotransmitter type.

Dopamine regulation of DARPP-32 phosphorylation

The state of phosphorylation of DARPP-32 is regulated in D_1-dopaminoceptive neurons by the neurotransmitter dopamine, which acts through increases in cAMP levels and activation of cAMP-dependent protein kinase (see Chap. 11). It seems likely that some of the effects of dopamine, acting at D_1-dopamine receptors, are mediated through the phosphorylation and activation of DARPP-32 [18]. Two types of physiological actions that might be achieved in this way are illustrated in Fig. 5. First, DARPP-32, phosphorylated and activated in response to dopamine and cAMP (as first and second messengers, respectively), can act as a positive feedback signal for these messengers by reducing the dephosphorylation of other substrates for the same protein kinase. Second, DARPP-32 can reduce the dephosphorylation of substrate proteins for other protein kinases and, in so doing, can mediate the effects of first- and second-messenger systems on one another.

Relationship of DARPP-32 to dopaminoceptive neurons

The restricted distribution of DARPP-32 makes it a uniquely useful tool for the identification and

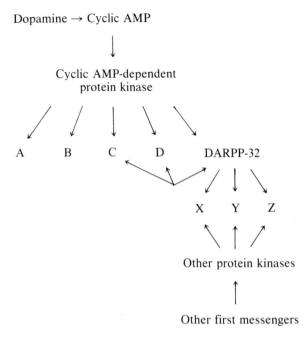

Dopamine → Cyclic AMP

Cyclic AMP-dependent
protein kinase

A   B   C   D   DARPP-32

X   Y   Z

Other protein kinases

Other first messengers

FIG. 5. Diagram of proposed roles that DARPP-32, a protein phosphatase inhibitor, may play in the regulation of neuronal function. The first messenger, dopamine, acting through cAMP and cAMP-dependent protein kinase, stimulates the phosphorylation of several proteins (A–D, DARPP-32) in an individual target neuron. The phosphorylation of A, B, C, and D leads directly to certain of the physiological effects of dopamine in this neuron. The phosphorylation of DARPP-32 converts it to an active phosphatase inhibitor. Activated DARPP-32 then decreases the dephosphorylation of some proteins (C and D) that are substrates for cAMP-dependent protein kinase, and of other proteins (X, Y, and Z) that are substrates for other protein kinases. By reducing the dephosphorylation of C and D, DARPP-32 represents a positive feedback signal through which dopamine modulates its own actions. By reducing the dephosphorylation of X, Y, and Z, DARPP-32 represents a mediator through which dopamine modulates the actions of other first messengers. (From Nestler et al. [24].)

ultrastructural study of the D_1 subclass of dopaminoceptive neurons throughout the nervous system and for the morphological analysis of the dendritic and axonal projections of these cells (Fig. 6). Immunocytochemical studies of DARPP-32 using high-resolution light microscopy and electron microscopy have made it possible to visualize medium-size spiny neurons in the neostriatum, which represent about 96 percent of all neurons in this region, and the projections of these neurons to the globus pallidus and substantia nigra (see Chap. 42). That part of the ventral pallidum that receives fibers from the ventral striatum can be visualized with unequaled clarity and definition by DARPP-32 staining. DARPP-32 has also yielded valuable information about the phylogenetic development of dopaminoceptive neurons, particularly in the basal ganglia. The regional distribution of DARPP-32 in the brains of several mammalian and nonmammalian vertebrates corresponds to that of dopamine and probably reflects the different locations of dopaminoceptive neurons in these various species. Finally, DARPP-32 can be used to study the pathophysiology of, and to develop diagnostic tests for, various neuropsychiatric disorders that appear to involve dopaminoceptive neurons in the basal ganglia, such as Huntington's disease, Tourette's syndrome, and tardive dyskinesia [18,24] (see also Chap. 42).

CELLULAR MESSENGER SYSTEMS INTERACT AT VARIOUS LEVELS OF PROTEIN PHOSPHORYLATION PATHWAYS

cAMP, cGMP, Ca^{2+}, and the numerous extracellular signals that act through these second messengers are known to regulate many of the same physiological processes

It is interesting that such actions are often synergistic or antagonistic. Furthermore, many other cellular messengers, for example, prostaglandins, phosphatidylinositol and its derivatives, and various growth factors, also influ-

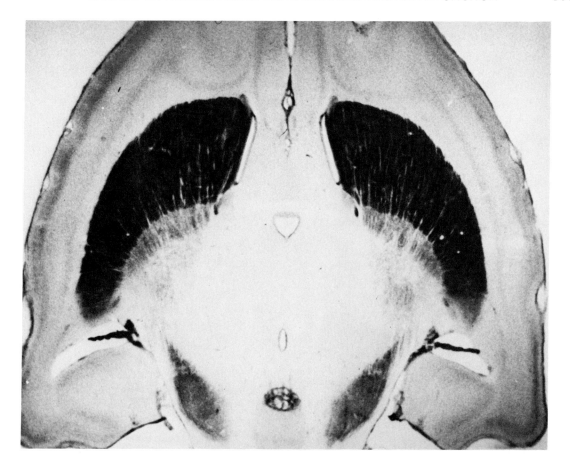

FIG. 6.   Horizontal section through a rat brain showing the immunocytochemical localization of DARPP-32. This phosphoprotein is enriched in the D_1 subclass of dopaminoceptive neurons throughout the brain, including those in the basal ganglia, which stain prominently here. DARPP-32 is one of a number of phosphoproteins that have been shown to be enriched in particular neuronal cell types and that appear to play an important role in regulating the function of those neurons. (C. C. Ouimet, H. C. Hemmings, Jr., and P. Greengard, *Science* 225 (4668) (cover), 1984.)

ence those same processes. Thus, rather than being generated through a single molecular pathway, most physiological responses represent the complex product of the coordinated actions of multiple cellular messengers involving multiple molecular pathways. One important question in such cases is: At which level or step(s) do the molecular pathways mediating the actions of these cellular messengers converge?

It is now apparent that such pathways frequently converge at various levels of protein phosphorylation systems. The cAMP, cGMP, and Ca^{2+} second-messenger systems are each known to interact with each other and with other prominent cellular messenger systems. These interactions have been shown to occur at multiple levels of protein phosphorylation pathways. Thus, such interactions occur at the level of the intracellular concentration of second messengers, at the level of protein kinases, at the level of protein phosphatases, at the level of the same substrate protein, and at the level of different substrate proteins. These interactions, too numerous to elaborate here, have been reviewed elsewhere [1]; some illustrative examples are now presented.

Concentration of cellular messenger

As examples of interactions at the level of the concentration of cellular messengers, adenylate cyclase and guanylate cyclase, which are the synthetic enzymes for cAMP and cGMP, respectively, are each regulated by Ca^{2+}, and cAMP and cGMP appear to alter cellular Ca^{2+} levels by regulating the flux of Ca^{2+} into neurons and the sequestration of Ca^{2+} by intracellular organelles. Prostaglandins also regulate cellular levels of cAMP and cGMP. Diacylglycerol, derived from the breakdown of phosphatidylinositol, allows the activation of Ca^{2+}/diacylglycerol-dependent protein kinase to occur at lower Ca^{2+} concentrations. In addition, cyclic nucleotides and Ca^{2+} have been reported to regulate the generation of these lipid messengers.

Protein kinase

As examples of interactions at the level of protein kinases, cAMP-dependent protein kinase phosphorylates certain Ca^{2+}/calmodulin-dependent protein kinases and thereby alters their catalytic activity, and protein tyrosine kinases are regulated by both cAMP-dependent and Ca^{2+}/diacylglycerol-dependent protein kinases.

Protein phosphatase

As an example of interactions at the level of protein phosphatases, DARPP-32, a phosphatase inhibitor activated by cAMP-dependent protein kinase, may produce physiological effects by inhibiting the dephosphorylation (i.e., increasing the state of phosphorylation) of substrate proteins for other protein kinases (Fig. 5). As another example, calcineurin, a Ca^{2+}/calmodulin-dependent protein phosphatase, is known to dephosphorylate a number of substrates for cAMP-dependent protein kinase.

Substrate proteins

As examples of interactions at the level of the same substrate protein, many phosphoproteins are phosphorylated at the same or at distinct residues by more than one protein kinase, as discussed above for tyrosine hydroxylase, the nicotinic acetylcholine receptor, synapsin I, and MAP-2. Indeed, multi–site phosphorylation of proteins appears to be the rule rather than the exception. This type of interaction includes the numerous substrates, such as the nicotinic acetylcholine receptor, that are phosphorylated on serine residues by second-messenger-dependent protein kinases and on tyrosine residues by protein tyrosine kinases. Finally, interactions can occur at the level of different substrate proteins, with substrates for cAMP-dependent, Ca^{2+}-dependent, and protein tyrosine kinases each regulating one physiological process. Proteins involved in the regulation of cellular motility and growth are examples of this type of interaction.

The extraordinary complexity in biological systems underscores the difficulty in determining the precise molecular basis of a physiological process. The central role of protein phosphorylation as a regulatory mechanism that mediates the actions of many individual cellular messengers and of interactions among them imbues the study of protein phosphorylation with a unique potential: to provide an experimental framework within which to unravel the layers of molecular steps that underlie and regulate cell function.

CONCLUSIONS

Twenty-five years ago, there was little information available concerning the molecular machinery by which chemical and electrical stimuli produce diverse physiological responses in various types of neurons. In fact, there was not even a conceptual framework available by which one could approach this subject. As a result of work over the past 20 years, it has become apparent that the study of protein phosphorylation provides such an approach. The injection of protein kinases and protein kinase inhibitors into neurons has demonstrated a direct causal relationship between the activation of specific protein kinases and the generation of specific physiological responses to extracellular signals in the nervous system. A diversity of substrate proteins for the kinases has been found in nervous tissue. In some instances, the identity and functional role of these phosphoproteins have already been established.

The protein kinase/protein phosphatase system, by controlling the phosphorylation state of substrate proteins of every conceivable category, provides the flexibility required for regulating a variety of neuronal processes having widely different temporal characteristics

By studying protein phosphorylation mechanisms, it should be possible to build a progressively more complete understanding of the molecular basis of innumerable types of neurophysiological phenomena, from the shortest-lived to the longest-lived, and from the most simple to the most complex.

REFERENCES

1. Nestler, E. J., and Greengard, P. *Protein Phosphorylation in the Nervous System.* New York: Wiley, 1984.

2. Rosen, O. M., and Krebs, E. G. (eds.), *Protein Phosphorylation.* Cold Spring Harbor, NY: Cold Spring Harbor Laboratory, 1981. [Cold Spring Harbor Conf. Cell Proliferation, Vol. 8.]

3. Hunter, T., and Sefton, B. M. Protein kinases and viral transformation. *Mol. Aspects Cell. Reg.* 2:337–370, 1982.

4. Corbin, J. D., and Hardman, J. G. (eds.), *Methods Enzymol.* 99F, 1984.

5. Nairn, A. C., Hemmings, H. C., Jr., and Greengard, P. Protein kinases in the brain. *Annu. Rev. Biochem.* 54:931–976, 1985.

6. Nishizuka, Y. Turnover of inositol phospholipids and signal transduction. *Science* 225:1365–1370, 1984.

7. Ono, Y., Kikkawa, U., Ogita, K., Fujii, T., Kurokawa, T., Asaoka, Y., Sekiguchi, K., Ase, K., Igarashi, K., and Nishizuka, Y. Expression and properties of two types of protein kinase C: Alternative splicing from a single gene. *Science* 236:1116–1120, 1987.

8. Nairn, A. C., Bhagat, B., and Palfrey, H. C. Identification of calmodulin-dependent protein kinase III and its major M_r 100,000 substrate in mammalian tissues. *Proc. Natl. Acad. Sci. U.S.A.* 82:7939–7943, 1985.

9. Nairn, A. C., and Greengard, P. Purification and characterization of Ca^{2+}/calmodulin-dependent protein kinase I from bovine brain. *J. Biol. Chem.* 262:7273–7281, 1987.

10. Greengard, P. Neuronal phosphoproteins: Mediators of signal transduction. *Mol. Neurobiol.* 1:81–120, 1987.

11. Kandel, E. R., and Schwartz, J. H. Molecular biology of learning: Modulation of transmitter release. *Science* 218:433–442, 1982.

12. Kaczmarek, L. K., and Levitan, I. B., (eds.), *Neuromodulation: The Biochemical Control of Neuronal Excitability.* Oxford: Oxford Univ. Press, 1986.

13. Llinás, R., McGuinness, T. L., Leonard, C. S., Sugimori, M., and Greengard, P. Intraterminal injection of synapsin I or calcium/calmodulin-dependent protein kinase II alters neurotransmitter release at the squid giant synapse. *Proc. Natl. Acad. Sci. U.S.A.* 82:3035–3039, 1985.

14. Paupardin-Tritsch, D., Hammond, C., Gerschenfeld, H. M., Nairn, A. C., and Greengard, P. cGMP-dependent protein kinase enhances

Ca^{2+} current and potentiates the serotonin-induced Ca^{2+} current increase in snail neurons. *Nature* 323:812–814, 1986.

15. Hammond, C., Paupardin-Tritsch, D., Nairn, A. C., Greengard, P., and Gerschenfeld, H. M. Cholecystokinin induces a decrease in Ca^{2+} current in snail neurones that appears to be mediated by protein kinase C. *Nature* 325:809–811, 1987.

16. Cohen, P. The role of protein phosphorylation in the neural and hormonal control of cellular activity. *Nature* 296:613–620, 1982.

17. Ingebritsen, T. S., and Cohen, P. The protein phosphatases involved in cellular regulation. 6. Measurement of type-1 and type-2 protein phosphatases in extracts of mammalian tissues; an assessment of their physiological roles. *Eur. J. Biochem.* 132:291–307, 1983.

18. Hemmings, H. C., Jr., Nestler, E. J., Walaas, S. I., Ouimet, C. C., and Greengard, P. Protein phosphorylation and neuronal function: DARPP-32, an illustrative example. In G. M. Edelman, W. E. Gall, and W. M. Cowan (eds.), *Synaptic Function*. New York: Wiley, 1987, pp. 213–240.

19. Greengard, P., and Kuo, J. F. On the mechanism of action of cyclic AMP. *Adv. Biochem. Psychopharmacol.* 3:287–306, 1970.

20. Nestler, E. J., and Greengard, P. Protein phosphorylation in the brain. *Nature* 305:583–588, 1983.

21. Rodnight, R. Aspects of protein phosphorylation in the nervous system with particular reference to synaptic transmission. *Prog. Brain Res.* 56:1–25, 1982.

22. Walaas, S. I., Nairn, A. C., and Greengard, P. Regional distribution of calcium- and cyclic AMP-regulated protein phosphorylation systems in mammalian brain. I. Particulate systems. *J. Neurosci.* 3:291–301, 1983.

23. Walaas, S. I., Nairn, A. C., and Greengard, P. Regional distribution of calcium- and cyclic AMP-dependent protein phosphorylation systems in mammalian brain. II. Soluble systems. *J. Neurosci.* 3:302–311, 1983.

24. Nestler, E. J., Walaas, S. I., and Greengard, P. Neuronal phosphoproteins: Physiological and clinical implications. *Science* 225:1357–1364, 1984.

25. Tachikawa, E., Tank, A. W., Yanagihara, N., Mosimann, W., and Weiner, N. Phosphorylation of tyrosine hyroxylase on at least three sites in rat pheochromocytoma PC12 cells treated with 56 mM K^+: Determination of the sites on tyrosine hydroxylase phosphorylated by cyclic AMP-dependent and calcium/calmodulin-dependent protein kinases. *Mol. Pharmacol.* 30:476–485, 1986.

26. Stryer, L. Cyclic GMP cascade of vision. *Annu. Rev. Neurosci.* 9:87–119, 1986.

27. Benovic, J. L., Mayor, F., Jr., Somers, R. L., Caron, M. G., and Lefkowitz, R. J. Light-dependent phosphorylation of rhodopsin by β-adrenergic receptor kinase. *Nature* 321:869–872, 1986.

28. Gilman, A. G. Receptor-regulated G-proteins. *Trends Neurosci.* 9:460–463, 1986.

29. Huganir, R. L., Delcour, A. H., Greengard, P., and Hess, G. P. Phosphorylation of the nicotinic acetylcholine receptor regulates its rate of desensitization. *Nature* 32:774–776, 1986.

30. Middleton, P., Jaramillo, F., and Schuetze, S. M. Forskolin increases the rate of acetylcholine receptor desensitization at rat soleus endplates. *Proc. Natl. Acad. Sci. U.S.A.* 83:4967–4971, 1986.

31. De Camilli, P., and Greengard, P. Synapsin I: A synaptic vesicle-associated neuronal phosphoprotein. *Biochem. Pharmacol.* 35:4349–4357, 1986.

CHAPTER **20**

Eicosanoids

Leonhard S. Wolfe

Basic Neurochemistry: Molecular, Cellular, and Medical Aspects, 4th Ed., edited by G. J. Siegel et al. Raven Press, Ltd., New York, 1989.
Correspondence to Leonhard S. Wolfe, Donner Laboratory of Experimental Neurochemistry, Montreal Neurological Institute, McGill University, Montreal, Quebec, Canada H3A 2B4.

The generic name eicosanoids (or icosanoids) was introduced by Corey in 1980 to encompass the increasing number of oxygenated products derived enzymatically from 20-carbon polyunsaturated fatty acids, such as eicosatrienoic acid, eicosatetraenoic acid (arachidonic acid), and eicosapentaenoic acid (EPA). The essential fatty acid linoleic acid, or all-*cis*-9,12-octadecadienoic acid, is converted successively by a Δ^6-desaturase, a two-carbon-chain elongation reaction, and a Δ^5-desaturase to arachidonic acid, or all-*cis*-5,8,11,14-eicosatetraenoic acid, which is the most important precursor of prostaglandins, thromboxanes, leukotrienes, and hydroperoxy- and hydroxyeicosatetraenoic acids in human and animal tissues. Polyunsaturated fatty acids derived from the N-3 family (named from the number of carbons from the ω end of the fatty acid, where the first *cis* double bond occurs) can also be either precursors or competitive inhibitors of prostaglandin and leukotriene synthesis.

Fatty acids, such as all-*cis*-5,8,11,14,17-EPA and all-*cis*-4,7,10,13,16,19-docosahexaenoic acid, important constituents of fish oils, are now coming into prominence as dietary agents that can modify the production of eicosanoids in human tissues. These substances may affect pathophysiological responses in a number of human diseases, such as myocardial infarction and rheumatoid arthritis. It is important to appreciate that polyunsaturated fatty acids, besides being precursors of eicosanoids, have roles in the structural and functional properties of the plasma membrane and in the maintenance of normal phospholipid metabolism. Suppression of hypercholesterolemia; maintenance of a normal healthy skin and normal brain growth; determination of the responses to inflammation, immune reactions, platelet activity, and resistance of the vascular endothelium to platelet aggregation and thrombus formation are also affected by polyunsaturated fatty acids [1,2].

GENERAL PROPERTIES AND BIOSYNTHETIC REACTIONS

The general field of eicosanoids is now very complex, but there are a number of general features that can help us to understand the importance of these varied and potent biologically active substances. Eicosanoids are formed by virtually every tissue in the body and are widely distributed in the animal kingdom, being found in invertebrates, such as coral, sea urchins, and arthropods, and even in plants. The biological activities of individual prostaglandins vary from organ to organ in a given species and may differ markedly from species to species. Even in different stages of development or in different phases of organ function (as occurs, for example, in the uterus), an individual prostaglandin may have different biological effects. Two main types of enzyme reactions initiate stereospecific oxygenations of arachidonic acid from molecular oxygen: fatty acid cyclooxygenase and lipoxygenases. The latter enzymes lead to the formation of stereospecific hydroperoxy and hydroxy compounds at the C-5, C-12, and C-15 positions. More recently, cytochrome P-450 monooxygenases (mixed-function oxidases) have been found to form a series of arachidonic acid epoxides that, via the action of epoxide hydrolases, can be transformed to hydroxyeicosenoic acids with all *cis* double bonds. These compounds also have a variety of biological activities. The fatty acid cyclooxygenase reaction requires activation by very small amounts of hydroperoxides; however, the reaction is self-limiting by the oxygen radicals that are generated in the catalysis. In the basal resting state in tissues including the brain, arachidonic acid is rapidly esterified by coenzyme A-dependent acylations to the sn-2 position of lysophospholipids, particularly phosphatidylcholine and phosphatidylinositol and its phosphate esters, and thus basal tissue levels of free arachidonic acid are very low. The release of arachidonic acid from phospholipids follows a wide variety of stimuli to receptors on cells—hormones, neurotransmitters, antibodies, growth factors, proteins and peptides, and toxins, as well as pathological conditions, including vascular shock, burns, brain trauma, hypoxia, ischemia, and seizures. Eicosanoids themselves can stimulate arachidonic acid release in specific organs. The release of arachidonic acid and its transformation into metabolites is local, and the effects of the eicosanoids occur in the immediate vicinity of their formation. At the sites of their formation the compounds rarely act in isolation but reinforce, sensitize, or antagonize many ongoing cellular processes, particularly stimulus-secretion-coupled events. There are many enzyme reactions in such tissues as liver, lung, and kidney (dehydrogenases, desaturases, β- and ω-oxidases, reductases, acetylases) that convert the parent eicosanoids into biologically inactive compounds that are then excreted as multiple metabolites in the urine. Thus, the naturally active compounds are not found in significant concentrations in the systemic circulation. Once formed, the compounds act as bioregulators of responses to second messengers, such as cyclic adenosine monophosphate (cAMP), inositol trisphosphate, inositol tetrakisphosphate, and their cyclic derivatives, and diacylglycerol, which affects calcium mobilization, specific protein binding, and the activity of protein kinases. Although we are just beginning to understand the genes coding for the specific enzymes, it is clear that their evolutionary origin is ancient and involves both the animal and plant kingdoms [3–6].

HISTORICAL DEVELOPMENT OF EICOSANOID CHEMISTRY AND PURIFICATION

The discovery of prostaglandins dates back to 1933, when von Euler and Goldblatt described active principles in human seminal fluid and in extracts of seminal vesicular glands of sheep that stimulated isolated intestinal and uterine muscle and lowered the blood pressure in intact animals. It was shown that these activities were due to highly potent acidic lipids, and von Euler proposed the name "prostaglandin" because initially they were thought to derive from the prostate gland. Subsequently, this proved to be incorrect; however, the name has persisted. It is of interest that two New York gynecologists in 1930 studied the influence of human seminal fluid on the uterus and the effect on the state of contraction of uterine strips. The effects observed turned out to have been due to prostaglandin E_2 and $F_{2\alpha}$. In the older literature one finds many names given independently to lipid extracts of tissues that affect the contractility of intestinal smooth muscle [*Darmstoff*, intestinal stimulant lipids, irin, menstrual stimulant, vasodepressor lipid, medullin, slow-reacting substance C (SRS-C), slow-reacting substance A (SRS-A)], which are now known to owe much of their biological activity to the presence of one or more of the eicosanoids.

Initial attempts to purify prostaglandins were carried out in 1947 by Bergstrom. With the development of more advanced chromatographic purification methods, intensive work on the purification and elucidation of the structure of these active principles was carried out by Bergstrom and his team in Sweden over the years 1956 to 1963. Two classes of prostaglandins were separated by solvent partition between ether and phosphate buffer. The compounds more soluble in ether were called prostaglandin E, and those more soluble in the phosphate buffer were called prostaglandin F (after *Fosfat*). Approaches involving chemical degradation and the powerful technique of gasliquid chromatography combined with mass spectrometry were also being developed simultaneously in Sweden and resulted in elucidation of the structures of this new group of compounds, even though only a few milligrams of the purified materials were then available. The prostaglandins were found to be a family of 20-carbon cyclopentane carboxylic acids in which individual members differ in the positions of oxygenation and unsaturation.

Immediately after the structures were established, their origin from the essential fatty acids was demonstrated by two groups of scientists (Bergstrom in Sweden and van Dorp in Holland) who showed that microsomal fractions from sheep seminal vesicular glands bioconverted $\Delta^{5,8,11,14}$-all-*cis*-eicosatetraenoic acid (arachidonic acid) into prostaglandin E_2 (PGE$_2$). Subsequently, it was shown that prostaglandin $F_{2\alpha}$ (PGF$_{2\alpha}$) was also formed from arachidonic acid; that $\Delta^{8,11,14}$-eicosatrienoic acid (homo-γ-linolenic acid) was the precursor of prostaglandin E_1 (PGE$_1$) and prostaglandin $F_{1\alpha}$ (PGF$_{1\alpha}$); and that $\Delta^{5,8,11,14,17}$-EPA was the precursor of prostaglandin PGE$_3$ (PGE$_3$) and prostaglandin PGF$_{3\alpha}$ (PGF$_{3\alpha}$) (see articles in Holman [2]).

In the mid-1960s to early 1970s, a number of interesting new biological activities of the primary prostaglandins were recognized. These included the ability to increase cAMP levels in cells, oxytocic and abortifacient activities, inhibition of catecholamine-induced lipolysis, and sedative and pyretic effects in the nervous system. During this period, biochemical studies on the biosynthesis of prostaglandins were being carried out by Samuelsson and his co-workers. A landmark occurred in 1971 when Vane discovered that aspirin inhibited prostaglandin synthesis, and this laid the foundation for understanding the action of nonsteroidal anti-inflammatory drugs.

Isolation of the prostaglandin endoperoxides by Hamberg and Samuelsson in 1973 to 1974 led to the discovery of an exceedingly short-lived compound named thromboxane A$_2$, which was found to be a potent platelet aggregant produced by platelets following stimulation by thrombin and collagen and a potent vasoconstrictor [7]. This compound

had been previously named "rabbit aorta contracting substance" by Vane and Piper. In 1976 Vane and his colleagues discovered a platelet antiaggregatory and vasodilator principle formed by aortic tissue, particularly the endothelium. Its chemical structure was soon confirmed by studies carried out by chemists at the Upjohn Company, aided by chemical studies carried out six years earlier by Pace-Asciak and Wolfe [4,6,8]. The principle was found to be a novel bicyclic acid-labile enol-ether prostaglandin called prostacyclin, later renamed prostaglandin I$_2$ (PGI$_2$). At the time of the discovery of thromboxane A$_2$ and its nonenzymatic hydrolysis product thromboxane B$_2$, platelets were found to synthesize 12(S)-hydroxy-5,8,14-*cis*-10-*trans*-eicosatetraenoic acid (12-HETE) by a 12-lipoxygenase not inhibited by nonsteroidal anti-inflammatory drugs.

Extension of these studies in polymorphonuclear leukocytes led to the characterization in the late 1970s of 5(S)-hydroxy-6-*trans*-8,11,14-*cis*-eicosatetraenoic acid (5-HETE) by a 5-lipoxygenase reaction and a dihydroxy arachidonic acid derivative that was identified as 5(S),12(R)-dihydroxy-6,14-*cis*-8,10-*trans*-eicosatetraenoic acid, called leukotriene B$_4$ (LTB$_4$) because of its conjugated triene structure, which absorbs in the 280-nm region. This compound confers potent chemotactic and chemokinetic properties on leukocytes. The conjugated triene structure suggested an unstable intermediate formed by 5-lipoxygenase, and further chemical studies by Samuelsson, Borgeat, and Corey led to the discovery of leukotriene A$_4$ (LTA$_4$) as the 5,6-epoxide precursor for LTB$_4$ synthesis (see articles in Holman [2]; see also [5,9–11]).

Of considerable historical interest is that these studies coincided with attempts to unravel the structure of the slow-reacting substances of anaphylaxis and immediate hypersensitivity reactions. From 1938 to 1940, Feldberg, Kellaway, and Threthewie described SRS-C and SRS-A obtained from guinea pig lungs challenged by cobra venom and specific antigens. The work of Brocklehurst in the 1960s showed that SRS-A was different from other mediators, leading to the suggestion that it could be an unsaturated fatty acid. Austen and Orange and also Morris described another compound with absorption at 280 nm, like LTB$_4$. Stimulated by these clues, in 1979 to 1980, Murphy and Samuelsson and their colleagues isolated from mastocytoma cells, basophil leukemia cells, and guinea pig lung a peptidoarachidonic metabolite that was found to be 5(S)-hydroxy-6(R)-sulfidoglutathionyl-7-cis-9,11-$trans$-14-cis-eicosatetraenoic acid named leukotriene C$_4$ (LTC$_4$). It was formed from LTA$_4$ by the action of glutathione-S-transferase, and it could be converted successively by γ-glutamyl transpeptidases and aminopeptidases into cysteinylglycine, cysteinyl, and cysteinylglutamate derivatives [leukotriene D$_4$ (LTD$_4$), leukotriene E$_4$ (LTE$_4$), and leukotriene F$_4$ (LTF$_4$), respectively]. These substances are powerful bronchoconstrictors and increase vascular permeability [5,9–11]. LTD$_4$ appears to be the most biologically active. The Nobel Prize in Physiology and Medicine was awarded to Sune Bergstrom, Bengt Samuelsson, and John Vane in 1982 for their pivotal role in eicosanoid biochemistry and pharmacology and in elucidating the clinical importance of eicosanoids.

In 1985 to 1986 a new class of arachidonic acid metabolites was detected in leukocytes by Samuelsson's group in Sweden and chemically studied also by Rokach's group in Montreal. Lipoxin A and B are tetraene arachidonic acid metabolites absorbing in the 300- to 315-nm region and derived by the combined interactions of 5- and 15-lipoxygenases through a tetraene epoxide intermediate (see Holman [2] and Samuelsson [5]). Figure 1 summarizes the known ways in which arachidonic acid can be converted into oxygenated derivatives identified at the present time.

RELEASE AND METABOLISM OF ARACHIDONIC ACID

Cell receptor activation by physiological and pathophysiological reactions stimulates arachidonic acid release by several mechanisms. Many studies now indicate that receptor stimulation coupled in the membrane through a G protein rapidly activates phospholipase C, a specific phosphodiesterase that cleaves phosphatidylinositol biphosphate into inositol trisphosphate and diacylglycerol. Inositol polyphosphates containing more than three phosphate groups, e.g., inositol tetrakisphos-

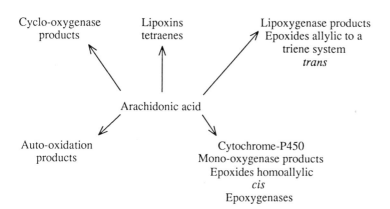

FIG. 1. Scheme of the various ways in which arachidonic acid can be oxygenated.

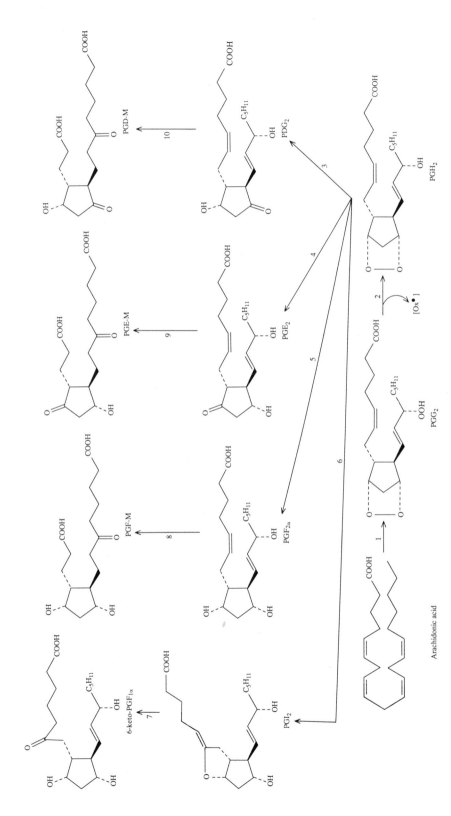

FIG. 2. Pathways in the synthesis of prostaglandins from arachidonic acid. PGF-M, PGE-M, and PGD-M represent metabolites formed by dehydrogenation at C-15, saturation of the 13,14 double bond and β- and ω-oxidations, and excreted in the urine.

phate, may also be formed and can activate calcium entry into cells. The inositol phosphates are second messengers that affect calcium mobilization. Diacylglycerol in association with phosphatidylserine activates protein kinase C. The phorbol esters [e.g., tetradecanoyl phorbol acetate (TPA)] can substitute for diacylglycerol in the activation of protein kinase C (see Chap. 16 and [3,6,9]). Arachidonic acid can be released from diacylglycerol by a diacylglycerol lipase; however, this pathway is probably of minor significance in most cells, since diacylglycerol is rapidly phosphorylated into phosphatidic acid. Of more importance is an associated activation of phospholipase A_2, which releases arachidonic acid from the sn-2 position of membrane phosphatidylinositol or phosphatidylcholine. Steroids can induce at the nuclear level the synthesis of a protein(s) (termed lipomodulin or macrocortin, which is probably the same protein as calpactin) that bind calcium and actin and associate with phospho-

lipids. These proteins inhibit phospholipase A_2, probably by inactivation of the enzyme by selective limited proteolysis. Thus, they also inhibit arachidonic acid release, and this is the basis of their anti-inflammatory action.

SYNTHESIS OF PROSTAGLANDINS, THROMBOXANES, AND LEUKOTRIENES

The metabolic pathways in the formation of prostaglandins, thromboxanes, and leukotrienes are shown in Figures 2 to 4 [4,5,9,12]. Fatty acid cyclooxygenase is a particulate enzyme that when purified has a molecular weight of 71 to 72 kilodaltons (kDa). It is a bifunctional enzyme that contains heme and has both prostaglandin endoperoxide-synthesizing activity, to form prostaglandin G_2 (PGG$_2$), and prostaglandin peroxidase activity, to form prostaglan-

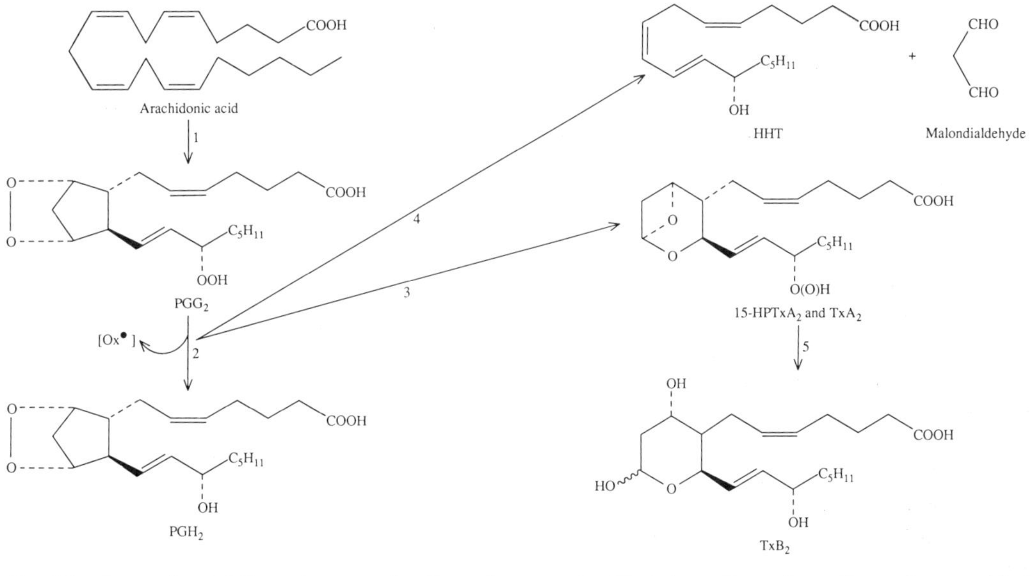

FIG. 3. The formation of thromboxanes by thromboxane A_2 (TxA$_2$) synthase from the endoperoxide PGH$_2$ and its nonenzymatic hydrolysis to thromboxane B_2 (TxB$_2$). In this reaction a 17-carbon hydroxy heptadecatrienoic acid (HHT) is formed by cleavage of the cyclopentane ring of PGH$_2$ to form malondialdehyde in equimolar amounts.

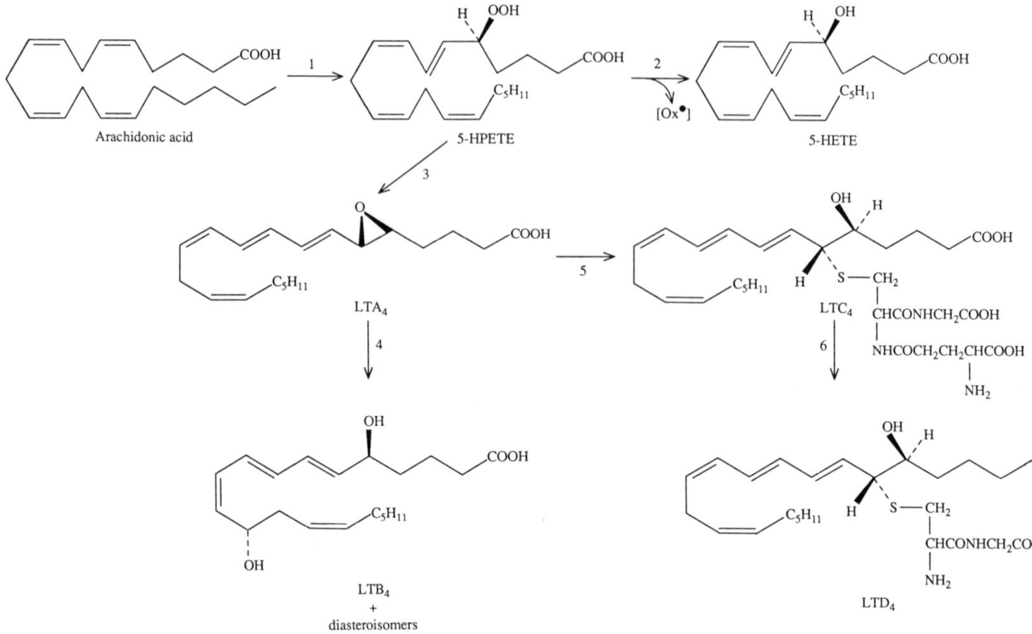

FIG. 4. Pathways in the formation of leukotrienes through the intermediates 5-(*S*)-hydroperoxyeicosate-traenoic acid and the 5,6-epoxy derivative LTA$_4$, which is the precursor for synthesis of LTB$_4$ and the peptidoleukotrienes (LTC$_4$ and LTD$_4$). The leukotrienes LTE$_4$, the 6-(*R*)-cysteinyl compound, and LTF$_4$, the 6-(*R*)-cysteinylglutamate compound, are not shown. The 5-(*S*)-hydroxyeicosatetraenoic acid (5-HETE) is derived from the hydroperoxy precursor by the elimination of an active oxygen radical.

din H$_2$ (PGH$_2$). The initial reaction is the removal, by a lipoxygenase-like reaction, of a prochiral hydrogen in the *S* configuration at C-13 of the polyunsaturated fatty acid substrate. The double bond at the C-11 position isomerizes into the C-12 position, and molecular oxygen is inserted at C-11 to form 11-peroxy eicosaenoic acid. Attack of the oxygen radical at C-9 leads to cyclization to form the cyclopentane ring and initiates the addition of molecular oxygen at C-15 to form PGG$_2$. Prostaglandin hydroperoxidase activity of the cyclooxygenase that transforms PGG$_2$ to PGH$_2$ was formerly thought to be catalyzed by glutathione peroxidase; however, the purified enzyme is free of glutathione peroxidase activity, and a wide variety of compounds can act as hydrogen donors.

Thromboxane A$_2$ synthase has recently been purified from human platelets and found to be a cytochrome P-450 protein. The enzyme forms thromboxane A$_2$, 12-L-hydroxy-5,8,10-heptadecatrienoic acid (HHT) and malondialdehyde in equimolar amounts. Pyridine and imidazole derivatives are thromboxane synthase inhibitors. PGE$_2$ synthase is an unstable microsomal enzyme that requires glutathione as a coenzyme. PGI$_2$ synthase is a microsomal enzyme that is inhibited by hydroperoxides. In the brain it is concentrated in cerebral blood vessels, cerebral capillaries, and the choroid plexus.

The origin of PGF$_{2\alpha}$ (9-α,11-α-PGF$_2$) in brain as well as in other tissues is more complex. It can be formed by enzyme-catalyzed reduction of the endoperoxide PGH$_2$, but it also appears that a different enzyme can stereospecifically form the 9-α,11-β- or the 11-epi-PGF$_2$ isomer by an NADPH-dependent reductase reaction from prostaglandin D_2 (PGD$_2$). A useful method to distinguish the PGF$_2$ isomers is the formation of the *N*-butylboronate derivatives, which will only form in the 9-α,11-α-PGF$_2$ configuration. Of considerable interest is the observation that 9-α,11-β-PGF$_2$ constricts blood vessels and inhibits platelet aggregation. PGD$_2$ synthetase is a cytosolic enzyme that has been partially purified from rat brain. It requires sulfhydryl compounds and, interesting to note, is inactivated by the PGH$_2$ endoperoxide isomerase reaction.

In addition to leukocytes and mast cells, many tissues including the brain contain a 5-lipoxygenase, which leads to the synthesis of leukotrienes. This enzyme is an unstable hydrophobic 80-kilodalton protein that requires calcium ions and ATP. Like fatty acid cyclooxygenase, it is a bifunctional enzyme that catalyzes the formation of 5-hydroperoxyeicosatetraenoic acid and has LTA$_4$ synthase activity [13].

CATABOLISM OF PROSTAGLANDINS AND OTHER EICOSANOIDS

Degradation of prostaglandins and other eicosanoids is complex and involves a number of enzymes [4,14]:

1. Oxidation of the allylic alcohol group at C-15 to the 15-ketoprostaglandins by specific NADH-dependent 15-hydroxyprostaglandin dehydrogenases. The highest activities of these enzymes are found in the lung, spleen, and kidney cortex and the lowest in brain.
2. Reduction of the Δ^{13} double bond to form dihydro compounds. There is much variability in the activity of the reductase in different tissues among animal species and with the stage of development.
3. β-Oxidation occurs principally in the liver to form *dinor* or *tetranor* prostaglandins.

4. ω-Oxidation by microsomal enzymes transforms the metabolites further into ω_1 and ω_2 hydroxylated compounds and then to dicarboxylic acids.
5. Interconversion of PGE prostaglandins to PGF prostaglandins by 9-ketoreductases or the reverse reactions by 9-hydroxyprostaglandin dehydrogenases.
6. PGI$_2$ and thromboxane A$_2$ are nonenzymatically hydrolyzed to 6-keto-PGF$_{1\alpha}$ and thromboxane B$_2$, respectively. These can also be subsequently modified by enzymatic oxidation reactions.

Measurement of the most important blood and urine metabolites of eicosanoids is the basic method of determining total body eicosanoid formation under normal physiological conditions or in pathological states. Specific radioimmunoassay and gas chromatography-mass spectrometry methods are the bases for measuring eicosanoid metabolites. Because little catabolism takes place in brain, the biologically active compounds can be measured directly in the cerebrospinal fluid.

PROSTAGLANDINS, THROMBOXANES, LEUKOTRIENES, AND HYDROXYEICOSATETRAENOIC ACIDS IN BRAIN

Release of prostaglandins into superfusates of cerebral cortex, cerebellum, and spinal cord and into the cerebral ventricles *in vivo* and increased synthesis and release after stimulation of neural pathways have been clearly demonstrated. The basal content of prostaglandins in quick-frozen cerebral neocortex (rat, gerbil, human) is at the limit of detection measured by specific gas chromatography-mass spectrometry analyses, or even by radioimmunoassay. However, Hayaishi and his colleagues found the highest basal levels in the olfactory bulb and pineal gland, followed by the hypothalamus (see articles in Samuelsson [5]; see also [15,16]). Other brain regions had low levels similar to those seen in the neocortex.

Interpretation of the meaning of basal levels of prostaglandins is controversial. Endogenous synthesis of prostaglandins can occur in dissected brain regions, even in the cold. The brain regions most difficult to dissect have the highest content, and this raises the question of whether this reflects actual basal levels or biosynthesis from endogenously released arachidonic acid post-mortem. There is good documentation that incubated intact brain tissue can synthesize prostaglandins (PGE_2, $PGF_{2\alpha}$, PGI_2, PGD_2) and thromboxane B_2 during short incubation periods (Table 1). In rodent brain, PGD_2 is quantitatively the most important fatty acid cyclooxygenase product. The cat brain differs in that $PGF_{2\alpha}$ and thromboxane B_2 are the principal products and that PGD_2 formation is undetectable or exceedingly small. In human cortex and hypothalamus, PGD_2 is apparently formed in only very small amounts. These results are in contrast to the results of biochemical and physiological studies in rats of Hayaishi's group [5]. Basal levels of eicosanoids in brain tissue may not represent the real concentrations of the compounds at the neuronal or glial cell level or in synaptic regions where the concentrations may be considerably higher. Furthermore, in human brain, PGD_2 may be rapidly converted enzymatically into epi-$PGF_{2\alpha}$ (9-α,11-β-PGF_2) by a NADPH-11-ketoreductase reaction. This reaction has been found to take place in human neocortex and may account for the very low levels of PGD_2 formed in human brain. Other human tissues can form PGD_2 in very significant amounts.

In the brain, regional differences of PGD_2, PGE_2, and PGF_2 synthetic enzyme activity do occur. Induction of seizures in convulsion-prone gerbils or in rats by electroshock or convulsant drugs (metrazol, bicuculline) markedly increases arachidonic acid release and formation of PGE_2, PGD_2, and $PGF_{2\alpha}$. The cerebral cortex and hippocampus show by far the largest increases, with considerably less effect observed at the level of the hypothalamus.

The leukotrienes (LTB_4, LTC_4, LTD_4) and monohydroxyeicosatetraenoic acids (HETEs) are synthesized by lipoxygenase pathways in brain, and these products are not derived from contamination with leukocytes or other blood elements (Table 2) [4,9,17]. Most of these studies have used either radioimmunoassay or reverse-phase high-performance liquid chromatography (HPLC) separation methods for the separation of HETEs monitored by absorption at 235 nm and LTB_4 and the 6-sulfidopeptide leukotrienes monitored at 275 to 280 nm. Mass spectrometry has been used to identify the specific HETEs and LTB_4; however, LTC_4, LTD_4,

TABLE 1.   Biosynthesis of prostaglandins[a] by brain tissue[b]

Brain tissue	$PGF_{2\alpha}$	PGE_2	PGD_2	6-Oxo-$PGF_{1\alpha}$	Thromboxane B_2
Rat neocortex basal levels (no incubation)	1.4	1.1	2	ND[c]	ND
Rat neocortex	141	45	720	9	361
Rat hypothalamus	262	70	320	—	—
Cat neocortex	660	203	ND	12	423
Human cortex, biopsy	51	18	4	7	72
Human hypothalamus, autopsy	102	22	5	9	—

[a] Formation, ng/g tissue/15 min.
[b] Results show the means of at least three tissue samples, incubated in phosphate-buffered saline, pH 7.4.
[c] (ND) not detectable.

and LTE_4 have usually been identified by comparing retention times to those of synthetic standards and by bioassay on guinea pig lung strips. The concentrations of LTC_4 in brain are in the picomolar range, with the highest concentration in the hypothalamus, median eminence, nucleus accumbens, and olfactory bulb. LTC_4 is reported to mediate luteinizing hormone release specifically from rat anterior pituitary cells at concentrations of 10^{-14} to 10^{-11} M. There is no effect on release of growth hormone. The effect of LTC_4 appears to differ from the action of hypothalamic luteinizing hormone-releasing hormone (LHRH). LTC_4 action is rapid, whereas LHRH action is much slower. Indeed, LTC_4 acts in leukocytes as a secretogogue [18]. Furthermore, by immunocytochemical methods, a specific group of LTC_4-reacting neurons has been found in the median eminence. LTC_4 action may be related to the immediate release of preformed stored hormone, whereas LHRH peptide action is directed to synthesis of new hormone at the nuclear level. There is no doubt that these studies are uncovering unexpected new roles for leukotrienes in brain in modulation of neurohormone and, possibly, neurotransmitter release. An efficient transport system for LTC_4 has been found in the choroid plexus. A further development in the leukotriene story in brain is the finding of increased LTB_4-, LTC_4-, and LTD_4-like immunoreactivity in the gerbil brain after ischemia and reperfusion and after brain injury and subarachnoid hemorrhage [5,6,19]. Since LTC_4 is a potent vasoconstrictor and increases vascular permeability, particularly in the lung, it is possible that it may be an important initiator of the formation of cerebral ischemic edema and may constrict small cerebral blood vessels. Some caution is needed, however, before jumping to the conclusion that LTC_4 is the important chemical that triggers development of vasogenic edema in brain following injury. Although some workers have reported that LTC_4 or arachidonic acid injected directly into the brain parenchyma induces breakdown of the blood-brain barrier (BBB), and that inhibition of arachidonic acid conversion to leukotrienes prevents vasogenic edema, other investigators employing open cranial window techniques could find no effect on the BBB, even at pharmacologic concentrations. Nevertheless, leukotrienes do cause venous and arterial vasoconstriction. What is clear is that 5-lipoxygenase activity is present in brain, which can lead to the synthesis of 5-hydroperoxy- and 5-hydroxyeicosatetraenoic acids, as well as the biologically active leukotrienes. (Brain ischemia and edema are discussed in Chap. 40.)

Tissue slices of cerebral cortex and homogenates from mouse and rat brain synthesize a number of HETEs. After addition of the calcium ionophore A23187 and arachidonic acid (75 µM), microgram amounts of 12-HETE are

TABLE 2. Biosynthesis of hydroxyeicosatetraenoic acids by rat brain tissue

	Eicosanoid formation[a] (ng/g tissue/10 min)		
	12-HETE	15-HETE	5-HETE
Endogenous formation stimulated by A23187 (5 µM)	195	50	<40
Added arachidonic acid (75 µM)	550	505	400
Added arachidonic acid (75 µM) plus A23187 (5 µM)	5,000	3,010	1,200

[a] 12-HETE, 15-HETE, and 5-HETE represent the individual eicosatetraenoic acids formed by lipoxygenase pathways.

formed far in excess of the formation of prostaglandins and thromboxanes (Table 2) (see Samuelsson [5]). The function of this eicosanoid in brain is unknown. The formation of 12-HETE is particularly high in the rat pineal gland, and it is also formed in the bovine retina. 12-HETE is synthesized by mouse neuroblastoma cells in culture, suggestive of a neuronal origin. Also of interest is that 12-HETE is formed in human skin and increases in hyperproliferative diseases such as psoriasis.

PROSTAGLANDINS AS NEUROMODULATORS IN THE NERVOUS SYSTEM

Stimulation of sympathetic or parasympathetic nerves is associated with release of prostaglandins, principally PGE_2 and $PGF_{2\alpha}$. The release rate is, in general, related to the stimulus frequency, and it decreases to spontaneous levels when stimulation ceases. The postsynaptic effector cell membrane is the most likely site of synthesis because receptor blockade by drugs (hyoscine, atropine, phenoxybenzamine, dibenzyline) inhibits prostaglandin release. Addition of neurotransmitter also stimulates prostaglandin release. Investigations by Hedqvist and coworkers on stimulation of sympathetic nerves to various organs (heart, oviduct, spleen, vas deferens) have revealed that effector responses are inhibited by PGE_1 and PGE_2 but not by the PGF series of prostaglandins. Such inhibition can be produced by picogram to nanogram amounts well within the range seen physiologically. Hedqvist proposed that endogenous PGE_2 formed and released from the postsynaptic effector membrane during stimulation inhibits the release of norepinephrine from presynaptic terminals; however, there is evidence both for and against the role of prostaglandins in inhibiting the exocytotic release of norepinephrine from sympathetic nerve endings [6,16,20].

Release of PGE_2 in the central nervous system may also be involved in the regulation of neurotransmitter release. The stimulated release of norepinephrine and dopamine from rat cerebral cortex and neostriatum *in vitro* is reduced by PGE_2. The disappearance time of dopamine histofluorescence in the neostriatum of rats pretreated with a tyrosine hydroxylase inhibitor decreases when PGE_2 is infused into the carotid artery. The physiological significance of prostaglandins at peripheral and central noradrenergic synapses is still far from clear. PGE prostaglandins can reduce calcium conductance, and this may underlie an inhibitory action on transmitter release [16,20].

In rat brain, PGD_2 administered by intracerebral or intraventricular injection induces sedation, catalepsy, sleep, and hypothermia in a dose-related manner. It also potentiates hexobarbitone hypnosis and has an anticonvulsant action. Intraventricular administration of PGD_2 also has a suppressive effect on the pulsatile release of luteinizing hormone (LH); however, *in vitro* studies in which the medial basal hypothalamus of the rat was superfused showed that PGD_2 has no effect on the release of LHRH but that it does induce release of LH from the pituitary gland. Of much interest is that PGD_2 also increases serotonin content and turnover in brain. In the rodent brain at least, a neuromodulatory action of PGD_2 appears to exist, particularly on serotoninergic neurons that are known to have widespread projections to the cerebral cortex. Various prostaglandins have modulatory effects on hormone release from the hypothalamic-pituitary axis by modulation of neurotransmitter release, particularly dopamine [21]. (See Chap. 14 for a discussion of these hypothalamic peptides.)

EFFECTS OF PROSTAGLANDINS ON CYCLIC NUCLEOTIDES

PGE prostaglandins stimulate cAMP formation in many tissues, including cerebral cortex slices *in vitro* (see Chap. 17). Which brain cell types (neurons or glial cells) are specifically affected has not yet been determined. Synergism of action on adenylate cyclase occurs with combinations of hormones and prostaglandins in intact brain tissue, but the meaning of these complex interactions is far from clear. Homogenization destroys this hormonal responsiveness. There is growing appreciation, however, that high concentrations of intracellular cAMP are associated with inhibition of cell growth in various cell lines in culture. Mouse neuroblastoma cells in culture respond to dibutyryl cAMP, PGE_1, and PGE_2 with a striking morphological differentiation and the development of neuritic processes. This may suggest that PGE prostaglandins play a role in cellular differentiation. Another aspect of the relationship between cAMP and PGE prostaglandins that is of particular relevance to the central nervous system is that morphine and related drugs inhibit the stimulation of cAMP formation by PGE prostaglandins. These studies raise the possibility that the pharmacologic effect of opiates is related to inhibition of the action of endogenously produced prostaglandins on cAMP levels in the brain. High activities of guanylate cyclase are present in brain and retina. Cholinergic agonists, serotonin, and PGF_2 may facilitate excitation of cholinergic and serotoninergic pathways in brain by activating guanylate cyclase [6,16,20].

PROSTAGLANDIN EFFECTS ON INTEGRATED CENTRAL NERVOUS SYSTEM FUNCTION

Direct intraventricular injection of PGE prostaglandins in laboratory animals has a marked sedative effect, which may progress to a stuporous and catatonic-like state. The effect of barbiturates is potentiated, and animals are protected to some degree against the convulsions produced by pentylenetetrazol or electroshock.

The effects of injected prostaglandins are prolonged and are present long after the injected prostaglandins have disappeared. The mechanism of such sedative effects is unclear but is probably triggered by a slowly reversible depression of neurotransmission in certain central pathways through the reduction of neurotransmitter release, as has been demonstrated in peripheral adrenergic pathways. PGE and PGF prostaglandins act on spinal cord reflexes and brain stem cardioregulatory and respiratory centers in complex ways. Inhibitory and excitatory responses have been found, but the results vary from species to species and by prostaglandin type [20].

A considerable body of evidence implicates PGE_2 in the genesis of fever by actions at the anterior hypothalamic level, most probably through effects on serotonin and norepinephrine release [5,6,16]. Although PGE_2 is hyperthermic after intraventricular infusion in rats, it is not involved in normal temperature regulation. There is continuing debate on the role of PGE_2 in the genesis of fever. PGE_2 still remains the best candidate for mediation of hyperthermic responses to leukocyte pyrogen, endotoxin, and interleukin-1; however, PGE_2 synthesis may also be initiated within brain capillaries. Endotoxin and interleukin-1 can gain access to the central nervous system at the organum vasculosum laminae terminalis and, within the anterior hypothalamic level, activate fatty acid cyclooxygenase to form PGE_2. Purified human leukocytic pyrogen induces a rapid increase in muscle proteolysis, and this is mediated by the synthesis of PGE_2. Both proteolysis and PGE_2 formation are blocked by indomethacin and by the thiol protease inhibitor Ep-475, which inactivates lysosomal cathepsins. It is possible that mediators formed by activated phagocytic cells entering the brain hypothalamic thermal regulatory centers have similar actions that lead to the release of vasopressin and prostaglandins, which can generate fever in pathological situations.

MECHANISMS OF CEREBRAL VASOSPASM

There is evidence linking PGE prostaglandins to the genesis of vascular headaches and to migraine in particular. Although certainly not the only mediator, PGE_2 is a potent hyperalgesic agent, and it potentiates induction of pain by tachykinins. It is also a potent dilator of peripheral vascular beds and could mediate temporal artery vasodilation [22]. PGE_2 has been shown in dogs to reduce cerebral blood flow and to cause vasoconstriction of cerebral arterioles. The release of thromboxane A_2 from activated platelets could also contribute to cerebral vessel vasoconstriction, thus adding to the neurological symptoms in the prodromal phase of migraine.

Cerebral vasospasm is an important cause of morbidity and mortality following subarachnoid hemorrhage in humans. Although vasospasm can occur immediately after hemorrhage, it usually develops considerably later. Possible chemical triggers responsible for cerebral vasospasm are numerous [23–25]. The prostaglandin or eicosanoid hypothesis of vasospasm is only one of several. Damaged brain and blood vessels and the changing chemical reactions within the hemorrhage itself (formation of heme; release of ferric ion; initiation of peroxidation of released polyunsaturated fatty acids; and formation of hydroperoxy radicals, leukotrienes, and HETEs) may all contribute over time to vasospasm. Indeed, cerebral vasospasm is almost certainly caused by multiple, interactive, and synergistic chemicals released from blood cells (erythrocytes, platelets, and leukocytes) and blood proteins during resolution of the blood in the subarachnoid space. Although there is no doubt that prostaglandins are released into cerebrospinal fluid following subarachnoid hemorrhage, brain surgery or trauma, encephalitis, and epilepsy, and in patients with stroke, there is little correlation with neurological symptoms or course of disease [6].

ROLE OF PROSTAGLANDINS IN BRAIN INJURY AND ISCHEMIA

It has been well established that brain injury causes gross damage to vascular elements and that the breakdown of the BBB gives rise to vasogenic edema. (These subjects are also discussed in Chap. 40.) After a focal freezing lesion to the parietal cortex of the rat, a functional disturbance occurs that leads to widespread depression of local cerebral glucose utilization. After a freezing injury to the brain, arachidonic acid is released, and PGE_2, PGD_2, and $PGF_{2\alpha}$ are formed in cortical regions adjacent to the injury. Nonsteroidal anti-inflammatory drugs, such as indomethacin and ibuprofen, which inhibit prostaglandin synthesis, significantly diminish the depression in cortical glucose utilization. These studies implicate the formation of prostaglandins in the sequence of events leading to the functional depression of glucose utilization. Dexamethasone also ameliorates some of the effects of trauma to the brain, but there is no direct evidence that this is due to inhibition of arachidonic acid release and the formation of prostaglandins. The underlying mechanism leading to widespread depression of glucose utilization is postulated to involve changes in biogenic amine neurotransmitter systems [14,19]. A significant increase in the turnover of serotonin on the side of the injury and a decrease in the concentration of norepinephrine but not dopamine have been observed in both hemispheres. Thus, both serotoninergic and noradrenergic neurotransmitter systems are perturbed following brain injury. A hypothesis linking brain injury to alteration in brain function through pathways involving arachidonic acid release, prostaglandin formation, and disturbances in neurotransmitter systems has been developed (Fig. 5). The demonstration that PGD_2 affects neuronal turnover and release of serotonin opens new possibilities for the therapeutic management of brain injury in humans.

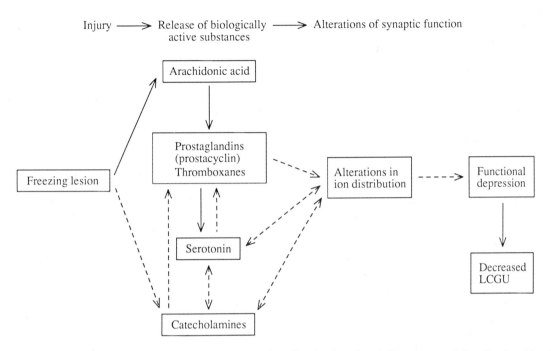

FIG. 5. A working hypothesis of the mechanisms underlying the functional disturbances following focal brain injury in the rat, which leads to widespread cortical decrease in local cerebral glucose utilization (LCGU): (*solid arrow*) demonstrated; (*dotted arrow*) postulated. (Courtesy of Dr. H. M. Pappius.)

The release of arachidonic acid and the formation of both fatty acid cyclooxygenase and lipoxygenase products occur following experimental cerebral ischemia in rodents, dogs, and cats [6,16,18]. PGI_2 has potent platelet antiaggregatory properties and is a vasodilator of many vascular beds including the brain. It also has fibrinolytic properties. These properties suggest that infusion of PGI_2 might be of therapeutic value in reversing the neurological impairment in humans after thromboembolic strokes. Studies do not support a beneficial effect on cerebral function after intravenous infusion of PGI_2 in patients with completed cerebral infarction (see articles in Holman [2]). It may be necessary to modify these studies so that PGI_2 can be given at the earliest stage of cerebral ischemia or given in combination with other drugs, such as the calcium channel block-

ers. The changes that take place over time in the brain in humans after stroke are very complex. Eicosanoids are certainly formed in the penumbral regions, but their specific effects have not been fully defined.

SELECTED REFERENCES

1. Holman, R. T. (ed.), *Essential Fatty Acids and Prostaglandins.* (*Progress in Lipid Research, Vol. 20*). Oxford: Pergamon Press, 1981.
2. Holman, R. T. (ed.), *Essential Fatty Acids, Prostaglandins and Leukotrienes.* (*Progress in Lipid Research, Vol. 25*). Oxford: Pergamon Press, 1986.
3. Majerus, P. W., Wilson, D. B., Connolly, T. M., Bross, T. E., and Neufeld, E. J. Phosphoinositide turnover provides a link in stimulus-re-

sponse coupling. *Trends Biochem. Sci.* 10:168–171, 1985.

4. Pace-Asciak, C., and Granstrom, E. *Prostaglandins and Related Substances.* (*New Comprehensive Biochemistry, Vol. 5*). Amsterdam: Elsevier, 1983.

5. Samuelsson, B. Leukotrienes and related compounds. In O. Hayaishi and S. Yamamoto (eds.), *Advances in Prostaglandin, Thromboxane and Leukotriene Research.* New York: Raven Press, 1985, Vol. 15, pp. 1–9.

6. Wolfe, L. S. Eicosanoids: Prostaglandins, thromboxanes, leukotrienes and other derivatives of carbon-20 unsaturated fatty acids. *J. Neurochem.* 38:1–14, 1982.

7. Hamberg, M., and Samuelsson, B. Prostaglandin endoperoxides. Novel transformations of arachidonic acid in human platelets. *Proc. Natl. Acad. Sci. U.S.A.* 71:3400–3404, 1974.

8. Moncada, S., and Vane, J. R. Pharmacology and endogenous roles of prostaglandin endoperoxides, thromboxane A_2, and prostacyclin. *Pharmacol. Rev.* 30:293–331, 1978.

9. Needleman, P., Turk, J., Jakschik, B. A., Morrison, A. R., and Lefkowith, J. B. Arachidonic acid metabolism. *Annu. Rev. Biochem.* 55:69–102, 1986.

10. Piper, P. J. (ed.), *SRS-A and Leukotrienes.* Chichester: Research Studies Press, 1981.

11. Sirois, P., and Borgeat, P. Mediators of immediate hypersensitivity. In P. Sirois and M. Rola-Pleszczynski (eds.), *Immunopharmacology.* Amsterdam: Biomedical Press (Elsevier), 1982, pp. 201–222.

12. Yamamoto, S. Enzymes in the arachidonic acid cascade. In C. Pace-Asciak and E. Granström (eds.), *Prostaglandins and Related Substances.* Amsterdam: Elsevier, 1983, pp. 171–202.

13. Rouzer, C. A., Matsumoto, T., and Samuelsson, B. Single protein from human leukocytes possesses 5-lipoxygenase and leukotriene A_4 synthase activities. *Proc. Natl. Acad. Sci. U.S.A.* 83:857–861, 1986.

14. Pappius, H. M., and Wolfe, L. S. Effect of drugs on local cerebral glucose utilization in traumatized brain: Mechanisms of action of steroids revisited. In K. G. Go and A. Baethmann (eds.), *Recent Progress in the Study of Therapy of Brain Edema.* New York: Plenum, 1984, pp. 11–26.

15. Ueno, R., Hayaishi, O., Inoue, S., and Nakayama, T. Prostaglandin D_2: A cerebral sleep regulating substance in rats. In O. Hayaishi and S. Yamamoto (eds.), *Advances in Prostaglandin, Thromboxane and Leukotriene Research.* New York: Raven Press, 1985, Vol. 15, pp. 581–583.

16. Wolfe, L. S., and Coceani, F. The role of prostaglandins in the central nervous system. *Annu. Rev. Physiol.* 41:669–684, 1979.

17. Bazan, N. G., and Birkle, D. L. Depolarization or convulsions increase the formation of HETE and prostaglandins in the central nervous system. In O. Hayaishi and S. Yamamoto (eds.), *Advances in Prostaglandin, Thromboxane and Leukotriene Research.* New York: Raven Press, 1985, Vol. 15, pp. 569–571.

18. Hulting, A.-L., Lindgren, J. Å., Hökfelt, T., Eneroth, P., Werner, S., Patrono, C., and Samuelsson, B. Leukotriene C_4 as a mediator of luteinizing hormone release from rat anterior pituitary cells. *Proc. Natl. Acad. Sci. U.S.A.* 82:3834–3838, 1985.

19. Wolfe, L. S., and Pappius, H. M. Arachidonic acid metabolites in cerebral ischemia and brain injury. In A. Bes, P. Braquet, R. Paoletti, and B. K. Siesjo (eds.), *Cerebral Ischemia.* Amsterdam: Elsevier, 1984, pp. 223–231.

20. Curro, F. A., Greenberg, S., and Gardiner, R. W. Effect of prostaglandins on central nervous system function. In S. Greenberg, P. J. Kadowitz, and T. F. Burks (eds.), *Modern Pharmacology-Toxicology.* New York: Marcel Dekker, 1982, Vol. 21, pp. 367–406.

21. Behrman, H. R. Prostaglandins in hypothalamo-pituitary and ovarian function. *Annu. Rev. Physiol.* 41:685–700, 1979.

22. Pickard, J. D., Macdonell, L. A., Mackenzie, E. T., and Harper, A. M. Prostaglandin induced effects in the primate cerebral circulation. *Eur. J. Pharmacol.* 43:343–351, 1977.

23. Maeda, Y., Tani, E., and Miyamoto, T. Prostaglandin metabolism in experimental cerebral vasospasm. *J. Neurosurg.* 55:779–785, 1981.

24. Robertson, J. C. Cerebral arterial spasm: current concepts. *Clin. Neurosurg.* 21:100–106, 1975.

25. White, R. P. Prostaglandins and cerebral vasospasm. In S. Greenberg, P. J. Kadowitz, and T. F. Burks (eds.), *Modern Pharmacology-Toxicology.* New York: Marcel Dekker, 1982, Vol. 21, pp. 341–365.

PART THREE

Molecular Neurobiology

CHAPTER 21

Gene Expression
in the
Mammalian Nervous System

Allan J. Tobin and Michel Khrestchatisky

This chapter is dedicated to the memory of Professor Edward Herbert, whose science and humanity continue to inspire his
former students and colleagues.

Basic Neurochemistry: Molecular, Cellular, and Medical Aspects, 4th Ed., edited by G. J. Siegel et al. Raven Press, Ltd., New York, 1989.
Correspondence to Allan J. Tobin, Department of Biology, University of California, Los Angeles, 405 Hilgard Avenue, Los Angeles, California
90024-1606.

In confronting the mammalian brain, molecular biology faces a seemingly impossible challenge: How do cells with the same genetic information come to have such diverse cellular phenotypes, each with the capacity to respond characteristically to changes in local environment and in the experience of the organism as a whole? The answers to this question must be based on an understanding of gene expression and its regulation, the subject of this chapter.

CELLULAR COMPLEXITY OF THE BRAIN

The human brain contains more than 10^{12} neurons. Each neuron is arguably unique, with a distinct size, shape, position, and pattern of connections, transmitters, and responses to chemical and electrical cues. But the human genome contains at most only enough information for about 10^6 genes. Even if all these genes were expressed in the brain, there would not be enough information to specify each neuron separately.

As in the case of the immune system, the key to understanding the complexity of the brain lies in combinations. Just as nine-digit zip codes specify each block in the United States, so could a relatively small number of genes specify the unique properties of every cell in the brain. In this chapter we discuss the general principles of gene expression in eukaryotes and show how variations in the processing of genetic information lead to the fantastic diversity of cells in the brain.

With its huge number of potential combinations of expressed genes, the brain has an extraordinarily high informational content. Flexibility in gene regulation in brain cells may explain the rapid spread of mammals into a wide variety of ecological niches. The relatively slow evolution of genetic adaptations, that is, the ability to express favorable gene combinations, has provided new opportunities for rapid phys-

iological adaptation to varying environments and, in the case of the human species, efficient cultural adaptation through learning and language. The brain, the organ in which regulatory complexity is greatest, has become the major agent for modifying the environment. More than any other organ, the brain illustrates the tight interaction between heredity and environment in the determination of phenotype, both of cells and organisms.

GENE EXPRESSION IN EUKARYOTES

The familiar central dogma of molecular biology states that information flows from DNA to RNA to proteins. Cells copy the information contained in the nucleotide sequence of DNA into corresponding nucleotide sequences of RNA. For structural genes—stretches of DNA that code for proteins—the carrier RNA is called messenger RNA, or mRNA. In eukaryotes, mRNAs are produced in the nucleus and travel to the cytoplasm. There, in association with the ribosomes and other synthetic machinery, each mRNA directs the synthesis of a single type of polypeptide chain, which directly or indirectly assembles into a mature protein [1,2].

DNA and RNA each consist of linear chains of four nucleotide building blocks. Information in DNA and RNA is thus contained in dialects of a single language, and the conversion of information from DNA into RNA is called transcription.

Each polypeptide consists of linear chains of 20 amino acid building blocks. The information in proteins is thus written in a different language, and the conversion of information from RNA to protein is called translation.

Structure of a eukaryotic mRNA

Each mRNA contains coding information that specifies the sequence of amino acid residues in a type of polypeptide chain. In addition, each mRNA contains noncoding information that includes control signals for translation: (a) an initiation site for translation, a sequence that dictates the starting site of the polypeptide, and the phase in which the triplet code is read; (b) a termination sequence that signals the end of the polypeptide chain; (c) a binding site slightly "upstream" from the initiation site that facilitates binding to ribosomes; and (d) other "upstream" and "downstream" sequences that contribute to the transport and stability of the mRNA. Most eukaryotic mRNAs also contain two additional structures that are added after transcription and are not copied from DNA: (a) an inverted "cap" at the 5' end; and (b) a "tail" of 50 to 150 residues of adenylic acid (poly A) at the 3' end of the mRNA. The sequence AAUAAA in the primary transcript is the usual signal for the addition of poly A some 20 bases downstream (Fig. 1).

Structure of a eukaryotic gene

The genes themselves contain still more noncoding sequences. Many of these contribute to the regulation of gene expression. In particular, some regulatory sequences specify the cells in which a given gene is expressed.

Molecular biologists are able to create specific alterations in DNA sequences of suspected function. They then can examine the effect of these changes on gene expression in a test system, e.g., *in vitro*, in cultured cells, or even in *transgenic* animals, in which altered genes are transferred to fertilized eggs and become part of the genome (see later). Among the sequences identified in this way are: (a) promoters, which specify the starting point and direction of transcription [3]; (b) enhancers, which facilitate the transcription of neighboring DNA, independent of orientation, and relatively independent of position [3]; and (c) termination signals [4].

Most eukaryotic genes also contain long stretches of DNA that are transcribed into RNA but are excised before the initial transcript matures into functional mRNA. These interruptions in the structural information for polypeptide synthesis are called *intervening sequences*, or *introns*. In contrast, the coding sequences are called *exons* (Fig. 2).

Mature mRNA usually results from an elaborate editing process. Introns are removed and exons spliced together, like so many pieces of film or magnetic tape. DNA and the primary RNA transcript also contain sequences that specify where the splices are to occur [5,6]. As we shall see, the pattern of splicing of a single transcript can vary from tissue to tissue.

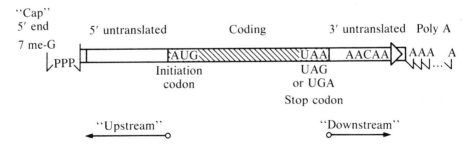

FIG. 1. Structure of a eukaryotic mRNA. A typical eukaryotic mRNA, reading from the 5' end ("upstream") on the left, to the 3' end ("downstream") on the right. The 5' untranslated region is usually 10 to 200 bases long, and the 3' untranslated region 50 to 2,000 bases long. The average size of the coding region in abundant mRNAs is about 1,500 bases.

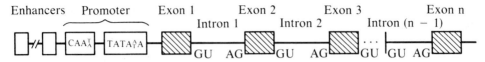

FIG. 2. Structure of a eukaryotic gene.

Post-translational events

After mRNAs are translated into polypeptides, still more information processing occurs, with attendant opportunities for developmental regulation. Polypeptides fold into specific conformations and assemble into complexes with other polypeptides. The creation of three-dimensional structures from linear polypeptides depends on the ionic conditions and pH of the surrounding cytosol, as well as on the concentrations of specific allosteric effectors. In addition, the covalent structure of each polypeptide may be altered by disulfide bond formation, protease cleavage, glycosylation, phosphorylation, methylation, fatty acid acylation, and covalent linkage to peptides or to membrane lipids. These covalent changes often affect the conformation of individual polypeptides, their association with other polypeptides, and their biological function.

The flow of information from DNA to functional protein is the same in the brain as in other organs. Until recently, however, researchers have avoided the brain for mechanistic studies because of its multiplicity of cell types and the complexity of gene expression. With the advent of recombinant DNA techniques for studying the expression of specific genes, many molecular biologists have undertaken detailed studies of the structure and expression of genes important to brain function.

Molecular hybridization techniques

The identification and quantification of specific sequences in DNA and RNA depend on duplex formation by polynucleotide strands with complementary base sequences. The stability of such duplexes depends on the length of the complementary sequences, the degree of matching between the two strands, the temperature, the salt concentration, and the presence of compounds such as formamide that interfere with the interactions of the two strands. Researchers can distinguish among exact and inexact matches by noting the temperature at which duplexes dissociate or "melt." Perfect or near-perfect matches maintain their double-strandedness under stringent conditions, that is, at high temperature and low salt concentration.

Formation of duplexes between previously associated DNA strands is called *reannealing*, or reassociation. Formation of duplexes between DNA and RNA, RNA and RNA, or between DNA sequences not originally associated, for example, between genomic and recombinant DNAs, is called *hybridization*.

Hybridization techniques are at the center of the technical repertoire of molecular biologists. Hybridization experiments allow researchers to identify DNA fragments, recombinant DNA molecules, and RNAs with specified base sequences. Such identification depends on the use of molecular "probes" of known sequence, usually recombinant DNAs or synthetic oligonucleotides.

Hybridization may be performed (a) in solution; (b) with blots of DNA or RNA onto various supports, most frequently nitrocellulose or nylon membranes; or (c) on tissue sections. Solution hybridization is the best understood and follows the kinetic course of simple bimolecular or pseudomonomolecular reactions. Hybridization to blots of DNA (Southern blots) or RNA (Northern blots, dot blots, and slot blots) are technically much simpler, however. Hybridization to extracted RNA allows researchers both to identify the sizes of specific mRNAs and their precursors and to estimate the amount of each RNA species in a given extract.

Hybridization of probes for specific mRNAs to tissue sections is called *in situ* hybridization or hybridization histochemistry [7]. *In situ* hybridization is especially useful for detecting the cellular distribution of mRNAs in heterogeneous tissues such as the brain. Most investigators now use RNA probes labeled with ^{35}S. These RNAs are transcribed *in vitro* from recombinant DNAs containing a sequence of interest attached to sequences that are recognized by specific bacteriophage RNA polymerases.

MULTIPLE RNAs FROM A SINGLE GENE

Most eukaryotic genes are mosaics of exons and introns. In the canonical picture of mRNA production, transcription begins at a single promoter and yields a single primary transcript containing all the introns and exons. All primary transcripts are immediately modified by the addition of a "cap" consisting of a 7-methylguanosine residue at the 5' end. Almost all transcripts that will eventually exit to the cytoplasm are further modified at their 3' ends by the addition of 200 to 250 adenylic residues (poly A). Polyadenylation occurs in the nucleus soon after the termination of transcription. Cytoplasmic nucleases subsequently nibble the poly A tail down to about 50 to 150 residues. Splicing machinery within the nucleus, including ribonucleoprotein particles containing small nuclear RNAs, then cut and splice the primary transcripts to produce mature mRNAs that lack introns.

Although many genes appear to produce only one primary transcript and a unique mature mRNA, other genes produce many alternative forms of primary transcripts and mature mRNAs. Primary transcripts may start or end

at different sites and may have more than one site for the addition of poly A; and different splicing events may string together different subsets of exons from a single primary transcript. A single stretch of DNA may thus encode a variety of polypeptides. Sometimes, a single cell may simultaneously express these different polypeptides; in other cases, the pattern of transcription and splicing is subject to developmental regulation. After geneticists spent decades arriving at the textbook definition, "one gene—one polypeptide chain," subsequent studies of gene expression conclusively showed that one gene can encode many different polypeptide chains, often with divergent functions.

Alternative transcription, splicing, and polyadenylation

The nervous system provides many examples of the same span of DNA encoding several polypeptide chains [1,2,6]. Two contrasting examples are especially instructive: (a) the multiple mRNAs for myelin basic protein, and (b) the alternative polyadenylation and splicing of a gene that encodes the Ca^{2+}-regulating peptide calcitonin in thyroid and a putative neurotransmitter called calcitonin gene-related peptide (CGRP) in brain.

Transcription of the gene for myelin basic protein appears to begin and end at single sites to yield a single primary transcript containing seven exons and six introns [8]. Alternative patterns of splicing yield at least five species of mRNA that encode five polypeptide chains of slightly different sizes. These polypeptides have common sequences at each end and slightly different sequences in the middle. No one knows whether these five polypeptides have different functions in myelin.

In contrast, the precursor of the mRNAs for calcitonin and CGRP contains six exons, five introns, and two sites for polyadenylation [9]. In the thyroid, the transcript is polyadenylated at the end of the fourth exon, whereas in neurons, poly A lies at the end of the sixth exon. Splicing in the thyroid yields calcitonin mRNA, which consists of exons 1, 2, 3, and 4; in neurons, however, exon 4 is removed, and exons 5 and 6 are attached to the mRNA. The two mRNAs each encode polypeptides that are precursors of the biologically active peptides. Exons 1 and 6 do not encode translated polypeptide sequence. Post-translational proteolytic processing in both thyroid and brain removes the amino acid sequences encoded by exons 2 and 3, so the final calcitonin peptide in thyroid derives entirely from exon 4, and CGRP in brain from exon 5.

Similar alternative patterns of polyadenylation and splicing occur for the common primary transcript for two tachykinin peptides: substance P and substance K. Each peptide results from the proteolysis of a larger peptide, respectively called α- and β-preprotachykinin. The primary transcript contains seven exons, and differential splicing of the primary transcript produces two mRNAs that either include or exclude exon 6, the coding region for substance K. The ratio of the two mRNAs varies among brain regions as well as between the extraneural sites of synthesis, the thyroid and intestine.

Modulation of mRNA translation and degradation

Once mature mRNAs arrive in the cytoplasm, they become subject to further regulation through alterations in the efficiencies of translation and in the rapidity of their degradation. The classic example of translational control of gene expression is the mRNA contained in the sea urchin egg prior to fertilization: The unfertilized sea urchin egg contains many apparently mature maternal mRNAs, but translation is extremely slow until after fertilization [10].

The egg yolk protein vitellogenin provides an excellent example of the regulation of mRNA

stability: Estrogen increases the half-life of vitellogenin mRNA by about 30-fold. No such changes have been shown in the development of neurons or glia, but studies of the processing and stability of brain RNAs are still in their infancy.

Alternative post-translational events

Even after the production of mature mRNA and its translation into a polypeptide, cells can still regulate the character and amount of biologically active gene products. The 134 amino acid residue polypeptide pro-opiomelanocortin (POMC), for example, is a precursor of at least seven biologically active peptides, including adrenocorticotropic hormone; β-endorphin; β- and γ-lipotropic hormones; and α-, β-, and γ-melanocyte-stimulating hormones (see Chaps. 13 and 14). The pattern of post-translational processing of POMC in turn is likely to depend on the activity of cell-type specific proteases, the products of other developmentally regulated genes.

Other post-translational processes are also subject to regulation. Among the most important and best studied of these are phosphorylations by a variety of kinases (see Chap. 19). Here we observe that specific post-translational modifications result from the action of extracellular signals, such as growth factors and neurotransmitters, acting through second messengers, such as cyclic AMP (cAMP), Ca^{2+}, or diacylglycerol. Furthermore, the proteins whose activity is modified by regulated phosphorylations may themselves regulate the expression of other genes.

Evolution of regulatory mechanisms

The many steps required for the production of a biologically active protein almost certainly result from the opportunism of evolution. The first genes were probably RNA rather than DNA, and present genes probably resulted from the combination of small coding regions. Like contemporary eukaryotic genes, the earliest genes, we now think, were mosaics of exons and introns. Because genomes continually rearranged in evolutionary time, the shuffling of exons allowed the sharing of useful domains by more than one gene [1].

Gene rearrangements

In the immune system, rearrangement of DNA occurs in the cytodifferentiation of both B and T cells. Whereas amplification, loss, and rearrangement of DNA occur during oogenesis in *Drosophila* and amphibia, no evidence of gene rearrangement in vertebrates presently exists outside the immune system.

Multigene families

Duplications and rearrangements of ancestral genes were instrumental in the evolution of the many gene families of the contemporary mammalian genome. Such duplications and divergent evolution allowed the refinement of functional differences in the final polypeptides and of the cell specificity of expression. The nervous system provides many examples of such families whose members differ in their function or their regulation. Among these families are

1. a G-protein superfamily that includes genes for the muscarinic acetylcholine receptor (see Chap. 10), the β-adrenergic receptor (see Chap. 11), and rhodopsin (see Chap. 7);
2. a ligand-gated channel superfamily that includes the four subunits of the nicotinic acetylcholine receptor (see Chap. 32), the γ-aminobutyric acid (GABA$_A$) receptor, and the glycine receptor (see Chap. 15); and
3. a conductance channel family that includes the voltage-dependent K^+- and Na^+-channel polypeptides (see Chap. 4).

COMPLEXITY OF GENE EXPRESSION IN THE MAMMALIAN BRAIN

Even before they could study the expression of specific genes in the brain, molecular biologists could address the question of the brain's transcriptional and translational repertoires. The question in these studies was, How many genes are expressed in the brain? The approach was to determine, by hybridization of appropriate DNAs and RNAs, the fraction of an organism's DNA that could form complementary duplexes with (a) mRNA—an index of how many genes were likely to be translated into protein; and (b) nuclear RNA (nRNA)—an index of how many genes are transcribed. As might be expected, much more of the informational capacity of the genome is expressed in the brain than in any other tissue [11,12].

The haploid genome of a mammal consists of about 3×10^9 nucleotide pairs. If all this DNA specified the amino acid sequences of polypeptides, it could encode 1 million polypeptides, each 1,000 amino acid residues long.

How many genes are expressed in the brain?

As discussed earlier, a typical eukaryotic gene contains much DNA that does not code for polypeptides. In fact, as much as 95 percent of an organism's DNA specifies introns, known regulatory sequences, and sequences of unknown function, both within and between genes. Some of the unexplained noncoding DNA may have a regulatory role; much of it, however, may represent DNA that makes no contribution to phenotype—such sequences have been called "selfish genes."

Molecular hybridization experiments permit one to determine the fraction of the genome that is expressed as mRNA. Such experiments show the complexity of gene expression in the brain: The brain contains about two to three times as much information in mRNA as other tissues. Similar experiments with nRNA show that the brain as a whole transcribes at least 30 percent of the sequences in genomic DNA.

Knowing the amount of DNA expressed in mRNA and the average size of mRNA, we can estimate the average number of genes expressed in the brain. The average size of brain-specific mRNAs is almost 5 kilobases (kb), two to three times the average size of the abundant mRNAs expressed in other tissues [13]. Present estimates range from about 30,000 to 200,000 different genes expressed in brain. We do not yet understand why brain-specific mRNAs should be longer than those of other tissues.

More complex brains do not depend on more genes

Cows, mice, and humans all have about the same amount of DNA per cell, but their brains differ dramatically in both cellular and intellectual complexity. A mouse brain, for example, contains about 5×10^6 cells, whereas a human brain contains about 10^{11} cells. The greater complexity of the human brain, then, apparently results from factors other than the overall amount of gene molecules. It seems likely that the complexity of the brain depends on combinations and interactions at the cellular level.

Does gene expression in the brain differ from that in other organs?

More mRNAs are expressed in the brain than in other organs, and brain-specific mRNAs appear to be larger than those elsewhere. Gene expression in the brain also differs from that in other tissues in the extent of polyadenylation of mRNA. In mammalian tissues other than the brain, more than 90 percent of mRNA molecules contain polyA tails of 100 to 250 residues at their 3' ends. Almost all mRNA in fetal rat and mouse brains also contains such poly A tails. In adult rodent brains, however, less than

50 percent of isolated mRNA (defined as polysomal RNA that is neither ribosomal RNA nor transfer RNA) contains poly A. RNA lacking poly A is termed (poly A)$^-$ RNA. In other tissues, (polyA)$^-$ RNA makes up less than 10 percent of the total mRNA. Several workers [11,12] have suggested that this reflects a large class of brain-specific (poly A)$^-$ mRNA that appears late in development.

An alternative explanation for the high level of (poly A)$^-$ RNA in the brain is that the late-appearing brain-specific mRNAs are substantially larger than the mRNAs expressed in fetal brain. The larger mRNAs are more sensitive to scission during isolation. If a 5-kb mRNA is cut in two, only the 3' portion will contain a poly A sequence. The 5' portion will appear to be a (poly A)$^-$ mRNA whose size is comparable to that of abundant mRNAs. Although a few mRNAs in higher organisms, notably those encoding the histones, are known not to contain poly A tails, there are at present no defined examples of brain-specific mRNAs that lack poly A. At this time, the significance of (poly A)$^-$ RNA is still unresolved.

Although gene expression in the brain is more complicated than in other tissues, it may not be fundamentally different. Rather, the complexity of the brain may result from the utilization of many mechanisms used more sparingly in other tissues.

Differences in gene expression in brain regions and in individual cells

Anatomical boundaries within the brain define regions of the brain that differ in organization, connections, and use of neurotransmitters. Ligand binding studies and immunocytochemistry have shown that specific neurotransmitter-related proteins are differentially distributed; for example, D_2 dopamine receptors are found in highest concentrations in the striatum (see Chap. 11), and the NMDA-type of glutamate receptors are found in highest concentrations in the hippocampus and dentate gyrus (see Chap. 15). Many neurodegenerative diseases preferentially affect specific regions of the brain, for example, the substantia nigra in Parkinson's disease, the striatum in Huntington's disease (see Chap. 42), and the basal forebrain in Alzheimer's disease (see Chap. 43).

Molecular hybridization experiments, however, have thus far failed to identify region-specific classes of mRNA. Individual brain regions are also similar in the total number of genes expressed [11,14].

On the other hand, immunocytochemistry, ligand binding studies, and *in situ* hybridization to mRNA within individual cells all indicate that various classes of cells differ in their expression of individual mRNAs. For example, the enzyme glutamic acid decarboxylase (GAD) and its mRNA are present in specific cell types in the cerebellum, hippocampus, cortex, thalamus, as well as in other regions of the brain [15]. Similarly, some randomly chosen (anonymous) mRNAs, whose translation products are unknown, are present in specific cell types in a number of brain regions [16]. Individual cell types, then, rather than anatomically defined regions, seem to be the units of developmental regulation of gene expression in the brain.

REGULATORS OF CELL-SPECIFIC TRANSCRIPTION

Many researchers are actively trying to identify the elements that control gene expression in individual cell types. A common strategy is to use recombinant DNA techniques to construct hybrid genes that contain a suspected regulatory region of one gene and the coding region of another gene [3]. The coding region of the second gene serves as a *reporter* of the ability of a given test sequence to regulate expression in a particular type of cell. The bacterial gene product chloramphenicol acetyltransferase is a valuable reporter, since it catalyzes a reaction not found in eukaryotic cells. The enzymatic activity of the reporter in cells containing a hybrid gene indicates the effectiveness of different test sequences in regulating gene expression. Other useful reporters include β-galactosidase and luciferase.

Test systems for regulatory sequences

Two principal test systems are employed for the expression of hybrid genes: (a) cell lines, and (b) transgenic mice. In the first case, hybrid genes are put into a continuous cell line, and the expression of the reporter gene is monitored. Some experiments measure the transient expression of hybrid genes in the hours or days that they have access to the host cells' machinery for gene expression. Other experiments examine the expression of hybrid genes that have become integrated into host DNA [17]. One goal of such experiments is to compare the ability of different DNA sequences to regulate gene expression in cell lines with different properties. A particularly interesting set of questions centers on gene regulation in different types of neurons. Why, for example, are tyrosine hydroxylase and dopamine-β-hydroxylase both expressed in the noradrenergic neurons of the locus coeruleus, but not in the dopaminergic neurons of the substantia nigra?

Cell lines

Expression of transient or stable hybrid genes in cell lines has allowed the identification of general and specific regulatory sequences for many genes. The paucity of cell lines with well-defined neuronal phenotypes, however, has limited studies of neuronal gene expression. Most of the cell lines used have derived from naturally occurring or chemically induced tumors. Recently, however, a number of laboratories have begun to generate neuronal cell lines by transforming neuronal precursors with oncogenes carried in engineered retroviruses. Potentially, the most valuable of these lines may contain stably integrated oncogenes whose activity is temperature sensitive: At a permissive temperature, e.g., 33°C, the oncogene product is active, and the cells proliferate as a neoplasm; at a restrictive temperature, e.g., 42°C, the oncogene product is inactive, and the cells revert to a specific neuronal phenotype.

Inserting DNA in cells presents another problem for studies of hybrid gene expression. Some cell lines readily take up DNA from coprecipitates with calcium phosphate. Other cell lines do not, and researchers need to use other methods, including the transient opening of the membrane with an electric pulse, known as electroporation; injection; or infection with engineered viruses, especially retroviruses.

Transgenic mice

The other general approach to the study of regulatory sequences takes advantage of the fact that it is possible to inject exogenous genes into mouse zygotes to produce transgenic mice. After a successful injection, an engineered *transgene* becomes part of the DNA in all cells, including the germ line. By examining the pattern of gene expression of the reporter gene by immunocytochemistry, for example, researchers can identify the elements that regulate cell-specific gene expression. As more laboratories gain the ability to produce transgenic mice, this approach will undoubtedly contribute much to our understanding of neuronal cytodifferentiation. It seems likely, however, that the cost and complexity of experiments with transgenic mice will make work with cell lines the more common approach.

cis-Regulatory sequences and *trans*-acting regulatory factors

Testing of hybrid genes in cell lines and transgenic mice has allowed the identification of sequences responsible for the expression of many genes in particular cells in specific environ-ments at precise times [3,17]. Because these sequences regulate the expression of adjacent structural genes, they are called *cis*-regulatory elements. In some cases, the regulatory sequences are in the immediate vicinity of the coding region; in other cases, they may lie 10 kb or more away.

Many neuronal functions are regulated by adenylate cyclase or by protein kinase C (see Chap. 19). Several groups have recently identified a specific 12-base *cis*-regulatory sequence present in several genes whose transcription is increased by cyclic AMP (cAMP) and phorbol esters.

Diffusible proteins, or *trans*-acting regulatory factors, interact with the *cis*-regulatory sequences to establish the pattern of gene expression within individual cells. Several methods can detect the specific binding of *trans*-acting factors to specific DNA sequences. These include experiments that measure the ability of bound proteins to prevent the chemical or enzymatic cleavage of specific DNA sequences ("footprinting"), and determination of lowered electrophoretic mobility of a specific DNA fragment when it is bound to a protein (gel retardation).

How *trans*-acting effector proteins interact with *cis*-regulatory DNA is still unknown. An *enhancer* could act in one of two ways: (a) It could transiently permit RNA polymerase to bind to the DNA; or (b) it could produce a stable change in chromatin structure, allowing continuous transcription. In the second case, the continuous presence of the *trans*-acting factor would not be required.

Stable changes in chromatin structure do occur during cytodifferentiation. Genes that are actively transcribed in a particular cell are often more susceptible to digestion by a variety of nucleases. In particular, accessibility to deoxyribonuclease I (DNase I) often parallels accessibility to RNA polymerase, so globin genes are preferentially digested by DNase I in chicken erythroid cells but not in oviduct.

In addition, DNA sequences that bind effector proteins, such as polymerase or an enhancer-binding protein, may have distorted structures that render them hypersensitive to DNase I digestion. Probes of chromatin structure thus suggest that the pattern of active genes within a given cell type depends on developmental history as well as on the expression of specific effectors at a given moment.

Regulation of gene expression by glucocorticoids

The regulation of gene expression by steroids provides an excellent example of the role of *trans*-acting factors in gene regulation (see also Chap. 47). Steroids diffuse across the plasma membrane and bind to specific cytoplasmic receptors. The steroid-receptor complex then diffuses into the nucleus, where it interacts with DNA and stimulates the expression of specific genes. Isolation of the gene for the glucocorticoid receptor has allowed the determination of the relationship between the structure and function of one such receptor [18]. The receptor consists of at least two domains, one of which binds glucocorticoids and another that consequently binds to an enhancer sequence.

Glucocorticoids and other steroids affect gene expression in many cells, including the nervous system. The action of steroids, however, differs among cell types. Glucocorticoids thus induce the synthesis of tyrosine aminotransferase in the liver and growth hormone in the pituitary, but decrease the synthesis of pro-opiomelanocortin in the pituitary and lead to the death of lymphocytes in the thymus. It seems likely that in each cell type, glucocorticoids act to alter gene expression through the same receptor. The differentiated state of each cell thus affects its susceptibility to regulation by the same effector. One possible set of mechanisms for these differences among cell types lies in the organization of DNA and proteins in chromatin:

A given gene may be more or less accessible to receptor in different cells.

ACKNOWLEDGMENTS

We are grateful to the following people for their helpful comments and suggestions: Dona Chikaraishi, Sophie Feldblum, William Hahn, Daniel Kaufman, Wendy Macklin, Gail Mandel, Roger Rosenberg, Joan Schwartz, Robert Snodgrass, and Gregor Sutcliffe.

REFERENCES

1. Darnell, J., Lodish, H., and Baltimore, D. *Molecular Cell Biology*. New York: Scientific American Books, 1986.
2. Lewin, B. *Genes III*. New York: Wiley, 1987.
3. Maniatis, T., Goodbourn, S., and Fischer, J. A. Regulation of inducible and tissue-specific gene expression. *Science* 236:1237–1244, 1987.
4. Platt, T. Transcriptional termination and the regulation of gene expression. *Annu. Rev. Biochem.* 55:339–372, 1986.
5. Green, M. R. Pre-mRNA splicing. *Annu. Rev. Genet.* 20:671–708, 1986.
6. Leff, S. E., Rosenfeld, M. G., and Evans, R. M. Complex transcriptional units: Diversity in gene expression by alternative RNA processing. *Annu. Rev. Biochem.* 55:1091–1117, 1986.
7. Uhl, G. R. (ed.). *In Situ Hybridization in Brain*. New York: Plenum, 1986.
8. Campagnoni, A. T., and Macklin, W. B. Cellular and molecular aspects of myelin protein gene expression. *Molec. Neurobiol. Rev.* 2:41–89, 1988.
9. Mayo, K. E., Evans, R. M., and Rosenfeld, G. M. Genes encoding mammalian neuroendocrine peptides: strategies toward their identification and analysis. *Annu. Rev. Physiol.* 48:431–446, 1986.
10. Davidson, E. H. *Gene Activity in Early Development, 3rd ed*. Orlando: Academic Press, 1986.
11. Chikaraishi, D. M., Brilliant, M. H., and Lewis, E. J. Cloning and characteristics of rat brain

RNAs: Rare brain specific transcripts and tyrosine hydroxylase. *Cold Spring Harbor Symp. Quant. Biol.* 48:309–318, 1983.

12. Chaudhari, N., and Hahn, W. E. Genetic expression in the developing brain. *Science* 220:924–928, 1983.

13. Sutcliffe, J. G. mRNA in the mammalian central nervous system. *Annu. Rev. Neurosci.* 11:157–198, 1988.

14. Wood, T. L., Frantz, G. D., Menkes, J. H., and Tobin, A. J. Regional distribution of messenger RNAs in postmortem human brain. *J. Neurosci. Res.* 16:311–324, 1986.

15. Wuenschell, C. W., Fisher, R. S., Tillakaratne, N. J. K., and Tobin, A. J. *In situ* detection of GAD mRNA in mouse brain. In G. R. Uhl (ed.), *In Situ Hybridization in Brain.* New York: Plenum, 1986, pp. 135–149.

16. Branks, P. L., and Wilson, M. C. Patterns of gene expression in the murine brain revealed by in situ hybridization of brain-specific mRNAs. *Mol. Neurobiol.* 1:1–16, 1986.

17. Palmiter, R. D., and Brinster, R. L. Germ-line transformation of mice. *Annu. Rev. Genet.* 20:465–499, 1986.

18. Giguere, V., Hollenberg, S. M., Rosenfeld, M. G., and Evans, R. M. Functional domains of the human glucocorticoid receptor. *Cell* 46:645–652, 1986.

CHAPTER 22

Molecular Probes for Gene Expression

Richard H. Goodman, Gail Mandel, and Malcolm J. Low

Basic Neurochemistry: Molecular, Cellular, and Medical Aspects, 4th Ed., edited by G. J. Siegel et al. Raven Press, Ltd., New York, 1989.
Correspondence to Richard H. Goodman, Division of Molecular Medicine, Tufts-New England Medical Center, 750 Washington Street,
Boston, Massachusetts 02111.

429

Studies of gene expression in the nervous system can be divided into two categories: (a) those directed toward identifying general aspects of gene expression that are unique to neural tissues, and (b) those focused on the expression of individual neural-specific genes. The first category was considered in Chapter 21. The present chapter deals with the second category, especially as it relates to the molecular pathology of inherited neurological diseases. Advances in our understanding of the molecular basis of ion channel, receptor, and transmitter physiology in the nervous system have become increasingly dependent on recombinant DNA technology. The generation of molecular probes for gene expression is inextricably associated with the construction, screening, and characterization of complementary DNA clones in gene libraries. In this chapter, we address the general approaches available for constructing such libraries and outline many of the techniques that have been used successfully to isolate neural-specific cDNAs.

STRUCTURE AND USES OF COMPLEMENTARY DNA

Complementary DNA is a double-stranded copy of messenger RNA and contains the same sequence information as RNA

A *complementary DNA* (cDNA) *library*, or cDNA bank, contains a representation of all of the messenger RNA (mRNA) molecules from a given cell or tissue source. In general, therefore, nonabundant mRNAs are infrequently represented. The differential representation of cDNAs in a cDNA library contrasts with a *genomic library*, which theoretically contains an equal representation of all genes. Another important difference between cDNA libraries and genomic libraries is that the former contain only transcribed sequences. Genomic libraries contain a large amount of nonstructural DNA, including intervening sequences (introns) and flanking DNA, that is never translated into protein (see Chap. 21). This nonstructural DNA can nonetheless be very important in controlling gene expression and can be the locus of pathological mutations associated with neurological disease (see Chap. 23). Thus, the issue of whether to screen a cDNA or genomic library for a neural-specific gene depends on the particular question being asked. In general, it is easier to isolate and characterize a cDNA clone, especially if the cDNA library can be constructed from a source that is rich in the desired mRNA. If an enriched source cannot be identified, it may be desirable to screen a genomic library directly. Regulatory elements that control gene transcription can only be isolated from a genomic library. Generally, in practice, genomic clones are isolated by using cDNA clones as hybridization probes.

The sequence of cDNA can provide information about proteins that is not available from protein analyses

All neuropeptides, for example, are synthesized as larger precursors. The N-terminals of these precursors invariably contain a signal sequence, 15 to 30 amino acids in length, that is removed during the process of translation. Thus, the structure of the primary translation product of a neuropeptide gene can only be deduced from the cDNA and can never be determined through biochemical analysis of proteins synthesized in intact cells. Additionally, many neuropeptides are synthesized as polyproteins, containing multiple bioactive peptides. Although the precursor (*prohormone*) forms of some neuropeptides have been identified immunochemically, the amounts isolated are often insufficient for structural analysis. Consequently, determining the sequence of a cDNA is frequently the only way to predict the primary structure of a precursor protein and to determine if multiple peptides are derived from a single precursor. Examples of novel neuroendocrine peptides predicted entirely through the analysis of cDNA clones include peptide histidine methionine (PHM-27) [1] and gonadotropin-releasing hormone-associated protein (GAP) [2]. Complementary DNA sequences have also been used to predict the functional domains of ion channels [3]; the ligand-binding regions of receptors [4]; and structural homologies among channels, receptors, and growth-regulating factors [5]. It is only through the analysis of cDNA sequences that many novel mechanisms for generating peptide diversity, such as exon-shuffling, have been discovered [6].

Cloned cDNAs are invaluable for studying the regulation of gene expression in the nervous system

The Northern blot technique, which allows the precise characterization and quantitation of specific mRNAs, utilizes radiolabeled cDNA molecules for hybridization to nucleic acids immobilized on a nitrocellulose or nylon membrane. *In situ* hybridization histochemistry allows a qualitative analysis of specific mRNA species in individual cells. The combination of these two methods provides a powerful technology for examining the molecular biology of gene expression in complex tissues such as the brain.

Cloned cDNAs are used in expression vectors to produce chemical amounts of neurobiological proteins

These vectors have been designed such that the cloned cDNAs can be expressed in either bacterial or animal cells, depending on the need to provide specific types of post-translational modifications. In some instances, bacterial cells are capable of providing all of the biosynthetic steps required for biological activity. For example, bacterial expression systems have been used to synthesize the C-terminal peptide (GAP) derived from the luteinizing hormone-releasing hormone precursor [2]. Other proteins require a complex series of processing events accomplished only by animal cells. The frog oocyte system has been particularly useful in determining the structure-function characteristics of ion channels and receptors [7].

Isolating a cDNA clone is frequently the first step toward isolating a gene

A cDNA provides an ideal probe for screening a genomic library because it contains long stretches of nucleic acids that are identical to the gene. Low-stringency hybridizations can be used to probe for related members of a multigene family or to screen for homologous sequences in other species. Eukaryotic genes can be highly complex, with multiple intervening sequences separating the individual protein-coding regions. Because a cDNA represents only the exon sequences, the structure of the cDNA allows an accurate assignment of the splice donor and splice acceptor sites. Indeed, determining the structure of a gene without knowledge of the cDNA sequence can be exceedingly difficult.

CONSTRUCTION OF cDNA LIBRARIES

Complementary DNA clones of neurobiological interest may be identified by hybridization, immunological or functional approaches

Hybridization approaches depend on the availability of a cDNA or oligonucleotide probe. Immunological approaches rely on specific antibodies to identify fusion proteins produced by an expression vector. Functional approaches depend on assays specific for particular biological features of the protein of interest. All of these methods require the construction of a cDNA library, although each method requires a library with slightly different features.

The first step in preparing a cDNA library is to isolate intact RNA

The most commonly used methods for isolation of RNA utilize chaotropic agents, such as guanidine isothiocyanate, to denature proteins that cause RNA degradation [8]. RNA is typically separated from DNA and protein by differential precipitation in lithium chloride or by centrifugation through cesium chloride. The polyadenylated fraction of RNA, which represents most of the mRNA pool but only approximately 1 percent of the total cellular RNA, can be purified by chromatography on a column containing oligodeoxythymidine (dT) cellulose. The polyadenylate tail at the 3' end of the RNA binds to the chain of deoxythymidine residues under high-salt conditions and can be eluted in low-salt buffer. A significant fraction of brain mRNA appears to be nonpolyadenylated and cannot be purified on oligo(dT) columns, however. Further enrichment for a particular species of mRNA can be achieved by sucrose gradient centrifugation or by denaturing agarose gel electrophoresis. In general, sucrose gradient centrifugation results in a lower degree of purification than gel electrophoresis but is technically easier and allows a greater yield of nondegraded RNA.

All methods for production of cDNA libraries utilize the enzyme reverse transcriptase to synthesize single-stranded DNA copies of mRNA molecules

Reverse transcriptase is an RNA-dependent DNA polymerase and requires a primer to initiate its activity. Typically, the primer used is a short chain of oligo(dT) residues, which hybridizes to the polyadenylate tail of the mRNA. Reverse transcriptase is a 5'- to 3'-directed polymerase. Therefore, the copy produced by the action of reverse transcriptase is complementary to the mRNA template and points in the opposite direction (antisense). If the mRNA sequence is partially known, synthetic oligonucleotide primers can be used instead of oligo(dT) to enrich the library for the desired cDNA. Similarly, either specific oligonucleotide or random hexanucleotide primers can be used to increase the likelihood of generating cDNA clones that represent the 5' end of the mRNAs, corresponding to the 5' untranslated region and the N-terminal of the protein.

Reverse transcriptase typically produces single-stranded cDNA molecules that have a hairpin loop at the 3' end. The original methods for cDNA cloning included steps to remove the mRNA template and to use the hairpin loop as a primer for second-strand synthesis. The second strand could be synthesized using reverse transcriptase, *Escherichia coli* DNA polymerase I (large fragment), or T4 DNA polymerase. Each of these enzymes catalyzes the polymerization of DNA in the 5'- to 3'-direction, producing a molecule that is open at one end and closed at the other. This structure is obvious when the double-stranded cDNA molecules are analyzed on denaturing and native agarose gels. Denaturation doubles the length of the cDNA molecules, indicating that they are covalently attached at one end. The closed end must be cleaved to generate a molecule that can be inserted into a plasmid or bacteriophage vector. This cleavage is accomplished by the enzyme S-1 nuclease, which is relatively specific for single-stranded DNA molecules. The hairpin loop is cleaved preferentially by the S-1 nuclease, leaving a double-stranded cDNA that is open at both ends. Unfortunately, S-1 nuclease also tends to degrade double-stranded nucleic acids, leading to a loss of sequences from the ends of the cDNA. Nevertheless, the S-1 nuclease procedure has been used successfully to clone many neuropeptides and receptors.

Several cloning approaches have been developed that avoid the need for S-1 nuclease digestion. The most sophisticated of these approaches was developed by Okayama and Berg [9]. This procedure utilizes a cloning vector that also serves as the primer for first-strand synthesis. By taking advantage of the property of the enzyme, terminal deoxynucleotide transferase, to catalyze the addition of nucleotides only to flush-ended or 3'-overhanging DNA, Okayama and Berg were able to select for clones that represent the full length of the mRNA. The mRNA template within the vector is replaced by DNA using a mixture of RNase H, DNA polymerase I, and DNA ligase.

Perhaps the most commonly used procedure for generating double-stranded cDNA is the method of Gubler and Hoffman [10]. This procedure utilizes reverse transcriptase to synthesize the first cDNA strand, but instead of removing the hybridized mRNA with alkali as in the classical method, the RNA is replaced with DNA by using RNase H and DNA polymerase I. This method has proven to be highly efficient, producing as many as 10^6 recombinants from each microgram of starting mRNA. Because S-1 nuclease treatment is avoided, the cDNA clones generated by the Gubler and Hoffman procedure are often full length.

Complementary DNA molecules introduced into bacteria would be rapidly degraded if not inserted into a suitable vector

Most early cDNA libraries utilized plasmid vectors, small circular molecules of DNA that contain multiple unique restriction sites and one or more antibiotic resistance markers. Plasmids exist within the bacterial cell as episomes and can be separated easily from the bacterial chromosomal DNA. Plasmids with relaxed replication characteristics can be amplified many times, increasing the relative amount of foreign DNA in the cell. Many libraries are now constructed in the bacteriophage vectors λgt10 and

λgt11. These bacteriophage vectors have a much higher cloning efficiency than plasmid vectors and offer several technical advantages.

The insertion of cDNA molecules into a vector can be accomplished either by annealing homopolymeric tails attached to both vector and cDNA or by using synthetic DNA linkers. Early cloning strategies primarily utilized the former approach; later strategies depend on the latter. Synthetic DNA linkers, typically small double-stranded fragments of DNA containing a single restriction site, can be added to the flush ends of cDNA molecules by using the enzyme DNA ligase. The blunt-ended linkers tend to add onto the ends of the cDNA as concatemers. By cleaving the "linkered" DNA with the appropriate restriction enzyme, a sticky-ended fragment of cDNA can be generated. This sticky-ended cDNA fragment can be inserted into a plasmid or bacteriophage vector at a site containing complementary sticky ends, sealed using DNA ligase, and passed in bacteria as a recombinant DNA molecule. To prevent the vector molecule from religating to itself without inserting a cDNA molecule, it is frequently necessary to dephosphorylate the ends of the vector. Alternatively, antibiotic selection or an easily assayed enzymatic activity can be used to identify bacterial clones containing recombinant plasmids. Recent advances in cloning strategies have utilized linkers that can insert a cDNA into a cloning vector in a particular orientation.

As mentioned above, screening bacteriophage libraries is far more efficient than screening plasmid libraries. While assaying 50,000 to 100,000 bacterial colonies is a tour-de-force, screening 10^6 bacteriophage plaques is relatively easy. Furthermore, genetic characteristics have been introduced into bacteriophage vectors to increase the ease of selecting recombinants; λgt10 is designed primarily for hybridization screening protocols. The cloning site in λgt10 interrupts the phage repressor gene (*cI*) such that only phages that contain a cDNA insert form clear lytic plaques on the appropriate bacterial strain. The cloning site in λgt11, a bacteriophage vector designed primarily for immunological screening, interrupts the *lacZ* gene. Consequently, recombinant λgt11 phage cannot metabolize the indicator X-gal (5-bromo-4-chloro-3-indolyl-β-D-galactoside) and form white plaques, whereas nonrecombinant phages form blue plaques.

SCREENING cDNA LIBRARIES

The procedures required for identifying a particular cDNA clone within a cDNA library depend on the abundance of the specific mRNA. To detect a rare cDNA, it may be necessary to screen as many as 10^6 independent clones. Abundant cDNAs can be identified by screening only a few hundred clones.

Very abundant clones are identified by screening the cDNA library with a radiolabeled cDNA probe generated from total polyadenylated RNA

In practice, this screening would be performed by using the colony hybridization procedure of Grunstein and Hogness [11]. Recombinant bacterial colonies would be grown on a nitrocellulose filter, replicated, and then lysed with alkali. The alkali also denatures the plasmid DNA and allows the DNA to become permanently attached to the filter. The filters are washed to remove the bacterial debris, baked to fix the DNA, and then incubated with the radiolabeled probe. Colonies that contain sequences complementary to the probe can be detected by autoradiography. If, for example, 10 percent of the mRNA molecules encode a single protein and the remainder of the mRNAs encode less abundant species, a cDNA probe generated from the total population of mRNAs would be enriched for the abundant molecule. Colonies detected with this probe are likely to encode the most abundant mRNA species.

For less abundant cDNAs, the hybridization arrest or hybridization selection procedures can be used

Both of these techniques, as originally designed, depend on the prior characterization of the cell-free translation product representing the protein of interest. The hybridization arrest procedure makes use of the observation that mRNAs hybridized to their complementary cDNA are inactive in cell-free translation assays. By mixing a particular cDNA with a population of mRNAs and determining which specific cell-free translation product is absent from a gel electrophoresis pattern, it is possible to associate the cDNA with a particular protein. The hybridization selection method is the converse of this procedure. For hybrid selection, cDNAs are immobilized on nitrocellulose, allowed to hybridize with the population of mRNAs, washed to remove nonhybridizing mRNA species, and eluted with low-salt buffer. The specifically hybridizing mRNAs are translated in a cell-free system and are analyzed by polyacrylamide gel electrophoresis.

The preferred hybridization method for detecting rare cDNA clones makes use of synthetic oligonucleotide probes

For isolating truly rare cDNAs, the hybridization arrest and selection procedures are too cumbersome for efficient screening. Frequently, the amino acid sequences of a protein or peptide fragment can be determined through biochemical techniques. Although the precise DNA sequence encoding the peptide might be unknown, it is nonetheless possible to synthesize a family of oligonucleotides representing all possible combinations of codons corresponding to any peptide sequence. Because of the degeneracy of the genetic code, the number of oligonucleotides required to represent every possible DNA sequence can be quite large. To decrease this number of possibilities, oligonucleotide probes are usually generated from peptide sequences rich in the amino acids methionine, tryptophan, phenylalanine, tyrosine, histidine, glutamine, asparagine, lysine, aspartic acid, glutamic acid, and cysteine, which are encoded by only one or two different codons. To reduce the number of ambiguous codons still further, several additional approaches have been utilized to generate probes. First, deoxyguanosine can be substituted for deoxyadenosine, and deoxythymidine can be used in place of deoxycytosine. These substitutions, which substantially decrease the complexity of an oligonucleotide mixture, can be made because guanosine and thymidine weakly base-pair in a double-stranded DNA molecule. By this simple maneuver, Touchot et al. [12] reduced the complexity of a mixed 20 *mer* from 512 to 61. Another approach to decreasing the complexity of a mixed oligonucleotide is to substitute deoxyinosine, which base-pairs with any of the four deoxynucleotides, at all ambiguous positions. The resultant probe has a low complexity but is not as specific as an oligonucleotide containing the normal nucleotide bases. Additionally, based on codon-usage tables that have been developed for different eukaryotic species, educated guesses can be made about the likelihood of a specific codon being correct [13].

Oligonucleotides synthesized for screening cDNA libraries are usually between 15 and 25 nucleotides long. By adjusting the stringency of hybridization by altering temperature and salt concentration, it is possible to distinguish among sequences that differ by as little as a single nucleotide. The specificity of oligonucleotide probes can be increased further by performing hybridization in the presence of tetramethylammonium chloride, which eliminates the preferential melting of adenine-thymine (A-T) base pairs. The use of two independent oligonucleotide probes representing

discrete portions of the cDNA is also a valuable method for increasing the specificity of hybridization.

Because hybridization between two nucleic acid sequences is a function of several independent parameters, including the degree of complementarity, the amount of guanine-cytosine (G-C) pairing, and the length of the hybridizing strands, it is often possible to overcome one deficiency of the probe by altering some other characteristic. Therefore an alternative approach for oligonucleotide screening is to use long probes (30–100 nucleotides long) containing a limited number of mismatches. Long probes that are only 80 percent homologous with the optimal sequence have been used to produce highly specific hybridization signals under conditions of low-stringency hybridization and washing [14]. In general, the hybridization conditions for long-probe screening need to be determined empirically to reduce background binding.

IMMUNOLOGICAL SCREENING IN BACTERIAL EXPRESSION SYSTEMS

Hybridization approaches to isolating cDNA clones require a great deal of prior information about the protein of interest. Often, especially for nonabundant proteins, it is difficult or impossible to determine the amino acid sequence of even a small peptide fragment. Immunological screening approaches in bacterial systems can obviate the need to obtain prior protein sequence information but depend on several assumptions. First, antibody recognition must not depend on post-translational modifications that are only accomplished by eukaryotic cells. This means that glycosylation, phosphorylation, sulfation, and particular patterns of proteolytic cleavage cannot be required for antibody binding. Second, the antibody recognition site cannot depend on the conformation of protein. Immunological screening approaches typically demand that the antibody recognize denatured proteins fused to a large bacterial product. Finally, the eukaryotic proteins expressed in bacteria must be protected from bacterial degradation and must not be toxic to the host bacterial cells.

An additional problem in any sort of expression-cloning, whether the screening procedure is immunological or functional, is the need to ensure that the cDNAs are translated in the proper reading frame and orientation. Because a DNA sequence theoretically can be translated in either orientation and in any of three reading frames, the random insertion of a cDNA into an expression vector has only one in six chances of encoding an authentic protein. Although there are methods for directing the orientation of a cDNA into a vector, it is often easier in bacterial systems to scale-up the number of colonies screened. This scaling-up requires a very efficient cloning strategy, however. Bacteriophage expression systems, such as the λgt11 system developed by Young and Davis [15], are far more efficient than plasmid cloning vehicles. Therefore, although cDNAs of neurobiological interest have been identified by immunological screening of plasmid libraries, the bacteriophage systems are probably more generally useful.

In the λgt11 vector, cDNA molecules are inserted into a unique restriction site near the end of the gene encoding the enzyme β-galactosidase. This approach provides three useful features. First, insertion of foreign DNA into the β-galactosidase gene inactivates enzyme activity and results in the production of white as opposed to blue plaques when the bacteriophages are grown in the presence of X-gal. This color screening allows an easy determination of the fraction of recombinant phage. Second, the foreign cDNAs are expressed as fusion proteins, linked to β-galactosidase. Fusion proteins constructed in this manner are less likely to be viewed as "foreign" by bacterial degradation systems. Finally, expression of the fusion pro-

teins can be controlled by isopropyl-β-D-thiogalactopyranoside (IPTG), an inducer of the β-galactosidase gene. Thus, it is possible to limit the expression of the potentially toxic fusion proteins until just before screening. Immunological screening consists of inducing the bacteriophage with IPTG, transferring the fusion proteins to a nitrocellulose filter, and then probing with specific antibody. In general, polyclonal antibodies have been preferable to monoclonals for library screening. Affinity-purified antisera, immunoabsorbed to remove antibodies to bacterial proteins, have been most useful. Binding of the specific antibody is detected by using iodinated staphylococcal protein A or by an alkaline phosphatase-based second-antibody technique.

Unfortunately, because immunological screening often depends on incompletely characterized antibodies and because the sequence of the protein of interest is typically unknown, it is often difficult to confirm that an immunopositive bacteriophage encodes the appropriate cDNA. It is essential, therefore, to devise a secondary screening procedure to eliminate false-positive cDNA clones. One approach that has been particularly useful for identifying neuropeptide cDNAs has been to combine immunological screening with *in situ* hybridization histochemistry [16]. This combination of methodologies is exemplified by the approach used to clone the cDNA encoding the precursor to thyrotropin-releasing hormone (TRH), a neuropeptide and hypothalamic releasing factor. Because TRH is only a tripeptide, oligonucleotides cannot recognize the three-amino-acid peptide unambiguously. Antisera directed toward the mature TRH molecule, modified at the N-terminal by cyclization of the glutamic acid residue and at the C-terminal by amidation of the proline residue, do not recognize the precursor form of the peptide. Lechan et al. [17] utilized an antiserum directed against a synthetic decapeptide, designed to represent an N- and C-terminal extended form of TRH, to screen a rat hypothalamic λgt11 expression library. Immunopositive clones detected using the antibody were then used in *in situ* hybridization assays of rat brain slices. Only the cDNAs that identified TRH-immunopositive neurons were considered to represent potential TRH precursors. The complexity of neuropeptide anatomy in the central nervous system, as assayed by *in situ* hybridization, appears to be a useful adjunct to the relatively nonspecific immunochemical expression cloning approaches.

EXPRESSION CLONING IN EUKARYOTIC SYSTEMS

As discussed above, bacterial expression systems do not accomplish the post-translational modifications that might be essential for immunological recognition or biological function. It is often necessary therefore to rely on eukaryotic expression systems for identifying cDNAs of neurobiological interest. These eukaryotic systems are particularly valuable for cloning cDNAs encoding large membrane proteins such as ion channels or receptors. Because sequences at the N-terminals of many proteins are essential for correct targeting, processing, and folding in eukaryotic cells, a prerequisite for expression cloning in animal cells is to construct a full-length cDNA library. Fortunately, several of the cloning strategies described earlier satisfy this requirement for providing full-length clones.

Fibroblast cells are a vehicle for DNA transfection

The earliest successes in eukaryotic expression-cloning resulted in the characterization of oncogenes. DNA-mediated gene transfer techniques were used to introduce high-molecular-weight DNA from human tumors into mouse fibroblast cell lines. Introduction of specific human DNA fragments led to altered growth of recipient cells, an effect that could be recognized by focus formation or growth in soft agar. Subsequent studies led to the precise characterization of many categories of oncogenes.

Neurobiologists use similar approaches to identify genes encoding cell-surface receptors. One of the most elegant examples of this approach was the cloning of the nerve growth factor (NGF) receptor by Chao et al. [18]. These workers introduced high-molecular-weight human genomic DNA into receptor-deficient mouse fibroblast L cells. Cotransfection of a gene encoding herpes virus thymidine kinase (TK) into the TK L-cell line allowed a selection for cells that had integrated the foreign DNA into their genome. TK$^+$ cells were screened for the expression of NGF receptors by an immunological erythrocyte rosette assay. To confirm that the transfected cells expressed an authentic NGF receptor, radiolabeled NGF-NGF receptor complexes were characterized by affinity cross-linking and polyacrylamide gel electrophoresis. Human DNA encoding the NGF receptor was identified by screening DNA from transfected NGF receptor-positive L cells with human repetitive sequence DNA.

Frog oocytes can be used for translation of mRNA

The most recent approaches to eukaryotic expression-cloning are actually very reminiscent of some of the early cDNA cloning strategies. The recent cloning of the serotonin [19] and substance K [20] receptors utilized several steps, including sucrose gradient centrifugation and denaturing agarose gel electrophoresis, to enrich a particular species of mRNA before beginning to construct a library. This emphasis on mRNA purification was a feature of the early approaches to cloning the cDNA encoding insulin.

A combination of two additional techniques, one old and one fairly recent, has proven to be particularly useful in cloning cDNAs encoding membrane proteins such as channels and receptors. The frog oocyte translation system, originally developed by Gurdon et al. [21], provides a means of translating mRNAs from almost any type of eukaryotic cell. More important, the frog oocyte has the ability to perform many of the post-translational modifications required for biological function of membrane proteins. Additionally, the oocyte provides a relatively simple cell system for performing electrophysiological or biochemical analyses of channels or transport proteins. Receptors that transduce signals through an inositol trisphosphate (IP_3)-based pathway are particularly easy to detect in oocytes. Increased levels of IP_3 liberate Ca^{2+} from intracellular storage pools in oocytes, as it does in many other types of eukaryotic cells. This increased level of Ca^{2+} opens a Ca^{2+}-activated Cl^- channel that can be detected by measurement of the voltage gradient or current across the oocyte membrane. Receptors coupled to a cyclic AMP-dependent signal transduction pathway are more difficult to assay in the frog oocyte system.

The RNA used in oocyte injection experiments can be isolated from cells or transcribed from cDNAs cloned into bacteriophage transcription vectors. By synthesizing a cDNA library from a source enriched for the mRNA of interest, transcribing the cloned cDNAs *in vitro*, and subsequently microinjecting the synthetic mRNAs into frog oocytes, one can test the activity of individual pools of cDNA clones. This functional method of cDNA screening requires that the cDNA inserts be full length and encode the entire protein. Depending on the length of the particular mRNA, this requirement can become an extremely difficult problem for cDNA screening strategies. If the membrane protein contains multiple subunits derived from separate mRNA species, cloning strategies based on oocyte expression become even more problematic. One approach to overcoming the full-length single-mRNA species requirement is

to use a procedure based on the hybridization arrest protocol. RNA from a tissue or cell line is allowed to hybridize to a pool of cDNAs in solution. Hybridized and nonhybridized RNA are separated by density gradient centrifugation and are tested in frog oocytes. By assaying sequentially smaller pools of clones, a single cDNA that encodes the receptor or transporter of interest can be identified. Once isolated, the individual cDNA can be used to screen a cDNA or genomic library by hybridization techniques. Proof that the isolated DNA sequences encode an authentic receptor or channel requires that RNA transcribed from the DNA produce a functional protein.

STRUCTURAL ANALYSIS OF cDNA CLONES

Complementary DNA molecules can be sequenced by either the chemical degradation method of Maxam and Gilbert [22] or by the enzymatic chain terminator method of Sanger et al. [23]. Many of the currently available cloning vectors contain restriction sites and primer regions that eliminate the need to subclone the DNA insert prior to sequencing. Consequently, it is now relatively easy to sequence one or two kilobases of DNA at a time. Details of the sequencing protocols can be found in many molecular biology manuals [24]. Sites of potential post-translational modification can often be predicted from nucleotide sequences of cDNA molecules. It is necessary to test these predictions in intact cells, however, because cell-specific factors are also important in determining which modifications are actually carried out.

HYBRIDIZATION ASSAYS USING cDNA PROBES

Complementary DNA probes can be used in four types of assays to quantitate gene expression in the nervous system. Three of these assays—the Northern blot, the RNase protection, and the *in situ* hybridization assay—utilize radiolabeled probes generated from the cDNA. Radiolabeled probes can be prepared by nick-translating the cDNA using DNase I and DNA polymerase I, by incubating the denatured cDNA with synthetic oligomers and the large fragment of DNA polymerase, or by transcribing the cDNA from the sense strand to produce an antisense RNA. In general, all three methods of producing radiolabeled probes are effective, but antisense RNAs have four particular advantages over DNA probes. First, it is easy to control the length of the labeled probe. Probes generated by labeling DNA are usually variable in length. Second, antisense RNA is single stranded. Consequently, back-hybridization to the sense strand does not compete for binding the probe to the target RNA. Third, the binding of RNA-RNA hybrids is stronger than RNA-DNA hybrids. Thus, it is possible to perform hybridizations under highly stringent conditions. Finally, nonhybridized antisense RNA can be digested with RNase, decreasing the background caused by free radiolabeled probe. Antisense RNAs are particularly useful for nuclease protection and *in situ* hybridization assays. (The interested reader is referred to a recent monograph that discusses these reactions and methodology in detail [25].)

Northern blot assays allow quantitation of specific species of mRNA and are typically performed by electrophoresing RNA on agarose gels containing formamide, glyoxal, or methylmercury, transferring the RNA to an inert support, such as nitrocellulose or nylon, by capillary or electroblotting and then hybridizing with a radiolabeled probe. Agarose gel electrophoresis provides the means of separating mRNAs of different size, but related RNAs of similar size cannot be distinguished. In general, the rules governing hybridization of nucleic acids in solution apply fairly well to RNAs immobilized on nitrocellulose filters. Hybridization is therefore dependent on the length of the

probe, G-C content, temperature, and salt concentration of the hybridization solution. Hybridizations using antisense RNA probes are usually performed under more stringent conditions than those using cDNA probes.

Occasionally, Northern blot assays are inadequate to distinguish among related mRNAs. The RNase protection assay can distinguish mRNAs that differ from each other by as few as one or two nucleotides. In this assay, radiolabeled antisense RNA is hybridized to RNA in solution, treated with a combination of ribonucleases, and then electrophoresed on a denaturing polyacrylamide gel. Ribonucleases A and T1 preferentially digest single-stranded RNA. Therefore, when the probe is completely hybridized to a complementary sequence of RNA, it is protected from digestion with RNase. Any divergence between the probe and target RNA allows the probe to be digested at the point of mismatch, resulting in a smaller fragment of radiolabeled RNA. Because the nonhybridized probe is completely degraded by RNase, the RNase protection assay is also an extremely sensitive and specific assay for the detection of low-abundance mRNAs.

Because neural tissues are so heterogeneous, Northern blot or RNase protection assays are often inadequate to detect differences in gene expression among individual neuronal nuclei. *In situ* hybridization assays coupled with densitometric analyses of grain counts allow crude quantitation of specific mRNAs in individual cells within the central nervous system. Probes for these assays include antisense RNA, oligonucleotides, or nick-translated cDNA. *In situ* hybridization assays have been used very effectively to evaluate the changes in neuropeptide mRNA levels after specific physiological events, to detect the expression of genes during development, and to distinguish receptor subtypes in different brain regions [25].

Northern blot, RNase protection, and *in situ* hybridization assays assess steady-state mRNA levels as opposed to providing a direct measure of gene expression. Messenger RNA levels are determined by both synthetic and degradative processes; therefore an alteration in specific mRNA content within a cell or tissue can reflect a change in RNA stability as well as a change in gene expression. To measure alterations in gene expression directly, the transcriptional runoff assay was developed. In this assay, isolated nuclei are incubated with radioactive ribonucleotides and allowed to transcribe *in vitro*. Radiolabeled transcripts are bound to specific cDNAs immobilized on a nitrocellulose or nylon filter. Because the elongation rate is constant, the amount of specific transcript produced is proportional to the transcriptional initiation rate for a particular gene. Unlike the previously described assays, transcriptional runoff studies do not utilize radiolabeled probe but instead are quantitated by filter hybridization of radiolabeled target RNA. Although runoff studies cannot be applied to neuronal cells *in situ*, recent attempts to detect mRNA precursors by *in situ* hybridization assays have provided encouraging results.

ACKNOWLEDGMENTS

Portions of this chapter have been adapted from a review previously published in *Neuropeptides* edited by G. Fink and T. Harmar, John Wiley, New York, 1988. [Ibro Handbook Series: Methods in the Neurosciences.]

REFERENCES

1. Itoh, N., Obata, K., Yanihara, N., and Okamoto, H. Human preprovasoactive intestinal polypeptide contains a novel PHI-27-like peptide, PHM-27. *Nature* 304:547–549, 1983.
2. Adelman, J. P., Mason, A. J., Hayflick, J. S., and Seeburg, P. H. Isolation of the gene and hypothalamic cDNA for the common precursor of gonadotropin-releasing hormone and prolactin release-inhibiting factor in human and rat. *Proc. Natl. Acad. Sci. U.S.A.* 83:179–183, 1986.
3. Salkoff, L., Butler, A., Wei, A., Seavarda, N., Giffen, K., et al. Genomic organization and deduced amino acid sequence of a putative sodium channel gene in *Drosophila*. *Science* 237:744–749, 1987.
4. Mishinal, M., Tobimatsu, T., Imot, K., Tanaka, K., Fujita, Y., et al. Location of functional regions of acetylcholine receptor alpha-subunit by site directed mutagenesis. *Nature* 313:364–369, 1985.
5. Hanley, M. R., and Jackson, T. Return of the magnificent seven. *Nature* 239:766–767, 1987.
6. Amara, S. G., Jonas, V., Rosenfeld, M. G., Ong, E. S., and Evans, R. M. Alternative RNA processing in calcitonin gene expression generates mRNAs encoding different polypeptide products. *Nature* 298:240–244, 1982.
7. White, M. M. Designer channels: Site-directed mutagenesis as a probe for structural features of channels and receptors. *Trends Neurosci.* 8:364–368, 1985.
8. Chirgwin, J. M., Przybyla, A. E., MacDonald, R. J., and Rutter, W. J. Isolation of biologically active ribonucleic acid from sources enriched in ribonuclease. *Biochemistry* 18:5294–5299, 1979.
9. Okayama, H., and Berg, P. High-efficiency cloning of full-length cDNA. *Mol. Cell. Biol.* 2:161–170, 1982.
10. Gubler, U., and Hoffman, B. J. A simple and very efficient method for generating cDNA libraries. *Gene* 25:263–269, 1983.
11. Grunstein, M., and Hogness, D. S. Colony hybridization: A method for the isolation of cloned DNAs that contain a specific gene. *Proc. Natl. Acad. Sci. U.S.A.* 72:3961–3965, 1975.
12. Touchot, N., Chardin, P., and Tavitian, A. Four additional members of the ras gene superfamily isolated by an oligonucleotide strategy: Molecular cloning of ypt-related cDNAs from a rat brain library. *Proc. Natl. Acad. Sci. U.S.A.* 84:8210–8214, 1987.
13. Grantham, R., Gautier, C., Gouy, M., Jacobzone, M., and Mercier, R. Codon catalog usage is a genome strategy for gene expressivity. *Nucleic Acids Res.* 9:r43–r74, 1981.
14. Jaye, M., de la Salle, H., Schamber, F., Balland, A., Kohli, V., et al. Isolation of a human anti-

hemophilic factor IX cDNA clone using a unique 52-base synthetic oligonucleotide probe deduced from the amino acid sequence of bovine factor IX. *Nucleic Acids Res.* 11:2325–2335, 1983.

15. Young, R. A., and Davis, R. W. Efficient isolation of genes by using antibody probes. *Proc. Natl. Acad. Sci. U.S.A.* 80:1194–1198, 1983.

16. Mandel, G., and Goodman, R. H. Using the brain to screen cloned genes. *Trends Neurosci.* 10:101–104, 1987.

17. Lechan, R. M., Wu, P., Jackson, I. M. D., Wolfe, H., Cooperman, S., Mandel, G., and Goodman, R. H. Thyrotropin-releasing hormone precursor: characterization in rat brain. *Science* 231:159–161, 1986.

18. Chao, M. V., Bothwell, M. A., Ross, A. H., Koprowski, H., Lanahan, A. A., et al. Gene transfer and molecular cloning of the human NGF receptor. *Science* 232:518–521, 1986.

19. Lubbert, H., Hoffman, B. J., Snutch, T. P., Van Dyke, T., Levine, A. J., et al. cDNA cloning of a serotonin 5-HT$_{ic}$ receptor by electrophysiological assays of mRNA injected *Xenopus* oocytes. *Proc. Natl. Acad. Sci. U.S.A.* 84:4332–4336, 1987.

20. Masu, Y., Nakayama, K., Tamaki, H., Harada, Y., Kuno, M., and Nakanishi, S. cDNA cloning of bovine substance K receptor through oocyte expression system. *Nature* 329:836–838, 1987.

21. Gurdon, J. B., Lane, D. C., Woodland, H. R., and Marbaix, G. Use of frog eggs and oocytes for the study of messenger RNA and its translation in living cells. *Nature* 233:177–182, 1971.

22. Maxam, A., and Gilbert, W. A new method for sequencing DNA. *Proc. Natl. Acad. Sci. U.S.A.* 74:560–564, 1977.

23. Sanger, F., Nicklen, S., and Coulson, A. R. DNA sequencing with chain-terminating inhibitors. *Proc. Natl. Acad. Sci. U.S.A.* 74:5463–5467, 1977.

24. Maniatis, T., Fritsch, E. F., and Sambrook, J. In *Molecular Cloning.* Cold Spring Harbor, NY: Cold Spring Harbor Laboratory, 1982, pp. 202–203.

25. Valentino, K. I., Eberwine, J. H., and Barchas, J. D. (eds.). *In Situ Hybridization Applications to Neurobiology.* New York: Oxford University Press, 1987, pp. 1–24; 126–145.

CHAPTER 23

Molecular Genetics of Inherited Neurological Degenerative Disorders

Roger N. Rosenberg

In recent decades advances have occurred in our understanding of the biochemical basis of inherited neurological diseases primarily through the detection of enzyme defects [1]. The pulse of research in this area has quickened considerably because of the introduction of re-

combinant DNA techniques discussed in detail in Chapters 21 and 22. This chapter discusses the implications of these techniques for clinical neurology.

The major increase in the number of diseases recognized as inheritable in mendelian

Basic Neurochemistry: Molecular, Cellular, and Medical Aspects, 4th Ed., edited by G. J. Siegel et al. Raven Press, Ltd., New York, 1989.
Correspondence to Roger N. Rosenberg, Department of Neurology, University of Texas, Southwestern Medical Center, 5323 Hines, Dallas, Texas 75235.

form is documented by the successive catalogs published by McKusick [2]. Between 1978 and 1982, nearly 200 newly identified dominant, 60 autosomal, and eight X-linked recessive disorders were recorded. Of the total 1,637 documented genetic disorders, over half exhibit an autosomal dominant pattern of inheritance. This pattern also characterizes most inherited neurological diseases. Paradoxically, our understanding of the origin of recessively inherited disease is more advanced. Many recessive disorders, such as aminoacidopathies (see Chap. 38), mucopolysaccharidoses, leukodystrophies, and gangliosidoses (see Chap. 37), are associated with the accumulation of a metabolite that can be related to specific enzyme defects. This scheme was pursued in deciphering the inherited gangliosidoses (2), in each of which a catabolic enzyme defect is associated with one or more accumulated metabolites (see Chap. 37).

DOMINANTLY INHERITED DISORDERS

In most dominantly inherited diseases, there are no obvious metabolic clues to indicate their potential biochemical bases

Diseases such as neurofibromatosis, myotonic dystrophy, Huntington's disease, the spinocerebellar degenerations, and tuberous sclerosis generally involve neuronal degeneration with a compensatory increase in glia. Even the finding of a specific protein abnormality or a specific change in mRNA in brain tissue in these cases does not permit distinction of a mutant product from the results of disease; different research strategies are therefore necessary. In autosomal dominant disorders (those present on chromosomes 1–22, i.e., not on the X or Y chromosome), two issues that must be addressed in each instance are (a) the molecular basis for the disorder, and (b) the molecular basis for the clinical variation in gene expression and pene-

trance. Because a dominant disorder can be inherited from one affected parent, early diagnosis is important for genetic counseling. It has been documented in several large families that the incidence of disease in the family will decrease significantly with good counseling. It is important to find ways to identify the children in such families who are affected, those who are at risk but do not show clinical signs, and those who are not at risk for the disease. The clinician must provide the pedigree information that is indispensable to the discovery of molecular markers for these diseases [3].

The molecular basis for clinical variation in dominantly inherited disease involves genetic polymorphism

The phenomenon of genetic polymorphism arises from the degeneracy of the genetic code: Sixty-four triplet codons are translated into 20 amino acids. Thus, phenylalanine may be represented by UUU or UUC. A mutation of either of these to UUA or UUG will cause substitution of leucine for phenylalanine. Mutations that result in the stop codons, UAA, UAA, and UGA can result from third base mutations in cysteine, tyrosine, or tryptophan codons and cause abortive peptide chain termination. This kind of background mutation occurs frequently [4]. It is estimated that about 100,000 proteins are expressed in brain. Codon point mutations provide genetic diversity in the normal population and, on occasion, effect directly the one mutation that causes a dominant disease. The expression of the abnormal gene can also be modified by genetic diversity that slightly alters other proteins that would otherwise function within a normal range, e.g., of enzyme activity, receptor binding affinity, or structure. Thus, different individuals express differently a range of normal enzyme activities in brain involving many different metabolic pathways. This enzyme heterogeneity is one factor that generates clinical variation within the same family: different family members expressing different features (expressivity) and severity (penetrance) of the same primary genetic mutation. These points will be discussed further.

In 1966, Harris [5] demonstrated genetic polymorphism in humans, altering the prevailing concept of a normal genotype. He showed that humans have marked variation in enzyme activity, i.e., enzyme polymorphism, in about one-third of the enzymes he assayed in normal individuals. These findings can be exemplified by two important brain enzymes: dopamine-β-hydroxylase (DBH) and catechol-O-methyl transferase (COMT). Each expresses its activity through two alleles; each allele is obtained from one parent. DBH^L-DBH^L or $COMT^L$-$COMT^L$ results in low activity; DBH^H-DBH^H or $COMT^H$-$COMT^H$ produces high-activity enzymes; and allelic heterozygosity, as seen in 50 percent of the population, manifests intermediate levels of these activities.

By extrapolating from these variations to the results of codon mutations involving up to 100,000 different proteins, one can envision the enormous number of combinations of biological activities that can affect the one mutation directly responsible for the dominant disease. The variations in severity of a given clinical manifestation of a disease is termed gene penetrance. The qualitative variation in the clinical features among affected individuals within a large pedigree with, presumably, the same genetic disease is termed genetic expressivity. Both of these properties must, in part, be explained by normal genetic diversity.

Genetic disease, whether recessive, dominant, or X linked, refers to a single gene defect. A second gene that has the ability to modify the penetrance or expressivity of the primary gene is termed a modifier gene. The best known modifier genes in humans are the ABO(H) blood groups. The ABO(H) antigens in secretions are determined by the secretor gene. Nonsecretors are homozygous *se/se* and secretors are either heterozygous *Se/se* or homozygous *Se/Se*. Thus, *Se* is a recessive suppressor gene. A modifier gene may be present in an autosomal dom-

inant spinocerebellar degeneration (Joseph's disease). This may be a typical determinant of the variations of penetrance and expressivity encountered in many common dominantly inherited disorders.

The occurrence of skipped generations in large pedigrees may also be caused by modifier genes. A possible example is the BA isozyme of erythrocyte acid phosphatase that was associated with the absence of clinically manifest disease in one family of a Joseph's disease pedigree. The location of the gene for this enzyme is chromosome 2,p23, where p refers to the short arm of the chromosome, and 23 refers to a specific locus on the p arm that has been defined by banding patterns. This locus is presumably near ("linked to") the locus of the proposed modifier gene. In an analysis of almost 200 families with Joseph's disease, 10 percent of the families were found to have significantly less than the expected 50 percent of affected children. Several of these families show classic skipped generations of this dominantly inherited disease, presumably because of the full suppression by the modifier gene acting on the primary mutant gene. The possibility that modifier genes may explain variations in penetrance and expressivity in dominantly inherited neurological diseases has not been fully explored; however, this postulate is more precise and directly assayable than the alternative proposal that clinical variations are caused by the normal background genetic heterogeneity involving many genes.

Dominantly inherited disease may result from defects in gene processing

Explanations of the molecular bases of dominantly inherited diseases require an understanding of the basic molecular structure of the genes and the biochemistry of their processing (see Chap. 21). Introns can make up a major proportion of the gene and of the unprocessed nuclear RNA. For example, the ovalbumin gene consists of some 7,000 bases, of which only

1,857 encode the protein. Most of the remaining bases are in seven introns [6,7]. It is thought that introns may regulate mRNA stability and thus increase the efficiency of message production and the level of the translated gene product. For example, one known intron mutation produces an in-phase termination codon sequence that prematurely terminates protein synthesis. This type of intron mutation also causes the mRNA for the β-globin gene to be unstable and this results in severe clinical thalassemia. It seems possible that similar frame shift mutations may become an important class of genetic neurological disease.

Genes occur in multiple copies

Genes coding for one function may occur as compact families of multiple copies on the same chromosome, such as the prolactin gene which occurs on chromosome 6 in a contiguous area. Families of genes may also be dispersed over several chromosomes, as has been found in the cases of argininosuccinate synthetase and β-tubulin genes. Not all of these genes may be transcribable: many can be defective copies, the so-called pseudogenes. Also, isogenic copies may have tissue specificities: For example, only one or two of several genes coding for isozymes of the same function may be expressed in brain. Multiple gene copies can also be expressed on "double-minute chromosomes," which are multiple copies of miniature chromosomes that have been found to amplify gene expression in some cells such as neuroblastomas [8]. Defects in interchromosomal regulation of multiple isogenic expression may occur and result in dominantly inherited neurological disorders.

DNA preparations that consist of single copies of each gene [single-copy DNA (scDNA)] can be used to assess gene expression by hybridization with RNA. When comparisons were made between the total nuclear RNA and the polyadenylated hnRNA fractions from whole newborn mice, hybridization with scDNA occurred to about the same extent. Similar degrees of gene expression represented in the polyadenylated hnRNA fractions prepared from brains of newborn and adult mice were also indicated; however, comparison of the degrees of hybridization of total brain hnRNA from newborn and adult mice demonstrated about one-third more hybridization by the adult preparation. This has been taken to indicate the existence of a unique nonpolyadenylated hnRNA in brain at a time when the brain is fully formed and functioning [9]. These findings raise the possibility that impairment in the processing of such a class of brain-specific RNA could be responsible for certain types of mental retardation syndromes in which the structure of the nervous system is entirely normal.

Some genes can exist as elements that can move from place to place within the chromosomes of a cell (transposons). Such elements were first described by McClintock in maize. They have now been identified in mammalian cells [10]. When incorporated into the linear DNA of the chromosome, transposons are transcribed, but when they appear as deleted elements in the nucleoplasm, they are not. Transposon activation-deactivation, gene shuffling, and rearrangements are emerging as important events in cell differentiation. Defects in these mechanisms may produce a class of dominantly inherited neurological diseases. Thus, dominantly inherited forms of brain tumors may be related to abnormal gene transpositions [11,12].

THE STUDY OF GENE LINKAGE

Characteristic patterns of DNA fragments produced by cutting DNA with restriction endonucleases provide an important basis for genetic linkage studies

Characteristic patterns of DNA fragments vary from individual to individual because of the normal variations in primary DNA sequences, as discussed above. Single base changes may introduce or delete sites sensitive to endonuclease cleavage (restriction sites). Sequence deletions, additions, or translocations affect the length of DNA between restriction sites. Some 20,000 polymorphic sites are estimated to exist in a human genome. Only a small fraction of these have been characterized so far. Restriction sites do not occur at random but are inherited and provide a means of identifying the mutation associated with a given disease [13].

The DNA fragment variations produced by restriction endonucleases are called restriction-fragment-length polymorphisms (RFLPs). Such fragments can be sorted according to molecular weight by electrophoresis on agarose gels. The patterns are usually preserved by blotting them onto nitrocellulose paper (Southern blots). Specific DNA sequences can be hybridized on these blots with radioactive DNA probes that are complementary to sequences of interest and identified by autoradiography.

A common phenotype may be associated with entirely different genotypes

The association of a common phenotype with an entirely different genotype has occurred in patients with Charcot-Marie-Tooth disease and also in one of the spinocerebellar degenerations in which linkage studies for specific biochemical markers have been positive in only some of the families that seem clinically identical. The close association of two genes is termed linkage. Linkage analyses can provide several important types of information:

1. Normal genes frequently can be used as linkage markers to segregate a pedigree with respect to the mutation responsible for a genetic disease and thus provide a precise means of documenting the genetic similarity or dissimilarity between two families that display a similar clinical phenotype.

2. Positive linkage between the presence of a genetic disease and a marker provides the means to develop cDNA probes to the marker locus that may segregate along with the disease genotype. The objective in such cases may be to find a probe that can be used to identify a specific RFLP that will be found only on gel blots from patient DNA associated with a particular disorder (Fig. 1).

3. Linkage studies can provide the crucial information for locating and ultimately isolating and sequencing a mutant gene.

Linkage studies have been successfully employed to characterize a number of important neurological diseases

Neurological diseases that have been mapped to a specific chromosome include those shown in Table 1. cDNA has been used to diagnose several nonneurological diseases *in utero*, using DNA from cells obtained by amniocentesis or by biopsy of chorionic villus tissue. Sickle cell anemia and noninsulin-dependent diabetes are two examples. The sickle cell mutation consists of a single base change that alters glutamate to valine in the sixth residue of the mutant β-globin peptide:

. . .CCT–GAG–GAG. . . →
    pro   glu   glu

        . . .CCT–GTG–GAG. . .
          pro   val   glu

The *MstII* endonuclease has been employed in this diagnosis because it has specificity for cleavage at sites containing the sequence CCTNAGG, where N is any base. The cloned normal gene is digested by *MstII* into two fragments of 1.15 and 0.2 kilobases (kb), respectively, whereas the cloned mutant gene resides in a single 1.35-kb fragment after this treatment. When the radioactive 1.15-kb cDNA is hybrid-

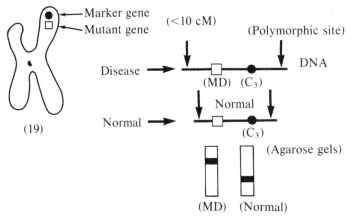

FIG. 1. Diagnostic application of a complementary DNA probe for a marker gene that is closely linked to the mutant gene for a dominantly inherited neurological disease. The DNA samples prepared from patient and control tissues are treated with restriction endonucleases that cleave at the points indicated by vertical arrows. Hybridization signals are detected on blots of agarose gel electrophoretic patterns that have been exposed to a radioactively labeled cDNA probe for a marker gene that is closely linked to the mutant gene of interest. In this instance, the mutant gene is for myotonic dystrophy (MD). The abnormal genotype for the mutant gene can be clearly identified as a hybridization pattern that segregates with affected patients but not with the "not-at-risk" persons in a given pedigree; (cM) centi-Morgans.

TABLE 1.   Neurological diseases mapped to specific chromosomes

Chromosome number	Disease
1	Charcot-Marie-Tooth disease
	Phosphofructokinase deficiency
3	GM$_1$ gangliosidosis
	Morquio's disease
4	Huntington's disease
5	Sandhoff's disease
6	Spinocerebellar degeneration
11	Acute porphyria
13	Familial retinoblastoma
15	Tay-Sachs' disease
	Prader-Willi's disease
17	Pompè's disease
	Neurofibromatosis
18	Amyloidotic polyneuropathy
19	Myotonic dystrophy
22	Metachromatic leukodystrophy
	Hurler-Scheie's disease
	Familial acoustic neuroma and meningioma
X	Duchenne's dystrophy
	Adrenoleukodystrophy
	Lesch-Nyhan syndrome
	Fragile X mental retardation

ized to the *MstII* RFLP gel blot from the homozygous sickle cell genotype, only the 1.35-kb fragment is detected, only the 1.15-kb fragment is seen in normal homozygotes, and both fragments are detected in DNA from heterozygotes.

With respect to neurological diseases, cDNA probes have been constructed for two X-linked disorders: Lesch-Nyhan syndrome and Duchenne's muscular dystrophy.

Lesch-Nyhan syndrome

HGPRT, the enzyme deficient in Lesch-Nyhan syndrome, has been cloned. A mutant enzyme from one Lesch-Nyhan patient was shown to have a single base change that altered the normal aspartate (residue 193) to asparagine, which resulted in an enzyme with very low substrate affinity. Many genotypes exist for Lesch-Nyhan patients due to different allelic mutations, deletions, or internal duplications in the HGPRT gene. At least 20 separate mutations have been found in individual patients. The RFLP technique has been used to detect another HGPRT mutant clinically associated with hyperuricemia and gout.

Duchenne's muscular dystrophy

Cloned fragments of the human X chromosome at Xp21 have been screened in search of linkage to Duchenne's dystrophy. Kunkel and colleagues [14] have determined the gene responsible for this disease. It is about 2,000 kb in length and comprises about 60 exons. There is a high rate of deletions with the majority concentrated in a single genomic segment corresponding to only 2 kb of the transcript. The gene codes for a protein, dystrophin, which is about 400 kDa and associated with the cytoplasmic face of the plasma membrane of skeletal muscle fibers and triads (junctures of transverse tubules and sarcoplasmic reticulum; see Chap. 31). Presumably, it functions to facilitate electromechanical coupling for muscle contraction (see also Chap. 31). Dystrophin is absent in Duchenne patient muscle extracts. Muscle of patients with Becker's muscular dystrophy contains normal amounts of a molecular weight variant of dystrophin. Duchenne and Becker forms of dystrophy are allelic mutations at Xp21.

Fragile X mental retardation syndrome

The fragile X mental retardation syndrome mutation occurs on the long arm of the X chromosome at a site very near the HGPRT and glucose-6-phosphate dehydrogenase loci, and probes for these latter sites as well as probes that identify RFLPs have been tested. At least one RFLP probe appears closely linked to the fragile X locus.

Huntington's disease

A systematic study of two families with Huntington's disease has been undertaken by Gusella and colleagues with the object of obtaining a definitive restriction fragment pattern that identifies the Huntington's disease gene. They have reported that the gene is linked to a DNA marker fragment that maps to human chromosome 4 from both families, and this has been further localized to the terminal band of the short arm of that chromosome, a region representing about 0.5 percent of the human genome. This assignment was made by examining DNA from patients with Wolf-Hirschhorn syndrome, a birth defect resulting from partial heterozygous deletion of the short arm of chromosome 4 [15].

Spinocerebellar degenerations

Hybridization studies have been initiated using genomic DNA obtained from brain and lymphocyte samples of patients with Joseph's disease, using cDNA probes obtained from several genes as well as probes generated from random DNA fragments. Another promising approach to the investigation of spinocerebellar degenerations may be the use of probes developed for the immune response genes that are also on chromosome 6. At least one form of olivopontocerebellar degeneration is linked to HLA antigens.

Myotonic muscular dystrophy

The myotonic muscular dystrophy mutation has been mapped to chromosome 19 by linkage studies associating the disease with the third component of complement (C_3). Roses and coworkers [16] are currently "walking" along the chromosome, beginning with a C_3 cDNA probe as a primer and adding adjacent segments of DNA to it in both directions from the C_3 locus, because it is not known on which side the myotonic locus lies.

Charcot-Marie-Tooth disease

The abnormal locus in some patients with Charcot-Marie-Tooth disease has been assigned to chromosome 1 by virtue of studies showing linkage to the Duffy blood group and to the antithrombin 3 locus.

Familial amyloidosis

Familial amyloidotic polyneuropathy (FAP) can be diagnosed by a Southern blot procedure because of linkage of a restriction site to a mutant prealbumin gene; FAP maps to chromosome 18. The DNA samples are digested by *NsiI* endonuclease and the blots are probed with radioactive human prealbumin cDNA. In the initial study, DNA digests from 10 disease-free individuals showed two labeled bands at 6.6 and 3.2 kb, whereas individuals with familial amyloidotic polyneuropathy exhibited two additional bands at 5.1 and 1.5 kb. Thus, the mutant prealbumin gene is associated with an additional *NsiI* restriction site. The defect resides in the protein transthyretin: Methionine appears in place of the normal valine at position 30. Transthyretin functions to transport vitamin A and thyroid hormone and is found at high concentration in the choroid plexus of the brain. The cause of amyloid deposition in peripheral nerve in patients with a mutant transthyretin peptide is not known.

ONCOGENES AND CARCINOGENESIS

Neuroblastoma and retinoblastoma are tumors of neuronal origin in which specific genetic defects may be the basis for malignant transformation

Both neuroblastoma and retinoblastoma have associated specific chromosomal deletions. This is consistent with the view that proto-oncogenes are activated through the loss of a suppressor element whose normal function is to turn off these embryonic genes and to allow these cells to become postmitotic neurons or retinal cells.

Neuroblastoma is associated with 20- to 40-fold amplification of a DNA domain (N-*myc*) in 24 of 63 untreated patients. Amplification was found in none of 15 patients with stage 1 or 2 disease and in 24 of 48 patients with advanced disease and is thus a marker of a poor prognosis. A similar correlation was found in a separate study. Thus, the genomic amplification of N-*myc* may play a key role in the aggressiveness

of neuroblastoma [17]. An additional characteristic of human neuroblastoma is the deletion of the distal short arm of chromosome 1, which has been identified in about 70 percent of both primary neuroblastomas and derived cell lines. Perhaps this deletion results in loss of the postulated suppressor gene (antioncogene) and subsequent activation and amplification of the N-*myc* oncogene on chromosome 2.

In situ hybridization studies have localized the amplified N-*myc* genes to homogeneously staining regions on different chromosomes. Gene amplification with the formation of homogeneously staining regions on chromosomes and of double-minute chromosomes can be induced experimentally in cultured neuroblastoma cells under the selective pressure of agents such as methotrexate [8].

A familial form of retinoblastoma has been recognized for many years. It is an autosomal dominant disease: 50 percent of the children of an affected parent will develop the disease, which occurs in the early years of life and involves both eyes. Nonfamilial, sporadic cases are unilateral and occur later in life.

A suggested explanation of the pattern of occurrence of the familial, bilateral disease is the Knudson model [18], which postulates that expression requires mutation of a specific site on both alleles of a single cell in the retina. In the inherited disease, one mutation has already occurred in each cell of the patient by virtue of a germ line mutation from the affected parent. Thus, a somatic mutation of the other allele in any retinal cell will initiate the malignancy. There is a high statistical probability for the second mutation to occur because there are about two million retinal cells, and a new mutation of a given gene occurs once in every million cell divisions. This model implies that familial retinoblastoma will produce a mendelian pattern of autosomal dominance clinically, even though expression of the defect, genotypically, is autosomally recessive.

The retinoblastoma gene is closely linked with the esterase D gene [19]. This gene was assigned to chromosome 13 band q14 by deletion mapping. In "deletion forms" of retinoblastoma this is exactly where the chromosome deletion occurs; however, "nondeletion forms" of the tumor also occur, which may have a submicroscopic mutation at the same site in both alleles.

Another study of 11 retinoblastoma patients showed that esterase D activity was 50 percent reduced in nontumor cells because of a systemic mutation. One female patient had 50 percent esterase D activity in normal cells, but these had no deletion at 13q14; however, stem cell lines of the retinoblastoma from this patient had a missing chromosome 13 and no detectable esterase D. Evidently, a total loss of genetic material at the 13q14 locus had occurred, which led to expression of the malignancy. Because the retinoblastoma gene is actually recessive, both alleles must be lost for tumors to develop. One 13q14 allele is deleted by the germ line mutation from the affected parent, and this is carried by all somatic cells of the precancerous patient. The second acquired mutation in this case was a complete loss of chromosome 13 from the tumor progenitor cell.

The hypothesis of Murphree and Benedict [20] is that production of the tumor is caused by loss of a suppressor element (antioncogene) at 13q14. They do not distinguish this hypothesis from the oncogene hypothesis. Actually, the two are closely related since by hypothesis, the loss of suppressor results in the activation of an oncogene. Oncogenes evidently may become activated by mutation, amplification, translocation, or suppressor deletion. Abnormal tyrosine phosphorylation of plasma membrane proteins, increased levels of cyclic AMP (cAMP) and other mechanisms may also be involved. In a rather short time, one molecular mechanism for carcinogenesis has been elucidated that applies to cells of neuronal origin. Similar molecular alterations may be operative in familial astrocytomas, meningiomas (chromosome 22), and the multiple tumor forms of neurofibromatosis (chromosome 17). Possibly,

this new knowledge of oncogene cellular transformation can be exploited to devise combinations of chemotherapeutic agents that can inactivate either oncogene transcription or the oncogene-specific protein kinase gene product.

Reiterated restriction fragments

A new gel hybridization method has been used to visualize and quantitate reiterated DNA restriction fragments (RRFs) without prior knowledge of their sequences. The patterns of EcoRI-cleaved DNA from 10 human tumors were compared with paired normal tissues from the same patients. In addition, patterns from 10 unpaired tumors and tissues from 20 noncancer patients were analyzed. Frequent two- to tenfold alterations in the relative apparent copy numbers of several RRFs were found in tumor-control comparisons. A 1.55-kb RRF was increased in five of eight tumors and decreased in none. Additional new RRFs were detected in a neuroblastoma (cytogenetically suggestive of gene amplification) and in a glioma. A 1.3-kb RRF was directly detectable in nine of ten cancer patient DNAs but in only 10 of 20 DNAs from individuals without cancer. These data suggest that frequent qualitative and quantitative alterations of specific reiterated DNA sequences may occur in human cancer and that possibly there are genomic differences between specific RRF levels of cancer and noncancer patients. Careful analysis of RRF patterns in such neural tumors as neuroblastoma and glioma, which can be a familial neoplasm, may provide insights into their molecular pathogenesis [21].

GENE THERAPY

Correction of genetic defects by gene therapy has been experimentally accomplished

Partial correction of expressed enzyme levels by use of viral vectors has been described for instances of cells deficient in HGPRT, galactose-1-phosphate uridyltransferase, and β-ga-lactosidase; however, because of a low frequency of transformation, this approach is inappropriate for patient treatment. A more practical approach was taken by Ley and colleagues [22] who utilized 5-azacytidine to increase fetal globin synthesis selectively in a patient with severe thalassemia. They treated a patient for 14 days, during which time there was considerable synthesis of fetal globin and suppression of the thalassemic β-globin gene product. Incorporation of 5-azacytidine into the patient's genomic DNA is hypothesized to have prevented DNA methylation and to have allowed gene transcription to occur. This approach might be useful in other diseases, such as Huntington's disease, spinocerebellar degeneration, tuberous sclerosis, and neurofibromatosis, if such diseases are the result of the normal inhibition of one isogene and the induction of another (mutant, in these cases) isogene at any of several stages of life. Such a genetic chronobiological hypothesis would imply that a whole series of isogenes become induced throughout life, analogous to the switches that occur between fetal and adult hemoglobin genes or between fetal and adult creatine phosphokinase genes. If enzymes, receptors, or structural protein isoforms may be expressed by a series of isogene inhibitions and inductions throughout life, reinduction of a repressed normal fetal gene to compensate for an adult mutant isogene might be a research strategy for the future.

The introduction of a desired gene into somatic cells has been successfully carried out by Palmiter and associates [23]. These workers fused the mouse metallothionein I gene with the rat growth hormone gene and injected the recombinant gene into fertilized pronuclei of mouse embryos so as to generate mice twice the size and weight of normal littermates (see Chap. 21). In addition to providing a means of investigating the regulation of the growth hormone gene, the success of this technique suggests a theoretical approach to the correction of gene mutations.

Recombinant DNA techniques have entered the arenas of clinical neurology and neurobiology and are providing a precise means of examining inherited neurological diseases. More generally, these techniques provide a profound new approach for understanding the regulatory events responsible for the development of the human brain.

ACKNOWLEDGMENTS

Portions of this chapter are modified and updated from reviews previously published in *Ann. Neurol.* 15:511–520, 1984, and in R. N. Rosenberg, *Neurogenetics: Principles and Practice*, Raven Press, New York, 1986, pp. 66–86; 87–93; 314–318.

REFERENCES

1. Rosenberg, R. Biochemical genetics of neurologic disease. *N. Engl. J. Med.* 305:1181–1193, 1981.
2. McKusick, V. *Mendelian Inheritance in Man*, 6th ed. Baltimore: Johns Hopkins Univ. Press, 1983.
3. Rosenberg, R. Recombinant DNA and neurological disease: The coming of a new age. *Neurology* 33:622–625, 1983.
4. Vogel, F., and Motulsky, A. In *Human Genetics*. Berlin: Springer-Verlag, 1982, p. 296.
5. Harris, H. Enzyme polymorphism in man. *Proc. R. Soc. Lond. (Biol.)* 164:298–310, 1966.
6. Alberts, B., Bray, D., Lewis, J., Raff, M., Roberts, K., and Watson, J. *Molecular Biology of the Cell*. New York: Garland Press, 1983.
7. Lewin, B. *Eucaryotic Chromosomes in Gene Expression*, Vol. 2, 2nd ed. New York: Wiley, 1980, pp. 797–799.
8. Baskin, F., Rosenberg, R., and Vaithilingham, D. Correlation of double-minute chromosomes

with unstable multidrug cross-resistance in uptake of neuroblastoma cells. *Proc. Natl. Acad. Sci. U.S.A.* 78:3654–3658, 1981.

9. Chaudari, N., and Hahn, W. Genetic expression in the developing brain. *Science* 220:924–928, 1983.

10. Shapiro, J. *Mobile Genetic Elements.* New York: Academic Press, 1983, p. 688.

11. Mushinski, J., Potter, M., Bauer, S., and Reddy, E. DNA rearrangement and altered RNA expression of the *c-myc* oncogene in mouse plasmacytoid lymphosarcomas. *Science* 220:795–798, 1983.

12. Weinberg, R. A molecular basis of cancer. *Sci. Am.* 249:126–142, 1983.

13. Botstein, D., White, R., Skolnick, M., and Davis, R. Construction of a genetic linkage map in man using restriction fragment length polymorphisms. *Am. J. Hum. Genet.* 32:314–331, 1980.

14. Koenig, M., Hoffman, E., Bertelson, C., Monaco, A., Feener, C., and Kunkel, L. Complete cloning of the Duchenne muscular dystrophy (DMD) cDNA and preliminary genomic organization of the DMD gene in normal and affected individuals. *Cell* 50:509–517, 1987.

15. Gusella, J., Tanzi, R., Bader, P., Phelan, M., Stevenson, R., Hayden, M., Hofman, K., Faryniarz, A., and Gibbons, K. Deletion of Huntington's disease-linked G8 (D4510) locus in Wolf-Hirschhorn syndrome. *Nature* 318:75–78, 1985.

16. Roses, A., Pericek-Vance, M., and Yamaoka, L. Molecular genetic studies in myotonic dystrophy. *Neurology* 33(Suppl. 2):79, 1983.

17. Schwab, M., Varmus, H., Bishop, J., Grzeschik, L.-H., Naylor, S., Sakaguchi, A., Brodeur, G., and Trent, J. Chromosome localization in normal cells and neuroblastomas of a gene related to *c-myc. Nature* 308:288–291, 1984.

18. Knudson, A., Mutation and cancer: Statistical study of retinoblastoma. *Proc. Natl. Acad. Sci. U.S.A.* 68:820–823, 1971.

19. Sparkes, R., Murphree, A., Lingua, R., Sparkes, M., Field, L., Fundervurk, S., and Benedict, W. Gene for hereditary retinoblastoma assigned to human chromosome 13 by linkage to esterase D. *Science* 219:971–973, 1983.

20. Murphree, A., and Benedict, W., Retinoblastoma: Clues to human oncogenesis. *Science* 223:1028–1033, 1984.

21. Baskin, F., Grossman, A., Bhaghat, S., Burns, D., Davis, R., Warmouth, L., Rosenberg, R. Frequent alterations of specific reiterated DNA sequence abundance in human cancer. *Cancer Genet. Cytogenet.* 28:163–172, 1987.

22. Ley, T., DeSimone, J., Anagnou, N., et al. 5-Azacytidine selectively increases fetal globin synthesis in a patient with beta⁺ thalassemia. *N. Engl. J. Med.* 307:1469–1475, 1982.

23. Palmiter, R., Brinster, R., Hammer, R., Trumbauer, M., Rosenfeld, M., Beinberg, N., and Evans, R. Dramatic growth of mice that develop from eggs micro-injected with metallothionein-growth hormone fusion genes. *Nature* 300:611–615, 1982.

PART FOUR

Cellular Neurochemistry

CHAPTER 24

Axonal Transport and the Neuronal Cytoskeleton

Richard Hammerschlag and Scott T. Brady

Basic Neurochemistry: Molecular, Cellular, and Medical Aspects, 4th Ed., edited by G. J. Siegel et al. Raven Press, Ltd., New York, 1989.
Correspondence to Richard Hammerschlag, Division of Neurosciences, Beckman Research Institute, City of Hope National Medical Center, 1450 East Duarte Road, Duarte, California 91010.

NEURONAL ORGANELLES IN MOTION

Perhaps the best introduction to axonal transport would be to watch the images produced with video-enhanced microscopy of neuronal organelles in motion [1] (Fig. 1). The patterns of movement, seemingly chaotic, but with an underlying order, are as engrossing as the ant farms of our childhood. The video images reveal an array of organelles moving down the axon toward the nerve terminal (anterograde) as well as back toward the cell body (retrograde), with some organelles gliding smoothly while others scurry in fits and starts. On closer examination, the organelles travel along wispy fibrils; those

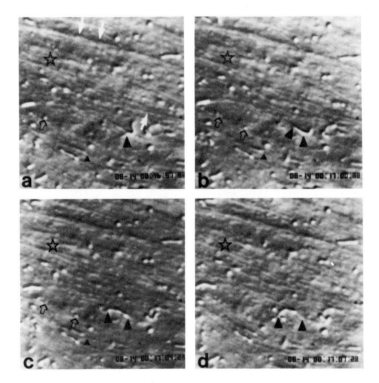

FIG. 1. Sequential video images of fast axonal transport in isolated axoplasm from the squid giant axon. In this preparation, anterograde axonal transport proceeds in the direction from *upper left* to *lower right* (from 10 o'clock toward 4 o'clock). The field of view in these stills is approximately 20 μm, and the images were recorded in real time on videotape. The large, sausage-shape structures (▲) are mitochondria. Medium-size particles (*open arrows*) most often move in the retrograde (right to left) direction. Most structures of this size are lysosomal or prelysosomal organelles. The majority of moving particles in these images are faint and moving rapidly (~2 μm/sec), so they are difficult to catch in still images; however, in the region above the *star*, a number of these organelles can be visualized in each panel. The entire field contains faint parallel striations (like those indicated by the *white arrows* in panel **A**) that correspond to the cytoskeleton of the axoplasm, primarily microtubules. The movement of membranous organelles is along these structures, although organelles can occasionally be seen to switch tracks as they move (see the mitochondrion indicated by *large triangles*). (From Brady et al. [5].)

moving downstream appear fainter and smaller but more numerous than those moving upstream. Occasionally, two organelles are seen to travel in opposite directions along the same fibril, avoiding head-on collision by seeming to pass through each other, while other organelles hop from one fibril to another.

Video images display many features of axonal transport previously demonstrated by biochemical and pharmacological approaches [2–4]

For example, the bidirectionality of transport, inferred from the accumulations of radiolabeled materials on both sides of a nerve crush, is directly apparent in the video images. Organelles traveling toward the nerve terminal transport newly synthesized materials from the cell body to their axonal destinations. Organelles traveling away from the terminal return axonal materials to the cell body for recycling and conveying information to the cell body about the axon and postsynaptic cells. Video microscopy also reveals that anterograde and retrograde rates of organelle movement are comparable to those detected for radiolabeled membrane-associated proteins. As a third example, organelle transport is seen to occur along fibrils, which have been shown by immunocytochemistry and electron microscopy to be microtubules, a cytoskeletal constituent of nearly all cell types. These findings confirm earlier studies in which transport of radiolabeled materials was inhibited by microtubule-disruptive agents.

As a final example, organelle movement continues in apparently normal fashion in axons isolated from their cell bodies. This implies that transport is driven by an energy-generating mechanism that exists locally in the axon. A similar conclusion had been drawn when application of a cold block or metabolic poisons, such as dinitrophenol or cyanide, to a discrete region of a nerve trunk was found to inhibit transport.

The dynamic features of axonal transport include more than the movements observed in video images

Anterogradely transported organelles are continually formed from vesicles that bud from the Golgi apparatus in the cell body. The vesicles are sorted and targeted to different destinations, including the axonal plasma membrane and the synaptic terminal. Retrogradely transported organelles are generated during endocytotic activity in presynaptic terminals. Even the cytoskeletal structures that give form to the axon and provide the tracks for organelle translocation are moving and being replaced.

Until recently, axonal transport was understood mainly at a descriptive level, in terms of the components, rates, and pharmacological sensitivities of the transport processes. In contrast, current research is beginning to probe the molecular mechanisms that underlie the movements detected both by direct video visualization and by radioactive tracer methods. The force-generating proteins that correspond to the transport "motors" are being isolated, and the molecules that ensure the correct sorting, routing, and arrival of transported materials are being sought. Such studies benefit both in design and interpretation from considering axonal transport in the broader cell biological context of contractile and intracellular transport phenomena. It may well be quantitative rather than qualitative features that make intraneuronal transport unique from transport in nonneuronal cells.

DISCOVERY AND CONCEPTUAL DEVELOPMENT OF FAST AND SLOW TRANSPORT

The concept that materials are transferred from cell body to axon was suggested by Ramón y Cajal and other eminent neuroanatomists during the early part of this century, but the first experimental evidence resulted from the renewed interest in peripheral nerve injuries during World War II. In the classic studies of Weiss and Hiscoe [6], surgical constriction of a branch of the sciatic nerve in test animals led to morphological changes in the nerve that implicated the cell body as the source of materials for axon regrowth. After several weeks, the axons were swollen just proximal to the constriction and shriveled distal to the dam. Following removal of the constriction, the bolus of accumulated axoplasm slowly moved down the nerve at 1 to 2 mm/day, very nearly the rate observed for outgrowth of a regenerating nerve. Weiss and His-

coe concluded that the cell body supplies a bulk flow of material to the axon, a view that would not be radically altered for two decades.

During the next few years, cell biologists provided a convincing argument for the necessity of this intracellular transport. Neuronal protein synthesis was almost completely restricted to the cytoplasm surrounding the nucleus, and ribosomes were undetectable in the axon. If proteins cannot be synthesized in the axon, it follows that axonal transport is not induced by axonal damage, but is an ongoing function of normal cells.

By the mid-1960s, the use of radioactive tracers confirmed the existence of a "bulk

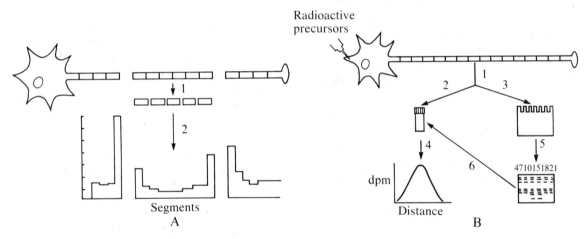

FIG. 2. Schematic diagram of two common methods for analyzing the various rate components of axonal transport. **A:** Accumulation of transported material can be studied at a focal block of axonal transport caused by a cut, a crush, a cold block or a ligature. This approach is a variation of that employed by Weiss and Hiscoe [6] and has been used most often in studies of fast axonal transport [2,8]. In this example, two cuts have been made in order to detect both anterograde and retrograde transport. After time for accumulation at the ends, the nerve segments are cut into uniform segments for analysis (*step 1*). Each segment is analyzed either for radioactivity in labeled nerves or for enzyme activity, and the rate of accumulation is estimated (*step 2*). **B:** With segmental analysis, the nerve must be pulse–labeled, usually with radioactive precursors. After an appropriate injection-sacrifice interval to label the rate component of interest, the nerve is also cut into segments (*step 1*). In some cases, only a single segment is used as a "window" onto the transport process. Each segment is analyzed both by counting the radioactivity in an aliquot (*step 2*) and by gel electrophoresis (*step 3*), where each lane corresponds to a different segment. The amount of radioactivity in different polypeptides can be visualized with fluorography (*step 5*) and individual bands cut out of the gel (*step 6*) for analysis by liquid scintillation counting. The distribution of either total radioactivity or radioactivity associated with a specific polypeptide can then be plotted (*step 4*); (dpm) disintegrations per minute. (For more details, see text and refs. [2], [3] and [8].) (Adapted from Brady [8].)

flow'' transport and soon demonstrated the existence of a faster rate. Using autoradiography, Droz and LeBlond [7] elegantly showed that systemically injected ^{3}H-amino acids were incorporated into nerve cells and transported along the sciatic nerve as a wavefront of radioactive protein. The surprising finding that expanded the concept of axonal transport was that portions of the radioactive materials move in both anterograde and retrograde directions at rates two to three orders of magnitude faster than the rate of bulk flow [2,3]. This faster moving material could be demonstrated by injection of radiolabeled amino acids into dorsal root ganglia or ventral spinal cord to reveal a wavefront of labeled protein traveling away from the cell body at close to 400 mm/day in mammals. A ''fast'' rate of transport was also inferred when acetylcholinesterase and norepinephrine were found to accumulate at a nerve constriction after only a few hours, well before the bulk accumulation of axoplasm. These two approaches for studying axonal transport—locating a radiolabeled wavefront by analysis of successive nerve segments and monitoring the accumulation of materials at a constriction (Fig. 2)—have yielded a large body of data concerning the kinetics and the metabolic and ionic requirements of axonal transport [2,3].

Fast and slow transport differ by their constituents in addition to their rates

Subcellular fractionation studies showed that fast-transport materials were predominantly membrane associated, whereas most of the slow-transport materials were recovered in the soluble fraction. Additional complexity was revealed when labeled polypeptides traveling down the axon were analyzed by polyacrylamide gel electrophoresis. Materials traveling away from the cell body could be grouped into five distinct rate components, each characterized by a unique set of polypeptides [9,10] (Fig. 3). As polypeptides associated with each rate class were identified, a new view of axonal

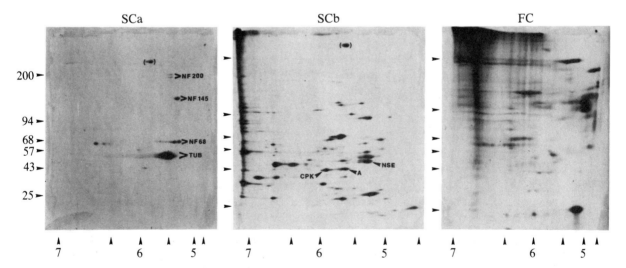

FIG. 3. Two-dimensional fluorographs showing the [^{35}S]methionine-labeled polypeptides in the three major anterograde rate components of axonal transport: (SCa) slow-component a; (SCb) slow-component b; (FC) fast component. Note that each rate component not only has a characteristic rate, but a characteristic polypeptide composition. The discovery that each rate component has a different polypeptide composition led to the Structural Hypothesis [10]. (From Tytell et al. [11]; illustration provided by Dr. Michael Tytell.)

TABLE 1. Major rate components of axonal transport

Component	Rate (mm/day)	Structure and composition
FAST TRANSPORT		
Anterograde	200–400	Small vesiculotubular structures, neurotransmitters, membrane proteins and lipids
Mitochondria	50–100	Mitochondria
Retrograde	200–300	Lysosomal vesicles and enzymes
SLOW TRANSPORT		
SCb	2–8	Microfilaments, metabolic enzymes, clathrin complex
SCa	0.2–1	Neurofilaments and microtubules

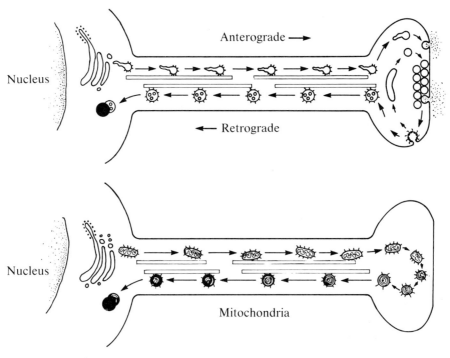

FIG. 4. Diagram illustrating the major features of fast axonal transport. Fast axonal transport can be seen as a continuing cycle in which membrane-associated proteins are synthesized on rough endoplasmic reticulum and assembled in the cell body after passage through the Golgi apparatus (see text and Fig. 6 for more details). Once these proteins are packaged into vesicular organelles (**upper**) or mitochondria (**lower**), the organelles are transported along microtubules in the axon to an appropriate destination, such as the presynaptic terminal. The microtubules have been drawn in as long rods to emphasize that movement of organelles requires a cytoskeletal substrate, but no tubulin or other cytoskeletal proteins are detectable in fast axonal transport. At its final destination, the organelle may contribute to the plasma membrane or form synaptic vesicles or function independently (i.e., mitochondria). In the distal regions of the axon and terminal, membranous structures are processed and eventually returned to the cell body via retrograde axonal transport. Movement in the retrograde direction also requires microtubules. The microtubule-based movement of membranous organelles in the axon has recently been shown to involve a previously unrecognized ATPase for motility [24]. (Adapted from Lasek and Katz [12].)

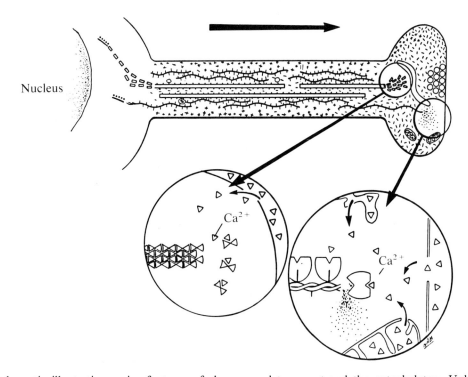

FIG. 5. Schematic illustrating major features of slow axonal transport and the cytoskeleton. Unlike fast transport, the slow components of axonal transport appear to be unidirectional, continuously moving away from the neuronal cell body.Constituents of slow axonal transport, including metabolic enzymes as well as elements of the cytoskeleton and the cytomatrix, are synthesized on cytoplasmic polysomes. These polysomes are often referred to as "free polysomes," but they are in fact attached to the cytoskeleton. Assembly of cytoskeletal structures appears to occur in the cell body soon after synthesis, and they are transported into the axon as intact cytoskeletal elements. The distribution and organization of the three major types of cytoskeletal structures are also illustrated. Actin microfilaments are shown as *short lines* or *crosses* near the axolemma, in association with microtubules, and are highly enriched in the synaptic terminal. Microtubules are the *long rods* with short sidearms that interact with other cytoskeletal structures. Axonal microtubules are relatively rigid and may be more than 100 μm in length but are not continuous back to the cell body. The neurofilaments are drawn as *wavy lines* with many sidearms that interact with other neurofilaments and microtubules. Both microtubules and neurofilaments are found in bundles in the axon and appear cross–linked to form a dense matrix in electron micrographs; however, these cross-bridges are dynamic and may be constantly forming and reforming. A few vesicles have been drawn in the axon and the terminal to emphasize that vesicles and cytoskeleton coexist in the axon. Moving vesicles must find a path through the matrix in order to move. As a result, large vesicles may be retarded in their movements by this matrix, producing a slower average velocity. **Insets:** Proposed fate of microtubules and neurofilaments that have reached the terminal. Each is evidently broken down by a Ca^{2+}-dependent mechanism. *Left inset*: Microtubule composed of tubulin dimers (the "figure eights") disassembling as a result of increased Ca^{2+} (△). It is not known whether the Ca^{2+} acts directly as shown here or is mediated by a factor such as calmodulin. *Right inset*: Helical neurofilament structure, which does not disassemble in physiological conditions. The neurofilaments appear to be degraded by a Ca^{2+}-activated protease, at least some of which may be associated with the neurofilament itself. Possible sources of Ca^{2+} include cisternae of the endoplasmic reticulum (left inset), mitochondria, or Ca^{2+} channels in the plasma membrane (right inset). (Adapted from Lasek and Katz [12].)

transport emerged: The Structural Hypothesis [10]. According to this view, proteins and other molecules move down the axon as component parts of discrete subcellular structures rather than as individual molecules (Table 1). The faster rates include only proteins that are preassembled into membranous organelles, including vesicles and mitochondria, or contained in the lumen of these organelles (Fig. 4). The slower rates include proteins that are part of cytoskeletal structures, including microtubules and neurofilaments, or are linked to these structures (Fig. 5).

Although five distinct rate components have been identified, the original broad categories of fast and slow transport remain useful. All of the membrane-associated proteins move in one of the fast rate components, while the cytoplasmic proteins move as part of the slow components. The synthesis and sorting of materials destined for transport in membrane-associated components utilize pathways that are completely different from those for soluble and cytoskeletal components. Current studies indicate that the several types of anterogradely transported organelles are driven down the axon by a common "motor" that is distinct from the mechanism(s) underlying the movement of cytoplasmic and structural elements of the axoplasm.

FAST AXONAL TRANSPORT

Newly synthesized proteins destined for the surface membrane travel by fast anterograde axonal transport

Fast-transport materials, including membrane and secretory proteins, together with membrane phospholipids, cholesterol and gangliosides, comprise a small portion of the total transported material but require a disproportionate amount of the total energy utilized for axonal transport [2,4]. (Fast axonal transport and the Na^+ pump may be the greatest users of ATPase-generated energy in the nervous system.) It is apparent

from video microscopy, and predicted by the Structural Hypothesis, that this transport is achieved by packaging fast-transport materials into organelles rather than by conveying them as separate molecules (see also Fig. 4). Clearly, an understanding of the mechanochemistry involved in moving these organelles is essential for fully appreciating fast transport. Equally important is an understanding of how these organelles are formed in the cell body and routed to the fast-transport system in the axon [4,13].

The well-characterized intracellular pathways of such secretory and membrane proteins as digestive enzymes in pancreas, acetylcholinesterase and acetylcholine receptor in muscle, and immunoglobulins in plasma cells have served as valuable models for examining the cell body or the initiation phase of fast axonal transport.

Proteins destined for the cell surface or for secretion are synthesized on polysomes bound to the endoplasmic reticulum

The role of endoplasmic reticulum organelles in fast transport is depicted in Figs. 4 and 6. In contrast, components of the cytoskeleton and enzymes of intermediary metabolism are synthesized on so-called free polysomes, which are actually associated with the cytoskeleton (Fig. 5). Secretory proteins enter the lumen of the reticulum, whereas membrane proteins become oriented within the bilayer of the reticular membrane. The newly formed membrane-associated proteins then pass via vesicles or direct membrane continuities to the Golgi apparatus for post-translational modification, including glycosylation, sulfation, and proteolytic cleavage, as well as for sorting. Their transport to the cell surface occurs via vesicles that bud off from the Golgi membrane, traverse the cytoplasm, and fuse with the plasma membrane. An important principle is that membrane and secretory proteins become membrane associated either during or immediately following their synthesis and

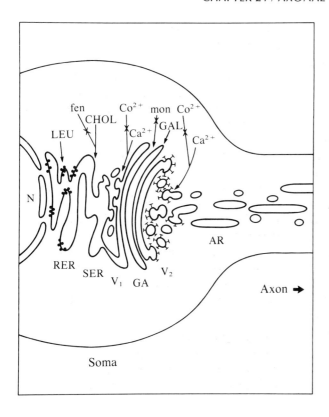

FIG. 6. Summary of pharmacological evidence indicating that newly synthesized membrane and secretory proteins in neurons reach the axons by a pathway similar to that utilized for intracellular transport in nonneuronal cells [4]. Incorporation sites are indicated for several precursors of materials in fast axonal transport: leucine (LEU) for proteins, choline (CHOL) for phospholipids, and galactose (GAL) for glycoproteins and glycolipids. Sites of action for several inhibitors are also indicated, including fenfluramine (fen), monensin (mon), and Co^{2+}. One possible site for Ca^{2+}-mediated vesicle fusion is at the transition from rough endoplasmic reticulum (RER) and smooth endoplasmic reticulum (SER) to the Golgi apparatus (GA) via one type of transition vesicle (V_1). The subsequent budding of vesicles (V_2) off the GA, presumably mediated by clathrin-coated vesicles, is a second site for Ca^{2+} involvement. The microtubule guides for the axonal vesiculotubular structures in transport and the axoplasmic reticulum (AR) are not shown.

maintain this association throughout their lifetime in the cell.

Evidence that a similar sequence of events occurs in neurons was first obtained by electron microscope autoradiography: Radiolabeled protein appeared to pass from the rough endoplasmic reticulum to the Golgi apparatus before entering the axon [14]. This pathway has been confirmed and expanded by pulse labeling proteins in the presence of pharmacological agents that inhibit particular events or disrupt selected structures on the intracellular pathway (Fig. 6) [4]. For example, inhibition of the synthesis of either protein or phospholipid leads to a proportional decrease in the amount of both fast-transport protein and phospholipid, whereas application of these inhibitors selectively to the axon has no effect on fast transport. This suggests that fast axonal transport depends on the

de novo synthesis and assembly of membrane components.

Passage through the Golgi apparatus is obligatory for newly synthesized proteins destined for fast transport

The role of the Golgi apparatus is demonstrated by pharmacological studies (Fig. 6). The Na^+ ionophore, monensin, selectively disrupts the stacks of the Golgi apparatus and depresses the amount of all fast-transport proteins entering the axon, including both glycosylated and nonglycosylated proteins. While all fast-transport proteins apparently traverse the Golgi, they may not all reach it by the same pathway. The antagonist of Ca^{2+}, Co^{2+} also depresses the amount of fast-transport proteins, but unlike monensin, proteins are differentially affected by

Co^{2+}. Those proteins with a molecular weight above approximately 35 kilodaltons (kDa) are predominantly glycoproteins and are inhibited to a greater extent than those proteins below this molecular weight, very few of which are glycoproteins.

Other studies suggest that fast-transport proteins pass through two Ca^{2+}-dependent steps: one prior to their entering the Golgi stacks and a second step during or after their exit from the Golgi. One explanation is that the nonglycosylated proteins pass through a single Ca^{2+}-dependent step, whereas the glycosylated set passes through both steps. Ultrastructural studies support this model. Passage of proteins from the endoplasmic reticulum to the Golgi apparatus may occur either by vesicles that bud off the reticulum and fuse with the Golgi or via membrane channels that appear to connect the two systems [4,13]. Although vesicle fusion is likely to be Ca^{2+} dependent, passage via continuous channels has no obvious Ca^{2+} requirement. The post-Golgi Ca^{2+} step, which would be common for all fast-transport proteins, may be the fusion of Golgi-derived vesicles to form the vesiculotubular organelles that appear to be transport vectors in the axon.

The post-Golgi transfer vesicle may well be the so-called coated vesicle

Coated vesicles mediate endocytotic retrieval from the plasma membrane as well as exocytotic transfers from the Golgi apparatus. When coated vesicles were isolated from [^{3}H]leucine-labeled dorsal root ganglia and the resulting ^{3}H-proteins coelectrophoresed on two-dimensional gels with [^{35}S]methionine-labeled fast-transport proteins from a separate preparation of sciatic nerve, approximately two-thirds of the ^{35}S-proteins were found to comigrate with coated-vesicle ^{3}H-proteins [15]. These results suggest that coated vesicles play a major, though not necessarily exclusive, role in the exit of fast-transport proteins from the Golgi apparatus. The pos-

sible existence of an alternate route of transfer is of interest because in nonneuronal cells, distinct subpopulations of newly synthesized proteins reach the plasma membrane via different vesicles [13]. Coated vesicles, however, are rarely observed in axons, and clathrin, the major coat protein, has been identified as a slow-transport protein [10]. Thus, it would appear that Golgi-derived coated vesicles shed their coats prior to undergoing fast transport, either as uncoated vesicles or as vesiculotubular fusion products that form from uncoated vesicles (Fig. 6). The transient involvement of coated vesicles in anterograde transport may well be similar to the role of these vesicles at synaptic terminals, where they transfer membrane-associated material from the plasma membrane to the retrograde transport system.

Retrograde axonal transport is demonstrated by placing two constrictions on a peripheral nerve trunk and observing the redistribution of transported material

An initial buildup on the proximal side of the constriction more distant from the cell body (indicative of anterograde transport) is followed by a buildup on the distal side of the constriction closer to the cell body [2,3]. This constriction-induced turnaround of transported material is believed to be similar to events at the presynaptic terminal that permit aging molecules or structures to be reprocessed, excess newly arrived materials to be recycled, and information about the periphery to be sent to the cell body. Presumably, plasma membrane from along the length of the axon is also periodically retrieved and recycled by this mechanism.

Exogenous molecules taken up into the nerve terminal by endocytosis are another important class of retrogradely transported materials. This is a route by which nerve growth factor and other neurotropic factors may reach their intraneuronal sites of action. It is also a means by which neurotoxins and viruses enter the nervous system. Numerous macromolecules, including horseradish peroxidase, ferritin, and a variety of fluorescent or radiolabeled lectins, have been used to examine the properties of retrograde transport. Many of these molecules bind to glycoproteins of the presynaptic membrane surface and ultimately arrive in the neuronal cell bodies. Studies of retrograde axonal transport led to the paradigm of applying a tracer molecule at the distal ends of nerves to map neuronal pathways [16].

Target cell-derived signals are likely to be important regulators of neuronal cell body metabolism. During neuronal development, for example, when an axonal growth cone makes its initial contact, a signal may be sent back to the cell body to trigger the synthesis and anterograde transport of the proteins required to establish a functional synapse. In mature neurons, the loss of target signals is a possible means by which the cell body learns that its axon has been damaged [17]. Loss of such target-derived factors has been proposed as a general neurological defect, contributing to Parkinsonism, amyotrophic lateral sclerosis, and Alzheimer's disease [18].

A range of velocities has been reported for retrograde transport, often approaching the fastest rates of anterograde transport. Other similarities between fast retrograde and fast anterograde transport include the materials transported (membrane-associated proteins, glycoproteins, and phospholipids) and the properties of the transport mechanism (involvement of microtubules and an energy-generating system present all along the axon). The major difference, as revealed by electron microscopic examination of material accumulated at focal blocks of transport, is in the nature of the organelles transported [19]. Anterogradely moving organelles are vesicles and vesiculotubular structures with relatively consistent diameters of 50 to 80 nm, whereas retrogradely moving organelles are larger and vary in morphology

and size, ranging from 100 to 500 nm in diameter. One class of retrograde organelles is multivesicular bodies that contain numerous vesicles in their lumens. Virtually all retrograde organelles resemble lysosomal or prelysosomal structures.

Molecular mechanisms of fast axonal transport are based on several models

For many years after the demonstration of a fast rate of axonal transport, most models of the transport mechanism were based on analogies to two well-studied systems of force-generated movement: actin/myosin-based contraction of muscle and dynein/microtubule-based beating of cilia [20,21]. An actomyosin-like or dynein-like ATPase was proposed to supply the energy to move membranous organelles (or to move a transport filament to which the organelles attach) through a relatively stationary axoplasm. Alternative models suggested that ATPases generate shear forces that create low-viscosity "microstreams" of axoplasm to convey the organelles. All models shared the feature that organelle transport occurs in close proximity to a cytoskeletal element, the most popular candidate being microtubules. A point of contention was whether direct, reversible interactions occur between the organelles and the cytoskeleton or whether the latter simply provides an orientation for the force-generating system. Progress made in the past few years has led to the understanding that anterograde translocation of membranous organelles in the axon represents a previously unrecognized type of intracellular motility, involving an ATPase that is unlike either actomyosin or dynein.

A new approach to the use of video in light microscopy, called Allen video-enhanced contrast (AVEC) microscopy [22] has facilitated such experimental advances. Analog and digital processing of the image generated by a high-resolution video camera have increased sensitivity and enhanced contrast to such an extent that structures below the theoretical limit of resolution for light microscopy (200 nm) can be detected (Fig. 1). Structures as small as individual microtubules (25 nm) and synaptic vesicles (40–70 nm) previously observable only via the electron microscope can now be seen in living cells.

The squid giant axon, often >500 μm in diameter, has provided an excellent preparation for AVEC microscopy [1,23]. The primary value of this preparation stems from the fact that the axoplasm of the squid giant axon can be extruded from its plasma membrane and connective tissue sheath while retaining both its cylindrical shape and ultrastructural organization. AVEC microscopy demonstrated that membranous organelles continue to move in the isolated axoplasm for hours after extrusion. Moreover, the characteristics of the movement of vesicles along microtubules were indistinguishable from transport in the intact axon. With this preparation, the mechanisms of transport became accessible to pharmacological manipulation since there was no plasma membrane to act as a permeability barrier.

A nonhydrolyzable analog of ATP, 5'-adenylyl imidodiphosphate, has provided insight into the transport mechanism

When 5'-adenylyl imidodiphosphate (AMP-PNP) at concentrations slightly higher than that of endogenous ATP, was perfused into isolated axoplasm, all anterograde and retrograde transport stopped [1]. Membranous organelles continued to attach to microtubules in AMP-PNP, but they did not move along or release from the microtubules until the inhibition was overcome by adding excess ATP. The affinity of both myosin and dynein-like ATPases for AMP-PNP is two to three orders of magnitude lower than their affinity for ATP, whereas AMP-PNP effectively inhibits organelle movement in the presence of near-stoichiometric levels of ATP.

In contrast with the effects of AMP-PNP on vesicles, both ATP and AMP-PNP induce myosin or dynein to release from microfilaments or microtubules. Thus, the motor for fast transport is fundamentally different from the ATPases associated with other types of cellular motility.

Kinesin

The use of AMP-PNP has also provided a means of identifying the polypeptide components of the fast-transport motor [24,25]. When brain microtubules are prepared in the presence of ATP, they contain tubulin as well as a number of microtubule-associated proteins (MAPs) (see Fig. 7 and discussion below). If, however, the ATP is replaced or supplemented with AMP-PNP, an additional polypeptide of approximately 130 kDa is associated with the microtubules (Fig. 7). Similar polypeptides have been identified in bovine, pig, rat, and chick brain, as well as in squid, sea urchin eggs, and *Drosophila*, suggesting that the mechanism underlying organelle movement is conserved in nature. Although reports from various laboratories show discrepancies concerning the properties and the polypeptide composition of the active fractions, the name *kinesin* has become generally accepted in referring to those proteins of 110 to 135 kDa that bind to microtubules in the presence of AMP-PNP but not in the presence of ATP. Kinesin appears to be a microtubule-activated ATPase having many properties in common with the fast-transport motor and interacting with both microtubules and vesicles.

Regulation of fast axonal transport

Routing of fast-transport proteins through the cell body to the axon and microtubule-mediated transport of organelles through the axon appear to be nonregulated or constitutive processes. Fast transport occurs continuously rather than in stimulus-dependent bursts. Under conditions where nerve stimulation increases protein synthesis, however, the amount of fast-transport

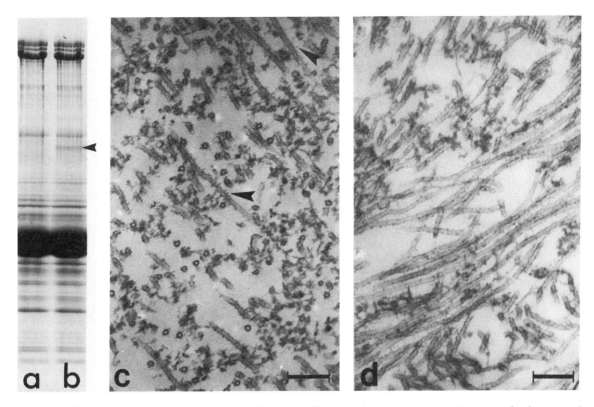

FIG. 7. The motor for fast axonal transport. Recent studies have demonstrated that the motor for fast axonal transport is a previously unrecognized mechanochemical enzyme. In the presence of the nonhydrolyzable analog of ATP, adenylyl imidodiphosphate (AMP-PNP), vesicles are frozen in place on microtubules. When microtubules from brain are assembled in the presence of ATP, electrophoretic analysis shows that the microtubules contain tubulin and an assortment of MAPs (**a**). When the same experiment is done in the presence of excess AMP-PNP (**b**), the electrophoretic pattern contains an additional polypeptide of molecular weight 120–130 kDa (*small arrowhead*). Comparison between electron micrographs of microtubule pellets made with AMP-PNP (**c**) and with ATP (**d**) reveals the presence of numerous small sidearms on the AMP-PNP microtubules (*large arrowheads*, **c**) that are not on the ATP microtubules (**d**). These sidearms are thought to correspond to the bridges between vesicles in transport and microtubules. Bars, 0.2 μm. (Electron micrographs adapted from Brady [24].)

protein increases, demonstrating that the fast-transport system can increase its normal capacity severalfold without altering the transport rate. In addition, the kinds of macromolecules in fast transport are subject to regulation.

Fast transport is responsive to the functional state of the axon. For example, transection of one branch of a bifurcating axon initially results in a diversion of transport such that the undamaged branch receives the total allotment of transmitter-containing vesicles [26]. This situation is corrected as the cell body reduces production of vesicles to the point where transport in the undamaged nerve is restored to normal. Moreover, when a severed axon regenerates, specific changes occur in the pattern of fast-transport proteins [28]. While many transported proteins are increased severalfold, a small number of acidic fast-transport proteins increase as much as 100-fold over normal. The latter proteins, called growth-associated proteins (GAPs), are associated with growth cones and, subsequently, with synaptic terminals and are also found in similarly high amounts in developing neurons. Down-regulation of GAPs generally occurs once synaptic contacts have been established, although recent intriguing evidence suggests that at least one of the GAPs is involved in synaptic modulation of mature neurons.

SLOW AXONAL TRANSPORT

Although the study of axonal transport began with a description of what is now considered slow transport (the nerve-dam paradigm of Weiss and Hiscoe), knowledge of the slow components of axonal transport initially lagged behind our understanding of fast transport, largely due to practical considerations. Studies of fast transport involve incubations lasting hours, whereas analyses of slow transport require experimental times of days and even months. Moreover, although fast transport involves the movement of well-defined membranous organelles, seen in electron micrographs to accumulate when transport is inhibited, the movement of structures representative of slow transport was not as readily detected. Thus, slow transport was long thought to represent the bulk flow of predominantly soluble axoplasmic materials.

Slow transport is a complex, multicomponent process

With the use of gel electrophoresis, coupled with autoradiography, three components of slow transport were detected that differ markedly in their rates of movement, protein composition and biochemical properties [9,10]. The slowest component, termed slow-component a

(SCa), or group V, moves at approximately 1 mm/day and has a relatively simple polypeptide composition; 70 to 80 percent of the material in this rate class is associated with only five polypeptides (Fig. 3). Two of these polypeptides were identified as α- and β-tubulin, the fundamental subunits of microtubules. Although the remaining three polypeptides did not correspond to any known proteins, the large volume of the axon occupied by neurofilaments (Fig. 8) led to the proposal that the remaining triplet (200, 145, and 68 kDa) represented the subunit proteins of this cytoskeletal structure [10]. Subsequent biochemical studies confirmed this proposal. Slow-component b (SCb), or group IV (2–4 mm/day), is considerably more complex, including more than 200 different polypeptides. These range from structural proteins like actin and clathrin to enzymes of intermediary metabolism, and, unlike SCa, no one polypeptide comprises more than a few percent of the total. Although SCb includes many readily solubilized proteins, all of the constituents move down the axon in a coherent wave. Thus, it is unlikely that they are freely diffusing in the axoplasm. Lasek and his colleagues proposed that the proteins of SCb travel in association with a heterogeneous structure that they called the *axoplasmic matrix*. This matrix includes some cytoskeletal proteins and enzymes of intermediate metabolism. By contrast with SCa and SCb, little is known about the polypeptides that comprise the remaining slow component (group III) except that they move at 4 to 8 mm/day and may include a myosin-like protein.

Slow-component a

Comparative studies have shown that the rates as well as the relative amounts and compositions of the two main classes of slow transport often vary between different populations of neurons, even in the same animal [29]. Thus, while slow transport is an invariant aspect of neuronal

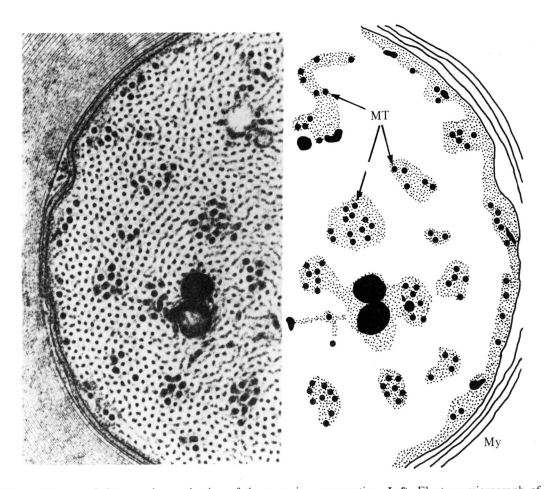

FIG. 8. The cytoskeleton and organization of the axon in cross section. **Left:** Electron micrograph of a myelinated toad axon in cross section taken near a Schmidt-Lanterman cleft; axon diameter is slightly reduced and the different domains within the axoplasm emphasized. **Right:** Diagram to highlight key features of the axoplasm. Portions of the myelin sheath surrounding the axon can be seen (My). Most of the axonal diameter is taken up by the neurofilaments (*clear area*). There is a minimum distance between neurofilaments and other cytoskeletal structures that is determined by the sidearms of the neurofilaments. (These sidearms are visible between some of the neurofilaments in the electron micrograph, **left**.) The microtubules (MT) (●) tend to be found in bundles and are more irregularly spaced. They are surrounded by a fuzzy material that is also visible in the region just below the plasma membrane (*stippled areas*, **right**). These areas are thought to be enriched in actin microfilaments and presumably contain other SCb proteins as well. The *stippled regions* with embedded microtubules are also the location of membranous organelles in fast axonal transport (*larger, filled irregular shapes*, **right**). Both microtubule and microfilament networks need to be intact for the efficient movement of organelles in fast transport. Electron micrograph provided by Dr. Alan Hodge; adapted from Hodge and Adelman [27].

activity, its properties appear to be modifiable to suit the requirements of different types of axons. For example, the rate of SCa may range from 0.2 to 0.5 mm/day in rat optic nerve to as much as 1 to 1.5 mm/day in sensory and motor neurons of the sciatic nerve in the same animal. In poikilotherms, where the rate of transport is dependent on ambient temperature, SCa has been measured as slow as 0.01 mm/day (in the optic nerve of goldfish kept at 15°C). The rate of SCa also changes during development of the nervous system, gradually slowing as neurons mature. In all cases, however, SCa is the slowest moving component and has a characteristic composition.

The polypeptides that serve as the signature proteins for SCa are the three neurofilament (NF) subunits, or the NF triplet. Although the tubulin subunits that constitute microtubules (see below) are also a major constituent of SCa, they are not as suitable a marker. For example, although essentially all the tubulin moving down adult mammalian optic nerves is associated with SCa, a substantial fraction of the tubulin traveling down sensory neurons in the same animal moves ahead of the NF triplet at a rate comparable to that of SCb proteins. In fact, tubulin may be the major labeled SCb protein detected in pulse-chase studies of transport in these neurons. Moreover, in fish and amphibian systems, tubulin is a prominent SCb protein, even in optic nerve. The minor protein components of SCa, such as the characteristic MAPs, are also unreliable markers of this rate class, again because they present no consistent pattern among various classes of neurons. Nevertheless, despite quantitative variations in tubulin and MAPs associated with SCa, this rate component always contains the tubulin doublet and a population of MAPs in addition to the NF triplet. As a result, SCa can be described as the *neurofilament-microtubule network* of the axon, a concept that is consistent with studies showing cross-bridges that link the two cytoskeletal structures.

Slow-component b

The peak of SCb in a pulse-chase study moves down the axon 4–10 times faster than SCa and includes a far greater number of different proteins [30]. Just as with SCa, the actual rate of SCb varies with the type of neuron, the temperature and the stage of development. Not surprisingly, the composition of SCb also exhibits considerable variability. Although only a few of the hundreds of polypeptides in this rate component have been identified, these known proteins provide insights into the organization and function of SCb. The structural correlate of SCb is termed the axoplasmic matrix and it includes both cytoskeletal proteins and metabolic enzymes.

Intermediary metabolism. Subcellular fractionation studies of axonally transported material indicate that many of the proteins in slow transport partition with the soluble fraction [30]. As a result, it is not surprising that many identified proteins in SCb are enzymes of intermediary metabolism, and are classically soluble proteins. Enzymes of glycolysis, such as enolase, aldolase, and pyruvate kinase, have been identified in SCb, and it is likely that the complete pathway of glycolysis is part of the SCb complex of proteins. In addition, other readily solubilized proteins involved in energy metabolism or regulation of metabolism are associated with SCb, for example, creatine phosphokinase and calmodulin. Although these proteins, when isolated from axoplasm, function well in free solution, axonal transport studies indicate that *in situ* they are organized as a complex.

Spectrin and clathrin. Among the many other proteins of SCb, two of particular interest are spectrin, an actin-binding protein, and clathrin, the coated-vesicle protein [30]. Spectrin (also called fodrin) is closely related to the spectrin of the erythrocyte membrane. It is particularly abundant near the plasma membrane but can also be detected throughout the axon. It is also the only polypeptide that is consistently detectable in more than one rate component, being present in SCa and SCb and, at very low levels, is even associated with mitochondria. Spectrin appears to be a linker protein and may be involved in the interconnection of microfilaments with membranous structures and with other cytoskeletal elements.

Clathrin is the major structural component that forms the lattice-like cage of coated vesicles. Although it appears to function in the cell body during formation of vesicles destined for fast axonal transport, coated vesicles are rarely seen in the axon, and clathrin itself moves with SCb. Once at the presynaptic terminal, clathrin plays a key role in the recycling of synaptic vesicles and in receptor-mediated endocytosis. In each case, the clathrin coat appears to be transiently involved in facilitating the budding-off of a vesicle from a membrane.

Growth cone extension reveals aspects of the slow transport mechanism

The one situation in which movement of the axonal cytoskeleton has been readily observed is the extension of the growth cone by the developing or regenerating neuron [31]. As the growth cone advances, its maximum rate of movement correlates with the rate of SCb, suggesting that the motor(s) for slow axonal transport is present in this rate component. Reports of myosin or myosin-like proteins in SCb raise the possibility that growth cone movement, and thus slow axonal transport itself, is an actomyosin-based form of motility, which would be consistent with movement of other cell types at similar rates. Although definitive mechanisms have not yet been established, two key points can be made. The cytoskeletal structures of the axon, including microtubules, neurofilaments, and axoplasmic matrix, are moved as assembled structures, and the motive force for their transport is generated locally along the axon, serving

to tow the various components and their associated cargo toward the presynaptic terminal.

The structures of slow axonal transport are apparently reorganized (e.g., microfilaments) or broken down (e.g., microtubules and neurofilaments) on entering the presynaptic terminal (see Fig. 5). Calcium ions appear to play an important role in regulation of the cytoskeleton at the synaptic terminal. For example, disassembly of neurofilaments seems to require a Ca^{2+}-activated protease and microtubules may also be very sensitive to Ca^{2+} levels. Unlike the proteins in fast axonal transport, the constituents of slow transport are not detectable in retrograde transport.

The physiological roles of slow transport are implicit in its composition

Since neurofilaments and microtubules are the primary structural elements of the neuron, it is not surprising that alterations in axonal caliber and length during development and regeneration can be correlated with changes in SCa [32]. For example, developing axons contain few neurofilaments until synaptogenesis is complete, at which time increased synthesis and transport of neurofilaments are accompanied by increases in axon caliber.

The contributions of SCb components to the structure of the neuron are most apparent in the growth cone, dendritic spines, and the synaptic terminal, regions of the neuron that are relatively poor in microtubules and neurofilaments (SCa elements) and rich in actin microfilaments (SCb elements). The distribution of microfilaments also suggests that SCb components play an important role in the formation and remodeling of synaptic connections. In addition, the presence of glycolytic enzymes implies that SCb contributes to the energy metabolism of the neuron. Finally, both SCa and SCb must be seen as contributing to the rich network of interconnections through which the axonal infrastructure is organized.

NEURONAL CYTOSKELETON

Neurofilaments make up the bulk of axonal volume in large myelinated fibers

Neurofilaments belong to the family of cytoskeletal structures known as intermediate filaments [33] (Fig. 8). All such filaments are long, unbranching fibrils approximately 10 nm in diameter and many micrometers in length. They share structural, biochemical, and immunochemical properties (including remarkable stability under physiological conditions), and their primary function is considered to be to confer form and mechanical strength to cells. Other examples of intermediate filaments include the keratins of skin and hair and the glial filaments of astrocytes in the central nervous system. Neurofilaments differ from other intermediate filaments in both the number and size of their subunits. Whereas nonneuronal intermediate filaments are composed of one or more different polypeptides in the range of 45 to 65 kDa neurofilaments—in species ranging from invertebrates to humans—have a single low-molecular mass subunit (60–70 kDa) and two or more high-molecular mass forms (130–200 kDa). A curious exception is found in the neurons of arthropods (insects and crustaceans), which contain no morphologically identifiable neurofilaments. Arthropod axons do contain large numbers of microtubules, but the properties of slow axonal transport have not been studied in these axons.

A unique feature of NF proteins is a tail region that contains numerous phosphorylation sites and glutamic acid residues. The glutamic acid-rich region appears to be responsible for the reaction of neurofilaments with the silver stains so useful in neuroanatomical studies. The tail regions of the high-molecular mass subunits appear to form the cross-bridges between neurofilaments as well as between neurofilaments and microtubules (see Fig. 8). These cross-bridges, which establish interfilament spacing, are presumably responsible for neurofilaments forming larger and more loosely packed bundles than are seen for glial and nonneuronal inter-

mediate filaments. Alterations in their packing density are associated with such pathological conditions as Alzheimer's disease (see Chap. 41) and chronic exposure to certain industrial toxins or neurotoxic drugs. Under physiological conditions, neurofilaments in the axon appear to exist only in the polymer form. This is consistent with the view that NF assembly occurs in the cell body, whereas disassembly is effected by Ca^{2+}-activated proteases at or near the nerve terminal (Fig. 5, inset).

The second major element of the neuronal cytoskeleton is the microtubule

Microtubules are 25 nm in diameter with walls usually composed of 13 protofilaments closely packed (Figs. 7 and 8) [34]. Each protofilament is in turn composed of globular α- and β-tubulin subunits. Axonal microtubules may be 100 μm or more in length but do not generally extend the length of the axon. Surprisingly, axonal microtubules are not continuous with the cell body. This is unusual, since in most nonneural cells—and even in neuronal dendrites—microtubules grow from a so-called microtubule-organizing center near the nucleus, associated with the centrosomal complex. Other mechanisms must be involved in regulating microtubules of the axon.

Microtubules include a number of accessory proteins. Highly purified tubulin can be induced to assemble into microtubules *in vitro* in the absence of other proteins; however, microtubules prepared by conventional methods using high-speed centrifugation in alternating cycles of cold (disassembly conditions) and warm (assembly conditions), with GTP and Mg^{2+} but little or no Ca^{2+}, contain small amounts of MAPs that cycle at a constant stoichiometry with the tubulin [34,35]. MAPs are a heterogeneous group of proteins that bind to microtubules (but not to tubulin dimers), altering their biochemical properties and linking them to other axoplasmic structures. The best characterized MAPs are those of high molecular weight (>300 kDa) and the tau proteins (55–70 kDa). Other proteins that interact with microtubules, either directly or indirectly, include neurofilaments and the motors that moves fast-transport membranous organelles along the microtubule (see Fig. 7). Curiously, tau MAPs, but not high-molecular-weight MAPs, have been detected in SCa. Immunochemical studies confirm the presence of tau proteins in axons and reveal that certain high-molecular-weight MAPs are located preferentially in dendrites [35].

Microtubules may differ, depending on their location in the nervous system [29,35]. The composition of MAPs varies from one class of neurons to the next and clearly differs when neurons are compared to glia and other non-neuronal cell types in the nervous system. Changes in the MAP composition of brain during development may reflect an additional level of regulation of neuronal microtubules. Biochemical specialization of neuronal microtubules extends to the tubulins as well. These proteins are a multigene family with six or more genes for both α- and β-tubulin. Several of these different gene products are enriched in nervous tissue and some may be preferentially located in axons. More than 20 distinct isotypes of tubulin have been detected in brain, a result of both differential gene expression and a number of post-translational modifications, including acetylation and tyrosylation.

The restriction of certain MAPs and isotypes of tubulin to particular regions of the neuron implies differential specialization of the neuronal cytoskeleton. Neurofilament variation also contributes to this regional uniqueness; axonal neurofilaments, unlike those in the cell body, are highly phosphorylated. The physiological functions of these specializations are currently being sought, but several conclusions are apparent: (1) the many variants in protein composition and posttranslational modification are highly regulated; (2) several of the specific protein variants are targeted for particular regions within the neuron; and (3) posttransla-tional modifications that occur in the cell body and in the axon may serve to coordinate interactions among the cytoskeletal components.

The third major cytoskeletal structure of all eukaryotic cells is the short filament, only 4 to 6 nm in diameter, generally referred to as the microfilament

Similar to the better studied microfilaments of skeletal muscle, nonmuscle microfilaments, including those of neurons, consist of two strands of globular actin molecules wrapped around each other in a helical fashion [36]. However, while the thin filaments of muscle may be more than 1 μm in length, nonmuscle microfilaments are typically much shorter, often comprising only a few dozen subunits. Moreover, nonmuscle cells contain different isoforms of actin as well as different actin-associated proteins; for example, their myosin is distinct, and they lack the troponin complex.

The brain is a rich source of nonmuscle actins and myosins and was one of the first tissues in which these proteins were identified. Within neurons, microfilaments are enriched and relatively well characterized in the presynaptic terminal and dendritic spines where they are the primary cytoskeletal elements, apparently providing both form and organization for these neuronal specializations. Within the axon, microfilaments are also enriched in a narrow layer (~50 nm) just below the plasma membrane, and they are presumed to be involved in the organization of the axoplasmic matrix, which represents the complex array of SCb proteins (see Fig. 8).

FUTURE DIRECTIONS

The rapid progress in clarifying the molecular basis of the fast-transport mechanism should soon produce a model of vectorial force generation that includes the anterograde and retrograde motors, their associated ATPases, and their role in the reversible formation of cross-bridges between organelles and microtubules. The generation of monoclonal antibodies to surface components of axonal organelles is another approach that is likely to identify molecules that interact with the transport motor [37]. Such studies of the surface of fast-transport organelles may also identify molecular markers that specify (1) which organelles undergo fast transport rather than remain in the cell body; (2) which organelles enter the axon rather than dendrites; (3) which are destined for sites along the axolemma; and (4) which will reach the presynaptic terminal [38]. The patterns of organelle movement revealed with AVEC microscopy, will eventually be understood in terms of molecular mechanisms, providing insights into the biochemical basis of directionality and regulation of neuronal development [23].

The near future also holds considerable promise for understanding the critical role of cytoskeletal elements in determining and maintaining the remarkable diversity among different classes of neurons [36]. Both translational and posttranslational regulatory mechanisms will continue to provide clues to the manner by which differing amounts and kinds of cytoskeletal elements are determinants of neuronal morphology [39]. Finally, many details of the mechanisms by which cytoskeletal elements act locally to promote such phenomena as axonal elongation and interneuronal connectivity remain to be determined [12].

ACKNOWLEDGMENTS

The collaborative efforts in preparing this chapter were supported by grants to R.H. from NIH (NS 18858), NSF (BNS 8545740), and the James Peters Research Fellowship administered through the Beckman Research Institute of the City of Hope; and to S.T.B. from NIH (NS 23320) and NS 23868) and from the Texas Neurofibromatosis Foundation.

REFERENCES

1. Brady, S., Lasek, R., and Allen, R. Fast axonal transport in extruded axoplasm from the squid giant axon. *Cell Motil.* 3(Videodisk Suppl. 1):Side 2, track 2, 1983. A companion paper is Brady, S., Lasek, R., and Allen, R. Video microscopy of fast axonal transport in extruded axoplasm: A new model for study of molecular mechanisms. *Cell Motility* 5:81–101, 1985.
2. Grafstein, B., and Forman, D. S. Intracellular transport in neurons. *Physiol. Rev.* 60:1167–1283, 1980; see also Weiss, D. G. (ed.). *Axoplasmic Transport* Berlin: Springer-Verlag, 1981.
3. Lasek, R. J. Protein transport in neurons. *Int. Rev. Neurobiol.* 13:289–321, 1970; Dahlström, A. Axoplasmic transport (with particular respect to adrenergic neurons). *Phil. Trans. R. Soc. London Ser. B* 261:325–358, 1971.
4. Hammerschlag, R., and Stone, G. C. Membrane delivery by fast axonal transport. *Trends Neurosci.* 5:12–15, 1982.
5. Brady, S., Lasek, R., and Allen, R. Fast axonal transport in extruded axoplasm from squid giant axon. *Science* 218:1129–1131, 1982.
6. Weiss, P., and Hiscoe, H. B. Experiments in the mechanism of nerve growth. *J. Exp. Zool.* 107:315–395, 1948.
7. Droz, B., and LeBlond, C. P. Migration of proteins along the axons of the sciatic nerve. *Science* 137:1047–1048, 1962.
8. Brady, S. Axonal Transport methods and applications. In A. Boulton and G. Baker (ed.), *Neuromethods, Vol. I: General Neurochemical Techniques.* Clifton NJ: Humana Press, 1986. pp. 419–476.
9. Baitinger, C., Levine, J., Lorenz, T., Simon, C., Skene, P., and Willard, M. Characteristics of axonally transported proteins. In D. G. Weiss (ed.), *Axoplasmic Transport.* Berlin: Springer-Verlag, 1982, pp. 110–120.
10. Lasek, R. J. Axonal transport: A dynamic view of neuronal structure. *Trends Neurosci.* 3:87–91, 1980.

11. Tytell, M., Black, M., Garner, J., and Lasek, R. Axonal transport: Each of the major rate components consist of distinct macromolecular complexes. *Science* 214:179–181, 1981.

12. Lasek, R., and Katz, M. Mechanisms at the axon tip regulate metabolic processes critical to axonal elongation. *Prog. Brain Res.* 71:49–60, 1987.

13. Kelly, R. B. Pathways of protein secretion in eukaryotes. *Science* 230:25–32, 1985.

14. Droz, B. Protein metabolism in nerve cells. *Int. Rev. Cytol.* 25:363–390, 1969.

15. Stone, G. C., Hammerschlag, R., and Bobinski, J. A. Involvement of coated vesicles in the initiation of fast axonal transport. *Brain Res.* 291:219–228, 1984.

16. LaVail, J. H. A review of the retrograde transport technique. In R. T. Robertson (ed.), *Neuroanatomical Research Techniques*. New York: Academic Press, 1978, pp. 356–384.

17. Bisby, M. A. Does recycling have functions other than disposal? In R. A. Smith and M. B. Bisby (eds.), *Axonal Transport*. New York: Alan R. Liss, 1987, pp. 365–383.

18. Appel, S. H. A unifying hypothesis for the cause of amyotrophic lateral sclerosis, Parkinsonism and Alzheimer's disease. *Ann. Neurol.* 10:499–505, 1981.

19. Tsukita, S., and Ishikawa, H. The movement of membranous organelles in axons: Electron microscopic identification of anterogradely and retrogradely transported organelles. *J. Cell Biol.* 84:513–530, 1980.

20. Weiss, D. G. The mechanism of axoplasmic transport. In Z. Iqbal (ed.), *Axoplasmic Transport*. Boca Raton: CRC Press, 1986, pp. 275–307.

21. Ochs, S. Fast axonal transport of materials in mammalian nerve fibers. *Science* 176:252–260, 1972.

22. Allen, R. D. New observations on cell architecture and dynamics by video-enhanced contrast optical microscopy. *Ann. Rev. Biophys. Biophys. Chem.* 14:265–290, 1985.

23. Brady, S. T. Fast axonal transport in isolated axoplasm from the squid giant axon. In R. S. Smith and M. A. Bisby (eds.), *Axonal Transport*, New York: Alan R. Liss, 1987, pp. 113–137.

24. Brady, S. T. A novel brain ATPase with properties expected for the fast axonal transport motor. *Nature* 317:73–75, 1985.

25. Vale, R. D., Reese, T. S., and Sheetz, M. P. Identification of a novel force-generating protein, kinesin, involved in microtubule-based motility. *Cell* 42:39–50, 1985.

26. Aletta, J. M., and Goldberg, D. J. Rapid and precise down regulation of fast axonal transport of transmitter in an identified neuron. *Science* 281:913–916, 1982.

27. Hodge, A., and Adelman, W. In D. Chang, I. Tasaki, W. Adelman, and H. Leuchtag (eds.), *Structure and Function in Excitable Cells*. New York: Plenum Press, 1983, pp. 75–111.

28. Willard, M. B., Meiri, K. F., and Johnson, M. I. The Role of GAP-43 in axon growth. In R. A. Smith and M. B. Bisby (eds.), *Axonal Transport*. New York: Alan R. Liss, 1987, pp. 407–420.

29. Oblinger, M., Brady, S., McQuarrie, I., and Lasek, R. Cytotypic differences in the protein composition of the axonally transported cytoskeleton in mammalian neurons. *J. Neurosci.* 7:453–462, 1986.

30. Lasek, R. J., Garner, J., and Brady, S. Axonal transport of the cytoplasmic matrix. *J. Cell Biol.* 99:212s–221s, 1984.

31. Lasek, R. J. Translocation of the neuronal cytoskeleton and axonal locomotion. *Phil. Trans., R. Soc. London B.* 299:313–327, 1982.

32. Hoffman, P., Griffin, J., and Price, D. Neurofilament transport in axonal regeneration: Implications for the control of axonal caliber. In J. Elam and P. Cancalon (eds.), *Axonal Transport in Neuronal Growth and Regeneration*. New York: Plenum, 1984, pp. 243–260.

33. Wang, E., Fischman, D., Liem, R., and Sun, T. (eds.), *Intermediate Filaments, Ann. N.Y. Acad. Sci.* Vol. 455, 1985.

34. Dustin, P. *Microtubules*. Berlin: Springer-Verlag, 1984.

35. Brady, S., and Black, M. Axonal transport of microtubule protein: Cytotypic variation of tubulin and MAPs in neurons. *Ann. NY Acad. Sci.* 466:199–217, 1986.

36. Schliwa, M. *The Cytoskeleton*. Berlin: Springer-Verlag, 1986.

37. Studelska, D. R., Oakes, S. G., and Brimijoin, S. Monoclonal antibodies to rapidly transported, particle-associated antigens of rat sciatic nerve:

Production and characterization. In R. S. Smith and M. A. Bisby (eds.), *Axonal Transport*. New York: Alan R. Liss, 1987, pp. 279–290.

38. Hammerschlag, R. How do neuronal proteins know where they are going? . . . Speculations of the role of molecular address markers. *Devel. Neurosci.* 6:2–17, 1983.

39. Matus, A. Neurofilament protein phosphorylation—where, when and why. *Trends Neurosci.* 11:291–292, 1988.

CHAPTER 25

Development of the Nervous System

Alaric T. Arenander and Jean de Vellis

Basic Neurochemistry: Molecular, Cellular, and Medical Aspects, 4th Ed., edited by G. J. Siegel et al. Raven Press, Ltd., New York, 1989.
Correspondence to Alaric T. Arenander, Departments of Anatomy and Psychiatry, Medical Retardation Research Center, Brain Research
Institute, School of Medicine, University of California, Los Angeles, California 90024.

Development is the study of the principles and processes that underlie growth and evolution of a biological organism [1,2]. Most developmental research has been devoted to studying the early periods of intense and extensive transformations that are associated with the unfolding of an organism from a single fertilized egg, through embryogenesis, to postnatal maturation. Change is one of the few constant aspects of the chemistry of the nervous system. This state of flux is seen across the entire spatial and temporal dimensions of the organism. This chapter examines the molecular and cellular processes in neural tissue that occur during these developmental periods from a neurochemical perspective.

Fundamental concepts of how the nervous system develops and functions molds this perspective. The dynamic interdependencies of (a) the genes and environment, and (b) the neuronal and neuroglial cells are two such concepts. During development, the systematic expression of the genetic blueprint can be seen in the creation and continuous molding of the environment at all levels of its hierarchical organization. The genetic machinery relies on feedback from the environment to function properly. This interaction creates a highly integrated, self-referential process that links the genetic information with the multitude of influences from all the different layers of the environment (Fig. 1). Biological interdependency is also dramatically displayed in the relationship of neurons and glia [3–5]. The intimate coupling of neuronal and glial cells, components of neural tissue, is a major locus of genetic and epigenetic interaction in determining the functioning and the morphological, chemical, and electrical development of the nervous system. Students learn that the neuron is the structural unit of the nervous system. The fundamental functional unit of the nervous system may be defined as the dynamic interaction of neuronal and glial cells (Fig. 2).

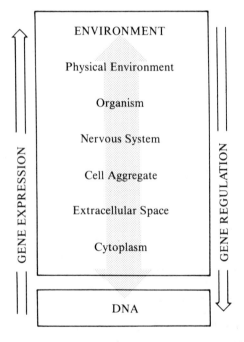

FIG. 1. Levels of genetic-epigenetic interaction. The development of each nerve cell occurs in a complex, changing environment. At the center of the cell is located the genetic material containing information necessary to form the nervous system. This information, as it is expressed, interacts with many hierarchical levels of the environment extending from the cell cytoplasm to the ecology of the organism. As gene expression alters the structure and function of the environment, the various levels of the environment influence the structure and function of the DNA through the process of gene regulation.

METHODOLOGY FOR THE STUDY OF NEURAL DEVELOPMENT

Cell culture techniques allow experimental control of developmental events

Cell culture techniques provide a powerful means of systematically studying complex nervous systems. The development of simple *in vitro* systems has had a great impact on neurochemistry, since it enables researchers to

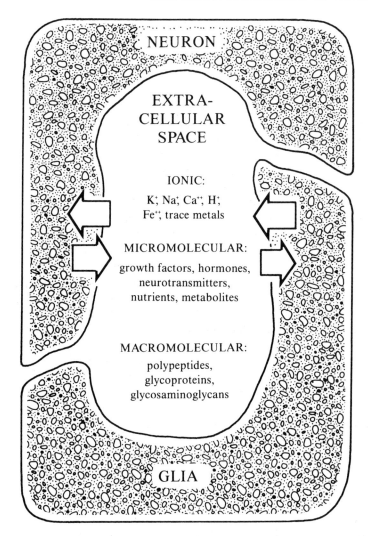

FIG. 2. Neuronal-neuroglial interaction represents a fundamental functional unit of the nervous system. Throughout neural development, neuronal and glial cells are shown to influence each others' physiology and behavior. The intercellular flow of materials and signals takes place within the extracellular space. This space, surrounding nerve cells, is heterogeneous. It is composed of ionic, micromolecular, and macromolecular elements contributed by neuronal, glial, endothelial, and ependymal cells. The various elements of this space represent the cellular microenvironment and exert considerable influence over the processes of neural growth and differentiation. (After Arenander and de Vellis [3].)

exert greater control over the chemical and cellular complexity of the nervous system [1,6,7]. Many cell cultures of developing nerve cells from vertebrate and invertebrate species are now available. As a result, the neurochemical dissection of development has greatly improved, revealing a growing spectrum of regulatory molecules and mechanisms that participate in neural development.

Vertebrate cell culture was developed in 1907 by Harrison. By placing fragments of frog embryo nervous tissue in a drop of clotted lymph, he was able to demonstrate that each nerve axon or dendrite is the extension of the neuronal cell body. This simple observation supported the neuronal doctrine at the expense of opponents who had claimed that nerve fibers were the product of fusion of many cells. Harrison's experiment was the prototype of the *explant cell culture* technique. In the 1960s, a second system, the *dissociated cell culture*, was introduced. In this method the tissue is dissociated mechanically or enzymatically to yield a suspension of single cells. The dispersed cells are usually cultured on the pretreated surface of a culture dish. A third system, *reaggregate cell culture*, was initiated by Moscona to provide a tissue-like environment for the cells. A few hours after dissociated cells are placed in a rotating flask, small, round aggregates are found floating in the media. These three systems, in which cultures are prepared directly from the tissues of an organism, are collectively termed primary cultures. Except for neuronal cells, it is possible to remove the primary neural tissue cells from the culture dish and establish secondary cultures and thus expand the population. Such cell preparations, e.g., of glia, can usually be passed successfully only a limited number of times due to either dedifferentiation or terminal differentiation of cells. A fourth system is that of *clonal cell culture* lines, established by culturing the progeny of a single cell. Neural cell lines come from endogenous tumors or from chemically or virally transformed cells.

Control of the physicochemical environment of the cells is possible *in vitro*. Substances can be added to or withdrawn from the culture medium, allowing precise temporal analysis of the sequence of events that occur, for example, in hormone action. Tissue culture also circumvents the problem of the blood-brain barrier and thus removes the endocrine and other signaling agents endogenous to the central nervous system. Furthermore, it also allows the study of a discrete nervous system area isolated from the normal *in vivo* homeostatic mechanisms.

Each of the tissue culture systems just described offers particular advantages. Dissociated cell cultures allow the visualization of individual living cells that can be monitored morphologically and electrophysiologically. It is possible to obtain and correlate biochemical, morphological, and electrophysiological data from a single cell. An alternative to observing and quantitating parameters at the single-cell level is to separate the cell types either prior to primary culturing if possible or after the culture is established. Ingenious methods developed in

different laboratories now make it possible to obtain cultures of all the cell types listed in Table 1 enriched 90 to 99 percent in one cell type. These pure cultures have become the system of choice for many neurochemists.

An advantage of using reaggregate cultures rather than dissociated cultures is the ability to provide a more structured, three-dimensional extracellular space that more closely approximates the *in vivo* conditions for cell growth and development. Such conditions may reduce the dilution of secreted cellular factors and increase the opportunity for morphological and biochemical differentiation to proceed more like *in vivo* events. The cells inside an aggregate are first distributed at random. They then sort out into patterns often resembling the organization seen *in vivo*. The importance of cell contact and histotypic organization is illustrated by the observation that glutamine synthetase, a marker of retinal glial Müller cells, is inducible by glucocorticoids in reaggregate but not dissociated cell cultures. Some laboratories are now using three-dimensional matrix cultures made from natural components, such as collagen and fibronectin, to obtain similar biological advantages.

Clonal cell lines, although tumoral in origin, have provided useful knowledge in neurochemistry over the past two decades. They provide homogeneous cell populations in large quantities in a very reproducible manner. The cell lines of choice are those which continue to express in culture the differentiated properties of their normal cell counterparts. The first such clonal cell line was the C6 glioma cell line established from a chemically–induced tumor in an adult rat; C6 cells possess differentiated properties of both astrocytes and oligodendrocytes. Like oligodendrocytes *in vivo* or in primary culture, C6 cells express glucocorticoid-inducible glycerolphosphate dehydrogenase and the myelin component 2',3'-cyclic nucleotide phosphohydrolase. They also display glucocorticoid-inducible glutamine synthetase and

TABLE 1. Cell markers for identifying major cell types[a]

Neurons
  Neurofilament
  Tetanus toxin
  A2B5*
  Enolase (γ, γ isozyme)
Oligodendrocytes
  Galactocerebroside (GC)
  Sulfatide (SULF)
  GD_3 ganglioside (GD3)
  Myelin basic protein (MBP)
  Myelin proteolipid protein (PLP)
  Myelin-associated glycoprotein (MAG)
  Glycerolphosphate dehydrogenase (GPDH)
  Cyclic nucleotide phosphohydrolase (CNP)
  Carbonic anhydrase II (CA)
  Cholesterol ester hydrolase
Meningeal cells
  Fibronectin
  Ran-2*
  Epen-1*
Fibroblasts
  Fibronectin
  Thy-1
Neuroepithelial stem cells
  Vimentin (VIM)
Astrocytes
  Glial fibrillary acidic protein (GFAP)
  Glutamine synthetase (GS)
  S-100 protein
  Ran-2*
Schwann cells
  217c*
  Ran-1
  Sulfatide (SULF)
  Glial fibrillary acidic protein (GFAP)
  Myelin basic protein (MBP)
  Laminin
  Galactocerebroside (GC)
Ependymal cells
  Cilia
  Ran-2*
  Epen-1*
Macrophages (microglia)
  MAC-1*
  MAC-3*
  Nonspecific esterase
  Labeled latex beads

[a] Most of the markers listed are available as both monoclonal and polyclonal antibodies. Since the antibodies are generated in different species, double labeling of cells is possible. The markers that are available only as monoclonal antibodies are marked by an asterisk. For these, the antigen is generally unknown, and the specificity is often species restricted, indicating that the epitope in the antigen was not conserved during evolution. Cell surface cilia of ependymal cells represent another type of marker. Macrophages readily phagocytose rhodamine-labeled latex beads, which then can be detected by fluorescence.

glial fibrillary acidic protein (GFAP), characteristic properties of astrocytes. C6 cells have been shown to conserve many of the regulatory control mechanisms and differentiated properties of glial cells and to provide large numbers of cells for experiments studying molecular mechanisms.

The PC12 clonal cell line was established from a rat pheochromocytoma, an adrenal medullary tumor [8]. PC12 cells have many properties in common with primary sympathetic neuron and chromaffin cell cultures. In response to nerve growth factor (NGF), they extend neurites and increase tyrosine hydroxylase (TH) activity. Useful clonal cell lines have also been established from mouse and human neuroblastoma. These cell lines express several neurotransmitter-synthesizing enzymes, which makes them good candidates for the study of regulation of gene expression as well as for the establishment of cDNA libraries.

Somatic cell hybrids resulting from the experimental fusion of two cells in culture can be cloned to obtain a hybrid cell line, provided that at least one of the parental cells is itself from an established cell line. This approach has been used to generate cell lines resulting from the hybridization of a normal neural cell and a tumoral cell line. For instance, an oligodendrocyte hybrid cell line produced by this method expresses myelin basic protein, a property of mature oligodendrocytes.

Cultured cells were originally maintained in the presence of biologically derived media, such as fetal calf serum. Chemically defined media are produced by replacing serum with pure growth factors, hormones, and adhesion molecules. These media have overcome the troublesome, uncontrollable, and undefined nature of sera and permitted the examination of the requirement of each cell type for survival, growth, and differentiation in culture. This has led not only to the discovery of the various target cells for different factors, but also of many new target cell-derived factors.

Molecular markers enable precise identification of cell types

Cell culture techniques in neurobiology expanded during the 1970s and increased the need for cell-type specific markers that would unambiguously identify all the cell types present in dissociated primary culture of neural tissue. The problem was most acute in developing systems because of the multiplicity of cell lineages and developmental stages, as well as the inadequacies of morphological criteria to identify population subsets. To develop neural cell markers, several neurobiologists turned to immunological approaches that were successful in analyzing lymphocyte subpopulations. Many cell markers are immunogenic molecules present in or on a single cell type and that can be detected with specific monoclonal or polyclonal antibodies. These two classes of antibody differ in specificity, sensitivity, and in the way in which they are generated. The generation of a polyclonal antibody requires purified antigen for the immunization of the appropriate mammal whose immune system responds by producing antibodies to specific sites, *epitopes*, on the antigen, resulting in a mixture of antibodies accumulating in the serum of the animal. Polyclonal antibodies have been generated against purified enzymes, peptides, and lipids, and many have gained acceptance as useful cell markers for cell culture and developmental studies (Table 1).

Monoclonal antibodies are produced by the hybridoma technique in which an antibody-secreting lymphocyte is fused with a myeloma cell to form a hybrid clonal cell line, secreting one monoclonal antibody that fits only a single epitope. Monoclonal antibodies have advantages and disadvantages over polyclonal antibodies. The most important advantage is that monoclonal antibodies can be generated against specific molecules present as a minor component of a complex impure mixture. The monoclonal antibodies can then be used to purify the antigen from the starting mixture. Because desirable hybridoma cell lines can be stored frozen and propagated indefinitely, monoclonal antibodies can provide potentially unlimited amounts of a standardized reagent. On the other hand, the absolute specificity toward one epitope may compromise their sensitivity and selectivity when compared to polyclonal antibodies. By recognizing several epitopes on a single antigen, polyclonal antibodies can bring more label to the target, increasing the sensitivity of detection. Furthermore, the occasional occurrence of a similar epitope on completely unrelated molecules reduces the selectivity of monoclonal antibodies.

Labeled nucleic acid probes represent another imaginative approach to help identify cell type. Specific nucleotide sequences can be labeled and used to detect corresponding mRNAs in cells in culture or *in situ*. In conjunction with immunocytochemistry, it is possible to analyze gene expression in relation to the cell's phenotype at the single-cell level.

General immunological markers used to identify each major cell type (Table 1) reflect the varying physiology of each cell type [9]. The difference in the protein composition of intermediate filaments among cells gave rise to the usefulness of the antibody to GFAP in the identification of astrocytes and of the antibody to one of the three neurofilament proteins to mark neurons. Embryonic cells of all classes have vimentin, which is retained only in adult radial glia, such as Müller cells in the retina and Bergmann glia in cerebellum. Because oligodendrocytes largely lack intermediate filaments, but produce abundant myelin, specific myelin-associated proteins and lipids provide numerous markers. Schwann cells placed in culture rapidly lose their myelin-associated markers. These cells were originally identified by the polyclonal antibody RAN-1, which is no longer available. Fortunately, the monoclonal antibody 217c has replaced it as a Schwann cell marker.

Functional or developmental specific subsets of neuronal populations require an array of appropriately restricted markers. Neurotransmitters, neurotransmitter-synthesizing enzymes, and neuropeptides have provided a great diversity of markers to identify specific neuronal subpopulations and to map neuronal networks. As more antibodies become available [1], multiple double-labeling immunohistochemical studies will enhance our ability to identify subpopulations of neurons and to determine developmental cell lineages. In addition, novel approaches using molecular biological techniques promise to increase the specificity of cell lineage analysis. One such method consists of using a retrovirus vector construct as a means of introducing foreign marker genes into cells at some specific stage of development.

DEVELOPMENT OF THE CENTRAL AND PERIPHERAL NERVOUS SYSTEMS

The nervous system originates from a rapid sequence of transformations of embryonic ectoderm

Genetic information contained in the single fertilized cell is capable of giving rise to the billions of neurons in the adult nervous system. Even though great diversity exists in the final neural design, due to variability in genetic and epigenetic influences, there exist basic transforming steps common to all vertebrates (Fig. 3). Early in embryogenesis, a sequence of transformations turns the zygote into a unilaminar sheet of ectoderm cells. A trilaminar embryo then appears that possesses the three primary "germ" layers: ectoderm, endoderm, and mesoderm. Neural ectoderm is then induced by interaction of the mesoderm with the overlying ectoderm. This region of ectoderm, the *neural plate*, is committed to develop into neural tissue, as can be demonstrated by transplantation experiments in which neural ectoderm placed in other parts of the embryo produce auxilliary neural tissue. In addition, local areas of the plate are predestined to develop into specific brain regions.

Migration of neural plate cells toward the midline and the acquisition of different shapes characterize the next major step (Fig. 4). The cells on the edge of the neural plate become narrower along their inner margin, whereas those more centrally located become narrower along their outer surfaces. As a result, the neural plate folds in to form the neural groove. The groove becomes deeper, and as the edges of the neural plate come in contact, the cells adhere to each other, and the groove "zips up" to form a tube of cells around a central fluid-filled space—the neural tube. As the tube closes, some cells on the margins of the plate migrate into the region between the surface ectoderm and the dorsal aspect of the neural tube to form the *neural crest*. Once the neural tube is formed, it is a pseudostratified epithelium undergoing proliferation. Increasing fluid pressure within the central canal leads to "ballooning" of the rostral end of the tube to form the three brain vesicles that define the major divisions of the brain: forebrain, midbrain, and hindbrain.

Neuroepithelium initially contains only one population of stem cells. These give rise to neuronal and glial stem cells from which originate all the types of neurons and glia (see Fig. 3). The neuronal stem cells continue to proliferate until some signal induces them to exit from the mitotic cycle. Once a cell becomes postmitotic it loses cytoplasmic contact with the ventricular surface and migrates away from it. This newly

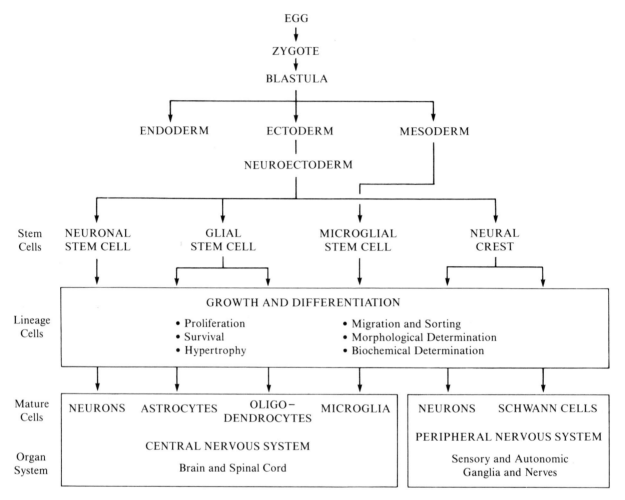

FIG. 3. Key developmental events leading to the mature nervous system. The fertilized egg goes through a series of transformations, leading to the formation of the trilaminar embryo, which possesses the primary germ layers: endoderm, ectoderm, and mesoderm. Except for the microglial lineage, the cells of the nervous system arise from the neuroectoderm. A number of events transform the neuroectoderm into the neural tube (not shown; see Fig. 4) and the neural crest, which structures then give rise to the neuronal and glial cells of the CNS and PNS, respectively. The large *central box* represents the periods of growth and differentiation of cells in the different lineages and lists the basic processes that interact to organize the individual and collective development of neurons. (Lineage pathways for astrocytes and oligodendrocytes are shown in Fig. 5 and for part of the neural crest in Fig. 7.)

formed layer of *mantle* cells continues to expand with incoming postmitotic neurons, and the progressive thickening of the walls of the neural tube become the future spinal cord and brain. A characteristic aspect of neurogenesis is that different subpopulations of neurons are generated in successive waves, with large neurons becoming postmitotic, i.e., "born," earlier than small neurons. Neuroepithelial cells give rise to the first neurons and glia at about the

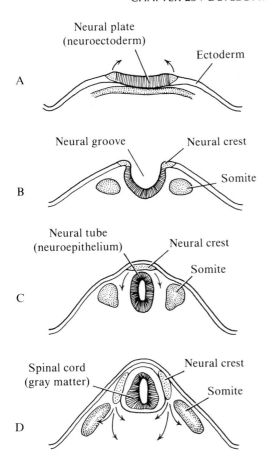

FIG. 4. Early embryonic development of the nervous system. The basic transformations of the neuroectoderm give rise to the cells that form the CNS and PNS. These cross-sectional views at the level of the future spinal cord illustrate some of the changes in the neuroectoderm (**A**) that lead to the formation of the neural groove (**B**) and neural tube (**C**), and the migration of neural crest cells (**C, D**). The somites forming in the mesoderm will become the vertebral column and segmental musculature. A migratory path of neural crest cell dorsal to the somites is not indicated. (See text for details.)

same time. Neuronal proliferation, however, ceases early in embryogenesis, whereas glial cells continue to divide, even into postnatal periods of development. The mechanisms controlling both the timing of birth and population size are not understood.

While all this change is occurring in the central nervous system (CNS), cells from the neural crest continue to proliferate even as they disperse by several migratory routes to form the melanocytes of the skin, endocrine cells, part of the muscles and bones of the face, and the sensory and autonomic ganglia of the peripheral nervous system (PNS) (see arrows in Fig. 4D).

Developmental decisions made by cells of each lineage are under the control of environmental factors

Lineages of glial cells (Fig. 5) are based on morphological and immunocytochemical studies [9]. In the neural tube, radial glial cells appear early and are morphologically easy to identify. Later in development, most radial glia detach their processes from the inner and outer surfaces of the neural tube wall to give rise to astrocytes. In the adult, radial glia (type III astrocytes; A2B5−, RAN-2−, VIM+) remain only in the retina and cerebellum.

A bipotential glial progenitor cell (Fig. 6; progenitor cell) has been identified in the rat optic nerve by Raff and his collaborators [10]. This cell (A2B5+) differentiates into either an oligodendrocyte (A2B5−, GC+), when placed in chemically defined medium, or a type II astrocyte (A2B5+, GFAP+), when placed in serum-containing medium. The progenitor cell is highly motile and migrates at embryonic day 16 into the optic nerve already populated with type I astrocytes. Up until postnatal day 7, the optic nerve contains only type I astrocytes, retinal ganglion cell axons, and the progenitor cells. After day 7, oligodendrocytes appear, and after day 15, two populations of astrocytes that differ morphologically, phenotypically, and developmentally are found in the optic nerve: type I astrocytes (A2B5−, RAN-2+), which are flat polygonal cells, and type II astrocytes (A2B5+, RAN-2−), which are process–bearing. Although type II astrocytes do not proliferate, type I astrocytes readily proliferate in culture in re-

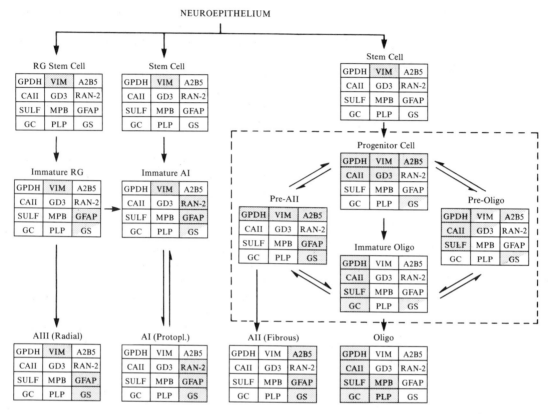

FIG. 5. Glial cell lineage pathways in the rat as defined by immunological markers. The neuroepithelium may contain a number of stem cells that are shown to pass through a series of specific developmental stages to become the four types of mature CNS macroglia: types I, II, and III astrocytes and mature oligodendrocytes. The lineage cell types are presently best identified by a series of 12 markers, which may be specific enzymes, structure support elements, or membrane components (see Table 1 for listing of markers and abbreviations). A specific pattern of these 12 markers distinguishes a given cell type: *stippling* indicates that the marker is present for a given cell type; *partial stippling* indicates that the marker is weakly expressed and not present in all cells of that type; *no stippling* indicates that the marker is not detected for the cell type. For simplicity, three stem cells are indicated, although they are presently indistinguishable using these markers. Note that types I and III astrocytes mature together and that the lineages for type II astrocytes and oligodendrocytes are intimately associated. For the latter cell types, a *large box* has been drawn around four of the precursor cell types to reinforce the current findings that these cells appear to reversibly cycle among the different stages depending on experimental conditions.

sponse to serum and most known mitogens. These observations have been extended to other areas of the brain. It is possible that this particular mode of gliogenesis may predominate throughout the developing CNS. Clearly, types I and II astrocytes diverge very early during development. For this reason, we have postu-

lated that they arise from two distinct populations of stem cells (see Fig. 5).

The oligodendrocyte lineage is marked by the sequential appearance of myelin-associated antigens allowing the distinction of three developmental stages (Fig. 5). The appearance of sulfatide and the decline of A2B5, VIM, and

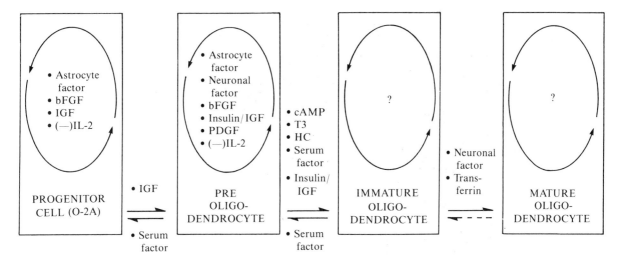

FIG. 6. Environmental factors influencing oligodendrocyte cell lineage. Mature oligodendrocytes originate from a stem cell that during development sequentially and transiently expresses a number of early cell phenotypes. Three specific developmental cell types have been identified based on immunological probes (see Fig. 5). Data suggest that none of these stages is irreversibly committed, since cells can shift back and forth between cell stages on the developmental trajectory by various environmental factors listed above and below the *arrows* located between the boxes. At least for the first two cell types, a cell stage-specific assortment of growth factors listed within the *large ovals* stimulate proliferation. It is interesting that only IL-2 inhibits proliferation. Thus, growth factors control cell proliferation as well as the sequence of cell differentiation.

GD3 define the preoligodendrocyte stage. Then, an immature oligodendrocyte type can be defined by the appearance of galactocerebroside and the complete loss of VIM, GD3, and A2B5. The mature oligodendrocyte expresses myelin basic protein and proteolipid protein and begins to make myelin membrane. Manipulations of the cell environment (Fig. 6) suggest that these developmental stages can be reversed by the presence or absence of certain signals [33].

A model of neural crest differentiation (Fig. 7) suggests that a small intensely fluorescent (SIF)-like precursor cell differentiates into each of the final neuronal phenotypes of the sympathoadrenal lineage depending on the timing and mixture of chemical signals in the environment. Hydrocortisone (HC), in a concentration-dependent manner, appears to induce these precursor cells to become either chromaffin or mature SIF cells. In cultures in the absence of HC, there is detected a neuron-like precursor

that can differentiate into sympathetic adrenergic neurons in the presence of NGF and further switch to cholinergic phenotype in the presence of adequate levels of cholinergic factor (CF). Additional molecular markers will help clarify the temporal sequence and environmental dependency of neural crest cell lineage [11].

DEVELOPMENTAL PROCESSES

Developing cells of the nervous system are embedded in complex fields of mechanical tension, biochemical diversity, and electrical current. These constantly changing patterns of spatial and temporal information for each cell are created in large part by the chemistry of the nerve cells themselves and are the major environmental forces that drive the sequence of developmental processes. The dynamic interaction between these environmental influences and the machinery of nerve cells force the cells

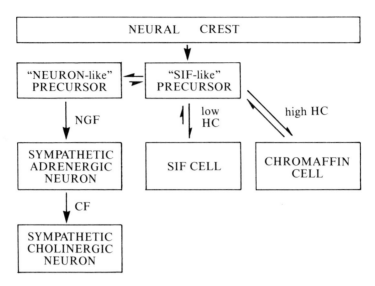

FIG. 7. Environmental factors influencing sympathoadrenal cell lineage. This schematic representation of neural crest differentiation indicates the importance of an early small, intensely fluorescent-like ("SIF-like") precursor cell in the generation of four mature neural crest cell types. Under conditions of high or low concentrations of hydrocortisone (HC), this precursor differentiates into chromaffin cells of the adrenal medulla or mature SIF cells of the sympathetic ganglia, respectively. In embryonic environments that supply NGF and little or no HC, a neuron-like precursor cell is thought to differentiate into an adrenergic phenotype. In turn, the presence of cholinergic factor (CF) switches transmitter phenotype to cholinergic. This model illustrates how regional and/or temporal differences in environmental factors can influence the final phenotypic assortment of neural crest cells.

to undergo considerable transformation during periods of growth and survival, migration and sorting, and morphological and biochemical differentiation.

Diffusible growth factors control the processes of proliferation and differentiation

Landmark events in the discipline of developmental neurochemistry include the discovery made in the early 1950s that developing chick nerve cells dramatically respond to a soluble tumor agent. Using an *in vitro* bioassay of sensory and sympathetic ganglia in proximity to fragments of mouse sarcoma, there was detected a soluble factor capable of inducing an extension of nerve fibers from each explant. The use of snake venom in the purification of the tumor factor revealed that snake venom was another, more potent source of nerve growth-promoting activity, mimicking the effects of mouse sarcoma extracts. Mouse submandibular salivary glands, the homolog of snake venom glands, were then screened using the *in vitro* bioassay and found to be an even more potent source of the factor. The salivary NGF was then identified and characterized as described below. Extensive *in vivo* and *in vitro* studies over the next 30 years elucidated a great deal about the chemical structure and the physiological mechanisms of actions of NGF. In 1986, Rita Levi-Montalcini and Stanley Cohen shared the Nobel Prize in Physiology and Medicine for their pioneering efforts in the discovery of NGF and in elucidating its role in development.

NGF [12] is isolated from male mouse salivary gland homogenates as a 131.5-kDa complex of three dissimilar subunits: α, β, and γ in a ratio of β:2α:2γ. The 44-kilodalton (kDa) β subunit appears to be the only neuroactive component of the three. The 26-kDa α subunit is closely related to γ and serine proteases but exhibits no proteolytic activity itself, and its function remains unknown. The γ subunit functions as an arginine peptidase, cleaving pro-β-NGF (307 amino acids) to the active β-NGF monomer of 118 amino acids. The standard Bocchini and Angeletti preparative method yields a smaller, 2.5S NGF dimer composed of two noncovalently linked β monomers. The amino acid sequence of this 26.5-kDa NGF molecule shares some homology with insulin and insulin-like growth factors. The NGF gene, which codes for the pro-β-NGF protein precursor, is highly conserved across species (human to chick).

NGF influences are thought to be initiated by the formation of NGF-receptor complexes on the cell surface and subsequent translocation of the complex into the cytoplasm. Responsive cells possess both high- and low-affinity receptors. Low-affinity receptors in the presence of NGF may cooperatively interact, cluster together, and be converted to high-affinity receptors as part of the biological response. In sympathetic nerve cells possessing axonal processes, NGF binds selectively to receptors at the axonal terminals, where it is internalized and transported along the axon to the cell body. A cascade of cytoplasmic and nuclear events occur within a temporal sequence ranging from seconds to days (Fig. 8). NGF treatment of PC12 cells, for example, leads to increased formation of cyclic AMP (cAMP) and hydrolysis of phosphoinositides, induction of Na^+ influx, and membrane ruffling. Within minutes there are changes in protein phosphorylation and increased expression of *transiently induced sequences* (TIS) of genes, such as the proto-oncogene *c-fos*. Intermediate events include increases in ornithine decarboxylase, choline acetyltransferase, and acetylcholinesterase activity; initial process outgrowth; and changes in

the levels of about 5 percent of cellular proteins. Late events are represented by extensive neurite outgrowth and the formation of functional synapses.

Physiological effects of NGF [12,14] can be classified as (a) an essential neurotrophic or nourishing influence during early development; (b) a potent influence on neuron differentiation; or (c) a strong neurotropic or guiding influence on direction of neurite growth. The main experimental strategy employed over the years to demonstrate the presence of the different activities of NGF has been to either block (via specific antibodies or drugs) or enhance (via addition of exogenous NGF) its actions.

Trophic effects on cell survival and development are evident in early "immunosympathectomy" experiments in which anti-NGF antibodies are added to cultures. In ganglia treated with both NGF and NGF antibodies, the normally luxurious halo-like nerve fiber outgrowth that occurs in the presence of NGF alone was prevented. When NGF antibodies were injected into neonatal mice, even more dramatic results were observed: Treated animals appeared normal and healthy but lacked nearly all sympathetic ganglia. Further support for a neurotrophic influence came from blocking experiments designed to study the effect of either chemical sympathectomy, resulting from the injection of axonal transport inhibitors, or surgical transection of ganglionic axons, to prevent the NGF internalized at nerve processes from reaching the cell bodies: Cells did not survive. In contrast, adding exogenous NGF *in vivo* or *in vitro* led to survival, with hypertrophy of target tissue and overcame many of the losses caused by blocking agents.

Differentiation of nerve cells is the second major activity of NGF. NGF can induce sympathetic neurons, chromaffin cells, basal forebrain cholinergic neurons, and PC12 cells to undergo biochemical and morphological differentiation. These changes include dramatic growth of neurites and changes in anabolic ac-

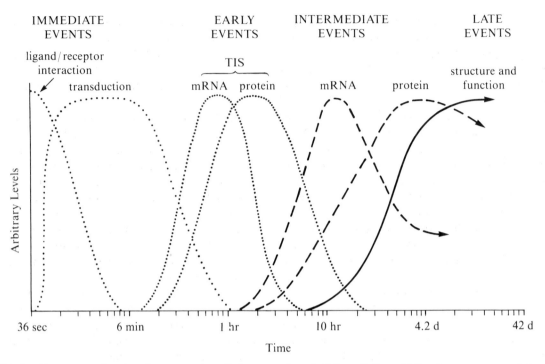

FIG. 8. Sequence of molecular events in cellular growth and differentiation. Following exposure of developing nerve cells to an agent, four major stages of the response are depicted. The pattern of physiological changes is graphed using a log time scale in order to cover the entire range of events stemming from immediate receptor-ligand interaction to long-term changes in cell structure and function. Transiently induced sequences (*TIS* genes) express distinct mRNAs whose levels rapidly and transiently increase following exposure of cells to a wide range of growth factors. The *TIS* genes may represent a subset of a larger family of early nuclear mechanisms by which growth factors control growth and differentiation. (From Arenander et al. [13].)

tivity and levels of neurotransmitter-synthesizing enzymes.

Tropic influences of NGF on cell process outgrowth are amply documented. *In vivo* and *in vitro* experiments have demonstrated that concentration gradients of NGF can function as an attractive guide for neurite outgrowth. In 1980, Campenot designed a simple yet elegant *in vitro* experiment to demonstrate the trophic and tropic effects of NGF in neural development. A three-chambered dish was constructed that allowed sympathetic neurons to grow in the central area separated by a grease barrier from lateral areas. The barrier prevented mixing of the media in different chambers but did not prevent cell processes from growing from the centrally located cell bodies into the lateral chambers. As a consequence, NGF added to a lateral chamber maintained neurites growing in these areas as well as the survival of centrally located parent cell bodies, presumably by retrograde transport of NGF. However, NGF added only to the central chamber permitted cells to survive and to grow neurites only within the confines of the central area; any preexisting neurites in the lateral chambers were retracted due to lack of local NGF. Thus, these experiments showed that the local concentration of NGF had a controlling influence on the maintenance of cell processes and that NGF could be retrogradely transported to support survival of the cell body lying some distance away in an environment lacking NGF.

Although these results are exciting, the neurite-promoting influence of NGF is not unique. In the past decade, the existence of many other such factors has been reported (Table 2), in particular, a family of closely related, small growth factors called fibroblast growth factors (FGF) derived from extracts of brain and pituitary [15].

FGFs were elusive until it was discovered that they shared high-affinity binding sites for heparin. Subsequent purification shows that the two molecules, acidic (aFGF) and basic (bFGF), had very different isoelectric points (pIs of 5.6 and 9.6) but were similar in mass (16 kDa) and shared a 55 percent amino acid sequence homology, well-conserved through evolution. Many studies have reported the existence of growth factors with trophic or tropic activities on neuronal and glial cells. Many of these factors are now recognized to be FGF. In addition to its possible influence during brain angiogenesis, FGF appears to have a number of other roles in development. It is proposed to act as a possible inducing factor during early embryonic transformations, as a survival and neurite-promoting agent for central neurons, and as a mitogen for astrocytes and oligodendrocytes. bFGF can increase levels of ornithine decarboxylase and process outgrowth and decrease protein phosphorylation in PC12 cells, actions similar to those reported for NGF. In fact, recent reports suggest that both FGFs may mimic all the short- and long-term influences of NGF on PC12 cells.

Epidermal growth factor (EGF) is another small but potent polypeptide mitogen (6 kDa, 53 amino acids) isolated originally by Cohen from male mouse salivary glands. EGF is a potent mitogen for many cells in culture, including astrocytes, and can also stimulate glial differentiation. Its effects are not limited to mitotic control. EGF can directly influence neuronal cell development. The survival and process outgrowth of cerebral neurons in culture, for example, are enhanced by EGF. In PC12 cells, EGF induces tyrosine phosphorylation, Na^+/H^+ exchange-mediated K^+ influx, membrane

TABLE 2. Growth factors affecting neural development

Growth factor	Molecular mass (kDa)	Target cells[a]	Tissue source
Brain growth factor	12	N	Brain
Cholinergic neuronotrophic factor	20	N	Eye, sciatic nerve
Epidermal growth factor	6	A, N	Submaxillary gland
Fibroblast growth factor (acidic)	16	A, N	Brain, retina, hypothalamus
Fibroblast growth factor (basic)	16	A, O, N	Brain, retina, pituitary, hypothalamus
Glial growth factor	31	A, S	Pituitary, caudate nucleus, neuroma
Insulin-like growth factor I	7	O, N	Liver, other cells
Insulin-like growth factor II	7		Fetal liver, fetal brain
Interleukin I (α, β)	16	A, O	Macrophages, astrocytes, microglia
Interleukin II	15	O	T cells
Nerve growth factor (βNGF)	26	N	Submaxillary gland, placenta
Neuroleukin	56	N	Submaxillary gland
Platelet-derived growth factor	32	A, O	Platelets, placenta, astrocytes

[a] (A) astrocytes; (N), neurons; (O), oligodendrocytes; (S), Schwann cells.

ruffling, and cell division. *In vivo* and *in vitro* studies demonstrate that EGF or EGF-like activity and its receptor can be found during embryonic development. EGF stimulates, for example, proliferation of neural crest cells and increases their release of hyaluronic acid and production of proteoglycans. These results suggest that EGF, by regulating the composition of the extracellular matrix and thereby influencing migration, may play a role in the morphogenesis of the neural crest.

Neuroactive factors, whether soluble or bound, seem to induce a variety of developmental processes depending on the cell type, stage of cell development, and environment [14]. A list of these factors can be found in Table 2. An example of the progress made to date in understanding and manipulating cell lineage is the growth factor control of oligodendrocyte development (Fig. 6). A number of factors have been reported to control the sequence of maturing cells in the oligodendrocyte lineage: Some can stimulate cells to either move forward or backward along a developmental trajectory; some can stimulate cells at a particular stage of development to enter the mitotic cycle.

Adhesion molecules also regulate proliferation and differentiation

A variety of substrate- and cell-attached factors can influence neural development by regulating adhesion properties of the cells. Interactions can occur directly between cells or between a cell and the *extracellular matrix* of the microenvironment. The molecules mediating these interactions have been implicated in regulating the specificity and timing of cell-cell adhesion. Hence they influence the ability of cells to migrate, sort themselves out, and to stabilize spatial relationships considered important for the process of differentiation [16,17]. These molecules have names such as cell adhe-

sion molecules (CAMs) and intercellular adhesion molecules (ICAMs).

Integrins are a family of structurally related cell surface glycoprotein complexes acting as receptors for a variety of cell and matrix adhesion molecules [18]. The integrin receptor is made up of noncovalently linked complexes of variable α and β subunits with large extracellular domains and small intercellular domains. These receptors may play a role in linking the cells' cytoskeleton and metabolism to the extracellular environment. There are also a number of intercellular adhesion molecules that may act as ligands for the various integrin receptors. The ICAMs, such as fibronectin and laminin, have been studied *in vivo* and *in vitro* and are considered to participate in many developmental processes, such as cell migration and neurite outgrowth. These molecules are part of the extracellular *basal lamina* surrounding the cells of the CNS and PNS. This lamina also contains collagen IV, polyanionic heparan sulfate proteoglycans, and entactin.

Laminin is the major noncollagenous component of the basal lamina and acts to link cell surfaces and the other matrix glycoproteins [19,20]. Each laminin molecule is composed of two similar but genetically and structurally different B chains, B_1 and B_2 (230 kDa), and a single large A chain (400 kDa). Several disulfide bonds hold the three subunits together in a cross-shaped design of about 900 kDa. Laminin also possesses a significant degree of glycosylation with complex oligosaccharides. The current model of laminin, derived from proteolytic digestion studies, amino acid, and DNA sequencing, suggests that it has multiple domains distributed among the helical and globular areas of its various arms. One proteolytic fragment, E8, a major lower part of the long arm, contains a sequence involved in promoting cell adhesion and spreading, neurite survival and outgrowth, and regulation of tyrosine hydroxylase activity. Antibody blocking experiments suggest that glia cells possess receptors for both E8 and another fragment, E4. These studies suggest that there may be a variety of laminin receptors on cells that are specific for different sites of the laminin molecule. Differential laminin binding by cells during development may thus contribute to the processes of cellular migration and intercellular sorting.

Fibronectin is another member of the ICAM family serving a variety of functions in the developing organism associated with intercellular and cell-matrix adhesion and cell mobility [21]. A single fibronectin molecule is composed of two polypeptide chains connected together by disulfide bonds at their C-terminal ends. The chains are very long (about 2,300 amino acids; 279 kDa), and either identical or similar chains can join together. Each chain possesses a complex linear arrangement of structural domains forming a number of functional domains with different biological properties. The diverse structure of fibronectin is known to arise from a combination of differential mRNA splicing and post-translational modification. Chain diversity probably alters fibronectin activity and its influence on cellular movement and intercellular aggregation and differentiation during neural development. Of special interest is the finding that a single tripeptide sequence (arg-gly-asp) represents a specific structural domain of fibronectin for cell binding. Thus, attachment of neurons and PC12 cells to fibronectin can be inhibited by a hexapeptide containing this cell-binding sequence. Two cell-binding domains on fibronectin appear to influence the adhesiveness and differentiation of human neuroblastoma cells. Domains also exist for binding with collagen, heparin, hyaluronic acid, and other matrix glycoproteins.

CAMs are another family of high-molecular-weight glycoproteins that possess morphoregulatory properties during neural development [16]. There are three well-characterized members of these cell surface glycoproteins.

Neural CAM (NCAM) [22] is the most thoroughly examined and is detected early in embryogenesis and throughout the development of the nervous system in both glia and neuronal cells. It is a cell surface glycoprotein mediating Ca^{2+}-independent homophilic binding and aggregation of neuronal cells. The liver CAM (LCAM) is a Ca^{2+}-dependent adhesion molecule important for epithelial intercellular binding. Neuronal-glial CAM (NgCAM) also displays Ca^{2+}-independent binding and is found only on neuronal cells and is probably involved in heterotypic binding between neuronal and neuroglial membranes.

NCAM may contribute to a variety of developmental processes, such as glial guidance of axonal processes, neurite fasciculation, axon-target cell interaction, and the creation and stabilization of cell position relationships. NCAMs are found in at least three different polypeptide forms. Whereas the extracellular domains appear to be identical in the three forms, the remaining C-terminal portions, however, vary greatly. The two large forms (180 and 140 kDa) span the cell membrane but have different intracellular lengths and presumably exert different influences on cell functions. The smallest form (120 kDa) does not have a plasma membrane-spanning region and is thought to be covalently linked to the outer membrane surface and/or is secreted into the extracellular environment. The large (682 amino acids) extracellular domains are antigenic and possess binding regions for both cellular and matrix elements. The conservation of the N-terminal extracellular sequences across the three classes of NCAMs and across vertebrate species suggests that all NCAMs can influence selective adhesion. Reported variations in NCAM activity may result from post-translational modifications. The extracellular domain has six possible sites of glycosylation and five pairs of cysteines, which may form secondary loop structures, similar to other putative mediators of cell adhesion, such as myelin-associated glycoproteins (MAGs). MAGs are considered to be responsible for glial-axonal interaction during myelination.

Sialylation during embryonic development is evident from the diffuse smearing between 170 and 250 kDa of the polypeptides during migration on sodium dodecylsulfate (SDS)-polyacrylamide gels. NCAMs were originally classified based on developmental correlations as either heavily sialylated, embryonic (E) form or lightly sialylated, adult (A) form. Since recent data suggest that the desialylated (A) form is also found during early embryogenesis; a nomenclature based on chemical characteristics may be more appropriate. Sialic acid content of the polypeptides range from less than 10 percent to 30 percent (wt/wt), hence the labels, NCAM-L (low) and NCAM-H (high), respectively. Discrepancies between amino acid sequence (predicting a 93-kDa polypeptide) and SDS-polyacrylamide gel analysis (yielding a desialylated 140-kDa form) suggest that significant post-translational modifications other than glycosylation occur.

In summary, interactions of cells with each other and with the extracellular matrix during development depend on the combined influence of several cell surface-ligand interactions. In the following sections, the major events of neural development are discussed in terms of the regulatory influences exerted by these neurochemical factors.

Cell proliferation and cell death during development determine the number and type of surviving neurons

A basic biologic tactic in creating complex systems is to generate an excess of elements and then, through a set of selective processes, determine which elements will participate in the final organizational pattern. This strategy is widely used in the construction of vertebrate nervous systems [23,24]. During development, the interaction between genetic and epigenetic forces is expressed as the balance between cell survival and cell death.

Invertebrate development depends a great deal on genetic instructions to control population size and diversity [1,17,25]. Perhaps because of the limited time available for development in a short life span and the relatively simple nervous system necessary to control the organism in a relatively constant ecological niche, the most reliable and economical approach is to depend on rapidly generated, simple, preprogrammed neuronal circuitry. The development of the nematode *C. elegans*, shown in studies pioneered by S. Brenner, is a prime example of cell lineage independent of environment. Precursor cells undergo cycles of stereotyped divisions, creating a restricted, preprogrammed cellular lineage. The little cell death that does occur appears to be due also to intrinsic instructions, which select specific pathways to terminate in senescence.

Vertebrate development represents the other extreme of the genetic/epigenetic continuum because of the numerous environmental cues used to direct cell activity, including the decision for survival, division, or death. Prolonged gestation and the plasticity inherent in allowing outside influences to guide developmental decisions permit the construction of large-scale highly interconnected circuitries.

Early experiments demonstrated that the presence and size of the target tissue are critical in determining the number and functions of the surviving nerve cells. Studies of early stages of limb bud development showed that removal of limb buds or transplantation of an extra limb bud resulted in predictable decreases or increases, respectively, of the innervating motor and sensory neurons. Each set of neuronal cells exhibits a characteristic degree of target-dependent cell death: some groups remaining quite stable in number while others lose up to two-thirds of the cell's progeny during development. What are the factors that influence the balance between cellular survival and death? One potential site of control over cell death is the nature of the cell microenvironment. Critical factors can also lie at a distance, at the level of the innervated target tissue. Research suggests that two features contribute to the regulation of cell death: (a) limited amounts of soluble factor(s) released by target cells, which leads to (b) competition among cells for the factor.

Cell death occurs at or shortly after the time of innervation of the target tissue in many cases. Innervating cells, by means of their axons, compete with each other for access to target factor(s) (Fig. 9). Neurons whose axons do not successfully compete for the limited amount of factor are unable to survive. This serves as a powerful selective mechanism capable of closely matching innervation requirements of corresponding neuronal and target populations, for example, motor neurons and muscle cells. In addition, this mechanism provides a powerful means of establishing the proper specificity of innervation in vertebrate systems, which exhibit considerable ambiguity and nonspecificity of innervation during early developmental stages. Thus, competitive mechanisms help shape not only the number of surviving cells and therefore the proper level of target innervation, but also select the proper cellular interconnections. An additional developmental mechanism for regulating the proper specificity and level of synaptic innervation is by a process referred to as pruning. This process determines the number of synaptic contacts each axon makes with its target, fine-tuning the interaction between source and target tissue needs [26,27] (Fig. 10).

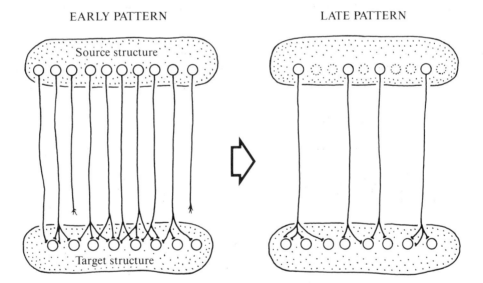

FIG. 9. Synaptic competition and cell death determine the extent and proper matching of synaptic relationships. Early in development, embryonic neurons schematically located in a source tissue (e.g., spinal cord) innervate a target tissue (e.g., muscle cells). A great number of synaptic elements influence the ability of source cells to compete successfully for sufficient amounts of a trophic factor produced by the target tissue in limited quantities. The result is the selective survival of source neurons. This process is responsible for matching the size of innervating source cell populations with the capacity of the target population. NGF and NGF-like molecules are examples of trophic factors released by target tissue. Note that late-arriving axonal processes may not compete successfully, thus controlling innervation specificity by eliminating mismatched cells. (After Cowan and O'Leary [26].)

NGF or NGF-like factors are released by innervated target cells [14]. Dependency on NGF during early embryonic periods is seen in the extent of survival and neurite outgrowth of sympathetic ganglia. NGF produced by target cells is taken up by specific synaptic or axonal terminal receptors and retrogradely transported to the cell body to support cell metabolism and developmental mechanisms. Interaction between soluble and bound factors is evident from laminin potentiation of NGF-enhanced neuronal survival.

Electrical activity is also important in determining neuronal survival. Toxin-induced blockage of electrical activity, for example, reduces the extent of naturally occurring cell death of spinal motor neurons *in vivo. In vitro* studies demonstrate that the effect of electrical activity blockade on neuronal survival can be modified by chemical factors found in conditioned media, such as vasoactive intestinal peptide (VIP). When these factors are added or removed, neuronal cell death is prevented or enhanced, respectively, during blockade of electrical activity. VIP may exert its effect in-directly by increasing glial production of a trophic factor that enhances neuronal survival.

At present, research has detected and characterized only a few of the many potentially active factors that impinge on the cell and its genetic blueprint to regulate survival, proliferation, and guidance along its developmental trajectory. Nevertheless, it is clear that during specific periods of early cell development, a factor, or factors, is necessary for it to survive and grow and enter the later stages of cell differentiation.

Migration of nerve cells is controlled by local concentration gradients of diffusible and bound neurochemical signals

Migration of cells plays a significant role in cytoarchitectural design. Neurons travel long distances through the complex extracellular terrain of the developing embryo to reach their final position. What mechanisms are used by neurons to move along the path, and what are the signals that are used to guide them? The most common

EARLY PATTERN   LATE PATTERN

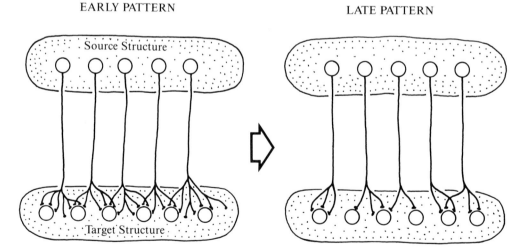

FIG. 10.   Process elimination alters the number of synaptic contacts made by each axon. The precision of synaptic innervation by source neurons (see Fig. 9) is increased by the "pruning" of synaptic contacts. (After Cowan and O'Leary [26].)

mechanism for cell translocation is a combination of (a) the extension of a cell process and its subsequent attachment to the substratum followed by (b) the pulling of the entire cell toward the point of attachment by means of contractile proteins associated with a cellular network of microfilaments.

Directional control of cell movement appears to be of two types: (a) cells moving along other "guide" cells arranged as a kind of scaffolding, and (b) cells moving across a multicellular terrain guided by a concentration gradient. Small molecules diffusing through the extracellular matrix may play a role in cell migration, but there is presently little supporting evidence. A dramatic example of the first mechanism is the sequential mass movements of young neurons from the inner proliferative or ventricular zone of the developing cerebral cortex to the outer cortical plate [28] (Fig. 11). In order to traverse these long distances, neurons migrate along a scaffolding comprising radially–oriented cell processes of cortical glial cells. These processes extend from the inner to the outer surface of the developing cerebral vesicle. Postmitotic neurons attach themselves to a nearby radial glial cell process and move along it away from the ventricular zone. Successive waves of neurons travel along the radial processes, following their lead process and moving at rates of 10 to 100 μm/day.

Molecular signals may permit neurons to distinguish radial glial processes from the other neuronal, glial, and endothelial surfaces that exist in the complex cerebral neuropil. Although the nature of these mediators is not clearly understood, one of the best candidates is NCAM [22]. During development, NCAM displays marked variation in its structure, and the sequence of expression of the various NCAMs suggests a role in cell migration and sorting out during morphogenesis and organogenesis. Chemical variants of NCAMs, for example, are closely correlated with developmental stages and with different areas of the developing nervous system. NCAMs can vary either in charge, determined primarily by polysialic acid content, or in polypeptide struc-

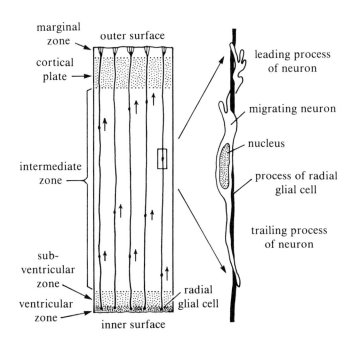

FIG. 11. The role of radial glial cells in the guidance of migrating cerebral neurons. **Left:** Postmitotic neurons migrate out of the ventricular zone by traveling along the radially oriented processes of glial cells that span the entire thickness of the neural tube wall. **Right:** An enlarged view of the neuronal/glial association illustrates a neuron cell body on a glial guide, extending a leading process in the direction of migration. (After Cowan [11].)

ture, determined primarily by the differences in the C-terminal intracellular domain. Although changes in the intracellular domain suggest differences in cellular transduction of homophilic binding, the changes in carbohydrate content and the possible consequences of varying sialylation are currently most easily interpreted.

The degree of surface charge on cells is directly correlated with ease of movement and inversely related to strength of adhesion of the cell and its processes. Such a relationship may exist *in vivo* and serve as a control over stability of cell-cell and cell-matrix interaction. For instance, periods of low sialic acid content (NCAM-L), observed during both very early embryonic transformation and late stages of neural differentiation, would enhance cell-cell adhesion and thus stabilize cell assemblies and minimize cell migration. In contrast, the increased expression of NCAM-H forms during the major portion of embryogenesis would create a state of increased charge repulsion and steric hindrance of possible homophilic binding. A condition of reduced intercellular adhesion may provide the necessary freedom for active morphogenetic movement. In fact, periods of high cell surface charge correlate with the major period of extensive cell migration and process outgrowth. Future studies will no doubt determine the molecules that confer specificity on the intercellular binding and the mechanisms by which the sequence of expression of the various NCAMs and other adhesion molecules is controlled.

A neuronal antigen, L1, with chemical and immunological properties similar to NgCAM, may mediate some aspect of neuronal migration in the cerebellum. In the development of the cerebellar cortex, postmitotic granule cells migrate along radially oriented Bergmann glial cells. L1 is never found on Bergmann glia in immunoelectron microscopic localization studies but is found on postmitotic, premigratory, and migratory granule cells, usually at points of interneuronal contact. In contrast, antibodies

raised to a mixture of all three NCAMs can be found localized during all phases of granule cell development at contact sites between Bergmann glia and the leading process and body of the granule cell. NCAM (180 kDa), however, is detected only late in development in the postmigratory phase, suggesting that large NCAM may, in cooperation with L1, contribute to the stabilization of cell contacts among postmigratory granule cells. Growth factors may also be important in these temporal relationships, since NGF can increase the expression of L1 but not NCAM on the cell surface during early PNS development. Thus, the temporal sequence of expression of several neural adhesion glycoproteins indicates that the control mechanisms of cell migration may rely on the coordinated interaction of multiple factors.

Neural crest cell migration is another well-studied model of molecular control of neural migration. The migration of the dorsal neuroepithelial cells [2] (see Fig. 4) into the spaces surrounding the neural tube depends on the nature of the extracellular matrix. In order to migrate over specific pathways, a number of signals must be regulated in a coordinated fashion both temporally and spatially. Unlike migration in the cortical systems, there are no glial cells to create highways for the crest cells. Instead, nearly all of the major components of the matrix, collagen, fibronectin, laminin, proteoglycans, and hyaluronic acid are involved in the regulation of the normal pattern of neural crest migration. Neural crest cell migration, for example, correlates with the appearance of high levels of hyaluronic acid. Hyaluronic acid produced by neural crest cells is considered to be important in the creation of space above the neural tube into which the cells migrate.

Migration also coincides with the distribution of fibronectin [16] (Fig. 12). *In vivo* and *in vitro* blocking studies using antibodies to fibronectin have demonstrated that the interaction of extracellular fibronectin and the neural crest cell surface is essential for migration. Note

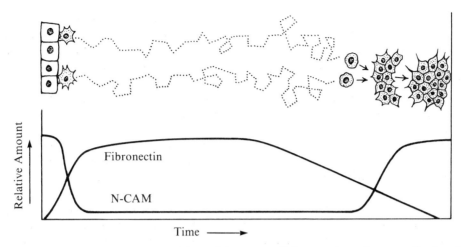

FIG. 12.   Correlation between the composition of the extracellular matrix and crest cell migration. **Upper:** During neural crest migration, cells detach from the neural tube (*left*) and individually move across the mesenchymal terrain in the developing embryo to join other cells at various final destinations and aggregate into autonomic and sensory ganglia (*right*). **Lower:** The rising and falling amounts of two components that help regulate crest cell movement are depicted. Note that periods of active cell movement are associated with high levels of fibronectin (and hyaluronic acid; see text) and low levels of NCAM, whereas stable cellular contacts during early and late phases of crest cell development are associated with high levels of NCAM. (After Edelman [16].)

that the temporal distribution of NCAM is observed to be inversely correlated with the amount of fibronectin. Laminin appears to be a preferred migratory substratum in experiments employing three-dimensional extracellular matrices. Addition of the small laminin cell-binding peptide of the B1 chain, but not the small fibronectin cell-binding peptide, completely inhibits the migration of crest cells from the neural tube. In addition, undersulfated chondroitin sulfate proteoglycans can restrict cell migration. Crest cells probably reach their final destination and cease migrating when the environment lacks fibronectin and hyaluronic acid, and the level of NCAM increases to stabilize intercellular contact (see Fig. 12). Growth factors can also modulate neural crest cell migration. Neural crest cells migrating out of explant cultures of neural tubes increase not only their rates of proliferation in the presence of EGF but also the release of hyaluronic acid and the production of proteoglycans. Together, these stud-

ies suggest that EGF may play a role in the morphogenesis of the neural crest by regulating both the number and state of differentiation of the cells, thereby controlling their migration by altering the composition of the extracellular matrix.

Control over cell process elongation and branching determines the cell's final morphological phenotype

One of the most important aspects of neural development is the laying down of the extensive network of intercellular contacts. On the average, each of the billions of nerve cells forms about 10,000 specific interconnections. This process of morphological differentiation requires the directed growth of a considerable number of cell processes to multiple specific targets, often at great distances from the cell body. It is likely that the various aspects of active elongation of a cell process creates the final size and geometry of the neuronal axon and dendritic tree [2,29]. What are the molecular mechanisms that control the progressive elongation of a cell process? What environmental signals are present to guide the processes through a complex, three-dimensional multicellular terrain? What mechanisms are used to determine the time and place of process branching? Are the molecules implicated in regulating cellular migration involved in controlling neurite outgrowth? This section examines some of the possible neurochemical cues and molecular mechanisms important to process elongation and branching. In general, many of the same soluble and matrix components that regulate cell proliferation, survival, and migration, as discussed above, have been shown to mediate process outgrowth *in vivo* and *in vitro*.

Growth cones are located at the leading edge of a neurite. When active they display motile structures called filopodia and lamellipodia. These delicate foot-like structures are important in pathfinding and outgrowth branching. Growth cone movement can be influenced by small diffusible molecules. Local concentration gradients of NGF, as described above, direct growth and movement. Specific neurotransmitters can alter neurite elongation and growth cone movements of neurons. Serotonin can inhibit neuronal outgrowth of specific subsets of neurons during development. Inhibition of neurite outgrowth can also be suppressed by electrical activity.

Adhesion molecules, either on the cell or in the extracellular matrix, may also play an important role in neurite outgrowth, since these molecules mediate neurite-neurite and neurite-glial interactions. The probability of outgrowth initiation, rate of elongation, and degree of branching of neurites are strongly influenced by the adhesive quality of the cells' substrata. Adhesion of growth cone structures may stabilize extensions. Growth cones may follow the path of greatest adhesiveness, leading to directional control over neurite outgrowth. Many

nonneuronal cells, e.g., heart and skeletal muscle cells and glial cells, condition their culture media and substrata with various basal laminae glycoproteins or with fibronectin, collagen IV, laminin, or heparan sulfate proteoglycan (HSPG). Neurite bioassays indicate that these matrix glycoproteins can increase neurite adhesion and outgrowth via a set of specific integrin adhesion protein receptors and may function *in vivo* as effectors of nerve fiber growth. Laminin and HSPG in the extracellular matrix can regulate neurite outgrowth [30]. Laminin induces extensive, highly branched neuronal processes. HSPG treatment of spinal cord neurons increases neurite elongation, whereas laminin-treated neurons display increased neurite branching. These effects could be blocked by specific anti-HSPG and antilaminin sera. Thus, we may speculate that laminin acts as a branch-promoting factor, inducing dendritic-like outgrowth, and HSPG may act as an elongation-promoting factor, inducing axon-like outgrowth.

Neuronal-glial interaction may also be involved in outgrowth. Sympathetic neurons grown in the absence of Schwann cells extend unbranched, axon-like neurites; in the presence of glial cells, however, process outgrowth is extensively branched and dendrite-like in form. In CNS preparations, this interaction is further characterized by the specificity of the astrocytic environment—glia from local homotopic regions give rise to branched neurites, and glia from heterotopic regions induce unbranched neurites. Although the actual chemistry of this interaction is not understood, it may be related to the composition of matrix glycoproteins or to regional differences in soluble factors.

Intracellular pathways are involved in the regulation of neurite outgrowth. cAMP and inositol phospholipids have been implicated as intracellular regulators, and work on the control of Ca^{2+} influx has proved to be successful in helping to establish a causal relationship with neurite outgrowth: Ca^{2+} influx can regulate both neurite elongation and growth cone movements [31]. Studies of invertebrate neurons and isolated growth cones suggest that in the presence of various agents that inhibit neurite outgrowth, e.g., serotonin and electrical activity, the level of free cytoplasmic Ca^{2+} is closely correlated with neurite outgrowth. Further support of Ca^{2+}-mediated control of neurite growth has been obtained from studies under conditions in which neurite outgrowth and Ca^{2+} influx could be directly manipulated. Data suggest that optimal levels of Ca^{2+} influx promote normal neurite elongation and movements of growth cones. Both of these activities are suppressed under either extremes of Ca^{2+} influx: high levels of Ca^{2+} influx stimulated by the Ca^{2+} ionophore A23187 and low levels of Ca^{2+} influx due to the presence of a Ca^{2+} channel blocker (La^{3+}). Moreover, these two components of neurite outgrowth are found to be differentially sensitive to intermediate ranges of Ca^{2+} influx. Under certain conditions, neurite elongation can occur in the absence of growth cone structures, a situation that enhances unbranched process geometry. Environment control over Ca^{2+} levels in different regions of the neurite may thus constitute a general mechanism of axonal morphogenesis.

In summary, a number of parameters of outgrowth initiation, elongation, branching, and cessation combine to generate axonal or dendritic geometry. These components can be modulated *in vitro* by a variety of soluble and substrate-bound factors, suggesting that *in vivo*, control over morphological differentiation is multifactorial.

Biochemical differentiation determines the neurotransmitter characteristics of the final neuronal phenotype

The path of differentiation that a cell follows is determined by epigenetic and genetic influences. A basic property of differentiated neuronal cells is the expression of neurotransmit-

ter. *In vivo* studies first demonstrated that the choice of neurotransmitter phenotype could be altered by the environment. Neural crest cells were studied because they give rise to a variety of cell types [11] (see Fig. 7), and their migration and final position can be followed by means of chimera transplantation. Two of the final neural crest cell phenotypes are sympathetic (mainly adrenergic) and parasympathetic (cholinergic) cells. Presumptive adrenergic neurons transferred to the presumptive cholinergic region of young embryos migrated along the path of vagal neural crest cells and became cholinergic instead of sympathetic. The nature of the environment could thus switch neurotransmitter phenotype. The inverse experiment also worked: Presumptive cholinergic cells become adrenergic when transferred to the adrenergic region.

Environmental factors are critical in determining neurotransmitter phenotype by altering existing cell properties and not by selecting different hypothetical subpopulations of neural crest cells. Over a period of several weeks, individual sympathetic neurons grown on heart-cell monolayers modify their biochemical, pharmacological, and electrical properties and shift from adrenergic to cholinergic phenotypes. Growing the neurons in heart-cell conditioned medium produces similar results, suggesting that nonneuronal cells, e.g., heart myoblasts or glial cells, release a soluble factor, now termed cholinergic factor (CF) (45 kDa). Since sympathetic ganglia cells normally grow *in vivo* in the presence of glial cells and become predominantly adrenergic, a second factor was sought in order to explain the discrepancy with the *in vitro* switch studies. Studies showed that physiological levels of hydrocortisone (HC) can modulate biochemical differentiation by blocking the shift from adrenergic to cholinergic phenotype. Data suggest that HC may act by inhibiting the synthesis and/or release of CF and thus decrease the amount of CF in the environment of developing sympathetic neurons.

Under these conditions, sympathetic neurons remain adrenergic, as *in vivo*. Electrical activity can also influence neurotransmitter phenotype *in vitro*. Cell depolarization appears to help overcome the effect of CF on adrenergic development. Manipulation of cell depolarization *in vivo*, however, fails to show this effect.

DEVELOPMENT AND PLASTICITY

The stability and complexity of neural tissue physiology that has developed by the postnatal stage provides a basis for later juvenile and adult stages of development, in which the dynamic interaction between the genes and the environment continues (see Fig. 1). Development is now less dramatic, observed predominantly in the structural and functional changes at the cellular and molecular levels. Environmental signals continue to produce lasting changes in neural structure and function in the adult nervous system. This genetic-epigenetic interaction leads to physiological and behavioral learning (see Chap. 48). External and internal events continue to regulate gene expression, and neuronal and glial cells continue to interact metabolically: In its broadest sense, development continues during adulthood. Neural plasticity can be defined as the long-lasting changes in neural structure and function following environmental perturbation (see Chap. 26). Thus the term is applicable to adult development. The molecular and cellular basis of adult neural plasticity has focused on environment-induced changes in neurotransmitter metabolism and synaptic structure and function. Two experimental models have proved to be most successful in delineating the neurochemical basis of plasticity: environmental control over catecholamine biosynthesis, and long-term potentiation.

Neurotransmitters serve to transduce electrical information from one cell to another, participating in the pattern of information flow in the nervous system. States of altered neurotransmitter metabolism can lead to changes in neuronal processing and physiological and behavioral control. Since the level of neurotransmitters in synaptic terminals is partly determined by the activity of rate-limiting synthesizing enzymes, which in turn depends on appropriate levels of mRNA transcription, environmental change can induce significant, long-lasting alterations in brain function by exerting transcriptional control over neurotransmitter-synthesizing enzymes [32,33] (see Fig. 8). Brief, excitatory perturbation of sympathetic neurons via electrical, pharmacological, or behavioral input can, for example, lead to long-term changes in the levels of colocalized neurotransmitters. These perturbing signals all lead to cell depolarization, which may be linked to the later events of enhanced transcriptional rates of tyrosine hydroxylase (TH), the rate-limiting enzyme in the synthesis of catecholamines and decreased transcriptional rates for the polypeptide precursor for substance P, a small putative peptide neurotransmitter colocalized with catecholamines. Thus, not only do neurotransmitter levels undergo long-lasting alterations following brief environmental stimulation, but neurotransmitters are differentially regulated by the same external stimuli.

CNS neurons show similar responsiveness, suggesting that the phenomenon is widespread and of fundamental importance in the development of adult function [35,36]. The locus coeruleus (LC) refers to a pair of small brainstem nuclei with extensive and diffuse axonal projections that are involved in controlling shifts in states of arousal, vigilance, and attention. *In vivo* and *in vitro* experiments demonstrate that a single, brief stimulation of the LC, leading to cell depolarization, results in increased amounts of mRNA and activity of TH. Increases in TH can still be observed for several weeks. It has been suggested that another, more subtle, consequence of environmental perturbation could be detected based on the extensive axonal domain of the LC. Since TH is synthesized in the cell body, the influence of induced levels of TH will be determined in part by the distance traversed by TH to reach the synaptic terminal and thus influence synaptic function. Because of the variable axonal path length and constant rate of axoplasmic flow (see Chap. 24), the initial environmental stimulation will result in maximal elevations of TH activity in the LC by 2 days; neurotransmitter activity, however, will peak in the cerebellum at 4 days and in the frontal cortex at 12 days. In this way, the genomic activation in a single location is expressed in an anatomically-dispersed temporal sequence. Thus, brief environmental stimulation of PNS and CNS neurons in the adult nervous system can lead to gene activation and long-lasting patterns of altered synaptic function. Another experimental model of neural plasticity, long-term potentiation (LTP) [34] is discussed further in Chap. 48.

In conclusion, throughout the life-span of an organism, environmental perturbation leads to alterations in neural structure and function. Therefore development can be viewed as a continual process of short- and long-term information storage whereby genetic and epigenetic interaction, at every step of development, becomes represented in the evolving structural and functional design of the nervous system.

ACKNOWLEDGMENTS

The authors thank Sharon Belkin and Maria Karras of the Mental Retardation Research Center Media Center for help in preparing the illustrations. The authors' research was supported by NIH Grant HD 06576, the Department of Energy contract DE-AC03-76-00012, and MIU Research Support Fund 011-705.

REFERENCES

1. Hunt, R. K. (ed.). *Neural Development, Pt. IV: Cellular and Molecular Differentiation.* New York: Academic Press, 1987. [Current Topics in Developmental Biology, Vol. 21.]

2. Purves, D., and Lichtman, J. W. *Principles of Neural Development.* Sunderland, MA: Sinauer Associates, 1985.

3. Arenander, A. T., and de Vellis, J. Frontiers of glial physiology. In R. Rosenberg (ed.), *The Clinical Neurosciences.* New York: Churchill Livingstone, 1983, pp. 53–91.

4. Fedoroff, S., and A. Vernadakis (eds.), *Astrocytes.* Orlando: Academic Press, 1987, Vol. 2.

5. Lauder, J., and McCarthy, K. Neuronal-glial interactions. In S. Fedoroff and A. Vernadakis, (eds.), *Astrocytes.* Orlando: Academic Press, 1987, Vol. 2., pp. 295–314.

6. Bottenstein, J., and G. Sato (eds.), *Cell Culture in the Neurosciences.* New York: Plenum Press, 1985.

7. Saneto, R. P., and de Vellis, J. Neuronal and glial cells: Cell culture of the central nervous system. In: A. J. Turner and H. S. Bachelard (eds.), *Neurochemistry—A Practical Approach.* Washington, DC: IRL Press, 1987, pp. 27–63.

8. Guroff, G. PC12 Cells as a model of neuronal differentiation. In J. Bottenstein and G. Sato (eds.), *Cell Culture in the Neurosciences.* New York: Plenum Press, 1985, pp. 245–272.

9. Raff, M. C., Fields, K. L., Hakomori, S.-I., Mirsky, R., Pruss, R. M., and Winter, J. Cell-type-specific markers for distinguishing and studying neurons and the major classes of glial cells in culture. *Brain Res.* 174:283–308, 1979.

10. Raff, M. C., Abney, E. R., and Miller, R. H. Two glial cell lineages diverge prenatally in rat optic nerve. *Dev. Biol.* 106:53–60, 1984.

11. Landis, S. C. Environmental influences on the development of sympathetic neurons. In J. Bottenstein and G. Sato (eds.), *Cell Culture in the Neurosciences.* New York: Plenum Press, 1985, pp. 169–192.

12. Yankner, B. A., and Shooter, E. M. The biology and mechanism of action of nerve growth factor. *Ann. Rev. Biochem.* 51:845–868, 1982.

13. Arenander, A. T., Lim, R., Varnum, B., Cole, R., Herschman, H. R., and de Vellis, J. Astrocyte response to growth factors and hormones: Early nuclear events. In P. Reirer, R. Bunge, and F. Seil (eds.), *Current Issues in Neural Regeneration Research.* New York: Alan R. Liss, 1988 (*in press*).

14. Thoenen, H., and Edgar, D. Neurotrophic factors. *Science* 229:238–242, 1985.

15. Gospodarowicz, D., Neufeld, G., and Schweigerer, L. Fibroblast growth factor: Structural and biological properties. *J. Cell. Physiol. Suppl.* 5:15–26, 1987.

16. Edelman, G. M. Cell adhesion molecules: A molecular basis for animal form. *Sci. Am.* 250:118–129, 1984.

17. Hay, E. D. (ed.). *Cell Biology of Extracellular Matrix.* New York: Plenum Press, 1982.

18. Hynes, R. Integrins: A family of cell surface receptors. *Cell* 48:549–554, 1987.

19. Davis, G. E., Varon, S., Engvall, E., and Manthorpe, M. Substratum-binding neurite-promoting factors: Relationships to laminin. *Trends Neurosci.* 8:528–532, 1985.

20. von der Mark, K., and Kuhl, U. Laminin and its receptor. *Biochem. Biophys. Acta* 8223:147–160, 1985.

21. Hynes, R. Molecular biology of fibronectin. *Ann. Rev. Cell Bio.* 1:67–90, 1985.

22. Cunningham, B. A., Hemperly, J. J., Murray, B. A., Prediger, E. A., Brackenbury, R., and Edelman, G. M. Neural cell adhesion molecule: Structure, immunoglobulin-like domains, cell surface modulation, and alternative RNA splicing. *Science* 236:799–806, 1987.

23. Berg, D. K. Cell death in neuronal development. Regulation by trophic factors. In N. C. Spitzer (ed.), *Neuronal Development.* New York: Plenum Press, 1982, pp. 297–331.

24. Cowan, W. M., Fawcett, J. W., O'Leary, D. D. M., and Stanfield, B. B. Regressive events in neurogenesis. *Science* 225:1258–1265, 1984.

25. Goodman, C. S., Bastiani, M. J., Doe, C. Q., du Lac, S., Helfand, S. L., et al. Cell recognition during neuronal development. *Science* 225:1271–1279, 1984.

26. Cowan, W. M., and O'Leary, D. D. M. Cell death and process elimination: The role of regressive phenomena in the development of the vertebrate nervous system. In K. J. Isselbacher (ed.), *Medicine, Science and Society.* New York: Wiley, 1984, pp. 643–668.

27. Cotman, C. W., and Nieto-Sampedro, M. Cell biology of synaptic plasticity. *Science* 225:1287–1293, 1984.

28. Cowan, W. M. The development of the brain. *Sci. Am.* 241:106–117, 1979.

29. Letourneau, P. C. Regulation of neuronal morphogenesis by cell-substratum adhesion. *Soc. Neurosci. Symp.* 2:67–81, 1977.

30. Ambriose-Hantaz, D., Vigny, M., and Koenig, J. Heparan sulfate proteoglycan and laminin mediate two different types of neurite outgrowth. *J. Neurosci.* 7:2293–2304, 1987.

31. Mattson, M. P., and Kater, S. Calcium regulation of neurite elongation and growth cone motility. *J. Neurosci.* 7:4034–4043, 1987.

32. Jonakait, G. M., and Black, I. B. Neurotransmitter phenotypic plasticity in the mammalian embryo. *Curr. Topics Dev. Biol.* 20:165–175, 1986.

33. Weingarten, D. P., Kumar, S., Bressler, J., and de Vellis, J. Regulation of differentiated properties of oligodendrocytes. In W. T. Norton (ed.), *Advances in Neurochemistry* New York: Plenum Press, 1984, pp. 299–338.

34. Teyler, T. J., and DiScenna, P. Long-term potentiation. *Ann. Rev. Neurosci.* 10:131–161, 1987.

35. Black, I. B., Adler, J. E., Dreyfus, C. F., Friedman, W. F., LaGamma, E. F., and Roach, A. H. Biochemistry of information storage in the nervous system. *Science* 236:1263–1268, 1987.

36. Black, E. B., Adler, J. E., Dreyfus, C. F., Jonakait, G. M., Katz, D. M., et al. Neurotransmitter plasticity at the molecular level. *Science* 225:1266–1279, 1984.

37. Manthorpe, M., Rudge, J. S., and Varon, S. Astroglial cell contributions to neuronal survival and neuritic growth. In S. Fedoroff and A. Vernadakis (eds.), *Astrocytes.* Orlando, FL: Academic Press, Vol. 2, pp. 315–376, 1987.

CHAPTER 26

Neural Plasticity and Regeneration

Carl W. Cotman and Kevin J. Anderson

Basic Neurochemistry: Molecular, Cellular, and Medical Aspects, 4th Ed., edited by G. J. Siegel et al. Raven Press, Ltd., New York, 1989.
Correspondence to Carl W. Cotman, Department of Psychobiology, University of California, Irvine, Irvine, California 92717.

POTENTIAL FOR REGENERATION IN BRAIN

For years, it had been assumed that the brain and spinal cord were "hard-wired," incapable of growth or repair processes. In the last several years, however, it has become clear that this is far from what can occur in the CNS—with the proper stimulus the brain has the capacity to regenerate its circuitry. The stimulus may be a perturbation, such as trauma or a metabolic insult, or it may be more subtle, such as learning a new task or behavior (see Chap. 48). The stimulus may also be a graft of neural tissue. We now know that central axons, previously thought incapable of regeneration, may grow through peripheral nerve or artificial "bridges" and form connections with denervated targets. In addition, whole neuronal networks can be replaced by transplanting embryonic or developing neurons into the adult brain.

In this chapter the major principles and advances in neural plasticity are reviewed and discussed. The study of plasticity in animal nervous system models, coupled with current methods has progressed to the point where it is realistic to examine the human CNS for neural plasticity-related events and to apply the lessons from these studies to clinical intervention. Indeed, work on neural transplants in animal models of disease has paved the way for clinical trials in the treatment of Parkinson's disease. One of the principal goals of research on synaptic plasticity and regeneration is to develop rational treatment strategies for disorders of the CNS.

Although this chapter is limited to mammalian nerve regeneration, there exists an extensive literature on nerve regeneration in avian and cold-blooded species as well as in invertebrates. Of particular note are the frog and the teleost—primarily the goldfish—visual systems, which have proven to be convenient experimental preparations. Unlike those of warm-blooded vertebrates, their central nervous systems regain full function after injury (see Chap. 48).

Axon sprouting and concurrent synapse turnover are ongoing plasticity processes in the mammalian CNS

Axon sprouting is defined as an outgrowth of processes from axons or terminals derived from undamaged neurons [1]; regeneration refers to the regrowth of damaged axons to their normal target. Axon sprouting is stimulated by injury in the mature and aged brain [1]. In several brain areas, however, sprouting and concurrent synapse turnover appear to be ongoing processes occurring in the absence of injury. Synapse turnover, or reactive synaptogenesis, refers to the loss and replacement of synapses that occurs in response to some stimulus that is not part of the normal developmental process.

These forms of synaptic plasticity may serve to mediate adaptive responses of the organism, and can be influenced by hormonal status, experience, and environmental changes as well as injury [2]. Axon sprouting can restore partially damaged circuits and can participate in functional recovery. In the peripheral nervous system, for example, collateral sprouting can restore function to partially denervated skeletal muscle until axons from damaged nerves eventually regenerate. In the CNS the situation is considerably more complex. Without experimental intervention, damaged projections usually fail to regenerate, resulting in the permanent loss of specific inputs. Most CNS targets receive inputs from a variety of sources, however, and sprouting from the remaining undamaged afferents often restores synaptic input to a denervated neuron. The functional significance of axon sprouting and synapse turnover in the CNS depends on the exact situation. If new connections are equivalent to those lost, or if they enhance the function of the remaining circuitry, then they might be functionally beneficial. Conversely, the formation of abnormal neuronal circuits may be functionally deleterious. Each case needs to be examined in its own context relative to the loss sustained. What general principles can be derived that elucidate the nature and significance of reactive synaptogenesis and axon sprouting?

REACTIVE SYNAPTOGENESIS

The response of the hippocampus to the unilateral removal of the entorhinal cortex provides an illustration of the general principles of reactive synaptogenesis

Fibers of the entorhinal cortex provide the major input to the dentate gyrus granule cells and terminate in the outer two-thirds of the dentate gyrus molecular layer (Fig. 1A). Following unilateral ablation of the entorhinal cortex, over 80 percent of the synapses in the outer molecular layer degenerate. Normal synapses disappear, and degenerative debris accumulates in

the denervated zone. New synapses begin to form within 2 to 4 days following the lesion, although clearance of degeneration products may take several weeks. The maximum rate of synapse replacement occurs between 10 and 30 days postlesion, and synaptic density is eventually restored to prelesion levels within a few weeks (Fig. 2).

The reactive fibers that participate in the reinnervation of the denervated zone have been described in detail [1,3]. Afferents from the ipsilateral and contralateral CA4 neurons (the commissural-associational [C/A] pathway) normally reside in the inner one-third of the dentate gyrus molecular layer. Following entorhinal lesion, these fibers sprout into the denervated zone, eventually occupying the inner one-half of the molecular layer. As these fibers sprout, their corresponding postsynaptic receptors also increase at locations of new fiber growth (Fig. 1B).

The cholinergic projection from the medial septum also sprouts in the denervated molec-

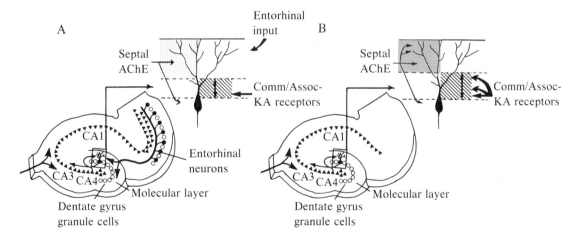

FIG. 1. Changes in the dentate gyrus molecular layer following a unilateral entorhinal lesion. **A:** Normal distribution of entorhinal input to the outer two-thirds of the molecular layer, commissural/associational (Comm/Assoc) inputs, and kainic acid (KA) receptors in the inner one-third of the molecular layer. Septal inputs, visualized with AChE histochemistry, occupy the outer molecular layer as well as a thin band of fibers in the supragranular zone. **B:** Following an entorhinal ablation, the septal afferents sprout, and AChE staining intensifies in the outer molecular layer. Commissural and associational afferents sprout and expand outward into the denervated zone. This is accompanied by an expansion of KA receptor distribution.

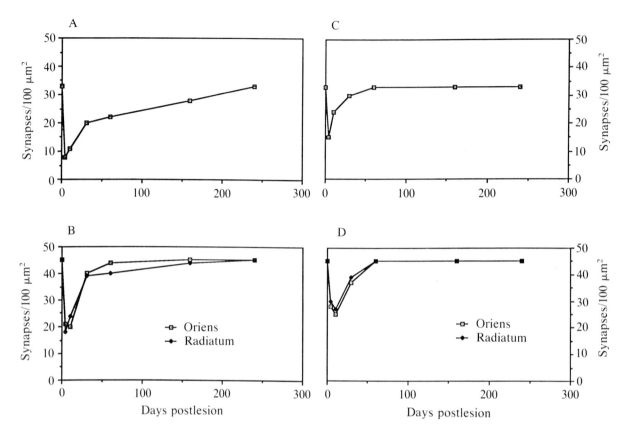

FIG. 2. Return of synaptic density in four lesion paradigms. **A:** Return of synapses following a unilateral entorhinal ablation. Synaptic density is restored by 120 days postlesion. **B:** Synaptic density in stratum oriens and radiatum following a commissural-associational lesion. **C:** Synaptic density in the dentate gyrus molecular layer following a commissural lesion. **D:** Synaptic density in stratum oriens and radiatum following a commissural lesion. Note that despite differences in the extent of initial synapse loss and the type of lesion involved, all regions are eventually repopulated so that synaptic density is restored to prelesion levels.

ular layer. These fibers normally reside in the outer molecular layer of the dentate gyrus and appear as a lightly staining fiber plexus in a section stained for acetylcholinesterase (AChE) activity (see Chap. 10). Following an entorhinal lesion, a dark, intensely staining AChE pattern is apparent, indicative of septal cholinergic sprouting. Direct biochemical measurements of AChE and choline acetyltransferase activity support the contention that septal input to the denervated molecular layer increases.

Fibers from the contralateral entorhinal cortex, normally sparse in the molecular layer, sprout extensively in the denervated zone after a unilateral lesion. These new synapses can drive the previously denervated dentate gyrus granule cells. Since the sprouted input from the contralateral cortex is essentially homologous to the lost entorhinal input, these sprouted fibers may thereby participate in the recovery of function following unilateral entorhinal ablation. A unilateral entorhinal lesion causes deficits in spontaneous or reinforced alternation tasks. The rate of behavioral recovery corresponds to the rate of sprouting by the contralateral fibers; a subsequent lesion of the sprouted pathway causes a loss of function that does not return.

It is surprising that fibers not in the primary denervated zone also reorganize in response to an entorhinal lesion. Synaptic density in the contralateral inner molecular layer as well as the ipsilateral hilus initially decreases, and the synapses are then gradually replaced over a period of 6 months. The synaptic changes take place in the absence of degenerating terminals within these zones. Thus, pronounced transneuronal changes may occur after major trauma to the CNS, suggesting that reactive synaptogenesis may adjust the functional integrity of complex circuit loops without a primary lesion. Further evidence to support this argument has been provided in other brain areas as well. In the hypothalamus, for example, synapse turnover elicited by hormonal changes does not appear to involve degeneration of old synapses; rather, they appear to withdraw or are engulfed by astroglia [4].

Aged animals retain the ability to replace damaged synapses

Reactive synaptogenesis may be most important in the aged brain where cumulative neuronal death occurs over the life span of the individual, and neurodegenerative diseases are most common. The brain of aged rodents demonstrates a remarkable capacity for sprouting and synaptogenesis [5].

In aged animals the reinnervation process is delayed, although it is eventually as complete as in younger animals (see Chap. 27). The diminished rate of synaptic replacement may be due to the rate at which degenerative debris is cleared from the neuropil. In aged rats there is a delay in the initiation of clearance of degenerative debris, although, once initiated, the process proceeds at the same rate as in younger

rats. Thus, the delay in the removal of debris may be related to the slower reinnervation response in the aged rats, which in turn may be related to their astrocytic hypertrophy and elevated corticosteroid levels. Recent evidence indicates that microglia also play an important role in the clearance of degenerative debris from the brain [6]. Their response to injury is inhibited by high levels of circulating corticosteroids, a result that supports a possible role for microglia in the response to brain injury during senescence.

Other brain areas demonstrate similar plastic responses following injury

Although the principles of reactive synaptogenesis have been most carefully defined in hippocampal formation, other regions of the CNS also have a remarkable capacity for synapse turnover after partial denervation [1]. The same basic rules that govern plasticity in the hippocampal formation also apply to areas such as the septal nuclei. If the fimbria-fornix or the medial forebrain bundle is transected, synapses lost by the medial septal neurons are replaced by heterotypic synapses from the remaining input. In the lateral septal nucleus, fimbria transection also causes reactive synaptogenesis; however, the lost input is preferentially replaced homotypically by fibers from the contralateral fimbria. With a bilateral fimbria transection, synapses are replaced in the septum by an unknown, presumably heterotypic, source of input.

CNS motor areas also demonstrate the principles of sprouting and reactive synaptogenesis. In the red nucleus, magnocellular neurons receive input from the ipsilateral motor cortex and the contralateral nucleus interpositus of the cerebellum (see Chap.42). The magnocellular neurons, in turn, project to spinal motor neurons. If the cerebellar input is interrupted, synaptic input to the magnocellular neurons is replaced by synapses from cortical afferents. Inputs from the cerebellum and motor cortex normally have distinct distributions along rubral neurons: Cerebellar afferents terminate on the soma and proximal dendrites; cortical afferents synapse on distal dendrites. Following lesion of the cerebellar-rubral pathway, both electrophysiological measurements as well as morphological observations demonstrate that the corticorubral afferents sprout to occupy the more proximal dendritic zone vacated by the damaged cerebellar afferents.

Synaptic rearrangements in the red nucleus can be induced in the absence of direct lesions, in response to cross-innervation of flexor and extensor nerves of the forelimb. Two to 6 months after cross-innervation of forelimb nerves, synaptic transmission is enhanced on red nucleus neurons, showing properties consistent with new synapses adjacent (proximal) to the soma. A similar effect is produced in response to the classical conditioning of elbow flexion in response to electrical stimulation of red nucleus neurons. The data suggest that cortical fibers innervating the distal dendrites of red nucleus cells sprout additional terminals that form synapses along regions of the dendrites more proximal to the cell bodies during the acquisition of learned responses.

These studies suggest that synaptic replacement elicited by lesions may share some of the same mechanisms as non-injury-induced synaptic turnover. It needs to be emphasized that these mechanisms occur naturally, and interventions that elicit regeneration take place against a background of reactive growth.

The general principles of reactive synaptogenesis have been derived from work on animal models

In summary, the hippocampus, in conjunction with other brain regions, displays a predisposition to organize or even repair its circuitry re-

gardless of the age of the animal. Based on this evidence, the following general principles can be stated:

1. Reinnervation proceeds until a normal, or near-normal, synaptic density is achieved in the denervated zone.
2. Aged animals also demonstrate lesion-induced neuronal growth, although the onset of reinnervation is delayed relative to young animals. The fact that aged animals can replace lost synaptic connections following a major ablation of afferent input suggests that aged animals can also replace synaptic connections due to a gradual loss of neurons over the animal's life span.
3. New synaptic connections are formed in response to a loss of synaptic input, and in most instances, a different circuitry is created when compared to the intact system; however, only those inputs already present on denervated neurons increase their abundance.
4. Homotypic input appears to have a preference in replacing lost synapses in several cases; for example, associational inputs selectively replace commissural inputs in the dentate gyrus and in area CA1. Homosynaptic reinnervation may compensate for lost synaptic terminals by an expansion of the remaining inputs. In these cases, circuit function per se may not be altered except for redundancy, which is decreased.
5. In the dentate gyrus, sprouting after entorhinal lesions is both homotypic and heterotypic. Heterotypic reinnervation in this case may also be compensatory, since the sprouted heterosynaptic input (C/A and septal inputs) can augment the residual (contralateral and/or ipsilateral entorhinal) pathways.
6. Reactive synaptogenesis may be the natural mechanism for restoring synaptic input after partial neuronal loss.

AXON SPROUTING AND REGENERATION

The hippocampus in Alzheimer's disease shows plasticity similar to that observed in the rodent brain after entorhinal lesion

Do the same rules derived from animal models apply to the human CNS? Research on animal models has progressed to the point where it is possible to predict what changes might occur in the human CNS following injury or insult.

A consistent feature of Alzheimer's disease is the severe cell loss in selected areas of the limbic system. Van Hoesen and colleagues have reported that Alzheimer's disease is accompanied by a selective loss of the layer II stellate cells of the entorhinal cortex as well as the pyramidal cells of the subiculum, producing a functional isolation of the hippocampal formation [7]. In essence, their findings suggest that Alzheimer's disease is characterized by a selective deafferentation of a brain region critical to memory storage and the major source of input to hippocampal formation (see also Chap. 43).

Does the cholinergic input to the human hippocampus sprout after loss of entorhinal neurons in Alzheimer's disease? One would not expect *a priori* that the Alzheimer's disease brain is incapable of sprouting because it is in a state of degeneration. On the contrary, AChE-positive fibers sprout in the hippocampus in Alzheimer's disease cases when the cholinergic input to the hippocampus is relatively intact (Fig. 3) [8]. As is evidenced in the rodent brain, AChE intensification is also seen in the outer molecular layer of the dentate gyrus, corresponding to the zone of perforant path deafferentation; however, in cases that exhibit AChE intensification, numerous AChE-positive senile plaques are also seen. It appears that sprouting may eventually contribute to senile plaque formation. C/A fibers also appear to sprout in the Alzheimer's disease brain in response to a pathologically induced neuronal loss, as evidenced by the expansion of kainic acid binding sites.

Generally, neuronal loss in the entorhinal cortex of Alzheimer's disease patients acts as a stimulus in a manner similar to that of entorhinal lesions in the rat brain. The selective loss of en-

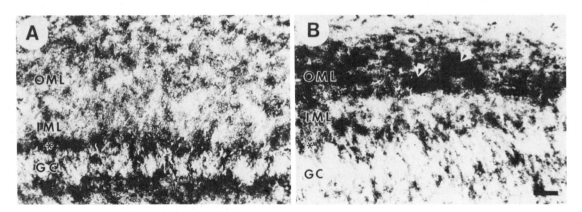

FIG. 3. AChE staining in the human hippocampal dentate gyrus. **A:** AChE staining from a control subject. Most AChE activity is seen in the regions adjacent to the granule cell layer (GC), e.g., the supragranular zone (*asterisk*). Less intense staining is seen in the outer (OML) and inner molecular layers (IML). **B:** AChE staining in the Alzheimer brain. Note the intensified AChE activity in the outer molecular layer and the presence of AChE-positive plaques (*arrowheads*); calibration bar, 25 μm.

torhinal neurons removes the perforant path input to the dentate gyrus, inducing a compensatory response from the adjacent C/A system and septal afferents. The observed expansion of a receptor field and the increase in the activity of a transmitter-metabolizing enzyme are in marked contrast to the numerous reports of reductions in transmitter-related parameters in Alzheimer's disease. Compensatory growth in the course of a degenerative disease indicates that the resultant circuitry cannot be simply considered a loss of neural elements.

In Alzheimer's disease brains, sprouting may constitute a natural compensatory mechanism. Cholinergic input facilitates hippocampal function by inhibition of a Ca^{2+}-independent K^+ current, producing an increase in excitability of hippocampal neurons [9]. Stimulation of cholinergic medial septal fibers *in vivo* when paired with commissural stimulation produces an augmentation of the non-cholinergic–evoked pyramidal field potential [10]. Stimulation of cholinergic medial septal fibers also produces an excitation of dentate granule cells [10a]. Thus, following entorhinal damage the resulting increase in cholinergic input may be beneficial with regard to hippocampal function. Also, since the association fibers form a recurrent loop to dentate granule cells, association sprouting may serve to amplify signals passing through this relay.

Axons retain the propensity to regenerate in adult animals

When CNS axons are severed, local connectivity may be reestablished by the growth of damaged cell processes or the extension of collateral sprouts from adjacent undamaged neurons. Whereas cut axons will regrow for long distances in the peripheral nervous system or in the CNS of fish and invertebrates, mammalian CNS axons rarely grow for more than a few millimeters through the injured area. The failure of CNS axons to grow for long distances was

attributed to the "inhospitable" CNS environment by Ramón y Cajal. In fact, it appears as though mammalian CNS axons have the ability to elongate for surprising distances when presented with the appropriate cellular milieu. The work of Aguayo and colleagues has demonstrated that severed central axons will grow for long distances when attached to a portion of peripheral nerve, suggesting that axon regeneration depends more on the nonneuronal environment of the growing fibers than on the origin of the parent cell bodies. Their observations have illustrated the influence of extrinsic conditions, such as growth factors and basal lamina, on the developing or regenerating axon.

The processes involved in CNS axon regeneration are best illustrated by recent work on the visual system [11]. Transection of the mammalian optic nerve results in the death of retinal ganglion cells and in the failure of the surviving cut axons to regenerate. When a cut optic nerve is sutured to a portion of autologous peripheral nerve, optic nerve axons will grow into the peripheral nerve graft (Fig. 4). As much as one-fifth of the surviving retinal ganglion neurons will grow axons into the graft. The regenerating fibers can grow for distances of up to 4 cm at the rate of 1 mm/day. Using electrophysiological techniques, it was demonstrated that the regenerated axons can respond to light in a manner similar to intact retinal ganglion cells, indicating that, functionally, the regenerated axons behave like native fibers. Illuminating the retina within discrete fields produces a discharge of ganglion cells that have regenerated into the graft. The onset or cessation of light is followed by changes in spontaneous electrical activity characteristic of normal retinal responses.

In addition to inducing a regenerative response in these neurons, the grafting of a peripheral nerve segment also exerts a neurotrophic effect on the axotomized retinal ganglion cells. Ganglion cell survival was greater in animals that had received a grafted

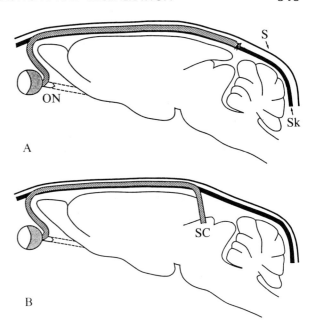

FIG. 4. Diagrams of adult rat brain in sagittal section showing peripheral nerve grafts (*cross-hatched*) used to replace the transected optic nerve (ON). **A:** One end of an autologous peroneal nerve graft was attached to the orbital stump of the ON transected close to the eye. The other end of the graft was ligated and left between the scalp (S) and the posterior part of the skull (Sk). **B:** Two to three months later, the distal end of the graft was reexposed and inserted into the superior colliculus (SC). (From Vidal-Sanz et al. [13].)

peripheral nerve, compared to nongrafted animals [12]. The source of the trophic activity is not known, but both short-term (2 weeks) and long-term (6 months) survival promotion occur, suggesting possible different trophic modes of action by the grafts.

Regenerating optic nerve axons will grow in the peripheral nerve graft for distances that often double the distance of the normal retinotectal projection. If the free end of a peripheral nerve graft to the optic nerve is placed in the superior colliculus of the host, the regenerated axons will arborize in the superior colliculus and penetrate it for distances of up to 500 μm [13]. Furthermore, the new axons will form synapses on neuronal elements within the superior colliculus.

NEURAL GRAFTS

Neural tissue transplants can partially restore damaged CNS circuitry

Axon regeneration experiments may provide the means of restoring point-to-point connectivity when specific pathways are interrupted. Are there measures to restore function when entire groups of neurons are lost? For example, Parkinson's disease and Huntington's disease involve two transmitter-specific groups of neurons (see Chap. 42). In Parkinson's disease, the dopaminergic neurons of the substantia nigra pars compacta die. This results in the loss of dopaminergic input to the striatum, resulting in motor abnormalities. In Huntington's disease, the cholinergic and, possibly, glutamatergic interneurons of the striatum are lost, also resulting in motor deficits. Do animal models of these disease states suggest rational therapeutic interventions?

Many of the most pressing questions concerning synaptic plasticity have been approached through the use of neural grafting techniques [14,15]. Fundamental problems that have been addressed by these techniques include survival properties of immature neurons with specific transmitter phenotypes, long distance growth of developing neurons within an adult host, guidance of axon growth to specific targets, and formation of specific synapses with host neurons. Reinnervation by transplant differs from reactive synaptogenesis in that new fibers entering a target region travel relatively long distances, whereas sprouting occurs only locally. Fiber outgrowth from CNS transplants has been shown to be extremely specific, both in the target, which it innervates, as well as in the fiber patterns and the synapses, which it ultimately forms [16].

The specific selectivity of transplant targets can be illustrated by two examples. Septal cholinergic neurons transplanted into the hippocampus, fimbrial cavity, or the entorhinal cortex will reproduce the normal pattern of cholinergic innervation to the hippocampus and entorhinal cortex following the removal of the native cholinergic inputs. Other adjacent areas that normally do not receive innervation from cholinergic fibers, for example, the inner molecular layer of the dentate gyrus, are not innervated by the transplant, even though these regions may be partially denervated during the transplantation process. Similarly, entorhinal cortex transplants selectively innervate specific regions of the host hippocampus and amygdala, the same areas to which the entorhinal cortex normally projects.

The pattern formed by transplant fibers on specific targets seems to be correlated to a degree with the transmitter phenotype of the innervating cells. Transplants of dopaminergic, noradrenergic, serotonergic, and cholinergic tissues into the hippocampus will each form a pattern of innervation that resembles the characteristic native innervation by each transmitter type. Furthermore, grafts of cholinergic neurons from the septum, habenula, or striatum into the hippocampus will each reproduce the native cholinergic fiber pattern in the hippocampus, although the propensity to innervate this target differs among the three graft types [17] (Fig. 5). Although septal grafts will densely innervate the hippocampus, habenular grafts show less robust innervation and striatal grafts

innervate only within 100 to 200 μm of the transplant-host interface.

The morphology of the synapses formed by transplanted neurons is also correlated to transmitter phenotype, at least to a first approximation. Transplanted serotonergic neurons form synapses with hippocampal targets that are characteristic of the normal serotonin innervation [18]. In particular, the ultrastructural features of serotonergic axons include the presence of large, nonsynaptic axonal dilations and a low proportion of synaptic terminals that are entirely asymmetrical. Septal, habenular, and striatal neurons form synapses with host targets that resemble the native types of cholinergic contacts [19]. Cholinergic fibers are devoid of axonal dilations, and the synapses are either symmetrical or asymmetrical in appearance. The reformation of synaptic connections by habenular and striatal transplants occurs despite the fact that the neurons are placed within an area of the brain that they normally would not innervate.

Transplant fibers innervate an adult brain against a competitive background of reactive synaptogenesis. Selective competition between host and transplant fibers has been demonstrated in several systems. For example, septal (cholinergic) transplants will reinnervate the hippocampus if the native cholinergic afferents are removed; however, the amount of reinnervation from grafts is limited if they are placed into intact hosts. Innervation is significantly impaired even when the target is massively deafferented by removal of other inputs. Similarly, entorhinal transplants fail to innervate the host hippocampus, even after denervation of the target by septal lesions, whereas the native entorhinal inputs remain intact. Thus, there appears to be competitive interaction between homologous transplant and host fibers.

Little is known about inputs from host to transplanted neurons. Grafted neurons receive synaptic input from local neurons, and cells within a graft probably innervate other graft

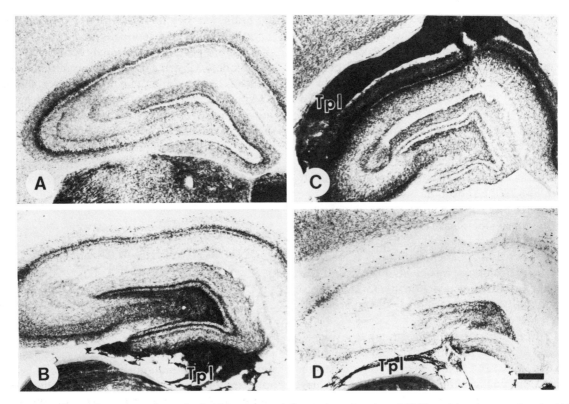

FIG. 5. Coronal sections through the hippocampal formation showing AChE-positive innervation in (**A**) unoperated control; (**B**) septal transplant; (**C**) habenular transplant; and (**D**) striatal transplant. Note that the staining intensity is greatest in areas adjacent to the transplant, and the laminar pattern of innervation produced is identical to the control subject [17]; (Tpl) transplant; calibration bar, 200 μm.

neurons. Entorhinal cortex transplants receive inputs from only three of the eight major projections that innervate the intact entorhinal cortex. It is interesting that none of these inputs are myelinated, suggesting that myelinated fibers may be associated with the difficulty in innervating transplants. However, entorhinal transplants will to a certain degree reform the perforant path to the dentate gyrus, a myelinated pathway. In addition, graft-derived cholinergic fibers have also been observed to be myelinated. Thus, when compared to the intact circuitry, transplants are incompletely integrated into injured networks.

Neural transplants can reverse behavioral deficits in animal models of human disease

Lesions of the ascending dopaminergic system have proven to be a useful model for Parkinson's disease [20]. Rats with unilateral 6-hydroxydopamine lesions of the substantia nigra exhibit stereotypic motor abnormality that results from loss of dopaminergic input to the ipsilateral striatum. Injections of apomorphine or amphetamine will cause rotational behavior away from or toward the side of the lesion, respectively. Transplants of fetal dopaminergic tissues into the CNS of adult rats ameliorate the sensorimotor asymmetries due to unilateral destruction of the nigrostriatal pathway [21]. Such grafts also reduce the severity of motor deficits associated with aging. In rats with unilateral lesions of the substantia nigra, transplants of fetal nigral tissue either within or adjacent to the denervated striatum will reduce apomorphine- and amphetamine-induced rotational behavior. Transplants of substantia nigra also reduce or eliminate other behavioral deficits associated with loss of the substantia nigra, including sensorimotor neglect and spontaneous locomotor asymmetry in a T maze. Functional recovery in this case appears to be related to transplant ability to increase dopaminergic input to the denervated striatum. Transplants placed into the lesioned substantia nigra do not promote behavioral recovery, since fibers will not grow the complete distance.

In a similar paradigm, septal transplants placed into the host hippocampus have been shown to improve spatial memory in animals in which the native cholinergic input to the hippocampus has been removed and in aged animals with spatial deficits [14]. As with dopaminergic transplants, the ability of septal transplants to restore function depends upon their ability to provide cholinergic innervation to the denervated areas of the host. These transplants do not reconstitute damaged circuits, but probably restore function by altering levels of cellular excitability and spontaneous activity within the denervated zones.

In the development of treatments for Parkinson's disease, and for any human application based on transplantation experiments, a major issue is the source of donor tissue. Ethical considerations as well as practical difficulties in obtaining human fetal brain tissue have led to the study of alternative sources of tissue. Adrenal chromaffin cells synthesize dopamine and will develop "neuron-like" characteristics when transplanted into the CNS; however, these cells show limited survival when transplanted into

the brain and they do not appear to reinnervate target neurons. The few cells that survive are sufficient to promote functional recovery in animal models. Grafting of autologous adrenal medulla has been attempted in human patients with Parkinson's disease, and these patients have shown improvement in their symptoms. With further advances in grafting methodology, application of these techniques to the treatment of Parkinson's disease and perhaps Huntington's disease remains a viable and attractive possibility.

NEUROTROPHIC AND GROWTH FACTORS

Functional recovery may be mediated by factors other than release of neurotransmitter

Does the return of function following a lesion require the reformation of point-to-point synaptic interactions? In many cases, behavioral improvement does not appear to require the precise reestablishment of specific circuitries. For example, following frontal cortical lesions, transplants of homologous cortex, purified astroglia, or Gelfoam from a lesion cavity can all increase the rate of recovery in a reinforced alternation task. In these cases, transplants probably provide some degree of trophic support to the injured brain, stabilizing the remaining neuronal circuitry.

The molecular basis of synaptic plasticity may involve specific trophic factors

In the developing, mature, and aged nervous system, the trophic support of neurons depends on a special class of growth factors, termed neurotrophic factors (see also Chap. 25). Some neurotrophic factors are specific to the nervous system, but others may interact with nonneural tissues. Neurotrophic factors are essential for the survival and growth of the brain's neurons. These molecules appear to be derived from the target cells of each neuron. Target cells nourish and sustain their input cells. Loss of axonal input or elimination of target cells during development deprives them of their trophic support, causing the remaining cells to become smaller and eventually degenerate.

It appears that injury to the CNS causes an increase in the activity of neurotrophic factors in injured parts of the CNS [3]. The increased amount of these factors may regulate sprouting and help maintain injured neurons. In the developing, mature, or aged rodent brain, injury causes an increase in the activity of these factors over time. After brain injury, extracts of both tissue and fluid around the injury show increased amounts of growth factor activity. In the tissue surrounding the wound, the maximal levels of trophic activity are successively higher in neonatal, adult, and aged animals. Neuro-

trophic activity is highest near the injury site and declines with distance. These injury-induced factors probably participate in axon and dendritic sprouting, in facilitating transplant survival, and even in saving cells from dying after their axons are cut [22].

Recently, it has been shown that delivery of an appropriate purified growth factor rescues damaged neurons from dying. If axons of the cholinergic neurons projecting to the hippocampus are cut, these neurons atrophy and die over a period of 1 to 2 weeks. Nerve growth factor (NGF) or fibroblast growth factor (FGF), however, prevents their degeneration [23,24] (Figs. 6 and 7). FGF can even be introduced several hours after injury to prevent neuronal loss and/or atrophy of cells, although the number saved declines with time after injury. In addition, FGF has been shown to prevent atrophy and degeneration of axotomized neurons in both the adult or aged brain. Growth-associated proteins

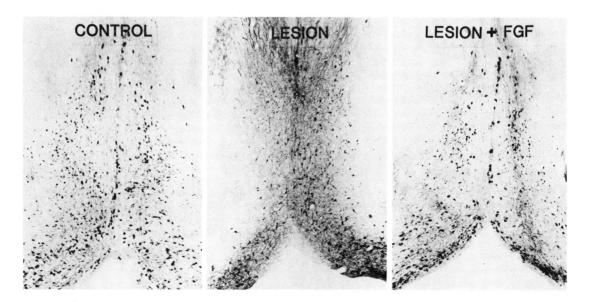

FIG. 6. Photomicrographs of AChE-stained neurons taken from a naive control animal (*control*), a lesion control subject (*lesion*), and a subject with a fimbria-fornix lesion that had received an infusion of FGF (*lesion + FGF*). All are shown 12 days after unilateral fimbria-fornix transection, and all are shown with the lesion side on the left. Note the prominent unilateral loss of neurons in the lesion subject. In the FGF-treated animals, neuronal death was prevented.

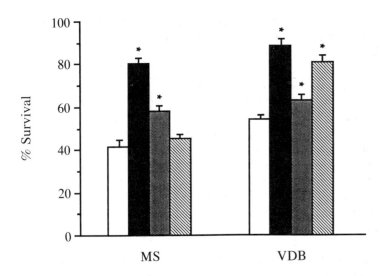

FIG. 7. Percent of cholinergic (AChE-positive) neurons in lesioned relative to unlesioned medial septum (MS) and vertical limb of the diagonal band (VDB) in FGF-treated and untreated (*control*) animals. In the FGF prelesion group, FGF administration began 2 days prior to transection of the fimbria-fornix. In FGF postlesion groups, FGF administration began 2 days after the lesion. All animals were sacrificed 12 days postlesion; *$p \leq$ 0.025 (Mann-Whitney). □, control; ■, FGF, prelesion (0.5 μg/ml); ▨, FGF, postlesion (0.5 μg/ml); ▨, FGF, postlesion (50 μg/ml).

(GAPs) (discussed in Chap. 24) may also turn out to have growth-promoting actions (see Chap. 48).

These data raise the prospect that specific growth factors may prove to be an appropriate therapeutic strategy for minimizing the effects of traumatic injury and perhaps even neuronal atrophy with age. The increase of growth factors after injury (see above) may act as a natural preventative mechanism to counteract degeneration. An adequate supply of growth factors may help minimize cell loss and pathology. This induction, however, requires several days to develop. Supplying factors earlier appears to improve their effectiveness. Recent data, in fact, suggest that NGF can improve the functional capacity of the normal aged brain when exogenously infused. Continuous infusion of NGF into aged, memory impaired rats, produces improvement in behavioral function in a spatial memory task [25]. Furthermore, cholinergic neurons in these rats were shown to be larger than in non-NGF-treated controls. It appears that NGF, by acting on the septal cholinergic system, can improve septohippocampal function much in the same manner as a septal transplant.

Work on growth factors is significant because it shows that damaged or even atrophied neurons can be rescued by pharmacological intervention. Although these factors work within the brain, they are large molecules that are prevented from entering the brain from the outside. Thus it is therefore not yet possible at this time to deliver them by oral or intravenous methods.

SUMMARY AND CONCLUSIONS

Research over the past decade has shown that the brain is highly plastic at the level of its circuitry. It is clear that central axons will sprout, and synapses turn over. It is also clear that by providing the proper stimulus, such as a piece of peripheral nerve or fetal transplant, mature neurons have the ability to regenerate. Given the proper environment—substrate and neurotrophic factors—the CNS has much more regeneration potential than was previously realized. The next major challenge is to translate findings from the cellular level to the molecular regulatory level.

REFERENCES

1. Cotman, C. W., Nieto-Sampedro, M., and Harris, E. W. Synapse replacement in the nervous system of adult vertebrates. *Physiol. Rev.* 61:684–784, 1981.
2. Cotman, C. W. (ed.). *Synaptic Plasticity*. New York: Guilford Press, 1985.
3. Cotman, C. W., and Nieto-Sampedro, M. Cell biology of synaptic plasticity. *Science* 225:1287–1293, 1984.
4. Hatton, G. I. In C. W. Cotman (ed.), *Synaptic Plasticity*. New York: Guilford Press, 1985, pp. 373–404.
5. Cotman, C. W., and Anderson, K. J. Synaptic plasticity and functional stabilization in the hippocampal formation: Possible role in Alzheimer's disease. *Adv. Neurol.* 47:313–336, 1988.
6. Vijayan, V. J., and Cotman, C. W. Hydrocortisone administration alters glial reaction to entorhinal lesion in the rat dentate gyrus. *Exp. Neurol.* 96:307–320, 1987.
7. Hyman, B. T., Van Hoesen, G. W., Damasio, A. R., and Barnes, C. L. Alzheimer's disease: Cell-specific pathology isolates the hippocampal formation. *Science* 225:1168–1170, 1984.
8. Geddes, J. W., Monaghan, D. T., Cotman, C. W., Lott, I. T., Kim, R. C., and Chui, H. C. Plasticity of hippocampal circuitry in Alzheimer's disease. *Science* 230:1179–1181, 1985.
9. Nicoll, R. A. The septo-hippocampal projection: A model cholinergic pathway. *Trends Neurosci.* 8:533–536, 1985.
10. Krnjević, K., and Ropert, N. Electrophysiological and pharmacological characteristics of facilitation of hippocampal population spikes by stimulation of the medial septum. *J. Neurosci.* 7:2165–2183, 1982.
10a. Wheal, H. V., and Miller, J. J. Pharmacological identification of acetylcholine and glutamate excitatory systems in the dentate gyrus of the rat. *Brain Res.* 182:145–155, 1980.
11. Aguayo, A. J., Vidal-Sanz, M., Villegas-Perex, M. P., Keirstead, S. A., Rasminsky, M., and Bray, G. M. Axonal regrowth and connectivity from neuron in the adult rat retina. In E. Agardh and B. Ehinger (eds.), *Retinal Signal Systems,*

Degeneration and Transplants. New York: Elsevier, 1986, pp. 257–270.
12. Villegas-Perex, M. P., Vidal-Sanz, M., Bray, G. M., and Aguayo, A. J. Influences of peripheral nerve grafts on the survival and regrowth of axotomized retinal ganglion cells in adult rats. *J. Neurosci. (in press)*.
13. Vidal-Sanz, M., Bray, G. M., Villegas-Perex, M. P., Thanos, S., and Aguayo, A. J. Axonal regeneration and synapse formation in the superior colliculus by retinal ganglion cells in the adult rat. *J. Neurosci.* 7:2894–2909, 1987.
14. Bjorklund, A., and Stenevi, U. Intracerebral neural implants: neuronal replacement and reconstruction of damaged circuitries. *Ann. Rev. Neurosci.* 7:279–308, 1984.
15. Gash, D. M., and Sladek, J. R. *Neural Transplants: Development and Function*. New York: Plenum Press, 1984.
16. Cotman, C. W., Gibbs, R. B., and Nieto-Sampedro, M. Synapse turnover in the central nervous system. In J.-P. Changeux and M. Konishi (eds.), *The Neural and Molecular Bases of Learning*. New York: Wiley, 1987, pp. 375–398.
17. Gibbs, R. B., Anderson, K. J., and Cotman, C. W. Factors affecting innervation in the CNS: Comparison of three cholinergic cell types transplanted to the hippocampus of the rat. *Brain Res.* 383:362–366, 1986.
18. Anderson, K. J., Holets, V. R., Mazur, P. C., Lasher, R. S., and Cotman, C. W. Immunocytochemical localization of serotonin in the rat dentate gyrus following raphe transplants. *Brain Res.* 369:21–28, 1986.
19. Anderson, K. J., Gibbs, R. B., and Cotman, C. W. Transmitter phenotype is a major determinant in the specificity of synapses formed by cholinergic neurons transplanted to the hippocampus. *Neurosci.* 25(1):19–25, 1988.
20. Freed, W. J., and Wyatt, R. J. Brain tissue transplantation in animal models of extrapyramidal motor dysfunction. In H. Y. Meltzer (ed.), *Psychopharmacology: Third Generation of Progress*. New York: Raven Press, 1987, pp. 471–479.
21. Bjorklund, A., Lindvall, O., Isacson, O., Brundin, P., Wictorin, K., Strecker, R. E., Clarke, D. J., and Dunnett, S. B. Mechanisms of action

of intracerebral neural implants: studies on nigral and striatal grafts to the lesioned striatum. *Trends Neurosci.* 10:509–516, 1987.

22. Nieto-Sampedro, M., and Cotman, C. W. In C. W. Cotman (ed.), *Synaptic Plasticity.* New York: Guilford Press, 1985, pp. 407–455.

23. Williams, L. R., Varon, S., Peterson, G. M., Wictorin, K., Fischer, W., Bjorklund, A., and Gage, F. H. Continuous infusion of nerve growth factor prevents basal forebrain neuronal death after fimbria fornix transection. *Proc. Natl. Acad. Sci. U.S.A.* 83:9231–9235, 1986.

24. Anderson, K. J., Dam, D., and Cotman, C. W. Basic fibroblast growth factor prevents death of cholinergic neurons *in vivo. Nature* 332:360–361, 1988.

25. Fischer, W., Wictorin, D., Bjorklund, A., Williams, L. R., Varon, S., and Gage, F. H. Amelioration of cholinergic neuron atrophy and spatial memory impairment in aged rats by nerve growth factor. *Nature* 329:65–68, 1987.

CHAPTER 27

Aging in the Nervous System

Carl W. Cotman and Christine Peterson

Basic Neurochemistry: Molecular, Cellular, and Medical Aspects, 4th Ed., edited by G. J. Siegel et al. Raven Press, Ltd., New York, 1989.
Correspondence to Carl W. Cotman, Department of Psychobiology, University of California, Irvine, California 92717.

Twenty-nine million Americans are 65 years of age or older. This represents approximately 11 percent of the total population (Fig. 1). Americans aged 85 and older are the fastest growing segment of the population, and this group, which is the most critical group in terms of health and social services, is expected to triple by the year 2020. These findings indicate that new emphasis must be placed on aging research to accommodate a growing aged population. In addition to the obvious human costs of aging, the elderly are also a financial concern, representing one-third of the nation's health costs. Fortunately, aging research is expanding, and progress is being made to elucidate the mechanisms that underlie the aging process.

HETEROGENEITY OF AGING PROCESSES

Most studies on aging emphasize age-related functional losses. Major deficits have been reported in such clinically relevant variables as hearing, vision, olfaction, glucose tolerance, immune response, endocrine function, sympathetic nervous system activity, learning, and memory. Losses are reported to occur in a number of central nervous system metabolic functions, which suggests that aging leads to a progressive decline in brain and body function.

Until recently, individual variability with respect to physiological or behavioral measures has been neglected. In nearly all aging studies, heterogeneity within the aged population increases. Some elderly subjects fall within the normal range for adult subjects, that is, they age successfully, whereas others show critical losses. Deviations may be due to illness or environmental factors rather than aging per se. In addition to variations in heredity, different lifestyles can either compromise or enhance vitality. Thus, heterogeneity may be an inherent characteristic of the aging process and its basis [1] provides new and exciting challenges for the neurochemist.

The characteristics of successful aging need to be defined. Functions that do not change may be just as important as those that do. Much of the recent neurochemical literature suggests that more functions and systems are maintained than might be predicted from the current dogma that aging is associated with an inevitable decline until death. Some individuals may show fewer deficits and/or possess better adaptive mechanisms in function that compensate for losses and preserve key functions. In this chapter, the issue of lost versus preserved function, at a cellular and molecular level, is examined. It is appropriate to start the discussion with a definition of aging.

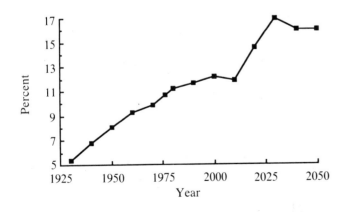

FIG. 1. Aged population as a percent of the total population. Values represent the number of elderly individuals (65 years of age or older) expressed as a percent of the total population. Source is the U.S. Bureau of the Census, *Current Population Reports*, series p-25, Nos. 311, 519, 614, 643, and 704. Data for years 1990 to 2060 are projections based on series II fertility assumption (2.1 children per woman; 400,000 net migration per year; slight mortality decline).

Aging is an irreversible process that begins at maturity and is characterized by increasing deviations from an ideal functional state

Aging is generally associated with an exponential rise in the presence of pathological changes; however, it is not a series of diseases whose cumulative effect leads to death. Increasing age causes predictable losses of certain biological functions. Proper biological function depends on a fine balance of neural and endocrine signals that sense internal and external environmental fluctuations and regulate cellular functions accordingly. The decline in adaptive or compensatory mechanisms with aging may predispose the individual to various diseases, compromise vitality, and shorten life span.

Aging research presents challenges beyond those of most disciplines in the neurosciences. Many changes in the central nervous system may not be primary to the aging process. Nerve cell degeneration, for example, can occur secondarily to deficits in the aging cardiovascular system. The critical challenge is then to design experiments that identify the primary versus secondary events. Another issue is to determine to what degree a deficit may occur before dynamic cell functions are compromised.

Neuron loss is not an inevitable consequence of aging, although it can occur

There are several noticeable gross changes in the aged human brain, such as a decline in brain volume and weight, enlargement of the ventricles, and narrowing of the gyri and sulci. It is surprising that the total number of neurons, neuronal density, and percentage of cell area in the cerebral cortex are unchanged with normal aging [2]. Large neurons appear to atrophy, with a consequent increase in the number of small neurons (Fig. 2A). After 55 years of age, there is a progressive increase in the number of atro-

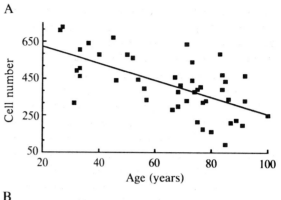

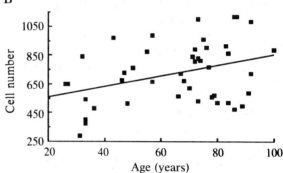

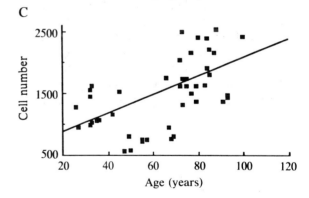

FIG. 2. Aging leads to alterations in neuronal and glial cell populations. Brains from a group of 51 individuals with normal cognitive function were used in this study. The brains were fixed and sectioned at 20 μm. After staining with cresyl violet, cortical cells were counted with a Quantimet 920. **A:** Large neurons (>90 μm) show a strong negative correlation with aging in all midfrontal, superior temporal, and inferior parietal areas of the neocortex. **B:** Small neurons (<90 μm but >40 μm) increase in number with advancing age. **C:** Glial cells (< 40 μm) increase with advancing age. (Data redrawn from Terry et al. [2].)

phied neurons, although there is wide variation within the population (Fig. 2B). The number of glial cells also increase with aging (Fig. 2C), reducing the neuron/glial cell ratio.

In contrast to cerebral cortex, the substantia nigra shows a progressive loss of dopaminergic neurons, beginning at approximately 30 years of age (Fig. 3) [3]. Thus, aging clearly does not affect all brain areas equally [4]. It should be noted that studies on neuronal density should be scrutinized closely, since earlier studies may not have used adequate volumetric methodologies, and some of the subjects may have had undetected diseases.

In aged rodents, there is surprisingly little evidence of major cell loss late in life. In the rat substantia nigra, cell loss is not as prominent as has been reported in man [5]. Cell loss is less than 20 percent, whereas in humans it can exceed 60 percent. Recent studies suggest that the nigral cell loss in humans may be related to environmental factors.

In the rodent hippocampus, neuronal loss does not exceed 20 percent, and synaptic density is also maintained. It appears that those specific subfields of the hippocampus (e.g., CA1 and CA3), which lose neurons during aging are also selectively vulnerable to metabolic encephalopathies, such as ischemia, hypoxia, and hypoglycemia. This suggests that selected neu-

rons are generally more susceptible to both aging and pathology. Theories of aging in the central nervous system should take into consideration such selective vulnerabilities.

Synaptic and dendritic plasticity may compensate for some cell loss in the aged brain

Some brain regions show very minor losses, whereas others show major losses. Despite these neuronal losses, however, the functional capacity of central nervous system circuits may be better preserved than might be predicted from cell loss alone. It has been suggested that the loss of neurons triggers the surviving cells to sprout and replace lost connections. This view is consistent with studies of reactive synaptogenesis in the injured aged brain [6]. In brain regions that show partial neuronal loss, dendritic arbors actually continue to grow between middle and old age (Fig. 4A) [7]. Thus, during aging, compensatory mechanisms of growth and remodeling, such as dendritic hypertrophy and synaptic growth, may be part of the lifelong program to maintain and adapt brain function. Only in very old age in humans does the dendritic tree appear to regress to that of mature younger adults (Fig. 4B and C).

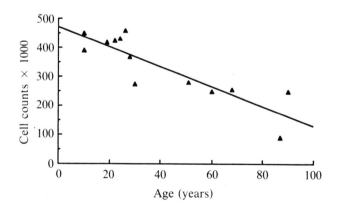

FIG. 3. Decreased cell number in the substantia nigra in humans as a function of age. The number of neurons in the substantia nigra is plotted against increasing age. (Data redrawn from McGeer et al. [3].)

A

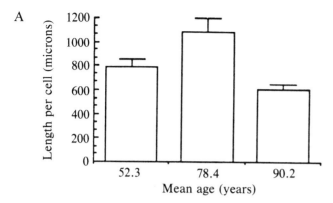

B

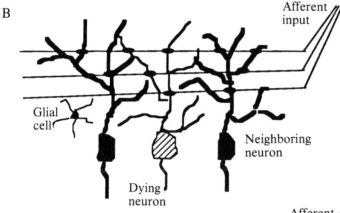

C

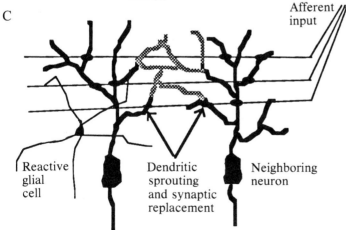

FIG. 4. Changes in granule cell dendritic length with increasing age. **A:** Total dendritic length per human dentate granule cell. The age-related changes are statistically significant. (Data are redrawn from Coleman and Flood [7].) **B:** Representation of reduced competition for an afferent supply consequent to the death of a neuron, which then leads to dendritic proliferation by surviving neurons. **C:** Surviving neurons increase their dendritic branching to fill in the areas vacated by the dead neuron. Astrocytes may increase their production of growth-promoting agents as they become reactive.

Synaptic transmission may show deficits in select parameters, but adaptive mechanisms may in some cases maintain function

In the aging brain it appears that much of the essential circuitry is present, and some of the functional losses may be compensated for by intrinsic mechanisms of synaptic plasticity. How then do these circuitries function at the level of the synapse? Studies on synaptic transmission may provide a focal point for neurochemical, electrophysiological, and behavioral studies.

In the central nervous system, acetylcholine is quantitatively a minor neurotransmitter; however, it is thought to play a key role in intellectual activity, including memory. Treatment of young subjects with scopolamine, an acetylcholine antagonist at the muscarinic receptor, produces memory deficits similar to those observed in elderly subjects. In the central nervous system, deficits in various cholinergic markers suggest a decline in cholinergic synaptic transmission. *In vivo* and *in vitro* acetylcholine synthesis, release, and choline uptake are depressed by aging despite no changes in either choline or acetylcholine content [8]. Acetylcholine metabolism is subject to rapid postmortem changes so that the most popular postmortem index of cholinergic neuron integrity is choline acetyltransferase activity. Reported age-related differences in choline acetyltransferase and acetylcholinesterase activities are inconsistent, although these enzymes markedly decline in Alzheimer's disease. With aging, muscarinic receptor number seems to decline, whereas receptor affinity is unaltered. The response of hippocampal pyramidal cells to iontophoretically applied acetylcholine decreases with age [9]. It would be expected that cholinergic transmission would be diminished, but direct electrophysiological evidence has not yet been reported. It is possible that various regulatory steps may compensate for loss of specific measures.

Pre- and postsynaptic dopamine metabolism are selectively altered by aging. Both the levels of dopamine and the number of midbrain dopamine-containing neurons decline (-50 percent) but not until very old age. This occurs even in the absence of neurological disease [5]. The density of dopamine D_2 receptors (autoreceptor for feedback inhibition of dopamine release) decreases (-40 percent), whereas D_1 receptors (the receptors linked to adenylate cyclase activity) are either increased (humans) or unchanged (rodents). The most consistent age-related decline is in striatal dopamine metabolism (e.g., content, synthesis, receptor binding). It has been suggested that the loss of D_2 receptors is related to reduced presynaptic input, whereas the D_1 receptor represents modest supersensitivity. Similar changes have been reported in rodents, although the losses are comparatively minor.

Norepinephrine shares several enzymes of synthesis and catabolism with dopamine. Thus, many of the age-related changes in the dopamine system also occur with norepinephrine. Depressed tyrosine hydroxylase activity decreases both norepinephrine and dopamine synthesis. The effect of age on serotonergic neurons has been studied less extensively than catecholamines, and the resulting reports are inconsistent. Relatively detailed studies on a number of neurotransmitter-related parameters have been performed on a variety of brain regions [4].

Neurochemical measures of transmitter-related parameters are limited in that they do not provide a direct index of function. It is possible that deficits in one or more aspects of neurotransmission may be compensated by changes in others. Studies on the function, structure, and chemistry of synaptic transmission at the neuromuscular junction serve as a useful model.

Synaptic transmission at the rat neuromuscular junction appears to be maintained over a wide range of stimulus conditions, perhaps through an adaptive integration of various aspects of cholinergic metabolism. Between 10 and 28 months of age, the average number of nerve terminals per end-plate increases by 34 percent (Fig. 5A). Resting acetylcholine efflux is greater in old rats (3.0 pmol/min) compared to young rats (2.0 pmol/min); this is probably related to the greater number of terminals. At rest, endogenous choline levels are unchanged; however, choline uptake is increased by +28 percent in aged rats.

Total acetylcholine release evoked by peripheral nerve stimulation (1–20 Hz) is similar in both young and old animals (Fig. 5B and C) [10], even though endogenous acetylcholine levels are reduced by −34 percent in aged rats. The lower acetylcholine concentrations appear to be due to enhanced leakage of acetylcholine from nerve terminals. To compensate for lower pools, choline incorporation into acetylcholine is faster in aged rats; that is, the time to half-maximal steady state is 2 min at 10 months of age, compared to 0.6 min by 28 months. There are no changes in choline acetyltransferase activity [10]. Thus, due to a series of integrated adaptations, neuromuscular synaptic transmission over a physiologically broad range of stimulus conditions can be retained with aging, although transmission does fatigue more readily at higher stimulation rates [11].

In the central nervous system, there are similar situations where adaptive mechanisms maintain synaptic transmission. Excitatory amino acids, such as glutamate, are the major neurotransmitters for excitatory pathways in the central nervous system. The role of excitatory amino acids in the aged brain is critical for normal function as well as for certain mechanisms of plasticity, such as long-term potentiation for which the *N*-methyl-D-aspartate (NMDA) receptor appears necessary (see Chap. 48). Moreover, long-term potentiation is maintained in aged rodent brain, even though binding to NMDA receptors declines [25].

In the aged brain, synaptic transmission actually appears to be enhanced in some pathways. The cortical input to the dentate gyrus in the aged rat appears to be potentiated even though there is modest cell loss within this circuit. It may be that increased transmitter release is due to additional terminals, enlargement of existing ones, more receptors, or other mechanisms. Part of the enhancement appears to be due to an increased electronic coupling between target cells, which makes it easier to fire more neurons to the same synaptic input [12].

Many issues remain unresolved in the study of synaptic transmission in the aged central nervous system. How much loss is needed before function is actually compromised? What pathways are most affected and which have preserved function? Partial neuronal loss may be compensated for by sprouting, adaptive increases in receptor number, or other mechanisms. Decreased transmitter release may be inconsequential during basal activity but may be inadequate during periods of peak activity. Since neurotransmitter systems act in concert it is possible that deficits in one transmitter may be compensated for by changes in another, but a decline in two interdependent transmitter systems may produce more than an additive decline. The current data suggest that age-related alterations need to be examined regionally, as well as according to cell type and transmitter system.

Calcium ion homeostasis in the aged nervous system may be a fundamental mechanism regulating age-related changes

The regulation of Ca^{2+} flux and its compartmentalization is essential to presynaptic (e.g., transmitter release) as well as postsynaptic events (e.g., excitability and second-messenger

A

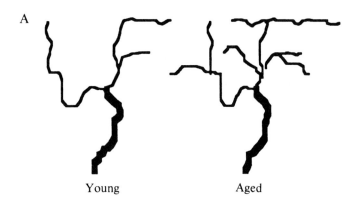

Young   Aged

B

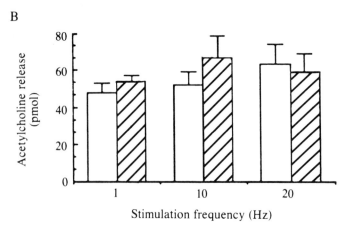

C

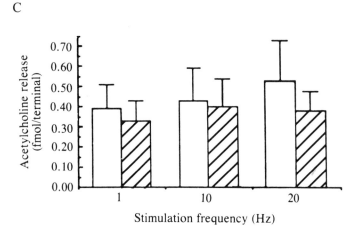

FIG. 5. Neuromuscular junction during aging. **A:** Neuromuscular junctions from a young and an aged rodent. Note the increased number of branches and longer terminals in the aged rodent. **B:** Total acetylcholine release. **C:** Acetylcholine released per nerve terminal. The values are the means ± SEM (Data are redrawn from Smith and Weiler [10].) Release of acetylcholine was evoked from a rat hemidiaphragm nerve preparation. The hemidiaphragm and phrenic nerve were isolated from the young (10 months of age) and old (28 months of age) male and female Fisher 344 rats. The stimulus (1, 10, or 20 Hz) was delivered for 15 min. □, 10 months; ▨, 28 months.

responses). Calcium ion homeostasis, in different brain compartments (e.g., pre- and post-synaptic) may respond differently to aging. Cytosolic free Ca^{2+}, which is the physiologically active pool of Ca^{2+}, is only 1/10,000th of total neuronal Ca^{2+}. Thus, alterations in the intracellular/extracellular Ca^{2+} ratio could produce deleterious changes in cell function. Alterations in Ca^{2+} homeostasis may influence a number of components that include, but are not restricted to, receptor mobility, the coupling of receptors with enzymes involved in phosphoinositide hydrolysis (see Chap. 16), the function of GTP-binding proteins, Ca^{2+} transport systems, Ca^{2+} binding proteins, and Ca^{2+}-activated proteases (for review see Gibson and Peterson [13]). For example, the brain contains an abundance of Ca^{2+}-activated proteases, such as calpain, which when either under- or overactivated can contribute to cellular damage. Calpain is present in high concentrations in selectively vulnerable neurons and also correlates with longevity [14]. In hippocampal brain slices from aged rats, repetitive stimulation appears to be associated with a prolonged Ca^{2+}-dependent K^+-mediated afterhyperpolarization [13]. These data indirectly suggest that in the aged rat, cytosolic free Ca^{2+} in hippocampal neurons is increased. Cytosolic free Ca^{2+}, however, has not been measured directly in the aged brain. In peripheral tissues, such as fibroblasts and lymphocytes, aging appears to decrease cytosolic free Ca^{2+} concentrations (Fig. 6) [15].

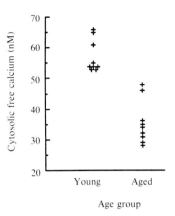

FIG. 6. Cytosolic free Ca^{2+} decreases with aging. Cultured skin fibroblasts from young (21 years) and aged (61 years) donors were used in these studies. Cytosolic free Ca^{2+} was determined with the Ca^{2+}-sensitive fluorescent dye Fura 2 in serum-deprived skin fibroblast from normal healthy individuals. The cells were examined at early passages to avoid complications due to *in vitro* aging. (Data from Peterson et al. [15].)

Brain energy metabolism may be preserved during aging in healthy individuals

Normal brain function depends critically on the ability of its neurons and glia to synthesize high-energy intermediates. Cerebral energy metabolism, such as cerebral blood flow, cerebral metabolic rate for oxygen, and cerebral metabolic rate for glucose, has been examined in animals and human subjects of various ages. In aged rats, which have only few age-related neuropathological changes, there are only slight declines in energy metabolism, and these changes are confined to sensory-related areas.

Positron emission tomography (PET) is a noninvasive technique that estimates local rates of glucose metabolism in humans. After [^{18}F]2-fluoro-2-deoxy-D-glucose is phosphorylated, it accumulates in the central nervous system in proportion to rates of glucose utilization (see Chaps. 29 and 44). Early PET scanning studies suggested that, with age, cerebral metabolic rate and cerebral blood flow were reduced either overall or in some brain regions at least; however, these changes may have been due to the inclusion in these studies of elderly subjects with various diseases. In a more detailed study [16], brain oxidative metabolism was measured in 40 healthy subjects (aged 21–83 years) selected for excellent cognitive ability and an absence of disease that could interfere with cerebral function. In 25 brain regions, brain oxidative metabolism does not change significantly with age when measured under conditions of reduced auditory and visual stimulation (Fig. 7). In elderly subjects, resting cerebral metabolism shows an increased coefficient of variation that implies heterogeneity in this population. No significant relationship could be found between resting cerebral metabolism and intelligence. There was no correlation between blood pressure and age in these subjects, although a significant positive correlation exists in the general population. These data underscore the importance of studying healthy subjects rather than using a representative sample of the general population. A decline in oxidative cerebral metabolism is thus not an inevitable consequence of aging.

Neuropathological examination reveals that aging is characterized by the appearance of abnormal protein structures

Structures called neuritic or senile plaques can accumulate with age in the neuropil in such brain regions as the frontal cortex or hippocampus. These plaques (~20–50 μm in diameter) consist of enlarged axonal and dendritic processes that appear to sprout and then degenerate. In many cases, the degenerating neurites surround a core of extracellular proteinaceous filaments called β-amyloid. Senile plaques are found in the brain of humans, primates, and several other species, such as dogs and polar bears, but not in rats. They accumulate with age and are present in even greater abundance in Alzheimer's disease (see Chap. 43).

Amyloid is an insoluble 4-kilodalton (kDa) protein with a high degree of a β pleated-sheet structure. The gene for the β-amyloid protein is on chromosome 21. Synthetic oligonucleotides based on the 4-kDa β-protein have been used to isolate the complementary deoxyribonucleic acid (cDNA) that encodes for the human β-amyloid protein. The amyloid gene is transcribed in the brain of humans and other species and, surprisingly, is also transcribed in almost all human tissues (e.g., kidney, heart, spleen, thymus, but not liver). Genetic mapping studies show that families with an inherited form of Alzheimer's disease have an abnormal gene that is located on chromosome 21. It appears that the amyloid gene is in the same region of the chromosome as the familial Alzheimer gene; however, it is unclear whether the amyloid gene or another closely associated gene product leads to Alzheimer's disease [17]. The β-amyloid protein is preferentially expressed in large pyramidal neurons of layers three and four of the prefrontal cortex and in CA1 hippocampal neurons that are

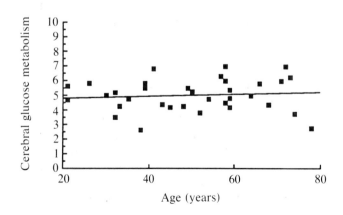

FIG. 7. Cerebral metabolic rate for glucose as a function of increasing age. Glucose utilization was measured by positron emission tomography with fluoro-2-deoxyglucose in carefully screened healthy individuals (aged 28–83 years). Values are expressed as the rate of glucose metabolized (mg) per 100 g tissue/min. (Data redrawn from Duara et al. [16].)

involved in degeneration in Alzheimer's disease. Apparently, some neuronal populations have a biochemical predilection for age-related pathologies, although not all neural groups with high amyloid levels are involved in the pathological accumulation of amyloid. The normal function of amyloid is unknown. β-Amyloid is derived from a large precursor protein that may have other functions. Isolation of a full-length cDNA indicates an open reading frame of 695 amino acids that contains the shorter β-amyloid protein of 42 amino acids near its carboxy terminus. There are some indications that amyloid is contained within a membrane receptor protein.

With advancing age, there is also an increase in intraneuronal inclusions known as neurofibrillary tangles. Ultrastructurally, neurofibrillary tangles are composed primarily of relatively insoluble proteins that assume a paired helical conformation. Although these structures are found in normal aged brain, they increase in number during the ninth and tenth decades of life. These structures are more commonly associated with the neuropathological diagnosis of Alzheimer's disease. Tangles are frequently located in the neuronal perikaryon and may enter the axon hillock or proximal dendrite. They are also found in axon terminals, where they contribute to the neuritic component of senile or neuritic plaques.

The role of senile plaques and neurofibrillary tangles in aging is unknown. The progressive accumulation of plaques and tangles associated with areas of specific neuron loss is diagnostic of a brain with Alzheimer's disease. Some have argued that Alzheimer's disease in fact is a form of accelerated aging, although this remains open to debate. (Further discussion is found in Chap. 43.)

Lipofuscin is an autofluorescent lipoidal pigment that is one of the most common features of aging in neurons. This product is considered to be formed from undegradable waste products that are derived from partially degraded membranes and other cell components [18]. Lipofuscin accumulates in the axon hillock, where it could interfere with the transport of materials within the axon. Certain neuronal groups within the motor system are especially prone to accumulate lipofuscin, including the larger pyramidal cells of the cerebral cortex, the anterior horn cells of the spinal cord, and the Purkinje cells. Lipofuscin accumulates as a linear function of age, but it does not appear to correlate with the presence or extent of dementia or with other clinical features of disease.

At a behavioral level, function in the elderly is either adequate, inadequate, or even improved, depending on the task and the individual

The proper integration of the brain's chemistry must ultimately be expressed as behavior. A detailed discussion of age-related changes in behavior is beyond the scope of this chapter (for discussion, see Rowe and Kahn [1]), but some general points should be emphasized. Elderly people perform well on tasks in which they can rely on well-established skills and knowledge. Word-finding difficulties are seldom observed in normal aging, and elderly subjects in fact perform certain tasks using verbal abilities better than young subjects. Elderly subjects do not perform as well as young individuals on timed tests of cognition and behavior; however, when given further time to respond, elderly subjects perform as well as young, which may also be due to lack of recent practice by the elderly subjects. After training, there is a substantial and retained improvement among individuals who were previously scored as cognitively impaired. In most studies there is variability within groups. Some elderly subjects show minimal or no cognitive losses when compared to younger counterparts.

Heterogeneity in learning ability has also been observed in rodent behavioral studies. For example, when aged (21–23 months) rats were tested for their ability to find a hidden underwater platform in a circular tank placed in a room with extramaze cues (e.g., windows, lamps), the older rats were much more variable in their performance than the young rats (Fig. 8) [19]. In animal studies, there have been various reports of age-related losses in behavior as well as no changes [9]. In behavioral studies of aging, it is essential that deficits in the animals' motivation, motor abilities, and sensory capacity not be misinterpreted for deficits in learning and memory. For example, visual or olfactory

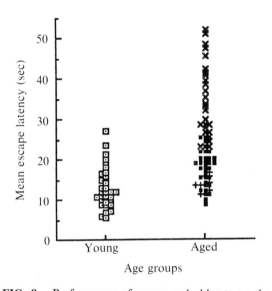

FIG. 8. Performance of young and old rats on the Morris water maze task. Nonbarrier-raised retired breeder female Sprague Dawley rats were used in these studies. Seventy-five old (21–23 months of age) and 31 young (3 months of age) rats were screened to select rats with impaired and nonimpaired performance. The water maze was a circular tank (140 cm diameter and 45 cm deep). The pool was located in the corner of a room filled with numerous extra maze cues that were available for the rats to use in locating the escape platform. The pool was filled to a depth of 30 cm, and water was made opaque by the addition of powdered milk. The aged animals showed a wider range of performance scores than those of younger animals. Some of the old rats performed as well as the young rats. □, Young; ■, aged; X, impaired aged; +, nonimpaired aged. (Data are redrawn from Gage and Bjorklund [19].)

impairments may be misinterpreted as learning difficulties in a task that requires searching for objects or food.

In general, theories of aging appear to have limited application to the central nervous system (for review, see Shock [20]. This can be illustrated by discussing three popular theories of aging. *In vitro*, many types of normal diploid cells, such as cultured fibroblasts, have a limited replicative life span, as in the Hayflick phenomena. How this theory applies to the brain is unclear, since neurons are postmitotic and glial cells divide infrequently. Another theory of aging suggests that free radicals generated in excessive amounts because of cellular reactions or environmental factors, such as ozone, radiation or drug administration, may damage cell membranes. The free radical theory of aging, however, does not explain why some brain cells are more vulnerable to influences of aging than others. Cells have a variety of mechanisms to protect the integrity of their deoxyribonucleic acid (DNA). Nevertheless, DNA damage can become fixed in the genome of a cell, either as a genetic mutation or chromosomal aberration. The DNA replication theory states that aging may result from a gradual accumulation of random errors with eventual functional and/or reproductive death of individual cells. The absence of a generally agreed-on set of age-related changes in nervous system function has made it difficult to evaluate specific theories for aging in the nervous system. These theories, however, may indirectly apply to brain, since the central nervous system interacts with and depends on various other systems in the body.

No specific factor leads to aging in the central nervous system, but a combination of deficits, imperfect compensatory mechanisms, and undetected disease may ultimately weaken function

The central nervous system detects signals both from the environment and from within the body and sends out signals that elicit proper responses. Unlike other tissues, brain cells operate in highly integrated networks. The total output must be meaningful, purposeful, and ultimately adaptive in response to an ever-changing environment. As described in the previous sections of this chapter, the nervous system can compensate for some losses that occur with age. When the contributions of disease or the compensations by mechanisms of plasticity are considered, few age-related changes are found to occur. Although the brain can compensate, at least partially, for some minor losses, less than perfect corrections may lead to computational errors and may predispose the system to further deficits.

Some deficits, either alone or in combination, make the system more vulnerable to further insult. With age there is an increased incidence of pathology. In many age-related disorders it appears that pathological characteristics of disease are present in normal aging, but to a much lesser degree. For example, the neuropathological changes that occur in Alzheimer's disease differ quantitatively but not qualitatively from normal aging: hence, it is reasonable to assume that there are some subtle neurochemical deficits that are ultimately followed by distinct pathology. It is not known, however, whether individuals that age successfully escape most pathology.

Thus, aging of the brain may result from a cumulative set of insults that ultimately lead to critical functional losses. Such losses may become particularly important when they are compounded. According to this notion, highly adaptive or plastic systems will be particularly susceptible to age-related losses. It is possible to illustrate how deficits can cause loss of function by examining the role of the hippocampus in learning and related functions.

As previously discussed, cholinergic function is partially reduced with normal aging and is even more extensive in Alzheimer's disease. Aged rodents have deficits in learning the Morris water maze (see previous section). One weak link in hippocampal function, which leads to learning difficulties, might be a loss of cholinergic function. If so, restoring cholinergic function should reverse the deficits. To test this hypothesis, fetal cholinergic neurons were transplanted into the hippocampus of aged rats [19]. Performance by behaviorally impaired aged rats that received cholinergic transplants was significantly better than pretransplant rodents. This suggests that the original learning deficit was not due to a global "aging mechanism" but, rather, a specific loss in a particular brain area and neurotransmitter system.

The precise mechanisms for the age-related decline in cholinergic function is unknown; however, trophic factors may be important. Trophic factors play a key role in development and cell death. Thus, they may be fundamental for the maintenance and repair of the injured or aged brain. The finding that axonal and dendritic sprouting occurs with age suggests that trophic mechanisms are operational, at least to a degree, since regenerative growth occurs until very old age. Cholinergic neurons appear to depend on nerve growth factor (NGF) for their trophic support. NGF levels and receptors may decline by as much as 50 percent with aging, which may underscore the potential role for such factors by making select systems more vulnerable in old age.

Cholinergic neurons also participate in neuritic plaque formation, which may further reduce function. The initial formation of plaque may be part of the sprouting response to compensate for cell loss [21]. Axon sprouts from cholinergic neurons appear to grow into a plaque as it develops. Neuritic plaques may originate from an abnormal sprouting reaction due to a local accumulation of neurotrophic molecules and generation of substrates that promote growth. Thus, sprouting, which can potentially rebuild and strengthen partially damaged circuits, may eventually contribute to age-related pathology. Amyloid accumulation may also be produced as a product of aberrant regeneration. β-Amyloid mRNA levels are very high in hippocampal fields in which sprouting is robust and plaque formation most abundant.

In the hippocampus, not only is cholinergic function decreased with aging, but some intrinsic cell groups also appear to be lost. Cell loss may not be due to aging per se but perhaps to interaction with the environment. It has been shown that prolonged (e.g., 3 months) exposure to glucocorticoid produces a loss of specific hippocampal neurons (e.g., area CA3), which have high concentrations of glucocorticoid receptors. In addition, within the population of the remaining cells, there are shifts in cell size so that there are more small neurons (Fig. 9). Rats treated chronically with glucocorticoids show shifts in CA3 neuron size similar to those observed in aged rats [22].

Loss of some CA3 neurons produces more damage when individuals are subjected to further stress. Circulating glucocorticoids feed back to the hippocampus to inhibit further steroid release from the adrenal gland. After hippocampal injury, steroid release is greater, since the hippocampal feedback inhibition is reduced; this causes more damage due to increased steroid levels. Glucocorticoids can also retard axonal sprouting, so compensation is further reduced. These data suggest that an age-related loss of CA3 neurons could be due to cumulative exposure to corticosterone, perhaps exacerbated by stress-related events. Thus, environmental factors may interact with the aging process in an autodestructive cascade.

Small losses may be more critical when they occur in highly overadapted systems. Ultimately, too many corrective mechanisms may cause more massive losses. Cholinergic deficits alone may be insufficient to reduce behavior, but in combination with cell loss they may lead to decreases that are greater than each individually. In the hippocampus, cholinergic synaptic transmission enhances the action of excitatory pathways. Thus, loss of intrinsic excitatory neurons, plus the mechanisms that augment their firing, may compromise the fine tuning of adaptive responses necessary for higher function.

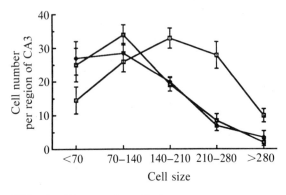

FIG. 9. Changes in cell size populations during chronic glucocorticoid treatment and normal aging. The chronic group represents rats (8 months old) that were treated for 3 months with glucocorticoids (5 mg/day). The aged group were male Fisher 344 rats aged 28 months. The outlines of all the cells that contained nuclei were traced, and the cell area was then determined by a computer program. The areas of the cells in the first 200 μm of the CA3 region, after the CA2-CA3 border, were calculated. Values are the mean ± SEM; $n = 3$ per experimental group. □, Control; •, chronic; ■, aged. (Data replotted from Sapolsky et al. [22].)

MODELS FOR THE STUDY OF AGING

Although some factors may decrease life span, other environmental influences may prolong it

Caloric restriction has been the most consistent method of extending life span in the laboratory animal. In the B6 mouse strain a reduction in body weight of 8 g leads to an increase in life span of approximately 6 months (Fig. 10) [23]. Reduced food intake can retard age-related changes in kidney function, fat metabolism, and muscle mass and decrease the incidence of spontaneously produced tumors. Dietary restriction also reduces brain serotonin levels, prevents age-related losses in striatal dopamine

A

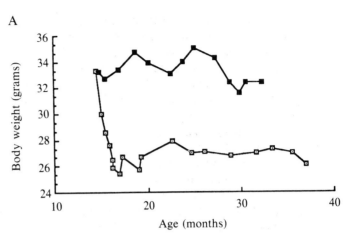

FIG. 10. Dietary food restriction prolongs survival. Mice were maintained on a diet of restricted foot intake, without malnutrition, starting at 12 months of age. **A:** Body weight of B6 mice fed *ad libitum* or a restricted diet. Mature B6 mice on the restricted diet stabilized at approximately 25 g after 2 months of underfeeding. Weights are plotted as the means for all mice alive at the indicated ages. **B:** Survival of B6 mice. Each point in the survival curve represents one mouse. Mean survival was 24.9 ± 0.9 months for all of the B6 mice fed *ad libitum*, as opposed to 29.9 ± 1.4 months for the B6 mice fed a restricted diet. Mean survival for the longest lived 10 percent of each B6 group (*n* = 3) was 31.5 ± 0.5 months for *ad libitum* and 38.2 ± 1.4 for the restricted diet groups, respectively. □, Restricted; ■, *ad libitum*. (Data are redrawn from Weindruch and Walford [23].)

B

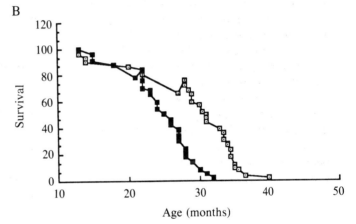

receptors, and improves maze learning performance in aged rats. Although the precise mechanism(s) for the effect of dietary restriction on extending life span remains to be discerned, it is interesting to note that reduced food intake leads to atrophy of the pituitary gland and diminished levels of pituitary hormones.

Aging studies require that careful attention be given to the subject selection and use of models

As discussed in this chapter, the conclusions that are drawn depend markedly on subject se-

lection. It is clear that literature on aging research can be quite contradictory and confusing in its own right. Heterogeneity may be an inherent factor in aging studies; however, it may also result from problems in experimental design. All aging studies generally make assumptions about methods, subjects, and the aging process that need to be considered when interpreting the literature and designing experiments. Differences in these parameters among laboratories can often alter the conclusions. Currently, the rate of aging is expressed chronologically, although this is recognized as a relatively weak marker of physiological age, since many individuals age at different biological rates. How old is old? Rodent strains most commonly used for aging studies live for over 2 years and have a maximum life span of approximately 30 months (Table 1) [24]. A rat 25 to 30 months old would be considered aged. Many investigators even disagree on when development ends and aging begins: A rat is not mature until approximately 3 months.

Rodents raised in a standard vivarium may be exposed to various diseases. In order to circumvent the potential problems associated with disease, the National Institute on Aging maintains a colony of aged rodents reared in germ-free environments. These animals are referred to as barrier raised. When rodents are reared in home colonies, information should be provided as to the breeding conditions used to produce the stocks, the health of the colony, the diseases to which they have been exposed, and the expected life span of the strain. Some aged-rat strains need to be studied with caution. For example, aged Sprague Dawley rats have spontaneously produced pituitary tumors and become obese with aging. Fischer 344 rats have been used more extensively; however, they are prone to testicular tumor formation. The use of

a single inbred strain does provide some "genetic control," although the results may not be generalizable to the species as a whole. Furthermore, single-strain studies do not adequately assess potential genotypic contributions to age-related alterations.

Autopsy tissue provides an approach to study the aged human brain

The study of the aged human central nervous system is an exciting and expanding area of research made feasible by the increased availability of autopsy tissues. Brain tissues from normal aged and subjects with age-related disease are routinely collected by various "brain banks." Detailed clinical data that describe the conditions just prior to death are essential. For example, a premortem condition known as the agonal state should be noted, since some patients that die in an agonal state suffer from respiratory or other problems that result in brain anoxia immediately prior to death. Some enzymes, transmitters, receptors, and high-abundance mRNA are surprisingly stable after death, so autopsy tissues can provide useful and important information; however, many dynamic cell processes, such as Ca^{2+} homeostasis, cannot be measured with postmortem tissue. The study of more accessible peripheral tissues like cultured fibroblasts and lymphocytes may help determine the general mechanisms that underlie the age-related alterations in the central nervous system as well.

TABLE 1. Commonly used rodent strains for aged animal studies

Rodent strain	Maximum life span[a]	
	Male	Female
A/HeJ mice	18.6	15.3
Balb/c mice	24.4	23.3
CBA/CA mice	27.1	24.4
C57B1/6 mice	25.6	25.6
DBA/2 mice	23.5	21.9
Fischer 344 rats	29.5[b]	

[a] Values are expressed in months. These rodents are commercially available through Charles Rivers Breeding Laboratories, which is under contract to the National Institute on Aging. Male and female rodents are virgins. (For review, see Abbey [24].)
[b] Rats housed one per cage have a mean life span of 22.7 months; however, when housed three per cage, life span increases to 28.5 months.

CONCLUSION

The process of aging in the central nervous system is an interaction of age-related losses, disease, and compensatory mechanisms that work to offset functional declines. Although most studies emphasize age-related losses, many properties of specific systems are preserved—

synaptic transmission in select brain pathways and oxidative cerebral metabolism. Neurochemical research on aging needs to be considered in the context of specific functions and the parameters most critical for those functions. Heterogeneity is one of the hallmarks of aging. Any molecular theory needs to account for the heterogeneity that exists among individuals and even among cell groups in the brain. Adaptive or plastic mechanisms probably play a key role in maintaining functions during aging. Brain aging probably is not due to a single factor but rather a series of interdependent mechanisms that ultimately compromise the precision and computational accuracy of the networks. This would first appear as an inability to cope with extreme challenges once easily managed. The speed at which select cognitive and noncognitive tasks can be accurately processed may slow down, perhaps because the brain needs more and more trials. Integrated multidisciplinary approaches appear essential in order to understand the process of aging. Indeed, as we learn more about aging, we may come to understand how to optimize the potential for successful aging.

ACKNOWLEDGMENTS

The authors thank Martina Klein for typing assistance and Danna Cotman for the artwork. This work was supported in part by NIA-AG00538, NIA-AG07855, the MacArthur Foundation and Research Program on Successful Aging, the Alzheimer's and Disease Related Disorders Association Faculty Scholar Award, the John Douglas French Foundation Fellowship, and the Wolf Memorial Fund.

REFERENCES

1. Rowe, J. W., and Kahn, R. L. Human aging: Usual and successful. *Science* 237:143–149, 1987.

2. Terry, R. D., DeTeresa, R., and Hansen, L. A. Neocortical cell counts in normal human adult aging. *Ann. Neurol.* 21:530–539, 1987.

3. McGeer, P. L., McGeer, G. G., and Suzuki, J. S. Aging and extrapyramidal function. *Arch. Neurol.* 34:33–35, 1977.

4. Rogers, J., and Bloom, F. E. Neurotransmitter metabolism and function in the aging central nervous system. In E. Schneider and C. E. Finch (eds.), *Handbook of the Biology of Aging.* New York: Van Nostrand Rheinhold, 1985, pp. 645–691.

5. Morgan, D. G., May, P. C., and Finch, C. E. Dopamine and serotonin systems in human and rodent brain: Effects of aging and neurodegenerative diseases. *J. Am. Gerontol. Soc.* 35:334–345, 1987.

6. Cotman, C. W., and Anderson, K. J. Synaptic plasticity and functional stabilization in the hippocampal formation: Possible role in Alzheimer's disease. In S. Waxman (ed.), *Physiologic Basis for Functional Recovery in Neurological Disease.* New York: Raven Press, 1988, pp. 313–336.

7. Coleman, P. D., and Flood, D. G. Dendritic proliferation in the aging brain as a compensatory repair mechanism. In D. F. Swaab, E. Fliers, M. Mirmiran, W. A. Van Gool, and F. VanHaaren (eds.), *Progress in Brain Research.* Amsterdam: Elsevier, 1986, Vol. 70, pp. 227–236.

8. Gibson, G. E., and Peterson, C. Interactions of calcium homeostasis, acetylcholine metabolism, behavior and 3,4-diaminopyridine during aging. In I. Hanin (ed.), *Dynamics of Cholinergic Function.* New York: Plenum Press, 1986, pp. 191–204.

9. Bartus, R., and Dean, R. L. Developing and utilizing animal models in the search for an effective treatment for aged-related memory disturbances. In C. Gottfries (ed.), *Physiological Aging and Dementia.* Basel: S. Karger Press, 1983, pp. 231–267.

10. Smith, D. O., and Weiler, M. H. Acetylcholine metabolism and choline availability at the neuromuscular junction of mature adult and aged rats. *J. Physiol.* 383:693–709, 1987.

11. Kelly, S. S., and Robbins, N. Sustained transmitter output by increased transmitter turnover in limb muscles of old mice. *J. Neurosci.* 6:2900–2907, 1986.

12. Barnes, C. A., Rao, G., and McNaughton, B. L. Increased electronic coupling in aged rat hippocampus: A possible mechanism for cellular excitability changes. *J. Comp. Neurol.* 259:549–558, 1987.

13. Gibson, G. E., and Peterson, C. Calcium and the aging nervous system. *Neurobiology of Aging* 8:329–343, 1987.

14. Baudry, M., Simonson, L., Dubrin, R., and Lynch, G. A comparative study of soluble calcium-dependent proteolytic activity in brain. *J. Neurosci.* 17:15–28, 1986.

15. Peterson, C., Ratan, R. R., Shelanski, M. L., and Goldman, J. E. Cytosolic free calcium and cell spreading decreases in fibroblasts from aged and Alzheimer donors. *Proc. Natl. Acad. Sci. U.S.A.* 83:7999–8001, 1986.

16. Duara, R., Grady, C., Haxby, J., Ingvar, D., Sokoloff, L., et al. Human brain glucose utilization and cognitive function in relation to age. *Ann. Neurol.* 16:702–713, 1984.

17. Barnes, D. Defect in Alzheimer is on chromosome 21. *Science* 235:846–847, 1987.

18. Oliver, C. Lipofuscin and ceroid accumulation in experimental animals. In R. S. Sohal (ed.), *Age Pigments*. New York: Elsevier/North-Holland, 1981, pp. 317–335.

19. Gage, F. H., and Bjorklund, A. Cholinergic septal grafts into the hippocampal formation improve spatial learning and memory in aged rats by an atropine-sensitive mechanism. *J. Neurosci.* 6:2837–2847, 1986.

20. Shock, N. W. Biological theories of aging. In J. R. Florini, R. C. Adelman, and G. S. Roth (eds.), *CRC Handbook of Biochemistry in Aging*. Boca Raton, Fl.: CRC Press, 1982, pp. 271–282.

21. Geddes, J. W., Anderson, K. J., and Cotman, C. W. Senile plaques as abberant sprout stimulating structures. *Exp. Neurol.* 94:767–776, 1986.

22. Sapolsky, R. M., Krey, L. C., and McEwen, B. S. Prolonged glucocorticoid exposure reduces hippocampal number: implications in aging. *J. Neurosci.* 5:1222–1227, 1985.

23. Weindruch, R., and Walford, R.L. Dietary restriction in mice beginning at 1 year of age: Effect on life-span and spontaneous cancer incidence. *Science* 215:1415–1418, 1982.

24. Abbey, H. Survival characteristics of mouse strains. In D. C. Gibson, R. C. Adelman, and C. E. Finch (eds.), *Development of the Rodent as a Model System of Aging*. DHEW Publ. No. (NIH) 79-161, 1978.

25. Peterson, C., Neal, J., and Cotman, C. W. Glutamate neurotoxicity during development and aging. *Soc. Neurosci.* 14:(*in press*).

CHAPTER 28

Intermediary Metabolism

Donald D. Clarke, Abel L. Lajtha, and Howard S. Maker

Basic Neurochemistry: Molecular, Cellular, and Medical Aspects, 4th Ed., edited by G. J. Siegel et al. Raven Press, Ltd., New York, 1989.
Correspondence to Donald D. Clarke, Chemistry Department, Fordham University, Bronx, New York 10458.

Although it is sometimes stated that the brain is unique among tissues in its high rate of oxidative metabolism, the overall cerebral metabolic rate for O_2 (CMRO$_2$) is of the same order as the unstressed heart and renal cortex [1]. Regional metabolic fluxes in brain may greatly exceed CMRO$_2$, however, and these are closely coupled to fluctuations in metabolic demand. (Alterations in energy and carbohydrate metabolism, which are produced by varying functional demands of the nervous system and by pathological conditions, are discussed in Chapters 29, 39, 40, and 41. Peripheral nerve metabolism is discussed in Chap. 35.)

ENERGY METABOLISM

ATP production in brain is highly regulated

Oxidative steps of carbohydrate metabolism normally contribute 36 of the 38 high-energy phosphate bonds ($\sim$P) generated during the aerobic metabolism of a single glucose molecule. Approximately 15 percent of brain glucose is converted to lactate and does not enter the Krebs (citric acid) cycle. There are indications, however, that this might be matched by a corresponding uptake of ketone bodies. The total net gain of high energy phosphate ($\sim$P) is 33 equivalents per mole of glucose utilized. The steady-state level of ATP is high and represents the sum of very rapid synthesis and utilization. On average, half the terminal phosphate groups of ATP turn over in approximately 3 sec; in certain regions, turnover is probably considerably

faster [2]. The level of $\sim$P is kept constant by regulation of ADP phosphorylation in relation to ATP hydrolysis. The active adenylate kinase reaction, which forms equal amounts of ATP and AMP from ADP, prevents any great accumulation of ADP. Only a small amount of AMP is present under steady-state conditions; consequently, a relatively small percentage decrease in ATP may lead to a relatively large percentage increase in AMP. Since AMP is a positive modulator of several reactions that lead to increased ATP synthesis, such an amplification factor provides a sensitive control for maintenance of ATP levels [3]. Between 37° and 42°C, brain metabolic rate increases at a rate of approximately 5 percent per degree.

The level of creatine phosphate in brain is even higher than that of ATP, and creatine phosphokinase is extremely active. The creatine phosphate level is exquisitely sensitive to changes in oxygenation, providing $\sim$P for ADP phosphorylation and thus maintaining ATP levels. The creatine phosphokinase system may also function in regulating mitochondrial activity. Shuttling high-energy phosphate produced by mitochondria to sites of utilization, such as membrane ATPase and axonal transport sites, in the form of creatine phosphate rather than ATP, sustains the ADP level and stimulates mitochondrial activity. In cells with a very heterogeneous mitochondrial distribution, such as neurons, the creatine phosphate shuttle may play a critical role in energy transport [4]. The BB isoenzyme of creatine kinase is characteristic of, but not confined to, brain. Thus, the presence of BB in body fluids does not necessarily indicate disruption of neural tissue.

Under ordinary conditions, the basic substrate for brain metabolism is glucose

The brain depends on glucose for energy and as the major carbon source for a wide variety of simple and complex molecules. Although other tissues can utilize glucose, it is not the primary metabolite of most. Heart, renal cortex, and even liver (the carbohydrate storehouse) derive most of their energy from fatty acids. During hypoglycemia these other tissues stop metabolizing glucose, making more available to the brain. Liver glycogen metabolism is under neural as well as hormonal control, allowing a sensitive response to the needs of the brain. Stimulation of a cholinergic pathway in the lateral hypothalamus causes increased liver glycogen synthesis and decreased gluconeogenesis (through the vagus nerve), and stimulation of the ventromedial hypothalamus causes increased glycogenolysis and gluconeogenesis by a process not mediated by cyclic AMP (cAMP).

A transient decline in the oxidative metabolism of glucose may lead to an abrupt disruption of brain function. Despite this dependence on glucose, the brain at rest extracts only approximately 10 percent of the glucose from the blood flowing through it [~5 mg (28 μmol) glucose/100 g/min]. If blood flow slows down, the brain takes up a relatively greater fraction of both the oxygen and glucose present in blood (see Chap. 29). The entry of most water-soluble substances into brain from blood is restricted. Specific mechanisms do exist, however, to carry certain important metabolites across the blood-brain barrier (BBB) (see Chap. 30). Many glycolytic metabolites, and substances that can be transformed into these metabolites, can sustain brain metabolism *in vitro*, but they fail to do so in the intact animal because they cannot penetrate into brain at sufficient rates. Although mannose may sustain brain metabolism *in vivo*, most other sugars, such as fructose, cannot be taken up rapidly enough to support brain metabolism. Fructose can in fact sustain metabolism in the immature brain, but this may be related to an incomplete BBB or to a lower metabolic demand before the brain matures.

Glucose crosses the BBB by a carrier mechanism (see Chap. 30) that regulates the rate of glucose entry into brain and helps to maintain the concentration of glucose lower in brain than in structures lacking this barrier, for example, sympathetic ganglia or peripheral nerve terminals [5]. The regulation of entry is governed by the Michaelis constant (K_m) of glucose uptake which is 7 to 8 mM in mammalian brain, approximately the level of plasma glucose. With a concentration at or below the K_m of the system, small changes in plasma glucose cause significant changes in the amount transported. Thus, within limits, glucose and glycogen levels in brain vary directly with blood glucose concentrations. The rate of influx of glucose increases linearly to approximately 7 mM plasma glucose and at a lower rate to approximately 20 mM. Brain glucose is always lower than blood glucose. There is, then, no safety device to supplement such a small carbohydrate reserve during hypoglycemia.

Beyond the BBB, brain cells take up glucose much more avidly. Glucose can be taken up into nerve terminals by carrier processes that possess an affinity for glucose 30 times higher than that of the BBB. These terminals may be able to function despite low overall brain glucose levels. Brain tissue beyond the BBB is apparently sensitive to insulin, and an increase in glucose uptake and glycogen storage by insulin can be demonstrated *in vitro*. Although at present there is no report of a definite effect of circulating insulin on the intact brain, insulin has been detected in cerebrospinal fluid (CSF). Insulin receptors are present in brain, and the metabolism of isolated brain tissue can be affected by insulin; however, the significance of these effects is unknown.

Although brain glucose levels vary (within limits) with plasma levels, the affinity of hexokinase for glucose is much greater than the apparent affinity of the capillary transport system, and under normal conditions glycolysis is regulated by hexokinase activity and not by glucose transport into brain [6]. Regionally, the influx may be independent of local glycolytic rates; for example, the cerebellum has a higher influx rate than cerebral cortex despite having a lower glycolytic rate.

In this respect brain differs from other tissues in which various insulin-dependent and insulin-independent transport systems modify glycolytic flux. Glucose influx becomes important under conditions of increased demand, such as seizures, or hypoglycemia (<50 mg/100 ml plasma glucose).

Brain also differs from other tissues by actually decreasing rather than increasing glucose transport across the BBB during hypoxia, perhaps an adjustment to prevent accumulation of potentially toxic lactate (see also Chap. 40). In contrast, heart and skeletal muscle, which increase glucose transport during hypoxia, have a much greater lactate efflux and accumulate much less lactate than brain. The low lactate transport capacity may be an adaptation to protect brain from the high plasma lactate levels that occur during strenuous exercise. Brain lactate efflux is more rapid in the neonate, possibly contributing to the resistance of neonatal brain to anoxia [6].

Glycogen is a dynamic, but limited, energy store

Although present in relatively low concentrations in brain (3.3 mmol/kg brain in rat), glycogen is a unique energy reserve that requires no energy (ATP) for initiation of its metabolism. As with glucose, glycogen levels in brain appear to vary with plasma glucose concentrations. Brain biopsies have shown that human brain contains much higher glycogen levels than rodent brain, but the effects of anesthesia and pathological changes in the biopsied tissue may have contributed to these high levels. Glycogen granules have been seen in electron micrographs of glia and neurons of immature animals but only in astrocytes of adults. Barbiturates decrease brain metabolism and increase the number of granules seen, particularly in astrocytes of synaptic regions; however, biochemical studies show that neurons do contain glycogen and that the enzymes for its synthesis and metabolism are present in synaptosomes. Astrocyte glycogen may form a store of carbohydrate made available to neurons by still undefined mechanisms. Associated with the granules are enzymes concerned with glycogen synthesis and, perhaps, degradation. The increased glycogen found in areas of brain injury may be due to glial changes or to decreased utilization during tissue preparation.

The accepted role of glycogen is that of a carbohydrate reserve utilized when glucose falls below need. However, there is a rapid, continual breakdown and synthesis of glycogen (19 μmol/kg/min). This is approximately 2 percent of the normal glycolytic flux in brain and is subject to elaborate control mechanisms. This suggests that, even under steady-state conditions, local carbohydrate reserves are important for brain function. If glycogen were the sole supply, however, the normal glycolytic flux in brain would be maintained for less than 5 min.

The enzyme systems that synthesize and catabolize glycogen in other tissues are also found in brain, but their kinetic properties and modes of regulation appear to differ [7]. Glycogen metabolism in brain, unlike in other tissues, is controlled locally. It is isolated from the tumult of systemic activity, evidently because of the blood-brain barrier. Although glucocorticoid hormones that penetrate the BBB increase glycogen turnover, circulating protein hormones and biogenic amines are without effect. Beyond the BBB, cells are sensitive to local amine levels; drugs that penetrate the BBB and modify local amine levels or membrane receptors thus cause metabolic changes.

Separate systems for the synthesis and degradation of glycogen provide a greater degree of control than would be the case were glycogen degraded by simply reversing the steps in its synthesis (Fig. 1). The level of glucose-6-phosphate, the initial synthetic substrate, usually varies inversely with the rate of brain glycolysis because of a greater facilitation of the phosphofructokinase step relative to glucose transport and phosphorylation. Thus, a decline in glucose-6-phosphate at times of energy need decreases glycogen formation.

The glucosyl group of UDP is transferred to the terminal glucose of the nonreducing end of an amylose chain in an α-1,4-glycosidic linkage (Fig. 1). This reaction is catalyzed by glycogen synthetase and is the rate-controlling reaction in glycogen synthesis [7]. In brain, as in other tissues, glycogen synthetase occurs in both a phosphorylated (D) form, which is dependent for activity on glucose-6-phosphate as a positive modulator, and as a dephosphorylated, independent (I) form sensitive to, but not dependent on, the modulator. Although in brain the independent form of the glycogen synthetase requires no stimulator, it has a relatively low affinity for UDP glucose. At times of increased energy demand, not only is there a change from the dependent to the independent form, but also an independent form with an even lower affinity for the substrate develops. The inhibition of glycogen synthesis is enhanced, and this increases the availability of glucose-6-phosphate for energy needs. Goldberg and O'Toole [7] hypothesize that the independent form in brain is associated with inhibition of glycogen synthesis under conditions of energy demand, whereas the dependent form is responsible for a relatively small regulated synthesis under resting conditions. Regulation of the dependent form may be responsible for reducing the rate of glycogen formation in brain to ap-

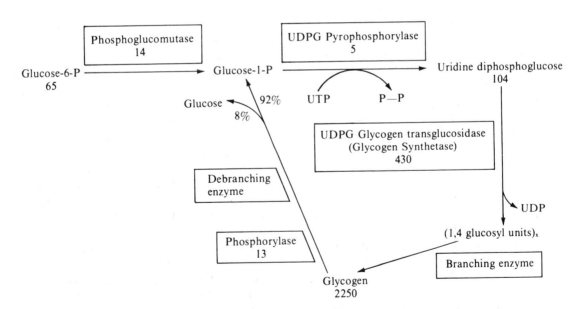

FIG. 1. Glycogen metabolism in brain. Enzyme data from mouse brain homogenates: *numerals* below each enzyme represent V_{max} at 38°C (in mmol/kg wet weight/min); metabolite levels from quick-frozen adult mouse brain in μmol/kg wet weight; (P) phosphate. (Metabolic data from J. V. Passonneau et al., *J. Biol. Chem.* 244:902, 1969; enzyme data from B. M. Breckenridge and P. D. Gatfield, *J. Neurochem.* 3:234, 1961.)

proximately 5 percent of its potential rate. In liver, where large amounts of glycogen are synthesized and degraded, the independent form of the synthetase is associated with glycogen formation. At the present time, it appears that the two tissues use the same biochemical apparatus in different ways in relation to differences in overall metabolic patterns.

Under steady-state conditions, it is probable that less than 10 percent of phosphorylase in brain (Fig. 1) is in the unphosphorylated *b* form (requiring AMP), which is inactive at the very low AMP concentrations present normally. When the steady state is disturbed, there may be an extremely rapid conversion of the enzyme to the *a* form, which is active at low AMP levels. Brain phosphorylase *b* kinase is indirectly activated by cAMP and by the micromolar levels of Ca^{2+} released during neuronal excitation (see Chaps. 17 and 18). Endoplasmic reticulum of brain, like that in muscle, is capable of taking up Ca^{2+} to terminate its stimulatory effect. These reactions provide energy from glycogen during excitation and when cAMP-forming systems are activated. It has not been possible to confirm directly, however, that the conversion from phosphorylase *b* to *a* is a control point of glycogenolysis *in vivo*. Norepinephrine and, probably, dopamine activate glycogenolysis through cAMP; but epinephrine, vasopressin, and angiotensin II do so by another mechanism, possibly involving Ca^{2+} or a Ca^{2+}-mediated proteolysis of the phosphorylase kinase.

Hydrolysis of the α-1,4-glycoside linkages leaves a limit dextrin that turns over at only half the rate of the outer chains (see also Chap. 33). The debrancher enzyme that hydrolyzes the α-1,6-glycoside linkages may be rate limiting if the entire glycogen granule is to be utilized. Because one product of this enzyme is free glucose, approximately one glucose molecule for every eleven of glucose-6-phosphate is released if the entire glycogen molecule is degraded (Fig. 1). α-Glucosidase (acid maltase) is a lysosomal

enzyme whose precise function in glycogen metabolism is not known. In Pompe's disease (the hereditary absence of α-glucosidase), glycogen accumulates in lysosomes in brain as well as in those elsewhere (Chaps. 33 and 37). The steady-state level of glycogen is regulated precisely by the coordination of synthetic and degradative processes through enzymatic regulation at several metabolic steps [8].

Brain glycolysis is regulated mainly by hexokinase and phosphofructokinase

Aerobic and anaerobic glycolysis have been historically defined as the amount of lactate produced under conditions of "adequate" oxygen and no oxygen, respectively. More recently, glycolysis refers to the Embden-Meyerhof glycolytic sequence from glucose (or glycogen glucosyl) to pyruvate. Glycolytic flux is defined indirectly—it is the rate at which glucose must be utilized to produce the observed rates of ADP phosphorylation.

Figure 2 outlines the flow of glycolytic substrates in brain. Glycolysis first involves phosphorylation by hexokinase. The reaction is essentially irreversible and is a key point in the regulation of carbohydrate metabolism in brain. The electrophoretically slow-moving (type 1) isoenzyme of hexokinase is characteristic of brain. In most tissues, hexokinase may exist in the cytosol (soluble), or it may be firmly attached to mitochondria. Under conditions in which no special effort is made to stop metabolism while isolating mitochondria, 80 to 90 percent of brain hexokinase is bound. In the live steady state, however, when availability of substrates keeps up with metabolic demand and end products are removed, an equilibrium exists between the soluble and the bound enzyme. Binding changes the kinetic properties of hexokinase and its inhibition by glucose-6-phosphate, so that the bound enzyme on mitochondria is more active. The extent of binding is inversely related to the ATP/ADP ratio, so that conditions in

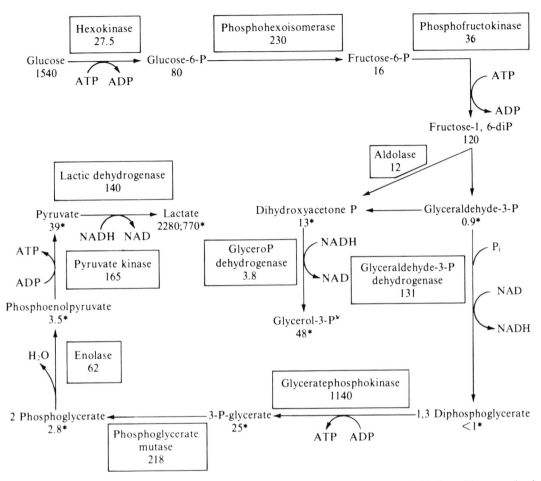

FIG. 2. Glycolysis in brain. Enzyme and metabolic data expressed as in Fig. 1; (∗) 10-day-old mouse brain (Matchinski, 1970). (Data from H. McIlwain, *Biochemistry and the Central Nervous System.* Boston: Little, Brown, 1966, pp. 1–26. F. M. Matchinski, *Adv. Biochem. Psychopharmacol.* 2:217–243, 1970.)

which energy utilization exceeds supply shift the solubilization equilibrium to the bound form and produce a greater potential capacity for initiating glycolysis to meet the energy demand. This mechanism allows ATP to function both as a substrate of the enzyme and, at another site, as a regulator to decrease ATP production through its influence on enzyme binding. It also confers preference on glucose in the competition for the $MgATP^{2-}$ generated by mitochondrial oxidative phosphorylation. Thus, a pro-

cess that will sustain ATP production continues at the expense of other uses of energy. Because energy reserves are rapidly exhausted postmortem, it is not surprising that brain hexokinase is found to be almost entirely bound.

The significance of reversible binding of other enzymes to mitochondria is not clear. The measured glycolytic flux, when compared with the maximal velocity of hexokinase, indicates that, in the steady state, the hexokinase reaction is 97 percent inhibited. Brain hexokinase is inhibited by its product, glucose-6-phosphate, and to a lesser extent by ADP and allosterically by 3-phosphoglycerate and several nucleoside phosphates, including cAMP and free ATP^{4-}. The ratio of ATP to Mg^{2+} may also have a regulatory action. In addition to acting on enzyme kinetics, glucose-6-phosphate solubilizes hexokinase, thus reducing the enzyme's efficiency when the reaction product accumulates. The sum total of these mechanisms is a fine tuning of the activity of the initial enzyme of glycolysis in response to changes in the cellular environment. Glucokinase (low-affinity hexokinase), a major component of liver hexokinase, has not been found in brain.

Glucose-6-phosphate represents a branch point in metabolism because it is a common substrate for enzymes involved in glycolytic, pentose phosphate shunt, and glycogen-forming pathways. There is also slight, but detectable, glucose-6-phosphatase activity in brain, the significance of which is not clear. The liver requires this enzyme to convert glycogen to glucose. The differences between liver and brain hexokinase and the differences between the modes of glycogen metabolism of these two tissues can be related to the function of liver as a carbohydrate storehouse for the body, whereas brain metabolism is adapted for rapid carbohydrate utilization for energy needs.

In glycolysis, glucose-6-phosphate is the substrate of phosphohexose isomerase. This is a reversible reaction (small free-energy change) whose 5:1 equilibrium ratio in brain favors glucose-6-phosphate.

Fructose-6-phosphate is the substrate of phosphofructokinase, a key regulatory enzyme controlling glycolysis [3]. The other substrate is $MgATP^{2-}$. Like other regulatory reactions, it is essentially irreversible. It is modulated by a large number of metabolites and cofactors whose concentrations under different metabolic conditions have a great effect on glycolytic flux. Prominent among these are availability of $\sim$P and citrate levels. Brain phosphofructokinase is

inhibited by ATP, Mg^{2+}, and citrate and is stimulated by NH_4^+, K^+, PO_4^{3-}, 5'-AMP, 3',5'-cyclic AMP, ADP, and fructose-1,6-bisphosphate.

When oxygen is admitted to cells metabolizing anaerobically, utilization of O_2 increases, whereas utilization of glucose and production of lactate drop (Pasteur effect). Modulation of the phosphofructokinase reaction can account directly for the Pasteur effect. In the steady state, ATP and citrate levels in brain apparently are sufficient to keep phosphofructokinase relatively inhibited as long as the level of positive modulators (or disinhibitors) is low. When the steady state is disturbed, activation of this enzyme produces an increase in glycolytic flux that takes place almost as fast as the events changing the internal milieu.

Fructose-1,6-bisphosphate is split by brain aldolase to glyceraldehyde-3-phosphate and dihydroxyacetone phosphate. Dihydroxyacetone phosphate is the common substrate for both glycerophosphate dehydrogenase, an enzyme active in NADH oxidation and lipid pathways (see Chap. 5), and triose phosphate isomerase, which maintains an equilibrium between dihydroxyacetone phosphate and glyceraldehyde-3-phosphate; the equilibrium strongly favors accumulation of dihydroxyacetone phosphate.

After the reaction with glyceraldehyde phosphate dehydrogenase, glycolysis in the brain proceeds through the usual steps. Brain enolase (D-2-phosphoglycerate hydrolase), which catalyzes dehydration of 2-phosphoglycerate to phosphoenolpyruvate, is present as two related dimers, one of which (γ) is specifically associated with neurons and the other (α) with glia. The neuronal subunit is identical to the neuron-specific protein 14-3-2. Immunochemical determination of the enolases makes them useful in determining neuron/glia ratios in tissue samples, but neuron-specific enolase is not confined to neural tissue. Brain phosphoenolpyruvate kinase controls an essentially irreversible reaction that requires not only Mg^{2+} (as do several other glycolytic enzymes) but also K^+ or Na^+. This step also may be regulatory.

Brain tissue, even when it is at rest and well oxygenated, produces a small amount of lactate, which is removed in the venous blood, accounting for 13 percent of the pyruvate produced by glycolysis. The measured lactate level in brain depends on the success in rapidly arresting brain metabolism prior to tissue processing. Five lactate dehydrogenase isoenzymes are present in adult brain, of which the one that moves electrophoretically most rapidly toward the anode (band 1) predominates. This isoenzyme is generally higher in those tissues that are more dependent on aerobic processes for energy; the slower moving isoenzymes are relatively higher in tissues such as white skeletal muscle, which is better adapted to function at suboptimal oxygen levels (see Chap. 31). The distribution of lactate dehydrogenase isoenzymes in various brain regions, layers of the retina, brain neoplasms, and brain tissue cultures and during development indicates that their synthesis might be controlled by tissue oxygen levels. Lactate dehydrogenase functions in the cytoplasm as a means of oxidizing NADH, which accumulates as the result of the activity of glyceraldehyde phosphate dehydrogenase in glycolysis. It thus permits glycolytic ATP production to continue under anaerobic conditions. Lactate dehydrogenase also functions under aerobic conditions because NADH cannot easily penetrate the mitochondrial membrane. The oxidation of NADH in the cytoplasm depends on this reaction and on the activity of shuttle mechanisms that transfer reducing equivalents to the mitochondria.

Glycerol phosphate dehydrogenase is another enzyme indirectly associated with glycolysis that participates in the cytoplasmic oxidation of NADH. This enzyme reduces dihydroxyacetone phosphate to glycerol-3-phosphate, oxidizing NADH in the process.

Under hypoxic conditions, levels of α-glycerophosphate and lactate increase initially at comparable rates, although the amount of lactate produced greatly exceeds that of α-glycerophosphate. The relative levels of the oxidized and reduced substrates of these reactions indicate much higher local levels of NADH in brain than are found by gross measurements. In fact, the relative proportions of oxidized and reduced substrates of the reactions that are linked to the pyridine nucleotides may be a better indicator of local oxidation-reduction states ($NAD^+/NADH$) in brain than is provided by the direct measurement of the pyridine nucleotides themselves [3,5].

An aspect of glucose metabolism that has led to much confusion among neurochemists is the observation that labeled glucose appears in carbon dioxide much more slowly than might be suggested from a cursory examination of the glycolytic pathway plus the citric acid cycle [10]. Glucose flux is 0.5 to 1.0 μmol/min/g wet weight of brain in a variety of species. The level of glycolytic plus Krebs cycle intermediates is 2 μmol/g. Hence, these intermediates might be predicted to turn over every 2 to 4 min, and $^{14}CO_2$ production might be predicted to reach a steady state in 5 to 10 min. This is not observed experimentally. In addition, large quantities of radioactivity are trapped in amino acids related to the Krebs cycle (70–80 percent) from 10 to 30 min after a glucose injection. This is due to the high activity of transaminase in comparison with the flux through the Krebs cycle, and the amino acids developed by transamination behave as if they were a part of the cycle. When the pools of these amino acids (~20 μmol/g) are added to the levels of Krebs cycle components plus glycolytic intermediates, the calculated time for $^{14}CO_2$ evolution is increased by a factor of 10, which agrees with the values observed experimentally.

In contrast, in tissues such as liver, the amino acids related to the Krebs cycle are present at much lower steady-state values, and

20 percent of the radioactivity from administered glucose is trapped in these amino acids at short times after injection. As a result, ignoring the radioactivity trapped in amino acids has a relatively small effect on estimates of glycolytic fluxes in liver but makes an enormous difference in brain. Immature brains more nearly resemble liver in this respect. The relationship of the Krebs cycle to glycolysis undergoes a sharp change during development, coincident with the development of the metabolic compartmentation of amino acid metabolism characteristic of adult brain.

The pyruvate dehydrogenase complex plays a key role in regulating oxidation

Pyruvate dehydrogenase (14 nmol/min/mg protein in rat brain), which controls the entry of pyruvate into the Krebs cycle as acetyl coenzyme A (acetyl-CoA), is actually a mitochondrial multienzyme complex that includes the enzymes pyruvate dehydrogenase (decarboxylase), lipoate acetyltransferase, and lipoamide dehydrogenase; the coenzymes thiamine pyrophosphate, lipoic acid, CoA, and flavine; and nicotinamide dinucleotides. It is inactivated by being phosphorylated at the decarboxylase moiety by a tightly bound $MgATP^{2-}$-dependent protein kinase and activated by being dephosphorylated by a loosely bound Mg^{2+}- and Ca^{2+}-dependent phosphatase. About half the brain enzyme is usually active. Pyruvate protects the complex against inactivation by inhibiting the kinase. ADP is a competitive inhibitor of Mg^{2+} for the inactivating kinase. Under conditions of greater metabolic demand, increases in pyruvate and ADP and decreases in acetyl-CoA and ATP make the complex more active. Pyruvate dehydrogenase is inhibited by NADH, decreasing formation of acetyl-CoA during hypoxia and allowing more pyruvate to be reduced by lactate dehydrogenase, thus forming the NAD necessary to sustain glycolysis. Several investigators have reported abnormalities of the complex

(particularly lipoamide dehydrogenase) in some hereditary ataxias, but not all studies have confirmed these findings, and the relationship remains tenuous. Pyruvate dehydrogenase defects do occur in several of the mitochondrial enzyme deficiency states (see below and Morgan-Hughes [9]). (These are also described in Chap. 33.)

Although acetylcholine synthesis is normally controlled by the rate of choline uptake and choline acetyltransferase activity (see Chap. 10), the supply of acetyl-CoA can be limiting under adverse conditions. Choline uptake is, however, independent of acetyl-CoA concentration. A cytoplasmic pyruvate dehydrogenase specifically associated with acetylcholine synthesis has been suggested. The mitochondrial membrane is not permeable to the acetyl-CoA produced within it, but there is efflux of its condensation product, citrate. Acetyl-CoA can then be formed from citrate in the cytosol by ATP citrate lyase. The acetyl moiety of acetylcholine is formed in a compartment with rapid glucose turnover, presumably the synaptosome. The cytosol of cholinergic endings is rich in citrate lyase, and it is probable that the citrate shuttles the acetyl-CoA from the mitochondrial compartment. During hypoxia or hypoglycemia, acetylcholine synthesis can be inhibited by failure of the acetyl-CoA supply.

Energy output and oxygen consumption in adult brain are associated with high levels of enzyme activity in the Krebs cycle

The actual flux through the Krebs cycle depends on glycolysis and acetyl-CoA production, which can "push" the cycle, the possible control at several enzymatic steps of the cycle, and the local ADP level, which is known to be a prime activator of the mitochondrial respiration to which the Krebs cycle is linked. The steady-state level of citrate in brain is about one-fifth that of glucose. This is relatively high compared with levels of glycolytic intermediates or with that of isocitrate.

As in other tissues, there are two isocitrate dehydrogenases in brain. One is active primarily in the cytoplasm and requires nicotinamide-adenine dinucleotide phosphate (NADP) as cofactor; the other, bound to mitochondria and requiring NAD, is the enzyme that participates in the citric acid cycle. The NAD-linked enzyme catalyzes an essentially irreversible reaction, has allosteric properties, is inhibited by ATP and NADH, and may be stimulated by ADP. The function of cytoplasmic NADP isocitrate dehydrogenase is uncertain, but it has been postulated that it supplies NADPH necessary for many reductive synthetic reactions. The relatively high activity of this enzyme in immature brain and white matter is consistent with such a role. α-Ketoglutarate dehydrogenase, which oxidatively decarboxylates α-ketoglutarate, requires the same cofactors as does the pyruvate decarboxylation step.

Succinate dehydrogenase, the enzyme that catalyzes the oxidation of succinate to fumarate, is tightly bound to mitochondrial membrane. In brain, succinate dehydrogenase may also have a regulatory role when the steady state is disturbed. Isocitrate and succinate levels in brain are little affected by changes in the flux of the citric acid cycle as long as an adequate glucose supply is available. The highly unfavorable free-energy change of the malate dehydrogenase reaction is overcome by the rapid removal of oxaloacetate, which is maintained at low concentrations under steady-state conditions by the condensation reaction with acetyl-CoA [8].

Malic dehydrogenase is one of several enzymes in the citric acid cycle that is present in both cytoplasm and mitochondria. The function of the cytoplasmic components of these enzyme activities is not known, but they may assist in the transfer of hydrogen from the cytoplasm into mitochondria.

The Krebs cycle functions as an oxidative process for energy production and as a source of various amino acids, for example, glutamate, glutamine, γ-aminobutyric acid (GABA), aspartate, and asparagine. To export net amounts of α-ketoglutarate or oxaloacetate from the Krebs cycle, the supply of dicarboxylic acids must be replenished. The major route for this seems to be the fixation of CO_2 to pyruvate or another substrate at this three-carbon level. Thus, the rate of CO_2 fixation sets the upper limit at which biosynthetic reactions can occur. This has been estimated as approximately 0.15 μmol/g wet weight brain/min in studies of acute ammonia toxicity in cats, or approximately 10 percent of the flux through the citric acid cycle. Liver, on the other hand, appears to have ten times the capacity of brain for CO_2 fixation, as is appropriate for an organ geared to making large quantities of protein for export. In brain, pyruvate carboxylase, which catalyzes CO_2 fixation, appears to be largely an astrocytic enzyme. Pyruvate dehydrogenase activity seems to be the rate-limiting step for the entry of pyruvate into the Krebs cycle from glycolysis.

The pentose shunt (hexose monophosphate) pathway is active in brain

Under basal conditions at least 5 to 8 percent of brain glucose is likely so metabolized in the adult monkey, and 2.3 percent in the rat [10]. Both shunt enzymes and metabolic flux have been found in isolated nerve endings. The pathway has relatively high activity in developing brain, reaching a peak during myelination. Its main contribution is probably to produce the NADPH required for the reductive reactions necessary for lipid synthesis (see Chap. 5). Shunt enzymes and metabolic flux are found in synaptosomes. Although the capacity of the pathway (as determined using nonphysiological electron acceptors) remains constant throughout the rat life span, activity with physiological acceptors could not be detected in middle-aged (18 months) and older animals. It is possible that the shunt serves as a reserve pathway for use under such stresses as the need for increased lipid synthesis, repair, or reduction of oxidative toxins. The shunt pathway also provides pentose for nucleotide synthesis; however, only a small fraction of the activity of this pathway would be required. As with glycogen synthesis, turnover in the pentose-phosphate pathway decreases under conditions of increased energy need, for example, during and after high rates of stimulation. Pentose phosphate flux apparently is regulated by the concentrations of glucose-6-phosphate, NADP, glyceraldehyde-3-phosphate, and fructose-6-phosphate. Since transketolase, one of the enzymes in this pathway, requires thiamine pyrophosphate as a cofactor, poor myelin maintenance in thiamine deficiency may reflect the failure of the pathway to provide sufficient NADPH for lipid synthesis [8].

Glutamate in brain is compartmented into separate pools

These pools, which subserve different metabolic pathways for glutamate, equilibrate with each other only slowly. This compartmentation is a vital factor in the separate regulation of special functions of glutamate and GABA, such as neurotransmission, and general functions, such as protein biosynthesis.

Glutamate metabolism in brain is characterized by the existence of at least two distinct pools; in addition, the Krebs cycle intermediates associated with these pools are also distinctly compartmented. A mathematical model to fit data from radiotracer experiments that require separate Krebs cycles to satisfy the hypotheses of compartmentation has been developed. A key assumption of the current models is that GABA is metabolized at a site different

from its synthesis. The best fit of kinetic data is obtained when glutamate from a small pool that is actively converted to glutamine flows back to a larger pool (8 μmol/g) that is converted to GABA. Of possible relevance, it has been shown that glutamic acid decarboxylase (GAD) is localized at or near nerve terminals, whereas GABA transaminase, the major degradative enzyme, is mitochondrial.

Evidence points to an inferred small pool of glutamate (2 μmol/g) as probably glial. Glutamate released from nerve endings appears to be taken up by glia (and by presynaptic and postsynaptic terminals, or both), converted to glutamine, and recycled to glutamate and GABA. Various estimates of the proportion of glucose carbon that flows through the GABA shunt (see Chap. 15) have been published, but the most definitive experiments show the value to be approximately 10 percent of the total glycolytic flux. Although this may seem small, that portion of the Krebs cycle flux that is used for energy production (ATP synthesis, maintenance of ionic gradients) does not require CO_2 fixation, but that portion used for biosynthesis of amino acids does. By recycling the carbon skeleton of some of the glutamate through glutamine and GABA to succinate, the need for dicarboxylic acids to replenish intermediates of the Krebs cycle is diminished when export of α-ketoglutarate takes place.

It is difficult to get good estimates of the extent of CO_2 fixation in brain, but estimates of the maximum capability obtained under conditions of ammonia stress, when glutamine levels increase rapidly, suggest that CO_2 fixation occurs at 0.15 μmol/g/min (in cat) and 0.33 μmol/g/min (in rat); that is, at about the same rate as for the GABA shunt.

For comparison, it should be pointed out that only approximately 2 percent of the glucose flux in whole brain goes toward lipid synthesis, and approximately 0.3 percent is used for protein synthesis. Thus, turnover of neurotransmitter amino acids is a major biosynthetic effort in brain.

Metabolic compartmentation of glutamate is usually observed when ketogenic substrates are administered to animals. It is interesting that acetoacetate and β-hydroxybutyrate do not show this effect, apparently because ketone bodies are a normal substrate for brain and are taken up into all types of cells. Acetate and similar substances, which are not taken up into brain efficiently, appear to be more readily taken up or activated in glia, or both. This may lead to the abnormal glutamate/glutamine ratio that is observed. Similarly, metabolic inhibitors like fluoroacetate appear to act selectively in glia and produce their neurotoxic action without marked inhibition of the overall Krebs cycle flux in brain. This difference in behavior between acetate and glucose has led to the suggestion that acetate and fluoroacetate may be useful markers for the study of glial metabolism by the technique of autoradiography [11].

A nonuniform distribution of metabolites in living systems is a widespread occurrence. Steady-state levels of GABA are well documented as varying over a five–fold range in discrete brain regions (2–10 mM), and it has been estimated that GABA may be as high as 50 mM in nerve terminals. Observations in brain indicate the existence of pools with half-lives of many hours for mixing, which is most unusual. The discovery of subcellular morphological compartmentation—different populations of mitochondria in cerebral cortex that have distinctive enzyme complements—may provide a somewhat better perspective by which to visualize such separation of metabolic function.

In addition to the phasic release of both excitatory and inhibitory transmitters, there may be a continuous tonic release of GABA, dependent only on the activity of the enzyme responsible for its synthesis and independent of the depolarization of the presynaptic membrane. Such inhibitory neurons could act tonically by constantly maintaining an elevated threshold in the excitatory neurons so that the latter would start firing when a decrease occurred in the continuous release of GABA acting on them. This is consistent with a known correlation between the inhibition of GAD and the appearance of convulsions after certain drug treatments. GABA levels have been observed to be depleted by some convulsant drugs and elevated by others.

The sine qua non *of brain metabolism is its high rate of mitochondrial respiration*

Brain mitochondria have an affinity for oxygen several times that of liver mitochondria and also react differently to osmolar changes both morphologically and biochemically. Because current methods of separating mitochondria from other cell components depend on sedimentation from homogenates, differences related to function and intracellular provenance are difficult to define. Furthermore, mitochondrial size and function do change during maturation. Therefore, functional heterogeneity among brain mitochondria may be related to their location in perikarya, synaptosomes, or various glial cells. Unexpectedly, the specific activities of mitochondrial energy and metabolic enzymes have been found to be higher in nonsynaptosomal than in synaptosomal mitochondria [12].

In the coupled, controlled state, the level of mitochondrial function depends on local concentrations of ADP. The entry of ADP into mitochondria is restricted insofar as it must exchange with intramitochondrial ATP. The high steady-state mitochondrial respiration in brain is related to local availability of substrates and the ratio of ADP to ATP. This may not be reflected in the average ratio of ADP to ATP in whole brain, which is quite low. Brain mitochondria also differ from those in other tissues because they contain higher concentrations of certain "nonmitochondrial" enzymes. Brain hexokinase, creatine kinase, and perhaps lactic dehydrogenase are partially mitochondrial. Hexokinase and creatine kinase may function to maintain local levels of ADP by transferring ~P from ATP to creatine or glucose [4].

Among the mitochondrial enzymes for which genetic information is carried in the small mitochondrial DNA complement are cytochrome C oxidase subunits I, II, and III and ATPase subunit 6 [9]. Defects in either the mitochondrial or the chromosomally specified enzymes or in their transport could lead to physiological dysfunction. Tissues with high rates of aerobic metabolism, such as brain, retina, and cardiac and skeletal muscle, are particularly vulnerable [9]. Several different clinical syndromes have been found to be due to defects in Krebs cycle metabolism: β-oxidase, carnitine and ATP metabolism, and the respiratory chain, including malfunction of the enzymes pyruvate dehydrogenase phosphatase, pyruvate decarboxylase, cytochrome C oxidase, and NADH-ubiquinone reductase (see Chap. 33).

The principal source of lipid carbon in brain is blood glucose

Carbohydrate intermediates and related metabolites, such as acetate (fatty acid and cholesterol), dihydroxyacetone phosphate (glycerol phosphate), mannosamine, pyruvate (neuraminic acid), glucose-6-phosphate (inositol), galactose, and glucosamine, supply the building blocks of the complex lipids (see Chap. 5). NADPH is also necessary for the reductive synthesis of lipids. When a few polyunsaturated fatty acids and sulfate are supplied, immature brain slices readily form all the lipids of myelin and cell membrane, using glucose as the only substrate. Energy supply through the carbohydrate pathways in the form of ATP is also required to supply nucleoside phosphates for lipid assembly [8].

Carbohydrate utilization varies with the brain's need for energy

The high functional requirement of nervous tissue for ~P is probably related to energy demands for transmitter synthesis, packaging, secretion, uptake, and sequestration; for ion pumping to maintain ionic gradients; for intracellular transport; and for synthesis of complex lipids and macromolecules in both neuronal and glial cells. The manner in which metabolism is coupled to function is conceptualized easily from the discussion of the regulatory mechanisms that control carbohydrate metabolism and can be illustrated by Na,K-ATPase, which functions in the Na^+-K^+ exchange pump so essential for maintaining electrolyte gradients (see also Chap. 3). This enzyme is particularly active in regions with high concentrations of synaptic membranes, for example, gray matter and synaptosomes. The ADP released intracellularly is an activating modulator for mitochondria and several rate-limiting reactions: glycolytic (hexokinase, phosphofructokinase), Krebs cycle (NAD-dependent isocitric dehydrogenase), and glycogenolytic (phosphorylase). Changes accompanying the consequently increased metabolic flux lead to inhibition of other pathways, such as that of glycogen synthesis and the pentose phosphate shunt, whereas lowered ~P and NADPH levels inhibit various synthetic reactions. Because the products of reactions that use ~P are accelerators of reactions leading to ~P formation, energy supply as ATP is regulated by utilization. The set-points of this regulation may be altered in certain toxic metabolic states. Under many adverse conditions, for example, hypoxia, energy utilization is decreased in brain, heart, and other tissues (see Chap. 40).

Although the linkage of neuronal function to energy metabolism has been emphasized, it should be pointed out that physiological failure during hypoxia, ischemia, or hypoglycemia in brain (and other tissues) begins before overall energy levels fall below those considered adequate to support function. Among the suggested causes of dysfunction are defects in acetylcholine (see Pyruvate Dehydrogenase Complex, above) and catecholamine synthesis. The affinity of tyrosine hydroxylase for oxygen is several orders of magnitude less than that of the mitochondrial enzymes; this makes amine synthesis relatively more vulnerable to hypoxia.

Regional differences in metabolism add a useful neurochemical dimension

There are two major techniques for studying regional metabolism. The first, developed by Lowry and Passonneau [3], measures changes in carbohydrate metabolites and energy cofactors during a few seconds of ischemia in microdissected samples and assumes that their rates of change reflect those before ischemia. The second (see Chap. 29) is based on the measurement of grain density by autoradiography of freeze-dried sections after isotopically labeled deoxyglucose has been administered and assumes instantaneous and sustained isotopic equilibrium throughout brain tissue and plasma.

Other methods have been developed. Nuclear magnetic resonance (NMR) can be used to quantitate separately the adenylate phosphates, creatine phosphate, sugar phosphates, and phospholipids, although these molecules cannot yet be used for anatomical mapping [13]. Chronically implanted surface coils in animal brain have been used to determine local changes in ~P during metabolic perturbations. Resonance detection of ^{13}C has made it possible to measure glycogen in rat glycogen storage disease after glucose loading. ATP distribution can be anatomically mapped in tissue sections by bioluminescence based on enzyme-linked reactions.

Metabolic mapping, with even greater anatomic resolution in tissue sections than methods based on autoradiography, has been based on the histochemical assessment of phosphorylase and detection of glycogen (reversal of the phosphorylase reaction). The normal glucose flux estimated by the former method is usually more than twice that of the deoxyglucose method. Estimates based on the Lowry technique are increased by the stimulation resulting from decapitation but are much closer to the glucose consumption calculated from oxygen consumption. Previous criticisms of the validity of the deoxyglucose method [14] have been amply and categorically refuted [15]. The deoxyglucose method of Sokoloff underestimates the true flux in that equilibrium conditions are not attained, but it gives accurate relative values in different regions. It is thus a practical method for comparing glucose phosphorylation in many different regions simultaneously and under different conditions (see Chap. 29).

In general, those regions of brain with higher metabolic requirements have both higher enzyme activity in the glycolytic series and the Krebs cycle and higher levels of respiration. Several glycolytic and mitochondrial enzymes are more active in regions with large numbers of synaptic endings (neuropil) than in areas rich in neuronal cell bodies. On the other hand, the activity of glucose-6-phosphate dehydrogenase (a rate-limiting enzyme of the pentose phosphate pathway) is high in myelinated fibers and tends to vary with the degree of myelination. Phosphofructokinase and phosphorylase are distributed in a relatively constant ratio in different brain regions; this suggests a relationship between glycolysis and glycogenolysis. Hexokinase distribution is more closely linked to mitochondrial enzymes than to glycolytic enzymes.

The oligodendroglial cell that maintains myelin in the CNS probably ranks, along with the neuron and its processes, as having the highest known metabolic requirements. Although the metabolism of neuronal terminals is high, that of their cell bodies may actually be lower than that of astrocytes, which appear to have a metabolic rate higher than early investigators had suggested.

Because of its stratified structure, the retina serves as a convenient model for the study of regional metabolism

The rabbit retina is avascular and depends almost entirely on diffusion from choroidal capillaries. The primate retina, however, is vascularized from the vitreal surface as far as the bipolar cell layer. The rabbit retina shows high rates of glucose and oxygen consumption and also of lactate formation. The high rate of aerobic lactate formation might be due to segregation of glycolytic and oxidative processes as well as to the adaptation of the poorly vascularized inner layers to a relatively anoxic existence. The rod cell inner segment contains packed mitochondria and has high levels of mitochondrial enzymes and hexokinase. This is the region closest to the choroidal nutrient supply.

In the vascularized inner layers of the monkey retina, hexokinase activity is almost twice that in the homologous layers of the rabbit retina. Several glycolytic enzymes, including phosphofructokinase and glyceraldehyde phosphate dehydrogenase, as well as lactic dehydrogenase and glycogen phosphorylase, tend to be higher toward the vitreous surface in rabbit than in monkey retina. The total energy reserves (especially high glycogen levels) and lactate levels increase as the avascular vitreous surface of the rabbit retina is approached. Malate dehydrogenase and NAD-dependent isocitrate dehydrogenase, the Krebs cycle enzymes, vary with the relative density of mitochondria, which is high in the layer of rod cell inner segments and in the synaptic layers. Data such as these suggest that adaptive changes occur in carbohydrate enzymes and metabolism and that these changes are dependent on the local availability of substrates and oxygen. As in brain,

however, continued electrical responsiveness of the retina depends on oxidative metabolism.

COMPOSITION OF FREE AMINO ACID POOLS

The brain depends on transport of essential amino acids from the blood

The carbon skeletons of certain amino acids, termed "essential," cannot be synthesized at a rate adequate to meet metabolic requirements. These amino acids must be derived from the diet and include arginine, histidine, isoleucine, leucine, lysine, methionine, phenylalanine, threonine, tryptophan, and valine. Tyrosine is formed in a single step from phenylalanine, and cysteine takes its sulfur from methionine. Those amino acids that can be made in the body of an animal appear to be synthesized in the brain as well. These "nonessential" amino acids are alanine, aspartate, and glutamate made by transaminations of α-keto acids; proline derived from glutamate; serine derived from 3-phosphoglycerate or from glycine; serine made from glycine plus tetrahydrofolate; glutamine from ammonia and glutamate; and asparagine from transamidation of aspartate (see Chaps. 15 and 38 for specific reactions).

Ammonia is taken up by brain when circulating ammonia levels are increased either experimentally or when liver function is impaired. Ammonia uptake from normal circulatory ammonia levels probably is sufficient to maintain the brain in nitrogen balance, although the proportion of nitrogen supplied as ammonia to that available as preformed amino acids is not well established.

Essential free amino acids in brain are present at low levels; their content in protein components is several hundred times higher. Because of this concentration difference, an incremental growth of less than 1 percent in brain protein would exhaust the available free amino acid content of the brain, were it not replenished from the circulation.

Neurochemists noted early that the composition of the free amino acid pool in the brain differs from that of other tissues; the biggest difference is the relatively high content of glutamate and related amino acids, including aspartate, glutamine, and GABA. Together they make up more than half the total free amino acid content in brain.

Glutamate uniquely supports the respiration of incubated slices of brain

Radioactivity rapidly accumulates in brain glutamate after the administration of radioactive glucose. Very rapid isotopic equilibration occurs via the Krebs cycle and oxoglutarate-glutamate amino transfer. For net synthesis of glutamate, CO_2 fixation must occur, and this process has been shown to be present in brain. Although many studies have measured changes in glutamate under hypoglycemic and ischemic conditions, the role of glutamate in energy production in the brain has not been clearly established. This concept led to unsuccessful trials of glutamate feeding as a treatment for mental illness. It was demonstrated that such feeding is unable to elevate cerebral glutamate levels because of an effective blood-brain barrier to the entry of this amino acid. Both under normal conditions and in acute ammonia toxicity, the conversion of glutamate to glutamine is the main form of removal of cerebral ammonia. This glutamine is formed from the small, rapidly turning-over glutamate pool. There seems to be little capacity for adaptation to hyperammonemia in the brain [16].

Active protein metabolism in the brain results in a high rate of exchange between free and protein-bound amino acids

The half-life of free amino acids through exchange to protein-bound forms in brain is usually a few hours. Since the amount of the amino acid in protein is much larger than its free concentration, when a labeled amino acid is given, most of the label will be in the protein-bound form in a short time.

The content of free amino acids in the brain is maintained at fairly constant levels

In general, three groups can be distinguished: (1) the essential amino acids, which are present at fairly low levels, close to those in plasma; (2) the nonessential amino acids, which are present at concentrations several times higher than the essential ones; and (3) compounds present in brain but absent or at very low levels in most other organs, such as GABA and N-acetylaspartate [17].

The composition of the free amino acid pool, as shown in Table 1, is similar in most species [18]. The amino acid level is much lower in CSF than in brain, although the amino acid concentration in brain interstitial fluid may be similar to that of CSF. CSF amino acid levels are also lower than those in plasma. The amino acid composition of CSF is not parallel to that of brain; for example, there are high glutamine and low glutamate levels in the CSF, and the brain/CSF concentration ratio for glutamate is approximately 800. The free pool in brain also does not reflect the amino acid composition of the cerebral proteins. The amino acids are present at much higher levels in the protein-bound than in the free form. The concentration ratio of protein-bound, to free, amino acids in brain varies from 10 for glutamic acid to 1,800 for isoleucine. The amino acids present at high levels (glutamate, taurine, GABA, and glycine) are the most active pharmacologically. The amino acids are not all evenly distributed in the brain; for example, taurine and glutamic acid are much lower, and glycine is much higher in the midbrain and pons than in other areas. There

TABLE 1. Levels of free amino acids and related substances[a]

	Brain				Human		
	Cat	Rat	Carp	Monkey	Brain	CSF	Plasma
Glutamic acid	600	1,160	550	1,100	600	0.8	2
Taurine	130	660	480	180	93	0.6	6
N-Acetylaspartate	600	560	80		490		0
Glutamine	400	450	770	540	580	50	60
Aspartic acid	150	260	350	240	96	0.02	0.2
γ-Aminobutyric acid	88	230		94	42		0
Glycine	62	68	62	48	40	0.7	22
Alanine	50	65	66	25	25	2.6	35
Serine	52	98	33	45	44	2.5	11
Threonine	17	66	36	13	27	2.5	14
Lysine	10	21	34	10	12	2.1	19
Arginine	9	11	14	10	10	1.8	8
Histidine	13	5	36	8	9	1.3	9
Valine	13	7	15	4	13	1.6	23
Leucine	8	5	22	4	7	1.1	12
Isoleucine	5	2	13	2	3	0.4	6
Phenylalanine	4	5	13	4	5	0.8	5
Tyrosine	5	7	9	4	6	0.8	5
Proline	13	8	12	7	10		18
Methionine	1	4		2	3	0.3	2
Ornithine	4	2	7	3	3	0.6	5
Phosphoethanolamine	93	200	62	150	110		0.2
Cystathionine	21	2	32	4	200		
Homocarnosine	0.4	6		59	23		0
Glutathione	170	260		220	200	0.3	

[a] Values presented are averages from many publications and are expressed as μmol amino acid/100 g brain, or 100 ml CSF or plasma.

are further indications of differences among various cells, but they are not easy to establish. The methods for separation and isolation of cells and of particulate fractions such as synaptosomes include procedures that result in losses or redistribution of the soluble amino acids. Most amino acids are stable; since the formation of GABA from glutamic acid is very rapid, GABA levels determined postmortem are not accurate. With sensitive techniques, the distribution of the nonessential amino acids has been measured in as many as 50 different brain structures, and concentration ratios between the highest and the lowest levels are 3 to 10, but with the majority of areas being close. Levels in synaptosomes are similar to those measured for whole brain. Although some attempts have been made with nonaqueous separation methods or microdialysis to measure the extracellular amino acid levels, the available data are difficult to interpret. (The physiological activity of amino acids is further discussed in Chap. 15; regional differences in transport are discussed later.)

Less is known about the distribution of certain peptides, mainly because methods are not as well developed for their separation and detection, and they are usually present at very low levels. Only a few peptides, such as glutathione, are present at high levels in the brain. Interest in this class of compounds is great because of their physiological activity (see Chap. 14). It is likely that a large number of peptides, still un-identified, are present in the brain. There are indications that a number of peptides are present exclusively in brain. Many γ-glutamyl peptides are found, including γ-glutamyl deriv-atives of glutamate, glutamine, glycine, alanine, β-aminoisobutyric acid, serine, and valine. These peptides are present at levels of 10 to 700 mg/g fresh tissue, and they may be formed by transpeptidation reactions from glutathione. *N*-acetyl-aspartylglutamate is present in fairly large amounts (~10–30 mg/100 g fresh brain). No function has been attributed to this peptide, but it is known that it forms the N-terminal se-quence of the actin molecule in muscle, and it may play a similar role in one or more brain proteins.

Homocarnosine and homoanserine, two peptides of histidine, are also unique to brain. Homocarnosine is γ-aminobutyrylhistidine, the homolog of the long-known muscle constituent, β-alanyl-L-histidine (carnosine). Homoanser-ine, the γ-aminobutyryl homolog of anserine (β-alanyl-1-methyl-L-histidine) is also present. These histidine peptides are at much higher lev-els in this tissue than are their more widely dis-tributed relatives carnosine and anserine. Car-nosine is restricted primarily to the olfactory areas of the brain; in the rest of the brain, mainly homocarnosine is present. Since destruction of nasal epithelium results in a marked decrease of olfactory bulb carnosine, this compound might have a role in olfaction.

The composition of the free amino acid pool in peripheral nerve is different from that in the brain

Most amino acids in mammalian nerve are lower than in brain. GABA is almost absent in ver-tebrate peripheral nerve. In some crustacean species, a few specific compounds, such as as-partate, glycine, and alanine, are at very high levels. In other species the levels of com-pounds, such as taurine, are 10 to 100 times higher in peripheral nerve than in brain.

Components of the free amino acid pool undergo complex changes during the maturation of the brain

These changes are not strictly parallel in all brain regions; some are illustrated in Table 2. Quantitatively, the greatest changes are a de-crease in taurine and an increase in glutamate. These changes are gradual compared with the rapid decrease in alanine near the time of birth. Although such changes indicate developmental changes in metabolism (in the relative rates of various metabolic pathways), the connection between substrate levels and metabolism is not clear. It is tempting to theorize that the decrease in essential amino acids parallels the decrease in the rate of protein turnover, for example, but one does not necessarily lead to the other. Al-though changes in amino acid levels, after low-protein diets, result in changes in protein me-tabolism in a number of organs, such as muscle and liver, brain protein metabolism seems to be resistant. Of special importance are altera-

TABLE 2. Changes in amino acid levels during development[a]

	Fetal (15 day)	Newborn (1 day)	Adult
Taurine	14	16	8.0
Glutamate	7.5	5.0	12
Aspartate	2.4	2.3	3.8
Threonine	4.3	0.90	0.56
Proline	0.89	0.57	0.15
Glycine	2.26	2.30	1.27
Alanine	5.08	0.80	0.56
Leucine	0.53	0.18	0.06
Tyrosine	0.24	0.20	0.08
Phenylalanine	0.24	0.13	0.07
γ-Aminobutyric acid	0.50	1.62	2.37
Arginine	0.45	0.14	0.11

[a] Values are from mouse brain, expressed as μmol amino acid/g brain tissue.

tions in the levels of amino acids, such as ty-rosine and tryptophan, that serve as precursors of neurotransmitters. Developmental changes in GABA levels may influence seizure sensitivity, and region-specific decreases in GABA levels have been reported [18].

Brain amino acids are in dynamic equilibrium, undergoing rapid metabolism and rapid exchange with plasma amino acids

Flux of the essential amino acids is especially high, with a half-life (time for half of the brain content to be exchanged) of a few minutes. Isotopic equilibrium is reached rapidly; this indicates that amino acids do not have an inaccessible, nonexchangeable fraction, although they remain relatively constant in level, as discussed above. Their distribution is heterogeneous: there are differences in transport rate, metabolic rate, and metabolic use in various compartments—cellular, subcellular, or regional—reflecting the enzymatic, morphological, and functional heterogeneity of the brain. As discussed in Chapter 30, the carriers responsible for transporting the amino acid classes between blood and brain are close to saturation, and therefore the selective increase in a single amino acid alters the transport of other members of its class [19].

Although a general increase (for example, after a meal) of all related amino acids does not increase their brain levels, a selective increase in the blood level of an amino acid that is a neurotransmitter precursor can result in an increase of the cerebral level of both that amino acid and its product, the neurotransmitter. For example, the increase in plasma tryptophan after meals is not reflected in brain, because other related amino acids also increase in plasma, competing for the same transport system and mutually inhibiting one another's uptake. However, a selective increase of tryptophan, especially when accompanied by a

decrease in the level of competing amino acids, increases the cerebral levels of tryptophan and its metabolic products, such as serotonin [20]. Although variations in the level of essential amino acids in the brain may occur under special or extreme conditions, the penetration of nonessential amino acids into brain is much slower, and no change in brain content occurs, even during large blood level alterations of these compounds.

In severe malnutrition, the changes of the brain amino acid pools are rather specific: There is a large increase in histidine and homocarnosine [21], whereas some amino acids, such as valine, serine, and aspartate, decrease. In insulin hypoglycemia, the major changes are decreases of nonessential amino acids; most likely this reflects changes in the activity of the citric acid cycle. Hyperthyroidism increases most of the nonessential amino acids. In general, relatively small changes in the reaction rates involved in carbohydrate or energy metabolism do not affect the levels of cerebral amino acids, whereas major changes do, with primarily glutamate, aspartate, alanine, and GABA affected. In ischemia, hypoxia, and hypothermia, glutamate and aspartate decrease and GABA increases. Similar changes may be found in hibernating animals; on arousal, levels return to normal.

The changes are somewhat different in convulsions. In human epileptogenic brain tissue, the most consistent changes reported were decreases in glutamate and taurine and an increase in glycine. These changes were localized in areas of pathological changes; in surrounding areas, aspartate and GABA levels were also reduced [22]. Such changes could be reproduced in experimentally induced convulsive states. On the administration of taurine, amino acid levels tended to return to normal. In induced convulsions, such changes also depend on the convulsant used: Pentamethylenetetrazole causes an increase in alanine (interference with the entry of pyruvate into the citric acid cycle); inhibitors of glutamic acid dehydrogenase (GAD) result in increased levels of glutamate.

Drugs have also been reported to affect the levels of nonessential amino acids. Chlorpromazine can lower glutamate, aspartate, and GABA; drugs, such as reserpine and 6-hydroxydopamine, that alter catecholamine metabolism have similar effects. Ethanol is reported to reduce GABA levels [18]. Some anticonvulsant drugs increase GABA levels, whereas some that inhibit GABA formation are convulsants [23].

Elevated levels of circulating ammonia are known to cause large increases in the level of brain glutamine. Loss of liver function in humans, which prevents the normal detoxification of ammonia, leads to ammoniagenic coma and increased levels of glutamine in the CSF. It has been suggested that this causes depletion of Krebs cycle intermediates in brain, thus leading to decreased oxidation and energy production; however, the demonstration that ammonia stimulates the flux of glucose through the Krebs cycle in brain contradicts this suggestion.

SPECIFIC AMINO ACID TRANSPORT SYSTEMS

The existence of transport classes is not specific for the brain, and many of the classes found in brain have the properties of these systems in other organs. In brain cells more than ten transport classes can be identified, with some overlap. Some of these have not yet been observed in other tissues. Some are specific for one type of amino acid: small neutral, large neutral, acidic, or basic. Others are fairly specific for a single amino acid: glycine, proline, GABA, taurine, or lysine [24]. *In vivo*, the transport by brain capillaries appears to utilize only three classes—large neutral, large basic, and acidic (see Chaps. 15 and 30). Diffusion of the nontransported amino acids into brain is a much slower process than transport, and it can occur

only in the direction from higher to lower concentration. The high rate of cellular transport for the nonessential amino acids, combined with low capillary transport of the same compounds, is specific for brain.

There is overlap among the classes because some amino acids have an affinity for more than one carrier. In substrate specificity, the transport classes in brain are similar, but not identical, to those described in other systems.

In addition to the transport classes discussed above, which have relatively low affinity, amino acid transport classes with high affinity and high substrate specificity have been described in brain. These classes have been found primarily in synaptosomal preparations. It was proposed that the low-affinity ($K_m \simeq 10^{-3}$ M), more generally distributed transport systems serve metabolic functions; the high-affinity ($K_m \simeq 10^{-5}$ M) systems remove the physiologically active (neurotransmitter) amino acids. This high-affinity transport was suggested as another criterion for assignment of neurotransmitter function. It was found for a number of amino acids in the brain, including glutamate, aspartate, GABA, glycine, proline, tryptophan, and taurine, each of which is also a substrate for low-affinity transport. Although the suggestion of high-affinity transport as a special mechanism for the removal of neurotransmitters in instances where metabolic inactivation is not sufficient is very attractive, there are indications of other functions for this process. The distribution of high-affinity systems does not seem to be highly specific; for example, high-affinity tryptophan uptake does not follow the serotonergic system or serotonin receptor binding, and a number of high-affinity systems, such as that for taurine, are present in glial and in neuronal cells. Furthermore, high-affinity uptake is found for such nonneurotransmitter amino acids as leucine and in other tissues as liver and heart. In spite of these findings indicating possible additional roles for the high-affinity uptake, the fact that these systems for the neurotransmitter amino acids are present primarily in synaptic or postsynaptic structures, and there they are the predominant transport system, indicates that they are likely to be a mechanism for amino acid removal.

Stereospecificity is not absolute: D amino acids are transported in most cases, but at considerably lower levels than are the L isomers. Despite this, some D amino acids can penetrate the brain. Although their uptake is slower, so is their exit, thus leading to slow accumulation. This again illustrates that both uptake and exit influence the levels of compounds. The amino acid concentration within brain cells is generally higher than in brain interstitial fluid. This indicates that transport into the cells occurs against a concentration gradient. Such transport requires energy. The primary source of the energy that fuels active amino acid transport is not known. Inhibitors of metabolic energy also inhibit amino acid uptake, and in many cases, but not all, the decrease in ATP levels is accompanied by a decrease in uptake. Such inhibition, however, may be indirect.

There is evidence that Na^+ electrochemical gradients may be a driving force for transport of selected amino acids. Not all compounds show the same dependence on Na^+: Diamine uptake is independent, and basic amino acid uptake is only partially dependent on Na^+ levels. Thus, lowering Na^+ does not affect all amino acids to the same degree. The Na^+ dependence of high-affinity uptake appears to be greater than that of low-affinity uptake. The Na^+ dependence of low-affinity systems is variable, those participating more in exchange having lower or no Na^+ dependence. Although other ions (probably K^+, possibly Ca^{2+}) may also influence transport, Na^+ seems to be a primary factor. The ion cotransport ratio was measured in GABA uptake in various neuronal, glial, and synaptosomal preparations, and some variations in the GABA-Na^+ cotransport coupling ratio were found, with 1:1 in astrocytes and 1:3

in neurons. The fact that several ratios were found indicates that GABA transport properties are modulated in different systems, but also that more than one GABA transport system may be present.

Transport of amino acids in brain changes during development

The composition of the brain, including the free amino acid pool, undergoes large changes during development as described earlier (Table 2). Permeability is generally greater in young than in adult brain. The developing brain therefore is not as well protected as the mature brain from fluctuations in plasma metabolite levels and from foreign substances, such as drugs. Although developmental changes in the free pool and in permeability to amino acids have been studied in detail, changes in amino acid transport are not as well documented.

Elevation of most amino acids in plasma causes a greater elevation of levels in brain in young, compared with adult, animals; however, barriers and transport processes are not entirely absent in the immature brain. For example, amino acid levels in fetal brain differ from those in fetal blood. As in adults, the barrier to nonessential amino acid penetration into the young brain is greater than the barrier to essential amino acids. Many transport processes develop rapidly and are present at early developmental stages. The transport systems for neurotransmitters develop somewhat later. Transport properties, such as apparent affinity (K_m), usually show no developmental alterations; GABA is an exception to this rule, with one GABA transport system present in immature cells that disappears during development. Capillary transport activity, like capillary permeability, is greater in the immature brain, perhaps reflecting the increased need for amino acid supply during growth.

Distribution, especially of nonessential amino acids, is heterogeneous within the brain

Only gross distribution has been studied, but there are indications that the amino acid pool in neurons is different from that in glia and that additional differences exist between nuclear and mitochondrial compartments. Lysosomes, in which protein degradation takes place, and the nerve-ending region, where release and removal of neurotransmitter amino acids take place, also represent special compartments. The indications are that GABA transport and glutamine transport in neurons are different from that in glial cells. Possibly, high-affinity glutamate uptake is present mostly in the glutamatergic cells or in glia near such cells.

Perhaps the most heterogeneous distribution of transport systems is represented by the high-affinity transport in synaptosomes. Synaptosomes containing the high-affinity glutamate system are distinct from those containing the GABA system; and synaptosomes from spinal cord, but not those from brain, contain the glycine system [25].

Amino acid transport may influence brain development

It seems that the period most sensitive to amino acid transport occurs when cell division takes place; this is also the period during which recovery can occur. Protein deficiency throughout the active mitotic period results in a permanent decrease in brain cell number and protein content [26]. Learning deficiencies are also seen; such deficiencies may carry over to the progeny, even if they are all well–nourished (see also Chap. 38).

In contrast, in adult protein deficiency, brain protein content is maintained despite the decrease of proteins in most other organs. This is thought to be the consequence of a more active amino acid transport in the adult brain that maintains the free amino acid pool to a greater degree than in other organs [17]. Pathological changes in protein metabolism could alter the free amino acid pool, since the major portion of amino acids is protein bound; for example, a net protein breakdown of 1 percent would increase most amino acids severalfold. An important, but still undecided, question concerns what effect an altered amino acid pool has on brain function. Brain protein synthesis in general is not sensitive to alteration of amino acid levels, and it is most likely that changes that alter neurotransmitters are of greater functional importance.

REFERENCES

1. Maker, H. S., and Nicklas, W. Biochemical responses of body organs to hypoxia and ischemia. In E. D. Robin (ed.), *Extrapulmonary Manifestations of Respiratory Disease.* New York: Dekker, 1978, pp. 107–150.
2. Gatfield, P. D., et al. Regional energy reserves in mouse brain and changes with ischaemia and anaesthesia. *J. Neurochem.* 13:185–195, 1966.
3. Lowry, O. H., and Passonneau, J. V. The relationships between substrates and enzymes of glycolysis in brain. *J. Biol. Chem.* 239:31–32, 1964.
4. Meyer, R. A., and Sweeney, H. L. A simple analysis of the "phospho creatine shuttle." *Am. J. Physiol.* 246:365–377, 1984.
5. Stewart, M. A., and Moonsammy, G. I. Substrate changes in peripheral nerve recovering from anoxia. *J. Neurochem.* 13:1433–1439, 1966.
6. Pardridge, W. M. Brain metabolism: a perspective from the blood-brain barrier. *Physiol. Rev.* 63:1481–1535, 1983.
7. Goldberg, N. D., and O'Toole, A. G. The properties of glycogen synthetase and regulation of glycogen biosynthesis in rat brain. *J. Biol. Chem.* 244:3053–3061, 1969.
8. Lehninger, A. L. *Biochemistry.* New York: Worth, 1982.

9. Morgan-Hughes, J. A. Mitochondrial disease. *Trends Neurosci.* 9:15–19, 1986.

10. Gaitonde, M. K., Evison, E., and Evans, G. M. The rate of utilization of glucose via hexose-monophosphate shunt in brain. *J. Neurochem.* 41:1253–1260, 1983.

11. Muir, D., Berl, S., and Clarke, D. D. Acetate and fluoroacetate as possible markers for glia metabolism *in vivo*. *Brain Res.* 380:336–340, 1986.

12. Leong, S. F., Lai, J. C. K., Lim, L., and Clark, J. B. The activities of some energy-metabolizing enzymes in non synaptic (free) and synaptic mitochondria derived from selected brain regions. *J. Neurochem.* 42:1308–1312, 1984.

13. Smith, F. W. Nuclear magnetic resonance in the investigation of cerebral disorder. *J. Cereb. Blood Flow Metab.* 3:263–267, 1983.

14. Cunningham, V. J., and Cremer, J. E. Current assumptions behind the use of PET scanning for measuring glucose utilization in brain. *Trends Neurosci.* 8:96–99, 1985.

15. Nelson, T., Lucignani, G., Goochee, J., Crane, A. M., and Sokoloff, L. Invalidity of criticism of the deoxyglucose method based on alleged glucose-6-phosphatase activity in brain. *J. Neurochem.* 46:905–919, 1986.

16. Cooper, A. J. L., Mora, S. N., Cruz, N. F., and Gelbard, A. S. Cerebral ammonia metabolism in hyperammonemic rats. *J. Neurochem.* 44:1716–1723, 1985.

17. Gaull, G. E., et al. Pathogenesis of brain dysfunction in inborn errors of amino acid metabolism. In G. E. Gaull (ed.), *Biology of Brain Dysfunction*. New York: Plenum, 1974, Vol. 3, pp. 47–143.

18. Perry, T. L. Cerebral amino acid pools. In A. Lajtha (ed.), *Handbook of Neurochemistry*. New York: Plenum, 1982, Vol. 1, pp. 151–180.

19. Miller, L. P., Pardridge, W. M., Braun, L. D., and Oldendorf, W. H. Kinetic constants for blood-brain barrier amino acid transport in conscious rats. *J. Neurochem.* 45:1427–1432, 1985.

20. Fernstrom, J. D., et al. Nutritional control of the synthesis of 5-hydroxytryptamine in the brain. In G. E. W. Wolstenholme and D. W. Fitzsimons (eds.), *Aromatic Amino Acids in the Brain (CIBA Foundation Symposium 22)*. New York: American Elsevier, 1974, pp. 153–173.

21. Enwonwu, C. O., and Worthington, B. S. Regional distribution of homocarnosine and other ninhydrin-positive substances in brains of malnourished monkeys. *J. Neurochem.* 22:1045–1052, 1974.

22. Perry, T. L., and Hansen, S. Amino acid abnormalities in epileptogenic foci. *Neurology* 31:872–876, 1981.

23. Seiler, N., and Sarhan, S. Drugs affecting GABA. In L. Battistin, G. Hashim, and A. Lajtha (eds.), *Neurochemistry and Clinical Neurology*. New York: Alan R. Liss, 1980, pp. 425–439.

24. Lajtha, A. Amino acid transport in the brain *in vivo* and *in vitro*. In *Aromatic Amino Acids in the Brain (CIBA Foundation Symposium 22)*. New York: American Elsevier, 1974, pp. 25–49.

25. Snyder, S. H., et al. Synaptic biochemistry of amino acids. *Fed. Proc.* 32:2039–2047, 1973.

26. Winick, M. Malnutrition and the developing brain. *Res. Publ. Assoc. Res. Nerv. Ment. Dis.* 53:253–261, 1974.

CHAPTER 29

Circulation and Energy Metabolism of the Brain

Louis Sokoloff

Basic Neurochemistry: Molecular, Cellular, and Medical Aspects, 4th Ed., edited by G. J. Siegel et al. Raven Press, Ltd., New York, 1989. Correspondence to Louis Sokoloff, Laboratory of Cerebral Metabolism, National Institute of Mental Health, 9000 Rockville Pike, Building 36, Room 1A-05, Bethesda, Maryland 20892.

The biochemical pathways of energy metabolism in the brain are in most respects like those of other tissues, but special conditions peculiar to the central nervous system *in vivo* limit full expression of its biochemical potentialities. In no tissue are the discrepancies between *in vivo* and *in vitro* properties greater or the extrapolations from *in vitro* data to conclusions about *in vivo* metabolic functions more hazardous. Valid identification of the normally used substrates and products of cerebral energy metabolism, as well as reliable estimations of their rates of utilization and production, can be obtained only in the intact animal; *in vitro* studies serve to identify pathways of intermediary metabolism, mechanisms, and potential, rather than actual, performance.

DIFFERENCES BETWEEN *IN VITRO* AND *IN VIVO* BRAIN METABOLISM

In addition to the usual differences between *in vitro* and *in vivo* studies that pertain to all tissues, there are two unique conditions that pertain only to the central nervous system. First, in contrast to cells of other tissues, individual nerve cells do not function autonomously. They are generally so incorporated into a complex neural network that their functional activity is integrated with that of various other parts of the central nervous system and, indeed, with somatic tissues as well. Any procedure that interrupts the structural and functional integrity of the network or isolates the tissue from its normal functional interrelationships would inevitably grossly alter, at least quantitatively and, perhaps, even qualitatively, its normal metabolic behavior. Second, the phenomenon of the blood-brain barrier selectively limits the rates of transfer of soluble substances between blood and brain (see Chap. 30). This barrier, which probably developed phylogenetically to protect the brain against noxious substances, serves also to discriminate among various potential substrates for cerebral metabolism. The substrate function is confined to those compounds in the blood which are not only suitable substrates for cerebral enzymes, but can also penetrate from blood to the brain at rates adequate to support the brain's considerable energy demands. Substances that can be readily oxidized by brain slices, minces, or homogenates *in vitro* and that are effectively utilized *in vivo* when formed endogenously within the brain are often incapable of supporting cerebral energy metabolism and function when present in the blood because of restricted passage through the blood-brain barrier. The *in vitro* techniques establish only the existence and potential capacity of the enzyme systems required for the utilization of a given substrate; they do not define the extent to which such a pathway is actually utilized *in vivo*. This can be done only by studies in the intact animal, and it is this aspect of cerebral metabolism with which this chapter is concerned.

STUDIES OF CEREBRAL METABOLISM *IN VIVO*

The variety of methods that have been used to study the metabolism of the brain *in vivo* vary in complexity and in the degree to which they yield quantitative results. Some require such minimal operative procedures on the laboratory animal that no anesthesia is required, and there is no interference with the tissue except for the effects of the particular experimental condition being studied. Some of these techniques are applicable to normal, conscious human subjects, and consecutive and comparative studies can be made repeatedly in the same subject. Other methods are more traumatic and either require killing the animal or involve such extensive surgical intervention and tissue damage that the experiments approach an *in vitro* experiment carried out *in situ*. All, however, are capable of providing specific and useful information.

Behavior and central nervous system physiology are correlated with blood and cerebrospinal fluid chemical changes

The simplest way to study the metabolism of the central nervous system *in vivo* is to correlate spontaneous or experimentally produced alterations in the chemical composition of the blood, spinal fluid, or both, with changes in cerebral physiological functions or gross central nervous system-mediated behavior. The level of consciousness, reflex behavior, or the electroencephalogram (EEG) is generally used to monitor the effects of the chemical changes on the functional and metabolic activities of the brain. For example, such methods first demonstrated the need for glucose as a substrate for cerebral energy metabolism. Hypoglycemia produced by insulin or other means altered various parameters of cerebral function that could not be restored to normal by the administration of substances other than glucose.

The chief virtue of these methods is their simplicity, but they are gross and nonspecific and do not distinguish between direct effects of the agent on cerebral metabolism and those secondary to changes produced initially in somatic tissues. Also, negative results are often inconclusive, for there always remain questions of insufficient dosage, inadequate cerebral circulation and delivery to the tissues, or impermeability of the blood-brain barrier.

Brain samples are removed for biochemical analyses

The availability of analytical chemical techniques makes it possible to measure specific metabolites and enzyme activities in brain tissue at selected times during or after exposure of the animal to an experimental condition. This approach has been very useful in studies of the intermediary metabolism of the brain. It has permitted the estimation of the rates of flux through the various steps of established metabolic pathways and the identification of control points in the pathways where regulation may be exerted. Such studies have helped to define more precisely the changes in energy metabolism associated with altered cerebral functions produced, for example, by anesthesia, convulsions, or hypoglycemia. Although these methods require killing the animal and analyzing tissue samples, they are *in vivo* methods in effect since they attempt to describe the state of the tissue while it is still in the animal at the moment of killing. These methods have encountered their most serious problems with regard to this point. Postmortem changes in brain are extremely rapid and are not always completely retarded, even by the most rapid freezing techniques available. These methods have proved to be very valuable, nevertheless, particularly in the area of energy metabolism.

Radioisotope incorporation can identify and measure routes of metabolism

The technique of administering radioactive precursors, followed by the chemical separation and assay of products in the tissue, has added greatly to the armamentarium for studying cerebral metabolism *in vivo*. Labeled precursors are administered by any one of a variety of routes. At selected later times the brain is removed, and the precursor and the various products of interest are isolated. The radioactivity and quantity of the compounds in question are assayed. Such techniques facilitate the identification of metabolic routes and the rates of flux through various steps of the pathway. In some cases, comparison of the specific activities of the products and precursors has led to the surprising finding of higher specific activities in the products than in the precursors. This is conclusive evidence of the presence of compartmentation. These methods have been used effectively in studies of amine and neurotransmitter synthesis and metabolism, lipid metabolism, protein synthesis, amino acid metabolism, and the distribution of glucose carbon through the various biochemical pathways present in the brain.

Radioisotope incorporation methods are particularly valuable for studies of intermediary metabolism that generally are not feasible by most other *in vivo* techniques. They are without equal for the qualitative identification of the pathways and routes of metabolism. They suffer, however, from several disadvantages. Only one set of measurements per animal is possible because the animal must be killed. Quantitative interpretations are often confounded by the problems of compartmentation. Also, they are all too frequently misused; unfortunately, quantitative conclusions are often drawn on the basis

of radioactivity data without appropriate consideration of the specific activities (ratio of radioactivity to pool size) of the precursor pools.

Oxygen utilization in the cortex is measured by polarographic techniques

The oxygen electrode has been employed for measuring the amount of oxygen consumed locally in the cerebral cortex *in vivo* [1]. The electrode is applied to the surface of the exposed cortex, and the local partial pressure for oxygen (P_{O_2}) is measured continuously before and during occlusion of the blood flow to the local area. During occlusion, the P_{O_2} falls linearly as the oxygen is consumed by the tissue metabolism, and the rate of fall is a measure of the rate of oxygen consumption locally in the cortex. Repeated measurements can be made successively in the animal, and the technique has been used to demonstrate the increased oxygen consumption of the cerebral cortex and the relation between the changes in the EEG and the metabolic rate during convulsions [1]. The technique is limited to measurements in the cortex and, of course, to oxygen utilization.

Arteriovenous differences identify substances consumed or produced by brain

The primary function of the circulation is to replenish the nutrients consumed by the tissues and to remove the products of their metabolism. This function is reflected in the composition of the blood traversing the tissue. Substances taken up by the tissue from the blood are higher in concentration in the arterial inflow than in the venous outflow, and the converse is true for substances released by the tissue. The convention is to subtract the venous concentration from the arterial concentration so that a positive arteriovenous difference represents net uptake and a negative difference means net release. In nonsteady states, as after a perturbation, there may be transient arteriovenous differences that reflect changes in tissue concentrations and reequilibration of the tissue with the blood. In steady states, in which it is presumed that the tissue concentration remains constant, positive and negative arteriovenous differences mean net consumption or production of the substance by the tissue, respectively. Zero arteriovenous differences indicate neither consumption nor production. This method is useful for all substances in blood that can be assayed with enough accuracy, precision, and sensitivity to enable the detection of arteriovenous differences. The method is useful only for tissues from which mixed representative venous blood can be sampled. Arterial blood has essentially the same composition throughout and can be sampled from any artery. In contrast, venous blood is specific for each tissue, and to establish valid arteriovenous differences, the venous blood must represent the total outflow or the flow-weighted average of all the venous outflows from the tissue under study, uncontaminated by blood from any other tissue. It is not possible to fulfill this condition for many tissues.

The method is fully applicable to the brain, particularly in humans, in whom the anatomy of venous drainage is favorable for such studies. Representative cerebral venous blood, with no more than approximately 3 percent contamination with extracerebral blood, is readily obtained from the superior bulb of the internal jugular vein in humans. The venipuncture can be made percutaneously under local anesthesia, and the measurements can therefore be made during the conscious state undistorted by the effects of general anesthesia. The monkey is similar, although the vein must be surgically exposed before puncture. Other common laboratory animals are less suitable because extensive communication between cerebral and extracerebral venous beds is present, and uncontaminated representative venous blood is difficult to obtain from the cerebrum without major sur-

gical intervention. In these cases, one can sample blood from the confluence of the sinuses (torcular Herophili), even though it does not contain fully representative blood from the brain stem and some of the lower portions of the brain.

The chief advantages of these methods are their simplicity and applicability to unanesthetized humans. They permit the qualitative identification of the ultimate substrates and products of cerebral metabolism. They have no applicability, however, to those intermediates that are formed and consumed entirely within the brain without being exchanged with blood, or to those substances that are exchanged between brain and blood with no net flux in either direction. Furthermore, they provide no quantification of the rates of utilization or production because arteriovenous differences depend not only on the rates of consumption or production by the tissue but also on blood flow (see below). Blood flow affects all the arteriovenous differences proportionately, however, and comparison of the arteriovenous differences of various substances obtained from the same samples of blood reflects their relative rates of utilization or production.

Combining cerebral blood flow and arteriovenous differences permits measurement of rates of consumption or production of substances by brain

In a steady state the tissue concentration of any substance utilized or produced by the brain is presumed to remain constant. When a substance is exchanged between brain and blood, the difference in its steady state of delivery to the brain in the arterial blood and removal in the venous blood must be equal to the net rate of its utilization or production by the brain. This relation can be expressed as follows:

$$CMR = CBF(A - V)$$

where $(A - V)$ is the difference in concentration in arterial and cerebral venous blood; CBF is the rate of cerebral blood flow in volume of blood per unit time; and CMR (cerebral metabolic rate) is the steady-state rate of utilization or production of the substance by the brain.

If both the rate of cerebral blood flow and the arteriovenous difference are known, the net rate of utilization or production of the substance by the brain can be calculated. This has been the basis of most quantitative studies of the cerebral metabolism *in vivo*.

The most reliable method for determining cerebral blood flow is the inert gas method of Kety and Schmidt [2]. It was originally designed for use in studies of conscious, unanesthetized humans, and it has been most widely employed for this purpose; but it also has been adapted for use in animals. The method is based on the Fick principle (i.e., the law of conservation of matter), and it utilizes low concentrations of a freely diffusible, chemically inert gas as a tracer substance. The original gas was nitrous oxide, but subsequent modifications have substituted other gases, such as ^{85}Kr, ^{79}Kr, or hydrogen, that can be measured more conveniently in blood. During a period of inhalation of 15 percent N_2O in air, for example, timed arterial and cerebral venous blood samples are withdrawn and analyzed for their N_2O content. The cerebral blood flow (in milliliters per 100 grams of brain tissue per minute) can be calculated from the following equation:

$$CBF = \frac{100\lambda V_T}{\int_0^T (A - V)\, dt}$$

where A and V are the arterial and cerebral venous blood concentrations of N_2O, respectively; V_T is the concentration of N_2O in venous blood at the end of a period of inhalation (i.e., time T); λ is the partition coefficient for N_2O between brain tissue and blood; t is variable time in minutes; T is the total period of inha-

lation of N_2O, usually 10 min or more; and $\int_0^T (A - V)\, dt$ is the integrated arteriovenous difference in N_2O concentrations over the total period of inhalation.

The partition coefficient for N_2O is approximately 1 when equilibrium has been achieved between blood and brain tissue; at least 10 min of inhalation are required to approach equilibrium. At the end of this interval, the N_2O concentration in brain tissue is about equal to the cerebral venous blood concentration.

Because the method requires sampling of both arterial and cerebral venous blood, it lends itself readily to the simultaneous measurement of arteriovenous differences of substances involved in cerebral metabolism. This method and its modifications have provided most of our knowledge of the rates of substrate utilization or product formation by the brain *in vivo*.

REGULATION OF CEREBRAL METABOLIC RATE

Brain consumes about one-fifth of total body oxygen utilization

The brain is metabolically one of the most active of all the organs in the body. This is reflected in its relatively enormous rate of oxygen consumption, which provides the energy required for its intense physicochemical activity. The most reliable data on cerebral metabolic rate have been obtained in humans. Cerebral oxygen consumption in normal, conscious, young men is approximately 3.5 ml/100 g brain/min (Table 1); the rate is similar in young women. The rate of oxygen consumption by an entire brain of average weight (1,400 g) is then approximately 49 ml O_2/min. The magnitude of this rate can be more fully appreciated when it is compared with the metabolic rate of the body as a whole. The average man weighs 70 kg and consumes

TABLE 1. Cerebral blood flow and metabolic rate in normal young adult man[a]

Function	Rate	
	Per 100 g brain tissue	Per whole brain[b]
Cerebral blood flow (ml/min)	57	798
Cerebral O_2 consumption (ml/min)	3.5	49
Cerebral glucose utilization (mg/min)	5.5	77

[a] Based on data derived from literature [3].
[b] Brain weight assumed to be 1,400 g.

approximately 250 ml O_2/min in the basal state. Therefore, the brain alone, which represents only approximately 2 percent of total body weight, accounts for 20 percent of the resting total body oxygen consumption. In children the brain takes an even larger fraction, as much as 50 percent in the middle of the first decade of life [4].

Oxygen is utilized in the brain almost entirely for the oxidation of carbohydrates [3]. The energy equivalent of the total cerebral metabolic rate is therefore approximately 20 watts, or 0.25 kcal/min. If it is assumed that this energy is utilized mainly for the synthesis of high-energy phosphate bonds, that the efficiency of the energy conservation is approximately 20 percent, and that the free energy of hydrolysis of the terminal phosphate of ATP is approximately 7 kcal/mol, this energy expenditure can then be estimated to support the steady turnover of close to 7 mmol, or approximately 4×10^{21} molecules of ATP per minute in the entire human brain.

The brain normally has no respite from this enormous energy demand. The cerebral oxygen consumption continues unabated day and night. Even during sleep there is only a relatively small decrease in cerebral metabolic rate; indeed, it may even be increased in rapid eye movement (REM) sleep (see below).

What are the energy-demanding functions of the brain?

The brain does not do mechanical work, like that of cardiac and skeletal muscle, or osmotic work, as the kidney does in concentrating urine. It does not have the complex energy-consuming metabolic functions of liver nor, despite the synthesis of some hormones and neurotransmitters, is it noted for its biosynthetic activities. Recently, considerable emphasis has been placed on the extent of macromolecular synthesis in the central nervous system, an interest stimulated by the recognition that there are some proteins with short half-lives in the brain. These represent relatively small numbers of molecules, and, in fact, the average protein turnover and the rate of protein synthesis in the mature brain are slower than in most other tissues except, perhaps, muscle. Clearly, the functions of nervous tissues are mainly excitation and conduction, and these are reflected in the unceasing electrical activity of the brain. The electrical energy is ultimately derived from chemical processes, and it is likely that most of the brain's energy consumption is used for active transport of ions to sustain and restore the membrane potentials discharged during the process of excitation and conduction (see Chap. 3).

Not all of the oxygen consumption of the brain is used for energy metabolism. The brain contains a variety of oxidases and hydroxylases that function in the synthesis and metabolism of a number of neurotransmitters. For example, tyrosine hydroxylase is a mixed-function oxidase that hydroxylates tyrosine to 3,4-dihydroxyphenylalanine (DOPA), and dopamine-β-hydroxylase hydroxylates dopamine to form norepinephrine. Similarly, tryptophan hydroxylase hydroxylates tryptophan to form 5-hydroxytryptophan in the pathway of serotonin synthesis. These enzymes are oxygenases, which utilize molecular oxygen and incorporate it into the hydroxyl group of the hydroxylated products. Oxygen is also consumed in the me-

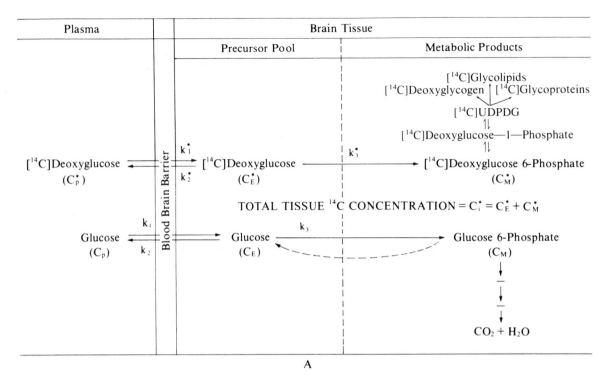

A

General equation for measurement of reaction rates with tracers:

$$\text{Rate of reaction} = \frac{\text{Labeled Product Formed in Interval of Time, 0 to T}}{\begin{bmatrix}\text{Isotope effect} \\ \text{correction factor}\end{bmatrix}\begin{bmatrix}\text{Integrated specific activity} \\ \text{of precursor}\end{bmatrix}}$$

Operational equation of [^{14}C]deoxyglucose method:

Labeled Product Formed in Interval of Time, 0 to T

Total ^{14}C in tissue at time T ^{14}C in precursor remaining in tissue at time T

$$R_i = \frac{C_i^*(T) - k_1^* e^{-(k_2^*+k_3^*)T}\int_0^T C_p^* e^{(k_2^*+k_3^*)t}\, dt}{\left[\dfrac{\lambda \cdot V_m^* \cdot K_m}{\Phi \cdot V_m \cdot K_m^*}\right]\left[\displaystyle\int_0^T \left(\frac{C_p^*}{C_p}\right)dt - e^{-(k_2^*+k_3^*)T}\int_0^T \left(\frac{C_p^*}{C_p}\right)e^{(k_2^*+k_3^*)t}\, dt\right]}$$

Isotope effect correction factor

Integrated plasma specific activity

Correction for lag in tissue equilibration with plasma

Integrated precursor specific activity in tissue

B

tabolism of these monamine neurotransmitters, which are oxidatively deaminated to their respective aldehydes by monamine oxidases. All of these enzymes are present in brain, and the reactions catalyzed by them utilize oxygen. When, however, the total turnover rates of the neurotransmitters and the sum total of the maximal velocities of all the oxidases involved in their synthesis and degradation are considered, it is clear that the oxygen consumed in the turnover of the neurotransmitters can account for only a very small, possibly immeasurable, fraction of the total oxygen consumption of the brain.

Continuous cerebral circulation is absolutely required to provide sufficient oxygen

Not only does the brain utilize oxygen at a very rapid rate, but it is absolutely dependent on continuously uninterrupted oxidative metabolism for maintenance of its functional and structural integrity. There is a large Pasteur effect in brain tissue, but even at its maximum rate anaerobic glycolysis is unable to provide sufficient energy to meet the brain's demands. Since the oxygen stored in the brain is extremely small compared to its rate of utilization, the brain requires the continuous replenishment of its oxygen by the circulation. If cerebral blood flow is completely interrupted, consciousness is lost within less than 10 sec, or the amount of time required to consume the oxygen contained within the brain and its blood content. Loss of consciousness as a result of anoxemia, caused by anoxia or asphyxia, takes only a little longer because of the additional oxygen present in the lungs and still-circulating blood. There is evidence that the average critical level of oxygen tension in the brain tissues, below which consciousness and the normal EEG pattern are invariably lost, lies between 15 and 20 mm Hg. This appears to be so whether the tissue anoxia is achieved by lowering the cerebral blood flow or the arterial oxygen content. Cessation of cerebral blood flow is followed within a few minutes by irreversible pathological changes within the brain, readily demonstrated by microscopic anatomical techniques. It is well known, of course, that in medical crises, such as cardiac arrest, damage to the brain occurs earliest and is most decisive in determining the degree of recovery.

The cerebral blood flow must be able to maintain the brain's avaricious appetite for oxygen. The average rate of blood flow in the human brain as a whole is approximately 57 ml/100 g tissue/min (see Table 1). For the whole brain this amounts to almost 800 ml/min, or approximately 15 percent of the total basal cardiac output. This level must be maintained within relatively narrow limits, for the brain cannot tol-

FIG. 1. Theoretical basis of radioactive deoxyglucose method for measurement of local cerebral glucose utilization. **A:** Theoretical model: (C_i^*) total ^{14}C concentration in a single homogeneous tissue of the brain; (C_p^*, C_p) concentrations of $[^{14}C]$deoxyglucose and glucose in the arterial plasma, respectively; (C_E^*, C_E) respective concentrations in the tissue pools that serve as substrates for hexokinase; (C_M^*) concentration of $[^{14}C]$deoxyglucose-6-phosphate in the tissue; (k_1^*, k_2^*, k_3^*) rate constants for carrier-mediated transport of $[^{14}C]$deoxyglucose from plasma to tissue, for carrier-mediated transport back from tissue to plasma, and for phosphorylation by hexokinase, respectively; (k_1, k_2, k_3) equivalent rate constants for glucose. $[^{14}C]$Deoxyglucose and glucose share and compete for the carrier that transports them both between plasma and tissue and for hexokinase, which phosphorylates them to their respective hexose-6-phosphates; *dashed arrow* represents the possibility of glucose-6-phosphate hydrolysis by glucose-6-phosphatase activity, if any. UDPDG, UDP-deoxyglucose. **B:** Functional anatomy of the operational equation of the radioactive deoxyglucose method: (T) time at the termination of the experimental period; (λ) ratio of the distribution space of deoxyglucose in the tissue to that of glucose; (Φ) fraction of glucose, which, once phosphorylated, continues down the glycolytic pathway; (K_m^*, V_m^*, K_m, V_m) familiar Michaelis-Menten kinetic constants of hexokinase for deoxyglucose and glucose, respectively; other symbols are as defined in **A**. (From Sokoloff et al. [7].)

erate any major drop in its perfusion. A fall in cerebral blood flow to half of its normal rate is sufficient to cause loss of consciousness in normal, healthy young men. There are, fortunately, numerous reflexes and other physiological mechanisms to sustain adequate levels of arterial blood pressure at the head level (e.g., baroreceptor reflexes) and to maintain the cerebral blood flow, even when arterial pressure falls in times of stress (e.g., autoregulation). There are also mechanisms to adjust the cerebral blood flow to changes in cerebral metabolic demand.

Regulation of the cerebral blood flow is achieved mainly by control of the tone or the degree of constriction or dilatation of the cerebral vessels. This, in turn, is controlled mainly by local chemical factors, such as P_{CO_2}, P_{O_2}, pH, and still unrecognized factors. High P_{CO_2}, low P_{O_2}, and low pH—products of metabolic activity—tend to dilate the blood vessels and increase cerebral blood flow; changes in the opposite direction constrict the vessels and decrease blood flow [5]. Cerebral blood flow is regulated through such mechanisms to maintain homeostasis of these chemical factors in the local tissue. The rates of production of these chemical factors depend on the rates of energy metabolism, and cerebral blood flow is therefore also adjusted to the cerebral metabolic rate [5].

Local rates of cerebral blood flow and metabolism can be measured by autoradiography and are shown to be coupled to local brain function

The rates of blood flow and metabolism presented in Table 1 and discussed above represent the average values in the brain as a whole. The brain is not a homogeneous organ, however; it is composed of a variety of tissues and discrete structures that often function independently or even inversely with respect to one another. There is little reason to expect that their per-

fusion and metabolic rates would be similar. Indeed, experimental evidence clearly indicates that they are not. Local cerebral blood flow in laboratory animals has been determined from local tissue concentrations, measured by a quantitative autoradiographic technique, and from the total history of the arterial concentration of a freely diffusible, chemically inert, radioactive tracer introduced into the circulation [6]. The results reveal that blood flow rates vary widely throughout the brain, with average values in gray matter approximately four to five times those of white matter [6].

A method has been devised to measure glucose consumption in the discrete functional and structural components of the brain in intact, conscious laboratory animals [7]. This method also employs quantitative autoradiography to measure local tissue concentrations but utilizes 2-deoxy-D-[1-^{14}C]glucose ([^{14}C]deoxyglucose) as the tracer. The local tissue accumulation of [^{14}C]deoxyglucose as [^{14}C]deoxyglucose-6-phosphate in a given interval of time is related to the amount of glucose that has been phosphorylated by hexokinase over the same interval, and the rate of glucose consumption can be determined from the [^{14}C]deoxyglucose-6-phosphate concentration by appropriate consideration of (1) the relative concentrations of [^{14}C]deoxyglucose and glucose in the plasma; (2) their rate constants for transport between plasma and brain tissue; and (3) the kinetic constants of hexokinase for deoxyglucose and glucose. The method is based on a kinetic model of the biochemical behavior of 2-deoxyglucose and glucose in brain. The model (diagrammed in Fig. 1) has been mathematically analyzed to derive an operational equation that presents the variables to be measured and the procedure to be followed to determine local cerebral glucose utilization.

To measure local glucose utilization, a pulse of [^{14}C]deoxyglucose is administered intravenously at zero time, and timed arterial blood samples are then drawn for the determination of the plasma [^{14}C]deoxyglucose and glucose concentrations. At the end of the experimental period, usually about 45 min, the animal is decapitated, the brain is removed and frozen, and brain sections, 20 μm in thickness, are autoradiographed on X-ray film along with calibrated [^{14}C]methylmethacrylate standards. Local tissue concentrations of ^{14}C are determined by quantitative densitometric analysis of the autoradiographs. From the time courses of the arterial plasma [^{14}C]deoxyglucose and glucose concentrations and the final tissue ^{14}C concentrations, determined by the quantitative autoradiography, local glucose utilization can be calculated by means of the operational equation for all components of the brain identifiable in the autoradiographs. The procedure is so designed that the autoradiographs reflect mainly the relative local concentrations of [^{14}C]deoxyglucose-6-phosphate. The autoradiographs are therefore pictorial representations of the relative rates of glucose utilization in all the structural components of the brain.

Autoradiographs of the striate cortex in monkey in various functional states are illustrated in Fig. 2. This method has demonstrated that local cerebral consumption of glucose varies as widely as blood flow throughout the brain (Table 2). Indeed, in the normal animals there is remarkably close correlation between local cerebral blood flow and glucose consumption [8]. Changes in functional activity produced by physiological stimulation, anesthesia, or deafferentation result in corresponding changes in blood flow and glucose consumption [9] in the structures involved in the functional change. The [^{14}C]deoxyglucose method for the measurement of local glucose utilization has been used recently to map the functional visual pathways and to identify the locus of the visual cortical representation of the retinal "blind spot" in the brain of the rhesus monkey [9] (Fig. 2). These results establish that local energy metab-

TABLE 2. Representative values for local cerebral glucose utilization in the normal conscious albino rat and monkey (μmol/100 g/min)

Structure	Albino rat[a] (mean ± SE; n = 10)	Monkey[b] (mean ± SE; n = 7)
GRAY MATTER		
Visual cortex	107 ± 6	59 ± 2
Auditory cortex	162 ± 5	79 ± 4
Parietal cortex	112 ± 5	47 ± 4
Sensory-motor cortex	120 ± 5	44 ± 3
Thalamus		
Lateral nucleus	116 ± 5	54 ± 2
Ventral nucleus	109 ± 5	43 ± 2
Medial geniculate body	131 ± 5	65 ± 3
Lateral geniculate body	96 ± 5	39 ± 1
Hypothalamus	54 ± 2	25 ± 1
Mammillary body	121 ± 5	57 ± 3
Hippocampus	79 ± 3	39 ± 2
Amygdala	52 ± 2	25 ± 2
Caudate putamen	110 ± 4	52 ± 3
Nucleus accumbens	82 ± 3	36 ± 2
Globus pallidus	58 ± 2	26 ± 2
Substantia nigra	58 ± 3	29 ± 2
Vestibular nucleus	128 ± 5	66 ± 3
Cochlear nucleus	113 ± 7	51 ± 3
Superior olivary nucleus	133 ± 7	63 ± 4
Inferior colliculus	197 ± 10	103 ± 6
Superior colliculus	95 ± 5	55 ± 4
Pontine gray matter	62 ± 3	28 ± 1
Cerebellar cortex	57 ± 2	31 ± 2
Cerebellar nuclei	100 ± 4	45 ± 2
WHITE MATTER		
Corpus callosum	40 ± 2	11 ± 1
Internal capsule	33 ± 2	13 ± 1
Cerebellar white matter	37 ± 2	12 ± 1
WEIGHTED AVERAGE FOR WHOLE BRAIN		
	68 ± 3	36 ± 1

[a] From Sokoloff and co-workers [7].
[b] From Kennedy and co-workers [10].

olism in brain is coupled to local functional activity and also confirm the long-held belief that local cerebral blood flow is adjusted to metabolic demand in local tissue. The method has been applied to humans by the use of 2-[^{18}F]fluoro-2-deoxy-D-glucose and positron

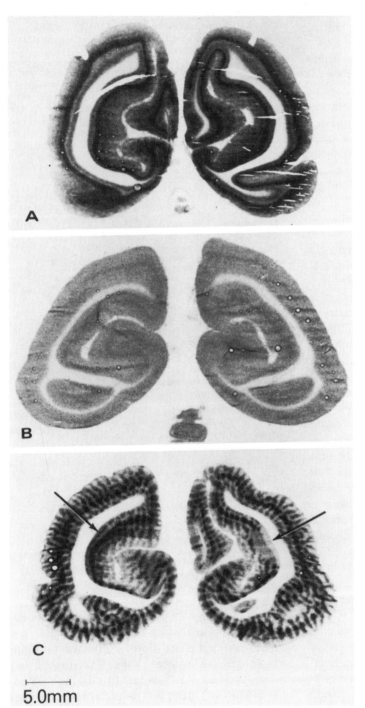

5.0mm

FIG. 2. Autoradiographs of coronal brain sections from rhesus monkeys at the level of the striate cortex. **A:** Animal with normal binocular vision. Note the laminar distribution of the density; the dark band corresponds to layer IV. **B:** Animal with bilateral visual deprivation. Note the almost uniform and reduced relative density, especially the virtual disappearance of the dark band corresponding to layer IV. **C:** Animal with right eye occluded. The half-brain on the left side of the photograph represents the left hemisphere contralateral to the occluded eye. Note the alternate dark and light striations, each approximately 0.3 to 0.4 mm in width, representing the ocular dominance columns. These columns are most apparent in the dark lamina corresponding to layer IV but extend through the entire thickness of the cortex. The *arrows* point to regions of bilateral asymmetry where the ocular dominance columns are absent. These are presumably areas that normally have only monocular input. The one on the left, contralateral to the occluded eye, has a continuous dark lamina corresponding to layer IV that is completely absent on the side ipsilateral to the occluded eye. These regions are believed to be the loci of the cortical representations of the blind spots. (From Sokoloff [9].)

emission tomography, with similar results (see Chap. 44).

SUBSTRATES OF CEREBRAL METABOLISM

Normally, the substrates are glucose and oxygen, and the products are carbon dioxide and water

In contrast to most other tissues, which exhibit considerable flexibility with respect to the nature of the foodstuffs extracted and consumed from the blood, the normal brain is restricted almost exclusively to glucose as the substrate for its energy metabolism. Despite long and intensive efforts, the only incontrovertible and consistently positive arteriovenous differences demonstrated for the human brain under normal conditions have been for glucose and oxygen [3]. Negative arteriovenous differences, significantly different from zero, have been found consistently only for carbon dioxide, although water, which has never been measured, is also produced. Pyruvate and lactate production have been observed occasionally, certainly in aged subjects with cerebral vascular insufficiency, but irregularly in subjects with normal oxygenation of the brain.

It appears, then, that in the normal *in vivo* state glucose is the only significant substrate for the brain's energy metabolism. Under normal circumstances no other potential energy-yielding substance has been found to be extracted from the blood in more than trivial amounts. The stoichiometry of glucose utilization and oxygen consumption is summarized in Table 3. The normal, conscious human brain consumes oxygen at a rate of 156 μmol/100 g tissue/min. Carbon dioxide production is the same, leading to a respiratory quotient of 1.0, further evidence that carbohydrate is the ultimate substrate for oxidative metabolism. The O_2 consumption and CO_2 production are equivalent to a rate of glu-

TABLE 3. Relationship between cerebral oxygen consumption and glucose utilization in normal young adult man[a]

Function	Value
O_2 consumption (μmol/100 g brain tissue/min)	156
Glucose utilization (μmol/100 g brain tissue/min)	31
O_2/glucose ratio (mol/mol)	5
Glucose equivalent of O_2 consumption (μmol glucose/100 g brain tissue/min)	26[b]
CO_2 production (μmol/100 g brain tissue/min)	156
Cerebral respiratory quotient	0.97

[a] Values are the median of the values reported in the literature. (From Sokoloff [3].)
[b] Calculated on the basis of 6 mol O_2 required for complete oxidation of 1 mol glucose.

cose utilization of 26 μmol glucose/100 g tissue/min, assuming 6 μmol of O_2 consumed and CO_2 produced for each micromole of glucose completely oxidized to CO_2 and H_2O. The glucose utilization actually measured is, however, 31 μmol/100 g/min, which indicates that glucose consumption is not only sufficient to account for the total O_2 consumption but is in excess by 5 μmol/100 g/min. For the complete oxidation of glucose, the theoretical ratio of O_2/glucose utilization is 6.0; the excess glucose utilization is responsible for a measured ratio of only 5.5 μmol O_2/μmol glucose. The fate of the excess glucose is unknown, but it is probably distributed in part in lactate, pyruvate, and other intermediates of carbohydrate metabolism, each released from the brain into the blood in insufficient amounts to be detectable in significant arteriovenous differences. Some of the glucose must also be utilized not for the production of energy but for the synthesis of other chemical constituents of the brain.

Some oxygen is known to be utilized for the oxidation of substances not derived from glucose, as, for example, in the synthesis and metabolic degradation of monoamine neurotransmitters, as mentioned above. The amount of oxygen utilized for these processes is, however, extremely small and is undetectable in the presence of the enormous oxygen consumption used for carbohydrate oxidation.

The combination of a cerebral respiratory quotient of unity, an almost stoichiometric relationship between oxygen uptake and glucose consumption, and the absence of any significant arteriovenous difference for any other energy-rich substrate is strong evidence that the brain normally derives its energy from the oxidation of glucose. In this respect, cerebral metabolism is unique because no other tissue, except for the testis [11], has been found to rely only on carbohydrate for energy. This does not imply that the pathways of glucose metabolism in the brain lead, like combustion, directly and exclusively to production of carbon dioxide and water. Various chemical and energy transformations occur between the uptake of the primary substrates, glucose and oxygen, and the liberation of the end products, carbon dioxide and water. Various compounds derived from glucose or produced through the energy made available from glucose catabolism are intermediates in the process. Glucose carbon is incorporated, for example, into amino acids, protein, lipids, and glycogen. These are turned over and act as intermediates in the overall pathway from glucose to carbon dioxide and water. There is clear evidence from studies with [^{14}C]glucose that the glucose is not entirely oxidized directly and that at any given moment some of the carbon dioxide being produced is derived from sources other than the glucose that enters the brain at the same moment or just prior to that moment. That oxygen and glucose consumption and carbon dioxide production are essentially in stoichiometric balance and no other energy-laden substrate is taken from the blood means, however, that the net energy made available to the brain must ultimately be derived from the oxidation of glucose. It should be noted that this is the situation in the normal state; as is discussed later, other substrates may be used in special circumstances or in abnormal states.

In brain, glucose utilization is obligatory

The brain normally derives almost all of its energy from the aerobic oxidation of glucose, but this does not distinguish between preferential and obligatory utilization of glucose. Most tissues are largely facultative in their choice of substrates and can use them interchangeably more or less in proportion to their availability. This does not appear to be so in brain. The present evidence indicates that, except in some unusual and very special circumstances, only the aerobic utilization of glucose is capable of providing the brain with sufficient energy to maintain normal function and structure. The brain appears to have almost no flexibility in its choice of substrates *in vivo*. This conclusion is derived from the following evidence.

Effects of glucose deprivation

It is well known clinically that a fall in blood glucose content, if of sufficient degree, is rapidly followed by aberrations of cerebral function. Hypoglycemia, produced by excessive insulin or occurring spontaneously in hepatic insufficiency, is associated with changes in mental state ranging from mild, subjective sensory disturbances to coma, the severity depending on both the degree and the duration of the hypoglycemia. The behavioral effects are paralleled by abnormalities in EEG patterns and cerebral metabolic rate. The EEG pattern exhibits increased prominence of slow, high-voltage delta rhythms, and the rate of cerebral oxygen consumption falls. In studies of the effects of insulin hypoglycemia in humans [12], it was observed that when the arterial glucose concentration fell from a normal level of 70 to 100 mg/100 ml to an average level of 19 mg/100 ml, the subjects became confused and their cerebral oxygen consumption fell to 2.6 ml/100 g/min, or 79 percent of the normal level. When the arterial glucose level fell to 8 mg/100 ml, a deep coma ensued and the cerebral oxygen consumption decreased even further to 1.9 ml/100 g/min

TABLE 4. Effects of insulin hypoglycemia on cerebral circulation and metabolism in humans[a]

	Control	Insulin-induced hypoglycemia without coma	Insulin-induced hypoglycemic coma
ARTERIAL BLOOD			
Glucose concn. (mg %)	74	19	8
O_2 content (vol %)	17.4	17.9	16.6
Mean blood pressure (mm Hg)	94	86	93
CEREBRAL CIRCULATION			
Blood flow (ml/100 g/min)	58	61	63
O_2 consumption (ml/100 g/min)	3.4	2.6	1.9
Glucose consumption (mg/100 g/min)	4.4	2.3	0.8
Respiratory quotient	0.95	1.10	0.92

[a] From Kety et al. [12].

(Table 4). These changes are not caused by insufficient cerebral blood flow, which actually increases slightly during the coma. In the depths of the coma, when the blood glucose content is very low, there is almost no measurable cerebral uptake of glucose from the blood. Cerebral oxygen consumption, although reduced, is still far from negligible, and there is no longer any stoichiometric relationship between glucose and oxygen uptakes by the brain—evidence that the oxygen is utilized for the oxidation of other substances. The cerebral respiratory quotient (R.Q.) remains approximately 1, however, indicating that these other substrates are still carbohydrate, presumably derived from the brain's endogenous carbohydrate stores. The effects are clearly the result of hypoglycemia and not some other direct effect of insulin in the brain. In all cases, the behavioral, functional, and cerebral metabolic abnormalities associated with insulin hypoglycemia are rapidly and completely reversed by the administration of glucose. The severity of the effects is correlated with the degree of hypoglycemia and not the insulin dosage, and the effects of the insulin can be completely prevented by the simultaneous administration of glucose with the insulin.

Similar effects are observed in hypoglycemia produced by other means, such as hepatectomy. The inhibition of glucose utilization at the phosphohexoseisomerase step with pharmacologic doses of 2-deoxyglucose also produces all the cerebral effects of hypoglycemia despite an associated elevation in blood glucose content. It appears, then, that when the brain is deprived of its glucose supply in an otherwise normal individual, no other substance present in the blood can satisfactorily substitute for it as the substrate for the brain's energy metabolism.

Other substrates in hypoglycemia

The hypoglycemic state provides convenient test conditions to determine whether a substance is capable of substituting for glucose as a substrate of cerebral energy metabolism. If it can, its administration during hypoglycemic shock should restore consciousness and normal cerebral electrical activity without raising the blood glucose level. Numerous potential substrates have been tested in humans and animals. Very few can restore normal cerebral function in hypoglycemia, and of these all but one appear to operate through a variety of mechanisms to raise the blood glucose level rather than by serving as a substrate directly (Table 5).

Mannose appears to be the only substance that can be utilized by the brain directly and

TABLE 5. Effectiveness of various substances in preventing or reversing the effects of hypoglycemia or glucose deprivation on cerebral function and metabolism[a]

Substance	Comments
Effective	
Epinephrine	Raises blood glucose concentration
Maltose	Converted to glucose and raises blood glucose level
Mannose	Directly metabolized and enters glycolytic pathway
Partially or occasionally effective	
Glutamate	Occasionally effective by raising blood glucose level
Arginine	
Glycine	
p-Aminobenzoate	
Succinate	
Ineffective	
Glycerol	Some of these substances can be metabolized to varying extents by brain tissue and could conceivably be effective if it were not for the blood-brain barrier
Ethanol	
Lactate	
Pyruvate	
Glyceraldehyde	
Hexosediphosphates	
Fumarate	
Acetate	
β-Hydroxybutyrate	
Galactose	
Lactose	
Insulin	

[a] Summarized from literature [3].

rapidly enough to restore or maintain normal function in the absence of glucose [13]. It traverses the blood-brain barrier and is converted to mannose-6-phosphate. This reaction is catalyzed by hexokinase as effectively as the phosphorylation of glucose. The mannose-6-phosphate is then converted to fructose-6-phosphate by phosphomannoseisomerase, which is active in brain tissue. Through these reactions mannose can enter directly into the glycolytic pathway and replace glucose.

Maltose also has been found to be effective occasionally in restoring normal behavior and EEG activity in hypoglycemia, but only by rais-

ing the blood glucose level through its conversion to glucose by maltase activity in blood and other tissues [3]. Epinephrine is effective in producing arousal from insulin coma, but this is achieved through its well-known stimulation of glycogenolysis and the elevation of blood glucose concentration. Glutamate, arginine, glycine, p-aminobenzoate, and succinate also are effective occasionally, but they probably act through adrenergic effects that raise the epinephrine level and, consequently, the glucose concentrations of the blood [3].

It is clear, then, that no substance normally present in blood can replace glucose as the substrate for the brain's energy metabolism. Thus far, the one substance found to do so—mannose—is not normally present in blood in significant amounts and is, therefore, of no physiological significance. It should be noted, however, that failure to restore normal cerebral function in hypoglycemia is not synonymous with an inability of the brain to utilize the substance. Many of the substances that have been tested and found ineffective are compounds normally formed and utilized within the brain and are normal intermediates in its intermediary metabolism. Lactate, pyruvate, fructose-1,6-bisphosphate, acetate, β-hydroxybutyrate, and acetoacetate are such examples. These can all be utilized by brain slices, homogenates, or cell-free fractions, and the enzymes for their metabolism are present in the brain. Enzymes for the metabolism of glycerol or ethanol, for example, may not be present in sufficient amounts. For other substrates, for example, D-β-hydroxybutyrate and acetoacetate, the enzymes are adequate, but the substrate is not available to the brain because of inadequate blood levels or restricted transport through the blood-brain barrier.

Nevertheless, nervous system function in the intact animal depends on substrates supplied by the blood and no satisfactory, normal, endogenous substitute for glucose has been found. Glucose must therefore be considered essential for normal physiological behavior of the central nervous system.

Brain utilizes ketones in states of ketosis

In special circumstances, the brain may fulfill its nutritional needs partly, although not completely, with substrates other than glucose. Normally there are no significant cerebral arteriovenous differences for D-β-hydroxybutyrate and acetoacetate, which are "ketone bodies" formed in the course of the catabolism of fatty acids by liver. Owen and co-workers [14] observed, however, that when human patients were treated for severe obesity by complete fasting for several weeks, there was considerable uptake of both substances by the brain. Indeed, if one assumed that the substances were completely oxidized, their rates of utilization would have accounted for more than 50 percent of the total cerebral oxygen consumption—more than that accounted for by the glucose uptake. D-β-Hydroxybutyrate uptake was several times greater than that of acetoacetate, a reflection of its higher concentration in the blood. The enzymes responsible for their metabolism, D-β-hydroxybutyric dehydrogenase, acetoacetate-succinyl-coenzyme A (CoA) transferase, and acetoacetyl-CoA-thiolase, have been demonstrated to be present in brain tissue in sufficient amounts to convert them into acetyl-CoA and to feed them into the tricarboxylic acid cycle at a sufficient rate to satisfy the brain's metabolic demands [15].

Under normal circumstances, when there is ample glucose and the levels of ketone bodies in the blood are very low, the brain apparently does not resort to their use in any significant amounts. In prolonged starvation, the carbohydrate stores of the body are exhausted, and the rate of gluconeogenesis is insufficient to provide glucose fast enough to meet the requirements of the brain; blood ketone levels rise as a result of the rapid fat catabolism. The brain then apparently turns to the ketone bodies as the source of its energy supply.

Cerebral utilization of ketone bodies appears to follow passively their levels in arterial blood [15]. In normal adults, ketone levels are very low in blood, and cerebral utilization of ketones is negligible. In ketotic states resulting from starvation, fat-feeding or ketogenic diets, diabetes, or any other condition that accelerates the mobilization and catabolism of fat, cerebral utilization of ketones is increased more or less in direct proportion to the degree of ketosis [15]. Significant utilization of ketone bodies by brain is, however, normal in the neonatal period. The newborn infant tends to be hypoglycemic but becomes ketotic when it begins to nurse because of the high fat content of mother's milk. When weaned onto the normal relatively high carbohydrate diet, the ketosis and cerebral ketone utilization disappear. The studies have been carried out mainly in the infant rat, but there is evidence that the situation is similar in the human infant.

The first two enzymes in the pathway of ketone utilization are D-β-hydroxybutyrate dehydrogenase and acetoacetyl-succinyl-CoA transferase. These exhibit a postnatal pattern of development in brain that is well adapted to the nutritional demands of the brain. At birth, the activity of these enzymes in brain is low; they rise rapidly with the ketosis that develops with the onset of suckling, reach their peak just before weaning, and then gradually decline after weaning to normal adult levels of approximately one-third to one-fourth the maximum levels attained [15,16].

It should be noted that D-β-hydroxybutyrate is incapable of maintaining or restoring normal cerebral function in the absence of glucose in the blood. This suggests that although it can partially replace glucose, it cannot fully satisfy the cerebral energy needs in the absence of some glucose consumption. One possible explanation may be that the first product of D-β-hydroxybutyrate oxidation, acetoacetate, is further metabolized by its displacement of the succinyl moiety of succinyl-CoA to form acetoacetyl-CoA. A certain level of glucose utilization may be essential to drive the tricarboxylic cycle and provide enough succinyl-CoA to permit the further oxidation of acetoacetate and hence pull along the oxidation of D-β-hydroxybutyrate.

AGE AND DEVELOPMENT INFLUENCE CEREBRAL ENERGY METABOLISM

Metabolic rate increases during early development

The energy metabolism of the brain and the blood flow that sustains it vary considerably from birth to old age. Data on the cerebral metabolic rate obtained directly *in vivo* are lacking for the early postnatal period, but the results of *in vitro* measurements in animal brain preparations and inferences drawn from cerebral blood flow measurements in intact animals [17] suggest that the cerebral oxygen consumption is low at birth, rises rapidly during the period of cerebral growth and development, and reaches a maximal level at about the time maturation is completed. This rise is consistent with the progressive increase in the levels of a number of enzymes of oxidative metabolism in the brain. The rates of blood flow in different structures of the brain reach peak levels at different times, depending on the maturation rate of the particular structure. In the structures that consist predominantly of white matter, the peaks coincide roughly with the times of maximal rates of myelination. From these peaks, blood flow and, probably, cerebral metabolic rate decline to the levels characteristic of adulthood.

Metabolic rate declines and plateaus after maturation

Reliable quantitative data on the changes in cerebral circulation and metabolism in humans from the middle of the first decade of life to old age are summarized in Table 6. By 6 years of age, the cerebral blood flow and oxygen consumption have already attained their high levels, and they decline thereafter to the levels of normal young adulthood [4]. Cerebral oxygen consumption of 5.2 ml/100 g brain tissue/min in a 5- to 6-year-old child corresponds to total oxygen consumption by the brain of approximately 60 ml/min, or more than 50 percent of the total body basal oxygen consumption, a proportion markedly greater than that occurring in adulthood. The reasons for the extraordinarily high cerebral metabolic rates in children are unknown, but presumably they reflect the extra energy requirements for the biosynthetic processes associated with growth and development.

Tissue pathology but not aging produces secondary change in metabolic rate

Despite reports to the contrary, cerebral blood flow and oxygen consumption normally remain essentially unchanged between young adulthood and old age. In a population of normal elderly men in their eighth decade of life—who were carefully selected for good health and freedom from all disease, including vascular disease—both blood flow and oxygen consumption were not significantly different from those of normal young men 50 years younger (see Table 6) [18]. In a comparable group of elderly subjects, who differed only by the presence of objective evidence of minimal arteriosclerosis, cerebral blood flow was significantly lower. It had reached a point at which the oxygen tension of the cerebral venous blood declined, which is an indication of relative cerebral hypoxia. Cerebral oxygen consumption, however, was still maintained at normal levels through extraction of larger than normal proportions of the arterial blood oxygen. In senile psychotic patients with arteriosclerosis, cerebral blood flow was no

TABLE 6. Cerebral blood flow and oxygen consumption in humans from childhood to old age and in senility[a]

Life period and condition	Age (years)	Cerebral blood flow (ml/100 g/min)	Cerebral O$_2$ Consumption (ml/100 g/min)	Cerebral venous O$_2$ tension (mm Hg)
Childhood	6[b]	106[b]	5.2[b]	—
Normal young adulthood	21	62	3.5	38
Aged				
Normal	71[b]	58	3.3	36
With minimal arteriosclerosis	73[b]	48[b]	3.2	33[b,c]
With senile psychosis	72[b]	48[b,c]	2.7[b,c]	33[b,c]

[a] From Kennedy and Sokoloff [4] and Sokoloff [18].
[b] Statistically significant difference from normal young adult ($P < 0.05$).
[c] Statistically significant difference from normal elderly subjects ($P < 0.05$).

lower, but cerebral oxygen consumption had also declined. These data suggest that aging per se need not lower cerebral oxygen consumption and blood flow but that when blood flow is reduced, it is probably secondary to arteriosclerosis, which produces cerebral vascular insufficiency and chronic relative hypoxia in the brain, or secondary to other tissue pathology that decreases function, as in dementia (see Chap. 43). Because arteriosclerosis and Alzheimer's disease are so prevalent in the aged population, most individuals probably follow the latter pattern.

CEREBRAL METABOLIC RATE IN VARIOUS PHYSIOLOGICAL STATES

Cerebral metabolic rate is determined locally by functional activity in discrete regions

In organs such as heart or skeletal muscle that perform mechanical work, increased functional activity clearly is associated with increased metabolic rate. In nervous tissues outside the central nervous system, the electrical activity is an almost quantitative indicator of the degree of functional activity, and in structures such as sympathetic ganglia and postganglionic axons,

increased electrical activity produced by electrical stimulation is definitely associated with increased utilization of oxygen. Within the central nervous system, local energy metabolism is also closely correlated with the level of local functional activity. Studies using the [^{14}C]deoxyglucose method have demonstrated pronounced changes in glucose utilization associated with altered functional activity in discrete regions of the central nervous system specifically related to that function [9]. For example, diminished visual or auditory input depresses glucose utilization in all components of the central visual or auditory pathways, respectively (Fig. 2). Focal seizures increase glucose utilization in discrete components of the motor pathways, such as the motor cortex and the basal ganglia (Fig. 3).

Convulsive activity, induced or spontaneous, has often been employed as a method of increasing electrical activity of the brain. Davies and Rémond [1] used the oxygen electrode technique in the cerebral cortex of cat and found increases in oxygen consumption during electrically induced or drug-induced convulsions. Because the increased oxygen consumption either coincided with or followed the onset of convulsions, it was concluded that the elevation in metabolic rate was the consequence of the increased functional activity produced by the convulsive state (see Chap. 41).

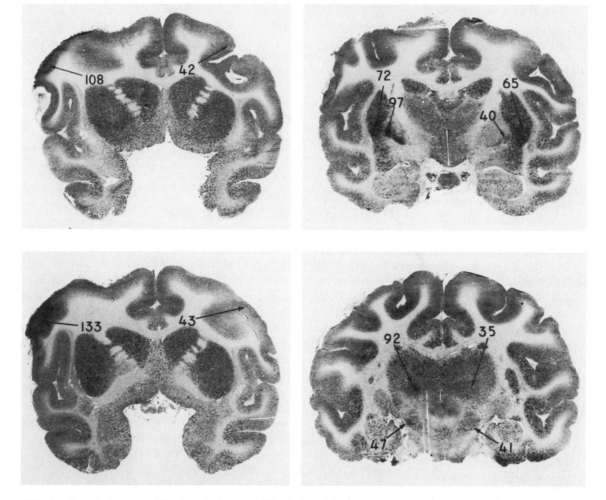

FIG. 3. Local glucose utilization during penicillin-induced focal seizures. The penicillin was applied to the hand and face area of the left motor cortex of a rhesus monkey. The left side of the brain is on the left in each of the autoradiographs in the figure. The numbers are the rates of local cerebral glucose utilization in μmol/100 g tissue/min. **Upper left:** Motor cortex in region of penicillin application and corresponding region of contralateral motor cortex. **Lower left:** Ipsilateral and contralateral motor cortical regions remote from area of penicillin applications. **Upper right:** Ipsilateral and contralateral putamen and globus pallidus. **Lower right:** Ipsilateral and contralateral thalamic nuclei and substantia nigra. (From Sokoloff [9].)

Metabolic rate and nerve conduction are directly related

Studies using the [^{14}C]deoxyglucose method have defined the nature and mechanisms of the relationship between energy metabolism and functional activity in nervous tissues. Studies in the superior cervical ganglion of the rat have shown almost a direct relationship between glucose utilization in the ganglion and spike frequency in the afferent fibers from the cervical sympathetic trunk [19]. A spike results from the passage of finite current of Na^+ into the cell and K^+ out of the cell, ion currents that degrade the ionic gradients responsible for the resting membrane potential. Such degradation can be expected to stimulate Na,K-ATPase activity to restore the ionic gradients to normal, and such ATPase activity would, in turn, stimulate energy metabolism. Indeed, Mata et al. [20] have found that, in the posterior pituitary *in vitro*, the stimulation of glucose utilization due either to electrical stimulation or opening of Na^+ channels in the excitable membrane by veratridine is blocked by ouabain, a specific inhibitor of Na,K-ATPase activity (see Chap. 3). Most, if not all, of the stimulated energy metabolism associated with increased functional activity is confined to the axonal terminals rather than to the cell bodies in a functionally activated pathway (Fig. 4) [21].

It is difficult to define metabolic equivalents of consciousness, mental work, and sleep

Mental work

Convincing correlations between cerebral metabolic rate and mental activity have been obtained in humans in a variety of pathological states of altered consciousness [22]. Regardless of the cause of the disorder, graded reductions in cerebral oxygen consumption are accompanied by parallel graded reductions in the degree of mental alertness, all the way to profound coma (Table 7). It is difficult to define or even to conceive of the physical equivalent of mental work. A common view equates concentrated mental effort with mental work, and it is also fashionable to attribute a high demand for mental effort to the process of problem solving in mathematics. Nevertheless, there appears to be no increased energy utilization by the brain during such processes. From resting levels, total cerebral blood flow and oxygen consumption

TABLE 7. Relationship between level of consciousness and cerebral metabolic rate[a]

Level of consciousness	Cerebral blood flow (ml/100 g/min)	Cerebral O_2 consumption (ml/100 g/min)
Mentally alert	54	3.3
Normal young men		
Mentally confused	48	2.8
Brain tumor		
Diabetic acidosis		
Insulin hypoglycemia		
Cerebral		
arteriosclerosis		
Comatose	57	2.0
Brain tumor		
Diabetic coma		
Insulin coma		
Anesthesia		

[a] From Sokoloff [22].

remain unchanged during the exertion of the mental effort required to solve complex arithmetical problems [22]. It may be that the assumptions that relate mathematical reasoning to mental work are erroneous, but it seems more likely that the areas which participate in the processes of such reasoning represent too small a fraction of the brain for changes in their functional and metabolic activities to be reflected in the energy metabolism of the brain as a whole.

Sleep

Sleep is a naturally occurring, periodic, reversible state of unconsciousness, and the EEG pattern in deep slow-wave sleep is characterized by high-voltage slow rhythms very similar to those often seen in pathological comatose states. As found in the pathological comatose states, cerebral glucose metabolism is depressed more or less uniformly throughout the brain of rhesus monkeys in stages 2 to 4 of normal sleep studied by the [^{14}C]deoxyglucose method [23]. There are no comparable data available for the state of paradoxical sleep (REM sleep) or for normal sleep in humans.

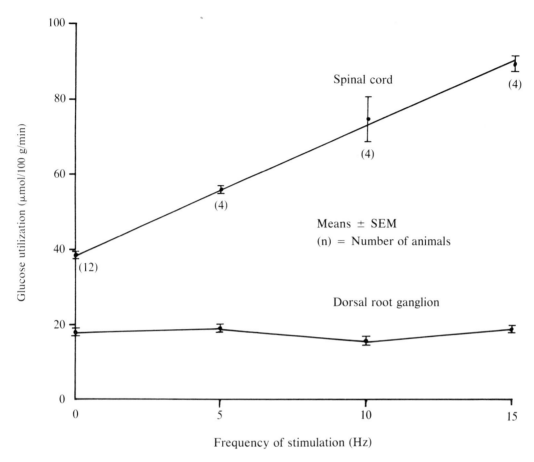

FIG. 4. Effects of electrical stimulation of sciatic nerve on glucose utilization in the terminal zones in the dorsal horn of the spinal cord and in the cell bodies in the dorsal root ganglion. (From Kadekaro et al. [21].)

CEREBRAL ENERGY METABOLISM IN PATHOLOGICAL STATES

Psychiatric disorders may produce effects related to anxiety

The cerebral metabolic rate of the brain as a whole is normally fairly stable and varies over a relatively narrow range under physiological conditions. There are, however, a number of pathological states of the nervous system and other organs that affect the functions of the brain either directly or indirectly, and some of these have profound effects on the cerebral metabolism.

In general, disorders that alter the quality of mentation but not the level of consciousness (e.g., the functional neuroses, psychoses, and psychotomimetic states) have no apparent effect on the average blood flow and oxygen consumption of the brain as a whole. Thus, no changes in either function are observed in schizophrenia [22] or LSD intoxication (Table 8) [22]. There is still uncertainty about the effects of

TABLE 8. Cerebral blood flow and metabolic rate in schizophrenia and in normal young men during LSD-induced psychotomimetic state[a]

Condition	Cerebral blood flow (ml/100 g/min)	Cerebral O$_2$ consumption (ml/100 g/min)
Normal	67	3.9
LSD intoxication	68	3.9
Schizophrenia	72	4.0

[a] From Sokoloff [22].

anxiety, mainly because of the difficulties in evaluating quantitatively the intensity of anxiety. It is generally believed that ordinary degrees of anxiety or "nervousness" do not affect the cerebral metabolic rate, but severe anxiety or "panic" may increase cerebral oxygen consumption [22]. This may be related to the level of epinephrine circulating in the blood. Small doses of epinephrine that raise heart rate and cause some anxiety do not alter cerebral blood flow and metabolism, but large doses that are sufficient to raise the arterial blood pressure cause significant increases in the levels of both.

Coma and systemic metabolic diseases depress brain metabolism

Coma is correlated with depression of cerebral oxygen consumption; progressive reduction in the level of consciousness are paralleled by corresponding graded decreases in the cerebral metabolic rate (see Table 7). There are almost innumerable derangements that can lead to depression of consciousness. Table 9 includes only a few typical examples that have been studied by the same methods and by the same or related groups of investigators.

Inadequate cerebral nutrient supply leads to decreases in the level of consciousness, ranging from confusional states to coma. The nutrition of the brain can be limited by lowering the oxygen or glucose levels of arterial blood, as in anoxia or hypoglycemia, or by impairment of their distribution to the brain through lowering cerebral blood flow, as in brain tumors. Consciousness is then depressed, presumably because of inadequate supplies of substrate to support the energy metabolism necessary to

TABLE 9. Cerebral blood flow and metabolic rate in humans with various disorders affecting mental state[a]

Condition	Mental state	Cerebral blood flow (ml/100 g/min)	Cerebral O$_2$ consumption (ml/100 g/min)
Normal	Alert	54	3.3
Increased intracranial pressure (brain tumor)	Coma	34[b]	2.5[b]
Insulin hypoglycemia; arterial glucose level			
74 mg/100 ml	Alert	58	3.4
19 mg/100 ml	Confused	61	2.6[b]
8 mg/100 ml	Coma	63	1.9[b]
Thiopental anesthesia	Coma	60[b]	2.1[b]
Postconvulsive state			
Before convulsion	Alert	58	3.7
After convulsion	Confused	37[b]	3.1[b]
Diabetes			
Acidosis	Confused	45[b]	2.7[b]
Coma	Coma	65[b]	1.7[b]
Hepatic insufficiency	Coma	33[b]	1.7[b]

[a] All studies listed were carried out by Kety and/or his associates [24], employing the same methods. For references, see Sokoloff [3,22].
[b] Statistically significant difference from normal level ($p < 0.05$).

sustain the appropriate functional activities of the brain.

In a number of conditions, the causes of depression of both consciousness and the cerebral metabolic rate are unknown and must, by exclusion, be attributed to intracellular defects in the brain. Anesthesia is one example. Cerebral oxygen consumption is always reduced in the anesthetized state regardless of the anesthetic agent used, whereas blood flow may or may not be decreased and may even be increased. This reduction is the result of decreased energy demand and not insufficient nutrient supply or a block of intracellular energy metabolism. There is evidence that general anesthetics interfere with synaptic transmission, thus reducing neuronal interaction and functional activity and, consequently, metabolic demands.

Several metabolic diseases with broad systemic manifestations are also associated with disturbances of cerebral function. Diabetes mellitus, when allowed to progress to states of acidosis and ketosis, leads to mental confusion and, ultimately, to deep coma, with parallel proportionate decreases in cerebral oxygen consumption (see Table 9) [24]. The abnormalities are usually completely reversed by adequate insulin therapy. The cause of the coma or depressed cerebral metabolic rate is unknown. Deficiency of cerebral nutrition cannot be implicated because the blood glucose level is elevated and cerebral blood flow and oxygen supply are more than adequate. Neither is insulin deficiency, which is presumably the basis of the systemic manifestations of the disease, a likely cause of the cerebral abnormalities since no absolute requirement of insulin for cerebral glucose utilization or metabolism has been demonstrated. Ketosis may be severe in this disease, and there is disputed evidence that a rise in the blood level of at least one of the ketone bodies, acetoacetate, can cause coma in animals. In studies of human diabetic acidosis and coma, a significant correlation between the depression of cerebral metabolic rate and the degree of ketosis has been observed, but there is an equally good correlation with the degree of acidosis [24]. Hyperosmolarity itself may also cause coma. It is possible that ketosis, acidosis, hyperosmolarity or the combination may be responsible for the disturbances in cerebral function and metabolism.

Coma is occasionally associated with severe impairment of liver function, or hepatic insufficiency. In human patients in hepatic coma, cerebral metabolic rate is markedly depressed (see Table 9). Cerebral blood flow is also moderately depressed but not sufficiently to lead to limiting supplies of glucose and oxygen. The blood ammonia level is usually elevated in hepatic coma, and significant cerebral uptake of ammonia from the blood is observed. Ammonia toxicity has therefore been suspected as the basis for cerebral dysfunction in hepatic coma. Because ammonia can, through glutamic dehydrogenase activity, convert α-ketoglutarate to glutamate by reductive amination, it has been suggested that ammonia might thereby deplete α-ketoglutarate and thus slow the Krebs cycle (see Chap. 28). The correlation between the degree of coma and the blood ammonia level is far from convincing, however, and coma has, in fact, been observed in the absence of an increase in blood ammonia concentration. Although ammonia may be involved in the mechanism of hepatic coma, the mechanism remains unclear, and other causal factors are probably involved.

Depression of mental functions and the cerebral metabolic rate has been observed in association with kidney failure, i.e., uremic coma. The chemical basis of the functional and metabolic disturbances in the brain in this condition also remains undetermined.

In the comatose states associated with these systemic metabolic diseases, there is depression of both the level of conscious mental activity and cerebral energy metabolism. From the available evidence, it is impossible to distinguish which, if either, is the primary change. It is more likely that the depressions of both functions, although well correlated with each other, are independent reflections of a more general impairment of neuronal processes by some unknown factors incident to the disease.

MEASUREMENT OF LOCAL CEREBRAL ENERGY METABOLISM IN HUMANS

Most of the *in vivo* measurements of cerebral energy metabolism described above, and all of those in humans, were made in the brain as a whole and represent the mass-weighted average of the metabolic activities in all the component structures of the brain. The average, however, often obscures the events in the individual components, and it is not surprising that many of the studies of altered cerebral function, both normal and abnormal, have failed to demonstrate corresponding changes in energy metabolism (see Table 8). The [^{14}C]deoxyglucose method [7] has made it possible to measure glucose utilization simultaneously in all the components of the central nervous system, and it has been used to identify the regions with altered functional and metabolic activities in a variety of physiological, pharmacologic, and pathological states [9]. As originally designed, the method utilized autoradiography of brain sections for localization, which precluded its use in humans. However, recent developments [25] with positron emission tomography have made it possible to adapt it for human use. (This is described fully in Chap. 44.)

REFERENCES

1. Davies, P. W., and Rémond, A. Oxygen consumption of the cerebral cortex of the cat during metrazole convulsions. *Res. Publ. Assoc. Nerv. Ment. Dis.* 26:205–217, 1946.
2. Kety, S. S., and Schmidt, C. F. The nitrous oxide method for the quantitative determination of cerebral blood flow in man: Theory, procedure, and normal values. *J. Clin. Invest.* 27:476–483, 1948.
3. Sokoloff, L. The metabolism of the central nervous system *in vivo*. In J. Field, H. W. Magoun, and V. E. Hall (eds.), *Handbook of Physiology-Neurophysiology*. Washington, D.C.: American Physiological Society, 1960, Vol. 3, pp. 1843–1864.
4. Kennedy, C., and Sokoloff, L. An adaptation of the nitrous oxide method to the study of the cerebral circulation in children; normal values for cerebral blood flow and cerebral metabolic rate in childhood. *J. Clin. Invest.* 36:1130–1137, 1957.
5. Sokoloff, L., and Kety, S. S. Regulation of cerebral circulation. *Physiol. Rev.* 40(Suppl. 4):38–44, 1960.
6. Freygang, W. H., and Sokoloff, L. Quantitative measurements of regional circulation in the central nervous system by the use of radioactive inert gas. *Adv. Biol. Med. Phys.* 6:263–279, 1958.
7. Sokoloff, L., Reivich, M., Kennedy, C., Des Rosiers, M. H., Patlak, C. S., Pettigrew, K. D., Sakurada, O., and Shinohara, M. The [^{14}C]deoxyglucose method for the measurement of local cerebral glucose utilization: Theory, procedure, and normal values in the conscious and anesthetized albino rat. *J. Neurochem.* 28:897–916, 1977.
8. Sokoloff, L. Local cerebral energy metabolism: Its relationships to local functional activity and blood flow. In M. J. Purves and L. Elliott (eds.), *Cerebral Vascular Smooth Muscle and Its Control* (Ciba Foundation Symposium 56). Amsterdam: Elsevier/Excerpta Medica/North Holland, 1978, pp. 171–197.
9. Sokoloff, L. Relation between physiological function and energy metabolism in the central nervous system. *J. Neurochem.* 29(5):13–26, 1977.
10. Kennedy, C., Sakurada, O., Shinohara, M., Jehle, J., and Sokoloff, L. Local cerebral glucose utilization in the normal conscious Macaque monkey. *Ann. Neurol.* 4:293–301, 1978.
11. Himwich, H. E., and Nahum, L. H. The respiratory quotient of testicle. *Am. J. Physiol.* 88:680–685, 1929.
12. Kety, S. S., Woodford, R. B., Harmel, M. H.,

Freyhan, F. A., Appel, K. E., and Schmidt, C. F. Cerebral blood flow and metabolism in schizophrenia. The effects of barbiturate semi-narcosis, insulin coma, and electroshock. *Am. J. Psychiatry* 104:765–770, 1948.

13. Sloviter, H. A., and Kamimoto, T. The isolated, perfused rat brain preparation metabolizes mannose but not maltose. *J. Neurochem.* 17:1109–1111, 1970.

14. Owen, O. E., Morgan, A. P., Kemp, H. G., Sullivan, J. M., Herrera, M. G., and Cahill, G. F., Jr. Brain metabolism during fasting. *J. Clin. Invest.* 46:1589–1595, 1967.

15. Krebs, H. A., Williamson, D. H., Bates, M. W., Page, M. A., and Hawkins, R. A. The role of ketone bodies in caloric homeostasis. *Adv. Enzyme Regul.* 9:387–409, 1971.

16. Klee, C. B., and Sokoloff, L. Changes in D(−)-β-hydroxybutyric dehydrogenase activity during brain maturation in the rat. *J. Biol. Chem.* 242:3880–3883, 1967.

17. Kennedy, C., Grave, G. D., Jehle, J. W., and Sokoloff, L. Changes in blood flow in the component structures of the dog brain during postnatal maturation. *J. Neurochem.* 19:2423–2433, 1972.

18. Sokoloff, L. Cerebral circulatory and metabolic changes associated with aging. *Res. Publ. Assoc. Nerv. Ment. Dis.* 41:237–254, 1966.

19. Yarowsky, P., Kadekaro, M., and Sokoloff, L. Frequency-dependent activation of glucose utilization in the superior cervical ganglion by electrical stimulation of cervical sympathetic trunk.

Proc. Natl. Acad. Sci. U.S.A. 80:4179–4183, 1983.

20. Mata, M., Fink, D. J., Gainer, H., Smith, C. B., Davidsen, L., Savaki, H., Schwartz, W. J., and Sokoloff, L. Activity-dependent energy metabolism in rat posterior pituitary primarily reflects sodium pump activity. *J. Neurochem.* 34:213–215, 1980.

21. Kadekaro, M., Crane, A. M., and Sokoloff, L. Differential effects of electrical stimulation of sciatic nerve on metabolic activity in spinal cord and dorsal root ganglion in the rat. *Proc. Natl. Acad. Sci. U.S.A.* 82:6010–6013, 1985.

22. Sokoloff, L. Cerebral circulation and behavior in man: Strategy and findings. In A. J. Mandell and M. P. Mandell (eds.), *Psychochemical Research in Man.* New York: Academic, 1969, pp. 237–252.

23. Kennedy, C., Gillin, J. C., Mendelson, W., Suda, S., Miyaoka, M., Ito, M., Nakamura, R. K., Storch, F. I., Pettigrew, K., Mishkin, M., and Sokoloff, L. Local cerebral glucose utilization in non-rapid eye movement sleep. *Nature* 297:325–327, 1982.

24. Kety, S. S., Polis, B. D., Nadler, C. S., and Schmidt, C. F. Blood flow and oxygen consumption of the human brain in diabetic acidosis and coma. *J. Clin. Invest.* 27:500–510, 1948.

25. Reivich, M., Kuhl, D., Wolf, A., Greenberg, J., Phelps, M., Ido, T., Casella, V., Fowler, J., Hoffman, E., Alavi, A., Som, P., and Sokoloff, L. The [18F]fluoro-deoxyglucose method for the measurement of local cerebral glucose utilization in man. *Circ. Res.* 44:127–137, 1979.

CHAPTER 30

Blood-Brain-Cerebrospinal Fluid Barriers

A. Lorris Betz, Gary W. Goldstein, and Robert Katzman

Basic Neurochemistry: Molecular, Cellular, and Medical Aspects, 4th Ed., edited by G. J. Siegel et al. Raven Press, Ltd., New York, 1989. Correspondence to A. Lorris Betz, Departments of Pediatrics and Neurology, University of Michigan, D3227 Medical Professional Building, Box 0718, Ann Arbor, Michigan 48109-0718.

CONSTANCY OF BRAIN INTERNAL ENVIRONMENT

In no other organ is constancy of the internal environment more important than in brain. Elsewhere in the body, the extracellular concentrations of hormones, amino acids, and potassium undergo frequent fluctuations, particularly after meals and exercise or during times of stress. In the central nervous system a similar change in the composition of the interstitial fluid could lead to uncontrolled brain activity because catecholamines and certain amino acids are centrally acting neurotransmitters and potassium influences the threshold for activation of synapses. The blood-brain-cerebrospinal fluid (CSF) barriers isolate brain cells from the normal variations in body fluid composition and thereby provide a stable environment for nerve cell interactions.

DEVELOPMENT OF THE CONCEPT OF BLOOD-BRAIN-CEREBROSPINAL FLUID BARRIERS

The concept of the blood-brain-CSF barriers was developed in the late nineteenth century when Ehrlich observed that vital dyes administered intravenously stained all organs except the brain. He concluded that the dyes had a lower affinity for binding to brain than to other tissues. In 1913, however, Goldmann disproved the binding hypothesis by administering trypan blue dye directly into the CSF. By this route, the dye readily stained the entire brain substance but was restricted to the brain and spinal cord and did not enter the bloodstream to reach other organs. The studies with vital dyes agreed well with the parallel work of Biedl and Kraus in 1898 using bile acids and Lewandowsky in 1900 using ferrocyanide. These compounds were not neurotoxic when administered by vein but caused seizures and coma when injected directly into the brain. These experiments estab-

lished that the central nervous system is separated from the bloodstream by blood-brain and blood-CSF barriers. The cellular basis for these barriers was not established until 50 years later when the development of electron microscopy permitted examination of the ultrastructure of the brain's microvasculature and the choroid plexus.

MEMBRANE TRANSPORT PROCESSES

Contemporary research has focused on how selected molecules are able to enter and leave the brain and how CSF is formed. This work had led to an appreciation of the important role played by membrane transport processes in the function of the blood-brain-CSF barriers [1]. (Monographs about the blood-brain and blood-CSF barriers are available for those readers interested in a more complete review of these subjects [2–4].)

Physical and biological processes determine molecular movement across membranes of the blood-brain-CSF barriers

These processes are diffusion, pinocytosis, carrier-mediated transport, and transcellular transport [5]. The types of carrier-mediated transport are described in Chap. 3.

Diffusion

Diffusion is the process by which molecules in solution move from an area of higher to one of lower concentration. With this type of transport, the net rate of solute flux is directly proportional to the difference in concentration between the two areas. In biologic systems, this process is an important mechanism for the movement of molecules within a fluid compartment; however, diffusion across a lipid membrane, (e.g., the cell membranes of the blood-brain barrier) is only possible when the solute is lipid soluble or when the membrane contains specialized channels. Diffusion is the primary mechanism for blood-brain exchange of respiratory gases and other highly lipid-soluble compounds. Although highly polar, water is able to diffuse rapidly across cell membranes and the blood-brain barrier by a process that is still not well understood.

Pinocytosis

In this process, extracellular fluid is engulfed by invaginating cell membranes, forming a vesicle which then separates from the membrane. This vesicle may move through the cell cytoplasm and release its contents on the other side of the cell layer by means of exocytosis. Under normal conditions, pinocytosis is thought to contribute little to the transport of molecules across the blood-brain barrier. Instead, the few vesicles that are observed within brain capillary endothelial cells are probably destined to fuse with lysosomes.

Transcellular transport

Transport across a layer of cells requires the presence of carrier or channel molecules (see Chap. 3) on luminal and antiluminal sides of the cells. Facilitated and active transport are defined in Chap. 3. In transcellular facilitated diffusion, the carriers on opposite sides of the cell are usually similar, and solutes are not moved against concentration gradients. Active transport across a cell layer, however, requires a special arrangement of transport proteins within the plasma membranes. The active transport system is found on only one side of the cell and is usually associated with a nonactive transport system on another side of the cell. With this arrangement, a solute accumulates within the cell by active transport through one membrane and subsequently leaves the cell by a channel or facilitated transport process through the opposite membrane. When plasma membranes of

two surfaces of a cell have different properties, that cell is said to be *polar*. Cellular polarity underlies active transcellular transport and secretion of fluid by epithelial cells in the choroid plexus.

When fluid is secreted at one site and absorbed at another, there is bulk flow of fluid. This means that solutes of various sizes move together with the solvent as a bulk liquid. This process is important in the circulation and absorption of CSF, which is secreted by the choroid plexus, circulates through the ventricular subarachnoid spaces, and is absorbed into the bloodstream.

Transport processes combine to provide stability for constituents of CSF and brain extracellular fluid

Bradbury and Stulcova [6] defined stability of the blood-CSF system as follows. If a substance is present in CSF at concentration C_{CSF} and in plasma at concentration C_{pl}, stability occurs when, as a result of a change in plasma concentration, a new steady state is reached so that

$$\Delta C_{CSF} < \Delta C_{pl}$$

At steady state, the flux of this substance from plasma to CSF, J_{in}, must equal its flux out, J_{out}, so that for any change in plasma concentration ΔC_{pl}, stability of CSF will occur when

$$\Delta J_{in}/\Delta C_{pl} < \Delta J_{out}/\Delta C_{csf}$$

where J_{in} and J_{out} represent transport processes that need not be identical. For instance, one might be passive and one active. If the carrier involved in J_{in} is saturated at the usual plasma concentration, then the ratio $\Delta J_{in}/\Delta C_{pl}$ will approach zero. Such carrier-mediated transport is probably the most common mechanism controlling the flow of water-soluble substances from the capillary lumen to the brain, but carrier systems have also been found to operate for outward flux. Here, the greatest stability is achieved when the carrier system operates well below saturation, so that the ratio $\Delta J_{out}/\Delta C_{CSF}$ is a positive number. Such asymmetric carrier mechanisms have been implicated in the maintenance of the control of the stability of K^+ in CSF and may also exist for other molecules.

BLOOD-BRAIN BARRIER

Endothelial cells in brain capillaries are the site of the blood-brain barrier

Studies of Reese and Karnovsky and Brightman and Reese demonstrated that brain endothelial cells differ from endothelial cells in capillaries of other organs in two important ways. First, continuous tight junctions are present between the endothelial cells that prevent transcapillary movement of polar molecules varying in size from proteins to ions. Second, there are no detectable transendothelial pathways. Thus, there is an absence of transcellular channels and fenestrations as well as a paucity of plasmalemmal and intracellular vesicles. As a result of these special anatomic features, the endothelial cells in brain provide a continuous cellular barrier between the blood and the interstitial fluid [7] (Fig. 1).

　　Not all areas of the brain contain capillaries that produce a barrier. In these nonbarrier regions, the morphologic features of the capillaries are similar to those of systemic microvascular beds. Thus, the tight junctions are discontinuous, there are more plasmalemmal vesicles, and some endothelial cells even exhibit fenestrations. Table 1 lists the brain regions that contain capillaries of this type. The absence of a blood-brain barrier in many of these regions may relate to their feedback role in the regulation of peptide hormone release.

　　Surrounding the capillary endothelial cell is a collagen-containing extracellular matrix. Embedded within this basement membrane are

pericytes whose function is unknown. Almost the entire outer surface of the basement membrane is covered with foot processes from astrocytes. This close association suggests an interaction between astrocytes and endothelial cells that is important for the function of the blood-brain barrier. Support for this hypothesis is found in brain tumors and nonbarrier regions of the brain, where a loss of the normal astrocyte-endothelial cell relationship is associated with the absence of a blood-brain barrier.

Substances with high lipid solubility may move across the blood-brain barrier by simple diffusion

Diffusion is the major entry mechanism for most psychoactive drugs. As shown in Fig. 2, the rate of entry of compounds that diffuse into the brain depends on their lipid solubility, as estimated by oil/water partition coefficients. For example, the permeability of very lipid soluble compounds, such as ethanol, nicotine, iodoantipyrine, and imipramine, is so high that they are completely extracted from the blood during a single passage through the brain. Hence, their uptake by the brain is limited only by blood flow, and this provides the basis for use of iodoantipyrine to measure cerebral blood flow rate. In contrast, polar molecules, such as acetylcholine and catecholamines, enter the brain only slowly, thereby isolating the brain from neurotransmitters in the plasma. The brain uptake of some compounds (e.g., phenobarbital

TABLE 1. Areas of brain without a blood-brain barrier
Pituitary gland
Median eminence
Area postrema
Preoptic recess
Paraphysis
Pineal gland
Endothelium of the choroid plexus

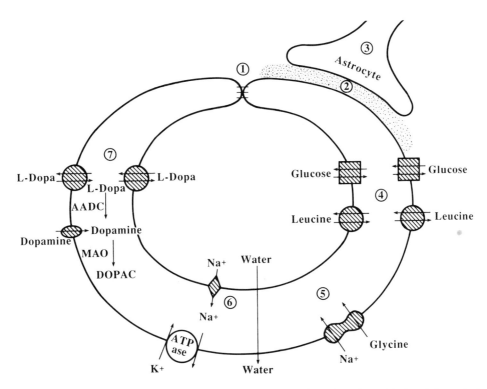

FIG. 1. Schematic diagram of brain capillary. The continuous tight junctions (1) that join endothelial cells in brain capillaries limit the diffusion of large and small solutes across the blood-brain barrier. The basement membrane (2) provides structural support for the capillary and, along with the astrocytic foot processes (3) that encircle the capillary, may influence endothelial cell function. Transport carriers (4) for glucose and essential amino acids facilitate the movement of these solutes into brain, while active transport systems (5) appear to cause indirectly the efflux of small, nonessential amino acids from brain to blood. Sodium ion transporters on the luminal membrane and Na,K-ATPase on the antiluminal membrane (6) account for the movement of Na$^+$ from blood to brain, and this may provide an osmotic driving force for the secretion of interstitial fluid by the brain capillary. The enzymatic blood-brain barrier (7) consists of the uptake of neurotransmitter precursors such as L-dopa into the endothelial cells via the large neutral amino acid carrier, and their subsequent metabolism to 3,4-dihydroxyphenylacetic acid (DOPAC) by aromatic amino acid decarboxylase (AADC) and monoamine oxidase (MAO) present within the endothelial cell. Neurotransmitters in the interstitial fluid may also be accumulated and metabolized by the brain capillary.

and phenytoin) is lower than predicted from their lipid solubility as a result of binding to plasma proteins.

Water

Water readily enters the brain by diffusion. Using intravenously administered deuterium oxide as a tracer, the measured half-time of the exchange of brain water varies between 12 and 25 sec, depending on the vascularity of the region studied. Although this rate of exchange is rapid compared with the rate of exchange of most solutes, it is limited both by the permeability of the capillary endothelium and by the rate of cerebral blood flow. In fact, the calculated permeability constant of the cerebral capillary wall to the diffusion of water is about the same as that estimated for its diffusion across lipid membranes.

As a consequence of its high permeability, water moves freely into or out of the brain as the osmolality of the plasma changes. This phenomenon is clinically useful, since the intravenous administration of poorly permeable compounds such as mannitol will osmotically dehydrate the brain and reduce intracranial pressure (see Chap. 40 on brain edema). For example, when plasma osmolality is raised from 310 to 344 mOsm, a 10 percent shrinkage of the brain will result, with half of the shrinkage taking place in 12 min.

Gases

Gases, such as CO_2, O_2, N_2O, Xe, and Kr, and volatile anesthetics diffuse rapidly into brain. As a consequence, the rate at which their concentration in brain comes into equilibrium with plasma is limited primarily by cerebral blood flow. Hence, inert gases (e.g., N_2O, Xe, and Kr) are used to measure cerebral blood flow.

An interesting contrast is found between CO_2 and H^+ with regard to their effects on brain pH. Since the blood-brain barrier permeability of CO_2 greatly exceeds that of H^+, the pH of brain interstitial fluid will reflect blood pCO_2 rather than blood pH. Consequently, in a patient with a metabolic acidosis and a compensatory respiratory alkalosis, the brain is alkalotic.

Carrier-mediated transport enables molecules with low lipid solubility to traverse the blood-brain barrier

Although glucose and mannitol are similar in size and structure, the brain extraction of glucose is 20- to 30-fold greater than that of mannitol (Fig. 2). This apparently anomalous relationship is also observed for other metabolically essential compounds (Table 2). The high permeability of these polar compounds is mediated by specific transport proteins (see Chap. 3) in the plasma membranes of the endothelial cells (Fig. 1).

Glucose

Glucose is the primary energy substrate of the brain, and its metabolism accounts for nearly all of the brain's oxygen consumption. Since entry of glucose into the brain is critical, mechanisms for glucose transport across the blood-brain barrier have been particularly well studied [11,12]. Highly specific carriers are present in brain capillary endothelial cells, and they mediate the facilitated diffusion of this polar substrate through the blood-brain barrier. The ac-

TABLE 2.   Blood-brain barrier transport systems[a]

Transport system	Representative substrate	Affinity (mM)	Maximal rate (nmol/g/min)
Hexose	Glucose	9.0	1,600
Monocarboxylic acid	Lactate	1.9	120
Large neutral amino acid	Phenylalanine	0.12	30
Basic amino acid	Lysine	0.10	6
Acidic amino acid	Glutamate	0.04	0.4
Amine	Choline	0.44	10
Purine	Adenine	0.027	1
Nucleoside	Adenosine	0.018	0.7
Thyroid hormone	T3	0.001	0.1

[a] From Pardridge [10].

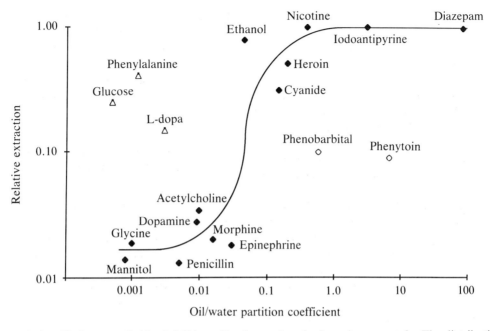

FIG. 2.   Relationship between lipid solubility and brain uptake of selected compounds. The distribution into olive oil relative to water for each test substance serves as a measure of its lipid solubility. Brain uptake is determined by comparing the extraction of each test substance relative to a highly permeable tracer during a single pass through the cerebral circulation. In general, the higher the oil-water partition coefficient, the greater the brain uptake (◆). Uptake of the two anticonvulsants, phenobarbital and phenytoin, is lower than predicted from their lipid solubility partly because of their binding to plasma proteins (◇). Uptake of glucose, phenylalanine, and L-dopa is greater than predicted by their lipid solubility because specific carriers facilitate their transport across the brain capillary (△). (Data are from Oldendorf [8,9].)

tivity of these carriers is sufficient to transport two to three times more glucose than is normally metabolized by the brain.

The stereospecificity of the glucose transport system permits D-glucose, but not L-glucose, to enter the brain. Hexoses such as mannose and maltose are also transported rapidly into the brain; the uptake of galactose is intermediate, whereas fructose is taken up very slowly. 2-Deoxyglucose is taken up quickly and will competitively inhibit the transport of glucose. Once within neurons and glia, 2-deoxyglucose is phosphorylated but not further metabolized. If 2-deoxyglucose is used in tracer quantities, the amount of the phosphorylated tracer in the brain reflects the rate of glucose metabolism (see Chaps. 29 and 44).

Monocarboxylic acids

Monocarboxylic acids, including L-lactate, acetate, pyruvate, and ketone bodies, are transported by a separate stereospecific system [12]. The rate of entry of these substances is significantly lower than that of glucose; however, they may become important metabolic substrates during starvation.

Neutral L-amino acids

The rate of movement of neutral L-amino acids into brain is variable [12]. Phenylalanine, leucine, tyrosine, isoleucine, valine, tryptophan, methionine, histidine, and L-dopa may enter as rapidly as glucose. These are supplied from protein breakdown and diet. Several are precursors for neurotransmitters synthesized in the brain. The transport of these large neutral amino acids into brain is inhibited by the synthetic amino acid 2-aminonorbornane-2-carboxylic acid (BCH), but not by 2-(methyl-amino)-iso-butyric acid (MeAIB); hence, the transport system in the blood-brain barrier is similar to the leucine (L) transport system defined by Christensen [5]. Since a single type of transport carrier mediates the transcapillary movement of structurally related amino acids, these compounds compete with each other for entry into the brain. Therefore, an elevation in the plasma level of one will inhibit uptake of the others. This may be important in certain metabolic diseases such as phenylketonuria (PKU), where high levels of phenylalanine in plasma reduce brain uptake of other essential amino acids (see Chap. 38).

Small neutral amino acids, such as alanine, glycine, proline, and γ-aminobutyric acid (GABA), are markedly restricted in their entry into the brain. These turn over continuously in the brain as intermediate metabolites (see Chap. 28), and several are putative neurotransmitters. This restriction is consistent with the inability of MeAIB to inhibit brain uptake of amino acids and suggests that the alanine (A) transport system [5] is not present on the luminal surface of the blood-brain barrier. In contrast, these small neutral amino acids appear to be transported out of the brain across the blood-brain barrier, suggesting that the A-system carrier is present on the antiluminal surface of the brain capillary [13]. Thus, essential amino acids that serve as precursors for catecholamine and indoleamine synthesis are readily transported into brain (L system), whereas amino acids synthesized by brain, including those amino acids that act as neurotransmitters, are not only limited in their entry but are actively transported out of the brain (A system).

Choline

Choline enters the central nervous system through a carrier-mediated transport process that can be inhibited by molecules such as dimethyl aminoethanol, hemicholinium, and tetraethyl ammonium chloride. Since choline cannot be synthesized by brain, it has been proposed that blood-brain barrier transport may regulate the formation of acetylcholine in the central nervous system [14].

Metal ions are exchanged between plasma and brain very slowly, compared to other tissues

Intravenously administered $^{42}K^+$, for example, exchanges with muscle K^+ in 1 hr, but K^+ exchange in brain is only half completed in 24 to 36 hr. The rate of K^+ flux into brain shows little change as plasma K^+ concentration is varied. Ca^{2+} and Mg^{2+} exchange in brain as slowly as does K^+. Na^+ exchange is somewhat faster, with half-exchange into brain occurring in 3 to 8 hr. Despite its relatively slow entry into the brain, Na^+ exchange across the blood-brain barrier appears to occur by mediated transport [15]. This occurs, in part, through brain capillary Na,K-ATPase, which is primarily located on the brain capillary antiluminal membrane of the endothelial cell (Fig. 1). Na,K-ATPase in the brain capillary may also mediate removal of interstitial fluid K^+ from brain and thereby maintain a constant brain K^+ concentration in the face of fluctuating plasma concentrations. In addition, the antiluminal location of Na,K-ATPase may underlie the proposed role of the brain capillary in extrachoroidal production of CSF [16].

Metabolic processes within the brain capillary endothelial cells are important to blood-brain barrier function

Most neurotransmitters present in the blood do not enter the brain because of their low lipid solubility and lack of specific transport carriers in the luminal membrane of the capillary endothelial cell. This is illustrated for dopamine in Fig. 2. In contrast, L-dopa, the precursor for dopamine, has affinity for the large neutral amino acid transport system and more easily enters brain from blood than would be predicted by its lipid solubility (Fig. 1). This is why patients with Parkinson's disease are treated with L-dopa rather than with dopamine (see Chap. 42); however, the penetration of L-dopa into the brain is limited by the presence of the enzymes L-dopa decarboxylase and monoamine oxidase within the capillary endothelial cell [17]. This "enzymatic blood-brain barrier" limits transendothelial passage of L-dopa into brain and explains the need for large doses of L-dopa in the treatment of Parkinson's disease. Therapy is currently enhanced by concurrent treatment with an inhibitor of peripheral L-dopa decarboxylase (see Chap. 42).

Intracapillary monoamine oxidase may also play a role in the inactivation of neurotransmitters released by neuronal activity, since monoamines are actively accumulated and metabolized by brain capillaries [17]. The fact that monoamines show very little uptake when presented from the luminal side suggests that the uptake systems are present only on the antiluminal membrane of the brain capillary endothelial cell (Fig. 1).

Blood-brain barrier undergoes development

Many of the features of the blood-brain barrier, including the presence of tight junctions in the capillary endothelium and the exclusion of protein molecules, are present in newborn animals [18]. In addition, the relationship between lipid solubility and barrier penetration is similar in adults and newborns; however, there is evidence for increased permeability of selected solutes. For example, concentrations of transferrin, α-fetoprotein, and albumin in the CSF of fetal and neonatal animals are disproportionately high, and this may be explained by receptor-mediated endocytosis in young, but not mature, animals. The increased uptake into immature brain of certain actively metabolized

substances such as organic acids is the result of an increase in transport capacity for these compounds.

BLOOD-CEREBROSPINAL FLUID BARRIER

CSF is formed by active transport of solutes across the epithelial cells in the choroid plexus

Since the concentrations of several constituents are maintained at levels different in CSF from those in plasma (Table 3), CSF is not simply a protein-free ultrafiltrate of plasma. The functional unit of the choroid plexus, composed of a capillary enveloped by a layer of differentiated ependymal epithelium, is diagrammed in Fig. 3. In normal subjects, the rate of CSF secretion is 0.3 to 0.4 ml/min, about one-third the rate at which urine is formed. Although the total volume of CSF cannot be precisely measured, it is estimated to be 100 to 150 ml in normal adults. This means that the CSF is totally replaced three or four times each day.

The major sites of CSF formation are the choroid plexus present in all cerebral ventricles (Fig. 4). This conclusion was first deduced from the observation that fluid accumulates and enlarges the ventricles if the aqueduct of Sylvius

TABLE 3. Typical plasma and CSF levels of various substances

Substance[a]	Plasma	CSF
Na	145.0	150.0
K	4.8	2.9
Ca	5.2	2.3
Mg	1.7	2.3
Cl	108.0	130.0
HCO_3	27.4	21.0
Lactate	7.9	2.6
PO_4	1.8	0.5
Protein	7,000.0	20.0
Glucose	95.0	60.0

[a] Protein and glucose concentrations are in mg/100ml; all others are in mEq/liter.

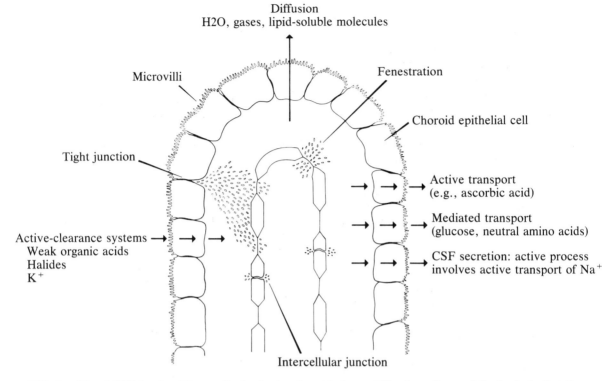

FIG. 3. Blood-CSF barrier. The capillaries in the choroid plexus differ from those of the brain in that there is free movement of molecules across the endothelial cell through fenestrations and intercellular gaps. The blood-CSF barrier is at the choroid plexus epithelial cells, which are joined together by tight junctions. Microvilli are present on the CSF-facing surface, and these may aid in secretion. Diffusion, facilitated diffusion, and active transport into CSF, as well as active transport of metabolites from CSF to blood, have been demonstrated in the choroid plexus.

is obstructed. Furthermore, neurosurgeons have reported seeing drops of fluid form on the surfaces of the choroid plexus.

Through histochemical and ultrastructural investigations, we now know that the choroid plexus epithelial cells have morphological features similar to those of other secretory cells, and there is abundant physiological data indicating that the choroid plexus is the primary site of CSF formation. However, extrachoroidal formation of CSF has also been demonstrated [16], and this may be the result of ion transport by brain capillaries, as discussed above.

Rate of formation of CSF can be measured by various means

A simple method of measuring the rate of formation of CSF is to measure the time it takes CSF pressure to recover after a known volume of CSF is removed. The rate in humans is 0.35 ml/min. A more accurate method of measuring CSF formation was introduced by Pappenheimer and co-workers [19]. With this method, simulated CSF is perfused between the ventricle and the cisterna magna, and inulin is added to the perfusion fluid. Because inulin diffuses very

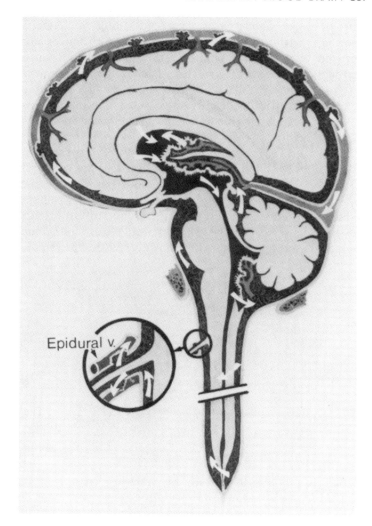

Epidural v.

FIG. 4. Circulation of CSF. CSF is secreted by the choroid plexus present in the cerebral ventricles and by extrachoroidal sources. It subsequently circulates through the ventricular cavities and into the subarachnoid space. Absorption into venous blood occurs through the arachnoid granulations in the superior sagittal sinus and along the spinal nerve root sheaths (*inset*). (From Fishman [4].)

slowly into tissue during such a perfusion, the dilution of inulin is taken as a measure of the rate of formation of new CSF. Therefore, if the perfusion at a rate of V_i ml/min is carried out until a steady state is reached, and if the initial concentration of inulin is C_i and the outflow concentration of inulin is C_o, the rate of formation of CSF (V_f) is given by

$$V_f = V_i(C_i - C_o)/C_o$$

Such perfusions have been carried out in a wide variety of species. Typical rates of CSF formation are as follows: rabbit, 0.001 ml/min; cat, 0.02 ml/min; rhesus monkey, 0.08 ml/min; and goat, 0.19 ml/min. In humans, the average value is 0.37 ml/min, and this corresponds rather closely to the value determined from drainage experiments.

By use of the ventriculocisternal perfusion method, it has been found that CSF formation decreases very little as intracranial pressure increases. Moreover, CSF is formed at a normal rate and osmolality, even when the fluid perfused through the ventricle is moderately hypertonic or hypotonic. When the perfused fluid is very hypotonic, however, CSF formation may cease. CSF formation is also reduced if serum osmolality is raised.

Carrier-mediated transport drives secretion of CSF

The movement of substances from the blood into CSF is, in many ways, analogous to that from blood into brain. There is free movement of water, gases, and lipid-soluble compounds from the blood into the CSF. Substances important for brain metabolism and maintenance of CSF electrolytes, such as glucose, amino acids, and cations, are transported by saturable carrier-mediated processes. Macromolecules such as proteins and most small polar molecules do not enter the CSF (Fig. 3).

The most important transport systems in the choroid plexus epithelial cells are those responsible for CSF secretion (Fig. 5). In most fluid-secreting epithelial tissues, transcellular movement of water is driven by active transport of Na^+ and Cl^+. The choroid plexus epithelium is no exception [20]; however, in contrast to the

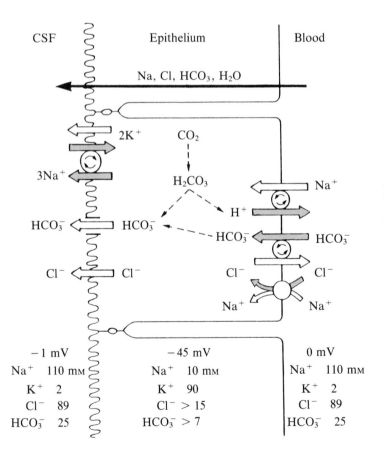

FIG. 5. Schematic diagram of ion transport mechanisms in the choroid plexus epithelial cell. Net transport of Na^+, Cl^-, and HCO_3^- across the choroid plexus epithelium results in the secretion of CSF. (From Saito and Wright [20].)

basolateral localization of Na,K-ATPase in other epithelia, this cation pump is found on the apical microvilli of the choroid plexus [21]. By pumping Na^+ out of the epithelial cell into the CSF, Na,K-ATPase maintains a low intracellular Na^+ activity. The active extrusion of Na^+ is associated with the downhill movement of Na^+ across the basolateral membrane mediated by both a coupled Na^+-Cl^+ symport system and a Na^+-H^+ antiport system (see Chap. 3). In addition, carrier-mediated exchange of HCO_3^- for Cl^- is an important step in the movement of anions from blood to CSF; by producing intracellular HCO_3^-, carbonic anhydrase within the choroid plexus epithelial cell also strongly influences secretion of CSF. The importance of these transport systems in CSF secretion was determined through the use of specific inhibitors such as ouabain for Na,K-ATPase, furosemide for coupled Na^+-Cl^+ symport, acetazolamide for carbonic anhydrase, and 4-acetamide-4'-isothiocyano-2,2'-disulfonic stilbene (SITS) for Cl^--HCO_3^- antiport. Acetazolamide and furosemide are used therapeutically to decrease the rate of CSF formation in hydrocephalus.

Other active transport systems in the choroid plexus are linked to the efflux of specific solutes [22]. For example, iodide and thiocyanate are transported from the CSF by saturable carrier mechanisms that can be competitively inhibited by perchlorate. This system must be active because the transport can be carried out against unfavorable electrochemical gradients. Another important transport system removes weak organic acids from the CSF. Among the molecules cleared by this mechanism are penicillin and neurotransmitter metabolites, such as homovanillic acid (HVA) and 5-HIAA. This clearance system, which transports against an unfavorable CSF to blood gradient, is saturable and inhibited by probenecid. Clearance of organic acids by a probenecid-sensitive transport mechanism may also occur across the blood-brain barrier in brain capillaries.

CSF circulates through the ventricles and over the surface of the brain

Choroid plexus pulsations are transmitted throughout the CSF and can be seen on the manometer at the time of lumbar spinal tap. The fluid circulation is from the lateral ventricles through the foramina of Monro into the third ventricle and then into the fourth ventricle. The fluid passes from the fourth ventricle through the foramina of Luschka and Magendie to the cisterna magna and then circulates into the cerebral and spinal subarachnoid spaces (Fig. 4). If obstructions are placed at the foramina between these ventricles, the ventricle upstream from the obstruction will enlarge significantly, producing obstructive hydrocephalus. Thus, if a foramen of Monro is obstructed, the ipsilateral ventricle will enlarge. If the aqueduct is obstructed, both lateral ventricles and the third ventricle will enlarge.

Occasionally, disease processes affect CSF removal. For example, obliteration of the subarachnoid space by inflammation or thrombosis of the sinuses will prevent clearance of fluid. When this occurs, CSF pressure increases, and hydrocephalus develops without obstruction of the ventricular foramina. This is called communicating hydrocephalus.

CSF is removed at villi and granulations over the large venous sinuses in the skull and at the cranial and spinal nerve root sheaths

There is evidence that absorption of CSF by the arachnoid villi occurs by a valve-like process, permitting the one-way flow of CSF from the subarachnoid spaces into the venous sinuses. CSF absorption does not occur until CSF pressure exceeds the pressure within the sinuses. Once this threshold is reached, the rate of absorption is proportional to the difference between CSF and sinus pressures. A normal human can absorb CSF at a rate up to six times the normal rate of CSF formation with only a moderate increase in intracranial pressure.

The combination of bulk absorption of solute and solvent together by the arachnoid villi and the selective removal of molecules by the choroid plexus is termed the sink function of the CSF. This implies that molecules reaching the interstitial fluid of the brain may diffuse into CSF and then be removed by either bulk absorption or active transport, or both mechanisms. This sink action helps maintain the low concentration of many substances in both brain and CSF, compared with plasma concentrations.

CEREBROSPINAL FLUID-BRAIN INTERFACE

The absence of tight junctions between some ependymal and pial cells permits diffusion of proteins and other hydrophilic molecules from the CSF into the interstitium of the brain, and vice versa. However, large molecules such as proteins and inulin penetrate poorly.

Quantitative studies of the movement of substances between CSF and brain suggest that the concentration of ions in the extracellular fluid in brain should be the same as that in CSF. This relationship has been directly demonstrated for K^+ using ion-specific electrodes placed in the brain's interstitial space. Brain interstitial K^+ concentration is approximately 3 mM, similar to that of CSF, and independent of the plasma K^+ concentration [23].

BYPASSING THE BARRIERS WITH DRUGS

A number of agents of potential therapeutic importance do not readily enter the brain because they have low lipid solubility and are not transported by the specific carriers present in the blood-brain barrier or choroid plexus. To overcome this limitation, schemes have been developed to enhance drug entry into the central nervous system [24].

The most obvious method of circumventing the barriers is to inject the agents directly into the CSF. Although ventricular or cisternal access sites may be used, intrathecal administration of antineoplastic agents is usually accomplished by intralumbar injection. Because of limited drug penetration into brain substance, these routes are most often used in patients with chronic meningitis and leukemia.

Enhanced delivery of drug into brain can be accomplished by raising its concentration in the blood, but this approach is often limited by the occurrence of systemic side effects. It is possible to achieve similar high concentrations of drug in the brain vasculature by infusing the drug directly into the carotid artery. In this way, the same total systemic dose produces a much higher concentration gradient across the blood-brain barrier and leads to greater uptake by the brain.

Another way to enhance delivery is to increase the permeability of the blood-brain barrier. The disease itself may produce this effect, and this is why the rate of penicillin passage into brain is highest early in the course of meningitis; however, when the capillaries are intact some intervention is necessary to open the barrier. The infusion of hyperosmolar solutions into the carotid circulation alters blood-brain barrier permeability in laboratory animals [25] and is used in treatment of patients with brain tumors. The change in permeability appears to be caused by separation of the tight junctions that normally seal together the endothelial cells in brain capillaries.

Designing drugs with high blood-brain barrier permeability is a more selective way to improve delivery into brain. In fact, most neuroactive drugs are effective because they dissolve in lipid and easily enter the brain. A good example of the importance of structure and lipid solubility is provided by comparison of the brain uptake of heroin and morphine [8]. These compounds are very similar in structure except for two acetyl groups that make heroin more lipid soluble. This greater lipid solubility of heroin explains its more rapid onset of action. Once within the brain the acetyl groups on heroin are removed enzymatically to produce morphine, which only slowly leaves the brain. By analogy, it would seem ideal to develop new therapeutic drugs that readily enter and then are trapped within the central nervous system. An understanding of transport processes is crucial to development of the next generation of drugs useful in treating various brain diseases.

REFERENCES

1. Goldstein, G. W., and Betz, A. L. The blood-brain barrier. *Sci. Am.* 254:74–83, 1986.
2. Katzman, R., and Pappius, H. M. *Brain Electrolytes and Fluid Metabolism.* Baltimore: Williams & Wilkins, 1973.
3. Bradbury, M. *The Concept of a Blood-Brain Barrier.* Chichester: John Wiley, 1979.
4. Fishman, R. A. *Cerebrospinal Fluid in Diseases of the Nervous System.* Philadelphia: W. B. Saunders, 1980.
5. Kotyk, A., and Janácek, K. *Cell Membrane Transport.* New York: Plenum Press, 1975.
6. Bradbury, M. W. B., and Stulcova, B. Efflux mechanism contributing to the stability of the potassium concentration in cerebrospinal fluid. *J. Physiol. (Lond.)* 208:415–430, 1970.
7. Brightman, M. W. Morphology of blood-brain interfaces. *Exp. Eye Res. (Suppl.)* 25:1–25, 1977.
8. Oldendorf, W. H. The blood-brain barrier. *Exp. Eye Res. (Suppl.)* 25:177–190, 1977.
9. Oldendorf, W. H. Clearance of radiolabeled substances by brain after arterial injection using a diffusible internal standard. In N. Marks and R. Rodnight (eds.), *Research Methods in Neuro-*

chemistry. New York: Plenum Press, 1981, Vol. 5, pp. 91–112.
10. Pardridge, W. M. Neuropeptides and the blood-brain barrier. *Annu. Rev. Physiol.* 45:73–82, 1983.
11. Lund-Anderson, H. Transport of glucose from blood to brain. *Physiol. Rev.* 59:305–352, 1979.
12. Pardridge, W. M. Brain metabolism: A perspective from the blood-brain barrier. *Physiol. Rev.* 63:1481–1535, 1983.
13. Betz, A. L., and Goldstein, G. W. Polarity of the blood-brain barrier: Neutral amino acid transport into isolated brain capillaries. *Science* 202:225–227, 1978.
14. Cohen, E., and Wurtman, R. J. Brain acetylcholine synthesis: Control by dietary choline. *Science* 191:561–562, 1976.
15. Betz, A. L., and Goldstein, G. W. Specialized properties and solute transport in brain capillaries. *Annu. Rev. Physiol.* 48:241–250, 1986.
16. Milhorat, T. H., Hammock, M. K., and Fenstermacher, J. D. Cerebrospinal fluid production by the choroid plexus and brain. *Science* 173:330–332, 1971.
17. Hardebo, J. E., and Owman, C. Barrier mechanisms for neurotransmitter monoamines and their precursors at the blood-brain barrier. *Ann. Neurol.* 8:1–11, 1979.
18. Saunders, N. R. Ontogeny of the blood-brain barrier. *Exp. Eye Res. (Suppl.)* 25:523–550, 1977.
19. Heisey, S. R., Held, D., and Pappenheimer, J. R. Bulk flow and diffusion in the cerebrospinal fluid system of the goat. *Am. J. Physiol.* 203:775–781, 1962.
20. Saito, Y., and Wright, E. M. Bicarbonate transport across the frog choroid plexus and its control by cyclic nucleotides. *J. Physiol. (Lond.)* 336:635–648, 1983.
21. Ernst, S. A., Palacios, J. R., and Siegel, G. J. Immunocytochemical localization of Na^+,K^+-ATPase catalytic polypeptide in mouse choroid plexus. *J. Histochem. Cytochem.* 34:189–195, 1986.
22. Lorenzo, A. V. Factors governing the composition of the cerebrospinal fluid. *Exp. Eye Res. (Suppl.)* 25:205–228, 1977.
23. Hansen, A. J., Lund-Anderson, H., Crone, C.

K^+-permeability of the blood-brain barrier, investigated by aid of a K^+-sensitive microelectrode. *Acta Physiol. Scand.* 101:438–445, 1977.

24. Riccardi, R., Bleyer, W. A., and Poplack, D. G. Enhancement of delivery of antineoplastic drugs into cerebrospinal fluid. In J. H. Wood (ed.), *Neurobiology of Cerebrospinal Fluid.* New York: Plenum Press, 1983, pp. 453–466.

25. Rapoport, S. I., Fredericks, W. R., Ohno, K., and Pettigrew, K. D. Quantitative aspects of reversible osmotic opening of the blood-brain barrier. *Am. J. Physiol.* 238:R421–R431, 1980.

PART FIVE

Medical Neurochemistry

CHAPTER 31

Biochemistry of Muscle and Disorders of Muscle Membranes

John Gergely and Frederick Samaha

Basic Neurochemistry: Molecular, Cellular, and Medical Aspects, 4th Ed., edited by G. J. Siegel et al. Raven Press, Ltd., New York, 1989.
Correspondence to John Gergely, Boston Biomedical Research Institute, 20 Staniford Street, Boston, Massachusetts 02114.

This chapter provides a brief summary of selected topics of muscle biochemistry in the context of ultrastructure, contraction, and relaxation, with a brief excursion into some membrane-related diseases. Topics related to those covered in other chapters have been omitted. The interested reader is referred to recent specialized works [1,2] for more detailed coverage. For a broad historical perspective, Dorothy Needham's *Machina Carnis* [3] cannot be surpassed.

STRUCTURE

Sarcomeres are the basis of the striation of muscle

Light microscopists have long known that the physiological unit of muscle, the cell or fiber, contains typical repeating structures along its length [1–4]. These repeating units are sarcomeres and are separated from each other by Z bands. Within each sarcomere, one can distinguish the A and I bands; the A band, lying between two I bands, occupies the center of each sarcomere and is highly birefringent. Within the A band, a central lighter zone, the H band, can be seen; and in the center of the H band is the darker M band. The Z disks are at the centers of the I bands. The contractile material is subdivided into smaller units—myofibrils separated by mitochondria and sarcoplasmic reticulum.

The muscle cell is surrounded by a plasma membrane, which, together with the various connective tissue elements and collagen filaments, forms the sarcolemma. The interior of the resting cell is maintained by the plasma membrane at an electrical potential about 80 mV more negative than the exterior. When the muscle is stimulated by its nerve, activation of the contractile machinery results in contraction and tension development. The coupling of excitation and contraction involves the transverse, or T, tubules, elements of the muscle cell that are continuous with the plasma membrane. These tubules are seen as openings on the surface of the muscle cell disposed either at the level of the Z bands or at the junction of the A and I bands, depending on the species; and the depolarization of the membrane spreads activity along the tubules to the interior of the fiber.

The electron microscope reveals two sets of filaments

The typical striation pattern of voluntary muscle can now be attributed to a regular arrangement of two sets of filaments (Fig. 1). The thin filaments (diameter, ~80 Å) appear to be attached to the Z bands and are found in the I band and in part of the A band. The second set of so-called thick filaments (diameter, ~150 Å) occupies the A band. The thick filaments seem to be connected crosswise by some material in the M band. In cross section, the thick filaments constitute a hexagonal lattice; in vertebrate muscle, the thin filaments occupy the centers of the triangles formed by the thick filaments.

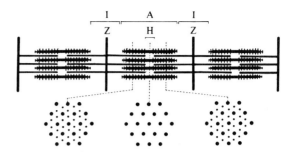

FIG. 1. Schematic representation of structure of striated muscle. Actin-containing thin filaments originate at Z lines. Note thick myosin-containing filaments that bear cross-bridges. The M disk lies in the center of the H band (see text). (From H. E. Huxley, The mechanism of muscle contraction. *Science* 164:1356, 1969.)

Contraction is due to the relative sliding of the filaments

With the acceptance of the existence of two sets of discontinuous filaments came the recognition that (a) the two kinds of filaments become cross-linked only on excitation; and (b) contraction of muscle does not depend on shortening the length of the filaments but rather on the relative motion of the two sets of filaments (sliding-filament mechanism). Thus the length of the muscle depends on the length of the sarcomeres, and in turn, the variation in sarcomere length is based on the variation in overlap between the thin and thick filaments. High-resolution electron micrographs have shown that cross-bridges emanate from the thick filaments, and it is thought that in active muscle, these structures are responsible for the links with thin filaments.

Distinct proteins are found in the two sets of filaments

Myosin is the chief constituent of thick filaments, and actin the chief constituent of thin filaments. Tropomyosin and a complex of three subunits subsumed under the name troponin are present in the thin filaments and play an important role in the regulation of muscle contraction. The proteins constituting the M and the Z bands have not been fully characterized. The presence of creatine kinase in the M line has been demonstrated, but its structural role is not clear, and the role of other components also remains to be elucidated. There is evidence, however, that α-actinin is present in the Z bands and in the rodlike bodies connected to

the Z bands that are found in nemaline myopathy. Another constituent of the Z band has been identified as desmin ($M_r \sim 50,000\ M$), the subunit of the so-called 10-nm filaments. Filaments in the 10-nm class have been found in a variety of cells and are considered part of the cytoskeleton. The existence of filaments that are continuous throughout the sarcomere (fibrillin) has long been suggested, but in view of the overwhelming evidence for the participation of the discontinuous myosin and actin filaments in the contraction process, the former have until recently not received much attention. Recent work has produced more information on a continuous elastic network surrounding the actin and myosin filaments [5,6]. Connectin, the main constituent of elastic protein filaments in muscle, appears to be identical with titin, a large myofibrillar protein. A related protein is nebulin. X-irradiation of a skinned rabbit fiber selectively destroys nebulin and titin, leading to disorganization of sarcomeres, and interferes with force development. Recent speculation connecting a possible defect in nebulin biosynthesis with the genetic basis of Duchenne dystrophy has not been supported by subsequent work [7,8] (see below; see also Chap. 23).

Nonmuscle motility involves proteins similar to those found in muscle

An important development that has taken place over the past few years is the recognition that all cells contain myosin, actin, and other components of the myofilaments and that a variety of cell functions, including cell motility and probably cell division, depend on these proteins (see, e.g., Warrick and Spudich [9]). An important difference between muscle and other tissue is that in nonmuscle, the myofibrillar proteins do not form the conspicuous structures found in muscle and the supramolecular complexes usually have a more fleeting existence. Nonmuscle cellular "contractile" proteins are discussed in Chapter 24.

PROTEINS

Actin forms the backbone of the thin filaments

The thin filaments of muscle contain slightly elongated, bilobar subunits, about 4×6 nm, arranged in helical structures, their longer dimension being roughly at a right angle to the filament axis [10,11]. These are identified with the protein actin, which can be extracted from muscle that has been treated with acetone. The molecular weight of actin is about 42,000. Variations in the amino acid sequence of actins in various cell types—skeletal muscle, cardiac muscle, brain, platelets—have been found in the same organism; however, amino acid replacements in actin are of a very conservative nature in that the character (charge and hydrophobicity) of the residue is preserved, even if species far from one another on the evolutionary scale are compared. This diversity reflects the existence of an actin multigene family leading to many isoforms. (See also several articles in Engel and Banker [1], and chapter by Gergely in Walton [2].)

Polymerization

On addition of salts to a solution of actin, a drastic change in viscosity results, and negatively stained electron micrographs reveal the presence of double-helical filaments that are essentially identical to the thin filaments in appearance. The two physical states of actin characterized by low and high viscosity are called, respectively, globular (G) and fibrous (F). The $G \rightarrow F$ transition is referred to as polymerization. The nucleotide in G-actin is ATP; that in F-actin is ADP. The transformation of ATP to ADP takes place during polymerization but is not involved in muscle contraction. This reaction presumably takes place when actin filaments are laid down in the course of development, growth, or regeneration.

A number of proteins interact with actin

There are a wide variety of proteins that interact with actin (actin-binding proteins), some of which are found in muscle, but many of which play an important role in nonmuscle cell motility [10]. They may affect the polymerization-depolarization of actin and are involved in the attachment of actin to other cellular structures, including the Z disks in muscle as well as membranes both in muscle and nonmuscle cells. The protein interacting with actin in the Z disk, α-actinin, is also a component of the rod-like bodies found in nemaline myopathy.

Myosin, the chief constituent of the thick filaments, is a multisubunit protein

Myosin is a highly asymmetrical molecule with an overall length of about 150 nm and a molecular weight of about 500,000 (Fig. 2) [1, p. 563; 4,12]. Its width varies between about 2 and 10 nm. In contrast to actin, which is made up of a single polypeptide chain, myosin consists of several peptide chains.

Recent years have seen a burst of activity in determining DNA sequences for various proteins [13]. It is clear that most muscle proteins are members of multigene families. Although there are differences among myosins (isozymes) in different muscle types (see below), the differences tend to be conservative, preserving the character of the structure. These differences are either due to the expression of different genes, which is the case for the heavy chain, or to so-called alternative splicing or similar mechanisms by which one gene may lead to several proteins (see Chaps. 21 and 22), as is the case for two of the light chains, LC_1 and LC_3 (see below).

Heavy chains

There are two heavy chains, each with a molecular weight of about 200,000, that run from one end of the molecule to the other. Along most of the length of the molecule, the two chains are intertwined to form a double-α-helix rod; at one end of the molecule they separate, each forming a somewhat elongated globular portion. Under appropriate conditions, a number of proteolytic enzymes, e.g., trypsin, chymotrypsin, papain, cleave the myosin molecule into well-defined fragments that retain various functional properties of the intact molecule. It has been possible to isolate the α-helical portions, including the whole rod and light meromyosin (LMM), which form the core of the thick filaments, fragments containing globular portions, the two-headed heavy meromyosin (HMM) and HMM subfragment 1 (S-1) corresponding to a single head. The two globular portions contain the sites responsible for the biological activity of myosin; that is, the ability to hydrolyze ATP and to combine with actin.

Light chains

In addition to the two heavy chains, each myosin molecule contains four light chains with molecular weights of about 20,000. Fast-twitch muscle contains three types of light chains, designated LC_1, LC_2, and LC_3, in order of increas-

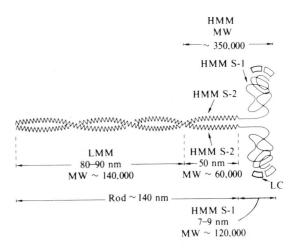

FIG. 2. Schematic representation of the structure of the myosin molecule. (Lowey, S., H. S. Slayter, A. G. Weeds, and H. Baker. Substructure of the myosin molecule. I. Subfragments of myosin by enzymatic degradation. *J. Mol. Biol.* 42:1, 1969.) The rod portion of the molecule has a coiled α-helical structure. Hinge regions postulated in the mechanism of contraction are at the junction of HMM S-1 and HMM S-2 and of HMM S-2 and LMM. It should be noted that HMM S-1 has one chief polypeptide chain, whereas other fragments have two. Note the light chains (LC) in the head region. The scheme suggests the presence of two different subunits in each HMM S-1. (From H. N. Walton (ed.), *Disorders of Voluntary Muscle*, 4th ed. Edinburgh: Churchill Livingstone, 1981.)

ing speed of migration on sodium dodecyl sulfate-polyacrylamide gel electrophoresis (SDS-PAGE). LC_1 and LC_3 are also referred to as A1 and A2, respectively, "A" indicating that they are removable by mild alkali. Myosin in cardiac and slow-twitch muscle contains only two types of light chains, whose mobilities are similar to, but distinguishable from, those of LC_1 and LC_2, respectively, of fast-twitch muscle myosin. The amino acid sequence of the myosin subunits is largely known. The rod portion exhibits a pattern characteristic of α-helical protein and bears many similarities to the sequence of tropomyosin, also an α-helical protein forming a coiled-coiled structure.

Each myosin molecule contains two LC_2 light chains. Some fast-twitch fiber myosin molecules contain pairs of either LC_1 or LC_3; others contain one LC_1 and one LC_3. In slow-twitch and cardiac muscle myosin, there are a pair of LC_1's and a pair of LC_2's per molecule. Light chains in the LC_2 mobility class seem to be related by their ability to undergo phosphorylation by a kinase whose activator is the ubiquitous Ca^{2+}-binding protein calmodulin (see Chap. 19). A light chain that can undergo phosphorylation has been implicated in the regulation of smooth muscle contraction. No direct evidence for the direct regulatory function for LC_2 has been found in skeletal muscle, although recently its phosphorylation and dephosphorylation *in vivo* during contraction and relaxation, respectively, have been reported. It is still not clear what possible role the two different non-phosphorylatable light chains, LC_1 and LC_3, may play, although differences in actin-activated ATPase, depending on which of the two chains is present, have been found under some conditions. Furthermore, the speed of *in vitro* contraction of single fast-twitch fibers shows correlation with the LC_1/LC_3 ratio.

Myosin is self-assembled into thick filaments

Myosin molecules have a tendency to form end-to-end aggregates involving the LMM rods, which then grow into larger structures (the thick filament) [4]. The polarity of the myosin molecules is reversed on either side of the central portion of the filament. The globular ends of the molecules form projections on the aggregates similar to those seen in electron micrographs of natural thick filaments. The central 0.2-μm portion of the thick filament is devoid of cross-bridges. Electron microscopic and X-ray data suggest that the headpieces are attached to the filaments by means of flexible hinges. Physicochemical studies have provided direct evidence for segmental flexibility within the

myosin molecule [14]. This has important implications for the possible molecular mechanisms of contraction, discussed below. According to X-ray data, the cross-bridges on the thick filaments are arranged in a helical fashion. The cross-bridges emerge at levels separated by 14.3 nm; the best evidence suggests that the number of bridges at each level is three. Of the proteins associated with myosin filaments *in vivo*, those found in the M-line region have already been mentioned. Other proteins, also known as C, X, and H proteins, whose role is not fully understood, form part of the thick filament.

Actin activates myosin ATPase

The discovery in 1939 by Engelhardt and Ljubimova (Needham [3]) of the ATPase activity of myosin led to the recognition of the important interrelations between the structural and functional aspects of this protein and its role in muscle contraction. The protein originally termed myosin was, in light of our current knowledge, a complex of actin and myosin. The ATPase activity of myosin itself is stimulated by Ca^{2+} and is low in Mg^{2+}-containing media. If purified actin is added to myosin at low ionic strength in the presence of Mg^{2+}, considerable activation of ATPase takes place. This activation is also accompanied by a remarkable change in the physical state of the system. Turbidity increases and, depending on the concentration, superprecipitation results. The latter refers to the appearance of a flocculent precipitate, which often shrinks into a contracted plug. Glycerol-extracted muscle fibers have also been found useful for studying the interaction of myosin and actin without destroying the spatial relation existing in intact muscle. These fibers lack the energy supply system and the excitation-contraction coupling mechanism of intact muscle. Addition of ATP, however, elicits contraction accompanied by the hydrolysis of the ATP.

The combination of actin and myosin can also be observed in solutions of high ionic strength, as indicated by an increase in viscosity. Addition of ATP to this system results in a lowering of viscosity and a decrease of light scattering by the actomyosin solution, both of which are attributable to the dissociation of actomyosin into actin and myosin. Myosin-catalyzed hydrolysis of ATP occurs in several steps [15]. There is an initial rapid formation of tightly but noncovalently bound products, namely, ADP and inorganic phosphate, (P_i), that are in equilibrium with bound ATP. The $ADP \cdot P_i$ complex of myosin undergoes a relatively slow transformation that is followed by the release of the products. In the presence of actin similar complexes are formed, and the rate of the conformational change is accelerated. It is now believed that *in vivo* tension development occurs following release of inorganic phosphate. The precise details of the conformational changes accompanying the hydrolysis of ATP and details of the mechanism by which the free energy of ATP is converted into mechanical work have not yet been fully elucidated.

Several proteins regulate the interaction of actin and myosin

Tropomyosin and troponin

Tropomyosin and troponin are proteins located in the thin filaments that, together with Ca^{2+} ions, regulate the interaction of actin and myosin [16,17]. Of these proteins, tropomyosin had been known for a long time, but its role in muscle contraction or its localization had not been elucidated. Tropomyosin is an α-helical protein consisting of two polypeptide chains; its structure is similar to that of the rod portion of myosin. The other component is troponin, a complex of three proteins (Fig. 3). If the tropomyosin-troponin complex is present, actin cannot stimulate the ATPase activity of myosin unless the concentration of free Ca^{2+} exceeds about 10^{-6} M. The system consisting solely of purified actin and myosin does not show the de-

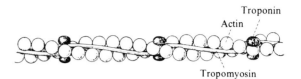

FIG. 3. Model of arrangements of actin, tropomyosin, and troponin in the thin filament. Note that troponin itself is a complex of three proteins. Tropomyosin is close to the groove of the actin filaments in relaxed muscle. Note that according to current views, the actin subunits are bilobar with their long axis more or less perpendicular to the filament axis [11]. The troponin complex also appears more elongated along the filament. (After G. N. Phillips, J. P. Fillers, and C. Cohen, Tropomyosin crystal structure and muscle regulation. *J. Mol. Biol.* 192:111, 1986; from S. Ebashi, M. Endo, and I. Ohtsuki, Control of muscle contraction. *Q. Rev. Biophys.* 2:351, 1969.)

pendence on Ca^{2+}. Thus the actin-myosin interaction becomes controlled by Ca^{2+} in the presence of the regulatory troponin-tropomyosin complex. This can be demonstrated readily *in vitro*; the Ca^{2+} concentration can be altered by varying the ratio of total Ca^{2+} added and of chelators such as EGTA. *In vivo*, the interaction of actin and myosin is regulated by the intracellular concentration of Ca^{2+}. It has been proposed that of the three proteins in troponin, one, TnT, anchors it to tropomyosin; one, TnC, is responsible for combination with Ca^{2+}; and the third, TnI, binds to a site made up of actin and tropomyosin when Ca^{2+} is absent. It has been found that the TnI and TnT subunits of troponin can undergo phosphorylation as well as can tropomyosin. At present it is not clear what role these phosphorylation processes play in the regulation of muscle contraction.

The Ca^{2+}-binding component of troponin

Troponin C (TnC), which binds Ca^{2+}, is closely related in structure to the ubiquitous Ca^{2+}-binding protein calmodulin that regulates cellular functions in many tissues, including the nervous system (see Chap. 19). X-ray crystallographic studies have shown that these Ca^{2+}-binding proteins consist of two globular domains connected by a long helical stretch [18,19]. This helical portion presumably interacts not only with TnI and TnT, but also with the doubly helical regulatory thin-filament protein tropomyosin. When Ca^{2+} binds to TnC, TnI is released, and as electron microscope and X-ray evidence indicates, tropomyosin changes its position within the thin filament to permit the combination of myosin with actin. There are actually two pairs of binding sites for Ca^{2+} on TnC. The pair of sites of higher affinity is specific for Mg^{2+}, and the other pair is specific for Ca^{2+}. It appears that the Ca^{2+}-specific sites play a crucial role in the regulatory process.

SARCOPLASMIC RETICULUM/ TRANSVERSE TUBULE SYSTEM

Excitation-contraction coupling depends on Ca^{2+} release from the sarcoplasmic reticulum

Motor nerve impulses cause the release of acetylcholine at the neuromuscular junction, initiating depolarization of the muscle cell membrane (see Chap. 32). Depolarization of the membrane penetrates the interior of the cell through the transverse (T) tubules that are continuous with the outer membrane (Fig. 4). The sarcoplasmic reticulum (SR) is a membrane system in close contact with, but distinct from, the T-tubules. Together they are the elements that, in appropriately oriented sections, form the so-called *triads* noted in electron micrographs. The SR stores Ca^{2+} in relaxed muscle and releases it into the sarcoplasm on depolarization of the cell membrane and the T-tubular system [20]. Much work has focused on the proteins present in the T-tubule SR junction. One of these may be the molecular counterpart of the so-called

feet seen in electron micrographs by Franzini-Armstrong and her colleagues [1, pp. 125 and 521] and may be identical to the Ca^{2+} channel through which Ca^{2+} is released [21]. Another component of the junctional region is a voltage-sensor protein that may act as intermediary between depolarization of the muscle membrane and the sarcoplasmic reticulum [22].

The free energy stored in ATP is used to keep Ca^{2+} low in resting muscle

The SR maintains the low intracellular Ca^{2+} concentration of resting muscle by means of an ATP-dependent Ca^{2+} pump, a Ca^{2+}-ATPase, located in the SR membrane (see Chap. 3). The free energy of ATP hydrolysis is utilized for the reuptake of Ca^{2+} into the SR vesicle via a phosphorylated enzyme intermediate. Application of the techniques of molecular genetics has made it possible to establish the sequence of the cDNA corresponding to the coding region of the ATPase gene, which has allowed the deduction of the amino acid sequence of the protein [23]. This in turn has created various tentative models of the tertiary structure of the Ca^{2+} pump protein and its relation to the lipid phase of the membrane. The mechanism of energy-coupled transport involves a switch of the enzyme from one conformation, denoted as E_1, to a second, E_2, differing in Ca^{2+} affinity (Chap. 3). The existence of these two states has been deduced from kinetic studies, and electron microscopic work on two-dimensional crystals has also afforded support for the view that the mechanism of Ca^{2+} transport involves cyclic alternation between the two main states of the enzyme [24].

Additional proteins affect Ca^{2+} uptake and storage

Phospholamban is prominent in cardiac muscle, where its phosphorylation participates in the control of Ca^{2+}-ATPase and Ca^{2+}-uptake ac-

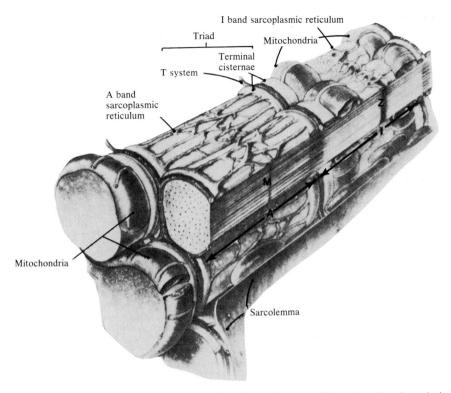

FIG. 4. A schematic drawing of part of a mammalian skeletal muscle fiber showing the relationship of the SR, terminal cisternae, T system, and mitochondria to a few myofibrils. (From B. R. Eisenberg, A. E. Kuda, and J. B. Peter, Stereological analysis of mammalian skeletal muscle. I. Soleus muscle of the adult guinea pig. *J. Cell. Biol.* 60:732, 1974.)

tivity. It is also present in slow-twitch muscle SR [25]. The precise mechanism of the interaction of phospholamban with Ca^{2+}-ATPase is not clear. Another protein of SR, calsequestrin [26,27], contains numerous low-affinity Ca^{2+}-binding sites; it is present in the lumen of the SR and is thought to participate in the Ca^{2+} storage function. Current work is exploring the possibility of the interaction of calsequestrin with those proteins that are involved in the initiation of Ca^{2+} release. Fast-twitch muscle contains a soluble Ca^{2+}-binding protein, parvalbumin [16], which is structurally related to TnC. Parvalbumin may play a role in regulating the Ca^{2+} level in the initial stages of relaxation.

Lipids modulate Ca^{2+}-ATPase

Lipid protein interactions play an important part in the activity of the Ca^{2+} pump of the SR, as shown by early work on the destruction of ATPase activity by phospholipase action. Changing the lipid composition modulates the ATPase activity, and it appears that the fluidity of the lipid is the key factor in regulating activity, possibly by affecting the mobility of the protein.

There has been recent active interest in the biosynthesis and assembly of the SR *in vitro* and *in vivo*. It appears that in the course of development, the ATPase enzyme is the last to be inserted into the membrane. A detailed knowledge of these processes is of potential interest for an understanding of various muscle diseases involving membranes.

DISEASES INVOLVING ABNORMALITIES OF MUSCLE MEMBRANES

Periodic paralyses are among those diseases that appear to be related to membrane and, possibly, metabolic abnormalities

Of interest here are the genetically determined, autosomally dominant, primary periodic paralyses, which can be classified according to the K^+ level in the serum during attacks of weakness as hyperkalemic (elevated K^+ in serum) and hypokalemic (lowered serum K^+); possibly a third type, normokalemic, may exist as a distinct entity, although it may have to be subsumed under the hyperkalemic type (Engel and Banker [1], pp. 1297, 1843).

These diseases are characterized, apart from their clinical symptoms, by morphological changes involving various membrane systems of the muscle, including the SR and the T tubules, as well as the plasma membrane; electrophysiological recordings show abnormal responses in the resting membrane potential to changes in extracellular K^+ and lack of propagation of the action potential, although the potential elicited at the endplate is normal. Possible metabolic disorders are suggested, although the latter have not been conclusively demonstrated.

The morphological changes were noted in the late nineteenth century by Goldflam using the light microscope and were described as large vacuoles replacing large portions of muscle fibers. More refined studies, particularly by A. Engel, have shown these to be characteristic of later stages of the disease. Early changes begin with dilation of the SR and the T tubules; the small initial vesicles grow into larger ones, including various inclusions; the vesicles undergo extensive remodeling and invaginations of the SR and mitochondria with irregular, curving membranous profiles. The vacuoles contain extracellular fluid, as shown by experiments with the enzyme peroxidase as tracer. As degenerative changes progress, the vacuoles rupture and admit the extracellular fluid to the myofibrils, causing contraction and eventual damage.

Both in patients with hypo- and hyperkalemic paralysis, muscle fibers show abnormal responses to changes in extracellular K^+, but motor end-plate potentials are normal during paralysis. In both types, there is failure of the paralyzed muscle sarcolemma to develop action potentials. Although reducing extracellular K^+ to 1 mM would normally lead to hyperpolarization and contraction, in patients with hypokalemic paralysis, depolarization ensues without excitation but with paralysis of the muscle. Slight depolarizations, to about -70 mV, have been reported to produce failure of the action potential to propagate. The paradoxical reaction to lowering K^+ has been attributed to an abnormally high Na^+ conductance which is not reversed by tetrodotoxin. As stated above, in hyperkalemic periodic paralysis there is also a failure to propagate the action potential. The abnormal depolarization induced by rising K^+ levels in this condition was blocked by tetrodotoxin. Abnormalities have been attributed to the Na^+ channel. The resting membrane potentials in paralyzed muscle in both types of periodic paralysis are decreased. Between attacks, membrane potentials have also been noted to be slightly decreased, more so in the hyper- than the hypokalemic form.

Insulin and glucose are known to exert opposite effects on hypokalemic and hyperkalemic forms. In the case of hyperkalemic paralysis, insulin and glucose have no effect, but an increase in serum K^+ induces an attack. Biochemical abnormalities of carbohydrate metabolism, involving perhaps a block in anaerobic glycolysis or glycogen synthesis, have been postulated as the primary cause in hypokalemic paralysis on the basis of adverse effects of glucose and insulin. This has not been fully substantiated. Agents such as insulin or epinephrine, which act on Na,K-ATPase, alter the biophysical properties of the plasma membrane of muscle rather than producing changes in metabolism.

Duchenne dystrophy is an inherited disease involving a protein of the sarcotubular triad

Although deficiencies in the function of SR Ca^{2+}-ATPase have also been reported in Duchenne dystrophy [28], the relationship to the genetic defect is unknown. (The molecular and genetic abnormalities are discussed in Chap. 23.) In further studies on SR membrane proteins, a decrease in the 100-kilodalton (kDa) band and an increase in the lower mass bands, with 55 and 45 kDa, were noted [29]. These studies suggested that the increased lower molecular weight proteins are probably derived from enzymatic digestion of the higher 100-kDa protein corresponding to the Ca^{2+}-ATPase. Further studies showed that there was an increased Ca^{2+}-activated neutral protease enzyme in Duchenne dystrophic muscle and that this protease was capable of cleaving the 100-kDa protein into smaller fragments. Enzymatic degradation of the 100-kDa protein occurring during its preparation could be considerably prevented by the addition of protease inhibitors to the initial homogenate. Because the ATPase protein is involved in Ca^{2+} transport, a decrease in it might be related to the decrease in Ca^{2+} transport in Duchenne dystrophy SR. Whether these observations are secondary or primary in relation to the cause of Duchenne dystrophy remains to be seen.

As mentioned, studies have identified a gene that is not expressed in Duchenne dystrophy (Chap. 23). The missing protein, named dystrophin [7], has been identified as present in the region of the sarcotubular junction [8], although no identity with any of the known SR or T-tubular proteins is yet apparent. It remains to be seen whether dystrophin is involved in some identifiable function of the SR or its interaction with the T tubules and whether biochemical changes in the SR system that have been described in the past may be related to the absence of dystrophin.

ENERGETICS OF MUSCLE CONTRACTION

Increased energy liberation is associated with mechanical change

The classic studies on the energetics of muscle contraction have shown that when muscle shortens under a load, extra energy is liberated in the form of work and that a certain amount of heat is inevitably evolved [1, p. 49; 30]. This extra energy liberation is known as the Fenn effect. A. V. Hill sought to describe the total energy liberated by a shortening muscle as the sum of three terms: (a) work; (b) activation heat, whose magnitude is independent of both the degree of shortening and the amount of work done; and (c) shortening heat, which is proportional only to the length changes and is independent of the load and, hence, of work. Subsequent studies by Hill himself have shown that this analysis of the energy balance may be somewhat oversimplified.

ATP is the immediate source of energy for muscle contraction

There is now general agreement that ATP hydrolysis accompanies muscle contraction and is the immediate source of its energy. In a series of contractions, the total energy liberated by a muscle, that is, heat and work, agrees well with the calculated energy release (based on *in vitro* data) from creatine phosphate breakdown. The latter continually rephosphorylates the ADP resulting from the hydrolysis of ATP. Discrepancies, however, still exist in the early stages of contraction between actual measured chemical energy changes and energy changes calculated from the heat content of compounds known to change during the early phase of contraction. Phosphorus nuclear magnetic resonance (NMR) has been found useful in the noninvasive study of the metabolism of P_i-containing compounds in living muscle, both normal and diseased [31,32].

MOLECULAR EVENTS IN CONTRACTION AND RELAXATION

Muscle contraction depends on molecular events involving the cross-bridges

The sliding-filament theory and the role of the cross-bridges in tension production are supported by the agreement between the experimentally determined tension of single muscle fibers as a function of length and the tension that would follow from the sliding-filament theory on the assumption that tension is proportional to the number of links formed between the thick and thin filaments [33].

X-ray diffraction [4] has shown that the position of cross-bridges of the thick filaments changes when the muscle is activated and develops tension. That the interaction of the cross-bridges with the actin filaments results in a unidirectional movement, contraction, seems to be based on two functions: First, the myosin filaments change their polarity in the middle of the sarcomere owing to the end-to-end aggregation of the constituent molecules; second, there is a built-in polarity in the actin filaments on each side of the Z band, as shown in electron micrographs by the "arrowheads" formed when

HMM or subfragment 1 complexes with actin. X-ray diffraction studies indicate that the distances among actin and myosin filaments increase as the sarcomere shortens. The flexible attachment of the myosin heads to the rod portions makes it possible for the cross-bridges to interact with actin across various distances.

Force generation is coupled to the hydrolysis of ATP

The site of force generation is most likely the interface between actin and the S-1 portion of the myosin molecule, although some conformational change induced by the interaction with actin and ATP in the myosin head itself cannot be excluded. The simple view that myosin heads (cross-bridges) are detached from actin in relaxed muscle and become attached to actin in contracting muscle has been challenged in recent years. Rather, it appears that even in relaxed muscle, some forms of myosin—those carrying bound ATP or ADP·P_i—are attached but undergo rapid detachment and reattachment. In contracting muscle there would be a shift to more tightly bound states rather than an absolute change in the number of attachments. Biochemically, the force-generating state is thought to be that resulting from the dissociation of P_i following hydrolysis of ATP [15,33,34].

Various schemes have been proposed to explain force generation

The pitch of the actin helix is slightly different from that of the cross-bridge helix, so a slight movement at an attached bridge would create a favorable situation for attachment of another bridge several actin units away on the same filament (Fig. 5). Several theoretical formulations of the cross-bridge model have been given [33]. In many models an elastic element is postulated in the link between the thick filament and the myosin head; in other schemes the connection is rigid, and the elastic element is either the

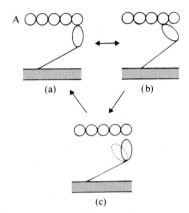

FIG. 5. Model of interaction of the myosin head with actin. (a) Attachment of myosin to actin, (b) tilting of the myosin head, (c) detachment produced by ATP followed by its hydrolysis. On the basis of *in vitro* kinetic studies, the myosin species present in (a) + (b) carried the ADP·P_i product complex. It is thought that P_i leaves before force is generated. The attached head may oscillate between positions (a) and (b), although conformational changes within the myosin head may also be important. (From J. N. Walton (ed.). *Disorders of Voluntary Muscle*, 4th ed. Edinburgh: Churchill Livingstone, 1981.)

myosin head or in the myosin-actin interface. It has generally been assumed that the basis of force development and contraction is a rotation of the myosin heads attached to actin with respect to the filament axis. Mechanisms involving shape changes within the myosin head are currently being investigated.

Activation of muscle by Ca^{2+} involves changes in the thin filaments

The mechanism by which the Ca^{2+}-induced changes in the thin filament lead to activation of muscle contraction is still not fully understood. Earlier views regarded the attachment of myosin heads to actin as the regulatory step. In contrast, later biochemical studies *in vitro* on myosin ATPase activated by regulated actin suggest that activation involves a shift among attached states from a state of weak binding to one of strong binding of myosin to actin [15,34]. There is also X-ray evidence for changed interactions between myosin and actin that lag some 15 msec behind the changes in the thin filament [35]. These have been interpreted as an indication of some attachment of myosin heads to actin; thus full reconciliation of structural and biochemical results requires further work. Time-resolved X-ray diffraction studies indicate that the first structural changes in the thin filaments may involve tropomyosin [30].

METABOLISM IN MUSCLE

Muscle utilizes energy made available in the form of ATP, which is hydrolyzed to ADP and P_i. The task of muscle metabolism, apart from the necessity of producing the specific constituents required for the construction of structural components, is to produce ATP. The metabolic pathways involved in the production of ATP in muscle are not essentially different from those present in other tissues, including nerve. There are, however, some features of muscle metabolism that are closely related to the mechanism by which contraction is initiated; others are subject to control by metabolites arising in the course of contraction. (See Chaps. 28 and 33; see also Engel and Banker [1] and Walton [2].)

Anaerobic metabolism

It has long been known that active muscle increases its metabolism by a factor greater than 100. This is particularly true in muscles that contain fast-twitch fibers that are involved in rapid bursts of activity. In these muscles, the chief source of energy is the anaerobic breakdown of glycogen, and the enzymatic control of glycogen metabolism furnishes a good illustration of the complex way in which regulation takes place. Apart from specific mechanisms discussed below, the increase in ADP and P_i itself serves to increase the rate of ATP synthesis by providing more substrate.

Phosphorylase

Phosphorylase catalyzes the breakdown of glycogen, and its properties have been clarified in considerable detail (see Chaps. 28 and 33). Phosphorylase *b*, the inactive form, is transformed into phosphorylase *a*, the active form, by means of phosphorylation. ATP is the phosphate donor, and the reaction is catalyzed by another enzyme, phosphorylase kinase (see Chap. 19).

As we have said, the onset of activity in muscle is mediated by the release of Ca^{2+} from the SR. Ca^{2+}, in roughly the same concentration as that required for the activation of the actomyosin system, also increases the activity of phosphorylase kinase by increasing the affinity for phosphorylase *b*. Thus, in parallel with the activation of the actomyosin system, phosphorylase kinase produces active phosphorylase *a* at a higher rate. As muscle activity proceeds, more phosphorylated glucose, which in turn is broken down through the glycolytic pathway, is made available from glycogen. Calmodulin, the Ca^{2+}-binding protein, which, as described above, is involved in the activation of myosin light-chain kinase, is also the Ca^{2+}-binding regulatory subunit of phosphorylase kinase. On the other hand, phosphorylase phosphatase, the enzyme that reverses the activation of phosphorylase, is inactivated by Ca^{2+}. This phosphatase is in turn controlled by an inhibitory protein, which is itself controlled by cyclic AMP (cAMP)-dependent phosphorylation.

Phosphorylase kinase can also be activated by phosphorylation catalyzed by a protein kinase. This enzyme in turn is activated by cAMP, which is formed from ATP under the influence of adenylate cyclase (see Chap. 17). The cyclase responds to hormones and neurohumoral agents, such as epinephrine (see Chap. 18).

As muscle activity proceeds, more phosphorylated glucose, which in turn is broken down through the glycolytic pathway, is made available from glycogen. Calmodulin, the Ca^{2+}-binding protein, which, as described above, is involved in the activation of myosin light-chain kinase, is also the Ca^{2+}1-binding regulatory subunit of phosphorylase kinase.

Glycogen synthetase

Glycogen synthetase catalyzes the biosynthesis of glycogen (see Chap. 28). It exists in two forms, one of which is active under physiological conditions, whereas the other is inactive (see Chap. 28). The same cAMP-dependent protein kinase that activates phosphorylase kinase also phosphorylates glycogen synthetase I. In this case, however, the dephosphorylated form (I) is active, and phosphorylation by the kinase converts it into an inactive (D) form. This ensures that when greater muscle activity requires increased release of phosphorylated glucose units from glycogen, the reverse process catalyzed by the synthetase is shut off. As in the case of phosphorylase, a phosphatase for converting the D to I form is regulated by an inhibitor that is controlled by cAMP-dependent phosphorylation.

Phosphofructokinase

Phosphofructokinase has an important role in regulating the rate of glycolysis. It introduces a second phosphate into the fructose-6-phosphate molecule prior to its breakdown into trioses, and it plays an important role in regulating the rate of glycolysis (see also Chaps. 28 and 33). Its activity is under the control of the concentration of various metabolites, such as P_i, AMP, ATP, and citrate, and even the enzyme's reaction product, fructose-1,6-bisphosphate. This regulation involves an allosteric mechanism, the binding of the so-called effectors taking place in activating and inhibitory sites different from the catalytic site. ATP and citrate are inhibitors; fructose-1,6-bisphosphate, P_i, 5'-ATP are activators. These regulatory processes are crucial for turning on the metabolism of the active muscle by a factor of several hundred and again reducing it to the resting level as the demand subsides.

Myokinase

Myokinase catalyzes the reversible reaction

$$2 \text{ ADP} \rightleftarrows \text{ATP} + \text{AMP}$$

This reaction assures better utilization of the energy stored in ATP by permitting the hydrolysis of both high-energy phosphate bonds.

Creatine kinase

Creatine kinase catalyzes the reaction

$$\text{Creatine phosphate} + \text{ADP} \rightleftarrows \text{ATP} + \text{creatine}$$

Because creatine phosphate is the chief store of high-energy phosphates in muscle, this reaction permits the rephosphorylation of ADP to ATP, the immediate source of energy in contraction. During rest, the metabolic processes, in turn, replenish the creatine phosphate stores. It is interesting that this reaction created considerable difficulty when attempts were made to demonstrate the breakdown of ATP during a single twitch because ADP was immediately rephosphorylated to ATP, and the small change in creatine phosphate could not be detected. The fact that creatine kinase can be blocked selectively by small amounts of dinitrofluorobenzene played an important role in showing that contraction is indeed closely coupled to a decrease in ATP and formation of ADP.

Oxidative metabolism

During sustained activity, particularly in those muscles that are rich in mitochondria and in heart muscle, oxidative processes dominate. These involve the oxidation of pyruvate through the Krebs cycle (see Chap. 28) and the oxidation of fatty acids, which, as has now been generally recognized, serve as the chief source of energy

in oxidative metabolism (see Chap. 33). Citrate, an intermediate in the Krebs cycle, is an allosteric inhibitor of phosphofructokinase, establishing a link between oxidative and anaerobic metabolism.

MUSCLE FIBER TYPES

It has been known for about 100 years that striated muscles differ in their velocity of contraction and that correlations exist among the color of the muscle, its velocity of contraction, and the stimulation frequency required to produce a tetanus. In general, red muscles are "slower" than white ones, and higher frequencies of stimulation are required to produce tetanus in red than in white muscles. However, hardly any muscle as a whole can be considered entirely red or white or slow or fast, and the properties of each individual muscle are determined by the distribution of various fiber types. There are wide differences when one compares various species. For instance, the soleus muscle in rabbit consists almost entirely of typically slow-twitch fibers, whereas in rat and humans, the soleus contains a mixture of fiber types. Differences in speed of contraction, unless one refers to the intrinsic shortening speed of the sarcomere, are partly due to differences in the contractile apparatus and partly to differences in the speed of Ca^{2+} release and uptake by the SR [1, p. 255].

Isozymes are involved in determining fiber type

Differences between types of muscle depend not only on the presence of certain enzymes in large or small amounts; different types of muscle may contain the same enzyme in different forms. The different forms of an enzyme catalyzing the same reaction have been called isoenzymes or isozymes. The first molecule thus identified was lactic dehydrogenase, which consists of four subunits. Each subunit can either be of the H type, which is predominant in heart muscle, or of the M type, predominant in fast-twitch skeletal muscle. A higher content of the H type has been found in embryonic muscle, although differences exist with respect to species and the muscles examined. Various muscles of the adult contain the two kinds of subunits in various proportions, again with species variations, and the complexes, of which there can be five, differ in their electrophoretic mobility.

As discussed before in connection with myosin, different muscles may contain different isoforms—products of a different gene or differently processed products of the same gene—of a given protein. This applies not only to myosin but also to proteins of the regulatory system, namely, troponin and tropomyosin. Recent studies have shown that in the course of development, transitional embryonic and neonatal isoforms of myosin appear.

Both innervation and muscle cell lineage are important for fiber differentiation

In muscles that contain fibers of different types, fibers innervated by the same motoneuron are of the same type, pointing to a close connection between fiber type and innervation. This view is further supported by early experiments involving cross-reinnervation and nerve stimulation, leading to type transformation (see below). The idea that the ontogenetic development of different fiber types is also determined by innervation has gained wide currency. Later work, however, provides strong evidence that differentiation occurs early in development, before contact with nerves is established, and that the role of cell lineage-dependent types has to be considered along with innervation-dependent modulation [36]. The role of hormones in the regulation of gene expression is the subject of current research.

Histochemistry helps in fiber classification

Variations in myosin stability at different pHs have become the basis for the histochemical classification of fast- and slow-twitch fiber types. The degree of correlation between staining for oxidative enzymes and the pH effect on myosin ATPase varies, depending on the species. Slow-twitch fibers are rich in mitochondria and, consequently, in mitochondrial enzymes. Most fast-twitch fibers are low in mitochondrial and high in glycolytic enzymes; but some fast-twitch fibers are rich in mitochondrial oxidative enzymes. Thus, on the basis of four histochemical assays, that is, assays of alkali–stable ATPase, acid-stable ATPase, succinic dehydrogenase (mitochondrial), and phosphorylase (glycolytic), in principle 16 classes of fibers might exist. By carrying out acid incubation at slightly different pH, fast-twitch fibers can be divided into at least two subgroups. The use of antibodies specific for slow- and fast-twitch types of myosin, coupled to a fluorescent dye has been found useful in identifying populations of fibers.

However, classification based on histochemistry alone appears to be oversimplified. Fibers that seem to belong to the same class histochemically may actually contain different isoforms of a given protein, e.g., myosin, in different muscles. Moreover, the same muscle may in different species contain proteins that are products of different genes [36].

Further refinements are to be expected from the use of monoclonal antibodies able to distinguish differences among fibers within the same (fast or slow) group, particularly when applied to single fibers, and the techniques of molecular genetics.

CHANGED INNERVATION AND ACTIVITY INDUCE CHANGES IN MUSCLE FIBER TYPE

Cross-reinnervation leads to muscle fiber type changes

Starting with the work of Eccles and co-workers, several authors have reported that when a fast muscle is cross-reinnervated by a nerve that originally supplied a slow muscle, it acquires properties characteristic of a slow muscle; reciprocal changes take place in a slow muscle that has been cross-reinnervated by a fast-muscle nerve [37,38]. Changes in contractile speed are accompanied by corresponding changes in both the myosin ATPase activity and the protein subunit pattern. Changes have also been observed in the pattern of metabolic enzymes and in the activity of the SR. These changes have been attributed to specific influences of fast- and slow-muscle nerves or to the elaboration of specific trophic substances by these nerves.

Innervation may exert a trophic effect

The trophic effects of nerve on muscle have been defined in three ways: (a) the formation of connections—the axons of a motor nerve must grow to and connect with a muscle cell through a neuromuscular junction; (b) the maintenance of integrity—failure of neuronal connection, whether functional or structural, will result in degenerative changes of the muscle; (c) the regulation of metabolic and physiological properties. In a phenomenological sense, such trophic effects cannot be denied. In the sense, however, that the nerve supplies specific trophic substances that not only maintain the integrity of the muscle, but also define its properties, such effects would be questionable, particularly in light of experiments that show changes in the character of the muscle whose nerve supply has been left intact.

Changed activity changes fiber type without change in innervation

The work of Salmons and Vrbova shows that even with undisturbed nerve-muscle connection, changes in physiological parameters can be brought about if the pattern of neuronal activity reaching the muscle is changed. When the motor nerve is stimulated continuously over a period of weeks, imposing on the fast muscle a pattern of activity similar to that normally reaching a slow muscle, a marked slowing of the time course of isometric contraction and relaxation ensues. Such stimulation also produces changes in the biochemical makeup of the fiber, including the type of myosin and other proteins that are expressed. The changes correspond to an essentially constant fast-slow transformation. The biochemical changes in myosin and other enzymes are reflected in the histochemical ATPase reaction, the glycolytic versus oxidative enzyme pattern and Ca^{2+} uptake by the SR. Perhaps the earliest changes, within the first few days, occur in the cytoplasmic Ca^{2+}-binding protein, parvalbumin, found in fast muscle. Studies on changes in the RNA level and their products suggest involvement of translational control in fiber transformation.

The changeover in muscle type is attributable to the transformation of the existing fibers by the switching on of normally inactive genes and the switching off of those that had been active, rather than to the destruction of the original fiber population and its replacement by new fibers. This is shown by the fact that early in the course of the transformation of fast muscle, antibodies against both fast and slow myosins react with the same fiber; in normal fast muscle, however, only the antibody against fast myosin reacts. After complete transformation, again, only one type of antibody reacts—that reacting with slow myosin. The same conclusion has been reached from SDS-PAGE studies on single fibers showing the transient presence of both the fast and slow types of myosin light chains. Clearly, the fact that changes in the activity pattern, with an undisturbed nerve-muscle connection, can alter the physiological and biochemical properties of a muscle raises many interesting questions concerning the trophic effects of the motor nerve. More work will be required to differentiate genuine neuronal effects related to the type of nerves from those effects that originate in the neuronal activity pattern.

ACKNOWLEDGMENTS

The preparation of this chapter was supported by grants from the National Institutes of Health (R37-HL-5949) and the Muscular Dystrophy Association.

REFERENCES

1. Engel, A. G., and Banker, B. O. (eds.). *Myology, Basic and Clinical.* New York: McGraw-Hill, 1986.
2. Walton, J. N. (ed.). *Disorders of Voluntary Muscle,* 5th ed. Edinburgh: Churchill, 1988.
3. Needham, D. M. *Machina Carnis.* Cambridge: Cambridge Univ. Press, 1971.
4. Squire, J. *The Structural Basis of Muscle Contraction.* New York: Plenum Press, 1981.
5. Maruyama, K. Connectin, an elastic filamentous protein of striated muscle. *Int. Rev. Cytol.* 104:81–114, 1986.
6. Wang, K. Sarcomere-associated cytoskeletal lattices in striated muscle. *Cell Muscle Mot.* 6:315–369, 1985.
7. Hoffman, E. P., Brown, R. H., Jr., and Kunkel, L. M. Dystrophin: The protein products of the Duchenne muscular dystrophy locus. *Cell* 51:919–928, 1987.
8. Hoffman, E. P., Knudson, C. M., Campbell, K. P., and Kunkel, L. M. Subcellular fractionation of dystrophin to the triads of skeletal muscle. *Nature* 330:754–758, 1987.
9. Warrick, H. M., and Spudich, J. A. Myosin structure and function in cell motility. *Annu. Rev. Cell. Biol.* 3:379–421, 1987.
10. Pollard, T. D., and Cooper, J. A. Actin and actin-binding proteins. A critical evaluation of mechanisms and functions. *Annu. Rev. Biochem.* 55:987–1035, 1986.
11. Egelman, E. H. The structure of F-Actin. *J. Muscle Res. Cell Motility* 6:129–151, 1985.
12. Harrington, W. F., and Rodgers, M. E. Myosin. *Annu. Rev. Biochem.* 53:35–74, 1984.
13. Emerson, C., Fischman, D., Nadal-Ginard, B., and Siddiqui, M. A. Q. (eds.). *Molecular Biology of Muscle Development.* New York: Alan R. Liss, 1986.
14. Gergely, J., and Seidel, J. C. Conformational changes and molecular dynamics of myosin. In L. D. Peachey, R. H. Adrian, and S. R. Geiger (eds.), *Handbook of Physiology.* Bethesda: American Physiological Society, 1983, pp. 257–274.
15. Hibberd, M. G., and Trentham, D. R. Relationships between chemical and mechanical events during muscular contraction. *Annu. Rev. Biophys. Biophys. Chem.* 15:119–161, 1986.
16. Leavis, P. C., and Gergely, J. Thin filament proteins and thin filament linked regulation of vertebrate muscle contraction. *CRC Critical Rev. Biochem.* 16:235–305, 1983.
17. Zot, A. S., and Potter, J. D. Structural aspects of troponin-tropomyosin regulation of skeletal muscle contraction. *Annu. Rev. Biophys. Biophys. Chem.* 16:535–560, 1987.
18. Herzberg, O., and James, M. N. G. Structure of the calcium regulatory muscle protein troponin C at 2.8 Å resolution. *Nature* 313:653–658, 1985.
19. Sundaralingam, M., Bergstrom, R., Strasburg, G., Rao, S. T., and Raychowdhury, P. Molecular structure of troponin C from chicken skeletal muscle at 3 Å resolution. *Science* 227:945–947, 1985.
20. Inesi, G., Mechanism of calcium transport. *Annu. Rev. Physiol.* 47:573–601, 1985.
21. Campbell, K. P., Knudson, C. M., Imagawa, T., Leung, A. T., Sutko, J. L., et al. Identification and characterization of the high affinity [^{3}H]yranodine receptor of the junctional sarcoplasmic reticulum Ca^{2+} release channel. *J. Biol. Chem.* 262:6460–6463, 1987.

22. Leung, A. T., Imagawa, T., Block, B., Franzini-Armstrong, F., and Campbell, K. P. Chemical and ultrastructural characterization of the 1,4-dihydropyridine receptor from rabbit skeletal muscle. *J. Biol. Chem.* 263:994–1001, 1988.

23. Brandl, C. J., Green, N. M., Korczak, B., and MacLennan, D. H. Two Ca^{2+}-ATPase genes: Homologies and mechanistic implications of deduced amino acid sequences. *Cell* 44:597–607, 1986.

24. Dux, L., Taylor, K. A., Ting-Beal, H. P., and Martonosi, A. Crystallization of the Ca^{2+}-ATPase of sarcoplasmic reticulum by calcium and lanthanide ions. *J. Biol. Chem.* 260:11730–11743, 1985.

25. Jorgensen, A. O., and James, J. R. Localization of phospholamban in slow but not fast canine skeletal muscle fibers. An immunocytochemical and biochemical study. *J. Biol. Chem.* 261:3775–3781, 1986.

26. MacLennan, D. H., Campbell, K., and Reithmeier, R. A. F. Calsequestrin. In R. A. F. Reithmeier (ed.), *Calcium and Cell Function.* New York: Academic Press, 1983, Vol. 4, pp. 151–173.

27. Franzini-Armstrong, C., Kenney, E., and Varriano-Martson, E. The structure of calsequestrin in triads of vertebrate skeletal muscle: A deep etch study. *J. Cell Biol.* 105:49–56, 1987.

28. Samaha, F. J., and Gergely, J. Biochemical abnormalities of the sarcoplasmic reticulum in muscular dystrophy. *N. England J. Med.* 280:184–188, 1969.

29. Nagy, B., and Samaha, F. J. Membrane defects in Duchenne dystrophy: Protease affecting sarcoplasmic reticulum. *Ann. Neurol.* 20:50–56, 1986.

30. Kushmerick, M. J. Energetics of muscle contraction. In L. D. Peachey, R. H. Adrian, and S. R. Geiger (eds.), *Handbook of Physiology.* Bethesda: American Physiological Society, 1983, pp. 189–236.

31. Radda, G. K. The use of NMR spectroscopy for the understanding of disease. *Science* 233:640–645, 1986.

32. Dawson, M. J. The relation between muscle function and metabolism studied by ^{31}P NMR spectroscopy. In S. Chien and C. Ho (eds.), *NMR in Biology and Medicine.* New York: Raven Press, 1986, pp. 185–200.

33. Huxley, A. F. Review lecture: Muscular contraction. *J. Physiol.* 243:1–43, 1974.

34. Eisenberg, E., and Hill, T. L. Muscle contraction and free energy transduction in biological systems. *Science* 227:999–1006, 1985.

35. Kress, M., Huxley, H. E., Faruqi, A. R., and Henrix, J. Structural changes during activation of frog muscle studied by time-resolved X-ray diffraction. *J. Mol. Biol.* 188:325–342, 1986.

36. Sanes, J. R. Cell lineage and the origin of muscle fiber types. *Trends Neurosci.* 10:219–221, 1987.

37. Jolesz, F., and Sreter, F. A. Development, innervation and activity-pattern induced changes in skeletal muscle. *Annu. Rev. Physiol.* 43:531–552, 1981.

38. Pette, D. Activity-induced fast to slow transitions in mammalian muscle. *Med. Sci. Sports Exercise* 16:517–528, 1984.

CHAPTER 32

Biochemical Pathology of the Neuromuscular Junction

Robert L. Barchi

Synaptic transmission requires the integrated activity of complex macromolecular systems at both the presynaptic and the postsynaptic level. In this serial system, defects in any of the elements can cause a degradation in synaptic efficiency and block the transmission of information. The neuromuscular junction (NMJ) is certainly the best studied vertebrate synapse

(Fig. 1). Since virtually all mammalian NMJs are of a uniform nicotinic cholinergic type, the system is simpler to analyze than synaptic junctions in the CNS. In addition, the outcome of synaptic failure at the NMJ is easily detected as muscle weakness, fatigability, or paralysis.

Since the NMJ represents the common link between the CNS and the initiation of motor

Basic Neurochemistry: Molecular, Cellular, and Medical Aspects, 4th Ed., edited by G. J. Siegel et al. Raven Press, Ltd., New York, 1989.
Correspondence to Robert L. Barchi, Mahoney Institute of Neurological Sciences, University of Pennsylvania School of Medicine, Philadelphia, Pennsylvania 19104.

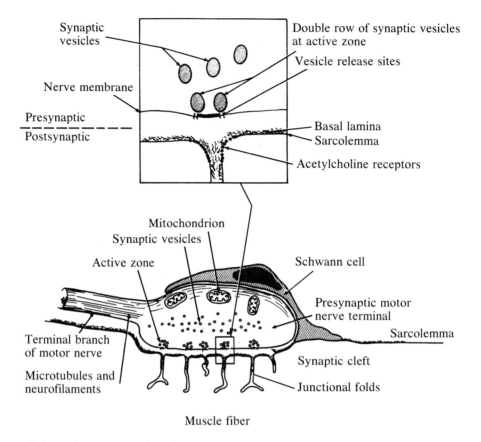

FIG. 1.   Schematic representation of the key presynaptic and postsynaptic elements at the NMJ.

activity, diseases that affect its function can have profound clinical consequences. It also provides an "Achilles heel," an optimal target for toxins produced by predators whose intent is to immobilize their prey. An unusual number of plant products and animal toxins affect the NMJ. In many cases, research into the pathophysiology of diseases and toxins affecting the NMJ has shed light on the underlying normal physiologic mechanisms as well as on the clinical conditions themselves.

In this chapter a number of toxins (Table 1) and several clinical disorders that specifically affect neuromuscular transmission are reviewed. The emphasis, however, is not on their clinical presentation or treatment, but on the mechanisms involved and the insights they can provide into the function of the normal junction. In addition, since toxins can be extremely useful tools for tinkering with the molecular machinery of the synapse, the biochemistry of these molecules is also discussed.

The process of synaptic transmission involves a sequence of events beginning with depolarization of the presynaptic nerve terminal membrane, continuing through transmitter release and interaction with the postsynaptic membrane, and culminating with modulation of

TABLE 1. Some toxins and diseases affecting the neuromuscular junction[a]

PRESYNAPTIC ACTION
Botulinum toxin
Black widow spider venom
Snake β-neurotoxins
Lambert-Eaton syndrome
JUNCTIONAL ACTION
Inhibitors of AChE
Congenital AChE deficiency
POSTSYNAPTIC ACTION
Snake α-neurotoxins
MG
Congenital defects of ACh receptor structure

[a] (AChE) acetylcholinesterase; (MG) myasthenia gravis; (ACh)acetylcholine.

postsynaptic events (see Chap. 8). In considering pathological events at the NMJ, the same conceptual sequence is followed: Toxins and disorders interfering with presynaptic mechanisms are considered first, followed by a discussion of those targeting events at the postsynaptic level.

NEUROMUSCULAR TOXINS ACTING AT THE PRESYNAPTIC LEVEL

The synthesis of acetylcholine (ACh) and its packaging into synaptic vesicles are prerequisites for normal neurotransmission. Subsequent release of ACh requires an influx of Ca^{2+} that follows depolarization of presynaptic membranes, the specific association of synaptic vesicles with release sites on the active zones, and the fusion of these vesicles with the membrane. Interference with any of these steps (discussed in Chaps. 8 and 10) will result in degradation of the fidelity of neuromuscular transmission. Several clinical disorders and a number of small polypeptide neurotoxins produce abnormalities in human neuromuscular function by interfering at this level.

Botulinum toxin blocks the release of synaptic vesicles from the presynaptic nerve terminal

Botulism is the clinical disorder that results from exposure to one of a family of exotoxins produced by strains of the bacterium *Clostridium botulinum* [1]. The botulinum exotoxin is one of the most toxic substances known; a dose of less than 50 μg can be lethal in humans. This toxin specifically blocks neuromuscular transmission. If not treated rapidly, ingestion of the toxin can result in widespread weakness and, ultimately, death due to paralysis of the muscles of respiration. In addition, botulinum toxin interferes with transmission at cholinergic parasympathetic terminals, producing autonomic symptoms.

Botulism usually results from the ingestion of foods contaminated with the anaerobic *Clostridium* organisms. This form of food poisoning typically produces symptoms over the first 6 to 36 hr after exposure. Infants between the ages of 3 weeks and 12 months can develop a milder and more insidious form of botulism from exotoxins produced by anaerobic bacteria colonizing their intestinal tract. Finally, although very rare, botulism can result from the contamination of a deep penetrating wound with the toxin-producing bacterium.

Clinically, individuals exposed to botulinum toxin develop progressive failure of neuromuscular transmission. When examined in its early stages in humans, this defect is characterized by an abnormally small electrical response in muscle after maximal stimulation of the motor nerve, although activation and conduction in the motor nerve itself are normal. Repeated stimulation of the motor nerve leads to an increase in the amplitude of the muscle response, in contrast to the decremental response seen in patients with myasthenia gravis (see below). These clinical findings point to a defect in the release of ACh from the presynaptic terminal, possibly one that can be overcome in part by the elevated intraterminal Ca^{2+} levels produced by repetitive depolarization.

Botulinum toxin is synthesized by the parent bacterium as an inactive protomer of approximately 150 kilodaltons (kDa) [2]. This protomer must be cleaved into two fragments of approximately 100 and 50 kDa before it becomes biologically active (Fig. 2). These two components, designated the heavy and light chains, are joined by a disulfide bridge; both chains are required for toxic activity.

At least eight related forms of botulinum toxin have been identified. A particular bacterial isolate will typically produce only one of these forms. The forms demonstrate strong sequence homology, and the group as a whole exhibits homology with the C-terminal region of the tetanus toxin produced by *Clostridium tetani*.

Although these toxins are produced by the *Clostridium* bacteria, their levels of synthesis do not correlate with the rate of growth of the parent microorganism itself. In fact, it is now clear that the toxin is the result of a lysogenic infection of the bacterium with a phage containing the genetic information encoding the toxin molecule. The form of toxin produced by a particular strain of bacteria reflects the nature of the phage with which it is infected rather than the genetic composition of the prokaryote itself. A strain cleared of its lysogenic infection will no longer produce toxin; reinfection with a different strain of phage results in the production of the toxin form characteristic of that phage.

Some forms of botulinum toxin are cleaved to the activated two-chain state by trypsin-like proteases produced by the bacterium in which they are made; others require processing in the host, often by an intestinal protease. Exposure of the mature molecule to papain can result in cleavage of a 50-kDa fragment from the C-terminal of the heavy chain; the remaining heavy-chain fragment disulfide linked to the light chain has no biological activity. The native toxin can also be inactivated by reduction of the disulfide bond joining the 50- and 100-kDa chains.

The mouse nerve-muscle preparation is paralyzed by picomolar concentrations of botulinum toxin. After a lag period of 20 to 40 min, the amplitude of the end-plate potential (EPP) falls, and transmission ultimately fails irreversibly after 70 to 100 min. Even after total block of stimulated transmitter release, a small amount of spontaneous release continues, although the amplitude of the miniature end-plate potentials (MEPPs) is shifted in a skewed distribution toward lower values. Paralyzed preparations are still capable of producing a burst of MEPPs in response to exposure to black widow spider venom (see below).

The initial step in toxin action involves the binding of the disulfide-linked light-chain–heavy-chain complex to specific receptors on the presynaptic membrane [3]. This binding occurs rapidly and is essentially irreversible. Binding probably involves the C-terminal portion of the large peptide; the heavy chain itself

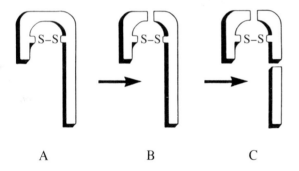

FIG. 2. Botulinum neurotoxin is synthesized as a single polypeptide chain of approximately 150,000 daltons (Da) that exhibits little toxic activity (**A**). When exposed to trypsin or trypsin-like enzymes, this protein is cleaved to yield a highly toxic two-chain complex whose fragments are held together through an interchain disulfide bond (**B**). The two chains have molecular masses of about 50,000 and 100,000 Da. Subsequent exposure to papain cleaves a 50,000-Da fragment from the C-terminal of the larger protein and inactivates the toxin (**C**). (From L. L. Simpson [2].)

is nontoxic, but can competitively block the effects of the intact toxin. Measurements of toxin binding have been carried out with synaptosomal membranes. Two classes of binding sites with apparent dissociation constant K_d of 5×10^{-10} and 5×10^{-8} have been identified. Binding to these high-affinity sites is specifically blocked by the 50-kDa C-terminal fragment of the heavy chain. Although the botulinum toxin receptor has not been identified, available evidence suggests that a membrane ganglioside is involved.

Molecules of toxin bound to the surface membrane must be internalized before they can exert their effect (Fig. 3). The lag time between toxin binding and its action on ACh release is strongly temperature dependent, in part reflecting the temperature sensitivity of this internalization process. At 37°C, antibodies against the toxin are effective in blocking its action only for a short period after binding of the toxin to membranes, suggesting that the toxin is hidden from access to external antibodies by internalization into lysosomal elements. In parallel experiments at low temperatures, internalization is blocked, and the toxin remains accessible to inactivation by antibody.

The toxin must cross the lysosomal membrane and enter the cytoplasm before it can interfere with transmitter release. Here, the N-terminal portion of the heavy chain plays a unique role. This half of the heavy chain is capable of forming a transmembrane channel in a lipid bilayer. The channel is large enough to allow an extended peptide chain to pass [4]. In artificial bilayers, channel-forming activity is pH dependent; it is most prominent when the side of the bilayer corresponding to the intralysosomal surface is at low pH (~4.5) and the cytoplasmic face is neutral (pH 7.0). The importance of pH to channel-forming activity is supported by the experimental observation that compounds, such as ammonium chloride or methylamine hydrochloride, and drugs, such as chloroquine, that prevent acidification of lyso-

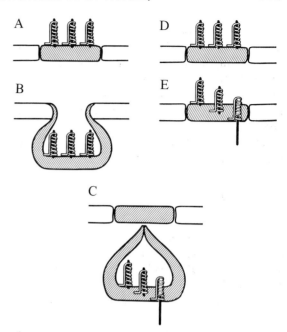

FIG. 3. Proposed mechanism for the translocation of botulinum toxin into presynaptic nerve terminals. The toxin binds to a specific class of receptors on the plasma membrane of cholinergic nerve terminals (**A**). The toxin is then internalized by the process of receptor-mediated endocytosis (**B**). The endocytotic vesicles become progressively more acidic as they approach the lysosome, and the fall in pH triggers a conformational change in the toxin molecule. A portion of the molecule, probably the N-terminal, partitions into the membrane and forms a channel. The light chain may then pass through this channel to reach the ultimate cytoplasmic site of action of the toxin (**C**). In an alternative mechanism, binding of the toxin complex to receptors on the cell surface (**D**) may lead directly to endocytosis when the tissue is exposed to a medium with low pH, triggering pH-dependent channel formation in the plasma membrane (**E**). (From L. L. Simpson [2].)

somes also block the pathologic action of the toxin.

Ultimately, the toxicity of botulinum toxin involves an effect of the 50-kDa light chain after it is released into the cytoplasm of the presynaptic terminal. A very small number of toxin molecules, probably less than 20, are capable of completely blocking all stimulus-induced transmitter release from a synapse, suggesting that an amplification step is involved. An attractive, but still unproven, possibility is that the toxin light chain is actually an enzyme, such as a kinase, which covalently modifies a specific protein involved in transmitter release. The ultimate site of action for this toxin may be the synaptic vesicle release site itself.

Black widow spider venom stimulates abnormal release of ACh

The bite of the black widow spider initially produces an increase in neuromuscular activity that leads to skeletal muscle spasms and rigidity. This phase of hyperexcitability is rapidly followed by progressive failure of neuromuscular transmission and paralysis.

In experimental preparations, the venom induces a transient but dramatic increase in spontaneous quantal release of ACh; at the peak of spontaneous release, MEPP frequencies of 500 to 1,000/sec can be seen. This is followed by a progressive decline and failure of both spontaneous and induced transmitter release. Nerve stimulation during the interval of increased spontaneous release produces EPPs of larger than normal amplitude, whereas direct nerve stimulation after the effect has developed fails to elicit any response.

The venom of the female black widow contains many distinct polypeptide components. The component responsible for its effects on the NMJ is a protein of 130,000 M_r, with an isoelectric point between 5.2 and 5.7 [5]. The purified active component, referred to as α-latrotoxin, is not glycosylated and contains no known enzymatic activity.

Exposure of experimental preparations to α-latrotoxin is followed by a latent period of several minutes during which transmission continues without change. Even at this time, however, it is impossible to remove the toxin and prevent its ultimate effect by washing the prepa-

ration. After this latent period, changes begin to appear. A progressive swelling of the nerve terminal is seen morphologically, with a parallel depletion of synaptic vesicles; other organelles within the terminals are not affected. The presynaptic membranes also exhibit an accumulation of characteristic large intramembranous particles that are thought to be the product of fusion of synaptic vesicles with the membrane.

Purified latrotoxin is capable of forming ion channels when applied to planar lipid bilayers [6]. The channel, with a conductance in excess of 100 pS, is permeant to Na^+, K^+, and Ca^{2+}, but not to anions. If α-latrotoxin has a similar effect on the presynaptic membrane, the result will be membrane depolarization and Ca^{2+} influx; depolarization alone could activate voltage-dependent Ca^{2+} channels, further adding to the influx of Ca^{2+}. The net effect of this activity would be the triggering of the fusion of synaptic vesicles with the plasma membrane, leading to transmitter release on a massive scale and eventually to depletion of the neurotransmitter stores in the terminal. Although other mechanisms of action may be involved, the ionophore activity of the toxin provides an attractive hypothesis to explain its effects.

If α-latrotoxin can produce cation channels in artificial lipid bilayers, how is its activity confined so exquisitely to the presynaptic nerve terminal *in vivo*? The answer may lie in the presence of a specific receptor for the polypeptide on the presynaptic membrane. Labeled toxin can be localized with the electron microscope to the extracellular surface of the presynaptic membrane [7]; in the same preparations, no binding is seen to muscle membrane or to the membrane of the unmyelinated terminal portions of the motor nerve at physiologically active concentrations of toxin. The apparent K_d for this binding site is approximately 3×10^{-10} M; about 2,500 sites are present per square micrometer of membrane.

The α–latrotoxin binding site in nerve membrane has been solubilized in nonionic detergents and purified by affinity chromatography on a column containing immobilized toxin [8]. The product is a single 200-kDa band on nonreducing sodium dodecylsulfate-polyacrylmide gel electrophoresis (SDS-PAGE); after reduction, two bands of 66 and 54 kDa are seen. The purified receptor can be reconstituted into liposomes. Subsequent exposure of these vesicles to purified α-latrotoxin results in depolarization and release of internal Ca^{2+} at concentrations of toxin that have no effect on vesicles not containing the receptor. Receptor-containing vesicles can also be fused with planar lipid bilayers, and the single-channel electrical activity produced by the application of α-latrotoxin can then be examined. In the presence of receptor, single-channel activity appears rapidly at low concentrations of toxin; in the absence of receptor, channels appear only very slowly, and higher concentrations of toxin are required [9]. The receptor itself produces no electrical activity in the bilayer.

Thus the effect of α-latrotoxin may involve the targeted binding of the toxin to a specific receptor protein in the presynaptic terminal membrane, followed by its insertion into the membrane to form a cation-specific ion channel. The normal function of this "toxin receptor" protein is unknown.

Some snake venoms contain β-toxins that interrupt presynaptic events at the NMJ

Many snake venoms contain polypeptide toxins that act on the NMJ. Some α-toxins act by interfering with the function of ACh receptors in the postsynaptic membrane; these toxins are considered later in this chapter. A second group, the β-toxins, interfere with neuromuscular transmission through their actions on the presynaptic nerve terminal. Although β-toxins are produced by a variety of crotalids, the β-bungarotoxin found in the venom of the krait

Bungarus multicinctus is the best studied of this group.

β-Bungarotoxin is a protein of 20,500 M_r, which on reduction proves to be a heterodimer consisting of a 13,500-M_r A chain and a 7,000-M_r B chain linked by at least one disulfide bond [10]. About 25 ng of this toxin is lethal in a mouse. The toxin inhibits the release of synaptic vesicles from motor nerve terminals and from some cholinergic autonomic terminals. Its onset of action is rather slow; 2 to 3 hr usually elapse between exposure of the terminal to toxin and complete block, although this interval can be shortened by repetitive stimulation of the motor nerve.

Both chains of the β-bungarotoxin molecule have been isolated and biochemically characterized. The native toxin exhibits phospholipase A_2 (PLA_2) activity, a feature found in all of the presynaptically acting snake toxins [11]. This activity is abolished by treatment with *p*-bromophenacyl bromide (BPB), which specifically modifies histidine residue 48 in the A chain. Both the A and B chains have been sequenced: the A chain exhibits extensive homology with other enzymes with PLA_2 activity, especially those from the porcine pancreas. Each of the other snake venom presynaptic toxins also contain one or more subunits homologous to the A-chain phospholipase, and this enzymatic activity is central to the action of all of the β-toxins. Treatment of β-bungarotoxin with BPB renders it biologically inactive. The sequence of the β-bungarotoxin B chain is not homologous with subunits of the other snake toxins, but has sequence homology with a number of protease inhibitors.

The physiological effects of β-bungarotoxin can be separated into three sequential stages [5]. In isolated nerve-muscle preparations, there is a slight reduction in EPP amplitude during the first few minutes after exposure to toxin. This is followed over the next 30 to 60 min by an augmentation of EPP amplitude, and finally by a slow but progressive fall in amplitude that ends in complete block of stimulated transmitter release. During the second stage, there is also a transient increase in the frequency of MEPPs, consistent with an increase in intraterminal free Ca^{2+}. The slight reduction in EPP amplitude characteristic of the first stage is seen with BPB-modified toxin, but all remaining effects require PLA_2 activity. Most recent work has focused on the relationship between this enzymatic activity and the onset of neuromuscular block; several potential sites of action have been identified.

β-Bungarotoxin depolarizes the presynaptic membrane in a Ca^{2+}-dependent manner. Although requiring intact PLA_2 activity, this depolarization does not depend on the action of released free fatty acids (FFA) and may be related to effects of the membrane lysophosphatides produced from phospholipid hydrolysis. This depolarization could result in an influx of Ca^{2+} and augmentation of transmitter release, but eventually will lead to block. Depolarization is partially blocked by preincubation of the terminal with dendrotoxin, another polypeptide toxin that lacks phospholipase activity, suggesting that it is mediated through binding of β-bungarotoxin to a specific receptor on the presynaptic terminal.

A presynaptic membrane protein that may qualify as the binding site for β-bungarotoxin has been isolated from chick brain membranes by affinity chromatography on a column of immobilized toxin [12]. Toxin binding to the purified protein is Ca^{2+} dependent and exhibits an apparent K_d of approximately 2×10^{-9} M. From physical measurements, the size of the binding protein is estimated to be 431 kDa, and there is speculation that it may represent a membrane ion channel.

The PLA_2 activity of these snake toxins also results in uncoupling of mitochondrial energy metabolism. This action is due to the effect of FFA released by the enzyme on mitochondria. This effect is prominent in the absence of albumin or other proteins that can bind FFA but

probably plays a minor role under physiological conditions. Finally, these toxins have an additional effect on synaptic vesicle function. They cause uncoupling of the vesicle membrane ATPase activity from the transport of ACh, resulting in failure of ACh accumulation with a parallel rise in ATPase activity.

Although the exact mechanism of action of these presynaptic toxins remains unclear, it seems that they, too, target the presynaptic membrane through specific binding to a normal membrane protein. Early effects may be due to the local action of the PLA_2, with direct interaction of phospholipid breakdown products with the target channel, increase in leakiness of the presynaptic membrane, Ca^{2+} influx, and depolarization. Effects on synaptic vesicle function and mitochondrial energy production may be caused by the FFA that are released during the hydrolysis of membrane lipids.

CLINICAL DISORDERS AFFECTING PRESYNAPTIC MECHANISMS

Autoimmune diseases can interfere with neurotransmitter release

Some patients with carcinoma, especially small-cell carcinoma of the lung, develop an unusual syndrome of muscle weakness associated with symptoms of autonomic dysfunction called the Lambert-Eaton myasthenic syndrome (LEMS). Complaints often begin with progressive proximal muscle weakness and fatigue; unlike myasthenia gravis, bulbar involvement is usually mild, and respiratory compromise is unusual. Autonomic complaints can include dry mouth, impotence, and orthostatic hypotension.

When examined electrophysiologically, a remarkable reduction is observed in the amplitude of the compound muscle action potential produced by a single supramaximal stimulus to the motor nerve of a resting muscle [13]. Repeated stimulation of the same nerve, however, results in progressive improvement in response amplitude, often returning to nearly normal levels. These clinical findings are indicative of a defect in presynaptic neurotransmitter release.

When analyzed at the level of the single cell, Lambert-Eaton syndrome is characterized by a dramatic reduction in the mean quantal content of the EPP, often to 10% or less of normal values. The amplitude of spontaneous MEPPs is normal, as is the frequency of MEPP, but the MEPP frequency does not increase with increasing extracellular Ca^{2+} concentration as it normally should. Repetitive stimulation results in a progressive increase in quantal content of the EPP consistent with the improvement seen in the compound muscle action potential.

Lambert-Eaton syndrome is an autoimmune disease. Patients respond clinically to medications that suppress their immune systems, and their clinical symptoms can be temporarily relieved by the removal of circulating immunoglobulin (IgG) molecules through plasmaphoresis. The salient features of the disease can be passively transferred to mice by injection of IgG from patients who have the disorder.

The target of the autoimmune reaction may be a Ca^{2+} channel in the presynaptic membrane. The Ca^{2+} dependence of neurotransmitter release in Lambert-Eaton junctions is shifted dramatically to the right, consistent with the disappearance of about 40% of the normally functioning Ca^{2+} channels. In freeze-fracture images of the presynaptic membrane, the normal organization of large intramembranous particles, which form the double rows of the active zones, is disrupted [14]. These particles are thought to represent Ca^{2+} channels associated with the specific release sites for synaptic vesicles. The number of arrays is reduced, with many particles found instead in irregular aggregates. Mice treated with IgG from LEMS patients demonstrate the same changes in intramembranous particle distribution. Finally, IgG from LEMS patients who also have small-cell carcinoma specifically reduced the depolarization-induced Ca^{2+} efflux from small-cell carcinoma cells grown in culture. It may be the cross-reactivity between this channel in the tumor cell and the related molecule in the normal presynaptic membrane that leads to the generation of symptoms at this seemingly unrelated site.

Of the patients who develop this syndrome, about 20% have no detectable tumor; some of these patients have been followed for more than 15 years without developing a malignancy. The nature of the initial antigenic stimulus in these patients remains an enigma.

TOXINS AND DISEASES ACTING AT THE POSTSYNAPTIC LEVEL

Acetylcholine released from the motor nerve terminal interacts specifically with acetylcholine receptor (AChR) molecules in the postsynaptic membrane (see Chap. 10). Molecules of acetylcholinesterase (AChE) in the junctional basal lamina compete for the transmitter and inactivate it by hydrolysis to acetate and choline. Successful transmission requires that a significant proportion of the ACh in each quantum reach receptors in the postsynaptic membrane prior to being hydrolyzed. This in turn depends on the relative number of functional AChR and AChE molecules present as well as their geometric organization relative to the release zones of the motor nerve terminal. The safety margin of transmission can be adversely affected, and junctional transmission blocked, by factors that modify either the number of AChRs, their functional ability, or their organization in the synapse, as well as by factors that alter the properties of the AChE.

α-Neurotoxins specifically bind to and block the activation of nicotinic AChRs

Toxins produced by snakes of the families Elapidae (cobras, kraits, coral snakes, mambas, etc.) and Hydrophidae (sea snakes) contain potent neuromuscular toxins. A major component in each of these toxins is a curarimimetic α-neurotoxin that produces a nondepolarizing block of the postsynaptic AChR [15]. When applied to the NMJ, these related small proteins block both EPPs and MEPPs. The frequency of MEPPs is not changed by a pure α-toxin, although crude venom, which contains β-toxins as well as α-toxins may have dramatic presynaptic effects (see above). The mean lethal dose (LD$_{50}$) for these toxins is typically 50 to 150 μg/kg in mice.

Exposure of humans to low doses of toxin, which produces partial blockade of junctional receptors, can produce a clinical picture of weakness and fatigability that resembles acquired myasthenia gravis. Repetitive stimulation results in a decremental response as the remaining receptors not complexed with toxin become desensitized. Exposure to higher doses of toxin can lead to complete neuromuscular block, paralysis, respiratory failure, and death.

The polypeptides responsible for this postsynaptic curarimimetic activity have been isolated from a number of snake venoms [15]. These α-toxins are low-molecular-weight basic proteins of 7 to 8 kDa with isoelectric points between pH 8 and 10. Chemically they fall into two groups: the long toxins, which have 71 to 74 amino acids and five internal disulfide bonds; and the short toxins, with 60 to 62 amino acids and four internal disulfide bonds. The α-toxins have approximately the same equilibrium dissociation constant for the AChR (6–8 × 10^{-10} M at pH 7.4, 20°C.), but they differ markedly in their binding kinetics. The short toxins have association rates five to six times faster and dissociation rates five to nine times faster than the long toxins. The binding of the short toxins can then be reversed by washing, whereas the long toxins bind essentially irreversibly under usual experimental conditions.

The α-toxins exhibit a high degree of homology when their primary sequences are aligned with respect to their cysteine residues. The eight cysteines of the short toxins that participate in disulfide bonds are invariant. In total, approximately 22 amino acid residues are conserved. Of these, three (trp-29, arg-37, and gly-38) appear to be conserved for functional reasons and are assumed to be components of the toxin binding site. The remaining invariant residues may be conserved to preserve the three-dimensional structure of these proteins.

Representative examples of these toxins have been crystallized and their tertiary structure determined [16]. These proteins are concave disks with a small projection at one end. Their elliptical dimensions are approximately 3.8 × 2.8 × 1.5 nm, and for the most part the structure is only a single polypeptide chain thick. The elliptical portion of the molecule is formed from six short peptide strands forming three side-by-side loops. Five of these strands form antiparallel β-pleated sheets, and the resultant structure is strongly stabilized by interchain hydrogen bonding. The reactive site of the protein is on the concave surface and involves the regions encompassed by residues 32 to 45 and 49 to 56, as well as isolated residues from other chains.

The α-neurotoxins bind specifically to sites on the α-subunits of the AChR; there is one binding site per subunit and thus two binding sites per receptor molecule (see Chap. 10). The toxin binding site sterically overlaps that for ACh, and binding of α-bungarotoxin prevents the interaction of ACh with the receptor. Electron diffraction studies suggest that the binding site for bungarotoxin is near the superior lip of the ion channel at the outermost surface of the α-subunit. Recent studies with synthetic oligopeptides implicate amino acid residues 153 to 241 in the formation of this site [17].

The relative irreversibility of the binding of the long α-neurotoxins to the AChR, especially that of bungarotoxin from the venom of *Bungarus multicinctus*, has made them valuable tools for the purification and characterization of this ion channel protein. Affinity columns formed from covalently immobilized toxin have been used to purify the receptor protein virtually to homogeneity from crude solubilized preparations of electroplax membranes.

In myasthenia gravis, an autoimmune response against the AChR leads to neuromuscular failure

Myasthenia gravis (MG), the prototypic human disorder of neuromuscular transmission, is an acquired autoimmune disease affecting AChRs in the postsynaptic membrane [18]. Clinically, the disorder is characterized by muscle weakness and abnormal fatigability. Most patients have circulating antibodies against the AChR in their serum.

Patients with MG typically show fluctuating symptoms; their weakness and fatigability may be worse in the evening and usually becomes more severe with exercise. Weakness may involve only the extraocular muscles, producing diplopia, or may be so extensive as to cause quadriparesis and respiratory compromise. Although spontaneous remissions can occur, the untreated disease is often progressive and can eventually lead to death from respiratory failure.

Myasthenia gravis is associated with abnormalities of the thymus gland in a high percentage of cases. About 15 percent of patients with MG have a thymoma, and an additional 65 percent exhibit hyperplasia of the germinal centers in the thymus. The incidence of associated autoimmune disease, such as rheumatoid arthritis, systemic lupus erythematosis, sarcoidosis, and autoimmune thyroid disease, is also high, with as many as 15 percent of patients with MG exhibiting symptoms of one or another of these disorders.

The classical electrophysiological observation in MG is a decrementing response in the extracellularly recorded bulk muscle action potential with repeated nerve stimulation (Fig. 4). Using intracellular electrodes, the amplitude of the MEPP is found to be decreased. The quan-

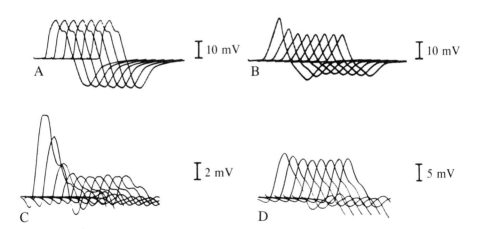

FIG. 4. Compound muscle action potentials recorded from the abductor digiti minimi of human subjects during repetitive stimulation of the ulnar nerve at three stimuli per second. (**A**) A recording from a normal individual shows no change in the amplitude of the muscle electrical response during the stimulation interval. (**B**) In a patient with MG, the same stimuli produce a 40 percent decrement in response amplitude over the first five stimuli, with a slow partial recovery during subsequent stimulation. Similar studies from a patient with severe MG before (**C**) and 2 min after (**D**) intravenous administration of 10 mg edrophonium. Note the change in amplitude scale between the two recordings and the reversal of the abnormal decrement by this short-acting AChE inhibitor.

tum content of the EPP is normal, although its amplitude is reduced as a consequence of a reduction in the amplitude of the MEPP. Noise analysis at myasthenic muscle end-plates reveals no difference in single-channel conductance or mean channel lifetime. It has now clearly been shown that the reduction in MEPP amplitude is not due to a reduction in the amount of ACh per quantum, but rather to a reduction in the number of AChR molecules present in the postsynaptic membrane, combined with a pathological alteration in the architecture of the postsynaptic membrane itself.

Evidence for a reduction in the density of AChR has been obtained from autoradiographic measurements with labeled bungarotoxin at the light microscopic level, as well as from quantitative electron microscopic measurements using peroxidase-labeled toxin [19]. Measurements of the density of AChR in homogenates of normal and myasthenic muscle have confirmed this finding. Receptor density in the myasthenic postsynaptic membrane may be as low as 20 percent of normal. In addition, the highly organized architecture of the postsynaptic membrane, with junctional folds immediately subjacent to presynaptic active zones and high densities of AChRs at the crests of these folds, is lost. The distance between pre- and postsynaptic membranes is often increased, and the postsynaptic membrane is highly simplified (Fig. 5).

The destruction seen at the postsynaptic membrane is mediated by antibodies directed against the AChR [20]. These antibodies can be detected in the serum of about 90 percent of patients with MG. Highest titers are seen in patients with MG associated with a thymoma; patients with MG limited only to the extraocular muscles may have no detectable circulating antibody levels. In general, however, the titer of serum antibodies against the AChR does not correlate well with the severity of the disease.

The antibody response to the AChR is polyclonal. Although antibodies against all four sub-

units of AChR can be detected, most of the response appears to be directed against a segment of the α-subunit designated the major immunogenic region (MIR). This region is thought to reside in an extracellular domain of the N-terminal portion of this subunit. Monoclonal antibodies against the MIR are capable of passively transferring a myasthenic syndrome to laboratory animals, although monoclonal antibodies against other portions of the AChR molecule have not been effective.

Although it is attractive to postulate receptor block by the antibodies as the primary mechanism through which transmission failure occurs, this does not seem to be the case. The major effects of anti-AChR antibodies seem to be twofold [21]. First, antibodies cross-link receptor proteins and increase their rate of endocytosis and lysosomal degradation. In the absence of an increased rate of receptor synthesis, this results in a net decrease in receptor density in the postsynaptic membrane. Second, these antibodies target the postsynaptic membrane for complement fixation and activation of the lytic phase of the complement reaction cascade. The presence of lytic C9 in the myasthenic postsynaptic membrane has been demonstrated both in humans and in animal models of MG.

A disease resembling MG, experimental autoimmune myasthenia gravis (EAMG), can be induced in animals by immunization with purified AChR protein. These animals develop elevated levels of circulating antibody to the AChR and express fluctuating muscular weakness and fatigue, along with a typical decrementing response to nerve stimulation. Intracellular recordings demonstrate abnormally small MEPPs, and the morphological changes are indistinguishable from those seen in the human disease.

Patients with MG can be effectively treated by suppressing the immune response. This can be done by administering adrenocortical steroids or cytotoxic drugs, such as cyclophosphamide or azathioprine. Transiently lowering

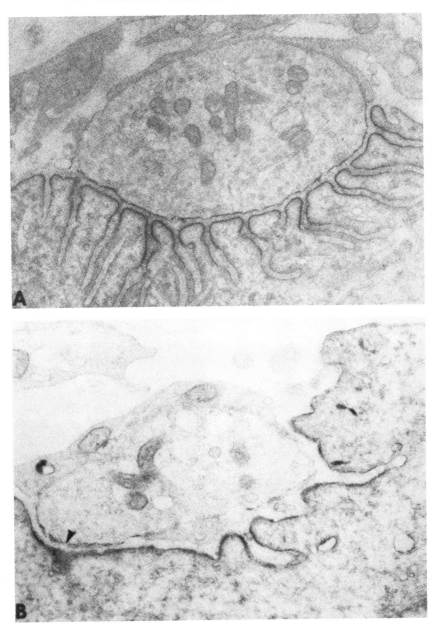

FIG. 5. Morphology of the NMJ in end-plates from normal human intercostal muscle (**A**) and from the intercostal muscle of a patient with MG (**B**). ACh receptors are localized with peroxidase-labeled α-bungarotoxin. In normal muscle, the AChR is associated with the terminal expanses of the junctional folds, and the architecture of the post-junctional membrane follows closely the distribution of active zones in the presynaptic membrane. In the myasthenic junction (**B**), the postsynaptic membrane is simplified, and its precise orientation with respect to the presynaptic membrane is lost. Only segments of the residual postsynaptic membrane are positively stained for AChR. (From A. Engel. The molecular biology of endplate diseases. In: M. Salpeter (ed.), *The Vertebrate Neuromuscular Junction*. New York: Alan R. Liss, 1987, pp. 361–424.)

the level of circulating IgG by plasmaphoresis also improves the clinical symptoms of MG.

Although the mechanism of ongoing neuromuscular damage in this disease has been defined, the nature of the initial triggering event is unclear. One hypothesis involves the role of myocytes, muscle-like cells that occur in the thymus gland. These cells have AChRs on their surface membranes. An initial inflammatory response in the thymus may trigger the generation of cross-reacting antibodies that subsequently target the muscle AChR. This hypothesis would help to explain the beneficial role of thymectomy in patients with MG. The diversity of predisposing and associated factors, however, suggests that a number of different triggering events may lead to the development of a common clinical picture.

Genetic abnormalities that affect ion channel structure or function can produce clinical disease

Given the central role of the AChR in neuromuscular transmission, it is reasonable to expect that mutations that affect channel function will also interfere with normal neuromuscular transmission. Defects that render the channel nonfunctional would be lethal, but milder alterations might be compatible with life.

Recently, investigators have described two genetic disorders in neuromuscular transmission that in some ways resemble MG as it is seen in infants. In one of these, an abnormally low density of AChR is found at the NMJ using assays with ^{125}I-bungarotoxin. In the other, the kinetics of channel opening appear abnormal, with a marked prolongation of the EPP and MEPP, which is further increased by the addition of inhibitors of AChE [22]. Although the quantum content of the EPP is normal, its amplitude is significantly reduced. Activity and kinetic properties of the AChE itself are normal. It is postulated that the defect in this disorder is an abnormally slow closing rate for the channel.

Abnormalities in AChE activity can interfere with neuromuscular transmission

At the NMJ, the duration of neurotransmitter action on the postsynaptic membrane is controlled by the rate of hydrolysis of ACh by AChE (see Chap. 10). This enzyme is associated with the basal lamina between the presynaptic membrane and the muscle plasma membrane [23]. Roughly one-third of the released ACh from each quantum is hydrolyzed by this enzyme before reaching the postsynaptic membrane. The remaining molecules interact with postsynaptic receptors but are rapidly inactivated after dissociation before having an opportunity for significant lateral spread. Thus, the site of action of released ACh is focused on a small disk under the point of release from the presynaptic active zone. Inhibition of AChE allows ACh to diffuse laterally out of the synapse and to interact with additional receptors. The result is a marked prolongation of the EPP. Also, since receptors are desensitized after exposure to their transmitter, prolonged exposure to ACh eventually leads to reduced sensitivity and to block of neuromuscular transmission.

Acetylcholinesterase exists in two forms in skeletal muscle: a globular form that is easily solubilized in low-salt solution, and an asymmetric form that requires high concentrations of salt for solubilization [24]. Both forms can be subdivided into two or three subspecies based on their sedimentation characteristics on density gradients. For the globular form, components with apparent sedimentation coefficients of 5 S, 7 S, and 11 S have been identified, corresponding to monomers, dimers, and tetramers of similar-size subunits. For the asymmetric form, sedimentation coefficients of 12 S, 15 S, and 16 to 18 S were found, corresponding to one to three globular tetramers joined by disulfide bonds to a common tail.

In most species, the globular subunit is between 70 and 80 kDa in size. It is a glycoprotein with approximately 15% w/w carbohydrate N-linked to asparagine residues. In the asymmetric form, one or more tetramers of globular subunits are linked together to a triple-stranded collagen-like tail. This tail contains hydroxyproline and hydroxylysine as well as the high concentrations of glycine and proline typical of collagen. The presence of other amino acids and protease-sensitive cleavage sites not characteristic of collagen suggests that the tail structure may also contain noncollagen domains.

Exposure of the asymmetric form of AChE to collagenase results in the generation of a single species of globular protein identical to that found in the globular form of the enzyme. This protein contains all the enzymatic activity found in the asymmetric form, suggesting that the collagen tail is merely required for immobilization or anchoring of the protein complex. The entire asymmetric AChE subunit from *Torpedo* electroplax has been sequenced. The molecule is homologous with the butyrylcholinesterase enzyme from erythrocytes but not with any of the subunits of the AChR. In muscle, about one-third to one-half of the active AChE molecules are localized on the cell surface. Most of the AChE at the NMJ is of the asymmetric collagen-tailed variety and is found associated with the basal lamina. A small amount may actually be located on the presynaptic membrane.

Acetylcholinesterase can be inhibited reversibly by a number of drugs useful in the clinical treatment of MG, such as edrophonium, neostigmine, and pyridostigmine. In addition, it is irreversibly inhibited by organophosphate insecticides such as parathion. These insecticides form covalent bonds at the active site of the enzyme, acting as suicide substrates. Inhibition of AChE with any of these compounds produces signs of cholinergic hyperactivity, initially with excessive motor activity, followed by skeletal muscle paralysis and autonomic dysfunction. Irreversible inhibitors of AChE are components of the early nerve gases, and accidental poisoning by organophosphate insecticides can be fatal.

Careful reduction of end-plate AChE activity following the administration of anticholinesterases can prolong the action of released ACh sufficiently to increase the amplitude of an abnormally low EPP above that required for successful neurotransmission. It is this effect that allows these agents to be used in the treatment of MG. Too much medication, however, will produce long-term postsynaptic depolarization, receptor inactivation, and block of neuromuscular transmission. It is difficult to differentiate at first glance between a patient with MG who has developed acute weakness and respiratory difficulty because of a marked exacerbation of this disease (called myasthenic crisis) from one who is in cholinergic crisis caused by overmedication with anticholinesterase agents.

In addition to the short-term effects of inhibition of AChE, there appear to be long-term effects that result from the prolonged exposure of the postsynaptic membrane to ACh. Animals treated chronically with reversible AChE inhibitors or acutely with single doses of irreversible anticholinesterase agents develop degenerative changes in their postsynaptic membranes and in the regions of the muscle fiber below the junctional complex. These effects may be mediated by increases of cytoplasmic Ca^{2+} concentrations secondary to increased influx of Ca^{2+} through open receptor channels or through voltage-activated Ca^{2+} channels. These increased levels of Ca^{2+} may activate Ca^{2+}-dependent proteases, leading to the observed degeneration.

A patient with an inherited disorder of AChE has been reported (25). This patient exhibited generalized weakness that increased with exertion as well as easy fatigability, which might have been mistaken for MG. His symp-

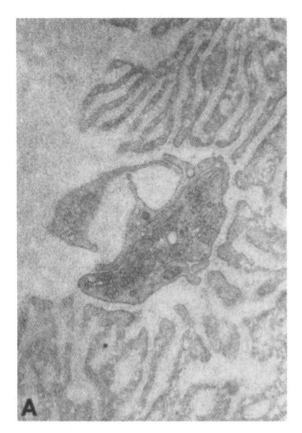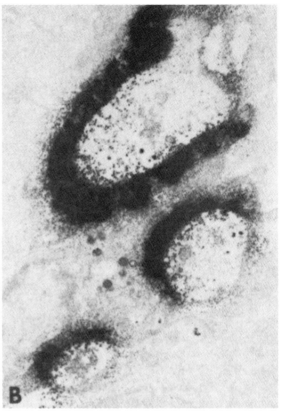

FIG. 6. Histochemical analysis of AChE activity in the end-plate of a patient with congenital cholinesterase deficiency (**A**) and a normal human NMJ (**B**). (From A. Engel et al. [25].)

toms, however, did not respond to treatment with inhibitors of AChE, and no anti-AChR antibody was present in the serum. Single supermaximal nerve stimuli produced multiple muscle action potentials, a response similar to that seen in patients who have been intoxicated with anticholinesterase drugs. With repetitive stimulation, the muscle action potential decreased in amplitude.

Electron cytochemistry of this patient's end-plates demonstrated a complete absence of AChE activity in the postsynaptic membrane (Fig. 6). Levels of AChE were only about 20 percent of that seen in homogenates of normal muscle. No 16 S asymmetric cholinesterase could be found, although small amounts of the 6 S globular component were present. It is likely that other patients with unexplained fatigue and muscle weakness may have similar or related defects in AChE activity at the NMJ.

REFERENCES

1. Sakaguchi, G. *Clostridium botulinum* toxins. *Pharmacol. Ther.* 19:165–194, 1983.
2. Simpson, L. L. Molecular pharmacology of botulinum toxin and tetanus toxin. *Ann. Rev. Pharmacol. Toxicol.* 26:427–453, 1986.
3. Hoch, D. H., Romero-Mira, M., Ehrlich, B. A., Finkelstein, A., DasGupta, B. R., and Simpson,

L. L. Channels formed by botulinum, tetanus, and diphtheria toxins in planar lipid bilayers: Relevance to translocation of proteins across membranes. *Proc. Natl. Acad. Sci. U.S.A.* 82:1692–1696, 1985.

4. Sathyamoorthy, V., and DasGupta, B. R., Separation, purification, partial characterization and comparison of the heavy and light chains of botulinum neurotoxin types A, B, and E. *J. Biol. Chem.* 260:10461–10466, 1985.

5. Howard, B. D., and Gunderson, C. B. Jr. Effects and mechanisms of polypeptide neurotoxins that act presynaptically. *Annu. Rev. Pharmacol. Toxicol.* 20:307–336, 1980.

6. Finkelstein, A., Rubin, L. L., and Tzeng, M. C. Black widow spider venom: Effect of purified toxin on lipid bilayer membranes. *Science* 193:1009–1011, 1976.

7. Valtorta, F., Madeddu, L., Meldolesi, J., and Ceccarelli, B. Specific localization of the alpha-latrotoxin receptor in the nerve terminal plasma membrane. *J. Cell Biol.* 99:124–132, 1984.

8. Scheer, H., and Meldolesi, J. Purification of the putative alpha-latrotoxin receptor from bovine synaptosomal membranes in an active binding form. *EMBO J.* 4:323–327, 1985.

9. Scheer, H., Prestipine, G., and Meldolesi, J. Reconstitution of the purified alpha-latrotoxin receptor in liposomes and planar lipid membranes. Clues to the mechanism of toxin action. *EMBO J.* 5:2643–2648, 1986.

10. Kondo, K., Narita, K., and Lee, C. Y. Amino acid sequences of the two polypeptide chains in beta-bungarotoxin from the venom of *Bungarus multicinctus. J. Biochem.* 83:101–115, 1978.

11. Kondo, K., Toda, H., and Narita, K. Characterization of phospholipase A₂ activity of beta-bungarotoxin from *Bungarus multicinctus. J. Biochem.* 84:1291–1300, 1978.

12. Rehm, H., and Betz, H. Solubilization and characterization of the beta-bungarotoxin binding protein of chick brain membranes. *J Biol Chem.* 259:6865–6869, 1984.

13. Newsome-Davis, J. Lambert-Eaton myasthenic syndrome. *Springer Semin. Immunopathol.* 8:129–140, 1985.

14. Fukunaga, H., Engel, A., Osame, M., and Lambert, E. Paucity and disorganization of presynaptic membrane active zones in the Lambert-Eaton myasthenic syndrome. *Muscle Nerve* 5:686–694, 1982.

15. Karlsson, E. Chemistry of protein toxins in snake venoms. In C. Y. Lee (ed.), *Snake Venoms.* Berlin: Springer-Verlag, 1979, pp. 159–204.

16. Low, B. W. The three-dimensional structure of post-synaptic snake neurotoxins: Considerations of structure and function. In C. Y. Lee (ed.), *Snake Venoms,* Berlin: Springer-Verlag, 1979, pp. 213–257.

17. Wilson, P. T., Lentz, T. L., and Hawrot, E. Determination of the primary amino acid sequence specifying the alpha-bungarotoxin binding site on the alpha subunit of the acetylcholine receptor from *Torpedo californica. Proc. Natl. Acad. Sci. U.S.A.* 82:8790–8794, 1985.

18. Lisak, R. P., and Barchi, R. L. *Myasthenia Gravis,* Philadelphia: W. B. Saunders Co, 1982.

19. Ashizawa, T., and Appel, S. Immunopathologic events at the endplate in myasthenia gravis. *Springer Semin. Immunopathol.* 8:177–196, 1985.

20. Lindstrom, J. Immunobiology of myasthenia gravis, experimental autoimmune myasthenia gravis, and Lambert Eaton syndrome. *Annu. Rev. Immunol.* 3:109–131, 1985.

21. Drachman, D. B., Pestronk, A., Stanley, E. F., and Adams, R. N. Mechanisms of acetylcholine receptor loss in myasthenia gravis. In: D. L. Schotland (ed.), *Disorders of the Motor Unit.* New York: Wiley, 1982, pp. 215–231.

22. Engel, A. G., Lambert, E. H., Mulder, D. M., et al. A newly recognized congenital myasthenic syndrome attributable to a prolonged open time of the acetylcholine-induced ion channel. *Ann. Neurol.* 11:553–569, 1982.

23. Massouli, J., and Bon, S. The molecular forms of cholinesterase and acetylcholinesterase in vertebrates. *Annu. Rev. Neurosci.* 5:57–106, 1982.

24. Rotundo, R. L. Biogenesis and regulation of acetylcholinesterase. In: M. Salpeter (ed.), *The Vertebrate Neuromuscular Junction.* New York: Alan R. Liss, 1987, pp. 247–284.

25. Engel, A. G., Lambert, E. H., and Gomez, M. R. A new myasthenic syndrome with endplate cholinesterase deficiency, swollen nerve terminals, and reduced acetylcholine release. *Ann. Neurol.* 1:315–330, 1977.

CHAPTER 33

Diseases of Carbohydrate, Fatty Acid, and Mitochondrial Metabolism

Salvatore DiMauro and Darryl C. De Vivo

Defects of energy metabolism cause profound disturbances in function of muscle or brain, or both. Such defects may present as myopathy, encephalopathy, or encephalomyopathy. Clinical features are best appreciated by having an understanding of the preferred oxidizable substrate for brain and muscle.

Muscle in the resting state utilizes fatty acids predominantly. The immediate source of energy for muscle contraction is ATP, which is

Basic Neurochemistry: Molecular, Cellular, and Medical Aspects, 4th Ed., edited by G. J. Siegel et al. Raven Press, Ltd., New York, 1989. Correspondence to Salvatore DiMauro, Columbia University College of Physicians and Surgeons, 630 West 168th Street, New York, NY 10032.

rapidly replenished at the expense of creatine phosphate by the phosphorylation of ADP by creatine kinase. During exercise of moderate intensity, the fuel choice depends on the duration of work. Initially, glycogen is the main fuel source; after 5 to 10 min, blood glucose becomes the more important fuel. As work continues, fatty acid utilization increases, and after approximately 4 hr, lipids are the primary source of energy. During high-intensity exercise, near maximal power, additional ATP is generated by the anaerobic breakdown of glycogen and by glycolysis. Intense exercise is performed in essentially anaerobic conditions, whereas mild or moderate exercise is accompanied by increased blood flow to exercising muscles, facilitating substrate delivery and favoring aerobic metabolism. This adaptation is known as the "second-wind" phenomenon.

Brain utilizes glucose predominantly in the postabsorptive state, with regional variations of the metabolic rate depending on the mental or motor task being performed. As with muscle, the immediate intracellular energy source is ATP butressed by the creatine phosphate stores. Glycogen provides very little energy reserve because brain concentrations are extremely low, approximating only one-tenth the amount found in muscle per gram wet weight. Therefore, brain is exquisitely sensitive to fluctuations in the blood glucose concentration. During starvation, the brain uses little if any fatty acids; however, fatty acids of varying chain lengths may be taken up by the brain, the efficiency of transport across the blood-brain barrier being much greater for short- or medium-chain fatty acids than for long-chain fatty acids. Ketone bodies represent the preferred cerebral fuel source during starvation when glucose supply is limited (these features of brain metabolism are discussed in Chap. 29). Defective fatty acid oxidation may therefore affect muscle directly, by blocking oxidation of this substrate, and brain indirectly, by limiting he-

patic ketogenesis. Elevated circulating free fatty acids may also have a direct toxic effect on brain, but the precise mechanisms are poorly understood (see Chaps. 39 and 40).

Energy metabolism has been studied extensively in skeletal muscle, and several metabolic disorders have been documented. Comparatively less is known about metabolic defects in cerebral energy metabolism—muscle tissue is accessible for biochemical analysis, whereas certain cerebral enzyme defects are presumed lethal.

DISEASES OF CARBOHYDRATE AND FATTY ACID METABOLISM IN MUSCLE

In muscle, disorders of glycogen or lipid metabolism cause two main clinical syndromes:

1. Acute, recurrent, reversible muscle dysfunction, with exercise intolerance and myoglobinuria (with or without cramps) is characteristic of phosphorylase, phosphofructokinase (PFK), phosphoglycerate kinase (PGK), phosphoglycerate mutase (PGAM), and lactate dehydrogenase (LDH) deficiencies among the glycogenoses and of carnitine palmitoyltransferase (CPT) deficiency among the disorders of lipid metabolism.

2. Progressive weakness is associated with acid maltase, debrancher enzyme, and brancher enzyme deficiencies among the glycogenoses, and with carnitine deficiency, some defects of β-oxidation, and other biochemically undefined lipid storage myopathies among the disorders of lipid metabolism. Figures 1 and 2 illustrate schematically the pathways of glycogen and fatty acid metabolism and indicate the sites of the biochemical lesions listed above.

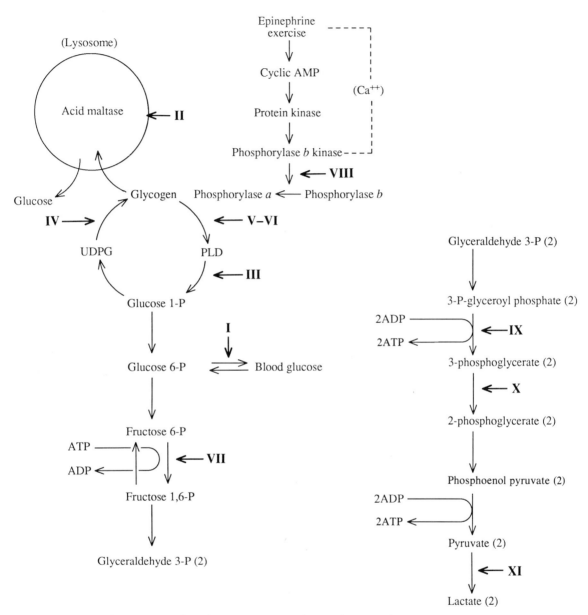

FIG. 1. Schematic representation of glycogen metabolism and glycolysis. *Roman numerals* indicate the sites of identified enzyme defects: (I) glucose-6-phosphatase; (II) acid maltase; (III) debrancher enzyme; (IV) brancher enzyme; (V) muscle phosphorylase; (VI) liver phosphorylase; (VII) phosphofructokinase; (VIII) phosphorylase kinase; (IX) phosphoglycerate kinase; (X) phosphoglycerate mutase; (XI) lactate dehydrogenase. (PLD) phosphorylase-limit dextrin; (UDPG) uridine diphosphate glucose; (P) phosphate.

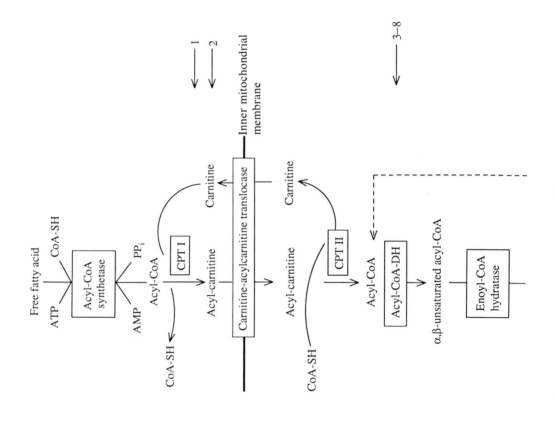

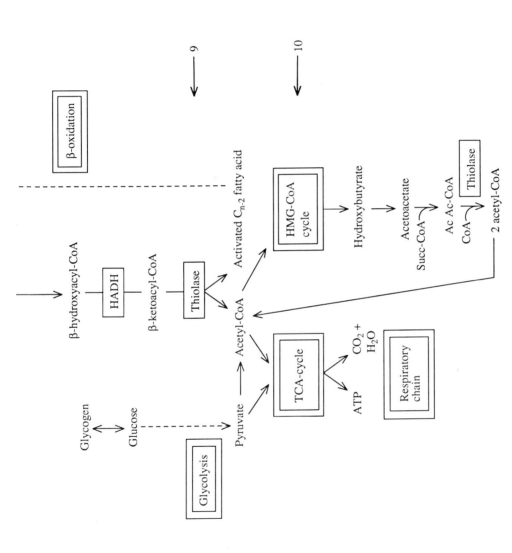

FIG. 2. Schematic representation of fatty acid oxidation and ketone body synthesis. *Numbers* indicate the sites of proved enzyme defects: (1) carnitine palmitoyltransferase; (2) carnitine; (3) long-chain acyl-CoA dehydrogenase; (4) medium-chain acyl-CoA dehydrogenase; (5) short-chain acyl-CoA dehydrogenase; (6) glutaryl-CoA dehydrogenase (glutaric aciduria I); (7) multiple acyl-CoA dehydrogenase (glutaric aciduria II); (8) isovaleryl-CoA dehydrogenase; (9) β-hydroxy-β-methyl-glutaryl-CoA lyase. (CoA-SH) coenzyme A, reduced; (PPi) pyrophosphate; (DH) dehydrogenase; (AMP) adenosine 5′-monophosphate; (CPT) carnitine palmitoyltransferase; (HADH) 3-hydroxyacyl-CoA dehydrogenase; (TCA) tricarboxylic acid; (HMG-CoA) hydroxymethylglutaryl-CoA; (succ-CoA) succinyl CoA; (AcAc-CoA) acetoacetyl CoA.

*Disorders causing recurrent
myoglobinuria and exercise intolerance*

Phosphorylase deficiency (McArdle's
disease; glycogenosis type V)

Phosphorylase deficiency is an autosomal recessive myopathy caused by a genetic defect of
the muscle isoenzyme of glycogen phosphorylase (Fig. 1). The gene encoding this enzyme has
been assigned to chromosome 11. There is a 2:1
predominance of affected males to females. Intolerance of strenuous exercise is present from
childhood, but onset is usually in adolescence,
with cramps after exercise. Myoglobinuria occurs in about one-half of patients. If they avoid
intense exercise, most patients can live normal
lives; however, about one-third of them develop
some degree of fixed weakness, usually as a
late-onset manifestation of the disease. In a few
patients, weakness rather than exercise-related
cramps and myoglobinuria characterizes the
clinical picture.

In patients with myoglobinuria, renal insufficiency is a possible life-threatening complication. Physical examination between episodes of myoglobinuria may be completely
normal or show some degree of weakness and,
occasionally, wasting of some muscle groups.

Even interictally, most patients have increased serum creatine kinase (CK) levels; forearm ischemic exercise causes no rise of venous
lactate level. This is a useful but nonspecific test
in McArdle's disease. The electromyogram
(EMG) at rest shows nonspecific myopathic features in about one-half of patients.

Muscle biopsy demonstrates subsarcolemmal blebs that contain periodic acid-Schiff-pos-
itive material (glycogen). The histochemical
stain for phosphorylase is negative, except in
regenerating fibers. Biochemical documentation of the enzyme defect requires muscle biopsy because the defect is not expressed in

more easily accessible tissues (leukocytes,
erythrocytes, cultured fibroblasts).

Phosphofructokinase deficiency (Tarui's
disease; glycogenosis type VII)

Phosphofructokinase (PFK) deficiency is an autosomal recessive myopathy caused by a genetic defect of the muscle (M) subunit of the
rate-limiting enzyme of glycolysis, PFK (Fig.
1). The gene encoding PFK-M is on chromosome 1. There is a 2.4:1 predominance of affected males to females. Presenting symptoms
are cramps after intense exercise, followed by
myoglobinuria in about one-half of patients. A
few patients may have mild jaundice, reflecting
excessive hemolysis, or typical symptoms and
signs of gout. In patients with typical presentation, fixed weakness appears to be less common than in phosphorylase deficiency. On the
other hand, in PFK deficiency, as in phosphorylase deficiency, a few patients have only
weakness, without cramps or myoglobinuria. In
addition to renal insufficiency due to myoglobinuria, other possible complications include
renal colic due to urate stones and gouty arthritis.

Physical examination may show slight jaundice. Neurological examination is normal.
Serum CK level is variably increased in most
patients. Forearm ischemic exercise causes no
rise of venous lactate level. Serum bilirubin
level is elevated in most patients, and the number of reticulocytes is increased. Serum uric
acid level is also increased in most patients.
EMG is usually normal. Muscle biopsy shows
focal, mostly subsarcolemmal, accumulation of
glycogen. In some patients a small portion of
the glycogen is abnormal: By histochemical
analysis, it is shown to be diastase resistant; by
electron microscopy, it appears finely granular
and filamentous in structure. The enzyme defect can be demonstrated by a specific histochemical reaction for PFK. Although a partial

defect of PFK activity is manifested in erythrocytes from patients, firm diagnosis usually requires biochemical studies of muscle.

Phosphoglycerate kinase deficiency

Phosphoglycerate kinase (PGK) deficiency is an X-linked recessive disease (type IX, Fig. 1). The most common clinical presentation includes hemolytic anemia with or without central nervous system involvement (see below). So far, only two patients, a 15-year-old boy and a 31-year-old man, have been described with a purely myopathic syndrome, characterized by exercise-induced cramps and myoglobinuria. Between episodes of myoglobinuria, physical and neurological examinations were normal. Forearm ischemic exercise caused contracture and no rise of venous lactate level.

Because the enzyme defect is expressed in all tissues except sperm, diagnosis can be made by biochemical studies of muscle, erythrocytes, leukocytes, or cultured fibroblasts.

Phosphoglycerate mutase deficiency

Phosphoglycerate mutase (PGAM) deficiency is an autosomal recessive myopathy caused by a genetic defect of the muscle subunit of the enzyme PGAM (type X, Fig. 1). Four patients with this enzyme deficiency have been identified so far, all black.

The clinical picture includes cramps and recurrent myoglobinuria following intense exercise. Aside from episodes of myoglobinuria, none of the patients was weak. Forearm ischemic exercise caused an increase of 1.5 to 2.0 times in venous lactate level, an abnormally low but not absent response. Muscle biopsy showed normal or only moderately increased glycogen concentration.

Because other accessible tissues, such as erythrocytes, leukocytes, and cultured fibroblasts, express a different isoenzyme, the diagnosis of PGAM-M subunit deficiency must be established by biochemical studies of muscle.

Lactate dehydrogenase deficiency

Lactate dehydrogenase (LDH) deficiency is an autosomal recessive myopathy caused by a genetic defect of the muscle subunit, which is encoded by a gene on chromosome 11 (type XI, Fig. 1). So far, only one patient with this disease has been described. The clinical picture is characterized by cramps and myoglobinuria after intense exercise.

Forearm ischemic exercise showed a subnormal rise of lactate level, contrasting with an increased rise of pyruvate. The diagnosis can be established by electrophoretic studies of LDH in serum, erythrocytes, and leukocytes, showing lack of subunit M-containing isoenzymes; it should nevertheless be confirmed by biochemical studies of muscle.

Carnitine palmitoyltransferase deficiency

Carnitine palmitoyltransferase (CPT) deficiency is an autosomal recessive myopathy caused by a genetic defect of the mitochondrial enzyme CPT (Fig. 2). The disease has been identified in about 50 patients, with a marked prevalence of affected men (male:female ratio, 5.5:1).

Clinical manifestations are limited to attacks of myoglobinuria, not preceded by contractures and usually precipitated by prolonged exercise (several hours in duration), prolonged fasting, or a combination of the two conditions. Less common precipitating factors include intercurrent infection, emotional stress, and cold exposure; but some episodes of myoglobinuria occur without any apparent cause. Most patients have two or more attacks, probably because the lack of muscle cramps deprives them of a warning signal of impending myoglobinuria.

For unknown reasons, some women seem to have milder symptoms, such as myalgia, after prolonged exercise without pigment in the urine. This has been observed in sisters of men with recurrent myoglobinuria. The only serious complication is renal failure following myoglobinuria.

Physical and neurological examinations are completely normal. Prolonged fasting at rest (to be conducted under close medical observation) causes a sharp rise of serum CK level in about one-half of patients. Also in about one-half of patients, ketone bodies fail to increase normally after prolonged fasting. Forearm ischemic exercise causes a normal increase of venous lactate level. Aside from episodes of myoglobinuria, serum CK level and EMG are normal. Muscle biopsy may appear completely normal or show variable, but usually moderate, accumulation of lipid droplets. Most patients with CPT deficiency benefit from a high-carbohydrate, low-fat diet, and the therapeutic response may serve as an indirect diagnostic clue. Because the enzyme defect appears to be generalized, tissues other than muscle (e.g., mixed leukocytes or isolated lymphocytes or platelets) can be used to demonstrate CPT deficiency, but the diagnosis should be confirmed in muscle.

One unresolved biochemical question is whether CPT deficiency affects specifically CPT I (the enzyme bound to the outer face of the inner mitochondrial membrane), CPT II (the enzyme on the inner face of the membrane), or both enzymes to the same extent. What is clear is that the mutation affects the kinetic properties of CPT, rendering the enzyme abnormally sensitive to substrate/product inhibition. These findings may explain why symptoms appear only when fat metabolism is stressed and why so little fat accumulates in muscle of patients.

Disorders causing progressive weakness

Acid maltase deficiency (glycogenosis type II)

Acid maltase deficiency (AMD) is an autosomal recessive disease caused by a genetic defect of the lysosomal enzyme acid maltase, an α-1,4- and α-1,6-glucosidase capable of digesting glycogen completely to glucose (Fig. 1). The gene encoding acid maltase has been localized on chromosome 17. Two major clinical syndromes are caused by AMD: a severe, generalized, and invariably fatal disease of infancy (Pompe's disease) and a less severe neuromuscular disorder beginning in childhood or in adult life. (Other lysosomal disorders are discussed in Chapter 37.)

Infantile, generalized cardiomegalic AMD (Pompe's disease). Pompe's disease usually becomes manifest in the first weeks or months of life, with failure to thrive, poor suck, generalized hypotonia, and weakness (floppy infant syndrome). Macroglossia is common, as is hepatomegaly, which, however, is rarely severe. There is massive cardiomegaly with congestive heart failure. Weakness of respiratory muscles makes these infants susceptible to pulmonary infection; death usually occurs before 1 year and invariably before 2 years of age.

Childhood- and adult-onset AMD. The childhood- and adult-onset forms of AMD cause signs and symptoms that are limited to the musculature, with progressive weakness of truncal muscles and of proximal more than distal limb muscles, usually sparing facial and extraocular muscle. In the childhood form, onset is in infancy or childhood, and progression tends to be rapid. In the adult form, onset is usually in the third or fourth decade but occasionally even later, and the course is slower.

The clinical picture in male children can closely resemble Duchenne-type muscular dystrophy; in adults it mimics limb-girdle dystrophy or polymyositis. The early and severe involvement of respiratory muscles in most patients with AMD is a distinctive clinical clue. Respiratory failure and pulmonary infection are the most common causes of death.

Serum CK level is consistently increased in all forms of AMD. Forearm ischemic exercise causes normal rise of venous lactate level in patients with childhood or adult AMD. The ECG is altered in Pompe's disease (short P-R interval, giant QRS complexes, and left ventricular or biventricular hypertrophy) but is usually normal in the later-onset forms. EMG shows myopathic features and fibrillation potentials, bizarre high-frequency discharges, and myotonic discharges.

Muscle biopsy shows vacuolar myopathy of very severe degree, affecting all fibers in Pompe's disease, but of varying degree and distribution in childhood and adult AMD. In adult AMD, biopsy specimens from unaffected muscles may appear normal by light microscopy. The vacuoles contain periodic acid-Schiff (PAS)-positive material (glycogen). Electron microscopy shows the presence of abundant glycogen both within membranous sacs (lysosomes) and free in the cytoplasm.

The enzyme defect is expressed in all tissues, and the diagnosis can be made by biochemical analysis of urine, lymphocytes (mixed leukocytes do not give reliable results), or cultured skin fibroblasts. Fibroblasts cultured from amniotic fluid can be used for prenatal diagnosis of Pompe's disease.

Debrancher enzyme deficiency
(glycogenosis type III; Cori's disease;
Forbes' disease)

Debrancher enzyme deficiency is an autosomal recessive disease caused by a genetic defect of the debranching enzyme (Fig. 1). In its more common presentation, debrancher enzyme deficiency causes liver dysfunction in childhood, with hepatomegaly, growth retardation, fasting hypoglycemia, and seizures. Myopathy has been described in about 20 patients. In most, onset of weakness was in the third or fourth decade. Wasting of distal leg muscles and intrinsic hand muscles is common, and the association of late-onset weakness and distal wasting often suggests the diagnosis of motor neuron disease or peripheral neuropathy. The

course is slowly progressive. In a smaller number of patients, onset of weakness is in childhood, with diffuse weakness and wasting. The association of hepatomegaly and growth retardation facilitates the diagnosis.

There is no glycemic response to glucagon or epinephrine (see Fig. 1), whereas a galactose load causes a normal glycemic response. Forearm ischemic exercise produces a blunted venous lactate rise or no response. Serum CK activity is variably, often markedly, increased. ECG shows left ventricular or biventricular hypertrophy in most patients. EMG may show myopathic features alone or associated with fibrillations, positive sharp waves, and myotonic discharges. This "mixed" EMG pattern in patients with weakness and distal wasting often reinforces the erroneous diagnosis of motor neuron disease. Motor nerve conduction velocities are moderately decreased in one-fourth of patients, suggesting a familial polyneuropathy.

Muscle biopsy shows severe vacuolar myopathy with glycogen storage. On electron microscopy, the vacuoles correspond to pools of glycogen free in the cytoplasm.

The enzyme defect is generalized, and it has been demonstrated in erythrocytes, leukocytes, and cultured fibroblasts. In patients with myopathy, the diagnosis is securely established by measurement of debrancher enzyme activity in muscle biopsy specimens or by studies of iodine adsorption spectra of glycogen isolated from muscle; there is a shift in the spectrum toward lower wavelengths, indicating that the polysaccharide has abnormally short peripheral branches.

Branching enzyme deficiency
(glycogenosis type IV; Andersen's
disease)

Branching enzyme deficiency is an autosomal recessive disease of infancy or early childhood typically causing liver dysfunction with hepatosplenomegaly, progressive cirrhosis, and chronic hepatic failure (Fig. 1). Death usually occurs in childhood. Although muscle wasting and hypotonia are mentioned in several reports, only three patients had severe hypotonia, wasting, contractures, and hyporeflexia, suggesting the diagnosis of spinal muscular atrophy.

There are no diagnostic laboratory tests. Muscle biopsy may be normal or show focal accumulations of abnormal glycogen, which is intensely PAS positive and partially resistant to diastase digestion. With the electron microscope, the abnormal glycogen is found to have a finely granular and filamentous structure.

Carnitine deficiency

Carnitine deficiency is a clinically heterogeneous disorder of multiple possible causes resulting in decreased concentration of carnitine in skeletal muscle (myopathic form) or in muscle, liver, blood, and various other tissues (systemic form).

Myopathic carnitine deficiency. Clinically, myopathic carnitine deficiency is characterized by generalized weakness, starting in childhood in most patients and affecting mainly proximal limb and trunk muscles but sometimes also facial and pharyngeal muscles. The course is usually slowly progressive, but weakness may fluctuate in severity.

Laboratory investigations show normal or near-normal serum carnitine levels (an important differential feature from systemic carnitine deficiency) and variably increased serum CK levels. EMG shows myopathic features with or without spontaneous activity at rest. Muscle biopsy reveals severe triglyceride storage, best seen with the oil red O stain in frozen sections. Myopathic carnitine deficiency seems to be transmitted as an autosomal recessive trait, and the primary biochemical defect may involve the active transport of carnitine from the blood into the muscle cell.

Systemic carnitine deficiency. Systemic carnitine deficiency probably does not exist as a primary condition. It can be secondary to other disorders causing excessive carnitine loss (renal Fanconi syndrome; chronic renal failure treated by hemodialysis) or decreased hepatic synthesis and dietary intake (cirrhosis with cachexia; kwashiorkor; total parenteral nutrition in premature infants), or it can be secondary to genetic defects of intermediary metabolism, such as organic acidurias, defects of β-oxidation, and defects of the respiratory chain. The mechanism of carnitine depletion in metabolic disorders appears to be mediated through excessive accumulation of acyl-coenzyme A (CoA) thioesters. These potentially toxic compounds are esterified to acylcarnitines and excreted in the urine, resulting in a loss of carnitine.

Regardless of the etiology, systemic carnitine deficiency usually presents in early childhood with recurrent episodes of encephalopathy closely resembling Reye's syndrome; in fact, in all cases thought to be recurrent Reye's syndrome, the diagnosis of systemic carnitine deficiency should be considered and serum carnitine concentration measured.

The episodes are often triggered by mild intercurrent illnesses and are accompanied by nausea, vomiting, confusion, or coma. A progressive neuromuscular disorder similar to that of the myopathic form is also known.

A special clinical presentation of systemic carnitine deficiency reported in two unrelated kindreds is dominated by cardiomyopathy rather than liver dysfunction; cardiomegaly and congestive heart failure occur in childhood.

Laboratory investigations show decreased levels of serum carnitine, variably increased serum CK activities, and, during attacks of encephalopathy, hypoglycemia, ketoacidosis, lactic acidosis, increased activities of serum glutamic:oxaloacetic and glutamic:pyruvic transaminases, and increased urinary excretion of dicarboxylic acids. EMG shows nonspecific myopathic features. Muscle and liver biopsy specimens show triglyceride storage and markedly decreased concentration of carnitine.

Oral administration of L-carnitine has proved to be beneficial in about one half of patients with hepatic symptoms. It has been particularly effective in the patients with cardiomyopathy.

Pathophysiology of symptoms

Of the nine glycolytic enzyme defects described above, six affect glycogen breakdown or glycolysis (phosphorylase, debrancher, PFK, PGK, PGAM, LDH deficiencies). The impairment of energy production from carbohydrate, which is the common consequence of these defects, should result in similar, exercise-related signs and symptoms. Except for debrancher deficiency, this is the case: Patients with phosphorylase, PFK, PGK, PGAM, or LDH deficiency have exercise intolerance manifested by premature fatigue, cramps, and myoglobinuria. As predicted by the crucial role of glycogen as a fuel source, patients are more prone to experience cramps and myoglobinuria when they engage in strenuous activities, such as lifting heavy weights or sprinting. Moderate exercise typically causes premature fatigue and myalgia, but these symptoms usually resolve after brief rest or slowing of pace; thereafter, patients find that they can resume or continue exercise without problems. This second-wind phenomenon seems to be due to early mobilization of fatty acids and to increased blood flow to exercising muscles.

Conversely, patients with CPT deficiency experience myalgia and myoglobinuria after prolonged, though not necessarily high-intensity, exercise. Fasting exacerbates these complaints. Thus, myoglobinuria occurs in CPT deficiency under metabolic conditions that favor oxidation of fatty acids in normal muscle. This observation suggests that impaired cellular en-

ergetics are the common cause of myoglobinuria in diverse metabolic myopathies.

Biochemical proof of energy depletion is still necessary. No abnormal decrease of ATP concentration has yet been measured in muscle of patients with McArdle's disease during fatigue (defined as failure to maintain the required or expected force) or during ischemic exercise-induced contracture. It cannot be excluded, however, that contracture (and necrosis) may involve only a relatively small percentage of fibers. Measurements of ATP and phosphocreatine in whole muscle might fail to detect loss of high-energy phosphate compounds in selected fibers. Additionally, ATP deficiency may affect a specific subcellular compartment.

The cause of weakness is also poorly understood. Chronic impairment of energy provision is unlikely because two of the three glycogenoses causing weakness involve a glycogen-synthesizing enzyme (branching enzyme deficiency) and a lysosomal glycogenolytic enzyme (acid maltase deficiency), neither directly involved in energy production.

A more likely explanation is that weakness may be due to a net loss of muscle fiber because regeneration cannot keep pace with the rate of degeneration. With fewer functioning fibers, the muscle cannot exert full force. Electromyography reinforces this interpretation: Motor unit potentials are of smaller amplitude and briefer duration than normal, due to loss of muscle fibers from a motor unit. Fibrillations are attributed to areas of focal necrosis of muscle fiber, isolating areas of the cell from the neuromuscular junction in a form of "microdenervation." Muscle fiber degeneration may be due to excessive storage of glycogen, as in acid maltase and debrancher enzyme deficiency, or lipid droplets, as in carnitine deficiency. In agreement with this hypothesis is the observation that in at least two of the glycogenoses causing weakness, infantile acid maltase deficiency and debrancher enzyme deficiency, glycogen storage is much more severe than in the glycogenoses causing cramps and myoglobinuria. Similarly, lipid storage is much more severe in carnitine deficiency than in CPT deficiency.

An additional cause of weakness may be involvement of the anterior horn cells of the spinal cord, which is very conspicuous in infantile acid maltase deficiency. All three glycogenoses causing weakness are in fact due to generalized enzyme defects, but histological signs of denervation are not evident.

DISEASES OF CARBOHYDRATE AND FATTY ACID METABOLISM IN BRAIN

The concentration of glycogen in the brain is small, approximately 0.1 g/100 g fresh tissue, compared to 1.0 g/100 g in muscle and 6 to 10 g in liver. The functional significance of glycogen in the brain is not completely understood, but it is generally assumed that it represents available energy to be tapped during glucose depletion; however, the limited glycogen reserve renders the brain vulnerable to injury within minutes of onset of hypoglycemia or hypoxia.

The role of fatty acids as oxidizable fuels for brain metabolism is negligible, but ketone bodies, derived from fatty acid oxidation, can be utilized particularly in the neonatal period. Diseases of carbohydrate and fatty acid metabolism may affect the brain directly or indirectly.

Diseases with enzyme defects found in brain

Acid maltase deficiency

Light microscopic studies of the nervous system show large amounts of glycogen in the perikaryon of glial cells in both gray and white matter, whereas cortical neurons contain much smaller quantities of glycogen. In the spinal cord, the neurons of the anterior horn appear ballooned and contain abundant PAS-positive

material that is digested by diastase (glycogen). Schwann cells of both anterior and posterior spinal roots and of peripheral nerves also contain excessive glycogen. By electron microscopy, the most striking feature is the presence of glycogen granules within membrane-bound vacuoles. These glycogen-laden vacuoles are particularly abundant in anterior horn cells, in neurons of brainstem motor nuclei, and in Schwann cells, whereas they are scarce in cortical neurons. Glycogen is increased in postmortem brain, and acid maltase activity is undetectable. The severe involvement of spinal and brainstem motor neurons, and the massive accumulation of glycogen in muscle, contribute to the profound hypotonia, weakness, and hyporeflexia seen in Pompe's disease.

Debrancher enzyme deficiency

As mentioned above, the debrancher enzyme defect appears to be generalized. Accordingly, although neither pathology nor debrancher enzyme activity has been reported, increased glycogen concentration has been observed in the brain of a patient. Thus, in debrancher enzyme deficiency, the nervous system seems to be involved biochemically, although clinical signs of brain dysfunction are limited to hypoglycemic seizures in childhood.

Branching enzyme deficiency

The branching enzyme also seems to exist as a single molecular form, and, accordingly, the enzyme defect has been described in multiple tissues, including the brain, from one patient. Although signs and symptoms of brain dysfunction are not prominent in brancher enzyme deficiency, deposits of abnormal polysaccharide, in the form of PAS-positive spheroids, were seen in subpial and perivascular zones of the brainstem and spinal cord but never within neurons. Electron microscopy showed that the spheroids were composed of branched osmiophilic filaments, 600 nm in diameter, and were located within distended astrocytic processes.

Phosphoglycerate kinase deficiency

The most common clinical presentation of phosphoglycerate kinase (PGK) deficiency includes nonspherocytic hemolytic anemia and central nervous system dysfunction. Neurological problems vary in severity: All patients show some degree of mental retardation with delayed language acquisition and behavioral abnormalities, and some have seizures. Although the enzyme defect has not been directly proved in the brain, the severe brain involvement can be explained by impairment of the glycolytic pathway. The lack of symptoms of brain dysfunction in some patients with PGK deficiency (for instance, the two patients with recurrent myoglobinuria described above) are probably attributable to the presence of sufficient residual enzyme activity to prevent severe energy shortage.

Lafora's disease and other polyglucosan storage diseases

In Lafora's disease and other polyglucosan storage disorders, there is accumulation of an abnormal glucose polymer resembling amylopectin (polyglucosan) in the central and peripheral nervous systems as well as in other tissues, but the biochemical defect(s) remains unknown.

Lafora's disease is transmitted as an autosomal recessive trait and is characterized by epilepsy, myoclonus, and dementia. Other neurological manifestations include ataxia, dysarthria, spasticity, and rigidity. Onset is in adolescence, and death occurs in most patients before 25 years of age.

The pathologic hallmark of the disease is the presence in the brain of Lafora's bodies: round, basophilic, PAS-positive intracellular inclusions varying in size from small "dustlike" bodies less than 3 nm in diameter to large bodies up to 30 nm in diameter. Lafora's bodies are typically seen in neuronal perikarya and processes, not in glial cells, and are more abundant in cerebral cortex, substantia nigra, thalamus, globus pallidus, and dentate nucleus. Ultrastructural studies have shown that Lafora bodies consist of two components: amorphous electron-dense granules and irregular branched filaments.

Although the storage material is histochemically and biochemically similar to the polysaccharide that accumulates in branching enzyme deficiency, brancher enzyme activity was normal in brain and muscle from one patient. A different form of polyglucosan body disease was described in 10 patients with a characteristic neurological syndrome consisting of progressive upper and lower motor neuron involvement, sensory loss, neurogenic bladder, and, in half of the patients, dementia without myoclonus or epilepsy. Onset is in the fifth or sixth decade, and the course varies between 3 and 30 years. Polyglucosan bodies are disseminated throughout the central and peripheral nervous systems in processes of neurons and astrocytes but not in perikarya. Other tissues are also affected, including liver, heart, and skeletal and smooth muscle.

Systemic metabolic diseases affecting the brain

Hypoglycemia may produce lethargy, coma, seizures, and brain damage in gluconeogenic and glycogen synthetase deficiencies.

Glucose-6-phosphatase deficiency (glycogenosis type I; Von Gierke's Disease)

Glucose-6-phosphatase deficiency results in hypoglycemia and excessive intracellular accumulation of glucose-6-phosphate (Fig. 1). As a result, there is formation of lactic acid, uric acid, and lipids. A second form of the disease (type Ib) has been described. The defect in this form involves the glucose–phosphate translocation system that is important in facilitating the movement of the substrate into the microsomal compartment for enzymatic conversion to glucose by glucose-6-phosphatase. The clinical features of type Ia and Ib are similar, but normal enzyme activity is present in type Ib. Hepatomegaly, bleeding diathesis, and neutropenia are present. The neurological signs result from the chronic hypoglycemia. Recent studies indicate that lactate may be used by the brain as an alternative cerebral metabolic fuel when hypoglycemia is associated with lactic acidosis. Nocturnal intragastric feeding and frequent daytime meals ameliorate most of the clinical and metabolic abnormalities of this condition.

Fructose-1,6-bisphosphatase deficiency

First described by Baker and Winegrad in 1970, fructose-1,6-bisphosphatase deficiency has now been reported in approximately 30 cases. It is more common in females and is inherited as an autosomal recessive disorder. Initial manifestations are not strikingly dissimilar from those of glucose-6-phosphatase deficiency. Neonatal hypoglycemia is a common presenting feature associated with profound metabolic acidosis, irritability or coma, apneic spells, dyspnea, tachycardia, hypotonia, and moderate hepatomegaly. Lactate, alanine, uric acid, and ketone bodies are elevated in the blood and urine. The enzyme is deficient in liver, kidney, jejunum, and leukocytes. Muscle fructose-1,6-bisphosphatase activity is normal, indicating its distinctness in this condition.

Fructose-1,6-bisphosphatase is an important rate-limiting step in gluconeogenesis. This gluconeogenic step antagonizes the opposite reaction that forms fructose-1,6-bisphosphate from fructose-6-phosphate and ATP (see Chap. 28). A futile cycle exists between these two enzymes, one forming fructose-1,6-bisphosphate and the other disposing of this substrate. Hers and associates have shown that small amounts of fructose-2,6-bisphosphate also are formed by the PFK reaction. This metabolite stimulates the PFK reaction and inhibits the fructose-1,6-bisphosphatase reaction. This finding nicely explains the subtle interplay between the key rate-limiting step in glycolysis (PFK) and the rate-limiting step in gluconeogenesis catalyzed by fructose-1,6-bisphosphatase.

Phosphoenolpyruvate carboxykinase deficiency

Distinctly rare and even more devastating clinically than deficiencies of glucose-6-phosphatase or fructose-1,6-bisphosphatase, phosphoenolpyruvate carboxykinase (PEPCK) activity is almost equally distributed between a cytosolic form and a mitochondrial form. These two forms have similar molecular weights but differ by their kinetic and immunochemical properties. The cytosolic activity is responsive to fasting and various hormonal stimuli. Hypoglycemia is severe and intractable in the absence of PEPCK. A young child with cytosolic PEPCK deficiency had severe cerebral atrophy, optic atrophy, and fatty infiltration of liver and kidney.

Pyruvate carboxylase deficiency

Pyruvate carboxylase (PC) deficiency has now been reported by numerous investigators. This enzyme, mitochondrial in location, catalyzes the conversion of pyruvate to oxaloacetate and is biotin dependent (see Chap. 38). The first report of PC deficiency involved an infant with subacute necrotizing encephalomyelopathy, or Leigh's disease. Subsequent reports have failed to confirm this relationship between PC deficiency and the neuropathologic features of Leigh's disease (see also pyruvate dehydrogenase deficiency, later). Leigh's disease has now been assigned to a respiratory chain defect discussed later in this chapter. Most infants with

PC deficiency present with failure to thrive, developmental delay, recurrent seizures, and metabolic acidosis. Lactate, pyruvate, alanine, β-hydroxybutyrate, and acetoacetate concentrations are elevated in blood and urine. Hypoglycemia is not a constant finding despite the fact that PC is the first rate-limiting step in gluconeogenesis. Robinson and colleagues described eight cases of isolated human PC deficiency. All patients had chronic lactic acidosis. Two patients presented with the added features of hyperammonemia, citrullinemia, and hyperlysinemia. These two patients failed to synthesize any immunologically cross-reacting material (CRM) corresponding to pyruvate carboxylase. Consequently, these investigators proposed that the different clinical manifestations of human PC deficiency resulted from two different mutations in the PC gene: one that results in the synthesis of a relatively inactive PC protein (CRM positive) and one that results in the lack of gene expression in the form of a recognizable protein (CRM negative). Prenatal and postnatal diagnoses can be made by enzyme assay of cultured amniocytes, fibroblasts, or white blood cells. Treatment remains symptomatic. Sodium bicarbonate is necessary to correct the acidosis; biotin supplementation is of no value.

Biotin-dependent syndromes

Infants may present with developmental delay and may demonstrate laboratory abnormalities resulting from the deficiencies of the four biotin-dependent carboxylases (see Chap. 38). Three of the carboxylases, located in the mitochondria, are involved in organic acid metabolism. Multiple carboxylase deficiency, when present in the newborn period, is the result of a deficiency of holocarboxylase synthetase, the enzyme that catalyzes the binding of biotin to the apocarboxylase. These infants often die shortly after birth. Older infants gradually develop neurological signs, with developmental delay and

seizures associated with alopecia, rash, and immunodeficiency. The responsible defect is a deficiency of biotinidase, the enzyme responsible for the breakdown of biocytin, the lysyl derivative of biotin, to free biotin. Biotinidase deficiency can be recognized at birth by measuring the serum activity. Biotinidase deficiency occurs in 1:41,000 live births, and it is eminently treatable by the oral administration of biotin.

Glycogen synthetase deficiency

Glycogen synthetase deficiency has been described in three families. It caused stunted growth and severe fasting hypoglycemia with ketonuria. Mental retardation was reported in the three affected children who survived past infancy. The liver was virtually devoid of glycogen and showed fatty degeneration in all cases. In two patients, the brain showed diffuse, nonspecific changes of the white matter (presence of reactive astrocytes and increased microglia), which were considered secondary to prolonged hypoglycemia or anoxia. Biochemical studies showed that glycogen synthetase activity was markedly decreased in liver but normal in muscle, erythrocytes, and leukocytes, suggesting the existence of multiple tissue-specific isoenzymes under separate genetic control. It is not known whether brain glycogen synthetase is different from that in liver.

In *liver phosphorylase deficiency* (glycogenosis type VI; Hers disease; Fig. 1) and in the two genetic forms of *phosphorylase kinase deficiency* (one X-linked recessive, the other autosomal recessive), hypoglycemia is either absent or mild, and symptoms of brain dysfunction do not usually occur (type VIII, Fig. 1).

In *systemic carnitine deficiency*, the drowsiness, stupor and coma that characterize the Reye's syndrome-like encephalopathy during acute crises is attributed to hypoglycemia and to the deleterious effects of toxic organic acids. Hypoglycemia is probably due to increased utilization of glucose by peripheral tissues with impaired ability to oxidize fatty acids and to inadequate gluconeogenesis (Fig. 2).

DISEASES OF MITOCHONDRIAL METABOLISM

Mitochondrial dysfunction produces three syndromes involving muscle and central nervous system

Although some energy can be quickly obtained from glucose or glycogen through anaerobic glycolysis, most of the energy derives from the oxidation of carbohydrates and fatty acids in the mitochondria. The common metabolic product of sugars and fats is acetyl-CoA, which enters the Krebs cycle. Oxidation of one molecule of acetyl-CoA results in the reduction of three molecules of NAD and one of FAD. These reducing equivalents flow down a chain of carriers (Fig. 3) through a series of oxidation-reduction events. The final hydrogen acceptor is molecular oxygen, and the product is water. The released energy "charges" the inner mitochondrial membrane, converting the mitochondrion into a veritable biological battery. This oxidation process is coupled to ATP synthesis from ADP and inorganic phosphate (P_i), catalyzed by mitochondrial ATPase. Considering the enormous amount of information collected since 1960 on mitochondrial structure and function, it is surprising that diseases of terminal mitochondrial metabolism (Krebs cycle and respiratory chain) have attracted the attention of clinical investigators only recently.

Initial clues that some diseases might be due to mitochondrial dysfunction came from electron microscopic studies of muscle biopsies showing fibers with increased numbers of structurally normal or abnormal mitochondria. These fibers have a "ragged red" appearance in the modified Gomori trichrome stain. Because the diagnosis was based on mitochondrial changes in muscle biopsies, these disorders were initially labeled mitochondrial myopathies. It soon became apparent, however, that many mitochondrial diseases with ragged red fibers were not confined to skeletal muscle but were multisystem disorders. In these patients, the clinical picture is often dominated by signs and symptoms of muscle and brain dysfunction, probably due to the great dependence of these tissues on oxidative metabolism. This group of disorders, often called mitochondrial encephalomyopathies, includes three distinctive syndromes (Table 1).

The first, Kearns-Sayre syndrome (KSS), is characterized by childhood onset of progressive external ophthalmoplegia and pigmentary degeneration of the retina. Heart block, cerebellar syndrome, or high cerebrospinal fluid protein may also appear. Almost all cases are sporadic. The second syndrome, myoclonus epilepsy with ragged red fibers (MERRF), is characterized by myoclonus, ataxia, weakness, and generalized seizures. Unlike KSS, MERFF is usually familial, and analysis of several pedigrees has suggested nonmendelian maternal inheritance. The third syndrome, mitochondrial myopathy, encephalopathy, lactic acidosis, and stroke-like episodes (MELAS), affects young children, who show stunted growth, episodic vomiting and headaches, seizures, and recurrent cerebral insults resembling strokes and causing hemiparesis, hemianopia, or cortical blindness.

Inheritance of mitochondrial DNA is from the ovum cytoplasm

What makes mitochondrial diseases particularly interesting from a genetic point of view is that the mitochondrion has its own DNA (mtDNA) and its own transcription and translation process unrelated to nuclear DNA (see Chap. 21). The mtDNA encodes only 12 to 13 polypeptides; nuclear DNA controls the synthesis of 90 to 95 percent of all mitochondrial protein. All known mitochondrially encoded polypeptides

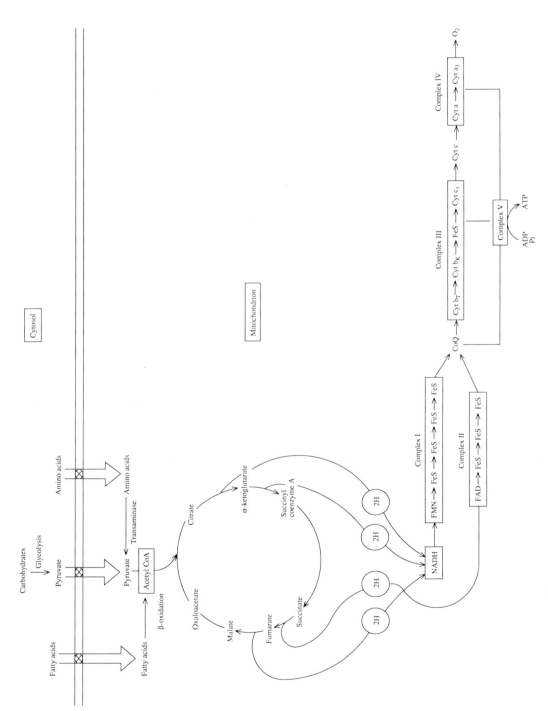

FIG. 3. Scheme of mitochondrial metabolism showing substrate transport, the Krebs cycle and the respiratory chain. (NADH) nicotinamide adenine dinucleotide, reduced; (FMN) flavin mononucleotide; (FAD) flavin adenine dinucleotide; (FeS) non-heme iron-sulfur protein; (CoQ) coenzyme Q (ubiquinone); (Pi) inorganic phosphate.

TABLE 1. Clinical and laboratory features in three syndromes with mitochondrial encephalomyopathy[a]

Features	KSS	MERRF	MELAS
Ophthalmoplegia	+	−	−
Retinal degeneration	+	−	−
Heart block	+	−	−
CSF protein >100 mg/dl	+	−	−
Myoclonus	−	+	−
Ataxia	+	+	−
Weakness	+	+	+
Seizures	−	+	+
Dementia	+	+	+
Short stature	+	+	+
Episodic vomiting	−	−	+
Cortical blindness	−	−	+
Hemiparesis, hemianopia	−	−	+
Sensorineural hearing loss	+	+	+
Lactic acidosis	+	+	+
Positive family history	−	+	+
Ragged-red fibers	+	+	+
Spongy degeneration	+	+	+

[a] (KSS) Kearns-Sayre syndrome; (MERRF) myoclonus epilepsy with ragged-red fibers; (MELAS) mitochondrial encephalopathy, myopathy, lactic acidosis, and stroke-like episodes; (CSF) cerebrospinal fluid; boxes highlight positive and negative differential features (see text).

are located in the inner mitochondrial membrane as subunits of the respiratory chain complexes. They include six subunits of complex I, the apoprotein of cytochrome b, the three larger subunits of cytochrome c oxidase (complex IV), and one subunit of ATPase (complex V).

In the formation of the zygote, almost all the mitochondria are contributed by the ovum cytoplasm. Therefore, mtDNA is transmitted by maternal inheritance in a vertical, nonmendelian fashion. Strictly maternal transmission of mtDNA has been documented in humans by studies of restriction-fragment-length polymorphisms (RFLPs) in DNA from platelets. Diseases of the mother caused by mutations of mtDNA should also be transmitted by maternal inheritance: An affected mother would pass the disease to all her children, but only her daughters would transmit the trait to subsequent generations.

Characteristics that distinguish maternal from mendelian inheritance include the following:

1. The number of affected individuals in subsequent generations is higher than in autosomal dominant disease
2. Inheritance is maternal as in X-linked diseases, but progeny of both sexes are affected
3. Because there are hundreds or thousands of copies of mtDNA in each cell, the phenotypic expression of a mitochondrially encoded gene depends on the relative proportions of mutant and wild-type mtDNAs within a cell
4. Because mitochondria replicate more often than do nuclei, the relative proportion of mutant and wild-type mtDNAs may change within a cell cycle
5. At the time of cell division, the proportion of mutant and wild-type mtDNAs in the two

daughter cells can shift, thus giving them different genotypes and, possibly, different phenotypes, a phenomenon called mitotic segregation.

Maternal inheritance has been suggested for chloramphenicol-induced blood dyscrasias and for Leber's optic atrophy. Among the mitochondrial myopathies, maternal inheritance has been confirmed in the MERRF syndrome and is suspected in the MELAS syndrome. A rational classification of the diseases of mitochondrial metabolism must be based on the identification of specific biochemical defects. Five major groups can be considered:

1. Defects of mitochondrial transport
2. Defects of substrate utilization
3. Defects of the Krebs cycle
4. Defects of oxidation-phosphorylation coupling
5. Defects of the respiratory chain

Defects of mitochondrial transport

Movement of molecules across the inner mitochondrial membrane is tightly regulated and controlled by specific translocation systems. One such system is modulated by CPT and carnitine and controls the translocation of acyl-CoA thioesters from the cytosol into the mitochondrial matrix. CPT and carnitine deficiencies have been described above.

Defects of substrate utilization

Alterations of pyruvate metabolism may be due to defects of pyruvate carboxylase, as discussed earlier, or the pyruvate dehydrogenase complex (PDHC).

Pyruvate dehydrogenase deficiency

Scores of patients have been described with disturbances of the pyruvate dehydrogenase com-

plex since the original report by Blass and colleagues in 1970. The clinical picture ranges from severe, devastating metabolic disease in the neonatal period to a milder encephalopathy, with intermittent ataxia in older children. There is considerable overlap clinically and biochemically with other disorders (see later).

The enzyme complex catalyzes the conversion of pyruvate to acetyl-CoA (Fig. 2) and is dependent on thiamine and lipoic acid as cofactors (see also Chap. 34). The complex has five enzymes: three subserving a catalytic function and two a regulatory role. Deficiencies have involved pyruvate dehydrogenase (E_1 component), lipoamide dehydrogenase (E_3 component), and pyruvate dehydrogenase phosphate phosphatase (or an associated activation defect). The reported enyme deficiencies have almost always been partial, attesting to the critical role of this complex in intermediary metabolism.

The affected newborn is critically ill with a severe metabolic acidosis. All patients have an elevated blood or cerebrospinal fluid lactate concentration. There is failure to thrive, seizures, optic atrophy, and microcephaly. Multiple brain abnormalities have been described, including dysmyelination of the cortex, cystic degeneration of the basal ganglia, ectopic olivary nuclei, hydrocephalus, and partial agenesis of the corpus callosum. Histopathologic features of subacute necrotizing encephalomyelopathy (see later) have also been described in several cases.

The older child presents with ataxia and encephalopathy. Unlike many progressive ataxic syndromes, PDHC deficiency is associated with a fluctuating course, often punctuated by severe deteriorations following metabolic or infectious stress. Cerebellar atrophy may be present on computed tomographic scan. Some patients also develop external ophthalmoplegia, ptosis, retinopathy, optic atrophy, and a central hypoventilation syndrome. PDHC deficiency has been proposed as the cause of Friedreich's ataxia, subacute necrotizing encephalomyelopathy (Leigh's disease), and glioneural dystrophy (Alpers' disease). This confusion indicates the overlap between the clinical and pathologic correlations of these clinical syndromes and PDHC deficiency.

Treatment is largely symptomatic, and the prognosis generally is poor. Thiamine, lipoic acid, ketogenic diet, and physostigmine have been tried in different concentrations and doses with equivocal results. Some patients with periodic ataxia associated with PDHC deficiency may respond to acetazolamide.

Fatty acid oxidation defects

Defects of β-oxidation may affect muscle exclusively or in conjunction with other tissues.

Glutaric aciduria type II. Glutaric aciduria type II (multiple acyl-CoA dehydrogenase deficiency; Fig. 2) usually causes respiratory distress, hypoglycemia, hyperammonemia, systemic carnitine deficiency, and nonketotic metabolic acidosis in the neonatal period, with death within the first week. A few patients with onset in childhood or adult life showed lipid storage myopathy, with weakness or premature fatigue.

Short-chain acyl-CoA deficiency. Short-chain acyl-CoA deficiency (Fig. 2) was described in one woman with proximal limb weakness and exercise intolerance. Muscle biopsy showed marked accumulation of lipid droplets. Although no other tissues were studied, the defect appeared to be confined to skeletal muscle, suggesting the existence of tissue-specific isozymes.

Defects of the Krebs cycle

Fumarase deficiency was reported in three children with mitochondrial encephalomyopathy. Two of them had developmental delay since early infancy, microcephaly, hypotonia, cere-

bral atrophy; one died at 8 months of age. The third patient was a 3½-year-old mentally retarded girl. The laboratory hallmark of the disease is the excretion of large amounts of fumaric acid and, to a lesser extent, succinic acid in the urine. The enzyme defect has been found in muscle, liver, and cultured skin fibroblasts.

Defects of oxidation-phosphorylation coupling

The best example of a disorder of oxidation-phosphorylation coupling is Luft's disease, or nonthyroidal hypermetabolism. Only two patients with this condition have been reported. Family history was noncontributory in either case. Symptoms started in childhood or early adolescence with fever, heat intolerance, profuse perspiration, resting tachypnea and dyspnea, polydipsia, polyphagia, and mild weakness. The basal metabolic rate was markedly increased in both patients, but all tests of thyroid function were normal. Muscle biopsies showed ragged-red fibers and proliferation of capillaries. Other tissues were morphologically normal. Studies of oxidative phosphorylation in isolated muscle mitochondria from both patients showed maximal respiratory rate even in the absence of ADP, an indication that respiratory control was lost. Respiration proceeded at a high rate independently of phosphorylation, and energy was lost as heat, causing hypermetabolism and hyperthermia.

Abnormalities of the respiratory chain

Identification of the different biochemical blocks in the respiratory chain is usually based on polarographic studies showing differential impairment in the ability of isolated intact mitochondria to use different substrates. For example, defective respiration with NAD-dependent substrates, such as pyruvate and malate, but normal respiration with FAD-dependent substrates, such as succinate, suggests an isolated defect of complex I (Fig. 3). However, defective respiration with both types of substrates in the presence of normal cytochrome c oxidase (complex IV) activity, localizes the lesions to complex III (Fig. 3).

Polarographic studies can be complemented by measurement of reduced-minus-oxidized spectra of cytochromes, showing decreased amounts of reducible cytochromes a and a_3 in patients with complex IV deficiency, and decreased concentration of reducible cytochrome b in many (but not all) patients with complex III deficiency (Fig. 3). Finally, electron transport through discrete portions of the respiratory chain can be measured directly. Thus, an isolated defect of NADH-cytochrome c reductase activity suggests a problem with complex I, while a simultaneous defect of NADH and succinate-cytochrome c reductase activities points to a biochemical error in complex III (Fig. 3). The function of complex III alone can be tested by measuring the activity of reduced coenzyme Q-cytochrome c reductase.

Defects of complex I

Defects of complex I have been described in about 25 patients and seem to cause two major clinical syndromes: pure myopathy, with exercise intolerance and myalgia presenting in childhood or adult life, and multisystem disorder. Patients with multisystem disorder are not clinically homogeneous: Some had a fatal infantile form of the disease, causing severe congenital lactic acidosis, hypotonia, seizures, respiratory insufficiency, and death before 3 months of age. Others had a less severe encephalomyopathy with onset in childhood or adult life and characterized by the association, in various proportions, of the following signs and symptoms: exercise intolerance, weakness, ophthalmoplegia, pigmentary degeneration of the retina, optic atrophy, sensorineural hearing loss, dementia, cerebellar ataxia, and pyramidal signs. This clinical heterogeneity is hardly sur-

prising when one considers the large number of proteins comprising complex I, but the molecular defect in most patients is not known (Fig. 3).

Defects of complex II

In the few reported patients with complex II deficiency, the biochemical defect has not been fully characterized, and the diagnosis has often been based solely on a decrease of succinate-cytochrome c reductase activity (Fig. 3). The clinical picture is characterized by severe infantile myopathy, with lactic acidosis in two cases, and by encephalomyopathy in three cases.

Defects of complex III

As in defects of complex I, the clinical picture of complex III disorders falls into one of two groups:

1. Myopathy, with onset in childhood or adolescence and with or without involvement of extraocular muscles
2. Encephalomyopathy, with exercise intolerance, fixed weakness, pigmentary degeneration of the retina, sensorineural hearing loss, cerebellar ataxia, pyramidal signs, and dementia

Biochemically, some patients show lack of reducible cytochrome b, whereas others have normal cytochrome spectra. In the patients with normal amount of reducible cytochrome b, the defect may involve the nonheme iron sulfur protein (Rieske protein) or coenzyme Q (Fig. 3).

In a young woman with complex III deficiency myopathy, the bioenergetic capacity of muscle was studied by ^{31}P nuclear magnetic resonance (NMR). The ratio of phosphocreatine to inorganic phosphate concentration (PC_r/P_i) was greatly reduced at rest, decreased further with mild exercise, and returned to preexercise values very slowly. Treatment with menadione (vitamin K_3) and ascorbate (vitamin C), two compounds whose redox potentials permit them to function between coenzyme Q and cytochrome *c* (Fig. 3), was associated with marked improvement of exercise capacity. NMR showed increased PC_r/P_i ratios at rest and improved rates of recovery after exercise.

Defects of complex IV

As seen with defects of complex I and complex III, the clinical phenotypes of complex IV [cytochrome oxidase (COX)] deficiency fall into two main groups: one in which myopathy is the predominant or exclusive manifestation and another in which brain dysfunction predominates (Fig. 3). In the first group, the most common disorder is fatal infantile myopathy, causing generalized weakness, respiratory insufficiency, and death before 1 year of age. There is lactic acidosis and renal dysfunction, with glycosuria, phosphaturia, and aminoaciduria (DeToni-Fanconi-Debre syndrome). The association of myopathy and cardiopathy in the same patient and myopathy and liver disease in the same family has also been described.

In patients with pure myopathy, COX deficiency is confined to skeletal muscle, sparing heart, liver, and brain. The amount of immunologically reactive enzyme protein is markedly decreased in muscle by enzyme-linked immunosorbent assay (ELISA) and by immunocytochemistry of frozen sections.

Benign infantile mitochondrial myopathy. In contrast, a few children with severe myopathy and lactic acidosis at birth improve spontaneously and are virtually normal by age 2 years. Benign infantile mitochondrial myopathy is due to a reversible COX deficiency. The enzyme activity is markedly decreased (<10 percent of normal) in muscle biopsies taken soon after birth but returns to normal in the first year of life. Immunocytochemistry and immunotitration show normal amounts of enzyme protein in all muscle biopsies. This finding differs from the virtual lack of CRM in patients with fatal infantile myopathy and may represent a useful prognostic test. The selective involvement of one or more tissues and the reversibility of the muscle defect in the benign form suggest the existence of tissue-specific and developmentally regulated COX isoenzymes in humans.

Subacute necrotizing encephalomyelopathy (Leigh's disease). Typifying the second group of disorders of complex IV, dominated by involvement of the central nervous system, Leigh's disease usually starts in infancy or childhood and is characterized by psychomotor retardation, brainstem abnormalities, and apnea. The pathological hallmark consists of focal, symmetrical necrotic lesions extending from thalamus to pons and involving the inferior olives and the posterior columns of the spinal cord. Microscopically, these spongy brain lesions show demyelination, vascular proliferation, and astrocytosis.

In these patients, COX deficiency is generalized, including cultured fibroblasts in most (but not all) cases: This may provide a useful tool for prenatal diagnosis in at least some families. Immunological studies show presence of CRM in all tissues.

Partial defects of COX. Partial defects of COX have been reported in patients with progressive external ophthalmoplegia and proximal myopathy and in patients with encephalomyopathy, but the precise pathogenic significance of COX deficiency in these disorders remains uncertain.

Defects of complex V (ATPase)

Two patients with muscle mitochondrial ATPase deficiency have been reported. One was a young woman with congenital, slowly progressive myopathy; the other was a 17-year-old boy who, at age 10, was found to have muscle carnitine deficiency. Later he developed a multisystem disorder characterized by weakness, dementia, ataxia, retinopathy, and peripheral neuropathy. In both patients, respiration of isolated mitochondria was decreased with all substrates but returned to normal after addition of the uncoupling agent 1,4-dinitrophenol. This finding suggested that the biochemical defect involved the phosphorylative pathway rather than the respiratory chain. ATPase activity was decreased and responded poorly to dinitrophenol stimulation.

ACKNOWLEDGMENTS

Some of the work discussed in this chapter was supported by center grants from the National Institute of Neurological and Communicative Disorders and Stroke (NS11766) and from the Muscular Dystrophy Association, and by USPHS grant NS17695. We are grateful to Ms. Mary Tortorelis and Ms. Alice H. Marti for typing the manuscript.

GENERAL REFERENCES

1. Blass, J. P. Inborn errors of pyruvate metabolism. In J. Stanbury, J. Wyngaarden, and D. Fredrickson (eds.), *The Metabolic Basis of Inherited Disease.* New York: McGraw-Hill, 1983, pp. 193–203.

2. De Vivo, D. C. The effects of ketone bodies on glucose utilization. In J. V. Passonneau, R. A. Hawkins, W. D. Lust and F. A. Welsh (eds.), *Cerebral Metabolism and Neural Function.* Baltimore: Williams & Wilkins, 1980, pp. 243–254.

3. DiDonato, S., Frerman, F. E., Rimoldi, M., Rinaldo, P., Taroni, F., and Wiesmann, U. N. Systemic carnitine deficiency due to lack of electron transfer flavoprotein: ubiquinone oxidoreductase. *Neurology* 36:957–963, 1986.

4. DiMauro, S., Bonilla, E., Zeviani, M., Nakagawa, M., and De Vivo, D. C. Mitochondrial myopathies. *Annu. Neurol.* 17:521–538, 1985.

5. DiMauro, S., Bonilla, E., Zeviani, M., Servidei, S., De Vivo, D. C., and Schon, E. A. Mito-

chondrial myopathies. *J. Inherited Metab. Dis.* 10(suppl. 1):113–128, 1987.

6. DiMauro, S., Bresolin, N., and Hays, A. P. Disorders of glycogen metabolism of muscle. *CRC Crit. Rev. Clin. Neurobiol.* 1(2):83–116, 1984.

7. DiMauro, S., and De Vivo, D. C. Disorders of glycogen metabolism. In A. Lajtha (ed.), *Handbook of Neurochemistry.* New York: Plenum Press, 1985, Vol. 10, pp. 1–13.

8. DiMauro, S., Servidei, S., Zeviani, M., DiRocco, M., De Vivo, D. C., DiDonato, S., Uziel, G., Berry, K., Hoganson, G., Johnsen, S. D., and Johnson, P. C. Cytochrome c oxidase deficiency in Leigh syndrome. *Annu. Neurol.* 22:498–506, 1987.

9. DiMauro, S., and Papadimitriou, A. Carnitine palmitoyltransferase deficiency. In A. G. Engel and B. Q. Banker (eds.), *Myology.* New York: McGraw-Hill, 1986, pp. 1697–1708.

10. Engel, A. G. Carnitine deficiency syndromes and lipid storage myopathies. In A. G. Engel and B. Q. Banker (eds.), *Myology.* New York: McGraw-Hill, 1986, pp. 1663–1696.

11. Fukuhara, N. Myoclonus epilepsy and mitochondrial myopathy. In G. Scarlato and C. Cerri (eds.), *Mitochondrial Pathology in Muscle Disease.* Padua: Piccin Medical Books, 1983, pp. 88–110.

12. Haymond, M. W. Hypoglycemia. In A. M. Rudolph (ed.), *Pediatrics,* 18th ed. Norwalk, CT: Appleton & Lange, 1987, pp. 262–270.

13. Morgan-Hughes, J. A. The mitochondrial myopathies. In A. G. Engel and B. Q. Banker (eds.), *Myology.* New York: McGraw-Hill, 1986, pp. 1709–1743.

14. Pavlakis, S. G., Phillips, P. C., DiMauro, S., De Vivo, D. C., and Rowland, L. P. Mitochondrial myopathy, encephalopathy, lactic acidosis, and stroke-like episodes: A distinctive clinical syndrome. *Ann. Neurol.* 16:481–488, 1985.

15. Robinson, B. H., Oei, J., Sherwood, W. G., et al. The molecular basis for the two different clinical presentations of classical pyruvate carboxylase deficiency. *Am. J. Hum. Genet.* 36:283–294, 1984.

16. Rosing, H. S., Hopkins, L. C., Wallace, D. C., Epstein, C. M., and Weidenheim, K. Maternally inherited mitochondrial myopathy and myoclonic epilepsy. *Ann. Neurol.* 17:228–237, 1985.

17. Rowland, L. P., Hays, A. P., DiMauro, S., De Vivo, D. C., and Behrens, M. Diverse clinical disorders associated with morphological abnormalities of mitochondria. In G. Scarlato and C. Cerri (eds.), *Mitochondrial Pathology in Muscle Disease*. Padua: Piccin Medical Books, 1983, pp. 143–158.

18. Rowland, L. P., Layzer, R. B., and DiMauro, S. Pathophysiology of metabolic muscle disorders. In A. K. Asbury, G. M. McKhann, and W. I. McDonald (eds.), *Diseases of the Nervous System*. Philadelphia: W. B. Saunders, 1986, pp. 197–207.

19. Schulz, H. Oxidation of fatty acids. In D. E. Vance and J. E. Vance (eds.), *Biochemistry of Lipids and Membranes*. Menlo Park, CA: Benjamin/Cummings Publ. Co., 1985, pp. 116–142.

20. Stansbie, D., Wallace, S. J., and Marsac, D. Disorders of the pyruvate dehydrogenase complex. *J. Inherited Metab. Dis.* 9:105–119, 1986.

21. Tzagoloff, A. *Mitochondria*. New York: Plenum, 1982.

22. Wolf, B., Grier, R., Parker, W. D., et al. Deficient biotinidase activity in late-onset multiple carboxylase deficiency. *N. Engl. J. Med.* 308:161, 1983.

23. Zinn, A. B., Kerr, D. S., and Hoppel, C. L. Fumarase deficiency: A new cause of mitochondrial encephalomyopathy. *N. Engl. J. Med.* 315:469–475, 1986.

CHAPTER 34

Vitamin and Nutritional Deficiencies

John P. Blass

That diet affects health has been known since Hippocrates, but only during the past century have the major foodstuffs, including the vitamins and other micronutrients, been characterized chemically. The minimum daily requirements of these nutrients were defined as the amount of each purified foodstuff that would easily prevent frank nutritional disease, typically in small numbers of otherwise healthy and well-nourished young men. This approach led to such public health triumphs as the effective eradication of pellagra (see below).

Common wisdom recognizes the existence of inherent variations among individuals in the

Basic Neurochemistry: Molecular, Cellular, and Medical Aspects, 4th Ed., edited by G. J. Siegel et al. Raven Press, Ltd., New York, 1989. Correspondence to John P. Blass, Cornell University Medical College, Burke Rehabilitation Center, 785 Mamaroneck Avenue, White Plains, New York 10605.

amounts of specific foodstuffs required or tolerated—"One man's meat is another man's poison." In a number of hereditary neurometabolic disorders, tailoring the diet to the individual is effective treatment. These disorders include several aminoacidopathies (discussed in Chap. 38) and a number of rare vitamin-dependency disorders, in which a genetic alteration in the utilization of a vitamin dramatically alters the amount required to maintain health. Environmental factors including intercurrent illnesses can require changes in the diet in order to maintain adequate nutrition.

MACRONUTRIENTS

Macronutrients comprise quantitatively the major portions of the diet: carbohydrates, fats, proteins, and water.

Protein and caloric deficiency during development reduces brain size

Protein and calorie deprivation in adult life are widely believed to have few, if any, lasting effects on laboratory animals and human brain. It is possible that malnutrition contributes to the premature atrophy of brain substance in adults with "concentration camp syndrome," but that is difficult to assess in light of all the other horrible stresses that accompany such experiences. The effect of protein and calorie malnutrition on the developing brain, however, has been controversial [1,2]. Calorie restriction during development clearly reduces body size and, concomitantly, brain size in laboratory animals and in humans. Brain/body ratios, however, typically increase. Extensive studies have documented a variety of neurochemical and histological changes that can be induced in undernourished animals, the functional significance of which is unclear. Loss of brain substance may represent in part lack of glia (which de-

velop postnatally in the rat) and adaptation to a smaller number of motor units. In laboratory animals, the well-documented effects of nutritional deprivation on performance appear to relate to motivational and attentional factors at least as much as to diminution in cognitive capacity [1]. Children who grow up poorly nourished and in poverty tend to do worse on IQ tests than do well-nourished children who grow up in comfort. The effects of nutrition are, however, difficult to isolate from the other effects of poverty.

By contrast, children malnourished as a result of specific gastrointestinal disease are often small but are rarely mentally deficient. There is a strong, direct relationship between nutrition and total body size for the same gene pool but no evidence that tall people are significantly smarter than short ones, even within the same gene pool. An approximation of a controlled experiment occurred in the Netherlands in 1944, when the Dutch population under the Axis powers starved while that under the Allies was well fed [3]. The cohort conceived or born during that period later entered compulsory national service, undergoing uniform physical examination and psychological testing (including Raven's matrices). There was a small reduction in height but none in intellectual performance. There may have been a small increase in personality problems. It appears that over the short term, the body spares nutrients for the nervous system. The effects of long-term malnutrition are harder to assess, since it usually occurs amid other problems.

Moderate caloric restriction during growth and development actually prolongs the lives of laboratory animals [4]. Because the conditions under which rodents and other laboratory animals are reared in captivity are artificial, the effect of restricted calories may result in the prevention of malignant obesity. Optimal nutrition during development is not the same as maximal nutrition.

Dietary variations can influence blood and brain concentrations of nutrients that are precursors of neurotransmitters

Tryptophan

Tryptophan is an obligatory precursor of 5-hydroxytryptamine (serotonin), because mammalian tissues lack the capacity to synthesize its indole moiety (see Chap. 12). This amino acid can also substitute, inefficiently, for vitamin B_3 (niacin; see below). Tryptophan is present in relatively small amounts in most proteins. It crosses the blood-brain barrier, like tyrosine, predominantly by the carrier system for long-chain neutral amino acids (see Chap. 30). As a result, a protein-rich meal can actually reduce the passage of tryptophan into the brain by elevating the levels of other amino acids competing for that carrier.

Therapeutically, pure tryptophan has been administered orally to depressed patients in amounts up to 4 g daily. Occasional depressed patients are reported to respond, even compared to placebo, in carefully controlled trials; these people may represent a biological subgroup of depressives. Tryptophan may aid about a third of geriatric patients to fall asleep, possibly by reducing sleep latency, and appears to be a sleep medication (hypnotic) without significant side effects. 5-Hydroxytryptophan has been reported anecdotally or in small series to calm hyperactive, self-stimulatory, or other self-destructive behaviors.

Tyrosine

Tyrosine or its precursor, phenylalanine, is an obligatory precursor of the neurotransmitters norepinephrine and dopamine, since they contain a phenyl moiety that mammals cannot synthesize (see Chap. 11). Both tyrosine and phenylalanine are present in relatively large amounts in ordinary dietary proteins. Tyrosine has been used therapeutically in depression, but less so than tryptophan. In laboratory animals, dietary loading with tyrosine may damp blood pressure oscillations that occur in response to stress.

Choline

Net choline synthesis in mammalian tissue, including brain depends on a series of reactions that require a dietary source of one-carbon groups (e.g., methionine, betaine; see Chap. 5). Blood levels of choline in both humans and laboratory animals, however, normally reflect the amount of choline ingested in recent meals. Intestinal bacteria can break down free choline; the resulting amines create a fishy odor in patients treated with choline itself. An efficient dietary precursor of blood choline is the phospholipid lecithin (phosphatidylcholine; see Chap. 5). The term lecithin is used in at least two different senses in nutrition. One is as a common name for phosphatidylcholine. The other is as a term for a mixture of phospholipids, often extracted from soybeans, in which phosphatidylcholine is a component. The mixture is commonly used as an emulsifying agent and is often sold in health food stores.

Increasing the amount of lecithin (choline is less well tolerated) in the diet under specific circumstances increases the levels of choline in the brain. Apparently, choline loading can increase the capacity of cholinergic neurons to synthesize acetylcholine in response to stimuli that increase their release of that neurotransmitter [5]. Under appropriate conditions of stimulation, a dramatic increase in the levels of acetylcholine can be measured in neural tissues or in the fluid bathing stimulated preparations.

Essential fatty acids are polyunsaturated fatty acids with double bonds either three or six carbons from the terminal methyl group

In laboratory animals, diets devoid of essential fatty acids (ω-3 or ω-6 linoleic acid) induce a syndrome in which dermatitis is prominent, but there is no disorder of the nervous system. Arachidonic acid can replace the dietary requirement for other essential fatty acids; however, in deficient animals, the fatty acid compositions of membranes do change—for example, hepatic mitochondria can become partially uncoupled. ω-6-Linoleic acid and its derivative, arachidonic acid, are precursors of the prostaglandins. Therefore the proportions of ω-3 and ω-6 fatty acids in the diet alter the proportions of specific prostaglandins and prostacyclins produced in response to activation of the prostaglandin/prostacyclin cascades (see Chap. 20).

A syndrome of absolute deficiency of essential fatty acids has not been convincingly established in humans. Increasing the amounts of ω-3 fatty acids (e.g., eicosapentaenoic, 20.5) in the diet to prevent or alleviate atherosclerosis, and therefore much of cerebrovascular disease, is a focus of research.

MICRONUTRIENTS

Micronutrients are present in the diet in small quantities but must be ingested in order to maintain health. They include vitamins and some minerals. Characterization of each micronutrient has required recognition of a syndrome associated with a deficiency of that nutrient in humans or in laboratory animals in which a model disorder could be standarized as a bioassay system [6].

Thiamine (vitamin B₁) was discovered as a treatment for beriberi

At the turn of the century brown husks from polished rice were found to cure the neurological syndrome of beriberi [6–8]. Funk introduced the term "vitamine" when he recognized that the active factor vital for life was an amine.

Biochemistry

Thiamine contains a pyrimidine linked to a thiazole moiety. Weak oxidants readily convert thiamine to an easily measured fluorescent derivative, thiochrome. The acidic carbon on the thiazole interacts readily with α-keto acids in both enzyme-catalyzed and nonenzymic reactions.

Thiamine appears to cross the blood-brain barrier both by diffusion and, more rapidly, by a carrier-mediated system that is inhibited competitively by the thiamine analog amprolium.

Thiamine is converted to the coenzyme form, thiamine pyrophosphate (TPP), or thiamine diphosphate (TDP), by a pyrophosphokinase that is active in brain. TPP is known to act as a coenzyme for four enzymes in the nervous system (see Chap. 28). Three are intramitochondrial multienzyme complexes that catalyze oxidative decarboxylation of α-keto acids to the coenzyme A (CoA) derivatives:

1. Pyruvate to acetyl-CoA, pyruvate dehydrogenase complex (PDHC)
2. α-Ketoglutarate into succinyl-CoA, α-ketoglutarate dehydrogenase complex (KGDHC)
3. α-Keto acids derived from the branched-chain amino acids to appropriate derivatives, branched-chain dehydrogenase complex (BCDHC)

The fourth enzyme requiring TPP in the nervous system is transketolase (TK), which carries out rearrangements of sugars in the pentose phosphate pathways (see Chap. 28). A kinase can convert a membrane-bound form of TPP to thiamine triphosphate (TTP), and a specific phosphatase hydrolyzes TTP to the diphosphate. TTP appears to play a role in nerve membrane function, notably in Na⁺ gating.

Experimental thiamine deficiency

Experimental deficiency of thiamine exists in several well-studied forms. The discovery of thiamine was due in part to its ability to cure weakness in chickens fed a diet of polished rice. The dramatic, thiamine-responsive opisthotonic posturing in pigeons was used as a bioassay. In cats made thiamine deficient, the earliest ultrastructural changes occur in synaptic regions including their mitochondria; dramatic changes in glia follow. Mink develop a thiamine-deficiency syndrome if fed raw fish, which contain a thiaminase. A syndrome of cerebrocortical necrosis in calves is due to dietary thiamine deficiency.

The most extensive studies of thiamine deficiency in laboratory animals are of rats and mice. Dietary thiamine deficiency is now conventionally induced with artificial diets complete in all foodstuffs except thiamine. Since the vitamin deficiency induces loss of appetite, each control must be "pair fed," which means it is allowed its complete diet only in the same (weighed) amount that a deficient animal consumes of a comparable diet missing thiamine. Otherwise, the effects of the vitamin deficiency are confused with the effects of general malnutrition. Weanling rodents fed a diet devoid of thiamine usually stop gaining weight after about 2 weeks and usually die within 4 to 5 weeks.

The thiamine antagonists oxythiamine and pyrithiamine are converted to catalytically inactive pyrophosphates that compete for TPP binding sites on enzymes. Oxythiamine does not cross the blood-brain barrier, and pyrithiamine can directly inhibit action potentials. Mice fed combinations of pyrithiamine with a low-thiamine diet develop abnormal neuropsychological responses within 5 to 7 days and gross neurological symptoms by day 8 or 9; death often occurs by day 10. In rats, abnormalities of motor performance occur by day 3, additional neurological symptoms by day 12, and death within 2 weeks.

Early neurochemical changes in experimental thiamine deficiency are greatest in regions of brain destined to show histological changes (see below and Chap. 39). The early biochemical changes are increases in glucose utilization with concomitant increases in lactate production; local decreases in pH; and local increases in intracellular Ca^{2+}. In late stages, decreases in oxidation of glucose can be detected in affected regions in *ex vivo* or *in vitro* studies. Levels of ATP and adenylate energy charge potential[1] (see Chap. 40) are maintained until very late stages of thiamine deficiency. In the affected areas, blood flow rises, but in animals successfully treated with thiamine, it falls below normal [9].

Experimental thiamine deficiency decreases the activities of at least three TPP-dependent enzymes: PDHC, KGDHC, and TK [10]. The activity of BCDHC has not been tested in experimental thiamine deficiency; urinary excretion of branched-chain amino acids does not rise. Levels of TTP are maintained in the brain even in terminal thiamine deficiency. The fall in TK activity in the brain persists after treatment with large doses of thiamine has abolished the frank neurological symptoms of pyrithiamine-induced thiamine deficiency. The decrease in KGDHC activity in pyrithiamine-induced deficiency parallels the fall in glucose oxidation. Cerebral pyruvate oxidation decreases in thiamine deficiency, but in preparations with intact mitochondria this effect can be secondary to decreases in the activity of KGDHC. A decrease in the activity of PDHC after lysis of mitochondria has been reported to occur in the brain stem of rats symptomatic with dietary thiamine deficiency [10].

Neuropharmacology

Cholinergic systems are exquisitely sensitive to thiamine deficiency, as they are to other conditions that impair carbohydrate oxidation [7].

---

[1] The energy charge potential is written as

$$\frac{[ATP] + 0.5[ADP]}{[ATP] + [ADP] + [AMP]}$$

Deficits in performance in the early stages of either dietary or antagonist-induced thiamine deficiency can be normalized by treatment with the cholinesterase inhibitor physostigmine. Thiamine deficiency reduces the turnover of acetylcholine in the brain, probably at least in part by effects on Ca^{2+}-dependent release. Serotonergic systems, including uptake mechanisms, are impaired in at least the later stages of thiamine deficiency. Catecholaminergic functions are impaired, as measured physiologically. The levels of glutamate and aspartate decrease, at least in the later stages, whereas decreases in γ-aminobutyric acid (GABA) have been more variable.

Disease in humans

In developed countries, clinically significant dietary deficiency of thiamine occurs most commonly in alcoholics but sometimes occurs in people malnourished for other reasons [8]. Thiamine deficiency is more common in developing countries where polished rice is the staple. The percentage increase in red cell TK activity on adding exogenous TPP *in vitro* is known as the TPP effect and has been used as a measure of thiamine nurriture in epidemiological studies.

A nonspecific neurasthenic syndrome developed within 5 to 6 days in healthy young adults eating an artificial diet deficient only in thiamine. The syndrome included lassitude, irritability, muscle cramps, and changes on the electrocardiogram.

Peripheral nerve damage (neuropathy) is a common consequence of thiamine deficiency (see Chap. 35). The neuropathy tends to be worse distally than proximally, involves myelin more than axons, and is often painful. The neuropathy is linked to multiple deficiencies in the group of water-soluble vitamins that often occur together in foods and are known for historical reasons as the vitamin B complex.

Wernicke's syndrome is characterized by the triad of staggering gait (ataxia), paralysis of eye movements (ophthalmoplegia), and confu-

sion (clouding of consciousness). Injections of thiamine can be lifesaving, with clinical improvement often evident within minutes. The syndrome is associated with small hemorrhages along the third and fourth ventricles. In human alcoholics with Wernicke's syndrome (see below), cerebral metabolic rate is reduced (as indicated by cerebral blood flow), particularly in the region containing the nucleus basalis [11]. Successful treatment restores blood flow to normal.

Korsakoff's syndrome is a striking loss of working memory with relatively little loss of reference memory (see Chap. 48). The patients characteristically confabulate, which means to make up stories in response to leading questions. Korsakoff's syndrome usually follows documented Wernicke's syndrome in the Wernicke-Korsakoff syndrome. Prompt treatment of Wernicke's syndrome with thiamine is believed to prevent the development of Korsakoff's syndrome, but the latter responds little if at all to treatment with thiamine. The characteristic pathological changes responsible for the memory deficits in Korsakoff's syndrome have been debated. Early views emphasized destruction of the mammillary bodies, which are the primary projection field of the hippocampus. Others emphasized damage to thalamic nuclei. Later studies indicated that cholinergic cells of the nucleus basalis of Meynert are as severely damaged in Korsakoff's syndrome as in Alzheimer's disease [11]. Animal models of thiamine deficiency show similar selective vulnerability, the chemical basis of which is still unknown [7–10].

Thiamine requirements

Thiamine requirements can be altered by genetic or environmental abnormalities. Among genetic disorders, thiamine-dependent maple syrup urine disease is a rare disease due to a reduced affinity of BCDHC for its coenzyme, TPP (see Chap. 38). A rare form of lactate acidosis appears to be due to a genetic defect in

PDHC affecting its affinity for TPP (see Chap. 33). Both disorders may respond to treatment with large doses of thiamine. Wernicke-Korsakoff syndrome is associated with a variant form of TK having a decreased affinity for TPP [12]. The variation may be more common in chronic alcoholics. People with this form of TK are at risk on a diet even marginally deficient in this thiamine.

Subacute necrotizing encephalomyelopathy (SNE) of Leigh is an uncommon autosomal recessive disorder, the pathology of which resembles that of Wernicke-Korsakoff syndrome. Dietary and tissue levels of thiamine are normal except for a reported deficiency in cerebral TTP attributed to an inhibitor of its biosynthesis. Most of the reported patients are children who die with elevated levels of lactate and pyruvate in their blood. A milder form with onset in the teens or later has been well documented, with damage to long tracts in the spinal cord as well as the characteristic changes of Leigh's disease. The nature of the primary genetic abnormality in Leigh's disease has been controversial. Some of these children appear to have a hereditary deficiency of PDHC, but deficiencies in cytochrome oxidase and in other enzymes have also been reported. TK appears normal. Studies at the molecular genetic level have not yet been done. Very large doses of thiamine have been reported to be of transitory benefit in many of these patients (see Chap. 33).

Environmental factors that modify thiamine requirements include ethanol ingestion (which impairs thiamine transport across intestinal mucosa), some raw fish, and certain teas [7,8]. Requirements rise with fever, presumably due to increased metabolism. Increasing the proportion of carbohydrates in the diet increases thiamine requirements.

Niacin (vitamin B_3) is the treatment for pellagra

The deficiency disease, pellagra, which includes mental symptoms, was recognized in the eighteenth century, shortly after the introduction of American corn (maize) into Europe [6].

Biochemistry

Niacin and niacinamide refer to nicotinic acid and its amide. Nicotinic acid is a pyridine derivative. The biosynthesis of nicotinic acid from tryptophan is carried out slowly in humans and other mammals, perhaps at least in part by intestinal bacteria. Approximately 60 mg dietary tryptophan provide the equivalent of 1 mg nicotinic acid/amide. Niacin is a vitamin because most diets do not contain enough tryptophan to fulfill the normal human requirement of 10 to 30 mg/day. Brain and other tissues incorporate nicotinic acid into the coenzymes nicotine adenine nucleotide and dinucleotide and their reduced equivalents (NAD^+, NADH, and $NADP^+$, NADPH). The NAD/NADP cofactors participate in multiple oxidation-reduction reactions (see Chap. 28). Cerebral tissues contain an active enzyme that hydrolyzes NAD and NADP and may play a role in metabolic regulation, since the enzyme acts on the oxidized but not reduced forms of the cofactors.

Experimental Niacin Deficiency

Experimental niacin deficiency usually requires a diet high in corn. Zein, the major storage protein of American corn, contains little tryptophan. Ingestion of corn can therefore be expected to raise the ratio, relative to tryptophan, of other long-chain neutral amino acids that compete for the same carrier. Corn-fed dogs develop "black tongue," with prominent abnormalities referable to the gastrointestinal system. Also, antiniacin compounds can induce deficiency states within days in rodents on a normal diet [13]. 6-Aminonicotinamide is converted by the brain to the enzymatically inactive NADP analog, and *N*-acetylpyridine is converted to inactive analogs of NAD and NADP. Neurological symptoms are more obvious in rats with antimetabolite-induced niacin deficiencies than in the corn-fed dogs.

Dietary niacin deficiency has been reported to reduce the levels of NAD and NADP coenzymes in the brain by 30% or more, with a higher proportion of NAD in the oxidized form and a slightly higher proportion of NADP in the reduced form. Changes in apoenzymes fit no clear pattern. Antimetabolite-induced niacin deficiency appears to have particularly strong effects on the dehydrogenases of the pentose shunt [14]. The inferior olivary nuclei are particularly susceptible to the actions of 3-acetylpyridine as studied histologically and biochemically [12].

Neuropharmacology

N-acetylpyridine poisoning can cause relatively localized decreases in the synthesis of acetycholine in the brain stem [12]. Administration of either 6-aminonicotinamide or 3-acetylpyridine can cause decreased levels of glutamate and GABA in brain.

Disease in humans

Dietary niacin deficiency (pellagra) was once common in areas where American corn was a dietary staple. Over 150,000 cases annually were reported in the southeastern United States. Addition of purified niacin to the diet has largely abolished the disorder. Pellagra is associated with the tetrad of dermatitis (particularly in areas exposed to the sun), diarrhea, dementia, and death. A chronic toxic delerium may precede the onset of other symptoms and may be the only clinical abnormality, at least early in the course. The delerium may resemble some forms of schizophrenia.

Niacin requirements

Niacin requirements can be modified by genetic and environmental factors. Hartnup syndrome is a hereditary disorder in which tryptophan transport is impaired and requirements for niacin increase. Phenylketonuria and hyperphen-ylalaninemia can increase niacin requirements by increasing the levels of amino acids that compete with tryptophan for transport systems (see Chap. 38).

Environmentally, the proportion of corn in the diet influences the requirement for niacin, as noted above. Alkalinization of corn meal flour, even by stone chips from primitive mortars, can apparently make niacin or tryptophan more available in the diet. Poisoning with vacor, a niacin antagonist, can induce widespread and persistant neurological dysfunction.

Pyridoxine (vitamin B₆) deficiency can produce neuropathy or seizures

Biochemistry

Pyridoxine is a pyridine derivative. Pyridoxol (alcohol), pyridoxal (aldehyde), and pyridoxamine (amine) are all active. The concentration in brain is normally about 100-fold that in the blood. In brain and other tissues, the vitamin is phosphorylated to the active coenzyme, pyridoxal phosphate, which readily forms Schiff bases. This coenzyme participates in decarboxylase reactions, including those forming the neurotransmitters GABA from glutamate, serotonin (5-hydroxytryptamine) from 5-hydroxytryptophan, and, probably, DOPA from dihydroxyphenylalanine. It is also a cofactor for transaminases. The conversion of tryptophan to nicotinamide requires pyridoxine as a cofactor, and the excretion of xanthurenic acid after a tryptophan load is widely used to test the adequacy of pyridoxine nurriture.

Experimental pyridoxine deficiency

Pyridoxine deficiency states have been induced in at least 12 mammalian species. Newborn animals are more sensitive to the dietary deficiency than weanlings; pups born to a rat deficient in pyridoxine show neuropathological damage including hypomyelination. A number of pyridoxine antagonists have been well characterized, including deoxypyridoxine and several hydrazides and oximes that can produce deficiency states.

Pyridoxine deficiency reduces cerebral metabolic rate, whereas addition of pyridoxal phosphate or substrate quantities of GABA restore the rate to normal in preparations of cat brain [7]. The activity of decarboxylases falls more than that of transaminases in deficient brain. Glutamic acid decarboxylase (GAD) activity falls as much as 70%.

Rats and dogs fed a pyridoxine-deficient diet first develop impairment in learning and conditioning. Irritability, seizures, and gait imbalance (ataxia) then develop, as well as anemia. The intensity of the seizures correlates with the extent of the fall in glutamate decarboxylase activity. The ataxia may relate to the demonstrated demyelination in long tracts and peripheral nerves. Antagonists induce more widespread disturbances, including skin disease, that nevertheless respond completely to treatment with pyridoxine.

Disease in humans

Pure pyridoxine deficiency has occurred in human infants fed a formula from which vitamin B_6 had been inadvertently omitted. The prominent finding was intractable seizures, which responded promptly to injections of the vitamin. Deficiency of pyridoxine can contribute to the polyneuropathy and other signs of B-complex deficiency (see Chap. 35).

Pyridoxine requirements

Like those of other nutrients, pyroxidine requirements can be altered by genetic or environmental factors and are increased in a number of nervous system disorders [6,15]. Genetically determined pyridoxine-dependent seizures occur in rare infants [15]. Doses of pyridoxine several hundredfold the normal daily requirement prevent the seizures. Maintenance with doses an order of magnitude greater than the normal requirement typically permits normal development if irreversible brain damage has not occurred. In a mentally retarded child with this syndrome who came to autopsy, levels of pyridoxine derivatives in the brain were about half normal [15]. The ratio of GABA to glutamate was decreased, although the activity of GAD was comparable to controls. Abnormalities were also evident in cystathionine, whose metabolism is also dependent on pyridoxine. This boy may have had a defect in the transport of pyridoxine into the brain. In another child with pyridoxine-dependent seizures, the cerebral metabolic rate for oxygen was reduced approximately 25% below normal, even during the seizures, and was restored to normal with vitamin treatment [16].

It is believed by some that mild forms of pyridoxine dependency may be a relatively common cause of intractable seizures and mental retardation, perhaps due to mutations in GAD that decrease its affinity for its pyridoxal phosphate coenzyme. In homocystinuria and cystathioninuria, two disorders of amino acid metabolism, some patients respond to large doses of pyridoxine. In those patients, the mutations appear to reduce the affinity of the relevant enzymes for the cofactor (see Chap. 38).

Environmentally, hydrazides and oximes can increase pyridoxine requirements. Large doses of pyridoxine are routinely given with the antituberculous medication isonicotinic hydrazide (INH) to prevent drug-induced neuropathy.

Biotin is a treatment for certain genetic diseases with carboxylase deficiency

Biotin consists of fused imidazole and thiophene rings [17]. The enzyme holocarboxylase synthetase links biotin covalently onto specific lysine residues of the proteins for which it acts as a coenzyme [18]. Those enzymes carry out carboxylation reactions, including acetyl-CoA carboxylase (forming acetyl-CoA from malonyl-

CoA in fatty acid synthesis); propionyl-CoA carboxylase (forming methylmalonyl-CoA from propionic acid); and pyruvate carboxylase (forming oxaloacetic acid from pyruvate in gluconeogenesis and as a primer for the tricarboxylic acid cycle).

Pure dietary deficiency of biotin is unknown, presumably because the intestinal flora of both humans and laboratory animals synthesize the small amounts required.

Genetic defects in biotin metabolism sometimes respond to large doses of the vitamin [17,18]. Defects include a form of lactic acidosis, due to deficiency of pyruvate carboxylase; a form of propionic aciduria, due to an abnormality in propionyl carboxylase; and a form of multiple carboxylase deficiency, due to a mutation in the holocarboxylase synthetase (see Chap. 33). A child with a proposed defect in intestinal absorption of biotin has also been described.

Addition to the diet of very large amounts of the egg white protein, avidin, which binds biotin avidly, induces a biotin-responsive syndrome in both laboratory animals and humans. Humans complain of malaise, but neurological signs are not particularly prominent.

Cobalamin (vitamin B$_{12}$) deficiency is associated with relatively common neurological syndromes

Biochemistry

The cobalamins are a series of porphyrin-like compounds. The active forms contain a cobalt ion covalently linked to one of the methylene groups. The cobalamins are synthesized by many microorganisms but not by higher plants or animals; the usual dietary source is meat, particularly liver. Effective absorption requires a series of transport proteins, including a glycoprotein *intrinsic factor* secreted by gastric parietal cells. Conversion to the active coenzymes

adenosylcobalamin and methylcobalamin requires at least two reductase reactions and an adenosyltransferase step. The reductases are flavoproteins that require NAD$^+$ as a cofactor. Stores of cobalamins in humans are normally large enough to maintain health for over 2 years without effective absorption from the diet [6,17].

Cobalamins have two well-established biochemical functions. Adenosylcobalamin is the cofactor for the mutase that converts methylmalonyl-CoA to succinyl-CoA (see Chap. 38, Fig. 2, reaction 9). This reaction is part of the pathway of metabolism of propionic acid, which itself derives from the metabolism of odd-chain fatty acids and from certain amino acids.

Methylcobalamin is the cofactor for the methyltransferase that converts homocysteine to the amino acid methionine. This reaction is important in folate metabolism as well. Its impairment appears to foster folate deficiency by an accumulation of N^5-methyltetrahydrofolate in a folate trap. Deficiency of either cobalamins or folate, or both, can restrict the supply of metabolically available one-carbon groups for pathways including those of nucleic acid synthesis.

Experimental cobalamin deficiency

Experimental deficiency of cobalamin has been difficult to induce. Poisoning with nitrous oxide or cycloleucine can induce conditions resembling the human disorder [19]. Pigs with a dietary deficiency provide another model.

Disease in humans

Cobalamin deficiencies are relatively common [6,17]. Pure dietary deficiency responding promptly to treatment with oral cobalamins has been described in a few children of strict vegan mothers. A more common syndrome, particularly in northern Europeans, is caused by failure of absorption due to an inadequate supply of the glycoprotein intrinsic factor, usually on an autoimmune basis. The most characteristic abnormality is pernicious anemia characterized by abnormal leukocytes called megaloblasts. Neurological symptoms occur in most of these patients and can precede the hematological changes.

Combined-system disease is the most common neurological syndrome [20]. These patients develop unpleasant tingling sensations (paresthesias), followed by loss of vibratory sensation, particularly in the legs and spastic weakness. The characteristic neuropathology is a spongy appearance of demyelination in the long tracts of the spinal cord, particularly prominent in the posterior columns. Combined-system disease responds poorly to treatment with cobalamin.

Cobalamin deficiency is characteristically associated with severe malaise that does respond dramatically to treatment, even before the hematological response is evident. Descriptions of B_{12} madness have appeared, but surveys of psychiatric populations have not revealed a significant proportion of B_{12}-responsive disorders.

Whether the neurological deficits relate more closely to the defect in methylmalonyl mutase or in the methyltransferase remains unsettled. Excretion of methylmalonic acid rises in cobalamin deficiency. Pure hereditary mutase deficiencies typically lead to psychomotor retardation, and odd- and branched-chain fatty acids have been found in the myelin of patients with combined-system disease. By contrast, patients with pure mutase deficiency do not develop the pathological or clinical hallmarks of combined-system disease. Clinically normal children with pure mutase deficiency are known. These include a patient who had a vitamin-dependent form of this disorder and stopped treatment at age 9 and developed normally until age 14 despite excreting massive amounts of methylmalonic acid. These observations suggest that methylmalonate accumulation need not be toxic in adults. Homocysteine excretion does not increase in patients with pernicious anemia, and children with homocystinuria and related disorders of amino acid metabolism from other causes do not develop the clinical or pathological stigmata of combined-system disease (see Chap. 38). An infant with apparent reduction in methyltransferase activity was clinically normal when reported at age 1 year. Patients with severe inherited deficiencies in the activities of both enzymes secondary to a defect in the metabolism of cobalamins do develop profound disease of the nervous system, with some characteristics of combined-system disease. Since the defect in methylmalonic acid metabolism in these children is not as profound as in those clinically less affected with pure mutase deficiency, the proposal has been put forward that the neurological disorder may be due primarily to the methyltransferase lesion [17].

Cobalamin requirements

Cobalamin requirements can be modified by genetic and environmental influences. Genetic factors apparently predispose to cobalamin deficiency secondary to intrinsic factor deficiency. At least six different inherited methylmalonic acidurias have been described [17]: absence of the mutase; decreased affinity of the mutase for adenosylcobalamin; deficiency of mitochondrial cobalamin reductase; deficiency of a mitochondrial cobalamin adenosyltransferase; and two distinguishable defects associated with abnormal cytosolic metabolism of cobalamins (see Chap. 38).

Environmental causes of increased cobalamin requirements include surgical removal of the stomach, excessive destruction of cobalamins in the gut by bacteria in a blind loop, or destruction by certain kinds of intestinal tape worm.

Abnormalities in the diet or in metabolism of a number of other vitamins can also damage the nervous system

Folic acid

Folic acid contains a pterin moiety linked to *para*-aminobenzoic acid, which is linked to one or more glutamate residues [21]. It plays a key role in the transfer of one-carbon (active methylene) groups, including the conversion of serine to glycine and the cobalamin-dependent transfer from homocysteine to methionine. Dietary deficiency of folate with normal cobalamin leads to anemia without significant neurological signs. On the other hand, both genetic and environmental disorders of folate metabolism have been associated with disease of the nervous system. (Genetic defects in the enzyme reactions are discussed further in Chap. 38.)

Genetically rare defects have been described in folate absorption, intraconversion, and utilization [21]. Children with a congenital inability to transport folate across their gut had severe megaloblastic anemia and profound psychomotor retardation with seizures. Injections of adequate amounts of folate reversed the anemia and the seizures but not the retardation. Psychomotor retardation with large ventricles and seizures has been associated with two disorders of folate intraconversion, putative deficiencies of $N^{5,10}$-methenyltetrahydrofolate cyclohydrolase and N^5-methyltetrahydrofolate: homocysteine methyltransferase. A boy with an apparent deficiency of hepatic dihydrofolate reductase activity had folate-responsive anemia without retardation. He was treated chronically with folate and developed a sociopathic personality disorder in his teens. A folate-responsive form of mental retardation with catatonia has been described in an adolescent girl with $N^{5,10}$-methylenetetrahydrofolic acid reductase deficiency. Her younger sister was mentally impaired with psychosis; an unrelated boy with a defect of the same enzyme had seizures and proximal muscle weakness without notable psychiatric problems. Most patients with glutamate formiminotransferase deficiency have had a syndrome of psychomotor retardation in infancy with seizures and large ventricles reminiscent of that in patients with disorders of folate intraconversions, but a few have been entirely normal clinically [21].

Environmentally, a number of common medications, including dilantin and certain antitumor agents, increase requirements for dietary folate. Folates and cobalamins can substitute for each other, although inefficiently, in the treatment of megaloblastic anemias, and treatment with folate can mask the hematological signs of cobalamin deficiency without affecting the progressive damage to the nervous system.

Pantothenic acid

Pantothenic acid is a substituted hydroxybutyric acid [22]. It is a constituent of CoA and thus plays a critical role in many acetylation and other acylation reactions. Experimental induction of pantothenic acid deficiency leads to signs of peripheral nerve damage—demyelination in laboratory animals and paraesthesias in humans [6,22]. Late signs of central nervous system damage in animals may relate as well to the adrenal failure that is a prominent part of the syndrome.

Carnitine

Not truly a vitamin, carnitine can be synthesized by mammalian tissues if dietary one-carbon sources are adequate (see Chap. 33). It participates in the transfer of acyl groups, including acetyl groups across mitochondrial membranes. Hereditary deficits in the ability to synthesize carnitine or in the long-chain carnitine acyltransferase have been associated with diseases of skeletal and cardiac muscle rather than of the nervous system (see Chap. 33). Large doses of carnitine have, however, been used to ameliorate the effects of damage to mitochondria in conditions that affect the nervous system, such as Reye's syndrome [23].

α-Tocopherol (vitamin E)

α-Tocopherol, a lipid-soluble vitamin, is an isoprenoid linked to a double-ring system. It is an effective antioxidant and can inhibit the peroxidation of polyunsaturated fatty acids. It was isolated as a factor that prevented infertility in rats, but the most common manifestation of deficiency in animals is skin disease. In humans, deficiency of vitamin E is usually secondary to malabsorption of fats (as in sprue or a-β-lipoproteinemias), but pure vitamin E deficiency secondary to deficiencies in absorption have been described. The typical syndrome in humans is a spinocerebellar degeneration, with loss of reflexes, ataxia, and impaired vibration and position sense [24].

Ascorbic acid (vitamin C)

Ascorbic acid is an unsaturated sugar derivative that is a potent reducing agent [6]. It probably participates in the hydroxylation of catecholamines. The uptake of ascorbic acid into synaptosomes requires glucose and oxygen; uptake into the brain appears to be via the cerebrospinal fluid rather than the blood. Fatigue and emotional changes are common in the full-blown deficiency disease scurvy, but diffuse disease of the small blood vessels with small hemorrhages is much more striking.

ACKNOWLEDGMENTS

It is a pleasure to thank Dr. Gary Gibson and other co-workers of the Dementia Research Service for helpful comments. Supported in part by Grant AG 03857 and the Will Rogers Institute.

REFERENCES

1. Dobbing, J. S. Infant nutrition and later achievement. *Nutr. Rev.* 42:1–7, 1984.
2. Wiggins, R. C., Fuller, G., and Enna, S. J. Undernutrition and the development of brain neurotransmitter systems. *Life. Sci.* 35:2085–2094, 1984.
3. Stein, Z., Susser, M., Saenger, G., Marolla, G. *Famine and Human Development.* New York: Plenum Press, 1974.
4. Harrison, D. E., and Archer, J. R. Genetic differences in effects of food restriction on aging in mice. *J. Nutr.* 117:376–382, 1987.
5. Wurtman, R. J., Hefti, F., and Melamed, E. Precursor control of neurotransmitter synthesis. *Pharmacol. Rev.* 32:315–335, 1981.
6. McIlwain, H., and Bachelard, H. S. Nutritional factors and the central nervous system. In *Biochemistry and the Central Nervous System*, 5th ed., London: Churchill Livingstone, 1985, pp. 244–281.
7. Sable, H. Z., and Gubler, C. J. (eds.). *Thiamin.* New York: New York Academy of Sciences, 1981.
8. Victor, M., Adams, R. D., and Collins, G. H. *The Wernicke-Korsakoff Syndrome.* Philadelphia: Davis, 1971.
9. Hakim, A. M. Effect of thiamine deficiency and its reversal on cerebral blood flow in the rat. Observations on the phenomena of hyperperfusion, "no reflow," and delayed hypoperfusion. *J. Cereb. Blood Flow Metab.* 6:79–85, 1986.
10. Butterworth, R. F. Cerebral thiamine-dependent enzyme changes in experimental Wernicke's encephalopathy. *Metab. Brain Dis.* 1:165–175, 1986.
11. Hata, T., Meyer, J. S., Tanahashi, N., Ishikawa, Y., Imai, A., Shinohara, T., Velez, M., Fann, W. E., Kandula, P., and Sakai, F. Three-dimensional mapping of local cerebral perfusion in alcoholic encephalopathy with and without Wernicke-Korsakoff syndrome. *J. Cereb. Blood Flow Metab.* 7:35–44, 1987.
12. Blass, J. P., and Gibson, G. E. Deleterious aberrations of a thiamine-requiring enzyme in four patients with Wernicke-Korsakoff syndrome. *New Eng. J. Med.* 297:1367–1370, 1977.

13. Gibson, G. E., and Blass, J. P. Oxidative metabolism and acetylcholine synthesis during acetylpyridine treatment. *Neurochem. Res.* 10:453–467, 1985.

14. Gaitonde, M. K., and Evans, G. M. The effect of inhibition of hexosemonophosphate shunt on the metabolism of glucose and function in rat brain *in vivo. Neurochem. Res.* 7:1163–1179, 1982.

15. Lott, I. B., Coulombe, T., DiPaolo, R. V., Richardson, E. P., and Levy, H. L. Vitamin B_6-dependent seizures: Pathology and chemical findings in brain. *Neurology* 28:47–54, 1978.

16. Sokoloff, L., Lassen, N. A., McKhann, G. M., Tower, D. B., Albers, W. Effects of pyridoxine withdrawal on cerebral circulation and metabolism in a pyridoxine-dependent child. *Nature* 183:751–753, 1959.

17. Rosenberg, L. E. Disorders of propionate and methylmalonate metabolism. In J. B. Stanbury, J. B. Wyngaarden, D. S. Fredrickson, J. L. Goldstein, and M. S. Brown (eds.), *The Metabolic Basis of Inherited Disease,* 5th ed. New York: McGraw-Hill, 1976, pp. 474–497.

18. Theone, J., Baker, H., Yoshino, M., and Sweetman, L. Biotin responsive carboxylase deficiency associated with subnormal plasma and urinary biotin. *New Eng. J. Med.* 304:817–821, 1981.

19. Hakim, A. M., Cooper, B. A., Rosenblatt, D. S., and Pappius, H. M. Local cerebral glucose utilization in two models of B_{12} deficiency. *J. Neurochem.* 40:1155–1160, 1987.

20. Rowland, L. P. (ed.). *Merritt's Textbook of Neurology.* Philadelphia: Lea & Febiger, 1984.

21. Erbe, R. W. Inborn errors of folate metabolism. *New Eng. J. Med.* 293:753–757, 807–812, 1975.

22. Bean, W. B., and Hodges, R. E. Pantothenic acid deficiency induced in human subjects. *Proc. Soc. Exp. Biol. Med.* 86:693–698, 1954.

23. Stumpf, D. A., Parker, W. D., and Angelini, C. Carnitine deficiency, organic acidemias, and Reye's syndrome. *Neurology* 35:1041–1045, 1985.

24. Krendel, D. A., Gilchrist, J. M., Johnson, A. O., and Bossen, E. H. Isolated deficiency of vitamin E with progressive neurologic deterioration. *Neurology* 37:538–540, 1987.

CHAPTER 35

Biochemistry of Neuropathy

David Pleasure

COMPARISON OF THE PERIPHERAL AND CENTRAL NERVOUS SYSTEMS

Disorders of the peripheral nervous system (PNS) are common and disabling and hence of considerable interest to physicians and neurobiologists. As a result of cellular and biochemical features that distinguish it from the central nervous system (CNS), the PNS is uniquely susceptible to certain disorders to which the CNS

Basic Neurochemistry: Molecular, Cellular, and Medical Aspects, 4th Ed., edited by G. J. Siegel et al. Raven Press, Ltd., New York, 1989.
Correspondence to David Pleasure, Neurology, Children's Hospital of Philadelphia, 34th and Civic Center Boulevard, Philadelphia, Pennsylvania 19104.

is not. Significant differences relate to the biology of myelin (see Chaps. 1 and 6), the capacity of the PNS far beyond that of the CNS for regeneration (see Chap. 26), and the evolution of special functions such as mechanical-electrical transduction in the PNS.

There are also many anatomical and metabolic similarities between the PNS and CNS. Somatic motor and sensory neurons giving rise to PNS axons maintain a large fraction of their total protoplasmic bulk within the CNS. Neurons of the enteric plexi and autonomic ganglia resemble certain classes of CNS neurons in neurotransmitter specificities, metabolism, and growth factor requirements. There are also similarities between PNS and CNS neuroglia. Phagocytic PNS microglia-like cells probably share with CNS microglia a common derivation from bone marrow. Although CNS macroglia develop from the neural tube and Schwann cells from the neural crest [1], some of their functions, such as regulation of conduction and neuronal trophic support, and the means by which these functions are accomplished, for example, by synthesis of myelin, are similar.

Still another resemblance between CNS and PNS is in the regulation of transfer of molecules between the bloodstream and neural extracellular space. The blood-nerve barrier, like the blood-brain barrier, is composed of capillary endothelial cells that, unlike the capillaries of most other tissues, are linked by interendothelial tight junctions. Endoneurial capillary endothelial pinocytosis is infrequent, but the cells express specific carriers to facilitate rapid passage of polar substrates and metabolites (see Chap. 30).

DISEASES AFFECTING BOTH THE PERIPHERAL AND CENTRAL NERVOUS SYSTEMS

Because of the similarities between the PNS and CNS, it is not surprising that many diseases affect both, and examples are given in Table 1. The clinical expressions of such diseases are variable and are sometimes restricted to the PNS. For example, patients with thiamine deficiency often display symmetrical distal sensorimotor polyneuropathy without accompanying Wernicke's or Korsakoff's syndrome (see Chap. 34); infection with human immunodeficiency virus (HIV) may cause early chronic demyelinative polyneuropathy and dementia months later; tertiary syphilis may destroy dorsal root ganglion sensory neurons without injuring neurons in the cerebral cortex; and sulfatidase deficiency (metachromatic leukodystrophy) may cause polyneuropathy initially, with CNS dysfunction occurring only later (see Chap. 37). In some instances, this apparent PNS specificity is simply an ascertainment artifact; that is, although both the CNS and PNS are involved, only the PNS component is detectable to the clinician in the early stages. In other cases, subtle host factors or etiologic variables yet unappreciated dictate the PNS selectivity.

DISEASES AFFECTING ONLY OR MAINLY THE PERIPHERAL NERVOUS SYSTEM

Some examples of disorders exclusively or predominantly of the PNS are listed in Table 2. Of these diseases, some are quite common, for example, diabetic neuropathy [2], Guillain-Barre

TABLE 1. Examples of diseases affecting both the PNS and the CNS

Infections (AIDS, syphilis)
Neurotoxins (acrylamide, triorthocresylphosphate)
Vitamin deficiencies (B_1, B_{12}, E)
Hormone deficiencies (hypothyroidism)
Arteritis (periarteritis nodosa)
Familial lipid storage disorders (sulfatidase deficiency, galactocerebrosidase deficiency, adrenoleukodystrophy)

syndrome [3], neurofibromatosis [4], whereas others occur very infrequently, (such as pyridoxine neuropathy). They are mentioned because they illustrate pathogenetic mechanisms. (Lambert-Eaton syndrome and botulism, disorders of cholinergic nerve terminals, are discussed in Chap. 32.) In some of the disorders listed in Table 2, the etiology is quite clear, but the mechanism of PNS degeneration remains obscure, for example, familial neuropathic amyloidosis [5]. In others, the specific involvement of the PNS is explicable on the basis of one or more of the following factors:

1. The PNS contains Schwann cells and fibroblasts, not oligodendroglia and astrocytes
2. There are regions of incompetence of the blood-nerve barrier that admit toxic macromolecules to endoneurium
3. Some PNS axons are extraordinarily long
4. The PNS is subjected to more physical stresses than is the CNS

FACTORS IN THE SPECIFIC INVOLVEMENT OF THE PERIPHERAL NERVOUS SYSTEM

The PNS differs from the CNS in cell type and in protein and lipid composition

Support cells of the PNS versus the CNS

In the CNS, oligodendroglia invest large axons in myelin, and type 2 astroglia provide metabolic support for these axons at nodes of Ranvier [6]; type 1 astroglia [7] regulate ion and metabolite concentrations in neuropil. In the PNS, all these functions are the responsibility of Schwann cells. Four Schwann cell phenotypes are recognized on morphological grounds:

1. Myelin-forming Schwann cells, ensheathing single axons greater than 1 μm in di-

TABLE 2. Some diseases affecting only the PNS[a]

Infections (leprosy, diphtheria)
Neurotoxins (pyridoxine, cisplatin, botulism)
Immune-mediated neuropathies (Guillain-Barré syndrome, EAN, neuropathy with IgM$_k$ anti-MAG, Lambert-Eaton syndrome)
Amyloidosis (familial neuropathic and myeloma-associated forms)
Hirschsprung's disease
Refsum's disease
Hereditary motor-sensory neuropathies
Diabetic neuropathy
Neurofibromatosis (central and peripheral forms)

[a] (EAN) experimental allergic neuritis; (MAG) myelin-associated glycoprotein.

ameter for hundreds of microns and synthesizing myelin-specific lipids and proteins
2. Nonmyelinating Schwann cells, investing multiple smaller axons [8]
3. Satellite Schwann cells surrounding the perikarya of neurons in ganglia
4. Tubular aggregates of Schwann cells ("bands of Bungner") in the distal segments of transected or crushed nerves.

These Schwann cell phenotypes are neuronally dictated and interconvertible. In addition, there are neuroglia within the plexi in the walls of viscera [9]. The relationship of these enteric glia to Schwann cells has not been established, nor has the role of these glia in the pathogenesis of such enteric denervating diseases as amyloidosis [5], Hirschsprung's disease [10], and diabetic autonomic neuropathy [2] been determined.

Immunohistological studies have demonstrated that both myelin-forming and nonmyelinating Schwann cells express a lipid characteristic of myelin, galactocerebroside (galC), on their surface [8] but that such expression is lost when the Schwann cells are deprived of axonal contact. Two other cell surface antigens are expressed in a fashion reciprocal to this. Nerve growth factor (NGF) receptor [11] and neural cell adhesion molecules [12] are displayed by axotomized Schwann cells, but such expression is down-regulated by axonal contact. Schwann cells investing small unmyelinated axons synthesize and express intracellular glial fibrillary acidic protein, as do enteric glia [9]; myelin-forming Schwann cells and axotomized Schwann cells do not.

There is no PNS neuroglial homolog of the type 1 astrocyte of the CNS, which articulates with capillary basal lamina [9], or of the ciliated ependymal cell, which delimits CNS neuropil from cerebrospinal fluid. In PNS, however, flattened, basal lamina-lined mesothelial cells of the perineurium delineate nerve fascicles, encircling the endoneurial contents and providing a barrier to movement of ionic compounds and macromolecules between nonneural tissues and endoneurium. Whether these perineurial cells have some other function in addition to restricting diffusion into endoneurium is unknown, but a neuronotrophic role is suggested by the observation that they, like Schwann cells, express a plasma membrane surface binding protein for NGF.

Fibroblasts constitute roughly 10 percent of total cells within endoneurium, and are the major cell type in epineurial connective tissue. Other cells in the PNS include epineurial adipocytes and occasional mast cells.

Protein and lipid composition of the PNS compared to that of the CNS

Myelin. PNS myelin contains a unique basic protein, P_2, the product of a gene distinct from that which codes for the family of myelin basic proteins shared by the CNS and PNS. Although the function of P_2 is not known, it has extensive sequence homologies with low-molecular-weight fatty acid binding proteins expressed in liver and other tissues [13]. PNS myelin contains a lower level of myelin-associated glycoprotein (MAG) (see Chap. 6) than

does CNS myelin but expresses another glycoprotein of very high apparent molecular weight, 170,000 M_r, unique to the PNS [14]. The major PNS myelin structural protein, P_0, is of much lower M_r (27,100) than MAG ($\sim$ 98,000) and contains an asparagine-linked carbohydrate moiety [15]. The major CNS myelin structural protein, lipophilin (proteolipid), is not glycosylated: rather, it contains covalently bound saturated fatty acid. Given that PNS myelin is devoid of lipophilin, the observation that Schwann cells actively synthesize lipophilin is unexpected.

The differences between the lipid composition of CNS and PNS myelin are less profound than the differences in protein (see Chap. 6). Molar ratios of cholesterol to phospholipid to galactosphingolipid are similar; however, human PNS myelin contains several sulfated glucuronyl glycolipids not expressed in adult human CNS myelin that cross-react with antibodies against carbohydrate epitopes of MAG [16].

Collagen. The collagens, a family of extracellular structural proteins characterized by a triple α helical configuration and a high content of hydroxyproline, hydroxylysine, and glycine are abundant in the PNS [17] but are much rarer in the CNS. In the CNS, collagen is encountered primarily in association with blood vessels and is virtually absent from the remainder of the neuropil. In the PNS, the collagens comprise 30 percent or more of total protein and are present in endoneurium both in the form of interstitial collagen fibrils and as a component of the basal lamina surrounding the processes of Schwann cells and perineurial cells, in addition to lining the outer aspect of endoneurial capillaries. Fibroblasts are responsible for the synthesis of the bulk of the interstitial collagen fibrils, whereas Schwann cells and, probably, perineurial mesothelial cells secrete the more heavily glycosylated basal lamina forms of collagen [18].

Blood-nerve barrier leaks at PNS nerve terminals and dorsal root ganglia

Both the CNS and PNS demonstrate local regions of incompetence of the respective blood-tissue barrier systems, and in both tissues these regions have specific physiological functions. In the CNS, for example, function of medullary chemosensory nuclei requires free passage of polar molecules from the blood. In the PNS, NGF gaining access to axon terminals that are not invested in a perineurial sheath becomes bound to specific nerve terminal receptors, and, after internalization, the NGF-NGF receptor complexes are transported retrograde to the neuronal perikaryon. Lectins and other proteins useful as anatomic tracers also gain access to the PNS at nerve terminals, and some viruses are able to penetrate at this site. In some species such as the rabbit, proteins gain access to endoneurium in the region of the dorsal root ganglia as well as at nerve terminals.

The length of PNS axons increases their vulnerability

PNS sensory and motor axons may exceed 1 m in length. Since PNS axons lack ribosomes, the supply of essential structural proteins and enzymes to distal regions derived from the neuronal perikaryon must be transported through the axons for great distances (see Chap. 24). The proteins that polymerize to form neurofilaments and microtubules, and many enzymes, move centrifugally at 1 to 10 mm/day. Organelles such as neurotransmitter vesicles and mitochondria, which are also derived from the neuronal perikaryon, are transported through axoplasm at velocities of more than 100 mm/day. Proteins internalized by the nerve terminal, such as NGF, are translocated toward the neuronal perikaryon at approximately 100 mm/day. Neurons with long axons are particularly vulnerable to disorders that compromise either perikaryal

synthesis of axonal proteins or the local axonal machinery that is responsible for axoplasmic transport.

Long axons are also more likely to sustain localized damage owing to trauma, ischemia, or other noxious influences. Further, since thousands of Schwann cells are required to myelinate such a long axon, the likelihood that a pathological process randomly compromising the capacity of Schwann cells to maintain myelin will interfere with saltatory conduction along such a fiber is high. Nonrandom distal segmental demyelination, owing to diminution in distal axonal caliber ("axonal dwindling"), is also most apt to occur in relation to the longest axons and has been observed in a variety of toxic, metabolic, and inherited polyneuropathies.

The clinical features of most polyneuropathies reflect this heightened vulnerability of the longest fibers. Typically, patients manifest symmetrical distal sensory disturbances, usually first in the feet, weakness of distal more than proximal muscles, and loss of distal prior to proximal tendon reflexes.

Repeated trauma in the PNS leads to Wallerian degeneration and segmental demyelination

Movements of the limbs subject nerves to repeated stretch. Although collagen fibrils afford tensile strength, and there is some waviness in the course of axons that permits a degree of nerve elongation without axonal ripping, stretch that is too great causes axonal disruption. Nerves in exposed regions, for example, the median nerve at the wrist, the ulnar nerve at the elbow, and the common peroneal nerve at the knee, are vulnerable to compression that, if sufficiently severe, can cause either demyelination or axonal transection. Such compression can also interrupt blood flow, causing nerve infarction. In addition to these mechanical injuries, superficial nerves experience considerable thermal fluctuations that can kill cells directly if sufficiently severe or predispose the nerves to damage by precipitation of cold-insoluble proteins or other mechanisms (see leprosy, for example, below).

A brief review of the responses of PNS to trauma-induced Wallerian degeneration or segmental demyelination will be helpful in suggesting why PNS is in general so much more successful in regenerating than is CNS.

Wallerian degeneration

Axotomized Schwann cells in the nerve segment distal to the axonal transection manifest a transient phase of intense proliferation and form tubular aggregates [19,20]. Mononuclear cells from the bloodstream enter the trauma zone and assist resident Schwann cells in catabolizing fragmented myelin. Schwann cells in the distal nerve segment cease to assemble basal lamina or to express cell surface galactocerebroside. Schwann cell levels of mRNA for myelin proteins fall markedly, and the smaller amount of myelin P_0 glycoprotein that is synthesized distal to axonal transection is degraded rapidly in lysosomes [15]. Expression of cell surface adhesion molecules is augmented [12], and there is also an increase in expression of cell surface NGF receptors that are believed to display NGF in a manner optimal for support of regenerating axonal sprouts [11]. Fibroblasts in the traumatized nerve segment and distal to it augment production of interstitial collagen, increasing the tensile strength of the damaged nerve and providing the collagenous framework required for axonal ensheathment by Schwann cells. This extracellular accumulation of collagen in the injured PNS [17] contrasts sharply with the astrogliosis and increased intracellular glial fibrillary acidic protein (GFAP) elicited by trauma in the CNS.

As regeneration proceeds, axonal growth cones penetrate the scar and extend into the tubular Schwann cell aggregates. On reestablishment of contact with axonal sprouts, the Schwann cells proliferate [20], assemble basal lamina, express surface galactocerebroside, and down-regulate surface NGF receptors and cell adhesion molecules. If the axon reaches a diameter sufficient to support myelination, the Schwann cell is induced to synthesize myelin-associated glycoprotein and, later, myelin P_0 and myelin basic proteins [21].

Segmental demyelination

Affected Schwann cells lose contact with the axon, proliferate, and participate in the catabolism of myelin fragments. If several successive internodes along an axon are demyelinated, nerve action potentials cannot be transmitted (conduction block). Data are not available about modifications in Schwann cell surface expression of galactocerebroside, adhesion molecules, and growth factor receptors or about rates of synthesis of myelin components during segmental demyelination. During subsequent remyelination, several Schwann cells usually participate in the remyelination of what was previously the territory of a single Schwann cell, giving rise to shortened internodes. During the initial period of remyelination, when the myelin sheath is very thin and its capacitance very high, the velocity of nerve conduction of action potentials is markedly below normal. Later, as the sheath approaches its normal thickness, conduction velocity rises. Excess Schwann cells generated during the phase of Schwann cell proliferation and not successful in establishing contact with an axon gradually disappear from the nerve. With repeated cycles of demyelination and remyelination, however, as can occur with repeated trauma or more commonly in certain inherited or chronic inflammatory demyelinative neuropathies, layers of redundant Schwann cells encircle demyelinated or partially remyelinated axons, forming "onion bulbs."

PATHOGENESIS OF DISEASES AFFECTING LARGELY OR SOLELY THE PERIPHERAL NERVOUS SYSTEM

Infections

The lepromatous form of leprosy is characterized by loss of cutaneous sensibility, a consequence of damage caused by the growth of Hansen's bacilli in Schwann cells in affected cutaneous nerves. Hansen's bacilli, fastidious organisms that proliferate only at temperatures below that maintained by most mammals, are able to grow in subcutaneous Schwann cells because these nerves are in an environment that is often cooler than the CNS and other deeper tissues.

Diphtheria causes a demyelinative neuropathy, initially affecting the cranial nerves and later the nerves to the limbs; whereas segmental demyelination is profound, axons are typically spared. *Corynebacterium diphtheriae*, a bacterium that colonizes the pharynx or, less commonly, the skin secretes a protein exotoxin that gains access to endoneurial fluid both at nerve endings and at the level of the dorsal root ganglia. The exotoxin has two functional domains, one of which permits binding of the toxin to the Schwann cell plasma membrane and the second of which is an enzyme that catalyzes the inactivation of one of the elongation factors required for protein synthesis by transfer to it of an ADP-ribose moiety derived from NAD^+. Remyelination subsequently occurs, largely owing to the activity of the new Schwann cells generated in the nerve as a consequence of the mitogenic stimulus associated with segmental demyelination.

Polio virus, which multiplies initially in the gut, binds to and selectively infects motor neurons of the anterior horns of the spinal cord and brainstem, producing inflammatory changes within the CNS, Wallerian degeneration of motor axons in the PNS, and motor deficits without accompanying sensory or autonomic dysfunction. Months later, surviving motor neurons reinnervate previously denervated muscle fibers, producing motor units (motor neurons and the muscle fibers that they innervate) that are much larger in size than normal. This reparative process produces partial or complete return of previously lost motor function.

Neurotoxins

Excessive ingestion of pyridoxine (vitamin B_6), usually the result of inappropriate self-medication, causes a progressive, purely sensory axonal polyneuropathy affecting predominantly the largest fibers, attributable to the toxic effect of the vitamin on dorsal root ganglion neurons. A similar purely sensory axonal polyneuropathy with dorsal root ganglion neuronopathy is seen in patients given cisplatin as a chemotherapeutic agent for the treatment of gynecologic or bladder carcinoma. In both instances, the toxin, after gaining access to endoneurial fluid, induces damage by binding covalently to macromolecules necessary for neuronal function (pyridoxine to proteins; cisplatin to DNA).

Immune-mediated neuropathies

Experimental allergic neuritis

Experimental allergic neuritis (EAN) can be elicited in Lewis rats and monkeys by immunization against myelin P_2 basic protein or in rabbits by immunization against the myelin glycolipid, galactocerebroside (galC). Although both types of EAN are primarily demyelinative, P_2-EAN is mediated by sensitized T-lymphocytes [22], whereas galC-EAN is mediated by galC antibodies. The reasons for PNS selectivity of the two EANs are also distinct. Although T-lymphocytes can penetrate the CNS as well as PNS, myelin P_2 basic protein is restricted to the PNS, and P_2-sensitized T-lymphocytes are therefore more likely to set up an inflammatory reaction in the PNS than the CNS. GalC, on the other hand, is a constituent of the plasma membranes of oligodendroglia as well as Schwann cells and of CNS myelin as well as PNS myelin, and PNS selectivity of galC-EAN seems to reflect more ready ingress of complement-fixing galC antibodies to the PNS than the CNS.

Guillain-Barré syndrome

Guillain-Barré syndrome, or acute idiopathic polyradiculoneuritis, often occurs 1 or 2 weeks after a variety of viral infections. Typically, no virus can be isolated from the PNS. If protected against hypoxemia, most patients recover completely, particularly if treated early in the course by plasmapheresis. Guillain-Barré syndrome resembles P_2-EAN both clinically and pathologically, being characterized by segmental demyelination and infiltration of endoneurium with lymphocytes. Probably due to an autoimmune mechanism [3], the responsible neural antigen has not yet been identified.

IgM$_k$ paraproteinemia

Elderly men with IgM$_k$ paraproteinemia caused by a plasma cell proliferative disorder occasionally develop a slowly progressive polyneuropathy characterized pathologically by focally abnormal compaction of PNS myelin lamellae. In such cases, the paraproteinemic immunoglobulin has been observed to bind to intact myelin and to MAG. The PNS specificity of this syndrome, despite the greater abundance of MAG in myelin of the CNS than the PNS, may be due to greater penetration of the paraprotein into the PNS than the CNS or, alternatively, to the presence in PNS myelin, but not in adult CNS myelin, of sulfated glucuronyl glycolipids that are recognized by the anti-MAG IgM$_k$ paraprotein [16].

Amyloidosis

Amyloid is the generic term applied to disorders characterized by abnormal deposition of pro-

tease-resistant protein aggregates in tissue. Three distinct types of neural amyloidosis have been recognized thus far. The most common is restricted to the CNS and is due to accumulation of a fragment of a trans-membrane glycoprotein and is seen in patients with Alzheimer's disease or Down's syndrome. The two other types predominantly affect the PNS. In one, patients with multiple myeloma or other plasma cell dyscrasias synthesize excessive immunoglobulin light chains. In the other, members of families with a point mutation in an exon coding for transthyretin deposit an abnormal form of this protein in the PNS [5]. In both types of PNS amyloid, the polyneuropathy that results, by a still uncertain mechanism, affects particularly unmyelinated sensory and autonomic fibers and the enteric plexi.

Hirschsprung's disease

Hirschsprung's disease presents in infancy with massive segmental dilatation of the colon, the result of absence from the affected segment of intrinsic innervation [10], due perhaps to failure of migration of neural crest cells [1] to this portion of the gut or to an abnormal gut wall microenvironment inhospitable to maturation of neural crest cells.

Refsum's disease

Refsum's disease is an autosomal recessively inherited peroxisomal defect in the α oxidation of dietary branched-chain fatty acids, most notably of phytanic acid (see Chap. 37). Patients with this disease manifest polyneuropathy with enlarged nerves, retinitis pigmentosa, scaly skin, and deafness. The polyneuropathy is largely demyelinative, and the nerve enlargement is due to the accumulation of excess Schwann cells in concentric periaxonal arrays, or "onion bulbs." Myelin isolated from the nerves of such patients contains excess amounts of esterified phytanic acid, and it is presumed that this accumulation causes a decrease in myelin stability. Removal of phytanic acid from the diet yields improvement in the polyneuropathy.

Hereditary motor and sensory neuropathy

Hereditary motor and sensory neuropathy (HMSN) is a heterogeneous group of human polyneuropathies with varying patterns of inheritance (dominant, recessive, or X-linked). Some families with HMSN (type 1 and type 3) are characterized by reduced velocity of nerve action potentials, prominent segmental demyelination, Schwann cell proliferation with onion-bulb formation, and distal axonal dwindling [23]; others (type 2) manifest chiefly distal Wallerian degeneration. Two murine models resembling HMSN types 1 and 3 are now available: the trembler mouse and transgenic mice expressing the 72-base-pair enhancer region of the SV40 viral genome [24].

Diabetic neuropathy

Diabetes mellitus is the most common cause of peripheral neuropathy in the United States. The usual clinical pattern is that of a slowly progressive, mixed sensorimotor and autonomic polyneuropathy, and the major structural change in the peripheral nerves of most patients is axonal degeneration [2].

Most of the work on pathogenesis of diabetic neuropathy has been done with rats that are hyperglycemic because of the administration of a pancreatic islet cell toxin (streptozotocin) or on a hereditary basis (in particular, the BB strain of rats) [2]. In such rats, nerve conduction velocities fall soon after the appearance of hyperglycemia, and this physiological deficit is temporally correlated with an accumulation of intracellular Na^+ within the endoneurium and the appearance of paranodal axonal swelling, disruption of the insertion of Schwann cell membrane loops on axolemma at the para-

nodes, proximal axonal dilatation, and atrophy of the distal regions of long axons.

Four pathogenetic mechanisms for diabetic neuropathy have been proposed: excess glycosylation of neural proteins; an alteration in nerve polyol metabolism induced by hyperglycemia; an abnormality in axoplasmic transport; and nerve hypoxia.

Nonenzymatic glycosylation of proteins is accentuated by hyperglycemia and is responsible for the increased glycosylation of hemoglobin and of collagen in poorly controlled diabetics. Excess glycosylation of PNS myelin and other nerve proteins has been demonstrated in diabetic rats. It is possible that an alteration in the structure and function of a vital neural protein by glycosylation is responsible for diabetic neuropathy, but there is still no evidence to support this hypothesis.

Because of the presence of aldose reductase in Schwann cells, hyperglycemia causes excess accumulation of sorbitol and fructose within the endoneurium, both in diabetic rats and in diabetic humans, although not to levels likely to cause damage because of osmotic disequilibrium. Hyperglycemia also diminishes endoneurial activity of plasma membrane Na,K-ATPase and inhibits carrier-mediated transport of myoinositol into endoneurium. Supplementation of the diet of diabetic animals with myoinositol or administration of an aldose reductase inhibitor partially prevents development of electrophysiological abnormalities in nerve.

The distal atrophy and degeneration of axons in diabetic neuropathy suggests that an alteration in axoplasmic flow is of pathogenetic significance. One laboratory observed diminished rapid transport of choline acetyltransferase in the nerves of diabetic rats. Other laboratories have reported that rapid axoplasmic flow is normal but that reverse axoplasmic flow of glycoproteins and of NGF is reduced. A defect in reverse axoplasmic flow of NGF might be of pathogenetic significance, since this protein is required for survival of sympathetic neurons. Slow axoplasmic flow has also been reported to be diminished, and it is possible that pooling of axonal cytoskeletal proteins near neuronal perikarya caused by such a flow defect is responsible for the proximal axonal engorgement as well as the distal axonal atrophy in streptozotocin-diabetic rats.

Endoneurial hypoxia has been demonstrated in diabetic rats, and, by limiting oxidative phosphorylation, could explain the slowing in axoplasmic flow and the diminution in Na,K-ATPase that occurs in the nerves of these animals. Certainly, hypoxia of the degree observed in these animals could account for the slowing of nerve conduction velocity in their nerves, since conduction velocity is also slowed in nerves of nondiabetic rats subjected to a partial pressure of oxygen low enough to produce a similar oxygen concentration in the endoneurium. The mechanism for endoneurial hypoxia in diabetes mellitus is unclear but could relate to hyperviscosity of the blood owing to dehydration, an abnormality in gas diffusion across the walls of endoneurial capillaries, or to an increase in neural arteriovenous shunting of blood. In this regard, morphometric studies of nerve biopsies from humans with diabetic neuropathy have shown thickening of the basal lamina surrounding endoneurial capillaries and a greater frequency of occluded endoneurial capillaries than in the nerves of patients without diabetes mellitus. Scattered infarctions of the proximal regions of peripheral nerves have been documented at autopsy in diabetic patients who during life had either mononeuropathy multiplex or what appeared overtly to be a symmetrical distal polyneuropathy.

Neurofibromatosis

Two distinct dominantly inherited disorders are referred to as neurofibromatosis. The central form, which is quite rare, is characterized by bilateral acoustic nerve Schwann cell tumors.

Patients with this condition are also at far greater risk than normal of developing Schwann cell tumors on spinal roots and have an increased incidence of meningiomas as well. The genetic basis for central neurofibromatosis is a partial deletion of chromosome 22, which is manifested both in the tumors and in other apparently normal tissues [25].

The peripheral form, or von Recklinghausen's neurofibromatosis, is quite common, with an incidence of about 1 in 2,000 persons in the United States. This disorder is characterized by multiple subcutaneous neurofibromas, the principal cell type of which, as in the acoustic nerve tumors in the central form, is the Schwann cell. Schwann cell tumors may also occur along the course of large nerves and nerve roots or cranial nerves, including the acoustic nerve. Although often enlarging relatively rapidly during puberty or pregnancy, at other times the Schwann cell tumors tend to be very slow-growing. In occasional patients, one of the tumors undergoes a malignant transformation, becoming locally invasive and capable of metastasis. Other characteristic features of the peripheral form are irregular areas of hyperpigmentation of the skin (café-au-lait spots) and iris (Lisch nodules), which are attributable to disturbed function of melanocytes; these pigmented cells, like Schwann cells, are of neural crest origin. Nonneural crest-derived cells are also occasionally affected, with an increased incidence of CNS glial tumors and of malformations of the skull, vertebral column, and long bones. The genetic defect in the peripheral form of neurofibromatosis is on chromosome 17, close to but distinct from the gene coding for NGF receptor [4]

REFERENCES

A text that describes many of the diseases mentioned in this chapter is Dyck, P. J., Thomas, P. K., Lambert, E. H., and Bunge, R., (eds.), *Peripheral Neuropathy*, 2nd ed. Philadelphia: W. B. Saunders Co., 1984, Vols. 1 and 2.

1. LeDouarin, N. M. Cell line segregation during peripheral nervous system ontogeny. *Science* 231:1515–1522, 1986.

2. Dyck, P. H., Thomas, P. K., Asbury, A. K., Winegrad, A. I., and Porte, D., Jr. *Diabetic Neuropathy.* Philadelphia: W. B. Saunders Co., 1987.

3. Pollard, J. D., Baverstock, J., and McLeod, J. G. Class II antigen expression and inflammatory cells in the Guillain-Barré syndrome. *Ann. Neurol.* 21:337–341, 1987.

4. Seizinger, B. R., et al. Genetic linkage of von Recklinghausen neurofibromatosis to the nerve growth factor receptor gene. *Cell* 49:589–594, 1987.

5. Sasaki, H., Sakaki, Y., Matsuo, H., Goto, I., Kuroiwa, Y., Sahashi, I., Takahashi, A., Shinoda, T., Isobe, T., and Takagi, Y. Diagnosis of familial amyloidotic polyneuropathy by recombinant DNA techniques. *Biochem. Biophys. Res. Commun.* 125:636–642, 1984.

6. ffrench-Constant, C., and Raff, M. C. The oligodendrocyte-type-2 astrocyte cell lineage is specialized for myelination. *Nature* 323:335–338, 1986.

7. Janzer, R. C., and Raff, M. C. Astrocytes induce blood-brain barrier properties in endothelial cells. *Nature* 325:253–257, 1987.

8. Jessen, J. R., Morgan, L., Brammer, M., and Mirsky, R. Galactocerebroside is expressed by non-myelin-forming Schwann cells in situ. *J. Cell Biol.* 101:1135–1143, 1985.

9. Jessen, K. R., and Mirsky, R. Astrocyte-like glia in the peripheral nervous system: An immunochemical study of enteric glia. *J. Neurosci.* 3:2206–2218, 1983.

10. Howard, E. R. Muscle innervation of the gut: Structure and pathology. *J. R. Soc. Med.* 77:905–908, 1984.

11. Yan, Q., and Johnson, E. M., Jr. A quantitative study of the developmental expression of nerve growth factor (NGF) receptor in rats. *Dev. Biol.* 121:139–148, 1987.

12. Daniloff, J. K., Levi, G., Grumet, M., Rieger, F., and Edelman, G. M. Altered expression of neuronal cell adhesion molecules induced by nerve injury and repair. *J. Cell Biol.* 103:929–945, 1986.

13. Lowe, J. B., Boguski, M. S., Sweetser, D. A., Elshourbagy, N. A., Taylor, J. M., and Gordon, J. I. Human liver fatty acid binding protein. *J. Biol. Chem.* 260:3413–3417, 1986.

14. Shuman, S., Hardy, M., and Pleasure, D. Immunochemical characterization of peripheral nervous system myelin 170,000-M_r glycoprotein. *J. Neurochem.* 47:811–818, 1986.

15. Brunden, K. R., and Poduslo, J. F. Lysosomal delivery of the major myelin glycoprotein in the absence of myelin assembly: Posttranslational regulation of the level of expression by Schwann cells. *J. Cell Biol.* 104:661–669, 1987.

16. Chou, D. K. H., Ilyas, A. A., Evans, J. E., Costello, C., Quarles, R. H., and Jungalwala, F. B. Structure of sulfated glucuronyl glycolipids in the nervous system reacting with HNK-1 antibody and some IgM paraproteins in neuropathy. *J. Biol. Chem.* 261:11717–11725, 1986.

17. Eather, T. F., Pollock, M., and Myers, D. B. Proximal and distal changes in collagen content of peripheral nerve that follow transection and crush lesions. *Exp. Neurol.* 92:299–310, 1986.

18. Carey, D. J., Eldridge, C. F., Cornbrooks, C. J., Timpl, R., and Bunge, R. P. Biosynthesis of type IV collagen by cultured rat Schwann cells. *J. Cell Biol.* 97:473–479, 1983.

19. Pellegrino, R. G., Politis, M. J., Ritchie, J. M., and Spencer, P. S. Events in degenerating cat peripheral nerve: Induction of Schwann cell S phase and its relation to nerve fibre degeneration. *J. Neurocytol.* 15:17–28, 1986.

20. Salzer, J. L., and Bunge, R. P. Studies of Schwann cell proliferation. I. An analysis in tissue culture of proliferation during development, Wallerian degeneration, and direct injury. *J. Cell Biol.* 84:739–752, 1980.

21. Martini, R., and Schachner, M. Immunoelectron microscopic localization of neural cell adhesion molecules (L1, N-CAM, and MAG) and their shared carbohydrate epitope and myelin basic protein in developing sciatic nerve. *J. Cell Biol.* 103:2439–2448, 1986.

22. Heininger, K., Stoll, G., Linington, C., Toyka, K., and Wekerle, H. Conduction failure and nerve conduction slowing in experimental allergic neuritis induced by P_2-specific T-cell lines. *Ann. Neurol.* 19:44–49, 1986.

23. Ouvrier, R. A., McLeod, J. G., and Conchin, T. E. The hypertrophic forms of hereditary motor and sensory neuropathy. *Brain* 110:121–148, 1987.

24. Messing, A., Chen, H. Y., Palmiter, R. D., and Brinster, R. L. Peripheral neuropathies, hepatocellular carcinomas and islet cell adenomas in transgenic mice. *Nature* 316:461–463, 1985.

25. Seizinger, B. R., Martuza, R. L., and Gusella, J. F. Loss of genes on chromosome 22 in tumorigenesis of human acoustic neuroma. *Nature* 322:644–647, 1986.

CHAPTER 36

Diseases Involving Myelin

Richard H. Quarles, Pierre Morell, and Dale E. McFarlin

Basic Neurochemistry: Molecular, Cellular, and Medical Aspects, 4th Ed., edited by G. J. Siegel et al. Raven Press, Ltd., New York, 1989.
Correspondence to Richard H. Quarles, National Institutes of Health, Room 425, Park Building, Bethesda, Maryland 20892.

The title of this chapter emphasizes that myelin cannot be considered an isolated entity because myelin-producing cells and neurons are interactive. For its maintenance in the peripheral nervous system (PNS), myelin depends on the normal functioning of a Schwann cell, and in the central nervous system (CNS), an oligodendrocyte. The integrity of myelin sheaths is also dependent on the viability of the axons that they ensheath and the neuronal cell bodies from which the axons emanate. It is well known, for example, that neuronal death inevitably leads to subsequent degeneration of axons and myelin. Although many conditions are recognized in which preferential loss of myelin occurs, damage to myelin is a common consequence of a multitude of unrelated pathological stigmata (e.g., genetically determined disorders, viral infection, toxic agents, neoplasia, trauma, and anoxia) that happen to affect various cells, including myelin or myelin-supporting cells.

GENERAL CLASSIFICATION

A deficiency of myelin can result either from failure to produce the normal amount of myelin during development or from demyelination. An inpediment of normal myelination is referred to as hypomyelination, or in some cases as dysmyelination. According to the definition of Poser, dysmyelination includes disorders in which "myelin initially formed is abnormally constituted, thus inherently unstable, vulnerable, and liable to degeneration" [25]. Diseases involving demyelination can be subdivided into primary and secondary categories on the basis of morphological observations. Primary demyelination involves the early destruction of myelin with relative sparing of axons; subsequently, other structures may be affected. Secondary demyelination includes those disorders in which myelin is involved after damage to neurons or axons. The classification scheme in this chapter is based on etiology as well as comparative neuropathology. Disorders causing hypomyelination and demyelination are both included in the four categories: (1) acquired allergic and infectious diseases; (2) genetically determined disorders; (3) toxic and nutritional disorders; and (4) disorders primarily affecting neurons with secondary involvement of myelin.

Biochemical changes in brain are similar in demyelinating diseases regardless of etiology

The most pronounced changes occur in white matter where there is a marked increase in the water content, a decrease of myelin proteins and lipids, and, in many cases, the appearance of cholesterol esters [1]. Table 1 details the results of demyelination caused by a genetically determined metabolic disorder, adrenoleukodystrophy (ALD), and of demyelination secondary to a viral infection, subacute sclerosing panencephalitis (SSPE) [2]. These changes can be explained by the breakdown and gradual loss of myelin, which is relatively rich in solids, and its replacement by extracellular fluid, astrocytes, and inflammatory cells. These cells are more hydrated, relatively lipid poor, and free of myelin-specific constituents. The frequent appearance of cholesterol esters in demyelinating diseases is apparently related to the fact that cholesterol is one myelin component that cannot be degraded to smaller units by phagocytes. Therefore, it is esterified and often remains in this form in phagocytes at the site of the lesion for some time. Since cholesterol esters are essentially absent from normal mature brain, their presence in myelin disorders is indicative of recent demyelination. Such compounds are also responsible for the neutral fat staining, or sudanophilia, demonstrated histochemically in many demyelinating diseases. The magnitude of the changes mentioned above varies considerably from specimen to specimen in the same

TABLE 1. Human white matter composition in two diseases compared with controls[a]

Component	SSPE		ALD	
	Control	Patient	Control	Patient
Water[b]	72	88.5	72.5	84.3
Proteolipid[c]			8.2	1.4
Total lipid[c]	60	23.4	56.3	34.7
Cholesterol	14	6.1	14.4	9.3
Cholesterol ester	0.2	1.8		9.9
Cerebroside	13	{0.8	{10.6	{0.8
Sulfatide	3.5	{3		
Total phospholipid	30	15	25	8.5
Ethanolamine phosphatides	10.2	4.7	7.9	1.3
Lecithin	7.5	4.8	7.3	2.7
Sphingomyelin	5.4	2.9	4.2	1.6
Serine phosphatides	5.9	1.7	5.0	1.6
Phosphatidylinositol	0.8	0.7	0.3	0.7

[a] (SSPE) subacute sclerosing panencephalitis; (ALD) adrenoleukodystrophy; source of data [2].
[b] Percentage of wet weight.
[c] Proteolipid, total lipid, and individual lipids as percentages of white matter dry weight.

disease depending on the severity, duration, and activity of the disease process.

ACQUIRED DISORDERS OF MYELIN HAVING AN ALLERGIC OR INFECTIOUS BASIS, OR BOTH

Nervous system damage in the acquired allergic and infectious demyelinating diseases is specifically directed against myelin or myelin-forming cells, and there is relatively little damage to other parenchymal elements. In most cases (except where noted otherwise), the lesions are inflammatory and are characterized by the following criteria:

1. Perivenular demyelination
2. Perivenular inflammation
3. Relative sparing of axons
4. Macrophage activity in the lesions
5. Disseminated lesions
6. Pia-arachnoid inflammation

7. Sudanophilic deposits, presumably products of myelin degradation

The extent to which these criteria are fulfilled depends on the particular type and phase of disease. Furthermore, it is not always clear whether the immunologic activity is autoimmune in nature or whether it is related primarily to an antecedent viral infection; nor is the extent of damage directly ascribable to putative viral agents known at the present time. (Most of the diseases discussed here are reviewed in more detail elsewhere [3].)

Multiple sclerosis is the most common demyelinating disease of the CNS in humans

Multiple sclerosis (MS) is usually chronic and is characterized by demyelinated areas called plaques in the CNS. The most typical onset of MS occurs in the second or third decade of life and is manifested by exacerbations and remissions over many years, but the disease is sometimes slowly progressive from the beginning. In a small number of patients, there is an acute form that rapidly progresses over weeks and months to death within a year. Lesions in the white matter can now be visualized and monitored by magnetic resonance imaging (MRI) in living patients. The diagnosis is based on classical clinical criteria, but MRI and cerebrospinal fluid abnormalities can be useful. (The interested reader is referred to other reviews [1,3–7] for more details on this major demyelinating disease in humans.)

At autopsy, plaques can be identified grossly. They are characterized by an absence or severe reduction of myelin and oligodendrocytes and the preservation of relatively normal-appearing axons. There is a strong tendency for plaques to be periventricular. Light microscopy of early lesions shows venules surrounded by lymphocytes, macrophages, and plasma cells. The greatest cellularity is found at the margins of acute lesions and is believed to be the location at which some of the earliest changes associated with myelin loss are occurring. Electron microscopy of such areas indicates that a major mechanism for myelin destruction is the direct removal of myelin lamellae from the surface of intact sheaths by macrophages. This involves the attachment of superficial lamellae to coated pits at the macrophage surface, implying the presence of receptors that bind to a ligand on the myelin. It may be that Fc receptors on the macrophages are binding immunoglobulins attached to the myelin, but this has not been established. For many years there has been discussion about whether the primary pathological effect in this disease is directed at oligodendrocytes or myelin sheaths, and, although this question may not be totally resolved, recent observations of apparently healthy oligodendrocytes in areas of active demyelination suggest that myelin sheaths themselves are the primary targets. Older chronic lesions are sharply defined and contain bare nonmyelinated axons and many fibrous astrocytes.

Biochemical analyses of MS lesions reveal an increase of catabolic enzymes and a severe loss of myelin proteins and lipids

Affected areas of MS white matter have the expected decrease of myelin constituents and a buildup of cholesterol esters (for review, see Norton and Cammer [1]). For example, polyacrylamide gel electrophoresis of homogenates of macroscopically normal-appearing white matter, outer periplaque, inner periplaque, and plaque show the expected decline of myelin basic protein (MBP) and proteolipid protein (PLP) in going from the normal-appearing white matter to the center of the plaque in both chronic and acute lesions (Fig. 1). There is a virtual absence of these myelin proteins in the center of the chronic plaque and an accumulation of glial fibrillary acidic protein (GFAP), indicative of astrogliosis. A plaque from a more acute lesion is not completely demyelinated, as indicated by the presence of some MBP and PLP, and there is no accumulation of GFAP indicative of astrogliosis. The more acute plaque contains albumin, indicative of breakdown of the blood-brain barrier. Immunocytochemical and quantitative biochemical analyses of myelin proteins have revealed that myelin-associated glycoprotein (MAG) is often decreased more than other myelin proteins at the periphery of plaques and suggests that this glycoprotein is involved early in the pathological events [1,8]. A number of biochemical studies have indicated that myelin constituents are significantly reduced, even in some areas of macroscopically normal-appearing white matter of MS brain in comparison to control white matter [1,8], and this is most likely explained by the presence of microlesions throughout the affected brain. Although the yield of myelin from MS tissue is

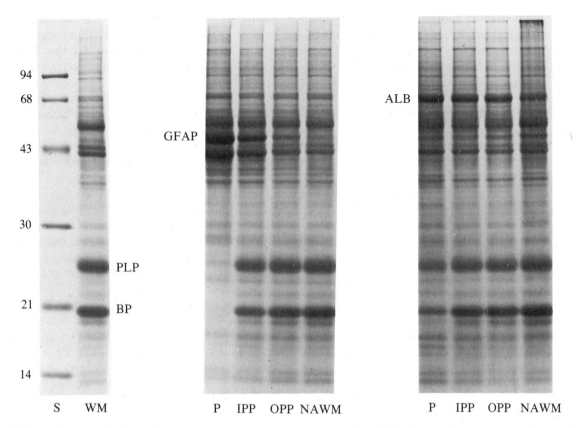

FIG. 1. Polyacrylamide gel electrophoresis of proteins in control and MS tissue. Total proteins of control and affected MS tissues were made soluble with a detergent (sodium dodecyl sulfate) and electrophoresed on a polyacrylamide gel system that separates proteins according to their size. After electrophoresis, the proteins were stained with Coomassie brilliant blue dye. **Left panel:** Molecular weight standards (S) labeled according to their size in kilodaltons and the proteins of control human white matter (WM). **Center panel:** Samples from a chronic MS plaque region. **Right panel:** Samples from an acute MS plaque region. Tissue samples: (P) plaque; (IPP) inner periplaque; (OPP) outer periplaque; (NAWM) macroscopically normal-appearing white matter. Proteins: (PLP) proteolipid protein; (BP) myelin basic protein; (GFAP) glial fibrillary acidic protein; (ALB) albumin. (From Johnson et al. [8].)

reduced, most studies indicate that there is no compositional difference between isolated MS and control myelin, suggesting that the etiology of MS is unlikely to be due to an underlying defect in myelin composition.

Plaque formation in MS tissue is thought to involve proteases and other catabolic enzymes [1]. MBP is highly susceptible to proteases even when present in myelin membranes. A neutral protease released by stimulated macrophages catalyzes the conversion of plasminogen to plasmin, which rapidly degrades MBP [1]. Acid proteinase and other acidic degradative enzymes, presumably lysosomal and of macrophage origin, are elevated in affected MS tissue and are likely to be involved in the breakdown of myelin proteins and lipids. In addition, protease activities intrinsic to myelin sheaths (such as Ca^{2+}-activated neutral protease) may facilitate myelin destruction [9,10]. Immunologically reactive, proteolytic fragments of MBP appear in the cerebrospinal fluid of MS patients during exacerbations of the disease [1,4] and presumably reflect myelin breakdown. Measurements of MBP-related material in cerebrospinal fluid, and possibly in urine, may be useful in monitoring the course of disease activity in patients; however, the presence of this material in the cerebrospinal fluid is not specific for MS, since it occurs in other conditions with myelin damage, such as stroke and encephalitis.

Although the cause of MS is unknown, genetic, immunological, and environmental factors are believed to contribute

Two types of studies have provided data that favor a genetic component [4]. The prevalence of MS varies among ethnic groups. It is quite rare among Bantu, Yakutes, Hutterites, and Inuit and is low in the Japanese and in Hungarian gypsies. The occurrence of MS in families is well known, and it is generally agreed that there is increased risk among first-degree relatives of individuals with the disease. Twin studies have shown a higher concordance in monozygotic twins than dizygotic twins. These observations have led to the conclusion that there is a significant genetic component and that two or more genes predispose to susceptibility in addition to an environmental factor. One group of genes linked to susceptibility includes those which code for histocompatibility molecules of the human leukocyte antigen (HLA) system. These molecules present antigen to immune cells. A number of diseases have been shown to be associated with various HLA genes, and in MS a strong association has been found with HLA molecules A3, B7, and DR-2 in patients of northern European Caucasian background; however, the presence of DR-2 is neither necessary nor sufficient to confer susceptibility to the disease. A second family of genes receiving considerable contemporary emphasis are those which encode for the T-lymphocyte receptor molecules involved in antigen recognition.

Epidemiological studies have provided data that support an environmental factor, possibly an infectious agent. The prevalence of MS is known to vary in different regions. A high prevalence is found above 40° north latitude, and a lower prevalence is found below 12°. Migrants from areas of different risks assume the risk of the region to which they migrate, provided that the age of migration is prior to age 15 years. After this age, the migrant essentially has the risk of the original area. This would be consistent with the involvement of an infectious agent acquired early in life. Finally, clusters of MS cases are well described. The best example is in the Faroe Islands, where there were no reports of MS prior to World War II. Clustering of cases after this time suggests that an environmental agent, possibly infectious and related to the arrival of the British troops, was important.

A viral etiology for MS has been proposed for decades [4,6,11]. Several indirect lines of evidence support this possibility. As indicated above, the data suggesting an environmental factor are consistent with it being a virus and suggest that the disease is related to childhood exposure, followed by a long latency. Next, there have been a number of naturally occurring experimental animal models in which the clinical disease caused by viruses have long incubation periods and evoke primary demyelination with sparing of axons. Although a possible viral etiology has stimulated an extensive amount of research, a definite causative agent has not been identified. Efforts to confirm a virus in the CNS of MS patients have included morphological studies and numerous attempts at isolation as well as transmission. To date, at least 12 agents have been proposed as candidates, and a human retrovirus has been the most recent addition. An agent of this type is attractive because retroviruses characteristically produce persistent infection and use virus-coded DNA polymerase (reverse transcriptase) to become incorporated into the host genome and, as such, hide in the cell.

Immunological mechanisms have been implicated in the pathogenesis of MS for many reasons [4,7]:

1. Perivenular infiltration of inflammatory cells seen in pathology specimens
2. Similarity of the pathology to the immune-mediated postvaccinial encephalomyelitis and experimental allergic encephalomyelitis (EAE) (see next section)
3. Abnormalities of immunoglobulin synthesis, resulting in oligoclonal bands in the CSF of most patients
4. Association with certain HLA types that are linked to immune-response genes
5. Variety of recently described abnormalities of cellular immune function
6. Clinical response seen after the administration of pharmacological agents that modify immune function, such as corticosteroids and immunosuppressants

It is also noteworthy that a recent trial of γ-interferon, which has the capacity to upregulate the immune response, seems to have accentuated exacerbations of the disease.

It should be emphasized that the above evidence suggesting an immune pathogenesis for MS does not exclude the likelihood of a viral etiology. It may be that an infectious agent somehow elicits an immune reaction that is responsible for the demyelination. For example, a coat protein of a virus might mimic some structural feature of the myelin sheath and thus induce an autoimmune reaction [11]: however, despite indications that immunological mechanisms are involved in the demyelination of MS, numerous attempts to identify a viral or brain antigen that is the target of a strong and meaningful humoral or cellular immune response in this disease have been unsuccessful [4,7]. Thus,

although it is widely thought that MS is an autoimmune disease instigated by an infectious agent, the putative antigen(s) and virus remain elusive.

Experimental allergic encephalomyelitis is an autoimmune model of demyelination

Shortly after Pasteur introduced rabies virus vaccination, it was noted that a small minority of individuals receiving this treatment developed an encephalomyelitis. Autopsy of fatal cases showed widespread lesions in the white matter that were somewhat similar to those in MS and quite distinct from features usually observed in rabies. Production of the vaccine involved growing the virus in CNS tissue, and this disorder was reproduced in monkeys by Rivers and co-workers by means of multiple injections of normal CNS tissue. Following the introduction of adjuvants by Freund, it was possible to produce this experimental model, EAE [4,12,13], with a single injection of CNS tissue. This prompted an extensive search for the responsible antigen in the hope of developing desensitization techniques that might be efficacious in the treatment of MS. The encephalitogen found was documented by Einstein, Kies, and co-workers to be MBP. EAE has subsequently been produced in many species, including monkeys, rabbits, guinea pigs, rats, and mice. A number of forms of EAE that vary clinically and pathologically have been described. The age and species of the animal under study, the inoculum, and the use of various adjuvants are important variables that may influence the clinical and pathological aspects as well as pathogenetic mechanisms.

MBP is a major component of myelin of all mammals, although there are some amino acid sequence differences among species, and within any one species MBP exists in a number of molecular forms. Much is known about the encephalitogenic epitopes of MBP that may vary in different species and even in different inbred strains of a given species, as summarized by Alvord [14]. For example, the portion of the molecule (residues 116–124) that causes EAE in strain 13 guinea pigs is conserved among various species. Consequently, EAE can easily be produced in this animal with MBP from virtually any vertebrate; however, the portion of the molecule (residues 74–87) that produces EAE in Lewis rats varies among different species. Consequently, the source of MBP is a critical variable in studies of EAE in Lewis rats. In SJL mice, the portion of the molecule that causes EAE resides in the C-terminal half of the molecule, whereas in some other strains exemplified by PL mice, the encephalitogenic epitope resides in the first nine N-terminal amino acids, including the terminal acetyl group.

Pathogenetic mechanisms responsible for autoimmune disorders have been investigated in EAE. Patterson demonstrated that the disease could be transferred from affected animals to normal animals with immune cells but not with serum from the affected animals. It is now established that the subset of T-lymphocytes responsible for the transfer of disease in mice, rats, and guinea pigs is analogous to the human CD4 subset. This subset recognizes antigen in association with class II major histocompatibility molecules (Ia). These molecules present antigen to T-cells and are under genetic control. In a number of species, the production of EAE is linked to these genes. Also, it seems likely that other genes make contributions to susceptibility, at least in some species. It is critical to determine where antigen recognition occurs and how this produces demyelination. Most workers agree that demyelination is largely mediated by macrophages, as originally described by Lampert. Electron microscopy of demyelinating lesions in EAE has shown the presence of macrophages binding myelin via coated pits in a manner indistinguishable from that occurring in MS, but the underlying mechanisms that direct macrophages to myelin are unknown (see Brostoff [12], Raine [13], and Alvord [14] for additional references).

Components of myelin other than MBP also show immunoreactivity. PLP has been reported to be encephalitogenic in some species. In some EAE models, antibodies to various myelin lipids such as galactocerebroside may contribute to the pathogenesis.

Chronic EAE and chronic relapsing EAE have been produced in animals [4,13]. These model diseases are of particular importance because they show closer resemblance to MS than acute EAE, both with regard to the clinical course of the disease and the extent of demyelination that occurs. Such models are important in the investigation of immune regulation, the pathogenesis of lesions in white matter, and in the use of experimental treatments for modification of disease. Initially, Stone, Raine, Wisniewsky, and colleagues showed that chronic relapsing EAE could be produced in guinea pigs by the injection of whole CNS tissue, in contrast to injection with MBP. Such experiments have led to speculation that the chronic disease was in part due to immune response against components of myelin other than MBP. This was supported by experimental data and the recent reports that PLP is encephalitogenic; however, in some species, including rats, monkeys, and mice, chronic relapsing disease has been produced in mice by the adoptive transfer of cells sensitized to MBP, and Zanvill and co-workers have produced chronic relapsing EAE in PL mice after transfer of T-cell clones, which react with a single epitope of MBP. These studies on chronic relapsing EAE illustrate two important points: (1) Immune reactivity to components other than MBP may significantly contribute to the clinical and pathological findings in some models; and (2) a clonal T-cell response to MBP is sufficient to give rise to chronic relapsing disease, at least in mice. Although the underlying mechanisms are not known, it is possible that the initial disease produced by T-cell reactivity to MBP leads to sensitization against other myelin components (see Goodman and McFarlin [4] and Raine [13] for references).

Landry-Guillain-Barré syndrome is an acute monophasic inflammatory demyelinating disease of the PNS, often preceded by a viral infection

Inflammatory demyelinating neuropathies also occur in chronic relapsing as well as acute forms [1,3,15]. With regard to Landry-Guillain-Barré syndrome (LGBS) and other demyelinating diseases of the peripheral nervous system (PNS), it should be kept in mind that PNS and CNS myelin, although morphologically related, differ significantly in chemical composition, especially in protein constituents (see Chap. 6). Immunocytochemical studies have indicated that all the PNS myelin proteins (P0, P1, P2, and MAG) are decreased or absent in demyelinated regions of nerve obtained at autopsy or biopsy [1]. Cumulative evidence suggests that the nerve injury is mediated by immunological mechanisms, but, as in MS, the role of the patients' cell-mediated and humoral responses in causing the demyelination has not been fully defined. Humoral immunity may play a role in the disease, as suggested by findings that sera from LGBS patients cause demyelination in appropriate test systems and that plasmapheresis is an effective therapy in some of these patients [15]. Although experimental allergic neuritis (EAN) is often considered to be a good animal model of this human disease, and the P2 myelin protein is implicated as an important antigen in this model (see Chap. 35), neither cellular nor humoral immunity to P2 has been detected consistently in LGBS [15]. Similarly, although antibodies to galactocerebroside have been shown to cause peripheral demyelination in laboratory animals, evidence for significant levels of antibodies to this glycolipid in LGBS is lacking

[15]. Recent investigations have detected high levels of antiganglioside antibodies in approximately 20 percent of LGBS patients [16], but the relevance of these antibodies to the pathology remains to be established. Since the P0 and P1 proteins of PNS myelin are degraded *in vitro* by enzymes secreted by activated macrophages in the presence of plasminogen, it has been speculated that early stages of myelin dissolution in LGBS may involve plasmin [1].

Demyelination of the PNS occurs in association with paraproteinemia

In contrast to the inability to demonstrate a strong immune response against a known myelin antigen in MS or in most LGBS patients, the presence of antibodies reacting with a myelin protein has been demonstrated clearly in a rarer type of demyelinating peripheral neuropathy. The paraproteinemia occurring together with this type of neuropathy results from the neoplastic expansion of a clone of plasma cells and leads to large amounts of a monoclonal antibody in the patient's serum. About half of the monoclonal IgM antibodies occurring in patients with this type of neuropathy have been shown to bind to MAG [10]. All of these human anti-MAG monoclonal antibodies bind to an antigenic determinant in the carbohydrate part of the MAG molecule, and this carbohydrate antigen is also present on some glycolipids and other glycoproteins that are present in the PNS but not the CNS [10,16]. The principal antigenic glycolipid has been identified as sulfate-3-glucuronyl paragloboside, and the sulfated glucuronic acid is an important part of the epitope. In other neuropathy patients, the monoclonal IgM antibodies do not react with MAG but often react with ganglioside antigens of nerve [16]. It may be that the monoclonal antibodies occurring in these patients cause the neuropathies by binding to myelin or Schwann cell antigens, but a causal relationship remains to be established.

Other acquired demyelinating disorders in humans may be secondary to viral infections, neoplasias, or immunosuppressive therapy

Acute disseminated encephalomyelitis

Acute disseminated encephalomyelitis, also called postinfectious or postimmunization encephalitis, represents a group of disorders of usually mixed viral immunological etiology. The condition is most commonly related to a spontaneous viral infection, of which major examples are measles, smallpox, and chickenpox [3,6].

Progressive multifocal leukoencephalopathy

Progressive multifocal leukoencephalopathy (PML) is a rare demyelinating disease that is usually associated with disorders of the reticuloendothelial system, neoplasms, and immunosuppressive therapy [3,6]. Lesions are noninflammatory and are apparently caused by infection of oligodendrocytes with a papovavirus.

Animal diseases are recognized in which inflammatory changes, primary demyelination, and, frequently, a viral infection are major components of the disease process

Canine distemper encephalomyelitis

Canine distemper encephalomyelitis is a viral-induced CNS demyelinating disease in dogs [6]. Lesions show a strong inflammatory response, and some similarities to acute disseminated encephalomyelitis exist.

Visna

Visna is a slowly progressive demyelinating disease of sheep caused by a retrovirus [6]. It is claimed by some to be of relevance to the study of MS, but other workers consider visna not specifically demyelinative in type.

Mouse hepatitis virus encephalomyelitis

Mouse hepatitis virus encephalomyelitis is caused by a neurotropic corona virus strain (JHM virus) [6]. This virus produces a direct infection of oligodendrocytes in mice and a chronic demyelinating disease [6,11]. Rats infected with JHM virus develop T-cell sensitization to both virus and myelin basic protein [11].

Theiler's virus encephalomyelitis

Theiler's virus encephalomyelitis is a picornavirus-induced disease of the CNS associated with demyelination [6]. It produces a persistent CNS infection in mice and inflammatory demyelinating lesions mediated by T-cells reactive with viral antigens [11].

Border disease

Border disease occurs in sheep as a result of prenatal infection with a pestivirus [17]. In contrast to the viral diseases described above that cause demyelination, this is a disease in which the virus interferes with myelin formation during development, resulting in a myelin deficit similar to that occurring in hypomyelinating genetic mutants, discussed next.

GENETICALLY DETERMINED DISORDERS OF MYELIN

There is a large group of genetically determined disorders of CNS white matter, most of which have their onset in humans before the age of 10 years. Morphologically, the diseases demonstrate a diffuse deficiency of myelin in white matter areas and are often termed leukodystrophies. Included among the human disorders of this type are some of the sphingolipidoses in which a specific lipid accumulates due to a genetic lesion in an enzyme that is involved in its catabolism [e.g., metachromatic leukodystrophy (MLD)]. Major points about MLD and other genetically determined human diseases leading to hypomyelination are summarized in Table 2. This category also includes the various hypomyelinating mutations in mice and other species that are of particular value to neurochemists because of their availability for experimentation aimed at elucidating molecular mechanisms of myelinogenesis. These mutants often have names relating to their characteristic tremor due to the myelin deficit (e.g., shiverer and jimpy mice), and the principal facts about some of the most important ones are given in Table 3. In many cases the primary genetic lesions are not known, but recent recombinant DNA techniques have led to identification of the primary genetic defects in some. (The genetically determined myelin disorders have been reviewed in detail elsewhere [1,3,18,20].)

The composition of myelin in genetically determined disorders can be normal, have a specific alteration reflecting the genetic lesion, or show a nonspecific pathological composition found in many myelin disorders

The composition of the small amount of myelin isolated from Krabbe's leukodystrophy is nor-

TABLE 2. Genetically determined disorders affecting myelin in humans

Disorder	Inheritance	Genetic lesion	Comments	Ref.
Metachromatic leukodystrophy	AR[a]	Aryl sulfatase A	Accumulation of sulfatide in brain; increased sulfatide in isolated myelin (see Table 4)	1, 3, 18; see also Chap. 37
Krabbe's leukodystrophy	AR	Galactocerebroside-β-galactosidase	Globoid cells contain galactocerebroside; small amount of myelin formed has normal composition	1, 3, 18; see also Chap. 37
Refsum's disease	AR	Oxidation of branched-chain fatty acids	Increase of branched-chain phytanic acid, especially prominent in PNS myelin	1, 3; see also Chap. 37
Adrenoleukodystrophy	X-linked	Peroxidation of long-chain fatty acids	Inflammation and lipid storage in CNS; myelin is of nonspecific pathological type	3, 18
Canavan's disease (spongy degeneration)	AR	Unknown	Widespread edema in white matter with diminished myelin; isolated myelin is nonspecific pathological type (see Table 4)	3
Pelizaeus-Merzbacher disease	X-linked	Likely to be PLP gene [19]	Severe hypomyelination; may be similar to jimpy murine mutant (see Table 3)	1, 3
Phenylketonuria	AR	Phenylalanine hydroxylase	White matter up to 40 percent deficient in myelin; hypomyelination may be caused by inhibition of amino acid transport or protein synthesis by high levels of phenylalanine	1, 3; see also Chap. 38

[a] (AR) autosomal recessive.

TABLE 3. Hypomyelinating murine mutants

Mutant	Inheritance	Genetic lesion	Comments
Shiverer [20]	Autosomal recessive	Large deletion in MBP gene	Severe hypomyelination of CNS with nearly normal myelination in PNS
			Almost complete absence of MBP in CNS and PNS
			Mutant phenotype corrected in transgenic Shiverer mice, with expression of 20 percent of normal amount of MBP [21]
			Myelin-deficient (MLD) mouse [20] also involves the MBP gene
Jimpy [20]	X-linked	Mutation in PLP gene resulting in deletion in mRNA due to aberrant splicing [22,23]	Severe hypomyelination of CNS, with normal PNS
			Nearly complete absence of PLP
			Other X-linked mutants with CNS specific hypomyelination, such as the myelin-deficient rat [20], shaking dog [20], and Pelizaeus-Merzbacher disease in man [19] probably also involve the PLP gene
Quaking [20]	Autosomal recessive	Unknown	Hypomyelination in CNS and PNS, with CNS more severely affected
			Possibly a defect in myelin assembly
Trembler [20]	Autosomal dominant	Unknown	Hypomyelination in PNS with normal CNS
			Primary defect is in Schwann cells

TABLE 4. Human myelin composition in three diseases compared with controls[a]

Lipids[b]	Control	Spongy degeneration	SSPE	MLD
Total lipid (% of dry weight)	70.0	63.8	73.7	63.2
Cholesterol	27.7	58.0	43.7	21.2
Cerebrosides	22.7	8.0	18.8	9.0
Sulfatides	3.8	2.0	2.8	28.4
Total phospholipids	43.1	33.4	36.6	36.1
Ethanolamine phosphatides	15.6	9.8	9.7	8.1
Plasmalogen[c]	12.3		9.1	5.3
Lecithin	11.2	11.3	10.4	10.7
Sphingomyelin	7.9	5.9	8.8	7.1
Serine phosphatides	4.8	5.5	4.6	3.8
Phosphatidylinositol	0.6	0.8	1.4	3.1

[a] (SSPE) subacute sclerosing panencephalitis; (MLD) metachromatic leukodystrophy; source of data [2].
[b] Individual lipids expressed as weight percentage of total lipid.
[c] Most of the plasmalogen is phosphatidyl ethanolamine and is also included in the ethanolamine phosphatides column.

mal, whereas that isolated from cases of MLD is enriched in sulfatide (Table 4). It is not known for certain whether the myelin formed in MLD is unstable because of the excess sulfatide and, thus, degenerates or whether the excess sulfatide in the isolated myelin fraction represents sulfatide micelles that are coisolated during the myelin purification. In some genetic disorders, such as adrenoleukodystrophy and Canavan's disease (spongy degeneration), as well as in a wide variety of disorders involving secondary demyelination, the myelin preparations have similar abnormal chemical compositions. This is shown in Table 4 for Canavan's disease and subacute sclerosing panencephalomyelitis (SSPE). Certain experimental disorders induced in animals by toxic agents show the same type of abnormality with respect to isolated myelin. In each case, the isolated pathological myelin has a grossly normal ultrastructural appearance; however, it has much more cholesterol, less cerebroside, and less phosphatidal ethanolamine than does normal human myelin. Myelin with this abnormal composition is referred to as the nonspecific pathological type and probably represents a partially degraded form. It is possible that the degradation involves macrophages. When a considerable accumulation of cholesterol esters are found in whole brain, such compounds are not in the myelin itself. The purification of myelin involves discontinuous sucrose gradients; and a light fraction, containing cholesterol esters, is separated from the denser myelin.

TOXIC AND NUTRITIONAL DISORDERS OF MYELIN

Diphtheria toxin causes fragmentation of myelin sheaths in the PNS

Diphtheritic neuropathy [1] is a possible complication of *Corynebacterium diphtheriae* infection and is characterized by vacuolation and fragmentation of myelin sheaths in the PNS. A similar disorder can be caused by injection of animals with the toxin, which may act by inhibiting protein synthesis of Schwann cells or by binding to myelin and producing channels in the membrane.

Organotins and hexachlorophene cause edematous demyelination, with splitting of myelin at the intraperiod line and without apparent damage to myelinating cells

A number of biochemical studies have been done on the triethyltin model, brought about by the inclusion of this compound in the drinking water of rats. Chronic administration of triethyltin may result in a loss of one-fourth to one-half of the total myelin, relative to untreated control animals. The myelin isolated is of the nonspecific pathological type with high cholesterol and low cerebroside, sulfatide, and ethanolamine plasmalogen. The massive myelin loss is not accompanied by inflammatory cells, and the levels of various proteinases are not elevated as they are in such disorders as EAE. The mechanism by which myelin is damaged under these conditions is unknown, but it clearly contrasts with the situation observed in the acquired demyelinating disorders. It is interesting to note that there may be almost complete recovery of myelin after triethyltin is removed from drinking water. Hexachlorophene is another agent that causes a similar reversible edematous demyelination and has been of clinical significance because it was used as an antiseptic agent for humans [1].

In neurochemical studies on edematous demyelination, loss of myelin is an operational term, since part of the myelin is converted to a form with different physical properties that is not isolated with normal myelin. Indeed, when animals are treated with triethyltin or with hexachlorophene, a somewhat lighter "floating fraction," containing many myelin components can be recovered [1]. This fraction probably represents degenerating myelin and does not contain cholesterol esters. It must be emphasized that this type of floating fraction is different from the cholesterol ester-rich floating fractions mentioned earlier that can be isolated in some of the hereditary diseases such as adrenoleukodystrophy.

Lead is a common environmental pollutant that is known to cause hypomyelination and demyelination

Suckling rats exposed to high doses of lead salts fail to myelinate normally in the CNS, apparently due to retarded growth and maturation of neurons; but the PNS is not affected. Trialkyllead administration to animals does not cause edematous demyelination, as is seen with trialkyltin, but it does inhibit myelinogenesis in rats when administered to developing animals. In addition, lead can cause segmental demyelination of the PNS in guinea pigs and humans. Effects of lead poisoning vary with species, age, dosage, and region of the nervous system [1].

Undernourishment leads to a preferential reduction in myelin formation

Much of the CNS myelin in mammals is formed during a relatively restricted time period, corresponding to the first few years of life in humans and days 15 to 30 in rats. Just before this rapid deposition of myelin, there is a burst of oligodendroglial cell proliferation. During these restricted periods of time, a large portion of the brain's metabolic activity and protein and lipid synthetic capacity are involved in myelinogenesis. This developmental phenomenon has practical input for the understanding of hypomyelination disorders. Any metabolic insult during the vulnerable period may lead to a preferential reduction in myelin formation. A model

system for such studies is obtained by limiting access of rat pups to the mother and thus inducing undernourishment. Starvation of rats from birth onward leads to a deficit in myelin lipids and proteins and a reduced amount of isolatable myelin compared with normally fed littermate controls. The size of whole brain is also somewhat reduced, but it is clear that the depression of myelin-specific lipids and proteins is greater than that of other brain components (see Smith and Benjamins [24] for review). The implication is that there is preferential depression in the synthesis of myelin-specific components during starvation, an interpretation that has been directly demonstrated by *in vivo* isotope incorporation experiments. Possibly, there is not only depression in the amount of myelin deposited (in part due to a lessened number of oligodendroglial cells), but the developmental program with regard to myelinogenesis is also somewhat delayed. The most vulnerable period appears to be the time of oligodendroglia proliferation, since animals deprived during this period have an irreversible deficit of myelin-forming cells and hypomyelination. Animals deprived at a later age, however, can often demonstrate significant catchup with regard to the amount of myelin when nutritional rehabilitation is initiated after a period of underfeeding.

Deficiencies of specific substances can cause myelin deficits

Failure to myelinate properly and demyelination are also associated with deficiencies of dietary protein, essential fatty acids, and several vitamins, including thiamine, B_{12}, and B_6 [3,24] (see Chap. 34). Hypomyelination also has been shown to be caused by copper deficiency in laboratory animals [24], and this model system may be an experimental analog of the sex-linked disorder called trichopoliodystrophy (Menkes' kinky hair disease), in which there appears to be disorder of copper metabolism.

DISORDERS PRIMARILY AFFECTING NEURONS WITH SECONDARY INVOLVEMENT OF MYELIN

A large number of disorders of the nervous system that preferentially cause lesions in gray matter, in particular neurons, and that are associated with ''accidental'' brain damage (infarcts, trauma, tumors, etc.) eventually result in regions of demyelination. Such diseases can be also of viral (SSPE), genetic (Tay-Sachs disease), or of unknown etiology (amyotrophic lateral sclerosis).

Secondary demyelination occurs in subacute sclerosing panencephalitis

The first human disease to be studied with respect to myelin composition during secondary demyelination was SSPE, a CNS disease caused by a defective measles virus infection [1]. It is probable that this disease involves destruction of both neurons and oligodendroglia. The brain white matter shows the typical changes for severe demyelination. The isolated myelin has a grossly normal ultrastructural appearance and a normal lipid-protein ratio; however, it was found to have the typical nonspecific changes with more cholesterol, less cerebroside, and less ethanolamine phosphatides than normal human myelin (Table 4). No cholesterol esters were found in the myelin, although they were abundant in the white matter. Such abnormal myelin has also been isolated from such sphingolipidoses as Tay-Sachs disease, generalized gangliosidosis, and Niemann-Pick disease (see Chap. 37).

The archetypical model for secondary demyelination is Wallerian degeneration

When a nerve (in the PNS) or a myelinated tract (in the CNS) is sectioned surgically, the proximal segment often survives and regenerates. In the distal segment, Wallerian degeneration occurs, with both axons and myelin disappearing rapidly. Debris is phagocytosed by neural cells and by macrophages. From such experiments, it is clear that the integrity of the myelin sheath depends on continued contact with a viable axon. Any disease that results in a general impairment of neuronal function will also result in axonal degeneration and cause onset of myelin breakdown secondary to the neuronal damage [1,24].

During Wallerian degeneration in the PNS, there is a rapid loss of myelin-specific lipids within a period of a week or two. Loss of myelin-specific proteins proceeds even more rapidly, and the disappearance of the major P0 glycoprotein may precede slightly the loss of the basic proteins. There is also a concomitant increase in many lysosomal enzymes. Between the second and fourth week after nerve section most of the myelin debris has been removed, and remyelination of regenerating axons begins.

Wallerian degeneration has been studied in the CNS by enucleating eyes in rats and examining the optic nerve at different times. The degeneration of CNS myelin is a much slower process than is PNS myelin degeneration and takes place within macrophages (not within the myelin-synthesizing cells, as in the PNS). By using this system, it has been demonstrated that the myelin isolated after enucleation, although present in decreasing amounts as degeneration progresses, does not differ significantly from control myelin in composition. It is not of the nonspecific pathological type encountered in other disease processes that lead to secondary demyelination. This may indicate a significant difference in the degenerative processes during surgically induced Wallerian degeneration and the secondary demyelination that follows naturally occurring disease processes (also generally referred to as ''Wallerian'' degeneration by neuropathological criteria). Another possible explanation is that the existence of the nonspecific pathological type of degraded myelin might be transitory and is not detected because of the morphological uniformity of the surgically lesioned nerve.

REMYELINATION

Much of this chapter has considered biochemical mechanisms of myelin loss, but it would not be appropriate to finish without some comments about the capacity of nervous tissue to repair the damage by remyelination [24]. It is well known that the capacity for remyelination is much greater in the PNS than in the CNS. Following nerve transection, as described in the previous section, myelination of the sprouting axons occurs soon after the final cleanup of myelin debris by Schwann cells. The Schwann cells that form the new myelin are probably not the same as those that phagocytose the debris but appear to arise by cell division. As expected, experiments have shown increased incorporation of radioactive precursors into myelin components during the remyelination phase. The difference in remyelinating ability between the PNS and the CNS may lie in the nature of the myelin-forming cells; that is, in the requirement for oligodendrocytes to myelinate many axons, in contrast to the single segments of myelin formed by Schwann cells. Under some circumstances, such as in EAE and MS, it has been demonstrated that Schwann cells will migrate into the spinal cord and remyelinate demyelinated CNS axons.

Despite the limited remyelination that generally occurs in the CNS, there is some capacity of oligodendrocytes to remyelinate. For example, it has been demonstrated that greater remyelination can be promoted in animals with chronic EAE by prolonged treatment with MBP and galactocerebroside [13]. In addition, careful observations of acute MS lesions have demonstrated the presence of healthy oligodendrocytes and regeneration of myelin in the presence

of myelin breakdown [5]. Such observations raise the possibility that management of patients with demyelinating diseases of the CNS may eventually involve treatments that stimulate the natural ability of the oligodendrocytes for remyelination.

REFERENCES

1. Norton, W. T., and Cammer, W. Chemical pathology of diseases involving myelin. In P. Morell (ed.), *Myelin*. New York: Plenum Press, 1984, pp. 311–335.
2. Morell, P., Borstein, M. B., and Raine, C. S. Diseases involving myelin. In G. J. Siegel, R. W. Albers, B. W. Agranoff, and R. Katzman. (eds.), *Basic Neurochemistry*, 3rd. ed., Boston: Little Brown and Co., 1981, pp. 641–660.
3. Traugot, U., and Raine, C. S. The neurology of myelin diseases. In P. Morell (ed.), *Myelin*. New York: Plenum Press, 1984, pp. 311–335.
4. Goodman, A., and McFarlin, D. E. Multiple sclerosis. *Curr. Neurol.* 7:91–128, 1987.
5. Prineas, J. W. The neuropathology of multiple sclerosis. In P. J. Vinken, G. W. Bruyn, H. L. Klawans, and J. C. Koetsier (eds.), *Demyelinating Diseases (Handbook of Clinical Neurology, Vol. 47)*. Amsterdam: Elsevier, 1985, pp. 213–258.
6. Johnson, R. T. Viral aspects of multiple sclerosis. In P. J. Vinken, G. W. Bruyn, H. L. Klawans, and J. C. Koestsier (eds.), *Demyelinating Diseases (Handbook of Clinical Neurology, Vol. 47)*. Amsterdam: Elsevier, 1985, pp. 319–336.
7. Reder, A. T. and Arnason, B. G. W. Immunology of multiple sclerosis. In P. J. Vinken, G. W. Bruyn, H. L. Klawans, and J. C. Koetsier (eds.), *Demyelinating Diseases (Handbook of Clinical Neurology, Vol. 47)*. Amsterdam: Elsevier, 1985, pp. 337–397.
8. Johnson, D., Sato, S., Quarles, R. H., Inuzuka, T. Brady, R. O., and Torutellotte, W. W. Quantitation of the myelin-associated glycoprotein in human nervous tissue for controls and multiple sclerosis patients. *J. Neurochem.* 46:1086–1093, 1986.
9. Banik, N. L., McAlhaney, W. W., and Hogan, E. L. Calcium stimulated proteolysis in myelin:

Evidence for a Ca^{2+}-activated neutral proteinase associated purified myelin of rat CNS. *J. Neurochem.* 45:1389–1405, 1985.

10. Quarles, R. H. Myelin-associated glycoprotein: Functional and clinical aspects. In P. J. Marangos, I. Campbell, and R. H. Cohen (eds.), *Functional and Clinical Aspects of Neuronal and Glial Proteins (Neurobiological Research, Vol. II)*. Petaluma, CA: Academic Press, 1988, pp. 295–320.

11. Waksman, B. H., and Reingold, S. C. Viral etiology of multiple sclerosis: Where does the truth lie? *Trends Neurosci.* 9:388–391, 1986.

12. Brostoff, S. W. Immunological responses to myelin and myelin components. In P. Morell (ed.), *Myelin*. New York: Plenum Press, 1984, pp. 405–440.

13. Raine, C. S. Experimental allergic encephalomyelitis and experimental allergic neuritis. In P. J. Vinken, G. W. Bruyn, H. L. Klawans, and J. C. Koetsier (eds.), *Demyelinating Diseases (Handbook of Clinical Neurology, Vol. 47)*. Amsterdam: Elsevier, 1985, pp. 429–466.

14. Alvord, E. C., Jr. Species restricted encephalitogenic determinants. In E. C. Alvord, Jr., M. W. Kies, and A. J. Suckling (eds.), *Experimental Allergic Encephalomyelitis: A Useful Model for Multiple Sclerosis*. New York: Alan R. Liss, 1984, pp. 523–537.

15. Hughes, R. A. C. Demyelinating neuropathy. In P. J. Vinken, G. W. Bruyn, H. L. Klawans, and J. C. Koetsier (eds.), *Demyelinating Disease (Handbook of Clinical Neurology, Vol. 47)*. Amsterdam: Elsevier, 1985, pp. 605–628.

16. Quarles, R. H., Ilyas, A. A., and Willison, H. J. Antibodies to glycolipids in demyelinating diseases of the human peripheral nervous system. *Chem. Phys. Lipids* 42:235–248, 1986.

17. Potts, B. J., Berry, L. J., Osborne, B. I., and Johnson, K. P. Viral persistence and abnormalities of the CNS after congenital infection of sheep with border disease virus. *J. Infect. Dis.* 151:337–343, 1985.

18. Moser, H. W., Leukoencephalopathies caused by metabolic disorders, In P. J. Vinken, G. W. Bruyn, H. L. Klawans, and J. C. Koetsier (eds.), *Demyelinating Diseases (Handbook of Clinical Neurology, Vol. 47)*. Amsterdam: Elsevier, 1985, pp. 583–604.

19. Koeppen, A. H., Ronca, N. A., Greenfield, E. A., and Hans, M. B. Defective biosynthesis of proteolipid protein in Pelizaeus-Merzbacher disease. *Ann. Neurol.* 21:159–170, 1987.

20. Hogan, E. L., and Greenfield, S. Animal models of genetic disorders of myelin. In P. Morell (ed.), *Myelin*. New York: Plenum Press, 1984, pp. 489–504.

21. Readhead, C., Popko, B., Takahashi, N., Shine, D. H., Saavedra, R. A., Sidman, R. L., and Hood, L. Expression of myelin basic protein gene in transgenic shiverer mice: Correction of the dysmyelinating phenotype. *Cell* 48:703–712, 1987.

22. Nave, K.-A., Lai, C., Bloom, F. E., and Milner, R. J. Jimpy mutant mouse: A 74-base deletion in the mRNA for myelin proteolipid protein and evidence for a primary defect in RNA splicing. *Proc. Natl. Acad. Sci. U.S.A.* 83:9264–9268, 1986.

23. Hudson, L. D., Berndt, J. A., Puckett, C., Kozak, C. A., and Lazzarini, R. A. Aberrant splicing of proteolipid protein mRNA in the dysmyelinating jimpy mouse. *Proc. Natl. Acad. Sci. U.S.A.* 84:1454–1458, 1987.

24. Smith, M. E., and Benjamins, J. A. Model systems for study of myelin metabolism. In P. Morell (ed.), *Myelin*. New York: Plenum Press, 1984, pp. 441–487.

25. Poser, C. M. Diseases of the myelin sheath. In J. Minckler (ed.), *Pathology of the Nervous System, Vol. 1*. New York: McGraw Hill, 1968, pp. 767–820.

CHAPTER 37

Genetic Disorders of Lipid, Glycoprotein, and Mucopolysaccharide Metabolism

Kunihiko Suzuki

Many neurological disorders occur as the result of genetically determined abnormal metabolism of lipids or of the carbohydrate moieties of glycoproteins or mucopolysaccharides. In most such disorders, underlying metabolic abnor-

malities exist in the catabolic pathways catalyzed by a group of enzymes commonly referred to as lysosomal enzymes (lysosomal disease). A series of genetic defects of enzymes normally localized in the peroxisome has also been at-

Basic Neurochemistry: Molecular, Cellular, and Medical Aspects, 4th Ed., edited by G. J. Siegel et al. Raven Press, Ltd., New York, 1989. Correspondence to Kunihiko Suzuki, Biological Sciences Research Center, CB# 7250, BSRC, University of North Carolina, Chapel Hill, North Carolina 27599-7250.

tracting increasing attention in recent years (peroxisomal disease). (The interested reader is referred to Scriver et al. [1] for the standard reference volume on the biochemical basis of these disorders.)

MOLECULAR GENETICS OF LYSOSOMAL AND PEROXISOMAL ENZYMES

Compared to some other genetic disorders, studies of most lysosomal and peroxisomal disorders are at an early stage of the application of recombinant DNA technology. The field is in transition from studies of gene products (enzymes, other proteins) to those of nucleic acids themselves. In a few instances, such as Gaucher's disease (glucosylceramidase), Tay-Sachs disease, and Sandhoff's disease (β-hexosaminidase, α and β), normal complementary DNA (cDNA) and genomic clones have been isolated and characterized, and at least some specific mutations identified. In addition, normal cDNA has been cloned for β-glucuronidase, α-fucosidase, α-galactosidase A, sulfatidase activator protein, and the protective protein for β-galactosidase-sialidase. As expected, the results obtained with these new tools show the complex genetic heterogeneity of these diseases, even when they appear to be homogeneous with regard to clinical manifestations, analytical biochemistry, and enzymatic defects.

DIAGNOSIS AND TREATMENT

Originally, diagnosis of this group of disorders was primarily based on clinicopathological findings and on identification of abnormally stored materials by analytical biochemistry. During the past two decades, however, emphasis has shifted to enzymatic assays [2], which provide relatively easy, noninvasive antemortem diagnosis because clinically available materials, such as serum, blood cells, and cultured fibroblasts, can be used. These procedures can generally be used, with varying degrees of reliability, to detect heterozygous carriers. Identification of affected fetuses during pregnancy is generally possible with similar procedures. The most commonly used material for prenatal diagnosis is cultured amniotic fluid cells. In recent years, biopsied chorionic villi are gaining popularity as the material of choice for prenatal diagnosis, because diagnosis can be done immediately after the procedure at a much earlier stage of pregnancy (7–8-week gestation vs. 18–20 weeks in cases of amniocentesis and cell culture). It can be anticipated that diagnostic procedures at the nucleic acid level will be forthcoming in the near future. Unlike enzymatic diagnosis, however, DNA diagnosis will not replace earlier procedures because DNA diagnosis is often too specific. It commonly requires prior information about the nature of the mutation in the family. One procedure based on a particular mutation may be useless for patients with the same enzymatic, and thus functional, defect but caused by another mutation. Enzymatic and metabolic procedures have an advantage in that they test for functionality of a particular metabolic step regardless of the nature of the abnormality.

Replacement of a defective enzyme with a normal one has been attempted through various routes, including direct injection of purified enzyme or transplantation of various normal organs or bone marrow. These trials have been at best partial successes. Long-term, pragmatic benefits to patients have been questionable in most cases. Identification of an affected fetus and termination of pregnancy remain the best that can be offered to families of identified patients. The situation could change dramatically in the next decade, however, when and if treatment at the level of genes becomes a reality.

Many of the genetic lysosomal diseases in humans have equivalents among other mammalian species [3]. Since most of the human diseases are rare, and since there are serious ethical constraints in studying human patients, these animal models provide useful tools for studying all aspects of these disorders, including the natural history of disease processes, pathogenesis, and therapeutic trials. Animal models, particularly smaller mammalian species, will probably be used more extensively in the near future as vehicles for recombinant DNA experiments.

THE LYSOSOME AND LYSOSOMAL DISEASE

The lysosome is the subcellular membrane-bound organelle responsible for digestion of cellular constituents

The lysosome, whose structure is described in Chap. 1, contains catabolic enzymes, generally glycoproteins themselves, that have very low pH optima for their function. Defective catalytic activity of any of these enzymes results in blockage of the intracellular digestive process that is essential for normal function. Hers originated the concept of lysosomal disease in the mid-1960s [4]. Using glycogenosis type II (Pompe's disease) as a model, Hers defined a category of genetic disease, called "inborn lysosomal disorder," that satisfied two major criteria: (1) An acidic hydrolase normally localized in the lysosome is genetically defective; (2) as a consequence, the substrate of the defective enzyme accumulates abnormally within pathologically altered secondary lysosomes. Over the years, several important groups of genetic disorders have been identified as inborn lysosomal diseases. Among them are the sphingolipidoses, mucopolysaccharidoses, and mucolipidoses. These disorders are often referred to as storage diseases because the abnormal storage of undigested substrates is often the most conspicuous clinical and pathological manifestation.

Lysosomal diseases are traditionally classified according to the nature of the material that accumulates abnormally. There is considerable overlap in substrate specificities of the enzymes and, consequently, classification is chiefly for convenience. For example, genetic β-galactosidase defects can result primarily in G_{M1}-ganglioside accumulation (sphingolipidosis) or bony abnormalities (mucopolysaccharidosis), depending on the nature of the mutation. In both instances, degradation of carbohydrate chains of glycoproteins are also impaired (glycoprotein disorder).

Sphingolipidoses are caused by genetic defects of a series of lysosomal hydrolases involved in degradation of lipids that contain sphingosine as the basic building block

Because the nervous system is rich in sphingolipids, many enzymatic defects manifest themselves as neurological disorders (see Chap. 5). Sphingolipids are degraded to ceramide by removal of the terminal moieties of the hydrophilic chain—sulfate, in the case of sulfatide; phosphorylcholine, in the case of sphingomyelin—and sequential removal of all the sugar moieties from the other sphingolipids. Ceramide is then hydrolyzed to sphingosine and fatty acid (Fig. 1). Genetic disorders are known in humans that affect almost every step of the degradative pathway (Table 1). The mode of inheritance is Mendelian autosomal recessive for all sphingolipidoses, except Fabry's disease, which is an X-linked disorder.

Farber's disease (ceramidosis, Farber's lipogranulomatosis)

Primary manifestations of Farber's disease are painful, progressively deformed joints and subcutaneous granulomatous nodules in infants. Nervous system involvement is usually moderate. The subcutaneous nodules, lung, and

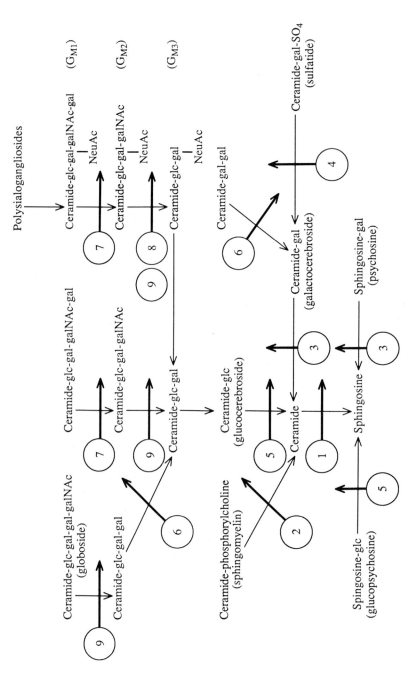

FIG. 1. Chemical and metabolic relationships among the major sphingolipids. Normal catabolic pathways are indicated by *arrows* connecting adjacent compounds. Biosynthesis of these lipids occurs in the reverse direction. *Large arrows with numbers* indicate locations of genetic metabolic blocks known in humans. (The numbers correspond to those in Table 1.)

TABLE 1. Major sphingolipidoses

Disease[a]	Clinicopathological manifestations	Affected lipid	Enzymatic defect
1. Farber's disease (lipogranulomatosis)	Mostly infantile disease; tender swollen joints; multiple subcutaneous nodules; later flaccid paralysis and mental impairment	Ceramide	Acid ceramidase
2. Niemann-Pick disease	Neuropathic and nonneuropathic forms; hepatosplenomegaly; foamy cells in bone marrow; severe neurological signs in the neuropathic form (type A)	Sphingomyelin	Sphingomyelinase
3. Globoid cell leukodystrophy (Krabbe's disease)	Almost always infantile disease; white matter signs; peripheral neuropathy; high CSF protein; loss of myelin; globoid cells in white matter	Galactosylceramide Galactosylsphingosine	Galactosylceramidase
4a. Metachromatic leukodystrophy	Late infantile, juvenile, and adult forms; white matter signs; peripheral neuropathy; high CSF protein; metachromatic granules in the brain, nerves, kidney, and urine	Sulfatide	Arylsulfatase A ("sulfatidase")
4b. Multiple sulfatase deficiency	Similar to metachromatic leukodystrophy, but additional gray matter signs; facial and skeletal abnormalities; organomegaly similar to mucopolysaccharidoses	Sulfatide; other sulfated compounds (see text)	Arylsulfatase A, B, C (see text)
4c. Sulfatidase activator deficiency	Similar to late-onset forms of 4a	Unknown	Sulfatidase activator
5. Gaucher's disease	Neuropathic and nonneuropathic forms; hepatosplenomegaly; "Gaucher cells" in bone marrow; severe neurological signs in the neuropathic form; also an intermediate form (type III)	Glucosylceramide Glucosylsphingosine	Glucosylceramidase
6. Fabry's disease	Primarily adult and nonneurological; angiokeratoma around buttocks; renal damage; X-linked	Trihexosylceramide (gal-gal-glc-cer) Digalactosylceramide	α-Galactosidase A (trihexosylceramidase)
7a. G_{M1}-gangliosidosis	Slow growth; motor weakness; gray matter signs; infantile form with additional facial and skeletal abnormalities and organomegaly; swollen neurons	G_{M1}-ganglioside Galactose-rich fragments of glycoproteins	G_{M1}-ganglioside β-galactosidase
7b. Galactosialidosis	Similar to late-onset form of 7a	Unknown	"Protective protein" (secondary defect in G_{M1}-ganglioside β-galactosidase and sialidase)
8a. Tay-Sachs disease	Severe gray matter signs; slow growth; motor weakness; hyperacusis; cherry-red spot; head enlargement; swollen neurons	G_{M2}-ganglioside	β-Hexosaminidase A
8b. Juvenile G_{M2}-gangliosidosis	Later onset, slower progression but otherwise similar to Tay-Sachs disease; milder pathology; some cases possibly B1 variant.	G_{M2}-ganglioside	β-Hexosaminidase A (partial defect)
8c. B1 variant	Similar to either 8a or 8b	G_{M2}-ganglioside	β-Hexosaminidase A
8d. AB variant	Similar to 8a	G_{M2}-ganglioside	β-Hexosaminidase A activator
9. Sandhoff's disease	Panethnic but otherwise indistinguishable from Tay-Sachs disease	G_{M2}-ganglioside; asialo G_{M2}-ganglioside; globoside	β-Hexosaminidase A and B

[a] Numbers correspond to the steps of metabolic blocks in Fig. 1.

heart are the main sites of abnormal accumulations of ceramide; however, ceramide levels are also increased in the central nervous system (CNS). A mild and probably nonspecific accumulation of simpler gangliosides in the brain is also commonly observed.

Niemann-Pick disease

Niemann-Pick disease is traditionally classified as types A, B, C, D, etc., primarily according to clinical phenotypes; however, only types A and B Niemann-Pick disease are allelic and caused by primary genetic sphingomyelinase deficiency. The term, Niemann-Pick, should be used only for these two types. Patients with either type A or B disease exhibit enormous hepatosplenomegaly and characteristic foamy cells in the bone marrow. Type A disease usually occurs in infants and is characterized by additional severe CNS involvement. Patients rarely survive beyond 5 years. On the other hand, type B form is more slowly progressive, occurring in older age groups. Despite similarly severe organomegaly, type B patients are normal in intellect and free of neurological manifestations. In both types, there is an enormous accumulation of sphingomyelin in the liver and spleen. Although available information is not extensive, a fewfold increase in sphingomyelin appears to occur in the CNS only in type A (neuropathic) patients. The degree of sphingomyelinase deficiency is similar in the two types; the reason that dramatically different phenotypes occur is not known.

The so-called Niemann-Pick types C, D, etc., are clinically similar in that patients exhibit organomegaly, slowly progressive CNS signs, and abnormal bone marrow cells. Liver and spleen show increased amounts of sphingomyelin; however, there are accompanying and usually even more severe increases in cholesterol and, sometimes, glucosylceramide. Sphingomyelinase activity is often, but not always, significantly lower than normal but not enough to account for the clinical picture. Recently, fibroblasts of Niemann-Pick type C and similar cases have been shown to be defective in esterifying cholesterol, exogenously added to the culture medium [5]. Since the abnormality is observed when cholesterol is given in the form bound to low-density lipoprotein (LDL), and since direct *in vitro* assays of cholesterol-esterifying enzyme are normal, the defect should be present anywhere between these two steps. It is likely that this is a heterogenous group of diseases with genetic defects at different steps in cholesterol uptake, intracellular routing, and esterification. These new findings further argue against the term, Niemann-Pick, for these diseases.

Globoid cell leukodystrophy (Krabbe's disease)

Globoid cell leukodystrophy and metachromatic leukodystrophy are two of the classical genetic myelin disorders simply because they involve abnormal degradation of two sphingolipids highly localized in the myelin sheath—galactosylceramide and sulfatide. The disease occurs mainly in infancy; however, exceedingly rare late-onset forms are also known. Clinicopathological manifestations are almost exclusively those of the white matter and the peripheral nerves. The unique globoid cells are hematogenous histiocytic cells that infiltrate the white matter in response to undigested galactosylceramide. Unlike all other storage diseases, the primary natural substrate of the defective enzyme, galactosylceramide, does not accumulate abnormally but it is almost always much lower than normal. On the other hand, a toxic metabolite, galactosylsphingosine (psychosine), does accumulate and appears to be responsible for the devastating pathology of the disease (psychosine hypothesis) [6,7]. Effects of psychosine, early cessation of myelination, and, possibly, overlapping substrate specificities between the two lysosomal β-galactosidases (galactosylceramidase and G_{M1}-ganglioside β-galactosidase) are important in understanding the pathogenesis of this disease.

Metachromatic leukodystrophy

The enzymatic defect in metachromatic leukodystrophy occurs one step before that in Krabbe's disease. Although these two diseases share many common features, as expected, there are significant differences that suggest different pathogenetic mechanisms. Clinically, a relatively large proportion of patients with metachromatic leukodystrophy have the early juvenile- or adult-onset form; others have the late juvenile-onset form. Pathologically, reduction in the number of oligodendrocytes is less severe. Remaining oligodendrocytes contain acid-phosphatase-positive lamellar inclusions that, on the light microscopic level, stain yellow-brown with cresyl violet at acidic pH (metachromasia). Unlike globoid cell leukodystrophy, the affected substrate (sulfatide) is always abnormally increased, including in the myelin sheath. There is no evidence for lysosulfatide, the equivalent compound to psychosine, even though the enzymatic machinery exists to synthesize it and even though degradation of exogenously added lysosulfatide is defective *in vitro*. The presence or absence of necessary intermediates (sphingosine for psychosine and psychosine for lysosulfatide) for biosynthesis appears to explain this difference. Bone marrow transplant treatment has been tried in this disease with some degree of positive effects. (See below for metachromatic leukodystrophy due to sulfatidase activator protein.)

Multiple sulfatase deficiency

Phenotypically, multiple sulfatase deficiency combines features of metachromatic leukodystrophy and mucopolysaccharidoses. In addition to clinical manifestations of metachromatic leukodystrophy, patients present with craniofacial abnormalities, skeletal deformities, and hepatosplenomegaly. There is abnormal urinary excretion of dermatan sulfate and heparan sulfate. Pathological findings can also be combinations of the two conditions. Inheritance is clearly Mendelian autosomal recessive. Nevertheless, activities of a series of sulfatases are deficient, including arylsulfatases A, B, C; steroid sulfatases; and sulfatases related to mucopolysaccharide degradation (see mucopolysaccharidoses, below). There is evidence that arylsulfatases A and B are qualitatively normal but are present in greatly reduced amounts. Defective synthesis or instability due to a gene defect that governs all sulfatases needs to be explored. Since some of the sulfatases involved, (e.g., arylsulfatase C) are not lysosomal enzymes, and since the primary genetic defect is not known, it is possible that multiple sulfatase deficiency may not be a lysosomal disorder as defined by Hers.

Gaucher's disease

Traditionally, Gaucher's disease is classified as three types: type I, mostly adult, nonneuropathic; type II, mostly infantile, severely neuropathic; and type III, intermediate phenotypes. Type I is highly prevalent in Jewish populations, whereas a large, distinct group of type III patients exists in Scandinavian countries. All types are allelic and are caused by defective glucosylceramidase activity. Glucosylceramide is present in great excess in the enlarged liver and spleen in all types. The brain, in which glucosylceramide is normally almost nonexistent, does not contain increased amounts. Analogous to Niemann-Pick disease, nonneuropathic patients are free of neurological involvement and survive for decades, whereas type II neuropathic patients die within a few years with severe CNS involvement. The difference in the pathogenetic mechanisms in these phenotypes is not known. Analogous to globoid cell leukodystrophy, glucosylsphingosine (glucopsychosine) may play an important role in the pathogenesis. The degree of CNS involvement is paralleled with the amounts of glucopsychosine in the brain. Some of these important questions may be answered in the near future, because normal cDNA and the gene for glucosylceramidase have been cloned and characterized [8,9]. Recently, a mutation possibly responsible for the neuropathic form (type II) has been reported [10]. A point mutation from leucine to proline was found at amino acid residue 444 that was more frequent in neuropathic forms (types II and III). No nonneuropathic patients were homozygous for this allele. The most intensive enzyme replacement therapy has been tried in patients with the nonneuropathic form of Gaucher's disease. In some patients, encouraging results were obtained, although long-term pragmatic benefits must be carefully evaluated. Complete correction of the enzymatic defect was reported in fibroblasts through retrovirus-mediated gene transfer [11].

Fabry's disease

Unlike most other sphingolipidoses, Fabry's disease is an X-linked disorder, occurring mostly in adults. It is also primarily a systemic disease, and neurological manifestations are largely secondary to kidney and vascular lesions. The affected lipids, trihexosylceramide (gal-gal-glc-ceramide) and digalactosylceramide, are essentially absent in the neural tissues in normal individuals. There are some accumulations of these lipids in the brain, thought to be contributed primarily by those in the blood vessels. Cerebrovascular pathology commonly results in secondary neurological symptoms; most patients succumb to renal failure and other vascular diseases. Transplantation of normal kidney had been tried as a treatment—a procedure frequently indicated because of renal failure—but the results were not encouraging enough to pursue further. The enzyme responsible for degradation of these sphingolipids with the terminal α-galactose residue is α-galactosi-

dase A, a mutation of which causes Fabry's disease. Normal cDNA coding for α-galactosidase A has been cloned [12]. No information is yet available about the mutant enzyme.

G_{M1}-gangliosidosis

The infantile form of G_{M1}-gangliosidosis shows, in addition to psychomotor retardation and other neurological manifestations, mucopolysaccharidosis-like clinical features. The late-onset form is relatively free of systemic signs. Genetically, Morquio disease type B probably should be considered an adult form of this disorder (see below). These pleomorphic phenotypes are consequences of the wide substrate specificity of the defective enzyme, G_{M1}-ganglioside-β-galactosidase, which hydrolyzes not only G_{M1}-ganglioside, asialo-G_{M1}-ganglioside, and lactosylceramide, but also terminal β-galactosyl residues of carbohydrate chains of various glycoproteins. Different mutations in the gene could differentially inactivate catalytic activity toward different substrates. Large accumulations of G_{M1}-ganglioside occur primarily in the brain of patients with the infantile and late-infantile forms of the disease. The major accumulated materials in the systemic organs are fragments of glycopeptides. It is not known whether or not G_{M1}-ganglioside accumulates in the brain in the adult form (Morquio B).

Tay-Sachs disease and variants

Classical Tay-Sachs disease, prevalent among the Ashkenazi Jewish population, is the prototype of human sphingolipidoses. It is caused by a mutation in the β-hexosaminidase α-subunit gene. Normally, the hexosaminidase α and β subunits form two catalytically active isozymes: β-hexosaminidase A (αβ) and B (ββ). A defect in the α subunit thus results in defective hexosaminidase A, with normal hexosaminidase B. Hexosaminidase A can hydrolyze all known natural substrates with terminal β-N-acetylgalactosamine or β-N-acetylglucosamine residues, whereas hexosaminidase B hydrolyzes all of these substrates except G_{M2}-ganglioside. As a result, a relatively specific accumulation of G_{M2}-ganglioside occurs in genetic hexosaminidase α-subunit deficiency states. A few genetic variants are known on the basis of clinical and enzymatic criteria. The juvenile form has a later onset and a slower course. When assayed with conventional artificial substrates, the juvenile form exhibits partial deficiency of hexosaminidase A. The B1 variant is characterized by apparently completely normal hexosaminidase A and B when assayed with the standard artificial substrates but completely defective hexosaminidase A against the natural substrate, G_{M2}-ganglioside, and recently developed artificial substrates, *p*-nitrophenyl- and 4-methylumbelliferyl glcNAc-6-sulfate. These enzymatic variants are all known to be caused by genetic defects in the hexosaminidase α-subunit gene. In contrast, the AB variant, which is phenotypically indistinguishable from the infantile hexosaminidase α-subunit defect, is caused by an entirely different genetic mechanism, a mutation in the activator protein (see below).

Although all of these phenotypic and enzymological differentiations have certainly been useful, molecular genetic understanding of these diseases is imminent. Normal cDNA and the gene for the hexosaminidase α chain have been cloned and characterized [13]. It is known that some forms of the disease lack the immunologically reactive α subunit, whereas others are cross-reacting material positive. Availability of cDNA has shown that the presence or absence of cross-reactive material largely corresponds to the presence or absence of messenger RNA (mRNA) for the subunit. Both classical Tay-Sachs disease and the phenotypically indistinguishable disease occurring in the French Canadian population are mRNA negative, whereas the B1 variant and some other unusual forms are mRNA positive. The French Canadian form showed a major deletion in the 5' end of the hexosaminidase α-subunit gene of

approximately 7 kilobases (kb) that spanned the putative promotor region to beyond the first exon into the first intron [14]. The first point mutation in the hexosaminidase α-subunit gene has been identified in a patient with the B1 variant form of the disease [15]. Normal arginine at residue 178 has been substituted by histidine. Computer analysis suggests that substantial changes occur in the secondary structure of the enzyme protein around the mutation, consistent with the unusual enzymological characteristic of this variant. Understanding being developed at the level of the gene is likely to render the traditional clinical and enzymatic classification of this disease obsolete.

Sandhoff's disease

When the hexosaminidase β-subunit gene is genetically defective, inactivation of both hexosaminidase A (αβ) and B (ββ) results. Although the typical infantile form of Sandhoff's disease cannot readily be distinguished clinically from infantile hexosaminidase α defect, histochemical and biochemical studies have disclosed an accumulation of materials other than G_{M2}-ganglioside in the brain. All sphingolipids with terminal β-hexosamine residue are affected, including G_{M2}-ganglioside, asialo-G_{M2}-ganglioside, and globoside (Fig. 1). Since globoside is primarily a systemic lipid, it also accumulates in systemic organs. cDNA and the gene for hexosaminidase β-subunit have also been cloned and characterized [16]. Despite localization on different chromosomes (α on chromosome 15 and β on 5), hexosaminidase α and β chains are highly homologous not only in the base and amino acid sequences of cDNAs but in gene organization as well. These two subunits appear to have been separated from a single gene relatively recently in the evolutionary time scale. No specific gene abnormalities have been reported for any forms of Sandhoff's disease; however, it has been determined that many patients with the infantile form are mRNA negative, whereas at least some with the late-onset form are mRNA positive [17].

Wolman's disease

Wolman's disease is not a sphingolipidosis but is described here for convenience. Clinical onset is within a few weeks after birth, with vomiting, diarrhea, and abdominal distention. Organomegaly is present. Calcified adrenals are commonly diagnostic. The disease rapidly progresses to cachexia and death within several months. The underlying genetic defect is a deficiency of acid lipase. As a consequence, cholesterol esters and triglycerides accumulate in visceral organs.

Activator and protective protein deficiencies

The concept of sphingolipidoses has been expanded to include a few genetic disorders that affect degradation of sphingolipids but do not fit the classical definition of lysosomal disease. Activator protein deficiencies and galactosialidosis are examples of such disorders.

In vivo degradation of the highly hydrophobic lipids often requires, in addition to the hydrolases, a third component, commonly referred to as activator proteins. They are generally small glycoproteins localized within the lysosomes but are not enzymes themselves. When such an activator is essential for *in vivo* degradation, and when it is genetically defective, the end results are very similar to deficiency of the enzyme itself. G_{M2}-gangliosidosis AB variant has been well characterized. It is caused by genetic absence of the activator required to hydrolyze G_{M2}-ganglioside. The degradative enzyme, *N*-acetylhexosaminidase A, is normal in these patients. A similar variant has been reported for metachromatic leukodystrophy in which an activator protein, rather than arylsulfatase A, is genetically defective. Normal cDNA coding for the sulfatidase activator protein has been cloned [18].

Galactosialidosis (combined sialidase-β-galactosidase deficiency)

Lysosomal β-galactosidase and sialidase appear to exist as a complex within the lysosome, along with a small protein, which protects both enzymes from being degraded by acid proteases also present in the lysosome. When this protein is absent, both enzymes are degraded rapidly. Genetic abnormality of the protective protein results in deficient activity of both sialidase and β-galactosidase [19]. Most commonly, galactosialidosis is a slowly progressive neurological disorder, resembling the late-onset form of G_{M1}-gangliosidosis.

Mucopolysaccharidoses are caused by genetic defects in the sequential degradation of the carbohydrate chains of glycosaminoglycans

Analogous to sphingolipidoses, genetic enzymatic defects in these lysosomal hydrolases result in accumulation of undegradable metabolites (Table 2). These materials are also excreted into urine in massive amounts. The standard classification of mucopolysaccharidoses is based on clinical manifestations and on the nature of the accumulated/excreted materials. The enzymatic classification does not necessarily correspond to the traditional classification. A single classical disease often consists of more than one nonallelic disorder, whereas two disorders classified earlier as different may be allelic. All mucopolysaccharidoses are inherited as autosomal recessive traits, except for Hunter's disease, which is X-linked.

Hurler's syndrome and Scheie's syndrome (mucopolysaccharidosis I and V)

Hurler's syndrome is the prototype of the mucopolysaccharidoses. Scheie's syndrome was once considered a separate disease and was classified as mucopolysaccharidosis V. It is

TABLE 2. Mucopolysaccharidoses

Disease[a]	Clinicopathological manifestations	Affected compound	Enzymatic defect
Hurler-Scheie syndrome (MPS I and V)	Craniofacial abnormalities; cloudy cornea; bone and other mesodermal tissue abnormalities; severe to mild psychomotor retardation; organomegaly; lysosomal storage in mesodermal organs, zebra bodies in neurons	Dermatan sulfate Heparan sulfate	α-L-Iduronidase
Hunter's syndrome (MPS II)	Generally similar to but milder than Hurler-Scheie but X-linked; corneal clouding rare	Dermatan sulfate Heparan sulfate	Iduronate sulfatase
Sanfilippo's disease (MPS III)	Four genetically distinct (nonallelic) types; similar clinicopathological manifestations; severe psychomotor retardation; relatively mild bone and other systemic involvement; zebra bodies in neurons	Heparan sulfate	Type A; heparan N-sulfatase Type B; N-acetyl-α-glucosaminidase Type C; N-acetyl-CoA: α-glucosaminide N-acetyltransferase Type D; N-acetyl-α-glucosaminide-6-sulfatase
Morquio's disease (MPS IV)	Two nonallelic forms; primarily bone abnormalities; corneal clouding; nervous system involvement secondary to bone changes; type B is probably allelic to G_{M1}-gangliosidosis	Keratan sulfate	Type A; N-acetyl-galactosamine 6-sulfatase Type B; β-galactosidase
Maroteaux-Lamy (MPS VI)	Severe to mild clinical types; bone and corneal changes; nervous system involvement generally mild	Dermatan sulfate	Arylsulfatase B (N-acetyl-galactos-amine-4-sulfatase)
α-Glucuronidase deficiency (MPS VII)	Organomegaly; bone abnormalities; mild to no psychomotor retardation; inclusions in leukocytes	Dermatan sulfate Heparan sulfate	β-Glucuronidase

[a] (MPS) mucopolysaccharidosis.

now known to be a milder allelic variant of Hurler's syndrome. Neurons in the brain are commonly distended and contain characteristic lamellar inclusions, known as zebra bodies. They are considered to be the site of abnormal ganglioside accumulation commonly found in this and other mucopolysaccharidoses. Although the increase occurs mainly in minor monosialogangliosides, commonly thought of as nonspecific abnormalities, the degree of increase is often substantial—50 to 100 percent above normal. Polysulfated mucopolysaccharides are inhibitory to some lysosomal enzymes *in vitro*. Similar inhibition *in vivo* might be responsible for the ganglioside increase. It is not known whether or not and to what extent the ganglioside accumulation and resulting neuronal distension contribute to the neurological manifestations of Hurler-Scheie syndrome.

Hurler's syndrome has an onset in infancy and leads to severe psychomotor retardation, skeletal and other organ abnormalities, and often death by the age of 10 years. Sheie's syndrome, at the opposite end of the spectrum, is compatible with normal life span and intelligence and near-normal stature.

Hunter's syndrome (mucopolysaccharidosis II)

Hunter's syndrome is an X-linked disorder, generally milder and slower in clinical features and course than Hurler's syndrome. Patients with Hunter's syndrome closely resemble those with Hurler's syndrome.

Sanfilippo's disease (mucopolysaccharidosis III)

An excellent example of a "disease," identified on the basis of clinicopathological criteria, Sanfilippo's disease has turned out to be a mixture of more than one genetically distinct disease. Four enzymatically different and nonallelic diseases are included under the eponym, Sanfilippo's disease. All four defective enzymes are involved at different steps of heparan sulfate degradation. Thus, the end results are essentially identical. Differential diagnosis cannot be established without appropriate enzyme assays.

Morquio's disease (mucopolysaccharidosis IV)

Unlike other mucopolysaccharidoses, Morquio's disease is primarily a skeletal disorder. Neurological involvement is almost always secondary to skeletal abnormalities. The most common neurological complications are traumatic lesions of the spinal cord at the cervical level due to vertebral deformity. Of the two genetically distinct types—type A (*N*-acetylgalactosamine-6-sulfatase deficiency) and type B (β-galactosidase deficiency)—type A disease is clinically more severe. The relationship of type B Morquio's disease to GM1-gangliosidosis has been mentioned above.

Maroteaux-Lamy disease (mucopolysaccharidosis VI)

Maroteaux-Lamy disease is another Hurler-like syndrome but can be differentiated from Hurler's syndrome by relatively well-preserved intellectual capacity. Urinary excretion of mucopolysaccharides is predominantly dermatan sulfate. Clinical severity and duration vary among apparently allelic cases.

β-Glucuronidase deficiency (mucopolysaccharidosis VII)

An exceedingly rare disease, the first case of β-glucuronidase deficiency was reported by Sly et al. in 1973 [20]. Although the general clinical picture is that of a mucopolysaccharidosis, the degree of severity of skeletal abnormalities, organomegaly, and nervous system involvement appears widely variable. β-Glucuronidase was one of the first lysosomal enzymes cloned [21]; however, no information is yet available concerning the mutation causing this disorder. Almost complete restoration of β-glucuronidase activity after allogeneic bone marrow transplantation has been reported in the liver and other organs of mice genetically deficient in glucuronidase activity [22]. The genetic β-glucuronidase deficiency state in the mouse is asymptomatic, however.

Glycoprotein disorders are caused by genetic defects in lysosomal glycosidases primarily involved in degrading carbohydrate chains of glycoproteins

When such lysosomal glycosidases are genetically defective, the results are accumulation and urinary excretion of undigested sugar chains and small glycopeptides, since the protein backbone is usually degradable by genetically normal proteases (Table 3).

TABLE 3. Glycoprotein storage diseases and mucolipidoses

Disease	Clinicopathological manifestations	Affected compound	Enzymatic defect
Sialidosis (Mucolipidosis I)	Two distinct phenotypes; mucolipidosis I (mucopolysaccharidosis-like features; severe to moderate psychomotor retardation) and cherry-red spot-myoclonus syndrome	Sialyloligo-saccharides	α-Neuraminidase (sialidase)
I-cell disease and Pseudo-Hurler polydystrophy (mucolipidoses II and III)	Mucopolysaccharidosis-like features; severe psychomotor retardation; characteristic inclusions in fibroblasts, mucolipidosis II is a milder allelic disease	Multiple (see text)	Primary defect in lysosomal enzyme-phosphorylating enzyme; secondary abnormality in multiple lysosomal enzymes (see text)
Mucolipidosis IV	Mucopolysaccharidosis-like features; relatively mild CNS involvement; conjunctival biopsy for characteristic inclusions can be diagnostic	Gangliosides? (see text)	Ganglioside sialidase? (see text)
α-Mannosidosis	Mucopolysaccharidosis-like features; severe to moderate psychomotor retardation	Oligosaccharides with terminal α-mannose	Acid α-mannosidase
β-Mannosidosis	Only one case known in humans; moderate psychomotor retardation; Sanfilippo-like general clinical features; apparently much milder than the goat disease	β-Mannosyl-glcNAc; heparan sulfate?	β-Mannosidase Heparan sulfamidase
α-Fucosidosis	Mucopolysaccharidosis-like features; severe to moderate psychomotor retardation	Fucose-containing oligosaccharides and glycolipids	α-Fucosidase

Sialidosis (neuraminidase deficiency; mucolipidosis I)

Apparently, two dissimilar phenotypes result from enzymatic defects in the same lysosomal α-neuraminidase (sialidase): Infantile and juvenile. The infantile form had been known as mucolipidosis I for many years because of the mucopolysaccharidosis-like appearance of patients. Neurological involvement is severe to moderate, including impaired intellectual capacity. In the juvenile type, three findings stand out: typical macular cherry-red spots, intract-able myoclonic seizures, and intact intellect. The α-neuraminidase deficient in sialidosis cleaves both α-2,6 and α-2,3 sialyl linkages but is apparently distinct from neuraminidase(s) that hydrolyzes sialic acid from gangliosides. Thus, patients accumulate and excrete excess sialic acid-containing materials derived from complex carbohydrate chains of glycoproteins. There is no evidence, however, for increased levels of gangliosides in the brain and elsewhere as the consequence of this genetic defect (see also galactosialidosis, above, and mucolipidosis IV, below).

I-cell disease (mucolipidosis II) and pseudo-Hurler polydystrophy (mucolipidosis III)

Among the disorders primarily affecting glycoprotein metabolism, I-cell disease and pseudo-Hurler polydystrophy are conceptually unique. These two disorders had been considered separate entities on the basis of phenotypic manifestations; however, they are now known to be allelic variants of the same disease. There is deficient activity of most, but not all, lysosomal hydrolases in solid tissues. Notable exceptions are glucosylceramidase and acid phosphatase. By contrast, their activity is generally much higher than normal in serum and other extracellular fluids, including the culture media in which patients' fibroblasts are grown. The primary genetic cause of the disease is not located in any specific lysosomal enzyme but occurs in UDP-glcNAc:lysosomal enzyme glcNAc phosphotransferase, which is localized in the Golgi apparatus and is essential for the normal processing and packaging of lysosomal enzymes. Without this enzyme, lysosomal enzymes cannot acquire the mannose-6-phosphate recognition marker that allows them to be properly routed to lysosomes. As the result, lysosomal enzymes are abnormally routed out of the cell with highly processed carbohydrate chains. Although lack of lysosomal enzyme activity must be the primary cause of clinicopathological manifestations, this disease does not satisfy the classical criteria of Hers for inherited lysosomal disease.

Mucolipidosis IV

Mucolipidosis IV occurs predominantly in the Jewish population. The genetic cause has not been unambiguously determined. Earlier, a sialidase deficiency presumably specific for ganglioside degradation had been proposed, based on moderately abnormal ganglioside patterns in cultured fibroblasts and reduced sialidase activity. The residual activity, however, was nearly half normal, much higher than usually expected for a disease-causing deficiency. Although two later studies reported much lower residual activities, another laboratory was unable to confirm the result on the same patient. Data have been presented to suggest that at least some of these ambiguities might result from assay procedures that are often used to measure total activity of a mixture of sialidases, only one of which is genetically affected in this disease. There is also some question as to whether or not a ganglioside sialidase deficiency is consistent with phenotypic expression. The accumulation of gangliosides in tissue seems much milder than expected in a genetic condition in which the ubiquitous G_{M3}-ganglioside cannot be degraded. Also, if polysialogangliosides cannot be degraded, we would expect much more severe neurological consequences than the relatively mild CNS involvement in this disease.

α-Mannosidosis

α-Mannosidases that participate in processing carbohydrate chains of glycoproteins are localized in the Golgi apparatus and are genetically intact in α-mannosidosis. The lysosomal α-mannosidase deficient in this disease degrades the carbohydrate chains. Therefore, abnormal accumulations and urinary excretion of undegraded oligosaccharides with terminal α-mannose residues derived from normally synthesized and processed glycoproteins occur as a consequence of the genetic defect. A plant toxin, swainsonine, inhibits α-mannosidases, and its chronic ingestion creates an experimental condition that mimics many aspects of genetic α-mannosidosis. This model is limited, however, in that swainsonine inhibits both lysosomal and Golgi α-mannosidases.

β-Mannosidosis

β-Mannosidosis is the only disorder among those discussed in this chapter that was discovered first in another mammalian species before an equivalent disease was found in humans. For several years, β-mannosidase deficiency was known in the goat. Affected goats show severe neurological signs almost from birth. Goat β-mannosidosis is rapidly fatal, and the almost complete lack of myelination is the unique feature of the neuropathology. A human patient with β-mannosidase deficiency has been reported [23]. Unlike the disease in goats, the clinical picture was relatively mild, presenting with Sanfilippo-like features. There was urinary excretion of a disaccharide, β-mannose-glcNAc, and heparan sulfate. The same disaccharide is excreted in the goat disease. It is thought to derive from the innermost mannose in the glycoprotein carbohydrate chains. The parents of the patient gave intermediate activities of the enzyme, consistent with the deficiency being the primary genetic defect. There was also a concomitant lack of heparan sulfamidase activity, which was normal in one parent and intermediate in the other. Clearly, the phenotypic expression of this human patient is entirely different from that of affected goats.

α-Fucosidosis

α-Fucoside residues are present in carbohydrate chains of both sphingoglycolipids and glycoproteins. Fucosylated glycolipids are quantitatively minor but are often functionally important tissue constituents. Many blood-group antigens are fucosylated glycosphingolipids. In patients with genetic α-fucosidase deficiency, accumulation and excretion of fucose-terminated oligosaccharides and fucosylated sphingolipids are observed. Consequences, if any, that result from genetic α-fucosidase deficiency in individuals with the blood groups expressed by the presence of fucosylated glycolipids have not been studied systematically. A partial cDNA for human α-fucosidase, still lacking the uppermost portion of the protein-coding sequence, has been cloned [24].

THE PEROXISOME AND PEROXISOMAL DISEASE

The peroxisome is a subcellular membrane-bound organelle specialized for oxidative reactions using molecular oxygen

The peroxisome had been known morphologically as a microbody before de Duve characterized it biochemically. Known functions of the peroxisome include metabolism of pipecolic acid, dicarboxylic acids, phytanic acid, and very long chain fatty acids and biosynthesis of plasmalogens and bile acids. Analogous to lysosomal disease, a group of inherited disorders are now recognized as being caused by genetic defects either in the peroxisomes themselves or in one of the enzymes normally localized in them [25]. Some disorders manifest themselves as primarily neurological and involve metabolic abnormalities in fatty acids (Table 4).

Zellweger syndrome (cerebrohepatorenal syndrome) is caused by the absence of peroxisomes

The Zellweger syndrome is the classical and the most severe genetic disorder due to peroxisomal dysfunction (Table 4). The specific genetic defect, which is autosomal recessive, has not been identified, but the most conspicuous finding is the almost total absence of peroxisomes, particularly in the hepatocytes and the proximal renal tubular epithelium. Consequently, there is a general failure of all metabolic functions normally associated with the peroxisome.

The disease is manifest at birth, with pronounced apathy, hypotonia, absence of reflexes, seizures, failure to thrive, cranial, and multiple organ abnormalities (Table 4). Most patients die within several months of birth, but some have been reported to have survived to several years. Consistent with absent peroxisomes, very long chain fatty acids, pipecolic

TABLE 4. Major peroxisomal diseases

Disease	Clinicopathological manifestations	Affected compound	Peroxisomal function
Zellweger syndrome	Craniofacial abnormalities; seizures; psychomotor retardation; severe hypotonia; hepatomegaly; rapid progression to death; hepatic cirrhosis; renal cysts	Rise in VLCFA[a], pipecolic acid, bile acid intermediate, phytanic acid; decreased plasmalogen content and synthesis	Absent peroxisomes; all peroxisomal functions defective
Neonatal adrenoleuko-dystrophy	Zellweger-like clinical features; extensive demyelination in the CNS; hepatic cirrhosis; adrenal insufficiency	As in Zellweger disease	Peroxisome decreases in number and size; all peroxisomal function defective
X-linked adrenoleuko-dystrophy	White matter and long tract signs; frequent visual impairment; seizures in late stage; adrenal insufficiency constant but of varying degrees; massive CNS demyelination; characteristic inclusions; clinical variant, adrenomyeloneuropathy, occurs in older patients	VLCFA in cholesterol esters and in some sphingolipids	Normal peroxisomes in size and number; defect in VLCFA oxidation? Peroxisomal functions otherwise normal?
Refsum's disease	Retinitis pigmentosa; cerebellar ataxia; hypertrophic neuropathy; high CSF protein	Elevated phytanic acid in serum and tissues	Normal peroxisomes in size and number; defect in phytanic acid α-hydroxylase

[a] (VLCFA) very long chain fatty acids ($>C_{22}$).

acid, intermediates for bile acid biosynthesis, and phytanic acid are all elevated in the tissue, whereas the plasmalogen content is decreased. Peroxisomal enzymes examined are all deficient in their activities.

Adrenoleukodystrophy is caused by defective oxidation of very long chain fatty acids?

The classical form of adrenoleukodystrophy (ALD) is an X-linked disorder, manifesting itself as a progressive neurological disorder in late infantile to juvenile boys. Severe, and often confluent, lesions of demyelination in the cerebrum, particularly toward the occipital region, are characteristic. There are varying degrees of

clinical and pathological signs of adrenal involvement. Most patients die in their adolescence. A clinical variant, adrenomyeloneuropathy, occurs in older individuals, with predominant spinal cord and peripheral nerve involvement. The clinical course is much slower than in typical ALD. Despite differences in phenotypes, adrenomyeloneuropathy is probably caused by the same mutation as in classical ALD, since both forms can occur in a single family. A significant proportion of female carriers show varying degrees of clinical signs of the disease. The most prominent biochemical finding is increased levels of very long chain fatty acids ($>C_{22}$) in the brain, adrenals, plasma, red cells, and cultured fibroblasts. These fatty acids are present mostly in the form of cholesterol esters, cerebrosides, gangliosides, and sphingomyelin. There are no indications of other peroxisomal dysfunction. The biochemical pathogenesis, which leads to massive demyelination, is unclear because even though the relative increase of very long chain fatty acids in tissue is large, the net amounts are still very small.

Neonatal (connatal, infantile) ALD is probably an entirely different disorder genetically. Unlike classical ALD, the neonatal form appears to be an autosomal recessive disorder. The disease occurs within a year of birth, with the clinical course rarely exceeding 5 years. In addition to clinical and pathological manifestations similar to but more severe than X-linked ALD, craniofacial dysmorphism reminiscent of Zellweger syndrome is usually present. Morphologically, peroxisomes can be greatly reduced in number and size. Consistent with peroxisome abnormality, biochemical and enzymatic findings show more similarity to Zellweger syndrome in that there are multiple abnormalities related to peroxisomal function.

Refsum's disease is caused by defective oxidation of phytanic acid

The classical form of Refsum's disease occurs as a recessive disorder in adults of both sexes, with hypertrophic polyneuropathy the most prominent manifestation (see Chap. 35). There is abnormal elevation of the methylated fatty acid, phytanic acid, which is a 20-carbon branched-chain fatty acid derived from chlorophyll in food and which, in the normal person, is oxidized to α-hydroxyphytanate. There is no indication of other peroxisomal dysfunction. Peroxisomes appear morphologically normal in size and number. Since phytanic acid is exclusively exogenous in origin, chlorophyll-free dietary treatment can be quite effective in alleviating the disease. An exceedingly small number of cases exist that have been reported to be the infantile form of Refsum disease. Clinical, pathological, and biochemical findings in these patients show substantial overlaps with Zellweger syndrome, as well as neonatal ALD. Whether infantile Refsum's disease represents a distinct genetic entity or is allelic to either Zellweger syndrome or ALD is not clear.

REFERENCES

1. Scriver, C. R., Beaudet, A. L., Sly, W. S., and Valle D. (eds.). *The Metabolic Basis of Inherited Disease,* 6th ed. New York: McGraw-Hill, 1989.
2. Suzuki, K. Enzymatic diagnosis of sphingolipidoses. *Meth. Enzymol.* 138:727–762, 1987.
3. Suzuki, K. ''Authentic animal models'' for biochemical studies of human genetic diseases. In M. Arima, Y. Suzuki, and H. Yabuuchi (eds.), *Proceedings of the Fourth International Symposium on Developmental Disabilities.* Tokyo: University of Tokyo Press, 1984, pp. 129–138.
4. Hers, H. G. Inborn lysosomal disease. *Gastroenterology* 48:625–633, 1966.
5. Pentchev, P. G., Comly, M. E., Kruth, H. S., Vanier, M. T., Wenger, D. A., Patel, S., and Brady, R. O. A defect in cholesterol esterification in Niemann-Pick disease (type C) patients. *Proc. Natl. Acad. Sci. U.S.A.* 82:8247–8251, 1985.
6. Miyatake, T., and Suzuki, K. Globoid cell leukodystrophy: Additional deficiency of psychosine galactosidase. *Biochem. Biophys. Res. Commun.* 48:538–543, 1972.
7. Svennerholm, L., Vanier, M. T., and Månsson, J.-E. Krabbe disease: A galactosylsphingosine (psychosine) lipidosis. *J. Lipid Res.* 21:53–64, 1980.
8. Sorge, J., West, C., Westwood, B., and Beutler, E. Molecular cloning and nucleotide sequence of human glucocerebrosidase cDNA. *Proc. Natl. Acad. Sci. U.S.A.* 82:7289–7293, 1985.
9. Tsuji, S., Choudary, P. V., Martin, B. M., Winfield, S., Barranger, J. A., and Ginns, E. I. Nucleotide sequence of cDNA containing the complete sequence for human lysosomal glucocerebrosidase. *J. Biol. Chem.* 261:50–53, 1986.
10. Tsuji, S., Choudary, P. V., Martin, B. M., Stubblefield, B. K., Mayor, J. A., Barranger, J. A.,

and Ginns, E. I. A mutation in the human glucocerebrosidase gene in neuropathic Gaucher's disease. *New Engl. J. Med.* 316:570–575, 1987.

11. Sorge, J., Kuhl, W., West, C., and Beutler, E. Complete correction of enzymatic defect of type I Gaucher disease fibroblasts by retroviral-mediated gene transfer. *Proc. Natl. Acad. Sci. U.S.A.* 84:906–909, 1987.

12. Bishop, D. F., Calhoun, D. H., Bernstein, H. S., Hantzopoulos, P., Quinn, M., and Desnick, R. J. Human α-galactosidase A: Nucleotide sequence of a cDNA clone encoding the mature enzyme. *Proc. Natl. Acad. Sci. U.S.A.* 83:4859–4863, 1986.

13. Myerowitz, R., Piekarz, R., Neufeld, E. F., Shows, T. B., and Suzuki, K. Human β-hexosaminidase α chain: Coding sequence and homology with the β chain. *Proc. Natl. Acad. Sci. U.S.A.* 82:7830–7834, 1985.

14. Myerowitz, R., and Hogikyan, N. D. Different mutations in Ashkenazi Jewish and non-Jewish French Canadians with Tay-Sachs disease. *Science* 232:1646–1648, 1986.

15. Ohno, K., and Suzuki, K. The mutation in G_{M2}-gangliosidosis B1 variant. *J. Neurochem.* 50:316–318, 1988.

16. O'Dowd, B. F., Quan, F., Willard, H. F., Lamhonwash, A.-M., Korneluk, R. G., Lowden, J. A., Gravel, R. A., and Mahuran, D. J. Isolation of cDNA clones coding for the beta subunit of human β-hexosaminidase. *Proc. Natl. Acad. Sci. U.S.A.* 82:1184–1188, 1985.

17. O'Dowd, B. F., Klavins, M. H., Willard, H. F., Gravel, R., Lowden, J. A., and Mahuran, D. J. Molecular heterogeneity in the infantile and juvenile forms of Sandhoff disease (0 variant G_{M2}-gangliosidosis). *J. Biol. Chem.* 261:12680–12685, 1986.

18. Dewji, N., Wenger, D. A., Fujibayashi, S., Donoviel, M., Esch, F., Hill, F., and O'Brien, J. S. Molecular cloning of the sphingolipid activator protein I (SAP-I), the sulfatide sulfatase activator. *Biochem. Biophys. Res. Commun.* 134:989–994, 1986.

19. d'Azzo, A., Hoogeveen, A., Reuser, A. J. J., Robinson, D., and Galjaard, H. Molecular defect in combined β-galactosidase and neuraminidase deficiency in man. *Proc. Natl. Acad. Sci. U.S.A.* 79:4535–4539, 1982.

20. Sly, W. S., Quinton, B. A., McAlister, W. H., and Rimon, D. L. β-Glucuronidase deficiency: Report of clinical, radiologic and biochemical features of a new mucopolysaccharidosis. *J. Pediatr.* 82:249–257, 1973.

21. Catterall, J. F., and Leary, S. L. Detection of early changes in androgen-induced mouse renal β-glucuronidase messenger ribonucleic acid using cloned complementary deoxyribonucleic acid. *Biochemistry* 22:6049–6053, 1983.

22. Slavin, S., and Yatziv, S. Correction of enzyme deficiency in mice by allogeneic bone marrow transplantation with total lymphoid irradiation. *Science* 210:1150–1152, 1980.

23. Wenger, D. A., Sujansky, E., Fennessey, P. V., and Thompson, J. N. Human β-mannosidase deficiency. *New Engl. J. Med.* 315:1201–1205, 1986.

24. Fukushima, H., de Wet, J. R., and O'Brien, J. S. Molecular cloning of a cDNA for human α-fucosidase. *Proc. Natl. Acad. Sci. U.S.A.* 82:1262–1265, 1985.

25. Schutgens, R. B. H., Heymans, B. S. A., Wanders, R. J. A., van den Bosch, H., and Tager, J. M. Peroxisomal disorders: A newly recognized group of genetic diseases. *Eur. J. Pediatr.* 144:430–440, 1986.

CHAPTER 38

Disorders of Amino Acid Metabolism

Virginia K. Proud, Yujen Edward Hsia, and Barry Wolf

Basic Neurochemistry: Molecular, Cellular, and Medical Aspects, 4th Ed., edited by G. J. Siegel et al. Raven Press, Ltd., New York, 1989.
Correspondence to Virginia K. Proud, University of Missouri Hospital, Columbia, MO 65212.

Amino acid metabolism involves many complex biochemical pathways (see Chapters 16 and 28). Genetic mutations, due to either altered structure or quantity of enzyme produced, can interrupt a single step in a metabolic pathway. Some disorders are the result of defective transport or receptor proteins. (The inheritance and molecular biology of genetic disorders are discussed in Chap. 23.)

Neurological disturbances result from altered amino acid metabolism when the biochemical pathway involved plays a role in brain metabolism, structure, or neurotransmitter function. A clear understanding of the consequences of such disorders is necessary for accurate diagnosis and effective treatment. In addition, knowledge about these disorders may help to elucidate normal biochemical pathways and neurophysiologic function. The interrelationships of inherited amino acid disorders and their organic acid intermediates are presented schematically in Figs. 1 to 3.

PATHOGENESIS OF CLINICAL FEATURES

Cognitive functions may be impaired by effects of abnormal transport and concentrations of amino acids

Mental retardation or impaired cognition, such as in minimal brain dysfunction, can result from a host of genetic, developmental, teratogenic, or metabolic insults to the central nervous system (CNS). Both extensive spongy degeneration and demyelination have been demonstrated in patients with severe aminoacidopathies. Whenever the concentration of a single plasma amino acid is significantly altered, the transport of related amino acids across the blood-brain barrier may be affected, producing abnormal structure, particularly during the period of brain development. Experimentally, uptake of labeled amino acids across the blood-brain barrier is unique for each amino acid, but is influenced by the concentrations of other similar amino

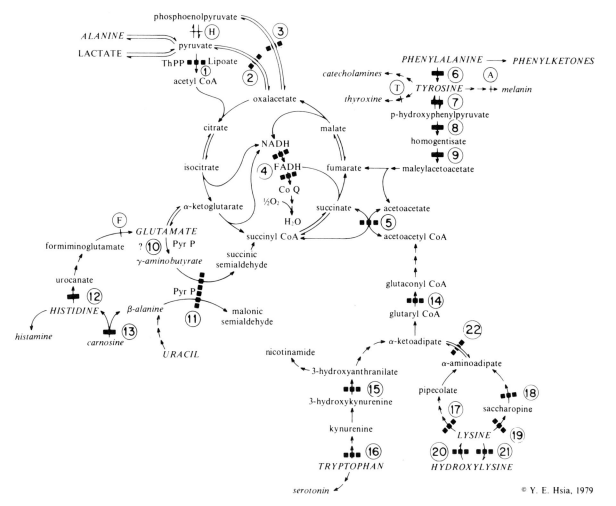

FIG. 1. Metabolic map of citric acid metabolism and related catabolism of some amino acids, indicating sites of inborn errors causing biochemical disturbances. The conversion of triose phosphates through pyruvate to acetyl-CoA (*top left*) leads to the citric acid cycle. The glutamate cycle, with its relation to formation of γ-aminobutyric acid is included, as well as β-alanine and its metabolism. The catabolism of phenylalanine and tyrosine are at the *top right*, indicating pathways of pigment and hormone formation from tyrosine; that of tryptophan and lysine are at the *bottom*, including the relation of serotonin, 5-hydroxytryptamine, to tryptophan. Within the citric acid cycle is diagramed the oxidative pathway of energy metabolism by which protons are transferred from NADH to molecular oxygen. The following abbreviations are used for coenzymes, which are included only when relevant to the cause or treatment of an inborn error: (CoA) coenzyme A; (CoQ) coenzyme Q; (FADH) reduced flavine adenine dinucleotide; (NADH) reduced nicotinamide adenine dinucleotide; (PyrP) pyridoxal phosphate; (ThPP) thiamine pyrophosphate; (A) sites of metabolic blocks causing albinism; (T) defects of thyroid hormone synthesis; (F) site of action of formiminofolate transferase on histidine catabolism (see Fig. 4). Enzymes: (1) pyruvate dehydrogenase complex; (2) pyruvate carboxylase; (3) phosphoenolpyruvate carboxykinase; (4) undetermined; (5) 3-ketoacid CoA-transferase; (6) phenylalanine hydroxylase; (7) cytosol tyrosine aminotransferase; (8) *p*-hydroxyphenylpyruvate dioxygenase; (9) homogentisate oxygenase; (10) glutamate decarboxylase; (11) ? β-alanine aminotransferase; ? γ-aminobutyrate aminotransferase; (12) histidase; (13) carnosinase; (14) ? glutaryl-CoA dehydrogenase; (15) kynureninase; (16) undetermined; (17) lysine dehydrogenase; (18) undetermined; (19) saccharopine dehydrogenase; (20) undetermined; (21) lysine hydroxylase; (22) ? α-aminoadipate aminotransferase.

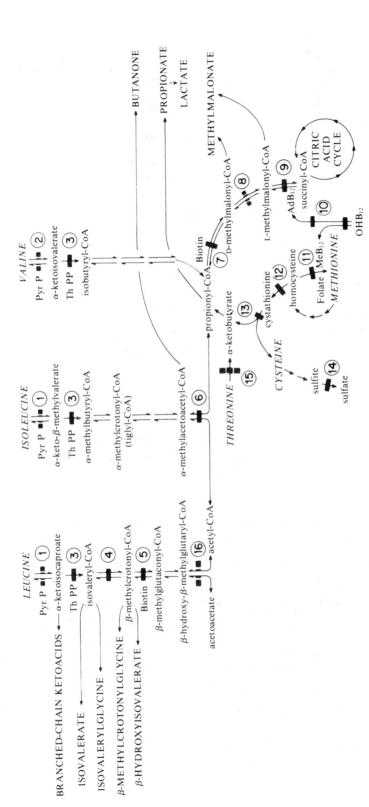

FIG. 2. Metabolic map of branched-chain amino acid and sulfur amino acid catabolism, indicating sites of inborn errors of metabolism. The catabolism of leucine, isoleucine, and valine descend to common intermediary metabolites from the *top*. Organic acids and other compounds excreted in these metabolic disorders are indicated on the *left* or *right*. The catabolism of threonine and methionine, with the pathways of vitamin B_{12} coenzyme synthesis, are *below*. Metabolic blocks at 6, 7, 8, 9, and 10 have all produced the syndrome of ketotic hyperglycinemia (see Tables 2 and 4): (PyrP) pyridoxal phosphate; (ThPP) thiamine pyrophosphate; (AdB$_{12}$) 5′-deoxyadenosyl-cobalamin; (MeB$_{12}$) methylcobalamin. Enzymes: (1) ? branched-chain amino acid aminotransferase; (2) ? valine-isoleucine aminotransferase; (3) branched-chain ketoacid decarboxylase complex; (4) isovaleryl-CoA dehydrogenase; (5) β-methylcrotonyl-CoA carboxylase; (6) β-ketothiolase; (7) propionyl-CoA carboxylase; (8) ? methylmalonyl-CoA racemase; (9) methylmalonyl-CoA mutase; (10) steps in B_{12} coenzyme synthesis; (11) homocysteine:methionine methyltransferase and steps in folate coenzyme turnover; (12) cystathionine synthase; (13) cystathionase; (14) sulfite oxidase; (15) ? threonine deaminase; (16) β-hydroxy-β-methylglutaryl-CoA lyase.

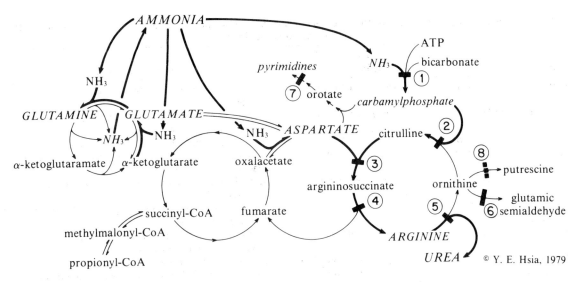

FIG. 3. Metabolic map of ammonia metabolism. The important relationships between ammonia, glutamine, glutamate, and aspartate are emphasized. The purine nucleotide cycle, which releases large amounts of ammonia from muscle, has been omitted. The relationship of the citric acid cycle to the arginine cycle is shown, as is the synthesis of pyrimidines from aspartate and carbamoyl phosphate. How disorders of propionate metabolism produce hyperammonemia is not clear. α-Ketoglutaramate, depicted on the *left*, has been found in the cerebrospinal fluid of patients with hepatic coma (see Tables 2 and 3). Enzymes: (1) carbamoyl phosphate synthetase; (2) ornithine transcarbamylase; (3) argininosuccinate synthetase; (4) argininosuccinase; (5) arginase; (6) ornithine transaminase; (7) orotidine-5′-phosphate pyrophosphorylase and orotidine-5′-phosphate decarboxylase; (8) ornithine decarboxylase. A transport defect of ornithine reentry into the mitochondrion is the probable cause of hyperornithinemia with homocitrullinemia.

acids that compete for the same carrier system (see Chaps. 28 and 30). For example, inverse relationship has been demonstrated between maternal plasma phenylalanine concentrations and the IQs of hyperphenylalaninemic children. Children with phenylketonuria had a mean of 10.5 lower IQ points per 25 mM increase in maternal plasma phenylalanine. Neuropsychological performance correlated inversely with plasma phenylalanine concentrations over 300 mM.

Metabolic acidosis, often with ketosis and lactic acidosis, arises from altered carbohydrate, organic acid, or amino acid metabolism

Acute acidosis arising from various conditions (Table 1) will cause symptoms of vomiting, ab-normal respiratory patterns, and decreased consciousness. Severe acidosis may produce irreversible brain damage. Chronic acidosis may also lead to general debilitation, malnutrition, and brain damage. Clinical experience with patients with pyroglutamic aciduria suggests that minimal neurotoxicity may occur with brief, moderately severe episodes of acidosis. In addition to the disorders of amino acid and organic acid metabolism listed in Table 1, ketoacidosis occurs in infants with type I glycogen storage disease, pyruvate carboxylase deficiency, and pyruvate dehydrogenase deficiency.

Lactic acidosis

Lactic acidosis can result from primary defects in the mitochondrial electron transfer chain, the pyruvate dehydrogenase complex, pyruvate

TABLE 1. Disorders of amino acids and organic acids that cause metabolic acidosis and are associated with neurological lesions[a]

Condition	Location of defective enzyme	Neurological lesions
Maple syrup urine disease	Fig. 2, reaction 3	Hypotonia, rigidity, retardation, failure of myelination
Isovaleric acidemia	Fig. 2, reaction 4	Drowsiness, cerebellar ataxia, hyperreflexia, psychomotor retardation
Biotin responsive multiple carboxylase deficiencies	Fig. 2, reactions 5, 7 Fig. 1, reaction 2	Prostration, irritability, lethargy, seizures, retardation, rash, and alopecia, hyperammonemia, lactic acidosis in some
β-Ketothiolase deficiency[b]	Fig. 2, reaction 6	Retardation, hyperammonemia in one; benign in the second
Acetoacetyl-CoA thiolase deficiency		Retardation, ataxia, chorea, hypotonia, in one girl with lactic acidemia
Propionic acidemia	Fig. 2, reaction 7	Lethargy, prostration, seizures, retardation; hyperammonemia in some
Methylmalonic acidemia	Fig. 2, reactions 8–10	As for propionic acidemia
Methylmalonic acidemia with homocystinuria	Fig. 4, reaction 6	May have cerebellar lesions, severe brain damage, convulsions
Pyroglutamic acidemia	Fig. 3, reaction 1	Retardation, athetosis, and tetraplegia in one of three known patients

[a] For disorders of carbohydrate metabolism and the hyperalaninemic lactic acidoses, see Chap. 33.
[b] Disorders described in only one or two families.

carboxylase, biotin holocarboxylase synthetase, or biotinidase, often accompanied by organic acidemia (see Chap. 33). Additional secondary causes of lactic acidosis include other organic acidemias, glycogen storage disease type I, diabetes, and fructose-1,6-bisphosphatase deficiency. Appropriate treatment of lactic acidosis depends on identifying the specific defect. Most will respond to a ketogenic diet, citrate, and vitamin supplementation (see also Chap. 34).

Abnormal organic acids accumulate as intermediates in specific enzymatic defects

Organic acids are intermediates in carbohydrate, lipid, steroid, and biogenic amine metabolism. Most organic acids are concentrated in the urine. Two hundred fifty different organic acids have been identified in the urine of normal individuals. Organic acid concentrations in plasma or urine may be modified by dietary change, environmental contamination, drug metabolism, and bacterial activity in the colon. Artifactual changes may occur during collection, storage, or processing of specimens. Therefore, analysis of tissue or body fluid organic acids depends on comparison with known standards. Gas-liquid chromatography and mass spectroscopy are particularly useful in the definitive identification and quantitation of abnormal organic acids.

Table 1 summarizes some of the disorders associated with abnormal urinary organic acids. Primary defects in organic acid metabolism are difficult to recognize and diagnose, but the presence of increased concentrations of abnormal organic acids may suggest a specific disorder or group of disorders.

Clinical features of these disorders include intermittent lethargy, vomiting, increased anion gap, ketonuria, hypoglycemia, hyperammonemia, hyperglycinuria, and seizures. Skin rashes, photosensitivity, hepatomegaly, and growth retardation are also common. A unique odor of sweat, urine, or breath of a patient is often a clue that strongly suggests the need for further evaluation of a possible organic acidosis.

Elevated ammonia, possibly in synergism with other metabolites, produces neurotoxicity

Ammonia concentrations are normally maintained within narrow limits in the blood and brain. Its metabolic turnover is closely regulated by the active enzymes that shuttle amino groups among glutamine, glutamate, and aspartate (Table 2; Fig. 3).

Severe hyperammonemia in infants produces vomiting, lethargy, hypertonia or hypotonia, a coarse tremor, coma, and a decerebrate state, with or without seizures. In older children, moderate hyperammonemia may have mild episodic manifestations and is often characterized by aversion to protein-rich foods. High protein intake, constipation, or intercurrent infections can exacerbate ammonia elevation in susceptible patients. Ammonia accumulates in liver disease (see Chap. 39), disorders of the urea cycle enzymes, a few organic acidurias, ketotic hyperglycinemia syndromes, and a few disorders of the dibasic amino acids.

A combination of metabolites can cause serious neurotoxic effects without marked elevation of any single agent. Some diamine derivatives of amino acids, such as putrescine (Fig. 3) have important neurochemical interactions that may increase with hyperammonia. Typical histological Alzheimer type II changes in astrocytes correlate with the degree of hyperammonemia in patients and laboratory animals.

Transient hyperammonemia of the newborn may be severe enough to cause coma and death unless treated aggressively. It may be due to delayed maturation of argininosuccinate synthetase, complicated by asphyxia or toxic effects of parenteral infusions.

THERAPY OF AMINO ACID METABOLIC DISORDERS

It is imperative to correct acute ketoacidosis with hydration and buffer infusion

Peritoneal dialysis, hemodialysis, or exchange transfusion may be needed to remove toxic organic metabolites and ammonia while helping to restore normal electrolyte and acid-base balance. Cardiorespiratory support is often required. The final outcome varies, from coma and death, or chronic neurometabolic impairment, to normal development with intermittent episodes caused by environmental stress such as diet, surgery, or infection. Often the outcome does not correspond to the actual degree of deficient enzyme activity.

Chronic treatment depends on maintaining diet and environmental stability

The patient with an aminoacidopathy who survives must be maintained in metabolic homeostasis by avoiding aggravating environmental factors and by receiving adequate nutrition. Dietary protein restriction must be sufficient to limit accumulation of toxic intermediates, yet liberal enough to permit adequate growth and development. In several specific conditions, supplementation with glycine (see isovaleric acidemia) or arginine, phenylacetate, and sodium benzoate (urea cycle defects) can facilitate removal of toxic intermediates and utilization of alternate metabolic pathways. Cofactor therapy (see below) may be the mainstay of therapeutic support in certain vitamin-responsive enzyme defects.

Gene therapy by somatic cell manipulation is being attempted. Bone marrow and liver

TABLE 2. Hyperammonemia caused by disorders of amino acid and intermediary metabolism

Condition	Location of defective enzyme	Comments
DISORDERS OF ARGININE-UREA CYCLE		
Carbamoyl phosphate synthetase deficiency[a]	Fig. 3, reaction 1	Several variants reported, ranging from lethal neonatal syndrome to milder syndromes; each variant was unique to one or two cases
Ornithine transcarbamylase deficiency	Fig. 3, reaction 2	X-linked dominant, variable severity in females; lethal in neonatal period in males; variants are known
Citrullinemia	Fig. 3, reaction 3	Variable severity, ranging from lethal neonatal syndrome to milder syndromes
Argininosuccinic aciduria	Fig. 3, reaction 4	Hyperammonemia is inconstant and moderate; neurological toxicity may be due to argininosuccinate, with ataxia; psychoses may occur
Argininemia[a]	Fig. 3, reaction 5	Variants reported; hyperammonemia is mild or absent; patients have all been retarded
DISORDERS OF DIBASIC AMINO ACID[b]		
Hyperornithinemia[a]	Fig. 3, reaction 8	One boy with mild hyperammonemia, myoclonic spasms, and moderate retardation; no hyperammonemia in other forms of hyperornithinemia
Hyperlysinemia[a]	Fig. 1, reaction 17	Moderate hyperammonemia, spasticity, seizures
Hyperlysinuria	? Transport defect	Postprandial hyperammonemia, severe mental retardation
Lysinuric dibasic aminoaciduria	? Transport defect	Variable hyperammonemia; episodic abdominal upset, with pain and distension; inconstant hyperammonemia
Hyperornithinemia and homocitrullinemia	Mitochondrial transport	Variable retardation, seizures, and ataxia in one family; severe retardation and stupor in another

[a] Disorders of branched-chain amino acids; see Table 2 and Fig. 2.
[b] Disorders described in only one or two families.

transplants have been attempted, but these are more appropriate in disorders with minimal neurological sequelae, since the blood-brain barrier remains a major obstacle to whole cell, enzyme, or gene replacement. A major limitation of these interventions appears to be that biochemical correction may not lead to clinical improvement. These procedures also have risks of grave morbidity and mortality. Because specific tissues need not express a given gene product, several conditions, such as phenylketonuria, are not amenable to bone marrow transplantation. Other approaches to enzyme replacement such as microencapsulated concentrates and fetal neural tissue transplantation, have been attempted with limited success. Most of these disorders are diagnosable prenatally. Ultimately, enzyme or gene manipulation during the early stages of zygote division may be possible.

BRANCHED-CHAIN AMINO ACIDS

Disorders of branched-chain amino acid catabolism (Fig. 2) are characterized by nonspecific symptoms of acute irritability, hypo- or hyper-tonicity, and drowsiness resulting from severe acidosis, hypoglycemia, or hyperammonemia. Brain damage may occur from failure of post-natal myelination. Cerebellar ataxia has been reported in some patients but not consistently. Specific organic acidemias are characteristic of several of these conditions.

Maple syrup urine disease is a disorder of branched-chain ketoacid dehydrogenase

Ketoacid dehydrogenase (Fig. 2, reaction 3), is a multienzyme complex analogous to pyruvate dehydrogenase in that the intermediate steps are similar and depend on the same cofactors: thiamine pyrophosphate, lipoic acid, nicotina-mide adenine dinucleotide, flavin adenine di-nucleotide, and coenzyme A (CoA). The defect results in elevated branched-chain amino acids and their ketoacid analogs in the blood, cere-brospinal fluid, and urine. Five variants are rec-ognized. Classic maple syrup urine disease is usually lethal in early infancy unless treated by restricting intake of leucine, isoleucine, and va-line. The source of the maple syrup odor, char-acteristic of this disease, has not been defined. Intermittent branched-chain ketoaciduria is a variant with a milder course, sometimes with ataxia. Patients may remain well except when stressed by infection or surgery, but it can be lethal. An intermediate type may not be ex-plained by a difference in enzyme activity. A fourth variant is thiamine responsive. Affected patients may escape all neurotoxicity if treat-ment is started early. A fifth variant is due to deficiency of dihydrolipoyl dehydrogenase, a component of the branched-chain ketoacid de-hydrogenase complex, and is associated with lactic acidosis. These variants make clinical di-agnosis difficult. Any child with hypotonia, in-termittent ketosis, and developmental delay must be evaluated for these abnormalities of branched-chain amino acid metabolism.

Newborn screening by blood-spot analysis for elevated leucine is effective in diagnosing the classic and intermediate forms. Intermittent and thiamine-responsive forms may not mani-fest in the newborn period. The incidence of the disorder is approximately 1 in 250,000 new-borns. Prenatal diagnosis is possible by analysis of branched-chain ketoacid dehydrogenase ac-tivity in cultured amniocytes. In addition to di-etary restriction, acute toxicity may require peritoneal dialysis or exchange transfusion. Thiamine supplementation should be initiated as soon as the diagnosis is suspected.

Isovaleric acidemia is a disorder of isoleucine metabolism

Two clinical types of isovaleric acidemia have been reported (Fig. 2, reaction 4): an acute, se-vere neonatal form and a chronic, intermittent form; however, true biochemical or genetic het-erogeneity has not been documented.

The acute form is characterized by severe ketoacidosis associated with an offensive odor of "pungent cheese" or "sweaty feet" due to excess isovaleric acid. Lethargy, poor feeding, vomiting, coma, and death occur in half of the patients. If a patient survives the neonatal pe-riod, the course is similar to the chronic, inter-mittent form with recurrent, often milder epi-sodes when stressed by surgery, infection, or a protein load. Common hematologic complica-tions include leukopenia, thrombocytopenia, and anemia.

Treatment by restriction of dietary leucine or protein has been beneficial. Administration of glycine enhances the formation and excretion of isovaleryl glycine.

KETOTIC HYPERGLYCINEMIC SYNDROMES

Organic acidemias due to enzyme blocks in iso-leucine and valine catabolism (Fig. 2, reactions

6–10) produce a common syndrome of keto-acidosis with intermittent hyperglycinemia, leukopenia, thrombocytopenia, hypoglycemia, and hyperammonemia. Affected children may exhibit acute metabolic imbalance in infancy, resulting in coma and death, or survival with episodic attacks of ketoacidosis or hyperammonemia, or both. As with many of the aminoacidopathies, a group of patients present later in life with seizures or moderate mental retardation but without serious metabolic disturbances.

Propionic acidemia is due to propionyl-CoA carboxylase deficiency

Lack of propionyl-CoA carboxylase (Fig. 2, reaction 7), usually causes ketoacidosis, hyperglycinemia, severe hyperammonemia, and lactic acidosis. Neonatal presentation may proceed to ketonuria, vomiting, coma, and death, but clinical expression has considerable variability. Some patients present at several years of age with developmental delay and seizures. One asymptomatic teenage girl had deficient enzyme activity indistinguishable from her symptomatic affected brother. Patients with apparent nonketotic hyperglycinemia should also be evaluated for propionyl-CoA carboxylase deficiency.

Neurotoxicity may arise from the hyperammonemia, the accumulation of organic acids, or odd-chain fatty acids. Synthesis of myelin and other brain lipids may be impaired. Patients have been found to have the potentially neurotoxic precursors and metabolites of propionate, tiglic acid, β-hydroxypropionate, and methylcitrate. Some patients had moderate mental retardation and seizures with intermittent hyperglycinemia without overt episodes of ketoacidosis. This raises the possibility that glycine is neurotoxic in these patients, as it is in primary defects of glycine catabolism; however, some patients were neurologically intact,

suggesting that elevation of glycine or propionate alone need not be neurotoxic. The affected sibling of one severely retarded athetotic child was treated by dietary restriction from birth and displayed superior intelligence at age 10 years. Several affected patients may have had secondary immune deficiencies.

Although propionyl-CoA carboxylase is a biotin-dependent enzyme, reports of successful treatment with biotin have not been verified. Dietary restriction of isoleucine, valine, threonine, and methionine is recommended. Any patient with hyperglycinuria on routine urine amino acid screening should be further evaluated by organic acid analysis. Since these patients, as well as those with other ketotic organic acidurias, often become carnitine deficient, carnitine supplementation is frequently beneficial.

Methylmalonic acidemia is due to deficient activity of methylmalonyl-CoA mutase or to defects in cyanocobalamin (vitamin B_{12}) metabolism

Primary methylmalonyl-CoA mutase deficiency (Fig. 2, reaction 9) and the vitamin B_{12}-responsive methylmalonic acidemias (Fig. 2, reaction 10) are ketotic hyperglycinemia syndromes (Table 1). The clinical picture is variable, but these diagnoses should be suspected in infants with acidosis and hyperglycinuria. The diagnosis is confirmed by organic acid analysis for excess methylmalonic acid in urine or plasma or by specific enzyme analysis in leukocytes or cultured cells. Homocysteine, vitamin B_{12}, and transcobalamin concentrations in plasma should be measured before a therapeutic trial of hydroxycobalamin injections. All affected patients should be given protein restricted diets. Episodes of severe ketosis may recur with stress, dietary excess, or infection. Thrombocytopenia and osteoporosis often occur.

Methylmalonic acidemia with homocystinuria results from defective formation of vitamin B_{12} and causes hypomethioninemia

Patients affected with methylmalonic acidemia with homocystinuria have normal serum cobalamin without hyperglycinemia or hyperammonemia (Fig. 4, reaction 6). At least ten patients have had neuropathological findings, including cerebral atrophy, histologic changes resembling those seen in pernicious anemia, and abnormal branched-chain and odd-chain fatty acids in the phospholipids of the brain, spinal cord, and sciatic nerve. Unusual neurological manifestations have been described in a teenage boy who was mentally retarded with psychosis, ataxia, increased deep tendon reflexes, and intention tremor. His 2-year-old, enzyme-deficient brother was asymptomatic; neither was anemic. Acquired vitamin B_{12} deficiency such as occurs in pernicious anemia (see Chap. 34) may produce degeneration of the long tracts of the spinal column, peripheral neuropathy, psychological deterioration, and even amblyopia due to metabolic blocks in both methylmalonate oxidation and homocysteine:methionine methyl transfer, resulting in methylmalonic aciduria. Sural nerve biopsies of patients with pernicious anemia have shown abnormal incorporation of propionate into odd-chain and branched-chain fatty acids.

β-Ketothiolase deficiency involves the final reaction in the conversion of isoleucine to propionyl-CoA

A variety of presentations have been described in children who lack β-ketothiolase (Fig. 2, reaction 6). There may be acute episodes of ketoacidosis when stressed or normal clinical and biochemical parameters. A single patient had hyperammonemia, hyperglycinemia, and developmental retardation. The marked clinical variability may be due to differences in the degree of enzyme deficiency or to differences in dietary and infectious stresses.

GLYCINE AND NONKETOTIC HYPERGLYCINEMIA

Glycine is abundantly present in most tissue fluids and cells; it participates in many metabolic reactions. In the nervous system, it can be formed from glyoxylate and serine and is formed slowly from glucose. Degradation in the brain is primarily by the glycine cleavage enzyme system (Fig. 4, reaction 7). Glycine, a putative inhibitory neurotransmitter, is present in very high concentrations in the inhibitory interneurons of spinal gray matter (see Chap. 15).

Sarcosine (*N*-methylglycine)

Sarcosine (*N*-methylglycine) is demethylated by sarcosine dehydrogenase to form glycine. Patients with sarcosine dehydrogenase deficiency may be asymptomatic with normal intelligence, but several children with mental retardation and multiple anomalies have been described. Growth delay, hypertonia, tremors, failure to thrive, and dysphagia have been reported (Table 3).

Nonketotic hyperglycinemia

Nonketotic hyperglycinemia may be caused by deficiency of an enzyme in the glycine-cleavage pathway (Fig. 4, reaction 7). It must be differentiated from other genetic and nongenetic causes of hyperglycinemia, including disorders of branched-chain amino acid catabolism (Table 3). Patients with defective glycine-cleavage enzymes have early infantile onset of lethargy, hypotonia, myoclonia, generalized seizures, hiccups, opisthotonus, and are unresponsive to anticonvulsant therapy but do not have ketoac-

TABLE 3. Other amino acid disorders with neurological lesions

Condition	Location of defective enzyme	Neurological lesions	Comments
BRANCHED-CHAIN AMINO ACIDS			
Hypervalinemia[a]	Fig. 2, reaction 2	Lethargy, retardation	
Hyperleucine-isoleucinemia[a]	Fig. 2, reaction 1	Retardation, seizures, retinal degeneration, deafness	Also had prolinemia type II
β-Hydroxy-β-methylglutaryl-CoA lyase deficiency	Fig. 2, reaction 16	Hypotonia in one, spasticity and stupor in another	Hypoglycemia in one
GLUTATHIONE			
Pyroglutamic acidemia	Fig. 6, reaction 1	Retardation, athetosis, tetraplegia in one adult	Severe acidosis
γ-Glutamylcysteine synthetase deficiency[a]	Fig. 6, reaction 2	Spinocerebellar degeneration, psychotic behavior in one patient; myopathy in the other	
Glutathionemia[a]	Fig. 6, reaction 3	Moderately retarded adult	
DIBASIC AMINO ACIDS			
Ornithinemia[a]	Fig. 3, reaction 6	Lethargy, ataxia, myoclonic seizures, retardation	
Gyrate atrophy with ornithinemia	? Fig. 3, reaction 6	Choroidoretinal degeneration	Hypoammonemia
Persistent hyperlysinemia[a]	Fig. 1, reaction 19	Two or three sisters were normal	No hyperammonemia
Hyperlysinemia:	?	Severe retardation, hypotonia	No hyperammonemia; lax ligaments
Saccharopinemia and lysinemia[a]	Fig. 1, reaction 18	Severe retardation	No hyperammonemia; cerebrospinal fluid lysine increased
Pipecolatemia[a]	?	Irritability, tremor, hypotonia, nystagmus, paralysis	Low brain homocarnosine
Cerebrohepatorenal syndrome	? Fig. 1, reaction 4	Hypotonia, retardation	Biochemical lesion might be in electron-transfer system
Hydroxylysinuria	Fig. 1, reaction 20	Retardation, myoclonic seizures	
α-Aminoadipic acidemia[a]	?	Borderline intelligence in one of two affected brothers	
TRYPTOPHAN AND METABOLITES			
Tryptophanemia[a]	Fig. 1, reaction 16	Retardation, cerebellar ataxia	Photosensitive rash
Xanthurenic aciduria	Fig. 1, reaction 15	Some patients had subnormal intelligence	One variant is responsive to vitamin B_6
Hydroxykynurenic acidemia[a]	Fig. 1, reaction 15	Mildly retarded girl	Unresponsive to vitamin B_6
α-Ketoadipic acidemia[a]	?	One of two affected brothers was retarded, selfabusive, and without speech	

TABLE 3. *(continued)*

Condition	Location of defective enzyme	Neurological lesions	Comments
Glutaric acidemia I	? Fig. 1, reaction 14; multiple acyl-CoA carboxylases	Dystonia, athetosis, retardation	
Glutaric acidemia II			
GLUTAMATE AND METABOLITES			
Glutamic acidemia	Nongenetic	? Neonatal susceptibility to neuronal necrosis and retinal degeneration	Also reported in Menke's syndrome
Pyridoxine-dependent seizures	? Fig. 1, reaction 10	Neonatal seizures, retardation	Dramatically responsive to vitamin B$_6$
β-Alaninemia[a]	Fig. 1, reaction 11	Somnolence, seizures	
Carnosinemia	Fig. 1, reaction 13	Retardation, seizures, lethargy, spasticity	
Homocarnosinosis[a]	?	Spastic tetraparesis retardation	
PHENYLALANINE AND TYROSINE			
Phenylketonuria	Fig. 1, reaction 6	Retardation, microcephaly, hyperactivity, occasional seizures, psychoses	Treatable by restricted dietary phenylalanine
Maternal phenylketonuria		Embryopathy and intrauterine brain damage	
Hyperphenylalaninemia variants	Fig. 1, reaction 6	Probably benign	
Dihydrobiopterin reductase deficiency[a]	Fig. 4, reaction 2	Early retardation, myoclonus, seizures, hypotonia, chorea	
Albinisms[a]: Cross syndrome	Fig. 1, reaction A	Microcephaly, retardation, athetosis; abnormal lateral geniculate bodies	Microphthalmia; other variants have no consistent neurological lesions
Tyrosine aminotransferase deficiency	Fig. 1, reaction 7	Agitation, tics, moderate retardation	Corneal ulcers, keratosis palmoplantaris
Neonatal tyrosinemia	Fig. 1, reaction 8	Risk of some retardation	Immature enzyme responsive to ascorbate
Hereditary tyrosinemia	Fig. 1, reaction 8	Irritability, mild retardation	Liver and kidney damage
Alcaptonuria	fig. 1, reaction 9	None	Urine turns black, arthropathy
SULFUR AMINO ACIDS AND METABOLITES			
Methioninemia[a]	Fig. 4, reaction 5	One healthy infant	
Homocystinemia	Fig. 2, reaction 12	Borderline retardation and mental instability in some patients	Marfanoid habitus, ectopia lentis, thromboembolic complications; vitamin B$_6$-responsive variant
Cystathioninemia	Fig. 3, reaction 13	Benign	Vitamin B$_6$-responsive variant
Cystinosis	? Lysosomal transport	Photophobia, retinopathy	Progressive nephropathy, aminoaciduria
Taurine deficiency[a]	?	Depression, insomnia, dysphagia, visual abnormality, parkinsonism, respiratory failure	Three brothers, their mother, and her brother were similarly affected

TABLE 3. (*continued*)

Condition	Location of defective enzyme	Neurological lesions	Comments
β-Mercaptolactate cysteine disulfiduria	? β-Mercapto-pyruvate sulfur-transferase	One retarded man with seizures, one retarded man without seizures, two sisters who were normal	Second man had ectopia lentis
Sulfite oxidase deficiency[a]	Fig. 2, reaction 14	Severe retardation, multiple abnormalities, decerebrate rigidity	Ectopia lentis
GLYCINE AND SARCOSINE			
Nonketotic hyperglycinemia	Fig. 4, reaction 7	Lethargy, hypotonia, myoclonus, seizures, severe retardation in survivors, hypertonia, and decerebrate rigidity	
Other glycinemic syndromes[a]	?	Extremely variable	
Sarcosinemia	Sarcosine dehydrogenase	Inconsistent association with retardation	May be benign
PROLINE AND HYDROXYPROLINE			
Type I hyperprolinemia	Proline oxidase	Possible retardation or seizures	Renal disease may be coincidental
Type II hyperprolinemia	Pyrroline carboxylate dehydrogenase	Retardation, seizures	
Hydroxyprolinemia[a]	? Hydroxyproline oxidase	Retardation in two of three known cases	
Iminopeptiduria[a]	Prolidase	Borderline intelligence	Abnormal collagen
FOLATE METABOLITES (AND HISTIDINE)			
Dihydrofolate reductase deficiency[a]	Fig. 4,	None	Megaloblastic anemia
Cyclohydrolase deficiency[a]	Fig. 4, reaction 3	Retardation	Probably nonexistent entity
Formimino-transferase deficiency	Fig. 4, reaction 4	Retardation, cerebral atrophy; another two were very clumsy; one was normal; three had speech problems	Histidine catabolism is blocked
Histidinemia	Fig. 1, reaction 12	Perhaps speech problems, mild retardation, and infantile spasms	
Homocysteine-methionine methyltransferase deficiency	Fig. 4, reaction 6	Retardation, cerebral atrophy	
$N^{5,10}$-methylene-tetrahydrofolate reductase deficiency[a]	Fig. 4, reaction 8	Two sisters were retarded; the third patient was hypotonic with seizures; one of the sisters had psychotic episodes	Patients had homocystinemia, the psychotic episodes appeared to respond to folate therapy

[a] Disorders described in only one or two families.

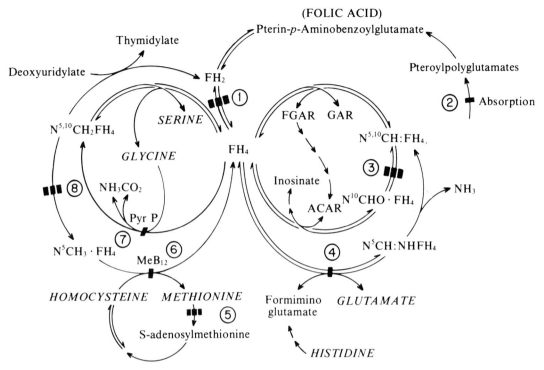

FIG. 4. Folate and glycine metabolism. The relationships of derivatives of FH_4 to glycine metabolism are indicated in the circle on the *left* and to purine biosynthesis in the circle on the *right*: (ACAR) 5-aminoimidazole-4-carboxyamide ribonucleotide; (FGAR), N-formylglycinamide ribonucleotide; (GAR) glycinamide ribonucleotide; (MeB$_{12}$) methylcobalamin; (PyrP) pyridoxal phosphate. Enzymes: (1) dihydrofolate reductase; (2) folate absorption; (3) cyclohydrolase; (4) formiminotransferase; (5) methionine adenosyltransferase; (6) homocysteine:methionine methyltransferase; (7) glycine cleavage enzyme; (8) $N^{5,10}$-methylene-FH_4 reductase.

idosis or hyperammonemia. Profound mental retardation affects those who survive beyond infancy. Hypertonia and decerebrate rigidity may occur in the later stages. Hyperglycinemia in the ketotic hyperglycinemia syndromes may be explained by secondary suppression of glycine-cleavage enzyme, but the mechanism of inhibition is not known.

Urine and blood glycine are markedly elevated in all the conditions causing hyperglycinemia, but brain and cerebrospinal fluid (CSF) glycine is markedly elevated only in patients with nonketotic hyperglycinemia. Patients with nonketotic hyperglycinemia have had undetectable glycine-cleavage enzyme activity in postmortem brain when liver enzyme activity was approximately 30 percent of normal. In these patients, every region of the brain had excess glycine. Strychnine or benzodiazepine administration has benefited a few patients, presumably by competitive binding to glycine receptors in the central nervous system (see Chap. 15).

GLUTARIC ACIDEMIAS

Glutaric acidemia type I

Glutaric acid is a normal intermediate in the oxidation of lysine, tryptophan, and hydroxylysine (Fig. 1, reaction 14). Infants with neurological deterioration and elevated concentrations of glutaric acid in urine and blood have been reported (Table 3). Dystonic posturing, choreiform movements, opisthotonus, and athetosis were noted in two siblings. Two other siblings exhibited developmental delay, seizures, chorea, dystonia, and progressive deterioration. Brain changes resembled those of Huntington's disease. Treatment has been with a diet low in tryptophan and lysine, supplemented with riboflavin and γ-aminobenzoic acid analogs.

Glutaric acidemia type II

Glutaric acidemia type II is an organic acidemia characterized by overwhelming dicarboxylic and glutaric acid elevations in serum and urine. Multiple acyl-CoA dehydrogenase deficiencies are found, suggesting that a common electron transport flavoprotein or enzyme is abnormal. Severe acidosis, hypoglycemia and, hypothermia occur in some children with a peculiar acrid odor. Dysmorphic facial features, including a high forehead, epicanthal folds, low-set ears, polycystic kidneys, and ventricular septal defect have been reported in several children. Although this disorder is generally fatal, a 19-year-old with hypoglycemia, elevated serum-free fatty acids, and organic acidemia, including glutaric acid, ethylmalonic acid, dicarboxylic acids, and isovalerylglycine, has been reported.

THE UREA CYCLE AND AMMONIA DETOXIFICATION

Ammonia detoxification occurs by reversible incorporation into glutamate, glutamine, aspartate, and asparagine and by fixation into urea through the Krebs-Henseleit arginine cycle (Fig. 3). Three enzymes, N-acetyl glutamate synthetase, carbamyl phosphate synthetase, and ornithine transcarbamylase are mitochon-

drial, whereas arginosuccinate synthetase, arginosuccinase, and arginase are cytosolic. The cycle synthesizes arginine, urea, and ornithine from ammonia, aspartate, and carbamyl phosphate mainly in the liver. In defects of the urea cycle enzymes, urea biosynthesis is never totally absent, perhaps because of continued urea production from arginine. Total block of urea biosynthesis is probably not compatible with fetal survival. Many infants succumb in the neonatal period. The major clinical findings in patients with defects of the urea cycle are neonatal coma from hyperammonemia and later protein intolerance with mental deficit.

Carbamyl phosphate accumulates in the mitochondria and leaks into the cytoplasm where it is converted to carbamyl aspartate, the rate-limiting step in pyrimidine biosynthesis. This stimulates orotate production; increased orotic aciduria is helpful in identifying carriers as well as affected patients.

Clinically suspect newborns or infants with a positive family history should have an immediate serum ammonia determination, with suspension of all milk feedings. Very strict protein restriction, ketoacid analog supplementation, arginine, sodium benzoate (to promote hippurate excretion), and phenylacetate supplementation are the main therapeutic modalities.

All the urea cycle enzyme deficiencies are autosomal recessive traits, except for ornithine transcarbamylase deficiency, which is X-linked and frequently lethal in males, but has variable expression in females. Prenatal diagnosis is possible by amniocyte enzyme assays for the cytosolic enzymes or DNA analysis in families at risk for ornithine transcarbamylase deficiency.

N-acetylglutamate synthetase deficiency

N-Acetylglutamate is an activator of carbamyl phosphatate synthetase. A male infant with N-acetylglutamate synthetase deficiency (Fig. 3, reaction 9) developed hyperammonemia without orotic aciduria on the third day of life. By

9 months of age, ataxia and slight retardation had occurred despite treatment with carbamyl glutamate, arginine, and dietary protein restriction.

Carbamyl phosphate synthetase deficiency

The hepatic mitochondrial enzyme, carbamyl phosphate synthetase I, preferentially accepts ammonia and is the primer for urea synthesis. A ubiquitous cytoplasmic enzyme, carbamyl phosphate synthetase II (Fig. 3, reaction 1), preferentially accepts glutamine as a substrate and is the primer for pyrimidine biosynthesis. Unless assays differentiate between these two enzymes, deficiency of the hepatic mitochondrial enzyme may be missed. Secondary deficiency of the mitochondrial enzyme may result from low-protein diets or from toxic inhibition, as in Reye's syndrome, which also may lead to misdiagnosis. Rectal or duodenal biopsy has been suggested for neonatal diagnosis.

All patients with complete or partial carbamyl phosphate synthetase deficiency show developmental delay, but with aggressive treatment, normal intelligence should be possible. Brain computerized tomography may reveal acute leukomalacia, and later, cortical atrophy or ventricular dilatation. Abnormal EEGs and recurrent seizures may occur. Hypotonicity and spasticity have been reported. One heterozygous mother had migraine attacks and another had protein intolerance.

Ornithine transcarbamylase deficiency

Ornithine transcarbamylase deficiency (Fig. 3, reaction 2) causes severe hyperammonemia and major CNS toxicity. Orotic aciduria may be seen; this is the most common urea cycle defect. Severe and mild clinical variants have corresponding variability in transcarbamylase activity. Brain pathology includes cortical atrophy, loss of white matter, edema, and glial reaction with proliferation of Alzheimer type II astrocytes similar to that seen in experimental hyperammonemia.

Many treatment protocols to counter the toxic effects of hyperammonemia have been tried, but few male patients have lived more than a few months. Female heterozygotes have ranged from severely brain damaged to completely asymptomatic. Treatment has consisted of daily phenylacetate, arginine, sodium benzoate, and a protein-restricted diet.

Citrullinemia

Caused by deficiency of arginosuccinate synthetase (Fig. 3, reaction 3), citrullinemia can be fatal in early infancy, due to acute liver failure, or may cause severe neurological dysfunction by late infancy. Many infants have lethargy, hypertonia, convulsions, and coma in the first few days of life. Plasma ammonia and citrulline were markedly elevated, but argininosuccinate was normal or low. Several patients developed acute hepatic necrosis. Others showed vomiting, irritability, and seizures at several months of age and later displayed severe mental retardation and ataxia. EEGs were often abnormal. Some patients had cerebral atrophy and hepatic necrosis or cirrhosis. Neurotoxicity seems to be due to the hyperammonemia. Since argininosuccinate synthetase is normally found in brain tissue, the huge excess of citrulline that occurs in brain and CSF may also be toxic; however, a number of patients have done well. A retarded adult and a neurologically intact boy have been reported, neither of whom had hyperammonemia. Treatment has been with ketoacids or essential amino acid supplements, protein restriction, arginine, and sodium benzoate.

Argininosuccinic aciduria

Argininosuccinic aciduria is due to deficiency of arginosuccinase (Fig. 3, reaction 4) but is not consistently associated with hyperammonemia. A neonatal form presents with acute seizures and intermittent ataxia. A common infantile form is characterized by failure to thrive, feeding difficulties, developmental delay, and seizures; and a benign form is associated with long-term asymptomatic survival not needing treatment. Abnormally brittle and fragile hair with trichorrhexis nodosa (microscopic nodular protusions on friable hair shafts) is found in about half of the cases. One infant's brain had elevated argininosuccinate and altered amino acid concentrations. Treatment has been with protein restriction and arginine supplementation.

Argininemia

Argininemia is caused by arginase deficiency in liver, red blood cells, white blood cells, and fibroblasts (Fig. 3, reaction 5). Patients have feeding problems, coma, and seizures in infancy, with subsequent severe mental retardation, spasticity, opisthotonus, convulsions, microcephaly, and cerebral atrophy. Some had extreme hyperammonemia. Orotic aciduria was reported in one patient with a normal blood ammonia concentration. Treatment has been a low-protein diet and restricted arginine.

HYPERORNITHINEMIA

Gyrate atrophy of choroid and retina

Gyrate atrophy of choroid and retina is caused by deficiency of ornithine ketoacid transaminase, a pyridoxine-requiring enzyme also called ornithine γ-aminotransferase (Fig. 3, reaction 6). Visual defects and night blindness with myopia may occur in childhood, together with chorioretinal atrophy (Table 3). Electroretinogram response is totally extinguished; posterior subcapsular cataracts are common by the second or third decade; blindness occurs by midlife. Electron microscopic abnormalities in liver and muscle mitochondria have been noted. Pyridoxine treatment or dietary arginine may reduce plasma ornithine and might improve the visual

symptoms. Administering lysine to promote ornithine excretion by the kidney has reduced plasma ornithine concentrations.

Hyperornithinemia with hyperammonemia, homocitrullinemia, and protein intolerance

Mental retardation and myoclonic seizures characterize hyperornithinemia (Table 3). Mitochondria containing "crystalloid structures" were described in skin fibroblasts reported to be deficient in ornithine decarboxylase (Fig. 3, reaction 8). Hepatic carbamyl phosphate synthetase (Fig. 3, reaction 1) was only 20 percent of normal in another affected patient. Neither of these enzymes is thought to be the primary defect. This disorder may be due to a defect in mitochondrial ornithine transport. Lysine loading facilitates renal clearance of ornithine, and ornithine supplementation has decreased the hyperammonemia.

Hyperornithinemia can also occur during isoniazid treatment, perhaps as a result of secondary pyridoxine deficiency. Spuriously elevated ornithine in blood samples held at room temperature results from conversion of arginine to ornithine by red cell argininase (Fig. 3, reaction 5).

LYSINE AND HYDROXYLYSINE

Glutaric aciduria can result from abnormalities in lysine or hydroxylysine metabolism. Lysine is an essential diamino acid that does not participate in the transamination reactions of the general amino acid pool. It can be carbamylated to form homocitrulline, which, in turn, can form homoarginine in a manner analogous to arginine formation from citrulline. Lysine is catabolized by at least two pathways (Fig. 1): one through ε-*N*-acetyllysine and pipecolate and the other through saccharopine. Both pathways form α-amino adipate, which then enters the degradative pathway for tryptophan and α-ketoadipate. No specific neurochemical action is known for lysine, hydroxylysine, or their derivatives, except that pipecolate is structurally similar to some hypnotic or cerebrotoxic agents, such as piperidine. Various forms of hyperlysinemia are listed in Table 3.

GLUTAMATE, GLUTAMINE, γ-AMINOBUTYRIC ACID, β-ALANINE, AND CARNOSINE

The metabolism and functional significance of glutamate and its derivatives are discussed in Chapter 15. Metabolic disturbances within this group have been reported in a few cases (Table 3).

Glutamic acidemia

Glutamic acidemia has been reported in Menkes' syndrome, but the relation of glutamate elevation to the disturbed copper metabolism, profound mental retardation, and seizures is obscure. Excessive ingestion of glutamate as a food additive (monosodium glutamate) causes acute symptoms similar to those induced by acetylcholine administration. Experimental, long-term administration of glutamate to young animals produces damage to retinal ganglion cells and results in neuronal necrosis in the hypothalamus, arcuate nucleus, and elsewhere in the developing brain, paradoxically without measurable increase in brain glutamate concentrations.

β-Alaninemia

β-Alaninemia (Table 3) has been reported in an infant who had somnolence from birth and seizures that were unresponsive to anticonvulsants. β-Alaninemia and γ-aminobutyric acid were present in high concentrations in the brain, CSF, blood, and urine of this patient. This is the basis for the postulate that β-alanine and γ-aminobutyric acid share the same transaminase (Fig. 1, reaction 11). Carnosine and β-alanylhistidine were also increased in the brain of this patient.

Carnosinemia

Carnosinemia, described in a few patients, is caused by deficiency of carnosinase (Fig. 1, reaction 13), a metalloprotein containing zinc. Carnosine is synthesized in the brain and muscle from β-alanine and histidine; the same enzyme synthesizes homocarnosine from γ-aminobutyric acid and histidine. The compound anserine, β-alanylmethylhistidine, is found in the muscle of many mammals but not in human tissues. The role of these dipeptides in brain and muscle is not known, although anserine and carnosine are both potent activators of muscle ATPase. Patients with carnosinemia are retarded and have myoclonic seizures, lethargy, and spasticity. Autopsy findings in one affected patient showed demyelinated white matter, loss of Purkinje fibers, cortical atrophy, unidentified "spheroids" in the cerebral gray matter, severe axonal degeneration, and atrophic fibrosis of muscle fibers (see also Chap. 33).

Homocarnosinemia

Homocarnosinemia is characterized by deficiency of homocarnosinase, a cobalt-dependent enzyme, in the brain. Homocarnosine is found only in the CNS and is converted to γ-aminobutyric acid and histidine by homocarnosinase. One woman had 10 to 20 times the normal concentration of homocarnosine in her CSF. Three of her children had spasticity.

TRYPTOPHAN CATABOLISM

Tryptophan, an essential amino acid, is hydroxylated and decarboxylated to yield the biogenic amine serotonin (see Chap. 12). It is catabolized through the kynurenines to α-ketoadipate, glutaryl-CoA, and eventually, ace-toacetyl-CoA (Fig. 1).

Table 3 lists several rare disorders in this group, including tryptophanemia, xanthurenic aciduria, hydroxylysinuria, α-aminoadipic acidemia, and α-ketoadipic acidemia. Although glutaric acidurias, types I and II, are disorders of tryptophan metabolism, they are described above with the organic acidurias. Hartnup disease is a disorder of tryptophan transport (see below).

AROMATIC AMINO ACIDS

The aromatic amino acids are of major significance neurochemically because they are precursors of catecholamines (see Chap. 11) and of thyroid hormone. Phenylalanine is hydroxylated to tyrosine. Tyrosine can be decarboxylated to tyramine, hydroxylated to dihydroxyphenylalanine (dopa), iodinated to the iodotyrosines and thyroid hormone, and catabolized through *p*-hydroxyphenylpyruvic acid to produce homogentisic acid and maleylacetoacetate (Fig. 1).

The hydroxylases for these aromatic amino acids and tryptophan have common properties: cross-specificity for aromatic amino acid derivatives, complex substrate- and product-inhibition behavior, and requirements for a reduced pteridine cofactor and molecular oxygen. Phenylalanine hydroxylase is a microsomal enzyme only expressed in liver, pancreas, and kidney but not in nervous tissue, white blood cells, or amniocytes. Tyrosine hydroxylase, present in noradrenergic and adrenergic neurons of the central and sympathetic nervous system, is the rate-limiting enzyme for catecholamine biosynthesis. Tryptophan hydroxylase, the rate-limiting enzyme for serotonin biosynthesis, is distributed in the brain in a pattern similar to that of serotonin, presumably localized in serotoninergic neurons.

The natural pteridine cofactor for phenylalanine hydroxylase is tetrahydrobiopterin (BH_4), which is recycled from dihydrobiopterin by dihydrofolate reductase or synthesized from pteridine precursors (Fig. 5, reaction 2). During the phenylalanine hydroxylase reaction, tetrahydrobiopterin is oxidized to the quinonoid form of dihydrobiopterin.

Phenylketonuria is due to deficiency of phenylalanine hydroxylase activity

Classic phenylketonuria (PKU) is one of the most common neurologically significant inborn errors of amino acid metabolism (Fig. 1, reaction 6). Prevalence is approximately 1 in 20,000 liveborn infants in the United States. The genetic defect is due to severe structural muta-

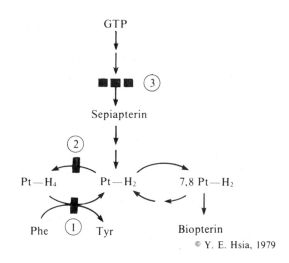

© Y. E. Hsia, 1979

FIG. 5. Generation and regeneration of tetrahydrobiopterin (Pt-H_4). The pterin cofactor for the aromatic amino acid is Pt-H_4, which is oxidized to the quinonoid form of dihydrobiopterin, Pt-H_2. Pt-H_2 spontaneously isomerizes to 7,8 Pt-H_2, which is oxidized to biopterin and excreted, or is salvaged by dihydrofolate reductase to yield Pt-H_4. *De novo* synthesis of Pt-H_2 is from guanosine triphosphate (GTP) through sepiapterin. Enzymes: (1) phenylalanine hydroxylase; (2) dihydrobiopterin reductase; (3) a step in sepiapterin synthesis.

tions in phenylalanine hydroxylase. PKU is detected in newborn screening by increased concentrations of plasma phenylalanine (>4 mg/dl) at 2 to 3 days of age, normal plasma phenylalanine response to BH$_4$ challenge, and absence of tyrosinemia.

The clinical features of PKU include microcephaly, hypertonicity, mental retardation, hyperactivity, aggressive behavior, seizures, eczema, hypopigmentation, and a pungent, "mousy" odor. Histochemically, there is generalized failure of myelination (dysmyelination) (see also Chap. 36).

Classic PKU was the first of the inborn errors of metabolism shown to be treatable by dietary restriction and for which large-scale, presymptomatic newborn screening has been effective. If PKU is confirmed, the patient is treated with a low-phenylalanine diet; serum phenylalanine concentrations are monitored to maintain the maximum between two and five times normal. In children with PKU, tyrosine becomes an essential amino acid and must be supplied in sufficient quantities to supply nutritional needs. When this regimen is rigorously followed, children with PKU are protected from severe brain damage. Dietary restriction may also ameliorate the hyperactive aggressive behavior of older retarded patients. Overzealous dietary restriction or imbalance can lead to malnutrition and secondary mental retardation.

A few adults with normal intelligence will have had all of the metabolic abnormalities of PKU. Unidentified innate biochemical differences or exceptional environmental factors may have protected these individuals during their period of rapid brain growth. Untreated adults have had major psychotic illness. Adult women with PKU, whether normal or retarded, are at a high risk for having miscarriages or infants with major malformations, such as microcephaly, congenital heart disease, and mental retardation. These defects might be prevented by dietary correction of serum phenylalanine concentration prior to conception and maintenance

of normal levels throughout pregnancy. Although phenylalanine restriction is often not maintained in adulthood, it is recommended to avoid aspartylphenylalanine methyl ester (aspartame), an artificial sweetener, since its ingestion raises the phenylalanine concentration in plasma without raising that of other amino acids of the L-transport system.

Heterozygote testing using phenylalanine:tyrosine ratios is often unreliable. Enzyme activity in the livers of carriers is usually approximately 10 to 30 percent of normal activity. Prenatal diagnosis and carrier detection using restriction fragment-length polymorphism or a DNA probe specific for the phenylalanine hydroxylase gene is feasible.

Many neurotoxic mechanisms could explain the brain damage in PKU. Unfortunately, experimental models for PKU have generally been unsatisfactory. A variety of abnormalities are found in the brains of affected individuals, including astrocytosis, structurally altered myelin, decreased brain lipids (especially galactolipids), decreased unsaturated:saturated fatty acid ratios, and decreased hydroxy fatty acids and sulfatides.

Atypical benign hyperphenylalaninemia

With newborn screening, patients with milder degrees of hyperphenylalaninemia have been identified. These seem to be due to milder structural variants at the phenylalanine hydroxylase locus. Neonatal hyperphenylalaninemia can be secondary to any cause of tyrosinemia, including prematurity; other hyperphenylalaninemia variants may be transient or more persistent but generally have a lower blood phenylalanine concentration than in classic PKU. Whether these variants are indeed benign has not yet been resolved. Whatever the neurotoxic mechanism might be in PKU, if it were directly proportional to the degree of hyperphenylalaninemia, the potential toxicity of the milder variants would be proportional to the blood phenylalanine concentration found during the vulnerable period of brain growth. In one survey, three of seventeen patients with an atypical form were mentally retarded. The activity of phenylalanine hydroxylase in liver was found to be 1.8 to 34.5 percent of that of normal individuals.

Severe PKU variants (malignant hyperphenylalaninemia)

From 1 to 3 percent of patients with hyperphenylalaninemia found on newborn screening will not respond to dietary treatment. These patients may develop intractable seizures and choreiform movements and all have had early, progressive mental retardation, despite apparent satisfactory dietary control of blood phenylalanine concentrations. Most patients had dihydropteridine reductase deficiency. Other patients had deficiencies in the synthesis of dihydrobiopterin. Since tetrahydrobiopterin (BH_4) is a cofactor for tyrosine hydroxylase and tryptophan hydroxylase, as well as phenylalanine hydroxylase, a block in the biosynthesis or regeneration of BH_4 (Fig. 5) will also interfere with catecholamine and serotonin formation. Deficient synthesis of these neurotransmitters provides a rational explanation for the refractory neurological disturbances in these children. All patients with hyperphenylalaninemia must be screened to exclude these variants. Treatment of these individuals with L-dopa, carbidopa, and 5-hydroxytryptophan has been attempted with variable success.

Neonatal tyrosinemia is found in premature infants

Approximately 1 percent of infants in newborn screening programs have had a benign transient tyrosinemia. It is most common in premature infants and may be associated with hyperphenylalaninemia (see above). This is mostly likely due to transient immaturity of liver hydroxyphenylpyruvate oxidase or tyrosine aminotrans-

ferase (a pyridoxine-dependent enzyme). Administration of ascorbic acid, a reducing substance that stimulates the oxidase enzyme, will usually correct the tyrosinemia. Decreased intelligence and acidosis have been reported in some tyrosinemic children, so whether it is truly benign is not clear.

Hereditary tyrosinemia type I is due to hepatic disease

This is a heterogenous group of disorders that may be secondary to viral infection, galactosemia, hereditary fructose intolerance, or other hepatic diseases associated with renal Fanconi syndrome. Some hypertyrosinemic patients with neurological findings, mental retardation, and a sweet or cabbage-like odor had decreased p-hydroxyphenylpyruvic oxidase. One was a 17-month-old girl with ataxia, hypotonia, and drowsiness. Another was a 35-year-old man who had tremor and ataxia. The disorder may be prevalent among French Canadians.

Hereditary tyrosinemia type II causes ocular, skin and neurological disease

The oculocutaneous form of hereditary tyrosinemia is due to tyrosine aminotransferase deficiency (Fig. 1, reaction 7), which causes tyrosinemia, painful dendritic corneal ulcers, keratosis palmoplantaris, agitation, tics, and moderate mental retardation. Lipid inclusion granules have been described in the stratum corneum layer of hyperkeratic skin. In the brain, tyrosine aminotransferase is mainly mitochondrial, and its role in tyrosine metabolism appears to be overshadowed by that of tyrosine hydroxylase. Therefore, degradation of tyrosine is superceded in the brain by catecholamine biosynthesis. It is not clear how neurotoxicity occurs in this condition, but dietary restriction to control blood tyrosine in the blood has improved at least the ocular and cutaneous manifestations of the disorder. The disorder has been treated with dietary restriction of tyrosine and phenylalanine, supplemented with pyridoxal phosphate.

Alcaptonuria is due to a deficiency of homogentisic acid oxidase

Alcaptonuria, a disorder in tyrosine metabolism, has no known neurological sequelae. The main complications are osteoarthritis and pigment accumulation in cartilage and sclera.

Albinism is due to defective synthesis of melanin

At least seven forms of oculocutaneous albinism have been described. Generally, they are associated with nystagmus, decreased visual acuity, photophobia, translucent irides, hypopigmented ocular fundi, and skin photosensitivity. Defective synthesis of melanin in the melanosome is sometimes due to tyrosinase deficiency (Fig. 1, reaction A). Curiously, melanin formation in the CNS, for example, substantia nigra, is never affected. Mammals have failure of decussation of the optic pathways to the lateral geniculate bodies. Deafness and faulty lateralization of visual or auditory stimuli have been reported. One form of oculocutaneous albinism (Cross syndrome), described in an Amish family, is associated with mental retardation, microphthalmia, choreoathetosis, and gingival fibromatosis. Another form, "bad locks, albinism, and deafness" syndrome has also been described with significant neurological findings and sensorineural deafness.

SULFUR AMINO ACIDS: METHIONINE, CYSTEINE, AND TAURINE

Methionine, an essential amino acid, has great biological significance, because *S*-adenosyl-methionine (Fig. 4) is the major methyl donor for many biochemical reactions. These include the synthesis of biogenic amines, such as choline and epinephrine, the inactivation of neurotransmitters, such as serotonin and the catecholamines, and the methylation of creatine, protein, and nucleotides. *S*-Adenosylmethionine may also be a precursor of polyamines. *S*-Adenosylhomocysteine, the demethylated donor, is recycled to methionine through homocysteine by homocysteine:methionine methyltransferase (Fig. 2, reaction 11; Fig. 4, reaction 6) or by hepatic betaine-homocysteine methyltransferase (see also Chap. 34) to regenerate methionine, an essential amino acid, using one-carbon fragments from serine and glycine (Fig. 4). Methionine excess has exacerbated the psychotic behavior of chronic schizophrenics. Hypermethioninemia occurs in acute liver failure and from blocked methionine or homocysteine metabolism.

Homocysteine reacts with serine to form cystathionine (Fig. 2, reaction 12), a compound with no known biological function, although it is found in high concentration in the brain, predominantly in white matter, and also in liver, kidney, and muscle. It is hydrolyzed by cystathionase to cysteine and homoserine (Fig. 2, reaction 13). Homoserine, like threonine, is a precursor of α-ketobutyrate and is catabolized through the propionate pathway (Fig. 2).

Cysteine is a component of proteins, glutathione, coenzyme A, and many other biologically active compounds. In cysteine catabolism, the sulfur radical is removed and oxidized (Fig. 2, reaction 14) to sulfate (which accounts for 80 percent of urinary sulfur); or the cysteine is oxidized to cysteinsulfinate, decarboxylated to hypotaurine, and oxidized to taurine. Taurine is found in very high concentrations in the cerebellar cortex, retina, muscle, and liver. It may act as an inhibitory modulator of synaptic transmission or as a transmitter. In the liver it forms bile salts that participate in fat absorption and are excreted in the stool.

Methioninemia

Several neurologically intact infants with methioninemia had hepatic methionine adenosyltransferase deficiency (Fig. 4, reaction 5). Because of the vital role of S-adenosylmethionine in transmethylation, it is surprising that this condition is compatible with survival, let alone with neurological normality. When detected by newborn screening for homocystinuria, hypermethioninemia is heterogeneous. Hypermethioninemia may also be associated with tyrosinemia, secondary to liver dysfunction, or hereditary fructose intolerance, a condition

called "oasthouse urine" disease, reported in a child with combined liver and renal abnormalities, and in two patients with complex neurological dysfunction, severe mental retardation, hypotonia, extensor spasms, seizures, diarrhea, and white hair (Table 4). They had the odor of burnt sugar or an oasthouse. The condition improved on administration of a low-methionine diet.

Homocystinuria

Deficiency of cystathionine synthase, a pyridoxine-dependent enzyme, (Fig. 2, reaction 12)

TABLE 4. Inherited abnormalities of amino acid transport

Condition	Location of lesion	Amino acids involved	Neurological features	Comments
Hartnup's disease	Intestine and kidney	Tryptophan and neutral amino acids	Ataxia, dementia, psychosis	Causes nicotinamide deficiency
Blue diaper syndrome[a]	Intestine	Tryptophan	Irritability	Hypercalcemia, indolyluria
Oasthouse urine disease[a]	Intestine and kidney	Methionine	Seizures, retardation, hyperapnea	White hair, odd smell, α-hydroxybutyric aciduria
Cystinuria	Intestine and kidney	Cysteine and dibasic amino acids	Possible liability to mental illness	Renal stones
Isolated cystinuria	Kidney	Cysteine	Probably benign	—
Pancreatitis and cystinelysinuria	Kidney	Lysine and cysteine	None	Hereditary pancreatitis
Lysinuric protein intolerance	Intestine and kidney	Dibasic amino acids	Abdominal cramps, hyperammonemia	Occasional growth retardation
Iminoglycinuria	Kidney	Proline, hydroxyproline, and glycine	Benign	—
Glycinuria	Kidney	Glycine	Benign	Kidney oxalate stones
β-Aminoisobutyric aciduria	Kidney	β-Aminoisobutyrate	Benign	A common normal variant
Hyperornithinemia and homocitrullinemia[a]	Mitochondria	Ornithine	Hyperammonemia	—
Folate malabsorption	Intestine	Pteroylglutamates	Retardation, athetosis, seizures	Megaloblastic anemia
Vitamin B_{12} malabsorption	Intestine	Vitamin B_{12}	Growth retardation, risk of brain damage	Megaloblastic anemia
Intrinsic factor deficiency	Intestine	Vitamin B_{12}	Growth retardation, risk of brain damage	Megaloblastic anemia
Transcobalamin II deficiency	Extracellular	Vitamin B_{12}	Growth retardation, risk of brain damage	Megaloblastic anemia

[a] Disorders described in only one or two families.

results in accumulation of homocysteine and methionine and depletion of cystathionine, with urinary excretion of homocysteine and traces of *S*-adenosylhomocysteine. Patients with homocystinuria may have congenital cataracts or developmental delay by 2 to 3 years of age. Affected newborn infants have been reported to have apnea, coma, and myoclonic seizures. Eye findings include downward subluxation of the lens, cataracts, central retinal artery occlusion, retinal detachment, and optic atrophy. A variety of neuropsychiatric symptoms, including muscle weakness, seizures, mental retardation, or schizophrenic-type emotional illness, may be present. Increased platelet adhesiveness and vascular fragility lead to multiple thromboembolic episodes. Marfanoid habitus with pectus excavatum in this disorder may be secondary to connective tissue disturbances.

The heterogeneity of homocystinuria indicates that a biochemical defect must be established before effective treatment can be started. Improvement following pharmacologic doses of pyridoxal phosphate has occurred in a proportion of patients. Low-methionine diet from infancy may delay or prevent its neurological complications. Supplemental dietary serine and cysteine to stimulate the reverse synthesis of homocysteine via cystathionase has been recommended.

Taurine deficiency

Taurine deficiency has been reported in three adult brothers, their mother, maternal uncle, and maternal grandfather who had mild depression, insomnia, anorexia, dysphagia, dyspnea, and loss of visual depth perception. They developed signs of parkinsonism and mental confusion; all three brothers died of respiratory failure. Biochemical investigations in one brother showed less than half of normal plasma taurine concentration and very low CSF taurine. At autopsy, taurine was reduced in all regions of brain tested, particularly the cerebellum, compared with controls or patients with Huntington's or Parkinson's disease. Other metabolites of sulfur amino acids and γ-aminobutyric acid were normal. Histologically, the substantia nigra was distinctly depigmented, with extensive neuronal loss and gliosis in his brain and in that of another brother. A younger sister was psychologically depressed and had low plasma taurine concentrations but showed no measurable abnormality in response to an oral taurine-loading test.

Taurine has inhibitory neurotransmitter properties in the CNS and retina. Dietary taurine deficiency produces a specific retinal degeneration in kittens. Because oral taurine in humans has no untoward effects and readily enters the CNS, taurine therapy should be attempted in taurine deficiency.

IMINO ACIDS: PROLINE AND HYDROXYPROLINE

Disorders of the imino acids proline and hydroxyproline are listed in Table 3. These disorders are heterogeneous, and each condition has been associated with normal intelligence.

ABNORMALITIES OF AMINO ACID TRANSPORT

Unique membrane-bound proteins transport solutes across membranes of all cells (see Chaps. 3 and 4). The proximal renal tubular cells and the intestinal mucosa have specialized microvillus membranes to increase surface area and facilitate transport. Highly specialized amino acid transport systems mobilize amino acids across the blood-brain barrier and maintain homeostasis between the body and the CNS. A number of abnormalities in amino acid metabolism are due to defects in these transport systems (Table 4).

Hartnup's disease

Hartnup's disease is characterized by a pellegra-like rash, reversible cerebellar ataxia, persistent headache, emotional liability, and a renal amino aciduria caused by defective neutral amino acid transport across the intestinal mucosa and renal tubule. The pellegra-like syndrome occurs because tryptophan malabsorption results in secondary nicotinamide deficiency. Therapeutic doses of niacin will reverse the cutaneous and neurological manifestations. One patient had cortical and cerebellar atrophy with severe generalized loss of neurons and Purkinje cells.

Lysinuric familial protein intolerance

Lysinuric familial protein intolerance has been described in several families, predominantly from Finland. The defect is in transport of dibasic amino acids by the renal and intestinal mucosa. Intestinal cramps, diarrhea, and vomiting after protein ingestion may be accompanied by hyperammonemia and obtundation. Affected patients may have short stature, enlarged liver, or mild mental retardation. Blood urea, lysine, and arginine are low; urinary lysine, arginine, and, sometimes, cystine are elevated. Arginine supplementation may be beneficial, suggesting that secondary arginine deficiency may be responsible for the hyperammonemia.

Cystinuria

Cystinuria is the most common aminoaciduria affecting between 1 in 2,000 and 1 in 15,000 individuals. The abnormal renal transport of cystine, lysine, ornithine, and arginine results in renal calculi from the less soluble cystine. The disorder is treated with large quantities of water and bicarbonate, to produce a dilute alkaline urine, and with D-penicillamine, to chelate cysteine, making it more soluble and less likely to form calculi.

Hyperglycinuria

Hyperglycinuria is a prominent feature of generalized aminoaciduria from any cause. Inherited transport defects of glycine alone are rare. The iminoglycinurias, due to defective shared renal transport mechanisms for proline, hydroxyproline, and glycine appear to be clinically benign.

Cystinosis

Cystinosis is due to an abnormality of lysosomal efflux of cysteine or its disulfide, cystine. The severe variant is nephrotoxic, with secondary generalized aminoaciduria, leading to renal failure by the second decade of life. Although there is patchy depigmentation of the retina and photophobia, with cystine crystal deposition in the cornea, it is otherwise neurologically benign. Unlike many other lysosomal storage diseases, the CNS is not involved.

AMINOACIDOPATHIES DUE TO COFACTOR DEFICIENCY

Many of the aminoacidopathies discussed above involve enzymes that require specific cofactors. The roles of biopterin, pyridoxal phosphate, thiamine, and cobalamin have already been discussed above and in Chap. 34.

The tripeptide glutathione is present in high concentrations in the brain

The enzyme γ-glutamyltransferase (Fig. 6, reaction 3) has high activity in the choroid plexus of the ventricles and in the ciliary bodies of the eye. γ-Glutamyltransferase has been found histochemically on the surface of certain neurons. Glutathione functions to protect red blood cells from oxidative hemolysis; however, the actual role of glutathione in the nervous system is unclear. The energy-dependent γ-glutamyl cycle, which serves to transport glutamate across membranes, depends on glutathione, a potent reducing agent. Neurologic abnormalities result from deficiencies at two sites of glutathione synthesis and at one site of glutathione degradation.

Pyroglutamic acidemia and aciduria

Pyroglutamic acidemia and pyroglutamic aciduria result in a chronic metabolic acidosis and, occasionally, neurological disorder. There is a generalized deficiency of glutathione synthetase (Fig. 6, reaction 1).

γ-Glutamylcysteine synthetase deficiency

γ-Glutamylcysteine synthetase (Fig. 6, reaction 2) deficiency was reported in one adult woman with mild hemolytic anemia, psychotic behavior, and signs of spinocerebellar degeneration. Her brother showed similar symptoms, except for the psychotic behavior, but he also had abnormal electromyographic changes. Both patients showed evidence of mental deterioration and exhibited generalized aminoaciduria. Unfortunately, the actual relation between the metabolic disorder and the neurological abnormality is not clear.

Glutathionemia

Glutathionemia has been described in three patients. The activity of the enzyme γ-glutamyl-transferase (Fig. 6, reaction 3) was reduced in body fluids. This transferase or transpeptidase may play a role in the transport of cerebral peptides, which are of psychiatric and behavioral significance.

Folic acid (pteroylglutamic acid) is present in food as polyglutamates

Polyglutamates are hydrolyzed to folate monoglutamate by the enzyme conjugase (Fig. 4). Folic acid is reduced intracellularly to tetrahydrofolate (FH_4), which serves as a cofactor to transfer one-carbon units at many sites of intermediary metabolism including glycine catabolism and purine biosynthesis (Fig. 4). Acquired folic acid deficiency in adults produces megaloblastic anemia resembling vitamin B_{12} deficiency but without the neurological consequences of pernicious anemia (see Chap. 34). CSF folate is normally three times its concentration in blood.

Congenital folate malabsorption

Congenital folate malabsorption (Fig. 4, reaction 2) presents in infancy with ataxia or athetosis, seizures, mental retardation, and megaloblastic anemia. The severe neurological damage in this disorder suggests that the developing brain is very susceptible to folate deficiency; but variable clinical findings and response to folate therapy suggest heterogeneity.

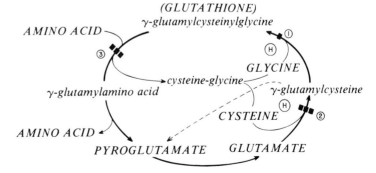

FIG. 6. Glutathione metabolism. Enzymes: (1) glutathione synthetase; (2) γ-glutamylcysteine synthetase; (3) γ-glutamyltransferase. γ-Glutamylcyclotransferase catalyzes the formation of pyroglutamate from γ-glutamylamino acid and also from γ-glutamylcysteine; (H) enzyme defects causing hemolytic anemia.

Formiminotransferase deficiency

Formiminotransferase deficiency (Fig. 4, reaction 4) blocks histidine catabolism and causes a large increase in urinary glutamate. A number of patients have had a variety of neurological symptoms, including mental retardation, hypotonia, clumsiness, abnormal EEGs, and cerebral cortical atrophy; but some had normal neurological development.

Methylene tetrahydrofolate reductase deficiency

Methylene tetrahydrofolate reductase deficiency blocks the synthesis of methyl-FH$_4$ (Fig. 4, reaction 8). One patient had psychiatric disturbances that improved with folic acid therapy. Two affected sisters and one unrelated male had elevated homocysteine in the urine and plasma and marginally low plasma methionine and folate, but cerebrospinal amino acids were not measured. One of the two mentally retarded sisters had an abnormal EEG and showed features of catatonic schizophrenia at age 14. Her mental status improved with pyridoxine and folate, but she developed peripheral neuropathy. She relapsed when therapy was stopped and improved again when it was reinstituted. The cofactors appeared to suppress homocysteine production. Their brother had proximal muscle weakness, seizures, and abnormal EEG but no mental instability. In these three siblings, enzyme activity in liver and cultured fibroblasts was less than 20 percent of normal. Flavin adenine dinucleotide doubled enzyme activity in cells from the sisters and controls, and stimulated it fivefold in cells from the affected male. Because methyl-FH$_4$ is a cofactor for the vitamin B$_{12}$-dependent regeneration of methionine from homocysteine (Fig. 4, reaction 6), its decrease in this condition would reduce the pool of *S*-adenosylmethionine for methyl-transfer reactions. Although degradation of methionine to sulfate in these patients was normal, their cultured cells did not grow in a medium when homocysteine was substituted for methionine, confirming that remethylation of homocysteine to methionine was impaired.

Biotin is the coenzyme for several carboxylases

Biotin is the coenzyme for pyruvate carboxylase, propionyl-CoA carboxylase, β-methylcrotonyl-CoA carboxylase, and acetyl-CoA carboxylase. Isolated deficiencies of the first three carboxylases have been reported. Several patients with these disorders have responded to biotin therapy, but further evaluation has either failed to verify this or revealed that the defect was a form of multiple carboxylase deficiency. Early-onset multiple carboxylase deficiency, due to a deficiency in holocarboxylase synthetase, usually responds to biotin supplementation. Biotin-responsive, late-onset multiple carboxylase deficiency is due to a defect in biotinidase, which is required for the recycling of biotin. These patients have all improved clinically when treated with biotin.

HEME METABOLISM

Heme is a tetrapyrrole ring with an activated central iron atom. It is a prosthetic group for many enzyme reactions involving mitochondrial electron transfer, oxygen transport, peroxide breakdown, and protein synthesis. Heme metabolism is diagrammed in Fig. 7. The first enzyme, δ-aminolevulinic acid (δ-ALA) synthetase, is rate-limiting and has a very short half-life of approximately 1 hr. δ-ALA is present in high concentrations in the hypothalamus, and it inhibits human brain Na,K-ATPase; porphobilinogen inhibits rat presynaptic transmission in the cat; the tetrapyrroles are potent photosensitizing agents. In degradation of heme, the porphyrin ring is broken to form biliverdin and bilirubin. In the liver, bilirubin conjugates with glucuronic acid, glycine, or taurine and is excreted mainly in the bile.

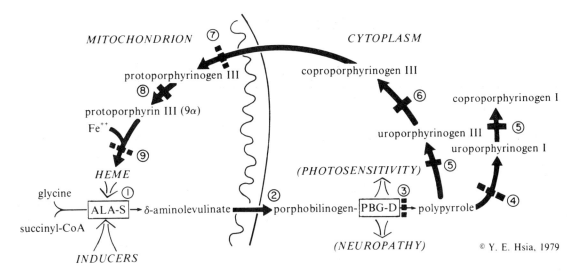

FIG. 7. Metabolic map of heme synthesis. The intramitochondrial generation of δ-aminolevulinate, shown at the *lower left*, is the rate-limiting step repressed by the end-product heme and induced by many agents. Two molecules of δ-aminolevulinate condense asymmetrically to form cyclic porphobilinogen; its deamination is thought to be a secondary rate-limiting step, overactivity of which produces excess of photosensitizing porphyrinogen products, and underactivity of which results in accumulation of neurotoxic precursors. Tetracyclic polymerization to the polypyrroles is followed by successive decarboxylations, reentry into the mitochondrion, oxidation of side chains, and finally insertion of the ferrous ion to form heme. The compounds on the *left* are excretion products found in some of the porphyrias (see Table 5): (ALA-S) δ-aminolevulinate synthetase (1); (PBG-D) porphobilinogen deaminase (3); (Fe^{2+}) ferrous iron. Enzymes: (l) δ-aminolevulinate synthetase; (2) δ-aminolevulinate dehydratase; (3) ? porphobilinogen deaminase; (4) ? urobilinogen I synthetase; (5) uroporphobilinogen III cosynthetase; (6) uroporphobilinogen decarboxylase; (7) coproporphyrinogen oxidase; (8) ? protoporphyrinogen oxidase; (9) ferrochelatase.

The porphyrias can result from toxins (lead and alcohol) and tyrosinemia and from inherited abnormalities of porphyrin synthesis

Unlike most other inherited enzyme abnormalities, the porphyrias are anabolic, and several are inherited as autosomal dominant traits (Table 5). These disorders may produce photosensitive rashes, hepatic dysfunction, or neurological and psychological manifestations, which are often precipitated by medication or other exogenous factors. Presumably, some intermediate metabolites are neurotoxic, whereas others are responsible for the photosensitivity.

Acute intermittent porphyria (Swedish type)

Acute intermittent porphyria (Swedish type) is associated with massive overproduction of porphyrins, increased δ-ALA synthetase activity, reduced porphobilinogen deaminase, or uroporphobilinogen I synthetase activities (Fig. 7, reactions 3 or 4) and decreased steroid 5-α-reductase activity. Patients become susceptible to acute attacks after puberty. Often, exacerbations are precipitated by inducers of δ-ALA synthetase, including barbiturates, alcohol, steroid hormones, particularly estrogens during the menstrual cycle, febrile illnesses, and starvation.

TABLE 5. The porphyrias

Type	Postulated metabolic block (Fig. 7)	Clinical features				
		Skin photosensitivity	Hemolytic anemia	Liver toxicity	Neurological involvement	Mode of inheritance
Acute intermittent prophyria (Swedish type)	3 or 4	None	None	None	Severe acute attacks	Autosomal dominant
Congenital erythropoietic porphyria (Günther's disease)	5	Bullous scarring	Usual	None	None	Autosomal recessive
Porphyria cutanea tarda	6	Bullous scarring	None	Frequent	None	Autosomal dominant
Hereditary coproporphyria	7	Mild	None	None	Milder acute attacks	Autosomal dominant
Variegate porphyria (South African type)	8 or 9	Mild scarring	None	None	Infrequent attacks	Autosomal dominant
Erythropoietic protoporphyria	9	Solar urticaria	Minimal	Present	None	Autosomal dominant

The unifying concept of the protean somatic symptoms in this disorder is that most are due to neuropathy. Autonomic nervous system dysfunction causes sweating, blood pressure lability, urinary retention, abdominal pain, and skin blanching. Other neurological manifestations include sensory or motor poly- or mononeuropathy, hypothalamic dysfunction, and inappropriate secretion of antidiuretic hormone; psychiatric disturbances occur in one-third of patients, including organic brain syndrome, depression, anxiety, and schizophrenia. Metabolically, δ-ALA and porphobilinogen are increased in the CSF and urine. Treatment is primarily the avoidance of precipitating factors such as known toxic drugs or starvation. Heme or hematin infusions to stimulate feedback inhibition of the porphyrin pathway have aborted acute attacks.

Variegate porphyria (South African type)

Variegate porphyria (South African type) appears to be due to a partial defect of protopor-phyrinogen oxidase (Fig. 7, reaction 8). Affected individuals may have neuropathic attacks and skin photosensitivity of variable severity, and urinary δ-ALA, porphobilinogen and coproporphyrins are intermittently increased with fecal coproporphyrins and protoporphyrins. These findings are compatible with blocked biosynthesis of heme from protoporphyrin and derepressed δ-ALA synthetase.

BILIRUBIN

Basal ganglia degeneration can be caused by many diseases, including toxic accumulation of bilirubin or copper (see Chap. 42). Neonatal hyperbilirubinemia due to immature hepatic conjugating systems is characterized by high serum concentrations of unconjugated bilirubin. When bilirubin penetrates the blood-brain barrier, it specifically stains the basal ganglia and cerebral cortex. Exchange transfusion, phototherapy, and phenobarbital to induce hepatic enzyme maturation, have all reduced the danger of basal ganglia degeneration and the resultant brain damage with acute opisthotonus, ataxia and seizures (kernicterus), late neural deafness, mental retardation and choreoathetosis, and cerebral palsy in survivors.

The Crigler-Najjar syndrome is a genetic deficiency of bilirubin conjugation that can cause kernicterus in infancy. Two patients were neurologically intact for 15 years and then developed movement disorders, myotonia, intellectual deterioration, and seizures. Autopsy showed neuronal loss and gliosis in the thalamus, the basal ganglia, and cerebellum. Although there was no staining in the brain, these patients may have had late-onset bilirubin neurotoxicity equivalent to neonatal kernicterus.

REFERENCES

1. Adams, R. D., and Lyon, G. *Neurology of Hereditary Metabolic Diseases of Children*. New York: McGraw Hill, 1982.
2. Ampola, M. G. *Metabolic Diseases in Pediatric Practice*. Boston: Little, Brown, 1982.
3. Bender, D. A. *Amino Acid Metabolism* (2nd ed.). Chichester: Wiley, 1985.
4. Bremer, H. J., Duran, M., Kanerling, J. P., Prvyrembel, H., and Wadman, S. K. *Disturbances of Amino Acid Metabolism: Clinical Chemistry and Diagnosis*. Baltimore: Irbin and Schwarzenberg, 1981.
5. Chalmers, R. A., and Lawson, A. M. *Organic Acids in Man: The Analytical Chemistry, Biochemistry and Diagnosis of the Organic Acidemias*. London: Chapman and Hall, 1982.
6. Cohn, R. M., and Roth, K. S. (eds.). *Metabolic Disease: A Guide to Early Recognition*. Philadelphia: Saunders, 1983.
7. Feuer, G., and de la Iglesia, F. A. *Molecular Biochemistry of Human Disease*. Vol I, Boca Raton: CRC Press, 1985.
8. Flannery, D. B., Hsia, Y. E., and Wolf, B. Current status of hyperammonemia syndromes. *Hepatology* 2:495–506, 1982.
9. Goodman, S. I., and Markey, S. P. *Diagnosis of Organic Acidemias by Gas Chromatography–Mass Spectrometry*. New York: Alan R. Liss, Inc., 1981.
10. Herrmann, K. M., and Somerville, R. L. (eds.). *Amino Acids: Biosynthesis and Genetic Regulation*. London: Addison-Wesley, 1983.
11. Holton, J. B. *An Introduction to Inherited Metabolic Diseases*. London: Chapman and Hall, 1985.
12. Hsia, Y. E., and Wolf, B. Disorders of amino acid metabolism. In G. J. Siegel, R. W. Albers, B. W. Agranoff, and R. Katzman (eds.), *Basic Neurochemistry* (3rd. ed.). Boston: Little, Brown, 1981, pp. 563–600.
13. Hsia, Y. E., and Wolf, B. Inherited metabolic disorders. In Avery, G. B., *Neonatology* (3rd ed.). Philadelphia: Lippincott, 1986, pp. 724–751.
14. Nyhan, W. L. *Abnormalities in Amino Acid Metabolism in Clinical Medicine*. Norwalk, CT: Appleton-Century-Croft, 1984.
15. Stanbury, J. B., Wyngaarden, J. B., Frederickson, D. S., Goldstein, J. L., and Brown, M. S. (eds.). *The Metabolic Basis of Inherited Diseases* (5th ed.) New York: McGraw-Hill, 1983.
16. Volpe, J. *Neurology of the Newborn*. Philadelphia: Saunders, 1987.
17. Wapnir, R. (ed.). *Congenital Metabolic Diseases: Diagnosis and Treatment*. New York: Marcel Dekker, 1985.

CHAPTER 39

Metabolic Encephalopathies and Coma

William A. Pulsinelli and Arthur J. L. Cooper

Basic Neurochemistry: Molecular, Cellular, and Medical Aspects, 4th Ed., edited by G. J. Siegel et al. Raven Press, Ltd., New York, 1989. Correspondence to William A. Pulsinelli, Department of Neurology, Cornell University Medical College, 1300 York Avenue, New York, New York 10021.

LEVELS OF CONSCIOUSNESS

Metabolic encephalopathy is defined as any disease process that disrupts cerebral metabolism sufficiently to alter consciousness. These may be acute or chronic processes with reversible or irreversible changes, but most if not all metabolic encephalopathies can cause permanent structural injury to the brain if left untreated.

Plum and Posner [1] define consciousness as "the state of awareness of self and environment" and describe two essential elements of consciousness: content of the mind and arousal state of the brain. Abstract thinking, attention, language, and memory are examples of the mind's content and collectively represent the brain's higher cognitive functions. The clinical consequences of metabolic encephalopathies on cognitive function range widely from relatively mild changes in attention to severe distortions of abstract thinking and loss of memory.

Arousal of the brain can fluctuate through several levels that are reflected by changes in a person's behavior or "appearance of wakefulness" [1]. Daily, the normal physiological effects of the sleep-wake cycle cause the arousal state of the brain to change from the fully alert to the coma-like state of deep sleep. Disturbances of cerebral metabolism may also affect the arousal state. Progression of such neurochemical abnormalities is associated with an orderly decline in the level of consciousness, with early signs of obtundation followed by signs of stupor and finally coma. The obtunded or lethargic patient is one who appears drowsy, has slowed thinking, and requires mild stimuli to maintain the appearance of wakefulness. The stuporous patient requires repeated, vigorous stimuli to remain awake, and the comatose patient is unarousable even with the most intense sensory stimuli.

Abnormalities of brain chemistry sufficient to cause encephalopathy and coma comprise a large and heterogeneous array of disorders. Vitamin and nutritional deficiencies (Chap. 34),

genetic diseases involving lipid (Chaps. 33 and 37), amino acid (Chap. 38), or carbohydrate metabolism (Chap. 33), substrate deficiencies (Chap. 40), and other still unclassified degenerative diseases (Chap. 43), may at an early or late stage disrupt the intricately balanced neurochemistry that subserves the integrative and arousal systems of the brain. It is beyond the scope of this chapter to review the metabolic abnormalities caused by each of these disorders or how such disturbances lead to encephalopathy and coma. In fact, although much is known about the primary neurochemical defects in most of these disorders, there are few definitive studies on how such changes cause altered cognition or arousal. Even in the often studied disorders of hypoxia and ischemia, hypoglycemia, hepatic encephalopathy, and uremia, which are the principal topics of this chapter, the precise pathogenesis of altered consciousness and cognition remains undefined. Accordingly, what follows is a descriptive account of the neurochemical and physiological changes that accompany the alterations of arousal and cognition in the more frequently encountered metabolic encephalopathies.

ANATOMICAL AND PHYSIOLOGICAL SUBSTRATE OF CONSCIOUSNESS

The content of consciousness is a consequence largely of the highly integrative activity of the neocortex. Arousal of the neocortex and other forebrain regions important for cognition is a physiological response mediated by several brainstem nuclei and fiber tracts that together constitute the ascending reticular activating system (ARAS). The anatomical and physiological limits of the ARAS remain undefined, but neurons within the brainstem reticular formation most directly responsible for arousal lie in the midline and extend from the middle of the pons rostrally through the midbrain and into the hypothalamus. Activating pathways ascend from the ARAS through thalamic synaptic relays to the neocortex.

Discrete structural lesions of the forebrain that cause deficits in language, memory, or motor function rarely affect in any clinically important manner the level of arousal unless the lesions are bilateral and involve extensive portions of the neocortex. In contrast, relatively small and localized lesions of the brainstem that interrupt the ARAS or its pathways are capable of altering consciousness through the full spectrum of lethargy to coma. Currently, most metabolic encephalopathies are thought to depress consciousness through diffuse disturbances of brain chemistry that act equally on forebrain and brainstem centers. Thiamine deficiency is one of the few proven exceptions to this general rule. The earliest encephalopathic symptoms of thiamine deficiency are caused by disturbances of specific brainstem, hypothalamic, and thalamic nuclei, which are particularly rich in the thiamine-dependent enzyme, pyruvate dehydrogenase (see Chap. 34). Future studies that focus on neurochemical changes in more discrete brainstem nuclei may reveal other metabolic encephalopathies that affect selective brainstem nuclei early in the course of the disease.

The diverse nature and location of the neurons that subserve arousal suggest an equally diverse family of neurotransmitters involved in this complex function. Although details of neurotransmitter physiology and its relationship to arousal mechanisms remain to be clarified, some evidence suggests a role for cholinergic and monoaminergic systems, including noradrenaline, dopamine, and serotonin.

HEPATIC ENCEPHALOPATHY

Human hepatic encephalopathy occurs in two forms. An acute form, fulminant hepatic failure (FHF), is associated with rapid onset of severe inflammatory and necrotic liver disease. The disease is characterized by progression of symptoms from an initial altered mental status and clouded consciousness to coma, usually within a matter of hours or, at most, days. At one time free fatty acids were considered contributors to the disease, but later work discounted this theory. Excessive ammonia may be a factor, but in some patients with FHF the blood ammonia concentration is found to be within normal limits at the onset of neurological symptoms; however, as the crisis progresses ammonia levels become elevated.

Much more common is chronic cirrhosis or recurrent hepatic encephalopathy, which accompanies chronic disease of the liver. In most cases, the cirrhosis is caused by alcoholism; in some cases, however, the disease may be due to infections, hemochromatosis, drugs, biliary obstruction, cardiovascular disease, genetic factors (see Chap. 38), or excessive exposure to certain organic solvents. Unless certain catastrophes occur, such as gastrointestinal bleeding or the ingestion of a heavy protein load (both of which lead to rapidly elevated blood ammonia levels), episodes of neurological dysfunction most often begin insidiously and develop slowly, nearly always requiring at least several days to reach a peak or to subside. Many patients recover from the neurological symptoms, at least temporarily; repeated bouts are common. Hypertension in the abdominal portal venous system characteristically accompanies chronic liver disease. Extrahepatic venous channels dilate, and the intravascular pressure shunts products of intestinal origin directly around the liver into the systemic circulation, bypassing the detoxification machinery of the liver (hence the alternative name, portal-systemic encephalopathy). In addition to extra hepatic shunting of potential toxins, the toxin-removing machinery of the liver itself may be depressed, further adding to the toxin load of the blood. Indeed, there is evidence that the urea cycle and glutamine synthetase activity may be depressed in cirrhotic livers.

In the following text we critically evaluate the various biochemical abnormalities thought to contribute to hepatic encephalopathy, keeping in mind that symptoms may be due to a combination of biochemical, morphological, energy, and physicochemical changes.

Elevated ammonia produces severe CNS toxicity

Many toxins are considered to contribute to the encephalopathy. These include ammonia, short-chain fatty acids, mercaptans, phenols, middle-molecular-weight compounds ($M_r \sim$ 2,000), and quinolinic acid. Although there is no doubt that each of these compounds (or class of compounds) at elevated concentrations is toxic to the CNS and may interact synergistically, much evidence suggests that ammonia is a major toxin in hepatic encephalopathy [2,3]. First, ammonia is a devastating toxin in infants born with defects of the urea cycle; the severity depends on the enzyme lesion. Most affected children must be treated as soon as possible with a regimen designed to lower blood ammonia. Abnormalities visible on computerized brain scans and IQ scores of surviving children correlate with the severity and length of neonatal hyperammonemia. Second, hyperammonemia is sometimes a complicating side effect in the treatment of epilepsy with valproate. In these patients, neurological symptoms occur without obvious liver damage. Third, ammonia is toxic to laboratory animals. However, acute hyperammonemia is somewhat different from that seen in patients with liver disease in that convulsions and hyperkinesia are seen rather than depression of CNS activity. Finally, crises in liver disease patients are induced by the administration of ammonium salts easily tolerated by healthy individuals and by ingestion of meals with a high ammonia-generating potential. Patients often respond, at least temporarily, to therapies designed to lower blood ammonia levels. On the negative side, it has been pointed out that blood ammonia concentrations do not always correlate with the degree of encephalopathy; however, blood ammonia concentration can fluctuate rapidly so that a single determination of the blood level is not necessarily a good predictor of brain ammonia levels. Better correlation exists between the degree of encephalopathy and concentration of glutamine (or its α-keto acid analog, α-ketoglutaramic acid) in the CSF of patients with hepatic encephalopathy.

Abnormalities may involve neurotransmitter amino acids

Ammonia metabolism is linked to the formation and turnover of a number of amino acids, two of which, glutamic and aspartic acid, are putative excitatory transmitters. Brain glutamate and aspartate are consistently lowered in hyperammonemic animals and in animals with experimentally induced liver disease. These changes in whole-brain glutamate and aspartate are usually modest; however, if the changes occur mostly in a select compartment, such as astrocytes or nerve endings, they could have a pronounced physiological effect. Some authors have proposed that glutamate neurotransmitter pools in the nerve endings are poorly repleted in the presence of excess ammonia, possibly by inhibition of glutaminase activity.

One widely publicized theory has suggested that hepatic encephalopathy is related to a defect in brain γ-aminobutyric acid (GABA) metabolism; however, this hypothesis is controversial and is not now widely accepted. GABA levels are usually normal in the brains of animals with experimentally induced liver failure and in biopsy specimens from patients dying with FHF; however, GABA receptor properties and density appear to be altered during hepatic encephalopathy.

Tryptophan, serotonin, and 5-hydroxyindole acetic acid (5-HIAA) are increased in the brains of rats with portacaval shunts. Serotonin and 5-HIAA are elevated in brains, and 5-HIAA is elevated in the CSF of patients with acute and chronic hepatic encephalopathy. Moreover, the serotoninergic receptor properties are altered by excess ammonia.

Fischer [4] has advanced the hypothesis that "false neurotransmitters" may contribute to the neurological changes associated with hepatic encephalopathy. False neurotransmitters are structural analogs of naturally occurring neurotransmitters that can occupy receptor sites blocking normal neurotransmitter function. Possible candidates include octopamine, tyramine, and β-phenylethanolamine. Evidence for the false-neurotransmitter hypothesis is as follows:

1. Patients in hepatic coma excrete increased amounts of tyramine and octopamine in their urine
2. Octopamine and β-phenylethanolamine are increased in brain and CSF of animals with liver failure
3. L-Dopa may lighten the coma of some patients with hepatic failure.

However, the effect of L-dopa may be peripheral in that it seems to enhance renal excretion of ammonia. Moreover, dopamine and norepinephrine in postmortem brains of patients with liver cirrhosis are not different from controls. In an experiment in which massive doses of octopamine were administered to rats, brain norepinephrine and dopamine were depleted 86 and 92 percent, respectively, with no discernible untoward effects on behavior.

In various animal models of liver disease, the concentration of tyrosine and phenylalanine is increased in the plasma, whereas the concentration of the branched-chain amino acids (valine, leucine, isoleucine) is depressed. The activity of the carrier of the neutral amino acids across the blood-brain barrier (BBB) is enhanced. These findings have prompted Fischer and colleagues [5] to suggest that in liver disease

an excessive influx of aromatic amino acids into brain causes an overproduction of monoamines. In patients with hepatic encephalopathy, changes in the plasma branched-chain amino acids (tyrosine and phenylalanine) ratio correlated inversely with the severity of symptoms. Fischer has advocated the administration of mixtures rich in branched-chain amino acids to decrease entry of aromatic amino acids into brain and to redress the imbalance in branched-chain amino acid uptake. Although most reports suggest that the treatment is effective, at least in the short term, some reports suggest no benefit, and the treatment remains controversial.

Hawkins and co-workers [6] investigated the effects of intravenous administration of glucose or glucose plus branched-chain amino acids on the brains of portacaval-shunted rats. Both treatments lowered the high concentration of brain tyrosine, phenylalanine, and tryptophan; neither treatment altered the high level of norepinephrine, but the glucose diet normalized the high level of serotonin and 5-HIAA. Hawkins et al. reported that brain glucose consumption [cerebral metabolic rate for glucose (CMRGlc)] was depressed 25 to 30 percent in all brain regions examined in the portacaval-shunted rat (but see below) and that neither treatment reversed this trend. It seems unlikely that excess monoamine transmitters in the brain are the primary cause of hepatic encephalopathy. One possibility for the beneficial effects of branched-chain amino acids is that they may help to normalize brain glutamate levels.

Abnormalities in protein synthesis are produced by ammonia and liver disease

Ammonia interferes with lysosomal protein degradation in rat hepatocytes and inhibits protein synthesis in brain slices from young rats. In rats 8 weeks after portacaval shunt, an acute ammonia load further depresses the *in vivo* incorporation of lysine into brain proteins; however, *in vivo* incorporation of tracer amounts of labeled leucine or flooding doses of valine into rat brain protein is unchanged 3 to 4 weeks after portacaval shunt. It is not clear whether impaired protein synthesis occurs after 4 weeks or whether rates of protein synthesis vary with different amino acids. There is evidence that the differences in incorporation of labeled amino acids into proteins may be related to the decreased capacity of the basic amino acid carrier of the BBB and the increased capacity of the neutral amino acid carrier in the portacaval-shunted rat. Acute administration of ammonium acetate to rats is associated with a decrease in brain protein. Protein content, particularly in gray matter, is depleted in autopsy specimens from patients dying with liver failure. The loss, which is largely neuronal, may severely compromise normal neuronal function in end-stage liver disease.

Elevated ammonia depresses metabolic energy reserves

In patients with hepatic encephalopathy, the cerebral metabolic rate for oxygen ($CMRO_2$) and cerebral blood flow (CBF) decline roughly in parallel with the decline of neurological function. In alert 8-week portacaval-shunted rats with chronic low-grade hyperammonemia, the addition of a superimposed ammonia load, that is, a load easily tolerated by normal animals, promptly led to electroencephalogram (EEG) abnormalities, stupor, and a marked reduction in $CMRO_2$ and CBF. There is some controversy, however, as to whether portacaval shunting raises or lowers CMRGlc of rat brain.

In acute as well as sustained low-level ammonia intoxication in rats, phosphocreatine (PCr) in the brain falls, whereas the adenylate pool (ATP + ADP + AMP) remains unchanged. In more persistent low-grade hyperammonemia, the total adenylate pool declines, but adenylate energy charge (see Chap. 40) remains unaltered. At ammonia levels of 1 to 3 mmol/kg (normal value, ~200 μmol/kg) in the

brain, both ATP and adenylate energy charge decline; the decline is especially notable in the brainstem [7].

Ammonia is known to stimulate glycolysis in brain extracts, probably by activating phosphofructokinase. Such stimulation could account for the apparent increase in CMRGlc reported for acutely hyperammonemic animals. Ammonia blocks oxidative metabolism of α-ketoglutarate and pyruvate by brain slices: Ammonia at concentrations of 0.5 to 1.0 mM markedly inhibits rat brain mitochondrial α-ketoglutarate dehydrogenase complex, a rate-limiting step of the tricarboxylic acid (TCA) cycle. Excess ammonia also inhibits isocitrate dehydrogenase in rat liver mitochondria, but its effect on the brain enzyme is unknown.

A theory formulated over 30 years ago proposes that ammonia is deleterious to the CNS because it stimulates reductive amination of α-ketoglutarate, draining TCA carbon. However, in hyperammonemic animals whole-brain levels of glutamate tend to be depleted, and α-ketoglutarate levels are either normal or elevated. Evidently, inhibition of the TCA cycle is not caused by withdrawal of five-carbon units but is due to a slowing of a key step of the cycle.

Several investigators have suggested that excess ammonia may stimulate glutamine synthetase, thereby draining ATP. This drain is likely to be small, however, and part of the increase in brain glutamine in hyperammonemic animals may be due to decreased glutamine breakdown. Nevertheless, hyperammonemia may cause a depletion of brain energy reserves (Fig. 1). D. D. Clarke (quoted in Berl [8]) has pointed out that the diversion of glucose carbon to glutamine could result in a loss of 28 to 38 equivalents of ATP that are potentially available through complete oxidation of glucose to CO_2.

In hyperammonemic rats both the cerebral lactate/pyruvate and cytoplasmic $NADH/NAD^+$ ratios are increased. The mitochondria are impervious to cytoplasmically generated NADH so that the electrons associated with this

NADH must cross the inner mitochondrial membrane via a shuttle system. Strong evidence suggests that the malate-aspartate shuttle (MAS) plays a major role in electron translocation in brain. The ammonia-induced changes in the lactate/pyruvate and cytoplasmic NADH/NAD^+ ratios suggest a block in the MAS [9], possibly by slowing of the glutamate-aspartate translocator and by decreased activity of the aspartate aminotransferases (Fig. 2). The block in

the MAS will further compromise energy metabolism.

Because CO_2 fixation and glutamine synthetase activity in brain are predominantly astrocytic, it is possible that at least a portion of the ammonia-induced cerebral energy deficit is in these cells. This deficit may contribute to the astrocytic pathology (Alzheimer type II changes) characteristic of hepatic encephalopathy in humans and laboratory animals.

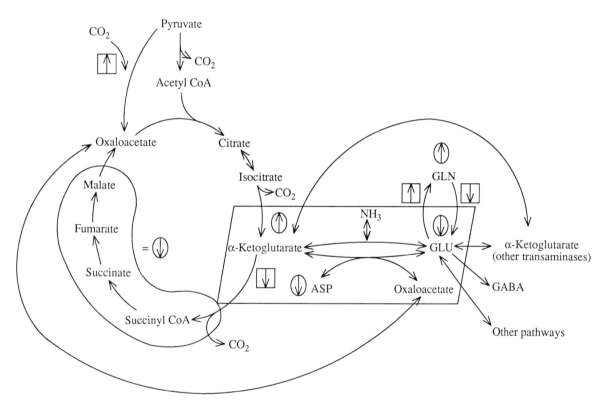

FIG. 1. Effects of excess ammonia on various substrates, TCA cycle, and related enzymes in brain where known. *Boxed arrows* indicate a stimulation or inhibition of an enzymatic reaction. *Encircled arrows* refer to ammonia-induced changes in metabolites. Note that most of the reactions depicted occur in the mitochondria but that changes shown refer to whole-brain metabolites (i.e., cytosol plus mitochondria). Excess ammonia strongly inhibits α-ketoglutarate dehydrogenase complex, impeding flux through the cycle toward malate, but strongly stimulates the anaplerotic pyruvate carboxylase reaction. Stimulation of carbon flow from CO_2 to glutamine will result in loss of ATP by (1) increasing ATP hydrolysis via pyruvate carboxylase and glutamine synthetase; (2) short-circuiting the TCA cycle (from α-ketoglutarate to malate); and (3) bypassing NADH formation at the pyruvate dehydrogenase reaction. Thus, the biochemical derangements induced by excess ammonia can be energetically expensive. (For further details see Berl [8].)

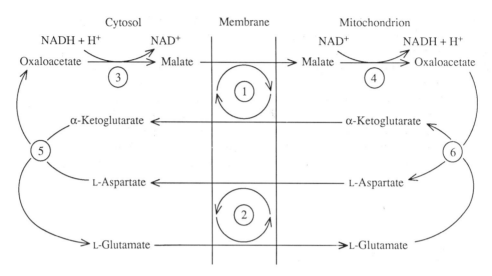

FIG. 2. The malate-aspartate shuttle for the transport of reducing equivalents between cytosol and mitochondrion: (1) α-ketoglutarate-malate carrier; (2) glutamate-aspartate carrier; (3) cytosolic malate dehydrogenase; (4) mitochondrial malate dehydrogenase; (5) cytosolic aspartate aminotransferase; (6) mitochondrial aspartate aminotransferase. The enzymatic steps are reversible, but a directionality is imposed via the energy-requiring one-way passage of aspartate from mitochondrion to cytosol. Glutamate and aspartate are consistently lowered in the brains of hyperammonemic animals. These changes may slow both the glutamate-aspartate exchange and flux through the transaminases. The mitochondrial enzyme may be particularly susceptible to changes in glutamate, since its apparent K_m for glutamate has been reported to be approximately 20 mM. (From Cooper and Meister [25]. Copyright © 1985 by John Wiley & Sons, Inc. Reprinted with permission.)

HYPOXIC ENCEPHALOPATHY

The metabolic consequences in brain of pure hypoxia as opposed to those of cerebral ischemia are best addressed separately, since ischemia causes, in addition to a reduced oxygen supply, loss of substrate and impaired removal of metabolic waste products. (For a detailed presentation of the metabolic changes that accompany cerebral ischemia, the reader is referred to Chap. 40.)

Graded hypoxia produces increasing CNS dysfunction

Pure hypoxic encephalopathy, uncomplicated by the effects of reduced CBF, occurs rarely in humans, since hypoxia-induced cardiac arrhythmias and systemic hypotension cause cerebral hypoperfusion. Hypoxic encephalopathy is encountered in patients who suffer pulmonary disease with ventilation-diffusion-perfusion defects, patients with severe anemia, and in normal individuals who are exposed acutely to high altitudes. In fact, the clinical manifestations of hypoxic encephalopathy in humans are best exemplified in experiments where healthy young individuals are subjected to rapid decompression hypoxia over a period of a few minutes. From the results of such experiments it is possible to define the partial pressures of ambient and arterial oxygen (Pao_2) at which neurological impairment occurs (Table 1). However, such Pao_2 threshold values may not directly apply to chronic or slowly developing hypoxia, where multiple compensatory mechanisms have suf-

TABLE 1. Hypoxic thresholds for CNS dysfunction

Simulated altitude (ft)	F_iO_2 (%)	PaO_2 (Torr)	Neurological status
Sea level	21	90	Normal
5,000	17	80	Impaired dark vision
8,000–10,000	15–14	55–45	Impaired short-term memory; difficulty learning complex tasks
15,000–20,000	11–9	40–30	Loss of judgment, euphoria, obtundation
>20,000	<9	<25	Coma

[a] Values derived from young volunteers subjected to acute (minutes) decompression hypoxia; (F_iO_2) fractional percentage of ambient oxygen.

ficient time to maintain cerebral homeostasis and brain function or where chronic changes have increased vulnerability.

Acute hypoxia, which is induced over a few minutes by breathing air equivalent to that found at approximately 5,000 ft (PaO_2 = 80 Torr), impairs the ability of retinal rods to adapt to the dark. At slightly higher altitudes, between 8,000 and 10,000 ft, which corresponds to PaO_2 = 55 to 45 Torr, difficulty with learning complex tasks and impaired short-term memory are encountered. At approximately 15,000 to 20,000 ft, which corresponds to PaO_2 = 40 to 30 Torr, cognitive function becomes more severely impaired, with loss of judgment, a sense of euphoria or delerium, and the onset of muscular incoordination. Acute hypoxia, equivalent to 20,000 ft or above, which corresponds to PaO_2 = 25 to 20 Torr, is associated with rapid loss of consciousness.

Energy failure in moderate hypoxia is not linear with partial pressure of arterial oxygen despite CNS dysfunction

The ultimate cause of encephalopathy associated with severe hypoxia (PaO_2 < 25 Torr) is a fall in the partial pressure of tissue oxygen to levels that no longer support mitochondrial respiration. Under such conditions loss of consciousness is readily explained by a rapid depletion of the high-energy organic phosphates,

PCr and ATP; however, the neurochemical basis for impaired cerebral function at PaO_2 > 25 to 20 Torr is less clear. Experimental studies indicate that energy metabolism remains normal at a time when mild to moderate hypoxia (PaO_2 = 25–40 Torr) has already markedly compromised cognition in human volunteers. Kety and Schmidt [10] and others [11] reported normal $CMRO_2$ in human volunteers at PaO_2 = 25 to 40 Torr; most showed either abnormal mental function or abnormal electrophysiological activity, a few temporarily lost consciousness despite a normal $CMRO_2$. Graded hypoxia in laboratory animals revealed that ATP levels remained normal above PaO_2 = 20 to 25 Torr [12] (Fig. 3), yet EEG in these animals showed slowing and attenuated sensory evoked responses.

Glycolysis is stimulated to maintain ATP levels under moderate hypoxia

Studies of laboratory animals have demonstrated several important changes in brain chemistry occurring at PaO_2 levels of approximately 50 Torr, an oxygen tension well above that necessary for blocking ATP synthesis. An increase in the cerebral lactate/pyruvate ratio and a decrease in brain tissue pH are the most consistent and earliest changes reported at PaO_2 = 45 to 50 Torr. Consistent with this increase in lactate production is a rise in the CMRGlc,

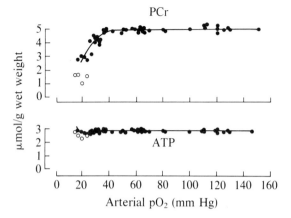

FIG. 3. Brain concentrations of PCr and ATP in rats anesthetized with 70 percent N_2O and subjected to graded hypoxia for periods of 15 to 30 min: (●) animals with ≤ 120 Torr mean arterial pressures; (○) animals with >80 Torr mean arterial pressure. (From Siesjö [12]. Copyright © 1978 by John Wiley & Sons, Inc. Reprinted with permission.)

which most certainly indicates accelerated glycolysis. The cytosolic redox potential as measured by the $NADH/NAD^+$ ratio shifts toward a more reduced state at approximately this same PaO_2. Phosphocreatine levels begin to decline slightly at $PaO_2 = 45$ to 50 Torr; they then fall more rapidly when PaO_2 falls below 20 Torr. The initial decline in PCr is probably related to the early increase in tissue lactic acid and the pH dependency of the creatine kinase equilibrium that favors the conversion of PCr to ATP. The later fall in PCr coincides with the decrease in ATP levels and undoubtedly reflects failure of mitochondrial respiration and oxidative phosphorylation.

To summarize the effects on energy stores, brain tissue oxygen content becomes limiting at PaO_2 in the neighborhood of 45 to 50 Torr. As a consequence, glycolysis is stimulated to a sufficient degree to maintain normal tissue ATP concentrations until the PaO_2 levels fall below 20 Torr. Paradoxically, cerebral dysfunction at 45 to 50 Torr is manifested by abnormal EEG activity and behavior, despite apparently normal energy stores.

Equally as puzzling as the abnormal EEG data is the rise of extracellular K^+ concentration at a PaO_2 of approximately 25 to 30 Torr. Since maintenance of Na^+ and K^+ concentration gradients is thought to rely largely on the activity of Na,K-ATPase, elevation of extracellular K^+ implies dysfunction of this enzyme pump or a hypoxic-dependent leakage of K^+ through membrane channels (see Chap. 3). In the presence of normal ATP levels, both mechanisms are difficult to understand.

One possible explanation for the early rise of the extracellular K^+ concentration is that the microregional concentration of ATP at the catalytic site of Na,K-ATPase is no longer sufficient for critical enzyme reactions. It is known that hypoxia will induce marked microregional heterogeneity of glucose [13] (Fig. 4) and oxygen [12] metabolism, and it is possible that measurements of ATP in milligram samples of brain are insensitive to similar microregional changes of ATP. Another possibility is that the available free energy ($\Delta G^{0'}$) of ATP hydrolysis becomes limiting with moderate hypoxia. A shift in the intracellular pH by one unit, that is, pH 7.2 to 6.2, which is fully attainable during hypoxic conditions in brain, will reduce the $\Delta G^{0'}$ of ATP hydrolysis by approximately 0.5 kcal/mol [14]. Although such changes in $\Delta G^{0'}$ appear insignificant in that they represent only 4 percent of the 12.5 kcal available per mole of ATP, it is conceivable that even small reductions in $\Delta G^{0'}$ may further alter the rate of critical enzyme reactions already affected by the hypoxic state.

Neurotransmitter abnormalities are found in moderate hypoxia

Hypoxia-induced changes in neurotransmitter chemistry may contribute in important ways to the symptoms of hypoxic encephalopathy. The synthesis and metabolism of norepinephrine, dopamine, and serotonin are oxygen dependent

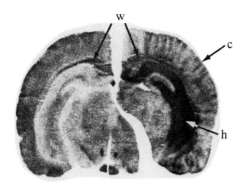

FIG. 4. Carbon-14 autoradiograph of a coronal brain section from a rat subjected to right common carotid artery ligation and hypoxia (Pao$_2$ = 28–32 Torr). The right cerebral hemisphere is shown on the right side of the photograph. Hypoxia raises CBF to the left hemisphere (patent carotid) to four times normal and to the right hemisphere (ligated carotid) to twice normal values. Note the alternating columns of high and low neocortical (c) metabolism (compared to the contralateral neocortex) and the increased glucose metabolism within the subcortical white matter (w) and hippocampus (h). (From Pulsinelli and Duffy [13]. Copyright © 1979 by the American Association for the Advancement of Science. Reprinted with permission.)

(Fig. 5). The rate-limiting reactions of dopamine, norepinephrine, and serotonin synthesis, which are catalyzed by the enzymes tyrosine hydroxylase and tryptophan hydroxylase, require molecular oxygen. Moreover, the conversion of dopamine via the enzyme dopamine-β-hydroxylase to norepinephrine also requires oxygen. The K_m of O$_2$ for these oxygen-dependent hydroxylases is approximately 12 μM (7 Torr). Brain tissue oxygen content is thought to vary between 2 and 25 μM (1–15 Torr); thus, small changes in tissue oxygen content may reduce monoamine synthesis [15]. At an arterial O$_2$ concentration of approximately 40 Torr, the turnover of catecholamines and serotonin, which reflect both synthesis and metabolism, is reduced by approximately 25 percent. Values for the tissue concentration of these monoamine neurotransmitters during hypoxia vary from one

laboratory to another, and interpretation of these data with regard to the cause of hypoxic encephalopathy are difficult, since both neurotransmitter synthesis and degradation are oxygen dependent.

The concentration of amino acid neurotransmitters and acetylcholine may also be sensitive to changes in tissue oxygen tension, since synthesis of these neurotransmitters is closely coupled to glycolysis and oxidative metabolism (Fig. 6). Arterial oxygen tensions of 50 to 60 Torr will reduce by 50 percent the incorporation of radiolabeled choline into acetylcholine but will not alter the tissue concentration of this neurotransmitter [16]. At similar arterial oxygen tensions, the incorporation of radiolabeled glucose into γ-aminobutyrate, glutamate, aspartate, serine, and alanine is reduced by approximately 40 to 60 percent, but as with acetylcholine, the tissue concentrations of these amino acids remain unchanged. The signifi-

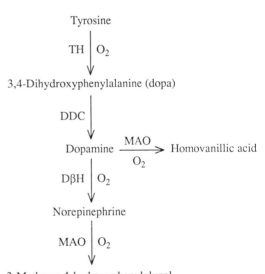

FIG. 5. Oxygen dependence of dopamine and norepinephrine synthesis and metabolism: tyrosine hydroxylase (TH); dopamine decarboxylase (DDC); dopamine β-hydroxylase (DβH); monoamine oxidase (MAO). (Modified from Gibson et al. [15].)

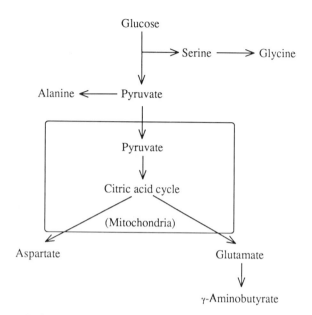

FIG. 6. The relationship between amino acid neurotransmitter synthesis and glycolysis and the TCA cycle (From Gibson et al. [15].)

cance of these hypoxia-induced changes in the pathogenesis of hypoxic encephalopathy remains problematic. Of note is the finding that alterations in metabolism of acetylcholine, catecholamine, and amino acid neurotransmitters occur at arterial oxygen tensions of 40 to 60 Torr, which are well above those that affect energy metabolism. Such changes may therefore partially explain the early signs and symptoms of hypoxic encephalopathy.

HYPERCAPNIC ENCEPHALOPATHY

Respiratory acidosis causes increased pH in the CNS

Although CO_2 is a normal metabolite, at elevated concentrations it is toxic; CO_2 is in equilibrium with carbonic acid (H_2CO_3) and bicarbonate (HCO_3^-) which is an important buffer of H^+ ions. Acute pulmonary or ventilatory insufficiency in humans if untreated rapidly leads to alterations in brain function resembling those of acute hypoxia and ischemia. Chronic pulmonary insufficiency is characterized by mild to moderate hypoxemia accompanied by varying degrees of CO_2 retention. Renal conservation of HCO_3^- usually buffers the hypercapnia, and blood pH is usually normal; however, the superpositioning of an added insult, such as infection, ingestion of a sedative, or fatigue, can further compromise lung function, resulting in even greater CO_2 retention and a disruption of the normal buffering mechanisms. The respiratory acidosis associated with CO_2 retention in blood causes an almost proportionate increase in [H^+] in systemic tissues including the CNS.

Hypercapnia produces increased CBF and variable effects on CMRO₂

Patients with chronic pulmonary insufficiency may exhibit lethargy, mental confusion, retrograde amnesia, and stupor. The combination of hypoxia and hypercapnia leads to cerebral vasodilation, increased CBF, and sometimes to increased intracranial pressure. The associated hypoxemia probably contributes to but is not the underlying cause of the neurological symptoms. Neurological symptoms correlate best with the degree of CO_2 retention. Acute, moderate hypercapnia (5–10 percent CO_2 in the inspired air) produces increased arousal and excitability; higher CO_2 concentrations (>35–40 percent) in the inspired air are anesthetic. Increased CO_2 levels are associated with a number of metabolic changes in the brain. In many studies, the arteriovenous (A-V) difference for oxygen across the brain is generally found to decrease in proportion to increases in CBF, leaving the CMRO₂ unchanged. In other studies, however, CMRO₂ is reported either elevated or depressed (range, 71–131 percent) [17]. The differences may be due to differences in species and methodology employed in the various studies. It is possible that at moderate concentrations, CO_2 stimulates the catecholamine system, thereby enhancing $CMRO_2$; at very high CO_2 concentrations, or when this system is blocked by drugs, CO_2 becomes a depressant.

In hypercapnia, CMRGlc is depressed, but the magnitude is variable

Some workers have reported a fall in CMRGlc that approximately parallels the fall in $CMRO_2$. Others have shown a proportionately greater decrease in CMRGlc. Glucose is the major fuel for the adult brain under normal circumstances; however, Miller [17] provided evidence that in acute hypercapnia (20 percent CO_2: 26 percent O_2: 54 percent N_2 in the inspired air for 10 min) in the adult rat, $CMRO_2$ is unchanged, but as much as a third of the inspired O_2 is used for the oxidation of other fuels, principally glutamate and lactate. To what extent this could continue in chronic hypercapnia is not known.

Several investigators have shown that acute hypercapnic acidosis results in an increase in cerebral glycolytic intermediates above the phosphofructokinase step and a decrease in metabolites below this step, possibly due to inhibition of phosphofructokinase activity by increased $[H^+]$. Despite continued acidosis and decreased CMRGlc, however, the components of the phosphofructokinase reaction gradually return to near-normal levels. The body temperature of the animals in these experiments was not monitored; it is possible that CMRGlc was decreased because of hypothermia.

Despite decreased CMRGlc during hypercapnia, cerebral ATP levels are generally found to be unaltered. Decreases in cerebral metabolism during hypercapnia are probably a consequence of decreased neuronal activity and not the cause of the encephalopathy. Possible factors contributing to hypercapnic encephalopathy include (1) depleted neurotransmitter glutamate pools; (2) decreased acetylcholine synthesis from pyruvate; (3) ammonia intoxi-

cation; and (4) interference with lipid metabolism.

HYPOGLYCEMIC ENCEPHALOPATHY

The large population of insulin-dependent diabetic patients explains the relatively high incidence of encephalopathy caused by hypoglycemia. Many of the earliest signs and symptoms of mild hypoglycemia reflect the workings of physiologic protective mechanisms initiated by hypothalamic sensory nuclei and effected through sympathetic and endocrine systems. If these early warning signals, which include diaphoresis, tachycardia, hunger, and anxiety, are unheeded, worsening hypoglycemia will lead to primary CNS symptoms similar to those of hypoxia. Loss of attention, confusion, delerium, seizures, lethargy, stupor, and, finally, coma are the consequences of progressively worsening hypoglycemia.

Less than 30 years ago insulin-induced hypoglycemic coma was an experimental therapy for psychiatric disease. In the course of such therapy Kety and colleagues [18] found that the CMRGlc fell to a greater degree than did $CMRO_2$ in patients subjected to hypoglycemic coma. The disproportionate decrease between $CMRO_2$ and CRMGlc was interpreted as evidence for the metabolism of substrates other than glucose by brain tissue. Experimental animal studies have corroborated the hypothesis that the brain is capable of metabolizing carbon sources other than glucose [19]. Despite the capacity for metabolizing alternative fuels, which include acetoacetate, β-hydroxybutyrate, and several amino acids, cerebral energy metabolism fails, and the concentrations of ATP and PCr fall in the total absence of glucose (see Chap. 29).

Under normal conditions the human brain consumes approximately 10 percent of the glucose delivered to it [20]. As blood glucose concentrations fall below 2.5 mM, CMRGlc and

$CMRO_2$ in laboratory animals begin to decline; $CMRGlc$ to a greater degree than $CMRO_2$ [21,22]. At this level of blood glucose, confusion or delerium is the initial sign of hypoglycemia in humans. The EEG initially shows an increase in amplitude and decreased frequency at approximately 2 mM blood glucose, and as the glucose falls further toward 1 mM, EEG amplitude and frequency decrease, and the patient becomes stuporous; below 1 mM, the EEG becomes isoelectric as coma develops.

Generalized energy failure does not account for CNS dysfunction in moderate hypoglycemia

Initially it was assumed that the onset of mental dysfunction and the early EEG changes associated with moderate (blood glucose, 1.5–2.5 mM) hypoglycemia were related to tissue energy failure, especially since they coincided well with changes in $CMRGlc$ and $CMRO_2$. However, many studies involving experimental animals show that the concentrations of high-energy organic phosphates remain entirely normal during the early stages of symptomatic hypoglycemia [12] (Fig. 7). As the blood glucose concentration falls to 1 mM and below, CNS symptoms are readily explained by a rapid decline in high-energy organic phosphates.

Generalized cerebral energy failure cannot account for the early neurological deterioration associated with moderate hypoglycemia, a situation similar to that encountered in mild symptomatic hypoxia. Since most studies of hypoglycemia correlated EEG activity and neurological behavior with measurements of PCr and ATP from tissue samples of either whole forebrain or neocortex, it is possible that site-specific changes in high-energy phosphates could account for altered consciousness. Indeed, results from McCandless and Abel [21] demonstrate that ATP levels in the reticular formation of the brainstem are decreased by approximately 30 percent and phosphocreatine by

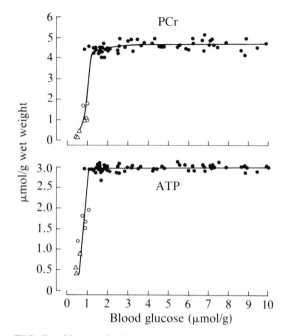

FIG. 7. Neocortical concentrations of PCr and ATP in rats subjected to graded hypoglycemia. Samples of frozen neocortex were used for these measurements. ●, EEG non-isoelectric; ○, EEG isoelectric for 3 minutes prior to freezing brain; △, EEG isoelectric for 6–28 minutes prior to freezing brain. (From Siesjö [12]). Copyright © 1978 by John Wiley & Sons, Inc. Reprinted with permission.)

55 percent during the precoma stages of hypoglycemia in animals.

Other mechanisms of hypoglycemic encephalopathy

Alternative explanations for the early metabolic encephalopathy associated with hypoglycemia include the accumulation of toxic products of nonglucose metabolism, such as ammonia and free fatty acids. Hypoglycemia enhances the accumulation of toxic levels of brain ammonia possibly derived from glutamate and aspartate, which decrease in hypoglycemia.

Other possible mechanisms that lead to deterioration of mental function during hypoglycemia include impairment of acetylcholine synthesis and changes in the concentrations of other putative neurotransmitters, such as glutamate, aspartate, and GABA [21].

UREMIC ENCEPHALOPATHY

Uremic encephalopathy is an acute or subacute syndrome that regularly occurs in patients in whom renal function falls below 10 percent of normal. Neurological symptoms include clouding of consciousness, motor hyperactivity, disturbed sleep patterns, nausea, decreased sexual activity, and bizarre behavior. Many patients suffer from transient hemiparesis and other focal neurological weaknesses. Amaurosis, nystagmus, vertigo, and ataxia are common. Some patients are prone to convulsions. EEG abnormalities occur in animals with experimentally induced uremic encephalopathy and in humans with the disease. Uremia is characterized by retention in the blood of urea, phosphates, proteins, amines, and a number of ill-defined low-molecular-weight compounds. It is interesting that despite acidemia, the pH of brain, muscle, leukocytes, and CSF appears to be normal. Since hemodialysis corrects the encephalopathy, low-molecular-weight compounds may be at least partially responsible. Urea, however, is nontoxic, even at elevated concentrations. In patients with acute renal failure, water, K^+, and Mg^{2+} are normal, whereas Na^+ is slightly decreased, and Al^{3+} increased; Ca^{2+} in the cerebral cortex is almost twice normal [23].

Uremia alters the characteristics of the blood-brain barrier

The permeability of the BBB toward insulin and sucrose is increased. Sodium ion transport is impaired, but potassium ion transport is enhanced; permeability toward weak acids tends to be decreased. The CBF in uremic patients has been reported to be elevated, but $CMRO_2$

and CMRGlc decline. Blood ammonia is normal or only slightly elevated in uremic patients; PCr, ATP, and glucose are increased in the brains of rats with acute renal failure, whereas AMP, ADP, and lactate are decreased. These changes are probably due to a reduction in cerebral energy demands. Osmolality increases to a similar extent in brain, CSF, and plasma (from ~310 to ~350 mOsmol/kg H_2O) in animals with renal failure. In acute renal failure all increase in brain osmolality is due to urea, whereas in the chronic model almost half the increase in brain osmolality is due to unknown molecules (idiogenic osmoles). The role of idiogenic osmoles in the uremia-induced encephalopathy is unknown.

Parathyroid hormone may be a factor in uremic encephalopathy and neuropathy

Circulating parathyroid hormone (PTH) ($M_r \sim$ 10,000) is not removed by hemodialysis. Administration of PTH (but not Ca^{2+} or vitamin D) to normal dogs induces EEG changes comparable to those found in uremic animals, whereas parathyroidectomy prior to induction of uremia prevents the EEG abnormalities and associated hypercalcemia.

Uremia also produces a chronic, peripheral neuropathy, usually in the lower extremities, that is not ameliorated by hemodialysis. The neuropathy cannot be attributed to nutritional or other complicating factors. Plasma PTH levels are often elevated in uremic patients, and such patients have significantly lower motor nerve conduction velocities than those of uremic patients with normal or moderately elevated levels of PTH.

Excess PTH in patients with hyperparathyroidism frequently produces psychiatric symptoms and EEG changes similar to those observed in uremic patients. In such patients, parathyroidectomy results in an improvement of both EEG and mental status. As with hyperparathyroid patients, parathyroidectomy or medical suppression of PTH improves the EEG and mental status of uremic patients. Teschan and Arieff [23] concluded that "PTH and/or a high brain calcium content are probably responsible, at least in part, for many of the encephalopathic manifestations of renal failure."

DIALYSIS ENCEPHALOPATHY

Dialysis disequilibrium syndrome

Repeated hemodialysis is now the standard treatment for many patients with chronic renal failure, but some patients develop neurological symptoms as a result of the dialysis. In extreme cases, seizure, coma, and death have resulted, but such incidences are now on the decline. Chronic renal failure occurs more commonly during rapid hemodialysis of patients with high blood urea levels. It was originally thought that the rapid drop of serum osmolality was responsible. It was argued that since osmotically active molecules (including urea) that have accumulated in the brain may be cleared relatively slowly from brain, water will shift from plasma to brain, causing brain swelling; however, Teschan and Arieff [23] have cautioned that some of the symptoms may be due to causes other than dialysis disequilibrium. Urea clearance from uremic dog brain parallels that of plasma during rapid hemodialysis. In both uremic dogs and humans, the CSF pH drops during rapid hemodialysis. Arieff suggests that an increase in brain [H^+] leads to secondary swelling.

Progressive dialysis encephalopathy

In some patients undergoing long-term hemodialysis therapy, a progressive, severe encephalopathy develops, which is almost always fatal. In some cases, a strong correlation exists with increased brain Al^{3+}; in other cases, brain Al^{3+} is not increased. Teschan and Arieff [23] suggest

that there may be several etiological agents and recognize three classes:

1. An epidemic form, possibly related to Al^{3+} in the dialysate
2. Spontaneous cases in which Al^{3+} is less likely to be causative
3. Dementia associated with congenital or early childhood renal disease

The last group includes some children who were never dialyzed or exposed to aluminum. Al^{3+} compounds placed on the brain surface are highly toxic. Interesting is the fact that Al^{3+} is increased in the brains of patients with Alzheimer's disease, hepatic encephalopathy, several forms of metastic cancer, and renal failure. The last group has the highest level of Al^{3+}; Al^{3+} concentration is greater in the brains of patients with chronic renal failure than those with acute renal failure and is greatest in patients with dialysis dementia (11 times normal in one study). Bone and tissues other than brain also contain increased Al^{3+} in uremic patients. Presumably, the source of at least some of this Al^{3+} is the $Al(OH)_3$ given to patients with chronic renal failure to control serum phosphate levels; untreated tap water used to prepare the dialysis fluids for patients on maintenance hemodialysis may be another source of Al^{3+}. The hypothesis that Al^{3+} may be a causative factor is controversial, although recent work by Alfrey [24] suggests that removing Al^{3+} from the dialysate greatly reduces the risk of dialysis encephalopathy.

REFERENCES

1. Plum, F., and Posner, J. B. *The Diagnosis of Stupor and Coma*. Philadelphia: F. A. Davis, 1980.
2. Duffy, T. E., and Plum, F. Hepatic encephalopathy. In I. M. Arias, H. Popper, D. Schacher, and D. A. Shafritz (eds.), *The Liver: Biology and*

Pathobiology. New York: Raven Press, 1982, pp. 693–715.

3. Cooper, A. J. L., and Plum, F. Biochemistry and physiology of brain ammonia. *Physiol. Rev.* 67:440–519, 1987.

4. Fischer, J. E. False neurotransmitters and hepatic coma. In F. Plum (ed.), *Brain Dysfunction in Metabolic Disorders. (Res. Publ. Assoc. Nerv. Ment. Dis., Vol. 53).* New York: Raven Press, 1974, pp. 53–73.

5. James, J. H., Jeppsson, B., Ziparo, V., and Fischer, J. E. Hyperammonaemia, plasma amino acid imbalance, and blood-brain amino acid transport: A unified theory of portal-systemic encephalopathy. *Lancet* 2:772–775, 1979.

6. Mans, A. M., Davis, D. W., Biebuyck, J. F., and Hawkins, R. A. Failure of glucose and branched-chain amino acids to normalize brain glucose use in portacaval shunted rats. *J. Neurochem.* 47:1434–1443, 1986.

7. Hindfelt, B. Ammonia intoxication and brain energy metabolism. In G. Kleinberger and E. Deutsch (eds.), *New Aspects of Clinical Nutrition.* Basel: Karger, 1983, pp. 474–484.

8. Berl, S. Cerebral amino acid metabolism in hepatic coma. In E. Polli (ed.), *Experimental Biology and Medicine (Neurochemistry of Hepatic Coma, Vol. 4).* Basel: Karger, 1971, pp. 71–84.

9. Hindfelt, B., Plum, F., and Duffy, T. E. Effects of acute ammonia intoxication on cerebral metabolism in rats with portacaval shunts. *J. Clin. Invest.* 59:386–396, 1977.

10. Kety, S., and Schmidt, C. F. The effects of altered arterial tensions of carbon dioxide and oxygen on cerebral blood flow and cerebral oxygen consumption of normal young men. *J. Clin. Invest.* 27:484–492, 1948.

11. Cohen, P. J., Alexander, S. C., Smith, T. C., Reivich, M., and Wollman, H. Effects of hypoxia and normocarbia in cerebral blood flow and metabolism in conscious man. *J. Appl. Physiol.* 23:183–189, 1967.

12. Siesjö, B. K. *Brain Energy Metabolism.* New York: Wiley, 1978, pp. 380–446.

13. Pulsinelli, W., and Duffy, T. E. Local cerebral glucose metabolism during controlled hypoxemia in rats. *Science* 204:626–629, 1979.

14. Alberty, R. A. Effect of pH and metal ion concentration on the equilibrium hydrolysis of adenosine triphosphate to adenosine diphosphate. *J. Biol. Chem.* 243:1337–1343, 1968.

15. Gibson, G. E., Pulsinelli, W., Blass, J. P., and Duffy, T. E. Brain dysfunction in mild to moderate hypoxia. *Am. J. Med.* 70:1247–1254, 1981.

16. Gibson, G. E. Hypoxia. In D. W. McCandless (ed.), *Cerebral Energy Metabolism and Metabolic Encephalopathy.* New York: Plenum Press, 1985, pp. 43–78.

17. Miller, A. L. Carbon dioxide narcosis. In D. W. McCandless (ed.), *Cerebral Energy Metabolism and Metabolic Encephalopathy.* New York: Plenum Press, 1985, pp. 143–162.

18. Kety, S. S., Woodford, R. B., Harmel, M. H., Freyhan, F. A., Appel, K. E., and Schmidt, C. F. Cerebral blood flow and metabolism in schizophrenia: The effects of barbiturate semi-narcosis, insulin coma and electroshock. *Am. J. Psych.* 104:765–770, 1948.

19. Hawkins, R. Cerebral energy metabolism. In D. W. McCandless (ed.), *Cerebral Energy Metabolism and Metabolic Encephalopathy.* New York: Plenum Press, 1985, pp. 3–23.

20. Plum, F., and Pulsinelli, W. Cerebral metabolism in hypoxic-ischemic brain injury. In A. K. Asbury, G. M. McKhann, W. Ian McDonald (eds.), *Diseases of the Nervous System.* Philadelphia: W. B. Saunders Co., 1986, pp. 1086–1100.

21. McCandless, D. W., and Abel, M. S. Hypoglycemia in cerebral energy metabolism. In D. W. McCandless (ed.), *Cerebral Energy Metabolism and Metabolic Encephalopathy.* New York: Plenum Press, 1985, pp. 27–41.

22. Ghajar, J. B., Plum, F., and Duffy, T. E. Cerebral oxidative metabolism and blood flow during acute hypoglycemia and recovery in unanesthetized rats. *J. Neurochem.* 38:397–409, 1982.

23. Teschan, P. E., and Arieff, A. I. Uremic and dialysis encephalopathies. In D. W. McCandless (ed.), *Cerebral Energy Metabolism and Metabolic Encephalopathy.* New York: Plenum Press, 1985, pp. 263–285.

24. Alfrey, A. C. Dialysis encephalopathy. *Kidney Int.* 29:S53–S57, 1986.

25. Cooper, A. J. L. and Meister, A. Metabolic significance of transaminations. In P. Christen and D. E. Metzler (eds.), *Transaminases.* New York: Wiley, 1985, pp. 534–563.

CHAPTER 40

Ischemia and Hypoxia

C. J. Flynn, A. A. Farooqui, and L. A. Horrocks

Basic Neurochemistry: Molecular, Cellular, and Medical Aspects, 4th Ed., edited by G. J. Siegel et al. Raven Press, Ltd., New York, 1989.
Correspondence to A. A. Farooqui, Department of Physiological Chemistry, Ohio State University, Columbus, Ohio 43210.

Insults to brain that interrupt its blood supply, as in ischemia, or its oxygen supply, as in hypoxia (low oxygen), and anoxia (zero oxygen), immediately cause cell dysfunction and rapidly lead to cell death (infarction). There are many causes of ischemia and hypoxia in the brain in humans, including diseases of the blood, heart, lungs, and blood vessels. The most prevalent cause of ischemic injury to brain is cardiovascular disease related to atherosclerosis and hypertension, which may produce interruption of cerebral blood flow as a result of abnormal cardiac output, occlusion of vessels by vasospasm, thrombi, atherosclerotic plaques, or emboli or rupture of vessels by hemorrhage. Sudden events are called cerebrovascular accidents (CVA) as in stroke. Cell damage may be transient, possibly reversible to some extent or sufficient to cause tissue death (infarction), depending on the duration and extent of the ischemia. The anatomical location and extent of ischemic damage depend on the blood vessels whose flow is thus limited and on the presence of collateral circulation. Ischemic events may be repetitive; they may involve single (focal) or multiple brain regions (multifocal). Ischemia and hypoxia may be rapid in onset (acute) or chronic and multifocal with cumulative deficits.

Damage due to focal or multifocal stroke commonly occurs in a graded fashion, due to collateral circulation partially perfusing the area surrounding the infarcted core. As blood flow to these areas drops to approximately 15 ml/100 g tissue/min, the tissue becomes electrically silent; at approximately 10 ml/100 g tissue/min, the transmembrane ionic gradient fails, and cell death results. Prior to this, the tissue is reversibly impaired for varying periods of time. The concept of partial or incomplete perfusion is important for two reasons:

1. The compromised status of these areas (termed the ischemic penumbra by Astrup et al. [1]) may be improved if effective early intervention is achieved.

2. To achieve such intervention, it is necessary to understand the complex biochemistry and pathophysiology of these areas.

In global ischemia, perfusion to the entire brain is interrupted with conditions such as cardiac arrest in which there is no collateral circulation; consciousness is lost immediately, and irreversible damage occurs within a few minutes. If circulation is reestablished promptly, cerebral damage due to global ischemia may be mild or absent.

ANIMAL MODELS OF CEREBRAL ISCHEMIA

Animal models and techniques for inducing ischemic brain injury for detailed study depends on several factors that elude complete control. First, the test insult should parallel as closely as possible the naturally occurring clinical insult. Although sophisticated means are available for achieving this, test animals do not readily develop the cardiovascular disease that commonly underlies stroke, nor do they duplicate the age, nutritional status, or drug history of most stroke patients. Further, test animals are usually anesthetized, curarized, and have undergone surgery, particularly craniotomy, all of which profoundly alters tissue response [2]. Second, test insults should elicit similar responses in each individual tested. This seldom happens because of anatomical and physiological variability, both within and among species. In general, larger animals, especially primates, exhibit greater similarity to humans because of similar brain size and structure. Animals with large brains can survive sizeable ischemic infarcts, as do humans, but such animals show more individual anatomical variability; some reproducibility is therefore sacrificed. Small-brained animals, such as rats and gerbils, suffer proportionately larger infarcts than do larger animals, so more of the smaller animals are lost

[2]. Newer methods and technology have overcome these limitations, and because rodents have more uniform cerebral vascularization, it is now possible to obtain more uniform responses to experimental hypoxic/ischemic injury. This, plus their lower cost, makes rats and gerbils especially useful. A third important factor requires that the experimental animal pathology be similar to that in humans. Nevertheless, results of test lesions induced by similar methods in various animal species have been very dissimilar in many cases; thus, caution is necessary before generalizing results to humans.

Experimental hypoxia/ischemia is induced in animals by occluding vessels to or within the cranium

Branches of the middle cerebral or the internal carotid arteries are commonly chosen sites for inducing hypoxia/ischemia in laboratory animals. The ischemic injury can be focal or global or restricted to one hemisphere so that the contralateral hemisphere serves as a control. There are several ways to occlude the vessels. Ligation or clipping for various lengths of time is the most common. Electrocoagulation has also been used. Microspheres made of metal or plastic can be injected into a vessel, following which the spheres lodge in several sites downstream, thus modeling multifocal ischemia. Less commonly used techniques include air and clot embolism and externally applied arterial cuffs. These methods of occlusion can be used in combination with other manipulations, such as the administration of drugs, glucose, arachidonate or the induction of hypoxia or hypotension. Rats, rabbits, gerbils, cats, dogs, several species of monkeys, pigs, and goats have been used to study ischemia [3]. The rat and gerbil models have been extensively developed, and a large base of neurochemical and histopathological data exists for these species. The mongolian gerbil is convenient because it has an incom-

plete circle of Willis, lacking connections between the vertebral arterial system and the internal carotids. However, some individuals have anterior communicating vessels linking both hemispheres, and some develop seizures. A highly successful model of ischemia has been developed using rats, where ligation of the vertebral arteries, followed by occlusion of one or both common carotids produces a graded, fairly reproducible hemispheral or global ischemia [4].

HISTOPATHOLOGY OF ISCHEMIC/ HYPOXIC BRAIN

Ischemia produces a characteristic sequence of alterations in structure, beginning with neuronal microvacuolation

There is agreement that biochemical alterations occur before histological changes appear. Some changes in cellular morphology may be observed only after irreversible progression toward cell death has ensued. Nevertheless, morphological changes are observable even after only a few minutes of ischemia or hypoxia. The degree of cellular disorganization progresses with injury of increasing severity and duration. Neurons show signs of degeneration earlier than do astrocytes or endothelial cells. Typically, an ischemic neuron initially undergoes mitochondrial swelling and disorganization of the cristae, as evidenced by microvacuoles in the cytoplasm. This is the stage of microvacuolation. This swelling, associated with ion gradient failure, is reversible with prompt reperfusion. Otherwise, the cell shrinks, the nucleus becomes displaced, and the cell stains more darkly. Lysosomes appear to be more resistant to hypoxia and ischemia than other structures. Eventually, chromatin clumping, microtubule fragmentation, and ribosomal dispersion occur, and electrodense encrustations around the cell bodies appear [5]. This process is accompanied by marked swelling of perineural and perivascular astrocytes and invagination of perikarya by swollen astrocytic processes, developing the edema that invariably accompanies ischemia and hypoxia.

The histological changes seen in other types of brain injury or disease, such as status epilepticus or hypoglycemia, have some features in common with hypoxic or ischemic changes, especially in the later stages. Earlier, some interesting distinctions can be made; for example, in hypoglycemia, mitochondria appear to shrink rather than swell. Identification of differential changes is helpful in distinguishing those due to ischemia from those that are nonspecific. Newer methods using perfusion fixation have improved the sensitivity of histological preparations, but the possibility of artifacts from tissue fixation, particularly immersion fixation, and staining requires cautious interpretation of results.

Some populations of neurons are selectively vulnerable

Several studies have shown that pyramidal neurons in the CA1, CA3, and CA4 areas of the hippocampus and the small and medium neurons of the striatum suffer more severe damage under conditions of global ischemia followed by reperfusion than do other regions of brain. Purkinje cells of the cerebellum and neurons of cortical layers 3, 5, and 6 are also vulnerable [6]. An associated phenomenon is the tendency of some of these neurons to undergo delayed autolysis. This "maturation" phenomenon occurs in cells that are functionally and morphologically intact immediately after reperfusion, the autolysis not appearing until hours to days later [7]. The factors involved in selective neuronal vulnerability could be either vascular or intrinsic to the neurons themselves. Although under certain circumstances, such as arterial hypo-

tension, there may be selective damage of neurons and white matter at arterial endfields, it appears that biochemical factors within the neuronal population, such as the presence of excitatory neurotransmitters, free radicals or Ca^{2+} ions may be more important.

LOCAL BLOOD FLOW REGULATION AFTER ISCHEMIA

Vasospasm may prevent reflow after reperfusion

Normally, arteriolar diameter is controlled mainly by vasoactive substances produced by the tissue, ensuring that local metabolic demand is met by the circulation (see Chap. 29). During ischemia and subsequent reperfusion, a progression of microcirculatory changes occurs that disrupts this balance, often for an extended period of time. At present, it appears that local vascular involvement in the reperfusion phase is an important determinant in the development of pathology. When a cerebral blood vessel is occluded, flow through the arterial bed is slowed, causing aggregation of the formed elements in the blood and increased blood viscosity. Vasospasm occurs in the ischemic area in response to the release and accumulation of vasoactive substances and ions. Which of these substances is most important is not completely known, but there is evidence supporting the involvement of neurotransmitters, eicosanoids (see Chap. 20), cyclic nucleotides, and increased concentrations of intracellular Ca^{2+} in the smooth muscle of the vessel walls.

After prolonged complete ischemia, particularly that complicated by hypotension, recirculation may not be possible, even if blood pressure is restored. This "no-reflow" phenomenon appears to be due to a combination of hemodynamic factors (sludging and coagulation), vascular compression due to edema and increased intracranial pressure, and vascular endothelial damage. Areas of no reflow may be distributed as patches in a reperfusing region.

Loss of local autoregulation leads to mismatch of metabolism and blood flow

After ischemia of shorter duration or lesser severity, reperfusion is accompanied by a brief period of vascular paralysis and hyperemia, followed by a delayed (30–60 min postocclusion) hypoperfusion in which blood flow may drop to 50 percent of normal [8]. The reason for delayed hypoperfusion appears to be multifactorial. The development of edema, hypoxia, and hypotension may contribute to the elaboration of eicosanoids and other metabolites, as well as to abnormal concentrations of neurotransmitters; Ca^{2+} may also be important, since Ca^{2+} channel blockers have been reported to attenuate the development of this condition [9]. The hyperemia and vasomotor paralysis may be due to the development of lactic acidosis and may be accompanied by hyperoxia because the tissue does not regain its normal metabolic rate; conversely, during delayed hypoperfusion, recovering tissue may become hypoxic. Thus, there is a considerable period with a mismatch between perfusion and metabolism that may be a significant factor in the development of damage beyond that of the original insult.

Nevertheless, the extent of damage is not exclusively dependent on defects of perfusion. Not only are there selectively vulnerable populations of cells whose damage does not correlate well with low reflows, but there are also regions of brain that are normally less densely vascularized and therefore more vulnerable. There is great variability in the capillary density of different regions of brain, and white matter has approximately 20 percent the blood flow of gray matter. White matter appears to suffer proportionately greater damage than gray matter during delayed hypoperfusion despite its lower metabolic rate.

DEVELOPMENT OF EDEMA

Edema accompanies many injuries and diseases, such as tumors, infections, trauma, and hormonal imbalances as well as ischemia and hypoxia. In any of these conditions, increased intracranial pressure and herniation of portions of the brain through the tentorium or other sites are serious complications. Edema is defined as the increase of tissue volume as the result of an increased water and Na^+ load (biochemistry of brain edema is discussed by Fishman [10]).

Cellular (cytotoxic) edema develops almost immediately following vascular occlusion (seconds to minutes) and, provided that circulation is promptly restored, is reversible. In this type of edema, neuronal and glial permeability to ions are increased, but capillary permeability is unchanged. Perivascular and perineuronal astrocytic processes swell, followed by swelling of neurons and endothelial cells. The extracellular space is reduced, and capillary permeability is unchanged. Large amounts of K^+ are lost from neurons to the extracellular fluid (ECF), and all cells take up water and NaCl. Glial cells may have a protective role in this process because they take up large amounts of K^+ as well as Na^+. Cellular edema affects both white and gray matter. The main cause is probably ATP depletion and failure of active transport.

Vasogenic edema develops if reperfusion is delayed or inadequate. It develops within hours to days after the ischemic or hypoxic episode and causes more damage to white matter than to gray. Endothelial damage results in increased capillary permeability, disrupting the blood-brain barrier, and there is extravasation of large proteins and other molecules and plasma filtrate to the extracellular compartment, expanding its size. This type of edema may result in vascular compression, increased intracranial pressure, and herniations of brain tissue. Cellular and vasogenic edema are the most common forms that accompany ischemia and are intrinsic to its pathology. Occasionally, an additional type, interstitial (hydrocephalic) edema, may be observed as a complication of hemorrhagic stroke, in which obstruction of the ventricular system forces CSF into periventricular areas.

ENERGY FAILURE, LACTIC ACIDOSIS AND CALCIUM IONS

No aspect of metabolism (Table 1) is spared in severe hypoxic or ischemic injury; therefore the key biochemical determinants of irreversible cell damage are not completely known. However, the interrelated factors of energy failure, lactic acidosis, and Ca^{2+} imbalance are presently viewed as critical steps leading to ischemic cell damage or death.

The adenylate energy charge drops in ischemia and hypoxia

In ischemia, glucose and glycogen stores are depleted, and oxygen deficiency impairs mitochondrial respiration. Cells metabolize residual stores of glucose anaerobically to lactic acid instead of CO_2 and water (see Chap. 28). ATP is utilized but production is decreased, thus leading to an increase in the proportionate amount of AMP that does not have high-energy phosphate bonds available for energy utilization. A parameter reflecting the ratio of high-energy phosphate bond production to consumption is the adenylate energy charge EC:

$$EC = \{[ATP] + \tfrac{1}{2}[ADP]\}/\{[ATP] + [ADP] + [AMP]\}$$

EC drops during the first minutes of complete ischemia, as the levels of ATP and the storage form of high-energy phosphate, phosphocreatine, fall to undetectable levels. The concentrations of adenine nucleotides reach a plateau ap-

TABLE 1. Major events in brain ischemia

EARLY CHANGES (sec–min)
Abolition of EEG
Ca^{2+} influx
Activation of lipolytic enzymes
Release of free fatty acids
Production of eicosanoids
Mitochondrial swelling
Increased NADH

INTERMEDIATE CHANGES (<10 min)
Increased glycolysis
Decreased glucose, glycogen
Increased lactate
Decreased energy charge
Failure of Na,K-ATPase
Development of edema
Neurotransmitter release
Increased cAMP

LATE CHANGES (>10 min)
Decreased protein synthesis
Increased proteolysis
Activation of lysosomal enzymes

proximately 10 min postinsult, and lactic acid levels reach a maximum at approximately 3 min [11]. The deamination and dephosphorylation of adenine nucleotides result in increased levels of adenosine and inosine, whereas adenylate cyclase stimulation results in increased levels of cyclic AMP (cAMP). As a result of these changes, the brain is exposed to altered levels of adenine nucleotides, whose concentrations regulate many enzymes of protein, carbohydrate, and lipid metabolism. Further, ATP-requiring processes are deprived of their energy supply.

Na,K-ATPase failure is a critical event

In particular, loss of ATP impairs the ATP-linked Na^+/K^+ pump of the plasma membrane, causing cells to lose K^+ and to take up Na^+ and Cl^- (Na,K-ATPase is discussed in Chap. 3). There is at first a gradual increase in K^+ conductance, followed by a more rapid phase of K^+ efflux, which probably represents true pump failure [12]. The mechanism of the initial gradual increase of K^+ conductance is not known. At approximately 15 μmol/g, extracellular K^+ depolarizes voltage-dependent Ca^{2+} channels, and as much as 95 percent of the extracellular Ca^{2+} enters the cell (see Chaps. 15 and 41). Without adequate ATP, the normal capacity of cells to sequester Ca^{2+} in the endoplasmic reticulum is overwhelmed, and the ability of mitochondria to transport it is impaired. Mitochondrial oxidative phosphorylation is uncoupled, due in part to futile Ca^{2+} cycling across the mitochondrial membrane. Free intracellular Ca^{2+} is known to activate lipolytic, proteolytic, and signaling cascades, which may irreversibly abolish the biochemical regulation of cellular metabolism (see Chaps. 16 and 19).

Lactic acidosis is associated with severe damage and edema

Lactic acid accumulation and increased pCO_2 cause acidosis, which can be severe, reaching pH values of approximately 6. Elevated concentrations of cAMP and decreased levels of ATP stimulate the activities of phosphofructo-kinase, glycogen phosphorylase, and hexokinase, further stimulating the rate of glycolysis. The severity of tissue damage both during an ischemic insult and in the recirculation phase has been shown to be related to the degree of lactic acidosis. Experiments on rats, cats, and monkeys whose blood glucose levels were altered by diet or glucose injections demonstrate a close correlation between lactic acid levels in brain and blood glucose levels; infarcts were more severe, and recovery was poorer in the fed/injected than fasted animals. The relationship between lactic acidosis and tissue damage accounts for the more severe damage observed after incomplete ischemia than in complete ischemia. Ordinarily, lactate levels generated from static blood reach approximately 15 μmol/g brain tissue. A trickle of blood to an ischemic area increases glucose availability, and lactate

levels may reach 40 μmol/g tissue. Poor outcomes are associated with lactate >20 μmol/g [13].

The specific pathogenetic mechanisms of lactic acidosis are not known. High concentrations of H^+ can denature proteins and alter the activities of enzymes whose activities are pH dependent. Low pH inhibits the reoxidation of NADH and the reuptake of neurotransmitters, promotes the formation of free radicals, prolongs or prevents the restoration of mitochondrial function, and delays the restoration of the EC. A major effect of lactate is enhancement of edema formation. The severity of glial and endothelial cellular edema appears closely related to the degree of acidosis present. Although the specific mechanism is not understood, it is possible that in combination with H^+, Na^+, and other metabolites, lactate increases intracellular osmolarity, thus drawing water from the ECF.

Recirculation after moderate periods of ischemia is accompanied by gradual resolution of ionic fluid and pH imbalances. During the recirculation phase, ATP levels and the energy charge remain depressed for some time, and adenosine levels remain relatively high. Regeneration of the energy charge lags, as some adenine and adenosine are lost to the circulation; thus, salvage pathways and *de novo* synthesis must augment rephosphorylation to replenish the ATP supply. Cerebral metabolism of glucose increases to several times normal after reperfusion and may remain elevated for several hours [13]. In conjunction with delayed hypoperfusion, accelerated glucose utilization may contribute to the postischemic progression of cell damage by prolonging the mismatch between circulation and metabolism.

Energy failure itself is not the determinant of cell death

As mentioned earlier, cells may die even after periods of time in which the energy metabolism of the area has been reestablished. It is the inability of cells to reestablish vital functions disrupted by transient energy failure that causes a gradual deterioration. Deregulation of such diverse processes as neurotransmission, protein synthesis, and membrane lipid metabolism are important in the continuation of pathologic processes triggered by Ca^{2+} influx.

NEUROTRANSMISSION FAILURE

A consequence of increased intracellular Ca^{2+} and decreased ATP supply is the derangement of neurotransmission

Calcium ion influx leads to the exocytosis of neurotransmitters and neuromodulators, whereas decreased levels of oxygen and ATP impair energy- and oxygen-dependent reuptake and biosynthesis. ATP, in addition, may have a regulatory effect on K^+ channels (see Chap. 41).

Extracellular accumulation of neurotransmitters is associated with receptor activation and cell stimulation at times when oxygen or glucose supply may still be impaired. Neurotransmitters also stimulate adenylate cyclase-linked receptors (see Chap. 18), leading to large increases in cAMP both during and after ischemia, which further contributes to metabolic deregulation. In addition, the vasculature is exposed to abnormal concentrations of neurotransmitters during ischemia and recirculation. The local imbalance in transmitter substances may contribute to dysautoregulation, which in turn impairs the matching or coupling of metabolism to blood flow during reperfusion.

Biogenic amines decrease in tissue and accumulate in the CSF during ischemia and hypoxia

Biogenic amines, such as norepinephrine (NE) and serotonin (5-HT) will cause edema, and 5-HT has vasoconstrictive and hemocoagulative effects. Possibly, these are factors in ischemic injury. Certain drugs, such as *p*-chlorophenylalanine, which blocks 5-HT synthesis, phenoxybenzamine, which blocks α-adrenergic receptors, and reserpine, which causes NE depletion, have been reported to prevent or attenuate ischemic damage [13]. Catecholamines in high concentrations may uncouple oxidative phosphorylation. Moreover, these amines may be auto-oxidized to highly reactive superoxide radicals (O_2^-) implicated in the peroxidation of lipids and cell membrane damage; O_2^- is also an intermediate in the reduction of O_2 to H_2O. Ordinarily, the enzyme superoxide dismutase catalyzes O_2^- reduction by H^+ to H_2O_2 and O_2. When O_2^- is produced, H_2O_2 and OH^- also are produced, all of which may damage cellular components (see also Chaps. 20 and 34).

Catecholamine uptake requires ATP, and its catabolism by monoamine oxidase requires oxygen. During ischemia and the immediate postischemic period there is therefore prolonged ligand-receptor interaction, causing decreased receptor sensitivity. In addition, energy-dependent resynthesis of neurotransmitters is sluggish, so that there is a prolonged period where normal intercellular communication is disturbed. These phenomena may underlie the disturbances of consciousness and mentation that accompany the postischemic period and explain why reestablishment of normal electrical and energetic parameters is not always accompanied by neurological recovery [13].

Accumulations of neuromodulatory substances such as adenosine also influence development of pathology

Adenosine, formed from the dephosphorylation of adenine nucleotides, is a potent vasodilator and neuromodulator. Adenosine receptors have been identified in selectively vulnerable cells of the hippocampus; adenosine also has been implicated in the development of edema. Ischemic conditions favor the oxidation of an adenosine metabolite, hypoxanthine, which is accompanied by the production of superoxide radicals and hydrogen peroxide, which appear to contribute to ischemia-induced membrane pathology, as mentioned earlier.

Excitatory amino acids may cause cell death

The accumulation of aspartate and especially glutamate (Glu) has been implicated in the selective vulnerability of some neurons in the hippocampus and cerebellum that receive input using these amino acids (see Chap. 15). They are known to cause edema and cell death at high concentrations, and several experiments have shown that anoxia enhances Glu release and that the CSF accumulates large amounts of Glu during ischemia. Glu induces a rapid accumulation of Na^+, Cl^-, and H_2O into cells after acute exposure; in the presence of Ca^{2+}, cells exposed to Glu for a brief period exhibit increased Ca^{2+} influx and delayed damage or death. Destruction of Glu input to the hippocampus or blockade of Glu receptors reduces ischemic damage [14].

PROTEIN METABOLISM

Complete ischemia and hypoxia decrease protein synthesis and degradation, although polyribosomal assemblies survive prolonged periods of ischemia and retain their synthetic capacity. They may disaggregate during the recirculation phase, during which time protein synthesis remains depressed, probably because of a chain-initiating defect. Recovery depends on the duration of the ischemic period. Selectively vulnerable areas of brain are reported to undergo a delayed suppression of protein synthesis after initial recovery; this interesting finding may be related to defects in Ca^{2+}-calmodulin-dependent phosphorylation, the effects of which require time to appear because the cell may have stores of proteins that maintain short-term function [6] (these phosphorylation reactions are discussed in Chap. 19).

PHOSPHOLIPID METABOLISM DURING ISCHEMIA

Other consequences of the rapid Ca^{2+} influx that accompanies ischemic injury to cells are (1) the activation of membrane phospholipases A_1, A_2, and C; (2) the breakdown of membrane phospholipids; and (3) the release of free fatty acids, including arachidonic and docosahexaenoic acids. The primary sources of free fatty acids are inositol, ethanolamine, and choline glycerophospholipids. (Lipid metabolism and phospholipases are described in Chaps. 5 and 16.)

After 30 min of severe incomplete ischemia and 30 min of reperfusion, ethanolamine glycerophospholipids are decreased by 6 percent, choline glycerophospholipids by 5 percent, and serine/inositol glycerophospholipids by 9 percent [15]. The arachidonic acid content of the glycerophospholipids of gerbil brain decreases very early during global ischemia. During the first 30 sec, arachidonic acid is released from the inositol glycerolipids. Ethanolamine plasmalogens are a source of arachidonic acid between 30 and 60 sec. Then, between 1 and 3 min of ischemia, choline glycerophospholipids are the primary source of the free arachidonic acid [16]. Plasmalogens are hydrolyzed either by a plasmalogenase/lysophospholipase pathway or by plasmalogen-specific phospholipase A_2/lysoplasmalogenase reactions. At present it is not clear which of the above pathways is activated during ischemia.

Ischemia reverses the synthetic reaction for phosphatidylcholine

Another pathway for the release of free fatty acids that may also be activated during ischemia is the reversal of the choline phosphotransferase reaction [17]. This Mg^{2+}-requiring enzyme catalyzes the transfer of phosphocholine to 1,2-diacylglycerol from CDP choline, with the release of CMP. Under normal conditions, the synthesis of phosphatidylcholine is favored as a result of the very rapid rephosphorylation of CMP to CTP, which requires ATP. During ischemia, when the ATP supply is depleted, CMP is not rephosphorylated. The transferase reaction is reversed, producing CDP choline and diacylglycerols, which are rapidly hydrolyzed by mono- and diacylglycerol lipases to free fatty acids and glycerol. In gerbil cerebral ischemia, arachidonic acid (see Chap. 20) is predominantly released from inositol-containing phospholipids by phospholipase C and diacylglycerol lipase pathways, rather than from phosphatidylcholine or phosphatidylethanolamine by phospholipase A_2 [18].

Free fatty acids have several harmful effects

Free fatty acids released as a result of ischemic insult are known to have a variety of detrimental effects on brain structure and function, primarily due to their ability to disrupt cell membranes. Free fatty acids are efficient uncouplers of oxidative phosphorylation and may cause the efflux of ions, such as Ca^{2+} and K^+, stored in the mitochondria. Tissue swelling has been observed in brain slices incubated with free fatty acids. Since free fatty acids have detergent properties, they may change the fluidity and permeability of membranes, influencing mechanisms dependent on membrane integrity [19].

Arachidonic acid, the substrate for eicosanoid production by monooxygenases (cyclo-oxygenase and lipoxygenase), is the precursor of several active compounds [20] (details of these reactions are given in Chap. 20). Eicosanoids (prostaglandins, thromboxanes, and leukotrienes) are vasoactive and may be involved in dysautoregulation. They may play a neuromodulatory role, and high levels produced in ischemia may damage cells further in still poorly understood ways. Reaction intermediates in the cyclo-oxygenase and lipoxygenase pathways that might have deleterious effects on the integrity of cell membrane structure and function are the endoperoxides, prostaglandin G_2 (PGG$_2$) and prostaglandin H_2 (PGH$_2$), and the hydroperoxides [21] (see also Chap. 20). These metabolites have a free radical character and may elicit a cascade of harmful reactions, including (1) peroxidation of polyunsaturated fatty acids in the cell membrane, irreversibly changing their properties; and (2) generation of free radicals in the hydrocarbon core of the cell membrane, possibly cross-linking proteins with phospholipids and altering the microenvironment and structure of proteins in the mitochondrial and plasma membranes [11].

PHARMACOLOGICAL INTERVENTION IN ISCHEMIA

The main classes of pharmacological agents used in the management of stroke injury in humans or in experimental work on animals are listed in Table 2. No agent has been shown to be of unequivocal value in all cases, and many are still highly experimental. A few are discussed briefly below.

CDP-amines have been reported to increase oxygen consumption, glucose incorporation into amino acids, and phospholipid and GABA synthesis. CDP-amines may cause a decline in lactate production and restoration of Na,K-ATPase activity; they may prevent accumulation of free fatty acids [17].

Calcium ion channel blockers are being investigated for the treatment of ischemia. By

TABLE 2. Proposed pharmacological strategies for stroke management

Agent	Proposed mechanism of action
CDP-choline	Induce phospholipid synthesis
CDP-ethanolamine	Reversal of CDP-ethanolamine phosphotransferase reaction
	Decrease production of free fatty acids
Ca^{2+} channel blockers Verapamil Nimodipine Flunarizine	Decrease Ca^{2+} entry
Antioxidants/free radical scavengers α-Tocopherol Ascorbic acid Mannitol Glutathione Catalase Superoxide dismutase	Protect lipids from peroxidation
Opiate antagonists Naloxone	Vasoregulation Antioxidant, anti-GABA activity
β-Adrenergic antagonists Propranolol	Decrease edema Lactic acid production Vasodilation
Gingko biloba derivatives [24]	Platelet activating factor antagonists Decrease platelet aggregation Decrease Ca^{2+} entry Free radical scavengers
Barbiturates	Membrane stabilizer Free radical scavenger Anticonvulsant
Prostacyclin (PGI₂)	Vasodilation Decrease platelet aggregation
Phosphodiesterase inhibitors [25] Aminophylline Dipyridamole Sulfinpyrazone	Vasoconstriction of nonischemic vessels Diverting blood to ischemic area
Phenothiazines Chlorpromazine Trifluoperazine	Inhibition of Ca^{2+}-calmodulin complex
Perfluorocarbons	Hemodilution O₂ carrier

TABLE 2. (*continued*)

Agent	Proposed mechanism of action
Excitotoxic amino acid blockers 2-Amino-7-phosphono-heptanoic acid	Decrease neuronal damage
Cyclooxygenase inhibitors Indomethacin Aspirin	Decrease prostaglandin synthesis
Fibrinolysis Streptokinase Urokinase Tissue plasminogen activator	Clot dissolution

blocking the entry of Ca^{2+} into cells, they may inhibit the essential role of this cation in the activation of lipolytic and other enzymes during ischemia. Increased blood flow, decreased lactic acidosis, and decreased infarct size have been reported following nimodipine treatment [22].

α-Tocopherol (Vitamin E), a well-known antioxidant (see Chap. 34), has been reported to have beneficial effects on brain edema and ischemia [23]. It inhibits both fatty acid release and lipoxygenase activity and plays a fundamental role in the stabilization of polyunsaturated fatty acid residues in membrane phospholipids. Vitamin E may also interact with cellular membranes and prevent lipid peroxide formation by acting as a hydrogen donor. Free-radical-induced damage in ischemia may also be prevented by the administration of mannitol and dimethylsulfoxide (DMSO), which possibly act as specific scavengers for hydroxyl radicals.

Use of the opiate antagonist, naloxone (see Chap. 13), for the treatment of ischemic insult is controversial [9]. Although endorphin levels are increased during ischemia, the beneficial effects of naloxone appear related to anti-inflammatory, antioxidant, and membrane-stabilizing properties [24]. The positive results obtained with this agent required higher doses than would be expected for opiate antagonist action alone. More research is needed to identify other important factors in the pathophysiology of ischemia and to point to more targets for intervention.

REFERENCES

1. Astrup, J., Siesjo, B. K., and Symon, L. Thresholds in cerebral ischemia—The ischemic penumbra. *Stroke* 12:723–725, 1981.

2. Molinari, G. F. Experimental models of ischemic stroke. In H. J. M. Barnett, B. M. Stein, J. P. Mohr, and F. M. Yatsu (eds.), *Stroke: Pathophysiology, Diagnosis and Management*. New York: Churchill Livingstone, 1986, Vol. 1, pp. 57–73.

3. Fieschi, C., and Lenzi, G. L. Experimental models of focal cerebral ischemia. In A. Bes, P. Braquet, R. Paoletti, and B. K. Siesjo (eds.), *Cerebral Ischemia*. Amsterdam: Excerpta Medica, 1984, pp. 57–62.

4. Pulsinelli, W., and Brierly, J. B. A new model of bilateral hemispheric ischemia in the unanesthetized rat. *Stroke* 10:267–272, 1979.

5. Pulsinelli, W. Selective neuronal vulnerability: morphological and molecular characteristics. In K. Kogure, K.-A. Hossmann, B. K. Siesjo, and F. A. Welsh (eds.), *Molecular Mechanisms of Brain Damage* (*Progress in Brain Research, Vol. 63*). Amsterdam: Elsevier, 1985, pp. 29–37.

6. Hossmann, K.-A. Post-ischemic resuscitation of the brain: Selective vulnerability versus global resistance. In K. Kogure, K.-A. Hossmann, B. K. Siesjo, and F. A. Welsh (eds.), *Molecular Mechanisms of Brain Damage* (*Progress in Brain Research, Vol. 63*). Amsterdam: Elsevier, 1985, pp. 3–17.

7. Kirino, T., Tamura, A., and Sano, K. Selective vulnerability of the hippocampus to ischemia— Reversible and irreversible types of ischemic cell damage. In K. Kogure, K.-A. Hossmann, B. K. Siesjo, and F. A. Welsh (eds.), *Molecular Mechanisms of Brain Damage.* (*Progress in Brain Research, Vol. 63*). Amsterdam: Elsevier, 1985, pp. 39–58.

8. Welsh, F. A. Role of vascular factors in regional ischemic injury. In K. Kogure, K.-A. Hossmann, B. K. Siesjo, and F. A. Welsh (eds.), *Molecular Mechanisms of Brain Damage* (*Progress in Brain Research, Vol. 63*). Amsterdam: Elsevier, 1985, pp. 19–27.

9. Welch, K. M. A., and Barkley, G. L. Biochemistry and pharmacology of cerebral ischemia. In H. J. M. Barnett, B. M. Stein, J. P. Mohr, and F. M. Yatsu (eds.), *Stroke: Pathophysiology, Diagnosis and Management*. New York: Churchill Livingstone, 1986, Vol. 1, pp. 75–90.

10. Fishman, Robert A. Brain edema. In G. J. Siegel, R. W. Albers, B. W. Agranoff, and R. Katzman (eds.), *Basic Neurochemistry*, 3rd ed. Boston: Little, Brown, 1981, pp. 681–691.

11. Siesjo, B. K. Cerebral circulation and metabolism. *J. Neurosurg.* 60:883–908, 1984.

12. Hansen, A. J., and Mutch, W. A. C. Water and ion fluxes in cerebral ischemia. In A. Bes, P. Braquet, R. Paoletti, and B. K. Siesjo (eds.), *Cerebral Ischemia*. Amsterdam: Excerpta Medica, 1984, pp. 121–130.

13. Nemoto, E. M. Brain ischemia. In A. Lajtha (ed.), *Alterations of Metabolites in the Nervous System* (*Handbook of Neurochemistry, Vol. 9*). New York: Plenum, 1985, pp. 553–588.

14. Rothman, S. M., and Olney, J. W. Glutamate and the pathophysiology of hypoxic-ischemic brain damage. *Ann. Neurol.* 19:105–111. 1986.

15. Rehncrona, S., Westerberg, E., Akesson, B., and Siesjo, B. K. Brain cortical fatty acids and phospholipids during and following complete and severe incomplete ischemia. *J. Neurochem.* 38:84–93, 1982.

16. DeMedio, G. E., Goracci, G., Horrocks, L. A., Lazarewicz, J. W., Mazzari, S., Porcellati, G., Strosznajder, J., and Trovarelli, G. The effect of transient ischemia on fatty acid and lipid metabolism in the gerbil brain. *Ital. J. Biochem.* 29:412–432, 1980.

17. Horrocks, L. A., and Dorman, R. V. Prevention by CDPcholine and CDPethanolamine of lipid changes during brain ischemia. In V. Zappia, E. P. Kennedy, B. I. Nilsson, and P. Galletti (eds.), *Novel Biochemical Pharmacological and Clinic Aspects of Cytidinediphosphocholine*. New York: Elsevier, 1985, pp. 205–215.

18. Abe, K., Kogure, K., Yamamoto, H., Imazawa, M., and Miyamoto, K. Mechanism of arachidonic acid liberation during ischemia in gerbil cerebral cortex. *J. Neurochem.* 48:503–509, 1987.

19. Siesjo, B. K. Cell damage in the brain: A speculative synthesis. *J. Cereb. Blood Flow Metab.* 1:155–185, 1981.

20. Samuelsson, B. Prostaglandins, endoperoxides and thromboxanes: Role as bioregulators. In F. O. Schmitt and F. G. Worden (eds.), *The Neurosciences: Fourth Study Program.* Cambridge: MIT Press, 1979, pp. 5–20.

21. Wolf, L. S. Eicosanoids: Prostaglandins, thromboxanes, leukotrienes, and other derivatives of carbon-20 unsaturated fatty acids. *J. Neurochem.* 38:1–14, 1982.

22. Meyer, F. B., Sundt, T. F., Jr., Yanagihara, T., and Anderson, R. E. Focal cerebral ischemia: pathophysiologic mechanisms and rationale for future avenues for treatment. *Mayo Clin. Proc.* 62:35–55, 1987.

23. Yoshida, S., Busto, R., Watson, B. D., Santiso, M., and Ginsberg, M. D. Postischemic cerebral lipid peroxidation *in vitro*: Modification by dietary vitamin E. *J. Neurochem.* 44:1593–1601, 1985.

24. Hosobuchi, Y., Baskin, D. S., and Woo, S. K. Reversal of induced ischemic neurologic deficit in gerbils by the opiate antagonist naloxone. *Science* 215:69–71, 1982.

25. Etienne, A., Chapelat, M.-Y., Braquet, M., Clostre, F., Drieu, K., DeFeudis, F. V., and Braquet, P. *In vivo* studies of free radical scavenging activity; relation to cerebral ischaemia. In A. Bes, P. Braquet, R. Paoletti, and B. K. Siesjo (eds.), *Cerebral Ischemia.* Amsterdam: Excerpta Medica, 1984, pp. 379–384.

26. Yatsu, F. M., Pettigrew, L. C., and Grotta, J. C. Medical therapy of ischemic strokes. In H. J. M. Barnett, B. M. Stein, J. P. Mohr, and F. M. Yatsu (eds.), *Stroke: Pathophysiology, Diagnosis and Management.* New York: Churchill Livingstone, 1986, Vol. 2, pp. 1069–1085.

CHAPTER 41

Epileptic Seizures

Claude Wasterlain

Epileptic seizures are characterized by paroxysmal, excessive, and hypersynchronous discharges of large numbers of neurons. Many causes can trigger abnormal discharges, and the behavioral manifestations of seizures depend on the type and location of the neurons involved. Epilepsy is a disease characterized by spontaneous, recurrent epileptic seizures in the absence of a known precipitating cause or illness. In addition, epileptic seizures are seen in many

Basic Neurochemistry: Molecular, Cellular, and Medical Aspects, 4th Ed., edited by G. J. Siegel et al. Raven Press, Ltd., New York, 1989.
Correspondence to Claude Wasterlain, Department of Neurology, School of Medicine, University of California, Los Angeles, California 90024.

illnesses that directly or indirectly involve the brain, including ionic and electrolyte imbalances; disorders of carbohydrate, amino acid, and lipid metabolism; infections; brain tumors; brain trauma; and elevations in body temperature in the young. A number of laboratory animal models of epilepsy with recurrent seizures have been studied. These include lesions of the cortex produced by alumina gel, penicillin, cobalt, and freezing; kainic acid-induced hippocampal lesions; genetic epilepsy, such as in baboons or audiogenic seizures in mice; and the kindling phenomenon, which is discussed later. Extensive surveys of this entire field have been compiled [1,2].

MECHANISMS OF EPILEPTOGENESIS

Repetitively firing neurons show a depolarizing shift in membrane potential

During seizures in humans and laboratory animals, the electroencephalogram records rapid changes in voltage as sharply angulated waves called spikes. Simultaneous extracellular recordings show the firing of many neurons; intracellular recordings show a depolarizing shift characteristic of a giant excitatory postsynaptic potential. These electrical changes correspond to the opening of specific ion channels in the neuronal membrane, although their precise sequence has yet to be defined. At the onset of the hypersynchronous discharge, the extracellular Ca^{2+} concentration falls, and slightly later, the extracellular K^+ rises. Changes in both extracellular Ca^{2+} and K^+ may participate in the large, progressive depolarizing shift in the membrane potential of neurons. Repetitive neuronal firing resulting from the depolarizing shift may release massive amounts of excitatory neurotransmitters at synapses, which, in turn, may result in an avalanche of excitation. Electrical coupling seems to play a less important role than chemical coupling in the process of hypersynchronous excitation.

Experimental seizures can be induced by electrical, metabolic, or pharmacologic mechanisms

The various means of producing seizures experimentally, while not reproducing human epilepsy, do have some counterpart in human pathology. These epileptogenic conditions may be grouped according to the following classification of mechanisms.

Alteration of membrane properties or membrane potential of neurons

Alteration of membrane properties or membrane potential of neurons include electrical depolarization, such as electroshock; ionic shifts, such as extracellular decreases in Na^+ or increases in K^+; alkalosis; hypoxia or hyperbaric O_2; hypoglycemia; poisons of glycolysis or respiration, such as fluoroacetate, which compromise the membrane potential by depleting ATP; inhibitors of cholesterol synthesis, ganglioside-binding substances and alterations of membrane lipids; and a variety of hormonal disorders that alter ion balance, for example, inappropriate secretion of antidiuretic hormone, causing water intoxication and hyponatremia [1].

Agonists of excitatory neurotransmitters

Kainic acid, quisqualic acid, ibotenic acid, and other excitotoxins that produce seizures directly bind to glutamate-aspartate receptors (see Chap. 15) that when activated lead to excitatory postsynaptic potentials (Chap. 4). Muscarinic agonists (see Chap. 10) and opioid peptides in large doses, such as met- and leuenkephalin (see Chap. 13), also produce seizures. A number of endogenous peptides and other neuroeffectors are released during seizures or have modulatory effects on seizures in various paradigms. Other convulsant agents (e.g., organophosphates, nerve gases that inhibit cholinesterase) interfere with the breakdown of excitatory neurotransmitters such as acetylcholine [1].

N-Methyl-D-aspartate (NMDA) binds to a particularly important subtype of glutamate receptor that commands postsynaptic ion channels through which Ca^{2+} enters neurons when the channels are open [3]. These channels can be blocked by Mg^{2+}, and hypomagnesemia has been reported to cause seizures. NMDA receptors only participate in synaptic transmission when the postsynaptic membrane is depolarized. These receptors are particularly prevalent in the hippocampus and may be involved in the kindling phenomenon (see later) and in long-term potentiation (LTP), which are associated with increased Ca^{2+} entry into neurons. The actions of NMDA receptors are strongly potentiated by glycine (nonstrychnine sensitive) and inhibited by drugs that bind to the σ (opiate) or phencyclidine (PCP) receptors, suggesting the existence of a molecular complex integrating these receptors and their ion channels. Such a complex may have a key role in excitatory transmitter actions and in epileptogenesis. (These receptors are discussed in Chaps. 13 and 15.)

Antagonists of inhibitory neurotransmitters

The neurotransmitter γ-aminobutyric acid (GABA) opens membrane ion channels permeable to Cl^-. The resulting Cl^- influx hyperpolarizes the neuronal membrane, raising its firing threshold and producing an inhibitory postsynaptic potential (see Chap. 4). Substances that block the GABA hyperpolarizing effect include bicuculline, which binds directly to the $GABA_A$ receptors for GABA (see Fig. 3 in Chap. 15); methyl-6,7-dimethoxy-4-ethyl-β-carboline-3-carboxylate (DMCM) and pentylenetetrazol, both of which block the benzodiazepine site linked to the $GABA_A$ receptor; picrotoxin, which alters the Cl^- channel regulated by the $GABA_A$-benzodiazepine receptor complex, thus reducing Cl^- entry; and strychnine, which blocks Cl^- channels linked to glycine receptors (see Chap. 15). All of these substances have in common the ability to increase excitability in some population of neurons and to induce seizures. Other epileptogenic substances or conditions (e.g., pyridoxal phosphate antagonists, pyridoxine deficiency) may prevent the synthesis of GABA by inhibiting glutamate decarboxylase (see Chaps. 28 and 34).

Drugs may prevent seizures through effects on transmitters, receptors, and ion channels

GABA is believed to play a particularly important role in seizure inhibition and in anticonvulsant drug action [4]. GABA agonists are often potent anticonvulsants. Benzodiazepines (e.g., diazepam and clonazepam) potentiate GABA binding to its receptor and are used clinically as anticonvulsants. Barbiturates bind to a site (termed the sedative-convulsant site) on the Cl^- channel (see Chap. 15). Barbiturates in therapeutic anticonvulsant doses also potentiate GABA effects on Cl^- influx [5]. GABA-, benzodiazepine-, and barbiturate-binding sites have allosteric interactions, providing an example of analog-type integration of neurotransmitter-receptor function at the molecular level (see Fig. 3, Chap. 15). This GABA receptor-benzodiazepine receptor-Cl^- channel complex is believed to play an essential role in recurrent inhibition, in some anticonvulsant drug actions, and in some genetic models of epilepsy [4].

Compounds that increase synthesis or release, or prevent reuptake or metabolism, of inhibitory transmitters, thereby potentiating their action, usually raise seizure thresholds. For example valproate, a potent anticonvulsant in clinical use, increases GABA levels in the brain and inhibits GABA transaminase, the enzyme that breaks down GABA [5].

However, GABAergic synaptic transmission may not be the only mechanism underlying anticonvulsant drug action. A number of clinically important anticonvulsants produce no demonstrable GABAergic enhancement but do reduce repetitive neuronal firing, which is believed to be related to effects on voltage-sensitive Na^+ channels. These include phenytoin and carbamazepine. Another group of anticonvulsants, previously mentioned, includes valproate, phenobarbital, and clonazepam, which both reduce repetitive firing and enhance GABAergic responses, but at different concentrations. These clinical anticonvulsants have different spectra of efficacy in various types of clinical and experimental seizures [5].

In addition, experimentally-used antagonists of excitatory neurotransmitters [e.g., the glutamate antagonists, 2-amino-7-phosphonoheptanoic acid (AP7), CCP, and MK801] have anticonvulsant activity (see Table 5 in Chap. 15). The Ca^{2+}-channel blockers (e.g., nimodipine, flunarizine), which reduce Ca^{2+} entry into presynaptic terminals and thereby reduce the amount of transmitter released, also have anticonvulsant action. Such features as blocking receptors for excitatory neurotransmitters, enhancing receptors for inhibitory neurotransmitters, and modifying ion channels are incorporated by investigators in the design of new anticonvulsant drugs.

METABOLIC HOMEOSTASIS IN SEIZURES

Epileptic seizures make the greatest metabolic demands on the brain and severely challenge its ability to maintain homeostatic mechanisms [6]. It is clear that between seizures, brain metabolism is normal in epileptic animals and that the ictal metabolic disturbances are the consequence, not the cause, of seizures. The release of large amounts of potentially excitotoxic neurotransmitters, large expenditures of energy, and major changes in ionic fluxes frequently result in brain damage when seizures are prolonged. It is likely that most of the energy expended during seizures serves to pump ions back across the membrane and to reestablish the resting membrane potential (see Chap. 3). At the same time, catabolic activities are greatly enhanced, and anabolic processes are profoundly inhibited, presumably to save energy essential for cell survival. A variety of adaptive mechanisms increase the supply of oxygen and glucose to the brain during seizures. These processes, while efficient for seizures of short duration, fail progressively when seizures are prolonged.

Cerebral blood flow is increased by seizures

Under normal circumstances, cerebral blood flow (CBF) is independent of blood pressure within very wide limits (see Chap. 29). This autoregulation of CBF is abolished by seizures, and since most generalized seizures result in massive catecholamine release and sympathetic excitation, the attendant increase in blood pressure results in large increases in CBF [7] (Table 1). This is not the only mechanism involved, since focal seizures result in focal increases in CBF independently of any changes in blood pressure.

During generalized convulsive seizures, hypoxemia from reduced ventilation results in impaired oxygen delivery to the brain despite the increased CBF, and oxygen content of cerebral venous blood is decreased. However, if hypoxemia is prevented by inducing paralysis and mechanically ventilating with oxygen, both in humans and animals, cerebral venous blood shows an increase in the partial pressure of oxygen, which indicates that the increase in CBF

TABLE 1. Indices of cerebral metabolism during generalized seizures[a]

Metabolic index	Relative increase
Glycolytic flux	Two- to eightfold
Oxygen consumption (CMRO$_2$)	0.6- to 2.5-fold
High-energy phosphate (~P) utilization	Two- to fourfold
Cerebral blood flow	1.5- to 9-fold
Glucose transport into brain	Approximately threefold
Respiratory quotient (RQ)	Rises above 1.0

[a] Scope of metabolic changes during generalized epileptic seizures. [From T. E. Duffy and F. Plum. In G. J. Siegel et al. (eds.), *Basic Neurochemistry*, 3rd. ed. Boston: Little, Brown, 1981, pp. 693–718.]

actually exceeds the increase in the metabolic needs of the tissue.

In status epilepticus, a state of nearly continuous seizures, lactic acidosis invariably develops, blood pressure frequently falls, and blood flow, which has become pressure dependent, falls with it. In addition, during status epilepticus, the ability of the tissue to utilize available oxygen may be compromised [8].

A peculiar situation occurs in neonates of some species, where immature cortical vessels appear unable to respond to seizures with an increase in blood flow commensurate with the increase in metabolic rate [9]; however, with the possible exception of those neonates and of prolonged status epilepticus, the increase in blood flow, provided that ventilation is not compromised, appears adequate to satisfy the metabolic needs of the tissue. These conclusions have been verified in humans with the use of positron emission tomography scanning or xenon measurements of CBF and metabolism (see also Chap. 44) [10,11].

Cerebral metabolic rates for glucose and oxygen are increased by seizures

Both animal and human studies show a large increase in cerebral metabolic rate for glucose

(CMRGl) and oxygen (CMRO$_2$) in all regions that participate in seizures [7]. During a single seizure, the rate of cerebral metabolism may increase 1.5- to fivefold (Table 1). Early studies showed a doubling of CMRO$_2$, and the first investigations in paralyzed oxygen-ventilated animals recorded a 60 percent increase in CMRO$_2$, with a two- to fourfold rise in CBF in generalized seizures in dogs and monkeys. Studies in humans undergoing electroconvulsive therapy (ECT) show a doubling of both CMRO$_2$ and CMRGl, with a rise in the respiratory quotient from 0.95 to 1.29, suggesting catabolism of lipids and/or amino acids in addition to carbohydrates as a source of energy.

The increase in glycolytic rate is the result of disinhibition of phosphofructokinase, the rate-limiting enzyme of glycolysis. This enzyme is activated by a fall in ATP or by an increase in ADP, AMP, inorganic phosphate, and cyclic AMP (cAMP), all of which are observed during epileptic seizures [2]. The increased rate of energy use results in increased lactate and decreased glucose and glycogen content. Associated decreases in ATP and phosphocreatine are severe in freely convulsing animals but mild if oxygenation is maintained (Fig. 1). Seizure termination is not due to this depletion of energy reserves, but reflects the activation of recurrent inhibitory circuits.

Lipids are actively metabolized in synaptic membranes during seizures

The synaptic plasma membrane, as other membranes, is composed of proteins, cholesterol, and phospholipids. A high proportion of polyunsaturated fatty acids may give the presynaptic membrane a high fluidity appropriate for its many exocytotic events. Seizures of several types result in dramatic changes in the lipid composition of membranes in brain [12] (Fig. 2). In rats, the first bicuculline-induced convulsion results in the doubling of cerebral free fatty acids and free arachidonic acid, but con-

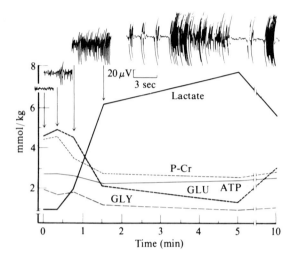

FIG. 1. Changes in metabolite concentrations of the mouse forebrain during status epilepticus. Animals were paralyzed and artificially ventilated with oxygen. Seizures were induced with pentylenetetrazole (150 mg/kg i.p.), and the mice were frozen after periods of continuous epileptiform activity in the EEG lasting up to 10 min. EEG tracings from control and treated animals at the time of freezing are shown at the *top* of the figure: (P-Cr) phosphocreatine; (GLU) glucose; (GLY) glycogen. (Data from Duffy et al. [20].)

tinuous convulsions produce increases of up to 17-fold. These changes are observed in paralyzed, oxygen-ventilated animals, so that they are not simply the result of hypoxia accompanying the seizure.

In addition, during seizures, phospholipase C is activated, and this enzyme generates diacylglycerol by catalyzing cleavage of the polar head groups of phospholipids. It is possible that diacylglycerol activates protein kinase C in this process (see Chap. 16). Released free arachidonic acid is metabolized by cyclooxygenase, which generates prostaglandins, and by lipoxygenase, which produces oxygenated metabolites (eicosanoids) and, possibly, leukotrienes (Fig. 2) (see Chap. 20). Both cyclo- and lipoxygenase can oxidize arachidonic acid in 5 to 10 mM oxygen, so that they can degrade membrane

lipids during ordinary seizures, and leukotrienes can generate free radicals that damage a variety of enzymes and membrane components (see also Chap. 40). These mechanisms may play an important role in seizure generation and spread and in the neuronal damage that repetitive seizures induce.

Seizures produce inhibition of protein and nucleic acid synthesis

Epileptic seizures disaggregate brain polysomes and inhibit brain protein synthesis independently of any hypoxia or systemic complication of seizures [13]. The inhibition of protein synthesis is so specific for the neuronal pathways occupied by the seizure that it has been used to map its anatomic spread. There may be several steps in protein synthesis that are inhibited, but only one has been studied in detail [14]. The first step of the translation of messenger RNA (mRNA) into protein involves the formation of a ternary complex between an initiation factor (eIF-II), the initiator species of methionyl-transfer RNA (tRNA), and GTP. The ternary complex then binds to the 40-S ribosomal subunit. Later steps include binding of the mRNA and, finally, of the 60-S ribosomal subunit (see Chap. 21). Formation of the ternary complex is severely inhibited when the ratio of GDP to GTP rises (Fig. 3). Through the action of nucleoside diphosphate kinase, the GDP:GTP ratio depends on the ratio of ADP to ATP, which increases dramatically during seizures. Since purine nucleoside diphosphate concentrations are only one-tenth of those of the respective triphosphates, the rise in ADP and GDP is relatively much greater than the fall in ATP and GTP. The resulting increase in the GDP:GTP ratio inhibits the initiation of protein synthesis. Seizures lasting over 30 min produce an inhibition of protein synthesis that is observable when extracted mRNA is translated in cell-free systems *in vitro*; therefore they must involve additional mechanisms of inhibition.

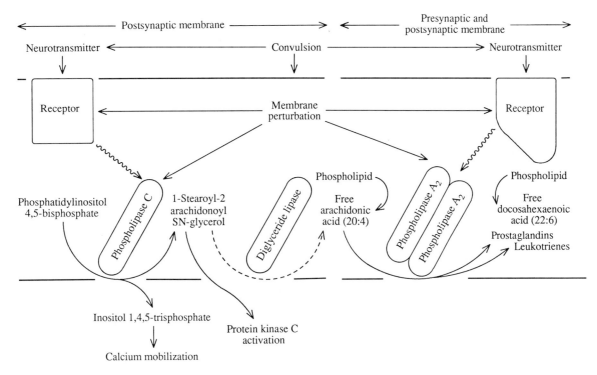

FIG. 2. Hypothetical scheme showing interaction of convulsive stimuli and brain lipid metabolism. (From Bazan et al. [12].)

DNA synthesis is also inhibited by seizures. This may be an important factor in the effects of seizures on brain development, since 80 percent of DNA in the human brain is generated postnatally [15]. Generally, inhibition or altered regulation of nucleic acid and protein synthesis is particularly crucial in the developing brain, which needs protein synthesis for growth, cell multiplication, and cell differentiation [16].

Second-messenger systems are activated in seizures

Electroconvulsive shock and a number of convulsants markedly elevate brain concentrations of cAMP [16]. This increase is observed also in focal seizures and in paralyzed, oxygen-ventilated animals. Anticonvulsants block or reduce the seizures together with the elevation of cAMP. Depletion of catecholamines by reserpine, destruction of the noradrenergic locus coeruleus, and administration of drugs that block β-adrenergic receptors or adenosine receptors reduce cAMP accumulation in response to seizures. These results indicate that the elevation of cAMP may be due to catecholamine release during the seizure.

The activation of noradrenergic release resulting in cAMP elevation in the cortex plays an important role in glycogen mobilization during seizures by stimulating cAMP-dependent phosphorylase kinase, which activates brain phosphorylase and leads to glycogen breakdown to glucose (see Chap. 28). Elimination of noradrenergic pathways renders the brain unable to mobilize glycogen in response to seizure activity.

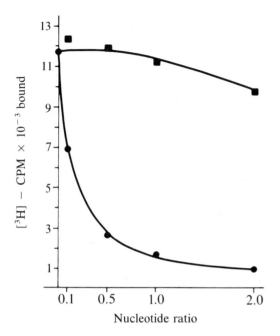

FIG. 3. Effect of GDP and GMP on GTP-dependent ternary complex formation. Ternary complex formation was assayed by retention of radioactivity on nitrocellulose filters. GTP was present in the assay mixture at 1.5 mM, and various amounts of GDP or GMP were added to give the desired concentration ratio. GTP-independent binding was subtracted from all measurements. ●, GDP/GTP; ■, GMP/GTP. (From Dwyer and Wasterlain [14].)

Epileptic seizures also elevate cyclic GMP (cGMP) concentrations in brain; the increase is prevented by anticonvulsants [2]. This elevation is also independent of hypoxia, since it is seen in focal seizures and in oxygen-ventilated animals, as is the increase in cAMP; however, the elevation of cGMP during seizures occurs earlier than that of cAMP. Dibutyryl cGMP injected into cortex is epileptogenic, suggesting a possible seizure-triggering effect of cGMP; but the time course for the elevation of cGMP in neurons is too slow to account for the rapid firing during seizures, and the role of cGMP in seizures is unknown.

Calcium ion moves from the extracellular space into neurons at or even before the onset of seizures. The probable second messenger, inositol-1,4,5-trisphosphate (IP3), is increased in response to glutamate binding to NMDA receptors in several types of neurons. The production of IP3 in response to glutamate and its agonists is greatly increased in brain slices from kindled animals (discussed later). This kind of effect, if present in seizures, could liberate more Ca^{2+} from intracellular stores (see Chap. 16).

Human epileptic foci may be hypometabolic interictally

Measurements of CBF and metabolism in human epilepsy have been made possible by positron emission tomography [10,17]. This method is described in Chapter 44. During generalized seizures, large increases in metabolic rate throughout the cerebral cortex have been measured (Fig. 4). In partial seizures, increases in LCMRGl are found in regions of brain corresponding to the seizure pathways. In the immediate postictal period, the metabolic rate of the cerebral cortex is reduced (see Fig. 4) [17].

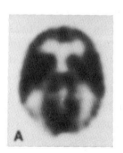
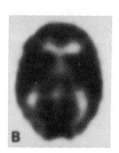
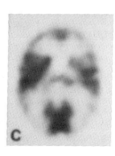

FIG. 4. Positron emission tomography scans of cerebral glucose metabolism using [¹⁸F]2-fluoro-2-deoxy-D-glucose. Scans were obtained during (B) and after (C) a generalized electroconvulsive seizure in a patient undergoing treatment for depression; control (A). (Data from Engel et al. [17].)

In patients with chronic partial complex seizures, the temporal lobe containing the epileptogenic focus frequently shows about 33 percent interictal reduction in LCMRGl compared to adjacent brain or contralateral temporal lobe [10,18]. During the seizure, the same region sustains a very large increase in metabolic rate (Fig. 5). The interictal reduction in LCMRGl [18] may be due partly to cell loss, but since the same region is very active during a seizure, there may exist some physiological mechanism to produce inhibition interictally. An interictal inhibitory process might function to retard seizure spread.

A

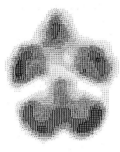

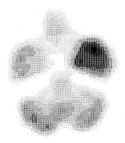
B

FIG. 5. [^{18}F]2-fluoro-2-deoxy-D-glucose positron emission tomography scan in a patient with complex partial seizures. **A:** Interictal scan showing slight temporal lobe hypometabolism (*right side* of images). **B:** Scan obtained seconds after onset of complex partial seizure (same patient as in **A**) showing focal hypermetabolism in temporal lobe and contralateral cerebellum and relatively reduced metabolic rate in other regions. The seizure was brief and postictal depression of activity during the 40-min tracer uptake period explains the reduced metabolic rate. (From Abou-Khalil et al. [18].)

MECHANISMS OF BRAIN DAMAGE FROM SEIZURES

Neuronal loss or subtle neuronal and astrocytic changes are frequently found around human epileptic foci, and it is sometimes difficult to know whether such changes represent a cause or a consequence of seizures or both. There is no experimental model closely resembling any of the primary epilepsies in humans, but various models reproduce some of the features or the metabolic consequences of epilepsy. The mechanisms by which seizures can produce brain damage and neuronal loss are under very active investigation.

What is the role of energy metabolism and blood flow in brain damage?

Meldrum and Brierly [19] demonstrated that status epilepticus in monkeys damages the brain, even in the absence of hypoxia or other complications of seizures. Many studies using bicuculline-induced status epilepticus in paralyzed oxygen-ventilated rats showed only a minimal decline in cerebral ATP and energy reserves [20], suggesting that brain damage from seizures is unrelated to energy failure. Subsequent studies [21], however, showed that most histopathological changes induced by this model of bicuculline-induced seizures are reversible. In neonates, status epilepticus is associated with depletion of cortical ATP and phosphocreatine [22].

Studies in rats have suggested that during late status epilepticus, CBF cannot keep up with metabolic demand and that this somehow results in brain damage [23]. A similar situation applies in newborn monkeys [9]. Other investigators have suggested that during late status epilepticus, oxygen is available to brain tissue but cannot be utilized [8]. Either effect would result in some degree of tissue hypoxia and, presumably, in energy failure.

Some regions of brain that sustain very high

metabolic rates during status epilepticus show tissue infarction (necrosis of all cell types in the region) associated with local accumulation of lactic acid above 20 mM [24]. A similar degree of lactate accumulation in ischemia has also been associated with tissue infarction (discussed in Chapter 40).

Excitatory amino acids can be neurotoxic

The putative amino acid neurotransmitters glutamate and aspartate and their analogs *N*-methyl-D-aspartate, quisqualate, and kainate have powerful excitatory and epileptogenic effects on many types of neurons. These substances also induce neuronal necrosis in association with those excitatory actions (see Chaps. 15 and 40). Excitatory amino acids such as glutamate are probably released during many types of seizures [25]. Some of their agonists open receptor-operated ion channels permeable to Ca^{2+}, the excess entry of which into neurons may be related to their death (see Chap. 40 and below). Through this or other action, excitotoxins may be responsible for some or all of the neuronal necrosis observed following repetitive seizures.

Rises in intracellular Ca^{2+} and in free radicals may be neurotoxic

During seizures, a number of processes may lead to increased intracellular Ca^{2+} in neurons: Receptor-operated Ca^{2+} channels open to allow influx of Ca^{2+}; receptor-stimulated phospholipase C catalyzes production of IP3, which releases Ca^{2+} from intracellular stores into the cytosol (see Chap. 16); microregional depletion of ATP at the membrane sites of Na,K-ATPase may limit Na^+ efflux (see Chap. 39); exchange of intracellular Ca^{2+} for extracellular Na^+ may be decreased because of reduced transmembrane Na^+ gradient; and Ca^{2+} efflux mediated by the Ca^{2+}-ATPase pump may fail if ATP is locally depleted. Since the Na^+-Ca^{2+} exchange

system has a high capacity and low affinity for Ca^{2+}, and Ca^{2+}-ATPase has a low capacity and high affinity for Ca^{2+}, the exchange is more crucial than is the pump to Ca^{2+} homeostasis under the condition of sustained high-Ca^{2+} influx, as in a seizure. Large Ca^{2+} accumulations have been observed inside brain mitochondria in status epilepticus [26]; however, such changes can be reversible, and their exact role in the mechanism of brain damage is still uncertain.

Peroxidation of membrane phospholipids has been shown to occur during seizures and may lead to leukotriene and to free radical formation [12,27]. Free radicals are atoms or molecules with one unpaired electron occupying an outer orbital. The superoxide anion radical (O_2^-), hydrogen peroxide (H_2O_2), and the hydroxyl radical (OH^-) are produced during the reduction of oxygen, during prostacyclin biosynthesis, and as a byproduct of leukotriene metabolism. These compounds have the capacity to initiate destructive chain reactions in biological membranes. The major natural defense is cytochrome oxidase, which in mitochondria of all respiring cells reduces oxygen without production of such intermediates. Many other enzymes, such as catalases and dismutases, specifically defend against free radical compounds. During status epilepticus, a massive increase in free radical species has never been demonstrated, but these elusive compounds are byproducts of normal metabolism and through increased rates of turnover may well play an important role in cell damage.

Certain neuronal populations are selectively vulnerable to seizures

Repeated stimulation of the perforant path in the hippocampus depolarizes the dentate granule cells, which show no ill effects. The granule cells, in turn, depolarize CA3 pyramidal cells, which are selectively necrosed if seizures are sufficiently long lasting [28]. Interneurons located in the hilus between these two types of cells have divergent fates: Somatostatin-containing interneurons are selectively vulnerable to relatively short seizure durations, whereas GABAergic interneurons are quite resistant despite high rates of firing; this selective vulnerability is not yet understood. In this experiment, the vulnerable cells lack, and the resistant cells possess, Ca^{2+}-binding protein (calbindin), which binds cytosolic Ca^{2+} and hence may prevent free Ca^{2+} inside neurons from reaching lethal concentrations.

Neonatal brain has a high risk of metabolic failure in seizures

Immature rats have a cerebral metabolic rate 10- to 20-fold lower than adults, but the rate in cortex increases at least twofold during seizures. Several factors contribute to imposing a great risk for metabolically-induced damage during seizures in newborn animals. These factors are the possible mismatch during seizures between CBF and metabolism (see Chap. 29); the need for DNA and protein synthesis, two energy-intensive processes in the neonatal period easily compromised by metabolic stress; the partial reliance for energy on ketone bodies that become unusable in anoxic states; the slow mobilization of glycogen reserves; and the limited glucose transport capacity of the blood-brain barrier in the neonate [29] (see also Chap. 30). The neonatal brain has sizable reserves of glycogen but very low concentrations of phosphorylase, phosphoglucomutase, and cAMP, which are needed to activate protein kinase and to transform phosphorylase B into its active form (phosphorylase A) (see Chap. 28).

The maximum rate of glucose transport across the immature blood-brain barrier has been estimated to be one-fifth the adult rate, probably as a result of lower capillary density in the neonatal brain. This transport rate appears to be lower than the maximal glycolytic rate in cortex and would therefore limit the metabolic response of the brain. Despite normal blood glucose concentrations, brain glucose falls rapidly after onset of seizures in newborn rats, rabbits, and marmosets. Since the K_m value of glucose transport into brain is about 7 mM, the carrier is less than half saturated at physiological blood glucose concentrations (5 mM). Glucose supplements, by increasing carrier saturation, reduce mortality and morbidity from seizures.

The healthy neonate's brain may obtain as much as one-third of its energy from ketone bodies, which become unavailable if there is anoxia during seizures, since the oxidation of ketone bodies requires molecular oxygen. Thus, anoxia enhances the dependence of the brain on glucose. Accumulation of lactic acid to levels observed in association with infarction is rarely seen in neonatal seizures. Lactate can easily be carried across the blood-brain barrier if circulation is intact because of the large amounts of monocarboxylic acid carrier present in the cerebral capillaries of suckling animals.

Biochemical changes are associated with kindling, a model of chronic focal epilepsy

Kindling is the progressive buildup, in response to intermittent low-intensity electrical or chemical stimulation of certain brain sites, of cellular discharges culminating in full-fledged seizures [30,31]. Kindling is very selective. For example, it is easily induced in most regions of the limbic brain but cannot be obtained in the cerebellum, no matter how long one stimulates. Few stimulations are needed to kindle a sensitive site such as the amygdala; however, reducing the interstimulus interval increases the number of stimulations needed to kindle. In the rat, the change in cerebral excitability acquired through kindling may persist for a lifetime.

In the electrically-stimulated hippocampus of kindled animals, extracellular Ca^{2+} concentration falls earlier and more severely than in the stimulated hippocampus of nonkindled control animals. This result indicates greater Ca^{2+} entry into hippocampal cells in the kindled brain. In nonkindled animals, glutamate receptors of the NMDA type, which admit Ca^{2+}, do not participate in the dentate granule cell responses to perforant path electrical stimulation; however, in kindled animals, these receptors respond massively to the same perforant path stimuli [32].

Other evidence of abnormal Ca^{2+} response in the hippocampus of kindled animals includes reduction in calbindin [33] and in Ca^{2+}-calmodulin kinase II activity [34]. The decrease in calbindin could amplify Ca^{2+} response in stimulated cells, and that in calmodulin kinase II might alter the level of phosphorylation of its natural substrate synapsin I (see Chap. 19). This protein in its native unphosphorylated form is attached to the wall of synaptic vesicles. Phosphorylation of the tail region of synapsin I by Ca^{2+}-calmodulin kinase II decreases the affinity of synapsin I for the vesicle surface. When synapsin I dissociates, the vesicle has an increased chance of fusing with the presynaptic membrane and releasing its neurotransmitter contents into the synaptic cleft [35]. Phosphorylation of synapsin I may also allow dissociation of vesicles from the cytoskeletal matrix and make them available for interaction with the presynaptic membrane.

The precise role, if any, of these biochemical changes in the kindling phenomenon and their relevance to human epilepsy remain unknown. Biochemical changes associated with the kindling phenomenon and other models of epilepsy are discussed further in several reviews for the interested reader [30,31].

REFERENCES

1. Delgado-Escueta, A. V., Ward, A. A., Jr., Woodbury, D. M., and Porter, R. J. (eds.). *Basic Mechanisms of the Epilepsies*. New York: Raven Press, 1986, pp. 3–55. [Advances in Neurology, Vol. 44.]

2. Wasterlain, C. G., Morin, A. M., and Dwyer, B. E. The epilepsies. In A. Lajtha (ed.), *Handbook of Neurochemistry*. New York: Raven Press, 1985, Vol. 10, pp. 407–409.

3. Monaghan, D. T., and Cotman, C. W. Identification and properties of *N*-methyl-D-aspartate receptors in rat brain synaptic plasma membranes. *Proc. Natl. Acad. Sci. U.S.A.* 83:7532–7536, 1986.

4. Olsen, R. W., et al. Benzodiazepine/barbiturate/GABA receptor-chloride ionophore complex in a genetic model for generalized epilepsy. In: A. V. Delgado-Escueta, A. A. Ward, D. M. Woodbury, and R. J. Porter, (eds.). *Basic Mechanisms of the Epilepsies*. New York: Raven Press, 1986, pp. 365–378. [Advances in Neurology, Vol. 44.]

5. Macdonald, R. L. and McLean, M. J., Anticonvulsant drugs: Mechanisms of action, In: A. V. Delgado-Escueta, A. A. Ward, Jr., D. M. Woodbury, and R. J. Porter (eds.). *Basic Mechanisms of the Epilepsies*. New York: Raven Press, 1986, pp. 713–736. [Advances in Neurology, Vol. 44.]

6. Chapman, A. G. Cerebral energy metabolism and seizures. In: T. A. Pedley and B. S. Meldrum (eds.). *Recent Advance in Epilepsy II*. New York: Churchill Livingstone, 1986, pp. 19–63.

7. Baldy-Moulinier, M., Ingvar, D. H., and Meldrum, B. S. *Current Problems in Epilepsy: Cerebral Blood Flow, Metabolism and Epilepsy*. London: John Libbey, 1983.

8. Kreisman, N. R., Rosenthal, M., La Manna, J. C., and Sick, T. J. Cerebral oxygenation during recurrent seizures. In: A. V. Delgado-Escueta, C. G. Wasterlain, D. M., Treiman, and R. J. Porter (eds.), *Status Epilepticus*. New York: Raven Press, 1983, pp. 231–239. [Advances in Neurology, Vol. 34.]

9. Fujikawa, D. G., Dwyer, B. E., Lake, R. R., and Wasterlain, C. G. Cerebral blood flow and metabolism during neonatal seizures. In: P. Vert and C. G. Wasterlain (eds.), *Neonatal Seizures*. New York: Raven Press (*in press*).

10. Ackermann, R. F., Engel, J. Jr., and Phelps, M. E. Identification of seizure-mediating brain structures with the deoxyglucose method: Studies of human epilepsy with positron emission tomography, and animal seizure models with contact autoradiography. In: A. V. Delgado-Escueta, A. A. Ward, D. M. Woodbury, and R.

J. Porter (eds.), *Basic Mechanisms of the Epilepsies.* New York: Raven Press, 1986. pp. 921–934. [Advances in Neurology, Vol. 44.]

11. Franck, G., et al. Regional cerebral blood flow and metabolic rates in human focal epilepsy and status epilepticus. In: A. V. Delgado-Escueta, A. A. Ward, D. M. Woodbury, and R. J. Porter (eds.). *Basic Mechanisms of the Epilepsies.* New York: Raven Press, 1986, pp. 935–948. [Advances in Neurology, Vol. 44.]

12. Bazan, N. G., Birkle, D. L., Tang, W., and Reddy, T. S. The accumulation of free arachidonic acid, diacylglycerols, prostaglandins, and lipoxygenase reaction products in the brain during experimental epilepsy. In: A. V. Delgado-Escueta, A. A. Ward, D. M. Woodbury, and R. J. Porter (eds.), *Basic Mechanisms of the Epilepsies.* New York: Raven Press, 1986, pp. 879–902. [Advances in Neurology, Vol. 44.]

13. Dwyer, B. E., Wasterlain, C. G., Fujikawa, D. G., and Yamada, L. Brain protein metabolism in epilepsy. In: A. V. Delgado-Escueta, A. A. Ward, D. M. Woodbury, and R. J. Porter (eds.). *Basic Mechanisms of the Epilepsies.* New York: Raven Press, 1986, pp. 903–918. [Advances in Neurology, Vol. 44.]

14. Dwyer, B. E., and Wasterlain, C. G. Regulation of the first step of the initiation of brain protein synthesis by guanosine diphosphate. *J. Neurochem.* 34:1639–1647, 1980.

15. Dobbing, J., and Sands, J. Quantitative growth and development of the human brain. *Arch. Dis. Child.* 48:757–767, 1973.

16. Wasterlain, C. G., and Dwyer, B. E. Brain metabolism during prolonged seizures in neonates. In: A. V. Delgado-Escueta, C. G. Wasterlain, D. M. Treiman, and R. J. Porter (eds.). *Status Epilepticus.* New York: Raven Press, 1983, pp. 241–260. [Advances in Neurology, Vol. 34.]

17. Engel, J. Jr., Kuhl, D. E., and Phelps, M. E. Patterns of human local cerebral glucose metabolism during epileptic seizure. *Science* 218:64–66, 1982.

18. Abou-Khalil, B. W., Siegel, G. J., Sackellares, J. C., Gilman, S., Hichwa, R., and Marshal, R. Positron emission tomography studies of cerebral glucose metabolism in patients with chronic partial epilepsy. *Ann. Neurol.* 22:480–486, 1987.

19. Meldrum, B. S., and Brierley, J. B. Prolonged epileptic seizures in primates: Ischemic cell change and its relationship to ictal physiological events. *Arch. Neurol.* 28:10–17, 1973.

20. Duffy, T. E., Howse, D. E., and Plum, F. Cerebral energy metabolism during experimental status epilepticus. *J. Neurochem.* 24:925–934, 1975.

21. Soderfeldt, B., Kalimo, H., Olsson, Y., and Siesjo, B. K., Bicuculline-induced epileptic brain injury. *Acta Neuropathol.* 62:87–95, 1983.

22. Fujikawa, D. G., Vannucci, R. C., Dwyer, B. E., and Wasterlain, C. G. Generalized seizures deplete brain energy reserves in normoglycemic newborn monkeys. *Brain Res.* 454:51–59, 1988.

23. Siesjo, B. K., Ingvar M., Folbergrova J., and Chapman A. G. Circulation and local cerebral metabolism in bicuculline-induced status epilepticus: Relevance for development of cell damage. In: A. V. Delgado-Escueta, C. G. Wasterlain, D. M. Treiman, and R. J. Porter (eds.), *Status Epilepticus.* New York: Raven Press, 1983 [Advances in Neurology, Vol. 34].

24. Ingvar, M., Folbegrova, J., and Siesjo, B. Metabolic alterations underlying the development of hypermetabolic necrosis in the substantia nigra in status epilepticus. *J. Cereb. Blood Flow Metab.* 7:103–108, 1987.

25. Chapman, A. G., Westerbrook, E., Premachandera, M., and Meldrum, B. S. Changes in regional neurotransmitter amino acid levels in rat brain during seizures induced by L-allylglycine, bicuculline, and kainic acid. *J. Neurochem.* 43:62–70, 1984.

26. Meldrum, B. S. Cell damage in epilepsy and the role of calcium in cytotoxicity. In: A. V. Delgado-Escueta, A. A. Ward, D. M. Woodbury, and R. J. Porter (eds.). *Basic Mechanisms of the Epilepsies.* New York: Raven Press, 1986, pp. 849–855. [Advances in Neurology, Vol. 44.]

27. Del Mastro, R. F. An approach to free radicals in medicine and biology. *Acta. Physiol. Scand.* (*Suppl*) 492:153–168, 1980.

28. Sloviter, R. S. Decreased hippocampal inhibition and a selective loss of interneurons in experimental epilepsy. *Science* 235:73–76, 1987.

29. Dwyer, B. E., and Wasterlain, C. G. Intermediary metabolism. In: H. H. Frey and D. Janz (eds.). *Antiepileptic Drugs.* Berlin. Springer-Verlag, 1985, pp. 79–100.

30. McNamara, J. O., Bonhaus, D. W., Shin, C., Carain, B. J., Gellman, R. L., and Giacchino, J. L. The kindling model of epilepsy: A critical review. *CRC Crit. Rev. Clin. Neurobiol.* 1:341–391, 1985).

31. Wada, J. *Kindling 3.* New York: Raven Press, 1985.

32. Mody, I., and Heinemann, U. *N*-Methyl-D-aspartate receptors of dentate gyrus granule cells become involved in synaptic transmission following kindling. *J. Neurophysiol. (in press).*

33. Bainbridge, K. G., and Miller, J. J. Hippocampal calcium-binding protein during commissural kindling-induced epileptogenesis: Progressive decline and role of anticonvulsants. *Brain Res.* 324:85–90, 1984.

34. Wasterlain, C. G., and Farber, D. B. Kindling alters the calcium/calmodulin-dependent phosphorylation of synaptic plasma membrane proteins in rat hippcampus. *Proc. Natl. Acad. Sci. USA* 81:1253–1257, 1984.

35. Llinas, R., et al. Intraterminal injection of synapsin I or calcium/calmodulin-dependent protein kinase alters neurotransmitter release at the squid giant axon. *Proc. Natl. Acad. Sci. U.S.A.* 82:3035–3039, 1985.

CHAPTER 42

Disorders of the Basal Ganglia

Theodore L. Sourkes

Some large, anatomically distinct masses of gray matter lie at the base of the brain, and certain of these (namely, the caudate nucleus, the putamen, and the globus pallidus) are collectively termed the basal ganglia. The first two constitute the striatum, or neostriatum, and the internal and external parts of the globus pallidus, or pallidum, are known as the paleostriatum. This striopallidal system is an integrative unit, the constituent parts of which have many connections to one another and to and from other regions of the brain. Some of the inter-

Basic Neurochemistry: Molecular, Cellular, and Medical Aspects, 4th Ed., edited by G. J. Siegel et al. Raven Press, Ltd., New York, 1989.
Correspondence to Theodore L. Sourkes, Department of Psychiatry, McGill University, 1033 Pine Avenue West, Montreal, Canada
H3A 1A1.

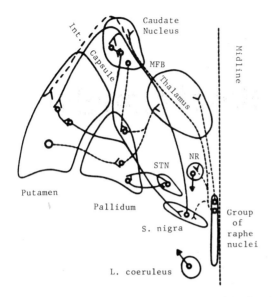

FIG. 1. Major subcortical connections of the basal ganglia and some associated structures. Nigral dopaminergic fibers pass upward in the medial forebrain bundle (MFB) to the caudate nucleus and putamen. These constitute the nigrostriatal tract. GABA-containing fibers pass from the striatum and pallidum to the substantia nigra (pars reticulata), where they exert inhibitory actions. Nondopaminergic fibers from the pars reticulata to the pars compacta exert a regulatory role. Cholinergic neurons (among others) that are intrinsic to the striatum serve as intermediaries between these two tracts. The major output of the basal ganglia is by way of the globus pallidus, to the lateral and anterior parts of the thalamus and other structures, by presumed cholinergic fibers. The thalamus, in turn, has direct connections with the motor cortex, so that the existence of a strial-pallidal-thalamic-cortical circuit, as well as connections to the thalamus from the motor cortex and the cerebellum, emphasize the fact that the basal ganglia are prominently involved in the regulation of motor phenomena. Fibers pass from the pallidum to the subthalamic nucleus (STN, corpus Luysii). The pallidum is reciprocally innervated by fibers originating in the STN. Noradrenergic neurons from the locus coeruleus innervate these and other regions of the brain. Serotonergic fibers from certain of the midline raphe nuclei reach the thalamus, striatum (by way of the MFB), substantia nigra, nucleus ruber (NR, red nucleus), and elsewhere. The nucleus ruber is important as an upper brain stem nucleus from which descending motor pathways, including the rubrotegmentospinal system, originate.

connections of the basal ganglia and related structures are shown in Fig. 1. The subcortical structures shown in Fig. 1 are equivalent to the extrapyramidal system, which includes the structures of the brain, apart from the cerebral cortex, that send efferent fibers to the spinal cord. Among the bodily functions regulated by the extrapyramidal system are the tone and posture of the limbs.

BIOCHEMICAL CHARACTERISTICS OF THE BASAL GANGLIA AND ASSOCIATED STRUCTURES

The basal ganglia are especially sensitive to carbon monoxide and to manganese. This sensitivity plays a role in the neurological complications that accompany intoxication with these chemicals. In infants, the predilection of bilirubin for basal ganglia cells may result in *kernicterus*, or jaundice of the nuclei of the brain. Historically, kernicterus was the first disease of the basal ganglia to be described. (It served as a model for S. A. K. Wilson in the classic study of hepatolenticular disease, a disease that carries his name.) When jaundice of the newborn is severe, kernicterus can be prevented by exchange transfusion.

The globus pallidus contains much iron, a property it shares with other nuclei of the extrapyramidal system: the subthalamic nucleus of Luys, the substantia nigra, the red nucleus (nucleus ruber), the dentate nucleus, and the inferior olive. It has been suggested that the metal is present in ferritin-like form.

The basal ganglia are richly innervated with cholinergic fibers. Although this is particularly evident in the caudate nucleus, other types of neurons, which are characterized by their content of substance P, γ-aminobutyric acid (GABA), serotonin, or enkephalin, have also been described.

The substantia nigra, the red nucleus, and the locus coeruleus each contain a distinctive pigment. The precursor of the pigmented material is thought to be 3,4-dihydroxy-L-phenyl-alanine (DOPA) or a catecholamine, but the specific pathways of pigment formation are not completely known. (The biochemistry of the basal ganglia and the changes found in extra-pyramidal disorders are described elsewhere [1–3].)

Dopamine is synthesized from tyrosine in the basal ganglia

A biochemical characteristic that has thrown much light on the functions of the basal ganglia and certain associated structures in humans and animals is the distribution of dopamine and of tyrosine hydroxylase, an enzyme found in catecholamine-containing neurons and cells. (The biosynthetic relationships of dopamine have been adduced in Chap. 11.) The starting point for dopamine synthesis is tyrosine, which is present in the whole brain at a level of approximately 1.2 mg/100 g fresh weight of tissue, or 70 μmol/kg. The first step is catalysis by tyrosine hydroxylase. This enzyme requires iron and a pteridine cofactor, tetrahydrobiopterin. The product of this oxidation is DOPA, which is normally present only in the most minute concentrations in the body because it is so readily decarboxylated to dopamine (3,4-dihydroxy-phenylethylamine), as catalyzed by the widely distributed enzyme DOPA decarboxylase or aromatic amino acid decarboxylase (AADC). Another important physiological substrate for it is 5-hydroxytryptophan, the immediate precursor of serotonin.

Like other amino acid decarboxylases, AADC requires pyridoxal phosphate as its coenzyme. It is inhibited by many compounds, a few of which have been used therapeutically. Some decarboxylase inhibitors are illustrated in Fig. 2. One of these, methyldopa (α-methyl-L-dopa), is used as an antihypertensive drug in humans. It is the only decarboxylase inhibitor known with such properties. Its action in essential hypertension is mediated through metabolites, either α-methyldopamine or α-meth-

ylnorepinephrine, formed, among other locations in the body, in the region of the vasomotor centers in the medulla oblongata, where these metabolites initiate their hypotensive action. Methyldopa has been widely used in biochemical and pharmacological studies because of its important effects on monoamine metabolism. Two other inhibitors of AADC are employed extensively when blockade of decarboxylation is required. These are carbidopa (the hydrazino analog of methyldopa) and benserazide [N^1-seryl-N^2-(2,3,4-trihydroxy-benzyl)]hydrazine. These two compounds are used with levodopa in the treatment of Parkinson's disease (see below). Neither one penetrates the blood-brain barrier significantly. A useful decarboxylase inhibitor in experimental work with animals is brocresine (*p*-bromo-*m*-hydroxybenzyloxyamine phosphate). Given parenterally, it inhibits AADC in nervous as well as nonnervous tissues.

Dopaminergic neurons form specific tracts

The formation of dopamine is the terminal step in biosynthesis in certain neurons of the brain. These neurons have been identified *in situ* by histochemical formation of derivatives of dopamine and other monoamines that emit specific fluorescence, as well as by immunofluorescent techniques. The principal dopaminergic fiber systems in the brain are the nigrostriatal—from the substantia nigra to the caudate nucleus and putamen; the mesolimbic—from the ventral tegmental area to the nucleus accumbens; the mesocortical—from the ventral tegmental area to the suprarhinal cortex; and the tuberohypophyseal—from the arcuate nucleus to the median eminence. Other dopamine fibers have been identified in brain, retina, and spinal cord. These neurons store dopamine in vesicles within the varicosities of the nerve terminations. In the case of nigrostriatal fibers, the intravesicular concentration of the amine may rise to as high as 1 to 10 mg/g fresh weight

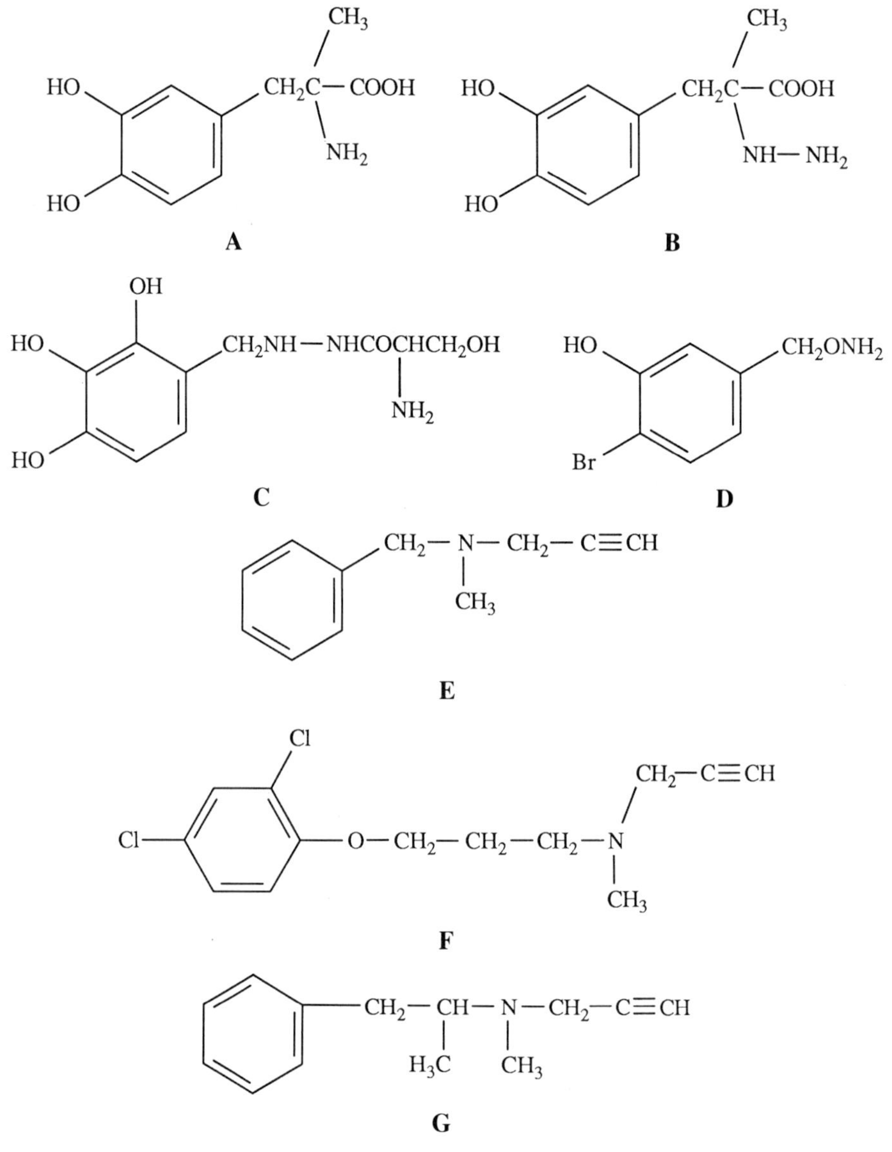

FIG. 2. Some frequently used inhibitors of aromatic amino acid decarboxylase (**A–D**) and monoamine oxidase (**E–G**). **A**: Methyldopa (L-α-methyldopa). **B**: Carbidopa, the hydrazino analog of α-methyldopa. **C**: Benserazide. **D**: Brocresine. **E**: Pargyline. **F**: Clorgyline. **G**: Deprenyl.

(i.e., in the range of amine concentration in chromaffin tissue).

Other types of brain neurons contain not only tyrosine hydroxylase and AADC but also dopamine-β-hydroxylase, which is found in the membrane and contents of the storage vesicles. These are the norepinephrine-containing fibers. There are also epinephrine-containing neurons in parts of the cerebral cortex. These contain, in addition to the enzymes already mentioned, phenylethanolamine-*N*-methyltransferase (PNMT). This catalyzes the transfer of the methyl group of methionine to norepinephrine. Under many circumstances, the biosynthesis of the catecholamines is limited by the slow flux through the stage of tyrosine hydroxylase because of the low turnover rate of that enzyme.

The regional distribution of dopamine in the central nervous system (CNS) is shown in Table 1. Dopamine and norepinephrine are irregularly distributed in the brain and spinal cord. Thus, dopamine is found in certain regions along with norepinephrine, but unlike norepinephrine, it is present in unusually high concentrations in some of the basal ganglia. By contrast, the locus coeruleus is very rich in norepinephrine but not dopamine. The highly uneven distribution of these two amines suggests specific neural roles for each.

Dopamine undergoes O-methylation and oxidation in the basal ganglia

The major metabolites of dopamine in the body are 3-*O*-methyldopamine (3-methoxytyramine) and homovanillic acid (HVA, or 4-hydroxy-3-methoxyphenylacetic acid). These are depicted in Fig. 3, which also shows the alternative pathways of metabolism of dopamine (see Fig. 2,

Chap. 11 for analogous reactions of norepinephrine). Some of the compounds shown in Fig. 3 have also been detected as conjugates of sulfate or glucuronate. The amine and its *O*-methyl derivative are both subject to the action of monoamine oxidase (MAO), a flavoprotein present in the outer membrane of the mitochondria. MAO exists in two forms: MAO-A is especially sensitive to the inhibitory drug clorgyline and is found in cell groups characterized by their content of catecholamines; MAO-B is sensitive to deprenyl and is prominent in serotonin-containing areas of the brain, such as the raphe nuclei. Pargyline acts on both MAO-A and MAO-B. These three propargylamine inhibitors are depicted in Fig. 2. Products of the MAO reaction include the aldehyde corresponding to the amine substrate, hydrogen peroxide, and ammonia. Most of the aldehyde undergoes further dehydrogenation to form, in the case of dopamine, 3,4-dihydroxyphenylacetic acid (DOPAC) or HVA. These acids, like the amines, are substrates for catechol-*O*-methyltransferase, an enzyme that catalyzes the transfer of the methyl group from *S*-adenosylmethionine to the *m*-hydroxyl group. This process appears to be very efficient in the brain because normally there are only very small quantities of DOPAC in the striatum but substantial amounts of HVA. A portion of the aldehyde undergoes reduction, catalyzed by alcohol dehydrogenase or a similar enzyme, with participation of reduced nicotinamide coenzyme. The alcoholic products that are formed are shown in Fig. 3; they are far less abundant than are the acidic metabolites of dopamine.

TABLE 1. Regional distribution of dopamine and HVA in the human CNS[a]

Brain region	Dopamine (μg/g fresh weight tissue)	HVA (μg/g fresh weight tissue)
Frontal cortex	<0.003	0.17
Caudate nucleus	2.4	4.0
Putamen	2.5	5.2
Hypothalamus	0.1	—
Substantia nigra		
Pars compacta	0.47	3.6
Pars reticulata	0.21	2.2
Nucleus accumbens	2.1	5.7
Spinal cord (lumbar)	0.008	0.11

[a] Data adapted from Scatton et al. [4].

PARKINSON'S DISEASE

Because the dopamine-rich regions of the brain are preeminently the basal ganglia and some associated structures (apart from the thalamus and hypothalamus), it is natural to investigate diseases of the basal ganglia for evidence of de-

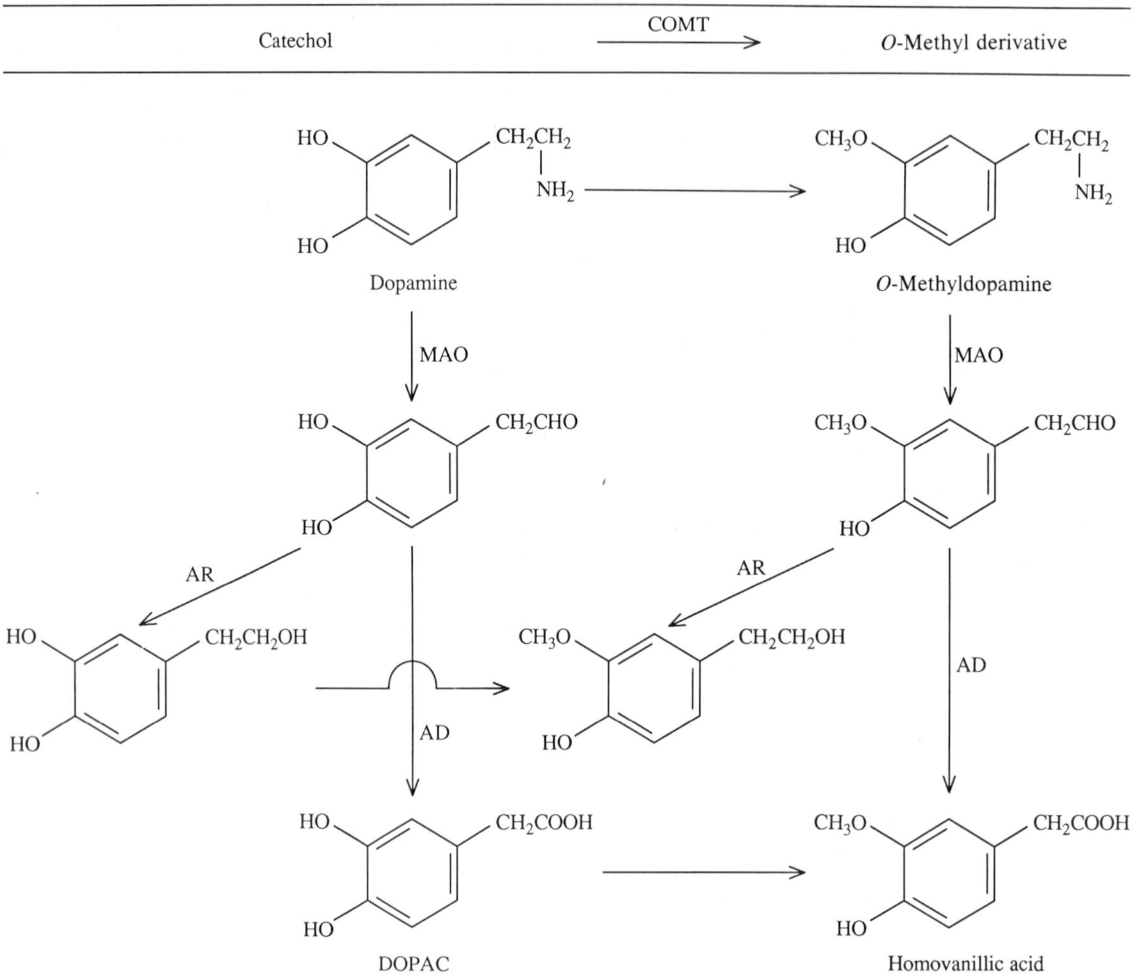

FIG. 3. Alternative pathways of dopamine metabolism: (COMT) catechol *O*-methyltransferase; (MAO) monoamine oxidase; (AD) aldehyde dehydrogenase; (AR) aldehyde reductase (alcohol dehydrogenase); (DOPAC) 3,4-dihydroxyphenylacetic acid. An analogous scheme can be drawn for norepinephrine; each compound then bears a β-hydroxyl group (see Chap. 11, Fig. 2).

ranged metabolism of catecholamines, in general, and dopamine, in particular. The search for such a faulty metabolism has been especially successful in Parkinson's disease, the "shaking palsy," which now stands as the paradigm of cerebral diseases that involve dysfunction of monoamine-containing fibers. This, the most prevalent disorder of the extrapyramidal system, was first described in 1817 by the London

physician James Parkinson. It is now recognized to stem from degenerative changes in the substantia nigra, a portion of the brain that has extensive connections with the striatum. Besides the shaking, or tremor, of the limbs, patients with Parkinson's disease may also exhibit muscular rigidity, which leads to difficulties in walking, writing, and speaking; masking of facial expression; and flexed posture. Some also suffer a loss of volitional movement that may progress to akinesia.

Chemical pathology of Parkinson's disease: Degeneration of nigrostriatal tract and reduced dopamine in striatum

Monoamines in the brains of patients dying of Parkinson's disease have been measured, and this has provided the principal evidence that there is a disturbance of monoamine metabolism [4,5]. This is now being supplemented by tomographic studies, in life, with positron-emitting analogs of levodopa, such as [18F]6-fluoro-L-dopa (see Chap. 44). The regional concentrations of catecholamines are shown in Table 2. The measured monoamines are all present in lower concentrations than monoamines observed under normal conditions, and the decrease of dopamine is greater than that of norepinephrine. Serotonin concentrations are abnormally low in the caudate nucleus of patients who have died of Parkinson's disease. Moreover, glutamate decarboxylase activity and concentrations of GABA in the substantia nigra are lower than in control cases. These results point clearly to some type of dysmetabolism of neurotransmitters, particularly dopamine, in an important disease of the brain. In fact, detailed studies of Parkinson's disease show that it stems from a striatal deficiency of

dopamine that in turn results from the loss of nigrostriatal fibers. The decreased ability of the diseased nigra to produce dopamine in Parkinson's disease is also reflected in lower concentrations of HVA and DOPAC in the caudate nucleus and putamen.

Some HVA normally diffuses into the cerebrospinal fluid (CSF), particularly from the caudate nucleus, and samples of CSF have readily detectable amounts of HVA. In Parkinson's disease the concentration of HVA is far below that found in patients with neurological disorders not involving the basal ganglia. This is clear from the data in Table 3. Within the category of Parkinson's syndrome the values are much lower in patients who present evidence of akinesia before death than in those without akinesia. This is also true for dopamine in the caudate nucleus.

CSF taken at the lumbar level has a much lower concentration of HVA than has the ventricular fluid (Table 3). The steep gradient is based on the important fact that most of the HVA originates in the brain, much of it in that portion of the caudate nucleus immediately adjacent to the lateral ventricles; that is, the parts lining the floor of the body and anterior horn and the roof of the inferior horn [6,7]. Of the remainder, some probably comes from dopamine-rich regions contributing HVA to the third and fourth ventricles and some from the spinal cord. Although the cerebral cortex also contains dopamine, HVA formed there and passing into the fluid bathing that region of the brain would probably not reach lower compartments of the CSF. Once HVA enters the CSF, an active transport mechanism works to remove it as well as other metabolic acids such as 5-HIAA (see Chap. 30). This mechanism is inhibited in a dose-dependent manner by probenecid (*p*-dipropylsulfamylbenzoic acid).

The concentration gradient of HVA in the CSF applies to Parkinson's disease as well (Table 3). The generally lower amounts of HVA in the fluid of the lumbar space, however, are

TABLE 2. Dopamine and HVA in brain in Parkinson's disease

Brain region	Dopamine[a]	HVA[a]
Frontal cortex	38	60
Caudate nucleus	15	30
Putamen	3	33
Substantia nigra		
Pars compacta	21	48
Pars reticulata	13	60
Hippocampus	30	52
Nucleus accumbens	40	60

[a] As percent of control values. Data adapted from Scatton et al. [4].

TABLE 3. Concentrations of HVA and 5-HIAA in CSF

	HVA (ng/ml)		5-HIAA (ng/ml)	
	No. of cases	Mean ± SE	No. of cases	Mean ± SE
LATERAL VENTRICLES				
Nonextrapyramidal disorders				
Various	15	447 ± 40	17	111 ± 12
Brain atrophy	3	62 ± 33		
Spasmodic torticollis	4	213 ± 60		
Extrapyramidal disorders				
Parkinson's disease	53	157 ± 17	17	46 ± 7
Akinesia present	6	52 ± 24		
Akinesia absent	41	169 ± 19		
Attitudinal tremor	21	230 ± 19	5	77 ± 9
LUMBAR SPACE				
Various neurological disorders	20	40 ± 5	20	26 ± 2
Parkinson's disease	5	15 ± 7	4	24 ± 9
Progressive supranuclear palsy	6	26 ± 9	6	20 ± 7
Epilepsy (partial complex seizures)	7	27 ± 5	7	20 ± 3
Huntington's chorea	15	23 ± 4	15	28 ± 3
Spasmodic torticollis[a]	8	15 ± 6	8	14 ± 2

[a] In this study, CSF was drawn from patients who had been recumbent overnight. Less of the metabolites are found under these conditions: The control group had a mean (±SE) of 18 ± 1.9 ng/ml for HVA (n = 10) and 23 ± 2.6 ng/ml for 5-HIAA (n = 21). (Data taken from various sources cited in Siegel et al. [27].)

also observed in patients with inflammatory and other disorders of the CNS. Attempts to differentiate these conditions have been made with probenecid. As long as this drug is present, the efflux of HVA and 5-HIAA is blocked, and their concentrations increase in the CSF. Parkinsonian patients tested with probenecid show less increase in HVA than do non-parkinsonian patients, suggesting a lower rate of dopamine synthesis in the former group. In interpreting this test one must recognize that the accumulation of the acidic metabolites may be significantly influenced simply by the level of probenecid attained in the CSF at the time of withdrawal of the fluid, regardless of other factors.

Clinicochemical studies of Parkinson's disease have also included the measurement of the urinary excretion of monoamines and some of their metabolites. Such investigations show that the excretion of epinephrine and norepinephrine is normal but that excretion of dopamine endogenously as well as after a bolus of levodopa is reduced and may be especially low in those patients with the greatest degree of akinesia [8]. The low values cannot be attributed to the use of anti-parkinsonian drugs, for the low urinary dopamine concentrations occur in untreated cases of Parkinson's disease as well [9].

Models of Parkinson's disease depend on interruption of nigrostriatal fibers

Neuropathological and necropsy findings by themselves cannot establish the precise biochemical defect that causes the loss of brain dopamine. Fortunately, one can prepare models in laboratory animals for comparison with the clinical state in humans. Cats, rabbits, rats, and other species have been used effectively in the identification of neurochemical events that accompany specific morphological changes. For the experimental study of motor disturbances directly relevant to human disease, however, it is necessary to carry out neurological and neuropharmacological investigations in those primate species with an extrapyramidal nervous system analogous to that of humans. In this way, it is possible to induce dyskinesias such as tremor and hypokinesia of the limbs opposite to a small unilateral lesion in the ventromedial tegmental area of the upper brain stem [10–12]. Histological study of the brains of such monkeys indicates that fibers from the substantia nigra to the striatum are interrupted, with consequent retrograde degeneration that entails loss of staining characteristics of the nigra, involving degeneration of cell bodies, and significant decreases in the concentration of catecholamines in the striatum, without involving its serotonin content. The disappearance of striatal monoamines is attributed to anterograde degeneration of these nigrostriatal fibers. The losses of cell bodies and of the dopamine in their axonal terminations parallel one another. Moreover, not only is dopamine lost from the striatum, but so also are DOPAC and HVA and neuronal enzymes such as tyrosine hydroxylase.

The lesion model has served to establish the existence of the nigrostriatal tract and its function and to explain the neuropathological and neurochemical (necropsy) findings in Parkinson's disease. Another important model is based on the predilection of the chemical N-methyl-4-phenyl-1,2,3,6-tetrahydropyridine (MPTP) for the pigmented neuronal cell bodies of the substantia nigra, which it causes to degenerate [13]. The action of MPTP is swift; drug users consuming it unknowingly as a contaminant of a novel synthetic heroin-like compound have rapidly developed severe akinetic parkinsonism [14]. Monkeys given MPTP exhibit an extrapyramidal syndrome, accompanied by decreases of dopamine and its metabolites and of

norepinephrine in the brain, but increased serotonin [15]. The pars compacta of the substantia nigra in both humans and monkeys is depigmented as a result of MPTP toxicity. In some species the syndrome has been prevented by prior treatment of the animals with pargyline or with deprenyl (Fig. 2). Thus, MPTP becomes toxic only after its intracellular stepwise oxidation to N-methyl-4-phenylpyridine (MPP^+) by MAO-B. The cause of most cases of Parkinson's disease is unknown, but the MPTP model suggests that some type of environmental toxicity plays a role. If so, research in Parkinson's disease should be directed toward identifying nigrally directed poisons and the means of blocking their effect, or of eliminating them altogether. Experience with MPTP indicates that an assessment of a preventive role of MAO-B inhibitors in patients manifesting the early stages of Parkinson's disease is in order. Of course, other mechanisms of environmental toxicity are not precluded.

Levodopa partially corrects loss of dopamine in treatment of Parkinson's disease

An important outgrowth of catecholamine studies has been the use of levodopa (L-DOPA) in the treatment of Parkinson's disease. In 1961, neuropharmacological studies in patients with the disease revealed that this amino acid exerts antirigidity and antiakinesic actions; that is, it influences the two most incapacitating symptoms of Parkinson's disease. Clinical experience shows that levodopa produces considerable improvement in most patients with Parkinson's disease, but although this treatment is considered the best available, as the disease progresses there may be some loss of efficacy of this substance [16].

It is generally assumed that the therapeutic role of levodopa lies in the ease with which it crosses the blood-brain barrier (see Chap. 30), in contrast to the exclusion of dopamine, and in its ability to replenish the supply of dopamine at appropriate sites. The passage of levodopa into the parenchymal tissue of the brain entails its transfer from blood through the endothelial cells lining the capillaries (see Chap. 30). These cells, like many other peripheral cells, contain considerable amounts of AADC, so that only a portion of a given amount of levodopa will eventually pass into the brain. For this reason the patient is also given an AADC inhibitor, such as carbidopa or benserazide (Fig. 2), in doses that affect only the peripherally located enzyme (including that of the brain capillaries) [5,17]. According to the commonly accepted hypothesis of its mode of action, when levodopa has crossed the blood-brain barrier, aided by an active transport mechanism, it must be converted to dopamine. Some question arises as to the source of the decarboxylase for this, for many of the dopaminergic neurons, including their content of AADC, have been eliminated. Studies with postmortem material have not yet revealed any cases with a total deficiency of AADC in the striatum: there has always been at least a small residue of enzyme activity. Moreover, cells of the striatum receive connections from many sources, including serotonin-producing raphe nuclei. Hence, levodopa could also be acted on by the decarboxylase within those neurons. Dopamine formed would then be available in the presynaptic space, although its path of diffusion to sensitive neurons might be longer than usual. Current developments in receptor studies with postmortem tissue indicate that the untreated parkinsonian patient has an elevated density of dopamine receptors of the D_2 type (those that are not linked to adenylate cyclase) in the striatum (see Chap. 11). This would represent a "supersensitive" state. Treatment with levodopa lowers the density to the same level as in control tissue.

The actions of levodopa in Parkinson's disease or of dopamine at receptor sites in the CNS are mimicked by certain compounds. Apomorphine, a semisynthetic catecholic alkaloid, has a brief dopaminergic action. It acts both pre- and postsynaptically, the presynaptic autoreceptors being particularly sensitive to this drug. Its best recognized action is at the dopamine receptor sites making up the trigger zone of the emetic center in the area postrema. Like levodopa, apomorphine is effective in certain neuroendocrine systems. In humans, subemetic doses provoke a great increase in the concentration of growth hormone in the plasma, presumably by an action of cells producing the appropriate releasing factor. In many species it depresses the concentration of serum prolactin. Another dopamine agonist, one which has found some practical use in the treatment of Parkinson's disease, is bromocriptine. This ergot alkaloid seems to act directly on postsynaptic dopamine receptors. Amantadine is used in treatment as an adjunctive therapy; its action favors the release of dopamine from residual intact neurons in much the same way as amphetamine does.

Among the most commonly used drugs in the treatment of Parkinson's disease, and the therapeutic mainstay before the advent of levodopa, are anticholinergic agents. They serve to restore the balance that is disturbed when striatal cholinergic neurons have been released from the inhibitory action of dopamine fibers that synapse with them.

A completely novel approach to treatment is based on the success of grafting dopamine-producing tissue (substantia nigra) into the neostriatum of rats previously injected in that region with the neurotoxin 6-hydroxydopamine [18]. Surgical intervention is now being carried out in patients with Parkinson's disease. In these cases, a homograft of the subject's own adrenal chromaffin tissue is introduced.

Parkinsonism may be induced by neuroleptics that antagonize dopamine

The introduction of the neuroleptics into the treatment of schizophrenia has led to the recognition of parkinsonian signs as unwanted effects of these drugs. The neuroleptics block the action of neurotransmitters, primarily catecholamines; their therapeutic effect seems related to action at dopamine receptors. However, they tend to act on dopamine systems without distinction, although for the antischizophrenia effect action at the limbic and cortical dopamine sites alone would probably suffice. Blockade of nigrostriatal dopamine receptors leads to the expression of parkinsonian features. Some newer neuroleptics are more selective. Thioridazine, clozapine, and molindone, for example, have electrophysiological effects in the limbic region of the brain, but little action in the nigrostriatal area.

Reserpine, a natural alkaloid, acts quite differently from the synthetic neuroleptics. It causes depletion of stored monoamines, including dopamine, by blocking vesicular uptake for storage. Its action also results in a form of chemical parkinsonism.

Patients who have received neuroleptics for long periods of time may develop a hyperkinetic disorder of the extrapyramidal system characterized by involuntary, purposeless movements affecting many parts of the body. Most commonly these are manifested in a syndrome involving abnormal movements of the tongue, mouth, and masticatory muscles. There are also choreoathetoid movements of the extremities. The mechanism of neurotransmitter disturbance in this tardive dyskinesia is the subject of much ongoing research [19,20].

HUNTINGTON'S DISEASE

Huntington's disease has been of special interest to the neurochemist because it is genetically transmitted by an autosomal dominant gene. Large cohorts of index patients and relatives have been investigated in Venezuela and the United States in the search for genetic markers. The disease is characterized by choreiform movements and progressive dementia. These features usually appear well into adulthood, but there are juvenile cases also.

Huntington's disease shows loss of cholinergic and GABAergic fibers in striatum

In some respects Huntington's disease is a biochemical mirror image of Parkinson's disease [21]. Postmortem studies have revealed the loss of many neurons in the striatum and globus pallidus, especially intrinsic cholinergic fibers. Long-standing cases show a decrease of cerebral choline acetylase as a result of this. In addition, there is a significant decrease in the number of muscarinic receptors, indicating that the cell bodies with which these interneurons normally synapse have also undergone some loss. There is a decrease of GABAergic neurons, characterized by reductions in the marker enzyme glutamate decarboxylase and in GABA. These striatal fibers appear to innervate the pars reticulata of the substantia nigra. The pars compacta of that structure retains normal pigmentation and cell population. Substance P-containing pallidonigral fibers are also targets for the degenerative process. Other peptidergic neurons such as those containing somatostatin and neuropeptide Y, are spared. The concentrations of dopamine and norepinephrine are increased in the basal ganglia. In the case of dopamine, the increase may represent overactivity of the nigrostriatal fibers. This concept is favored by experience with drugs having an ameliorative effect in that they act to diminish the effect of dopamine: reserpine and methyldopa, which lower the amounts of dopamine and some other monoamines in the brain; α-methyl-*p*-tyrosine, which inhibits the synthesis of catecholamines at the tyrosine hydroxylase step; and neuroleptics, which provide postsynaptic blockade of dopamine receptors.

If GABA normally exerts an inhibitory action over nigrostriatal function (see Fig. 1), then the deficiency of this transmitter in Huntington's disease could contribute to an overproduction of dopamine at striatal synapses. Reduced cholinergic function at the output from the basal ganglia could also favor dopaminergic dominance. Both these findings are consistent with the exacerbation of abnormal movements in Huntington's disease caused by the administration of levodopa.

Animal models of Huntington's disease have been sought through the use of specific neurotoxins. For example, kainic acid, a rigid analog of glutamate, when injected directly into the striatum, causes destruction of intrinsic GABA-containing and cholinergic neurons but spares fibers of passage. Ibotenic acid, another plant product, acts similarly. Quinolinic acid, a tryptophan metabolite found in brain and other tissues, has a more restricted neurotoxicity. Although it lowers cerebral GABA and substance P, unlike kainic acid it does not alter the amounts of somatostatin and neuropeptide Y. Thus, the quinolinic acid-treated animal would mimic the chemical pathology of the clinical state quite precisely [22].

HEPATOLENTICULAR DEGENERATION (WILSON'S DISEASE)

Wilson's disease is a combined brain-liver disorder characterized by progressive rigidity and intention tremor, stemming from lesions of the lenticular nucleus (putamen and pallidum), along with hepatic cirrhosis of the coarse type and recurrent hepatitis. Mental deterioration ultimately sets in. Renamed hepatolenticular degeneration in 1921, it is recognized as a familial disorder inherited in an autosomal recessive fashion. The frequency rate of the gene is estimated to be 1 in 500. Biochemically, hepatolenticular degeneration entails low concentrations of copper and ceruloplasmin in the serum, elevated excretion of the metal in the urine, and deposition of excess copper in the brain (especially in the basal ganglia) and in the liver and

kidneys. In some cases, copper is deposited in the cornea, where it is reduced, forming the "Kayser-Fleischer ring." This sign is virtually pathognomonic of the disease but appears also in occasional cases of primary biliary cirrhosis. In addition, there is a constant aminoaciduria, including excretion of some oligopeptides and, sometimes, abnormal excretion of monoamines and their metabolites. Amino acid levels in plasma are normal; thus, the urinary findings may simply result from a renal defect caused by histotoxicity of copper.

Transport of copper is regulated at liver, kidney, and blood-brain barrier

Adult humans require only 1 to 2 mg copper daily; most diets supply more than this. A primary requirement of copper is in the utilization of iron for hemoglobin synthesis and other functions, and in some species, copper deficiency readily results in anemia. In other animals, a neurological disturbance is prominent, such as swayback in cattle and posterior paralysis in swine. Myelination of nerve is delayed in lambs born of copper-deficient ewes [23].

The regulation of copper metabolism is achieved by an enterohepatic cycle. Much of the ingested copper is absorbed from the intestinal tract and reaches the liver in the portal circulation; some is utilized there, but most is excreted in the bile. Copper is present in the serum mainly in the form of ceruloplasmin in concentrations of 20 to 40 mg/100 ml. In hepatolenticular degeneration these amounts are reduced to half or less. A much smaller amount of copper, approximately 5 percent of the total, is present in the ionic state, loosely bound to serum albumin. This is the transport form of the metal. Only a minute fraction of dietary copper normally appears in the urine. The regulatory mechanism can be overwhelmed in laboratory animals by repeated parenteral administration of copper; the metal then accumulates in the liver, kidneys, and other organs.

Entry of copper into the brain is highly restricted, even under the aggravated conditions of copper loading, so that the net increase of copper in that organ is small and not at all of the proportions seen in hepatolenticular degeneration. A genetic disorder in Bedlington terriers also involves a disturbance of copper metabolism. Affected dogs have hepatic cirrhosis but of a different kind than in hepatolenticular degeneration. Moreover, brain copper is not consistently high. Ceruloplasmin seems to function in the metabolism of iron. Thus, when this protein is perfused through the isolated liver, there is a specific and rapid shift of transferrin from the organ to the perfusate. The vexing question of the pathogenesis of hepatolenticular degeneration remains on the research agenda. The excessive deposition of copper in the basal ganglia presumably is the cause of the neurological syndrome, but it is not known how the metal breaks through the rigorous regulation at the blood-brain barrier and what specific neuronal functions it damages.

Some metal-chelating agents have been tested therapeutically in hepatolenticular degeneration. The most effective in treatment has been D-penicillamine (3,3-dimethylcysteine). It is given in doses to approximately 3 g/day. Triethylene tetramine has also been used. Computerized tomographic studies show that the use of these chelating agents leads to improvement in the occurrence of hypodense areas in the basal ganglia [24], a common abnormality in this disease. Thus, the cytotoxicity of copper can be reversed.

CHRONIC MANGANESE POISONING

A small proportion of miners exposed to manganese dust develop manganism. The disease is ushered in by self-limited psychiatric symptoms, followed by permanent neurological changes. The manifestations are those of extrapyramidal disease and respond in some measure to treatment with levodopa.

ALS-PARKINSONISM-DEMENTIA OF GUAM

The Chamorro people of Guam have had a very high incidence of a syndrome resembling amyotrophic lateral sclerosis (ALS), but with elements of parkinsonism and dementia (25). This apparently developed prominently during the second World War. Then, as a result of food shortages, there was considerable dependence upon the seeds of *Cycas circinalis* (false sago), a source of β-*N*-methylamino-L-alanine, an amino acid with predilection for NMDA receptors and which, on chronic administration to monkeys, reproduces some of the features of ALS-parkinsonism-dementia (see Chap. 15 and [26]). Incidence of the disease has been decreasing since the introduction of other foods into the Chamorro diet. The chemistry of the cycad toxin reminds one that the toxic principle of the chick pea causing neurolathyrism is β-*N*-oxalyl-L-alanine.

ACKNOWLEDGMENT

Research in the author's laboratory is supported by a grant of the Medical Research Council of Canada.

REFERENCES

1. Fahn, S. Biochemistry of the basal ganglia. *Adv. Neurol.* 14:59–89, 1976.
2. Gauthier, S., and Sourkes, T. L. Anatomical and biochemical basis of the extrapyramidal disorders. *Prog. Neuropsychopharmacol. Biol. Psychiatry* 6:595–599, 1982.

3. Marsden, C. D. Basal ganglia disease. *Lancet* 2:1141–1147, 1982.

4. Scatton, B., Javoy-Agid, F., Montfort, J. C., and Agid, Y. Neurochemistry of monoaminergic neurons in Parkinson's disease. In E. Usdin, A. Carlsson, A. Dahlström, and J. Engel (eds.), *Catecholamines, Part C: Neuropharmacology and Central Nervous System—Therapeutic Aspects.* New York: Alan R. Liss, 1984, pp. 43–52.

5. Birkmayer, W., and Riederer, P. *Die Parkinson-Krankheit: Biochemie, Klinik, Therapie.* Vienna: Springer-Verlag, 1980.

6. Sourkes, T. L. On the origin of homovanillic acid (HVA) in the cerebrospinal fluid. *J. Neural Transm.* 34:153–157, 1973.

7. Garelis, E., and Sourkes, T. L. Sites of origin in the central nervous system of monoamine metabolites measured in human cerebrospinal fluid. *J. Neurol. Neurosurg. Psychiatry* 36:625–629, 1973.

8. Sourkes, T. L. Metabolism of monoamines in extrapyramidal disorders. In J. De Ajuriaguerra and G. Gauthier (eds.), *Monoamines, Noyaux Gris Centraux et Syndrome de Parkinson.* Geneva: Georg (Paris: Masson), 1971, pp. 129–141.

9. Hoehn, M. J., Crowley, T. J., and Rutledge, C. O. Dopamine correlates of neurologic and psychologic status in untreated parkinsonism. *J. Neurol. Neurosurg. Psychiatry* 39:941–951, 1976.

10. Sourkes, T. L., and Poirier, L. J. Neurochemical bases of tremor and other disorders of movement. *Can. Med. Assoc. J.* 94:53–60, 1966.

11. Goldstein, M., Battista, A. F., Ohmoto, T., Anagnoste, B., and Fuxe, K. Tremor and involuntary movements in monkeys: Effect of L-dopa and of a dopamine reception stimulating agent. *Science* 179:816–817, 1973.

12. Schultz, W. Recent physiological and pathophysiological aspects of parkinsonian movement disorders. *Life Sci.* 34:2213–2223, 1984.

13. Burks, T. F. (ed.) *Current Concepts in Dopamine Neurotoxic Features of MPTP. Life Sci.* 36:201–254, 1985.

14. Burns, R. S., LeWitt, P. A., Ebert, M. H., Pakkenberg, H., and Kopin, I. J. The clinical syndrome of striatal dopamine deficiency: parkinsonism induced by 1-methyl-4-phenyl-1,2,3,6-tetrahydropyridine (MPTP). *New Eng. J. Med.* 312:1418–1421, 1985.

15. Di Paolo, T., Bédard, P., Daigle, M., and Boucher, R. Long-term effects of MPTP on central and peripheral catecholamine and indoleamine concentrations in monkeys. *Brain Res.* 379:285–293, 1986.

16. Yahr, M. D. Limitations of long term use of antiparkinson drugs. *Can. J. Neurol. Sci.* 11:191–194, 1984.

17. Yahr, M. D. (ed.). *The Treatment of Parkinson's Disease: The Role of DOPA Decarboxylase Inhibitors (Advances in Neurology, Vol. 2).* New York: Raven Press, 1973.

18. Schmidt, R. H., Ingvar, M., Lindvall, O., Steveni, U., and Björklund, A. Functional activity of substantia nigra grafts reinnervating the striatum: neurotransmitter metabolism and [^{14}C]2-deoxy-D-glucose autoradiography. *J. Neurochem.* 38:737–748, 1982.

19. Baldessarini, R. J., and Tarsy, D. Dopamine and the pathophysiology of dyskinesias induced by antipsychotic drugs. *Ann. Rev. Neurosci.* 3:23–41, 1980.

20. Chouinard, G., and Steinberg, S. Type 1 tardive dyskinesia induced by anticholinergic drugs, dopamine agonists and neuroleptics. *Prog. Neuropsychopharmacol. Biol. Psychiatry* 6:571–578, 1982.

21. Spokes, E. G. S. The neurochemistry of Huntington's chorea. *Trends Neurosci.* 4:115–118, 1981.

22. Beal, M., Kowall, N. W., Ellison, D. W., Mazurek, M. F., Swartz, K. J., and Martin, J. B. Replication of the neurochemical characteristics of Huntington's disease by quinolinic acid. *Nature* 321:168–171, 1986.

23. Sourkes, T. L. Transition elements and the nervous system. In E. Pollitt and R. L. Leibel (eds.), *Iron Deficiency: Brain Biochemistry and Behavior.* New York: Raven Press, 1982, pp. 1–29.

24. Williams, F. J. B., and Walshe, J. M. Wilson's disease: An analysis of the cranial computerized tomographic appearances found in 60 patients and the changes in response to treatment with chelating agents. *Brain* 104:735–752, 1981.

25. Garruto, R. M., and Yase, Y. Neurodegenerative disorders of the Western Pacific: the search

for mechanisms of pathogenesis. *Trends NeuroSci.* 9:368–374, 1986.

26. Spencer, P. S., Nunn, P. B., Hugon, J., Ludolph, A. C., Ross, S. M., Roy, D. N., and Robertson, R. C. Guam amyotrophic lateral sclerosis-parkinsonism-dementia linked to a plant excitant neurotoxin. *Science* 237:517–522, 1987.

27. Siegel, G. J., Albers, R. W., Agranoff, B. W., and Katzman, R. (eds.). *Basic Neurochemistry*, 3rd ed. Boston: Little, Brown, 1981.

CHAPTER 43

Neurochemistry of Alzheimer's Disease

Robert Katzman and Leon J. Thal

ALZHEIMER'S DISEASE IS THE MOST COMMON CAUSE OF DEMENTIA

Alzheimer's disease is the most common of the neurodegenerative disorders of aging. The best current estimate is that 7 percent of persons over 65 years of age in the United States, that is about two million individuals, have Alzheimer's disease. This disorder was first described in 1907 by Alois Alzheimer, a psychiatrist and neuroanatomist, in a woman who had a 5-year progressive course with loss of memory and language ability. Because Alzheimer's patient was in her fifties the disease was considered for many decades to represent a presenile dementia. It is now recognized that Alzheimer's disease is in fact the most common cause of dementia in late life, accounting for almost two-thirds of cases of senile dementia. In fact, the occurrence of Alzheimer's disease rises dramatically with age. The incidence of new cases at ages 60 to 65 years is 0.1 percent/year but at ages 80 to 85 years, becomes 2 percent/year [1].

Basic Neurochemistry: Molecular, Cellular, and Medical Aspects, 4th Ed., edited by G. J. Siegel et al. Raven Press, Ltd., New York, 1989.
Correspondence to Robert Katzman, University of California, San Diego School of Medicine, La Jolla, California 92093.

Neuronal loss, neurofibrillary tangles, and neuritic plaques in a selective distribution characterize the pathology

The disorder, as described by Alzheimer, is a clinical-pathological entity. Clinically, it presents with progressive intellectual deterioration that involves not only memory, orientation, and language functions but other components of higher function as well, such as personality, judgment, problem solving, calculation, and visual-spatial and constructional abilities. Alzheimer patients remain alert until terminal stages, and changes in gait and motor abilities occur late in the course.

The pathological changes are distinctive and correlate quite well with the clinical symptoms [1,2]. On gross examination, there is atrophy of the brain, most marked in hippocampus and in association areas of cerebral cortex. The relative preservation of primary motor, auditory, somatosensory, and visual cortex is consistent with the relative preservation of motor and sensory functions. An exception is the involvement of olfactory bulb and olfactory cortex. The hallmarks of the disorder, however, are observed on microscopic examination: These include loss of neurons and the presence of neurofibrillary tangles (NFT) and neuritic plaques (NP). NFT (Fig. 1) are abnormal neuronal soma in which the cytoplasm is filled with unique submicroscopic filamentous structures, consisting of filaments approximately 10 nm in diameter that are wound around each other with a period

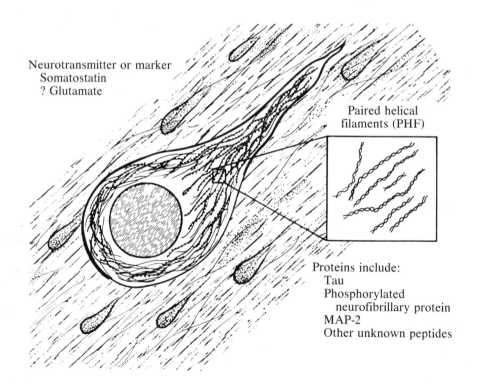

Neurotransmitter or marker
Somatostatin
? Glutamate

Paired helical filaments (PHF)

Proteins include:
Tau
Phosphorylated
    neurofibrillary protein
MAP-2
Other unknown peptides

FIG. 1. Neurofibrillary tangle.

of 800 nm in a helical fashion, the paired helical filament (PHF). The NP (Fig. 2) consist of clusters of degenerating nerve endings, both axonal and dendritic, with a central core that usually contains extracellular linear filaments that have the optical and ultrastructural characteristics of an amyloid protein. The NFT and NP are difficult to observe with ordinary hematoxylin and eosin stains but are displayed dramatically by the Bielschowsky organic silver dyes, as first observed by Alzheimer; today they are most easily detected using a fluorescent thioflavine stain. Other pathological changes often found in the Alzheimer brain include amyloid in arter-

ioles in meninges and cerebral cortex and inclusions, termed granulovacuolar bodies, in hippocampal neurons.

Projection nuclei of isodendritic core and large pyramidal neurons in the association and hippocampal cortex are most involved

The Alzheimer brain is characterized by a selective distribution of cell loss, although there is variability in the intensity of pathological changes in different areas in brains from differ-

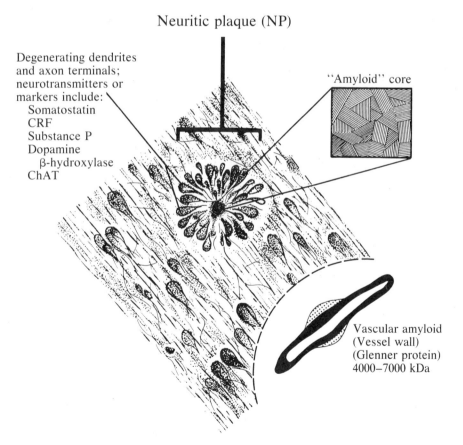

FIG. 2. Neuritic plaque.

ent patients. NFT, NP, and cell loss occur principally in the association cortex, hippocampus, entorhinal cortex, amygdala, olfactory bulb, olfactory cortex, and a limited number of subcortical cellular groups, in particular the basal nucleus of Meynert, locus coeruleus, dorsal tegmentum, lateral hypothalamus, and paramedian reticular formation. Within each area specific neurons are especially vulnerable; thus, about one-half of the large pyramidal cells in the association cortex are lost, whereas neurons under 90 μm^2 are relatively intact. In the hippocampus, the neurons that are particularly involved are the large pyramidal cells in CA1 and subiculum. In entorhinal cortex, the large pyramidal neurons in layer II [3] are the site of formation of NFT, whereas adjacent cells are spared. In subcortical nuclei, the cells that are involved appear to be those that project to the cerebral cortex and hippocampus: in the basal nucleus, the large cholinergic cells [4]; in the dorsal raphe, the serotoninergic cell bodies; in the locus coeruleus, the noradrenergic cell bodies.

The cholinergic, noradrenergic, and serotoninergic projection systems, each nucleus giving rise to groups of axons that project to the cerebral cortex and hippocampus, and, in addition, the paramedian reticular nucleus, which also sends axonal projections to cerebral cortex, have been described as the "isodendritic core" of the brain. One hypothesis concerning the pathogenesis of Alzheimer's disease has emphasized the importance of the involvement of these neuronal systems. It can be demonstrated that some axonal terminals of these systems participate in formation of NP. In contrast, another hypothesis suggests that the primary event occurs in the NP in the cortex and that the projection nuclei are secondarily involved. There is not direct evidence for either viewpoint, and it is equally likely that selectively vulnerable cells share a common cellular determinant such as a membrane receptor. The sequential pathophysiology of Alzheimer's disease is not understood at present; nor is the etiology or etiologies of this disorder known.

Biochemical changes involve multiple neurotransmitter systems

The cholinergic deficiency

The discovery of a cholinergic deficit in the Alzheimer brain has proven to be a turning point in research on Alzheimer's disease. In 1976 and 1977, three independent groups in Great Britain discovered that the biosynthetic enzyme choline acetyltransferase (ChAT) was markedly reduced in the cerebral cortex and hippocampus in Alzheimer brain [5,6]. This finding has subsequently been confirmed by more than 15 laboratories. The reduction in the levels of enzymatic activity as compared to brains matched for age and postmortem time varies from 50 to 90 percent. A significant loss of acetylcholinesterase, although not as great as the loss of ChAT, is found in Alzheimer brain. In contrast to this marked reduction of biosynthetic and degradative enzymes, the level of muscarinic cholinergic receptors in the cortex and hippocampus of the same Alzheimer brains is normal or only modestly reduced. Similarly, the level of ChAT in other regions of the Alzheimer brain, such as the basal ganglia, is little changed [7]. A significant reduction in ChAT levels in the cerebral cortex is found in surgical biopsy samples from Alzheimer patients, biopsies sometimes obtained during the first year of symptomatology.

The discovery of the ChAT deficiency in the Alzheimer brain has proven to be of importance not only in its own right but in terms of its impact on subsequent work on the chemical pathology of degenerative diseases and on our knowledge of the anatomy of cholinergic systems in the mammalian brain. An implicit assumption has been that certain structural elements, such as lipids, could be analyzed in post-mortem brain but not tissue enzyme activity, due to the effects of proteolysis. In fact, the immediate small drop in enzymatic activity during the first hour after death is followed by a very slow and gradual loss of activity. Therefore, brains frozen within 24 hr can be used in such analysis if properly matched with control brain. This success has led to the widespread use of postmortem brain tissue in neurochemical studies. It is important to note, however, that although many enzymes, peptides, and even amines can be studied successfully, the validity of the use of postmortem tissue must be demonstrated for each molecular species studied. It is known that certain enzymes, such as tyrosine hydroxylase, are more sensitive to postmortem changes. Moreover, immediate premortem events must be taken into account; for example, glutamic acid decarboxylase levels may be reduced if the patient had bronchopneumonia or was on a respirator for several days before death.

It is interesting to note the impact that neurochemical research on the cholinergic system has had on basic neuroscience. The chemical pathology of Alzheimer's disease has focused attention on the details of the neurotransmitter organization of the cerebral cortex. With curiosity aroused by the discovery of the reduced cortical ChAT in Alzheimer's disease, the projection of the basal nucleus to cerebral cortex was discovered. It was found that this system accounts for more than 70 percent of the ChAT in the cerebral cortex of rats [8]. In turn, immunohistochemical investigation of Alzheimer brain has shown that ChAT is present in some of the degenerating neurites that form cortical NP [9].

Biogenic amines

Although the involvement of the locus coeruleus and dorsal raphe clearly indicates that the noradrenergic and serotoninergic projection systems are also involved in this disorder, the neurochemical evidence is not as robust as in the case of the cholinergic system, due in part to the greater postmortem lability of their enzymatic markers (tyrosine hydroxylase, dopamine β-decarboxylase, and tryptophan hydroxylase). Some reduction in levels of norepinephrine and serotonin is found in postmortem Alzheimer brain, however; Bowen and colleagues [10] have also demonstrated reductions in serotonin uptake in brain biopsies.

In contrast, minimal loss or normal levels of dopamine are found in the Alzheimer brain. This is consistent with the pathological finding that the substantia nigra is not involved in the majority of Alzheimer brains; however, there are occasional Alzheimer brains in which NFT are found in the substantia nigra. To confound the situation, there may be increased incidence of Alzheimer changes in the brains of patients with both the classical clinical and pathological features of Parkinson's disease, a disorder in which the primary change is loss of dopamine. Some reports suggest that up to 30 percent of parkinsonian patients develop Alzheimer changes in their brain, but these series may have been subject to selection bias. It is uncertain at present whether the coincidence of Parkinson's disease and Alzheimer's disease is related to a shared unknown risk factor or simply represents joint occurrence of two common disorders of aging.

Inhibitory and excitatory amino acids

There is less specific information about the state of amino acid transmitters in the Alzheimer brain. Postmortem measurement of these transmitters and their enzymes is less satisfactory than in the case of amine or peptide transmitters. The γ-aminobutyric acid (GABA) biosynthetic enzyme glutamic acid decarboxylase (GAD) is especially labile (both to premortem disease and postmortem time), and great care must be used in selecting brains suitable for analysis. Also, glutamic acid serves a dual function in cells as part of the intermediate metabolism of neurons, as well as an excitatory neurotransmitter (see Chap. 15).

GABA is the major inhibitory amino acid neurotransmitter in the cerebral hemispheres. In primate cerebral cortex, GABA is present in more than one-quarter of all neurons and is especially localized in small interneurons. Many of these GABA interneurons also contain a neuropeptide or even two neuropeptides. If human neocortex is organized similarly, then there will be, for example, interneurons containing GABA plus peptides, such as somatostatin and substance P, that are affected by the Alzheimer process, whereas GABA neurons that contain other peptides, such as cholecystokinin (CCK), are not affected by the Alzheimer process. Thus, it is likely that a proportion of the GABA-containing cells will be lost. Hence, one might expect that levels of GABA would be slightly but not significantly reduced.

It is likely that the major excitatory amino acids in brain (glutamate and aspartate) play a central role in the Alzheimer process, but this is at present speculative. Many of the large pyramidal neurons in the association cortex, entorhinal cortex, and hippocampus (neuronal groups that are usually devastated in Alzheimer brain) are probably glutaminergic; yet there is little direct data in part because of the absence of a specific enzymatic marker. Also, glutamate may be the transmitter in many cells that are spared by Alzheimer's disease. The best evidence of glutamate involvement was obtained by Hyman and co-workers [11]. Using a microdissection technique, these investigators demonstrated an 80 percent reduction of glutamate in the terminal zone of the perforant pathway; the cells of origin of this pathway are layer II entorhinal cortical pyramidal cells, a neuronal group regularly devastated by Alzheimer's disease.

Neuropeptides

A decrease in the concentration of somatostatin in the neocortex and hippocampus in Alzheimer brain is a consistent finding; the reduction is almost as great as that of ChAT [12,13]. In monkey brain, over 90 percent of somatostatin cells contain GABA and its biosynthetic enzyme, GAD; most are interneurons. It is not yet clear whether the localization of somatostatin in human neocortex is entirely confined to GABA-containing interneurons or whether some medium or large neurons also contain this peptide. One investigator reported the presence of somatostatin in NFT, but others have not been able to replicate this; however, a number of investigators using immunohistochemical techniques have identified abnormal somatostatin terminals in NP [14]. Corticotropin releasing factor (CRF) is the other neuropeptide that is significantly reduced (by over 40 percent) in the neocortex [15]. Small but inconsistent reductions have been reported in substance P and neuropeptide Y (NPY). Both substance P and NPY immunoreactivity have been found in degenerating neurites in NP. In contrast, a number of neocortical peptides show little or no change in the Alzheimer brain. Most important among these are vasoactive intestinal peptide (VIP) and CCK, both present in significant amounts in human neocortex.

The relative integrity of VIP and CCK is consistent with the pathological finding of relative sparing of the small cortical interneurons in Alzheimer brain. It is interesting to note that in primate brain, VIP is located with ChAT in neocortical interneurons, and CCK is located with GABA. The major inconsistency in the peptide data is the loss of somatostatin, which in much greater than the loss of NPY. Monkey brain studies indicate that NPY is localized with somatostatin in over 80 percent of somatostatin cells and that this accounts for over 80 percent of NPY present. Perhaps the neurochemical anatomy of the human neocortex differs from the monkey neocortex in this regard.

Neurotransmitter changes are correlated with brain pathology and cognitive deficits

The discovery that the degree of dementia in Alzheimer patients measured during life with standardized mental status and functional scales is highly correlated (with correlation coefficients between 0.6 and 0.7) with the number of NP in the cerebral cortex has played a major role in the development of the consensus that Alzheimer pathology is indeed the principal cause of dementia in the elderly. The number of NP in the cerebral cortex in turn is correlated with the level of ChAT. The concentration of ChAT also correlates with dementia scores obtained during life. In one study, the highest correlation ($r = 0.78$) obtained was that of the level of hippocampal ChAT with the score on a simple memory task requiring the subject to recall the names of 10 common objects that had been touched, seen, and named [16]. This finding is consistent with the known role of the hippocampus in recent memory. On the other hand, somatostatin levels in Alzheimer brain have not correlated as well as ChAT with tests of cognition or function, although one group of investigators did find that the level of CSF somatostatin correlated with indices of intellectual impairment. Because the role of cortical somatostatin interneurons in cognition is not understood, the proper psychological tests may have not been carried out. These findings in Alzheimer's disease highlight our present limitations in the understanding of the functional role of neurotransmitters in the neocortex.

Cholinergic receptors

Following the demonstration of a marked loss of the synthetic enzyme ChAT in Alzheimer's disease, investigators began to search for the presence of alterations in muscarinic receptor levels. Using only a single concentration of ligand, early investigators failed to demonstrate alteration in receptor number (Table 1). One study, however, demonstrated a 57 percent decrease in muscarinic binding in hippocampus without a change in receptor number in other brain regions. A more recent study demonstrated a 35 percent decrease in receptor number in hippocampus and a 40 percent decrease in nucleus basalis. In cerebral cortex, small decreases have been reported. Mash et al. claimed that cortical muscarinic receptor loss in Alzheimer's disease is secondary to loss of M_2 or presynaptic receptors (see Chap. 10), with the number of postsynaptic receptors remaining intact. This work remains to be confirmed. Overall, muscarinic receptor changes in Alzheimer's disease appear to be small, averaging about a 25 percent decrease. Several processes may occur, including simultaneous loss of presynaptic receptors and increase in postsynaptic receptors secondary to denervation supersensitivity. It is not surprising that the net effect of these two processes might result in either no apparent change or only a small change in receptor number. Additionally, different rates of progression of these two processes in individual brains may well underlie the discrepancies reported in the literature. The evaluation of nicotinic receptors in this disorder remains in its infancy, with two reports of a 60 percent decrease in nicotinic receptor number in the cortex and one report of no change. Large decreases have also been reported in the putamen and nucleus basalis. The data on nicotinic receptor binding suggest that decreases will be found; however, the significance and extent of these decreases remain to be determined. Future work evaluating receptor changes will likely utilize autoradiographic techniques to obtain more precise localization of receptor change *in vitro* and the use of positron emission

TABLE 1. Receptor changes in Alzheimer's disease

Receptor type	Subtype (ligand)	Findings
Cholinergic	Muscarinic (QNB)	No changes in cortex or hippocampus[a]
		35–57% Decrease in hippocampus[b,c]
		20–30% Decrease in frontal cortex[d]
	Nicotinic (nicotine)	No change in cortex or hippocampus[c]
		60% Decrease in cortex[e,f]
		46% Decrease in putamen; 70% decrease in nucleus basalis of Meynert[c]
Serotoninergic	S$_1$ (serotonin)	40–50% Decrease in hippocampus, amygdala, temporal cortex[g]
	S$_2$ (ketanserin)	40–65% Decrease in cortex, hippocampus, amygdala[g]
Dopaminergic	D$_1$ (flupenthixol)	No change in putamen or caudate[h,i]
		30–35% Decrease in accumbens and substantia nigra[h,i]
	D$_2$ (spiperone)	25–35% Decrease in putamen[h,i]
		30–50% Decrease in caudate[b,j]
		30% Decrease in accumbens[i]
α-Adrenergic	α$_1$ (WB 4101; prazosin)	No change in temporal cortex[g,k]
		50% Decrease in hippocampus[k]
	α$_2$ (Rauwolscine; yohimbine)	No change in temporal cortex[g,k]
		50% Decrease in nucleus basalis of Meynert[k]
GABAergic	(Muscimol; GABA)	No change in temporal cortex[g]
		40–50% Decrease in caudate and frontal cortex[b]
Somatostatinergic	(Somatostatin-28 analog)	40–50% Decrease in hippocampus and cortex[l]
CRF	(CRF analog)	50–100% Decrease in cortex[m]

[a] Davies, P., and Verth, A. H. *Brain Res.* 138:385–392, 1978.
[b] Reisine, T. D., et al. *Brain Res.* 159:477–481, 1978.
[c] Shimohama, S., et al. *J. Neurochem.* 46:288–293, 1986.
[d] Mash, D. C., Flynn, D. D., and Potter, L. T. *Science* 228:1115–1118, 1985.
[e] Flynn, D. D., and Mash, D. C. *J. Neurochem.* 47:1948–1954, 1986.
[f] Whitehouse, P. J. et al. *Brain Res.* 371:146–151, 1986.
[g] Cross, A. J., et al. *Neurobiol. Aging* 7:3–7, 1986.
[h] Cross, A. J., et al. *Neurosci Lett.* 52:1–6, 1984.
[i] Rinne, J. O., et al. *J. Neurol. Sci.* 73:219–230, 1986.
[j] Rinne, J. O., et al. *J. Neural. Trans.* 65:51–62, 1986.
[k] Shimohama, S., et al. *J. Neurochem.* 47:1295–1301, 1986.
[l] Beal, M. F., et al. *Science* 229:289–291, 1985.
[m] De Souza, E. B., et al. *Nature* 319:593–595, 1986.

tomography (PET) to measure receptor changes *in vivo* in patients.

Other receptors

In addition to cholinergic receptors, many other receptors have been examined in Alzheimer's disease (Table 1). There is general agreement that cortical serotonin receptors including both S$_1$ and S$_2$ receptors are diminished in the hippocampus, cortex, and amygdala. Dopamine D$_2$ receptors are reported to be decreased in the caudate, putamen, and nucleus accumbens. In contrast, D$_1$ receptors are reported to be normal in the caudate and putamen. Both α$_1$- and α$_2$-adrenergic receptors are unchanged in the temporal cortex but α$_1$ receptors are decreased in the hippocampus, whereas α$_2$ receptors are decreased in the nucleus basalis. GABA receptors are decreased in the caudate and frontal cortex but not in the temporal cortex. Several other conventional neurotransmitter receptors have been examined, including β-adrenergic, histamine, benzodiazepine, and opiate receptors in the temporal cortex without any evidence of change. A 40 to 50 percent decrease in somatostatin receptors was found in the hippocampus and cortex, whereas a 50 to 100 percent increase in receptors for CRF was recently reported in the cortex of Alzheimer patients. Most striking, however, was the reciprocal relationship with increased CRF receptors and diminished CRF-like immunoreactivity in the same region. These reciprocal changes strongly suggest that CRF receptor concentration is modulated by CRF content.

Most of the data currently available suggest that there are widespread changes in serotonin, somatostatin, and CRF receptors in Alzheimer's disease. Receptor changes for most other systems await confirmation by additional investigators. Receptor alterations within the cholinergic system may be secondary to loss of only one subclass of receptor. The precise degree of receptor loss is not yet agreed on, nor is the physiological role of this receptor loss known.

Cerebral metabolic changes and PET findings parallel pathology

As Alzheimer's disease progresses, a significant decrease in oxygen and glucose utilization [measured with 2-^{18}fluoro-2-deoxyglucose (FDG)] is shown on PET scans (see Chap. 44). Although glucose metabolism is decreased *in vivo*, glucose metabolism of biopsy tissue measured in slices is increased. These findings are consistent with the hypothesis that the reduction in glucose metabolism *in vivo* reflects reduced activity of the brain rather than a change in cellular metabolic capacity.

PET has proven to be very useful in providing visual images of the evolution of the metabolic changes in the Alzheimer neocortex. A characteristic early deficit in glucose metabolism is seen in the parietal and temporal regions in Alzheimer patients, areas with particularly high numbers of NP [17]. In longitudinal studies it has been found that memory deficit may precede PET changes but that metabolic reductions in the parietal association cortex precede the impairment of such neocortical-mediated functions as language and visuospatial deficits [18]. In the first report of an autopsy carried out in an Alzheimer patient who had undergone PET, the regional variation in metabolic impairment measured with FDG paralleled the severity of neuronal loss.

Molecular constituents of abnormal fibrous proteins are being identified

One of the rapidly evolving areas of neurochemical research on Alzheimer's disease is that of identifying the chemical and molecular structure of the abnormal fibrous proteins found in the Alzheimer brain, particularly the amyloid in the core of the NP, the amyloid present in some blood vessels in Alzheimer brain and meninges, and the proteins that constitute the PHF. Interest in this research is heightened because it is likely that unraveling the protein chemistry will help explain the pathogenesis of Alzheimer's disease and perhaps offer a clue as to etiology.

Amyloid

Amyloid is a term used to describe extracellular protein fibrils with characteristic staining properties; that is, fibrils that become birefringent when stained with Congo red. This optical property results from the β-pleated configuration of amyloid proteins. Amyloid accumulations in various tissues are found in a number of different chronic diseases, and it has become apparent that there are several amyloid proteins. The protein present in the amyloid of meningeal blood vessels in Alzheimer's disease, isolated by Glenner and Wong [19], has been partially sequenced and found to be a unique peptide. There is good evidence that the amyloid present in the core of the NP is similar or identical to the cerebrovascular amyloid. The peptide present in the Alzheimer brain contains 42 or 43 amino acids. The gene that codes for a larger precursor protein is present in the normal human genome and is located on chromosome 21 [20,21]. This gene has been cloned and the full sequence of the precursor protein has been published [22]. This precursor molecule has been shown to have two forms, one form with an insert of a serine protease inhibitor [23]. The amyloid peptide is located in the transmembrane portion of the precursor protein, which may contribute to the extracellular matrix of the synapse [24]. There is considerable interest in the question of whether the amyloid peptide present in Alzheimer brain is synthesized locally or whether it is made in other tissue and crosses an altered blood-brain barrier in Alzheimer's disease.

Neuritic plaques with amyloid cores are found in small number in the brains of some aged primates and other species. In contrast, NFT are uniquely found in the human brain. Within the NFT are accumulations of masses of PHF that have an extraordinary periodicity on electron micrographs; these structures are approximately 200 Å at their widest, narrowing to 100 Å with a periodicity of about 800 Å. Use of a tilting-stage electron microscope has suggested that these structures are composed of two filaments wound around each other in a helical structure. Computerized image analysis of electron micrographs has been interpreted as suggesting that the filament arises by the stacking of a subunit that lies transversely across the axis of the filament and has a short axial length.

The isolation and purification of the protein constituents of PHF have been difficult because of the insolubility of the PHF in ordinary protein solvents [25]. It is not difficult, however, to isolate from the Alzheimer brain subcellular fractions highly enriched in PHF; such fractions are highly antigenic. Moreover, one can raise antibodies to known cytoskeletal or fibrous proteins and test their antigenicity against NFT in tissue sections and against purified PHF fractions. There is now agreement that antibodies to the phosphorylated higher molecular weight neurofilament peptides, to microtubule-associated protein (MAP)-2, and to tau protein react both with NFT and with purified preparations of PHF. Monoclonal antibodies to tau protein react with NFT and PHF preparations, and antibodies to PHF isolates react with tau protein, suggesting that this is a consistent component of PHF. Normally, tau proteins are found in axons in white matter in adult brain, whereas in Alzheimer brain the tau protein is in the soma of the NFT. Tau protein is ordinarily soluble but can be polymerized under unusual conditions. At this time, it is uncertain whether the tau protein present in PHF preparations is associated with another peptide in the formation of the PHF.

With regard to cytoskeletal abnormalities, it should be noted that aggregations of tubulin are found in the granulovacuoles often seen in hippocampal neurons in the Alzheimer brain. The Hirano body, an elliptical eosinophilic structure sometimes present in Alzheimer hippocampus, has been shown to be made up of actin fibrils. The state of phosphorylation of these proteins has not been determined.

Other protein abnormalities

An additional abnormal protein present not only in NFT but also in other cells that may be undergoing atrophic changes in the Alzheimer brain has been named A-68 by Wolozin and colleagues [26]. This phosphorylated soluble protein is the antigen for an antibody, Alz-50, obtained from a series of antibodies raised to various subcellular fractions of Alzheimer brain nucleus basalis and selected on the basis of its success in differentiating Alzheimer from normal age-matched brain [26].

The presence in Alzheimer brain of abnormally phosphorylated cytoskeleton constituents is an intriguing finding. Neuronal soma normally contain nonphosphorylated neurofilaments, whereas in normal axons these proteins are often phosphorylated; in Alzheimer brain, NFT contain phosphorylated neurofilaments. There is preliminary data suggesting that the tau protein in NFT is highly phosphorylated. Saitoh and Dobkins have described an increase in phosphorylation of a 60-kilodalton protein and a decrease in protein kinase C activity in Alzheimer brain [27]. It may be speculated that an abnormality in phosphorylation plays a central role in the pathogenesis of the structural abnormalities present in Alzheimer's disease.

REFERENCES

1. Katzman, R. Alzheimer's disease. *N. Engl. J. Med.* 314:964–973, 1986.
2. Terry, R. D., and Katzman, R. Senile dementia of the Alzheimer's type. *Ann. Neurol.* 14:153–176, 1983.
3. Hyman, B. T., Van Hoesen, G. W., Damasio, A. R., Barnes, C. L. Alzheimer's disease: Cell-specific pathology isolates the hippocampal formation. *Science* 225:1168–1170, 1984.
4. Whitehouse, P. J., et al. Alzheimer's disease and senile dementia: Loss of neurons in the basal forebrain. *Science* 215:1237–1239, 1982.
5. Davies, P., and Verth, A. H. Selective loss of central cholinergic neurons in Alzheimer's disease. *Lancet* 2:1403, 1976.
6. Perry, E. K., et al. Correlation of cholinergic abnormalities with senile plaques and mental test scores in senile dementia. *Br. Med. J.* 2:1457–1459, 1978.
7. Davies, P., and Verth, A. H. Regional distribution of muscarinic acetylcholine receptor in normal and Alzheimer's type dementia brains. *Brain Res.* 138:385–392, 1977.
8. Johnston, M. V., McKinney, M., and Coyle, J. T. Evidence for a cholinergic projection to neocortex from neurons in basal forebrain. *Proc. Natl. Acad. Sci. U.S.A.* 76:5392–5396, 1979.
9. Bowen, D. M. Biochemical assessment of neurotransmitter and metabolic dysfunction and cerebral atrophy in Alzheimer's disease. In R. Katzman (ed.), *Banbury Report 15: Biological Aspects of Alzheimer's Disease.* New York: Cold Spring Harbor Laboratory, 1983, pp. 219–231.
10. Armstrong, D. M., et al. Choline acetyltransferase immunoreactivity in neuritic plaques of Alzheimer brain. *Neurosci. Lett.* 71:229–234, 1986.
11. Hyman, B. T., Van Hoesen, G. W., and Damasio, A. R. Alzheimer's disease: Glutamate depletion in the hippocampal perforant pathway zone. *Annu. Neurol.* 22:37–40, 1987.
12. Davies, P., Katzman, R., and Terry, R. D. Reduced somatostatin-like immunoreactivity in cerebral cortex from cases of Alzheimer disease and Alzheimer senile dementia. *Nature* 288:279–280, 1980.
13. Beal, M. F., et al. Somatostatin: Alterations in the central nervous system in neurological diseases. In J. B. Martin and J. D. Barchas (eds.), *Neuropeptides in Neurologic and Psychiatric Disease (Association for Research in Nervous and Mental Disease, Vol. 64).* New York: Raven Press, 1986, pp. 215–258.
14. Morrison, J. H., et al. Somatostatin immunoreactivity in neuritic plaques of Alzheimer's patients. *Nature* 314:90–92, 1985.
15. Bissette, G., et al. Corticotropin-releasing factor-like immunoreactivity in senile dementia of the Alzheimer type. Reduced cortical and striatal concentrations. *JAMA* 254:3067–3069, 1985.
16. Katzman, R., et al. Significance of neurotransmitter abnormalities in Alzheimer's disease. In J. B. Martin and J. D. Barchas (eds.), *Neuropeptides in Neurologic and Psychiatric Disease (Association for Research in Nervous and Mental Disease, Vol. 64).* New York: Raven Press, 1986, pp. 279–286.
17. Friedland, R. P., Budinger, T. F., Koss, E., and Ober, B. A. Alzheimer's disease: Anterior-posterior and lateral hemispheric alterations in cortical glucose utilization. *Neurosci. Lett.* 53:235–240, 1985.
18. Haxby, J. V., et al. Neocortical metabolic abnormalities precede nonmemory cognitive deficits in early Alzheimer's-type dementia. *Arch. Neurol.* 43:882–885, 1986.

19. Glenner, G. C., and Wong, C. W. Alzheimer's disease: Initial report of the purification and characterization of a novel cerebrovascular amyloid protein. *Biochem. Biophys. Res. Commun.* 122:1131–1135, 1964.

20. Tanzi, R. E., et al. The genetic defect in familial Alzheimer's disease is not tightly linked to the amyloid β-protein gene. *Nature* 329:156–157, 1987. [letter].

21. St. George-Hyslop, P. H., et al. The genetic defect causing familial Alzheimer's disease maps on chromosome 21. *Science* 235:885–890, 1987.

22. Kang, J., et al. The precursor of Alzheimer's disease amyloid A4 protein resembles a cell-surface receptor. *Nature* 325:733–736, 1987.

23. Kitaguchi, N., Takahashi, Y., Tokushima, Y., Shiojiri, S., and Hirataka, I. Novel precursor of Alzheimer's disease amyloid protein shows protease inhibitory activity. *Nature* 331:530–532, 1988.

24. Schubert, D., Schroeder, R., LaCorbiere, M., Saitoh, T., and Cole, G. Amyloid β-protein precursor is possibly a heparan sulfate proteoglycan core protein. *Science* 241:223–241, 1988.

25. Selkoe, D. J., Ihara, Y., and Salazar, F. J. Alzheimer's disease: Insolubility of partially purified paired helical filaments in sodium dodecyl sulfate and urea. *Science* 215:1243–1245, 1982.

26. Wolozin, B. L., Pruchnicki, A., Dickson, D. W., and Davies, P. A neuronal antigen in the brains of Alzheimer patients. *Science* 232:648–650, 1986.

27. Saitoh, T., and Dobkins, K. Increased *in vitro* phosphorylation of a M_r 60,000 protein in brain from patients with Alzheimer's disease. *Proc. Natl. Acad. Sci. U.S.A.* 83:9764–9767, 1986.

CHAPTER **44**

Positron Emission Tomography

Kirk A. Frey

Basic Neurochemistry: Molecular, Cellular, and Medical Aspects, 4th Ed., edited by G. J. Siegel et al. Raven Press, Ltd., New York, 1989.
Correspondence to Kirk A. Frey, Mental Health Research Institute, The University of Michigan, Ann Arbor, Michigan 48109-0720.

839

In vivo determinations of biochemical and physiologic processes have provided unique insights into the integrated functioning of the central nervous system. Approaches to the study of brain function that rely on the use of intact experimental subjects are of particular value for several reasons. First, the metabolic relationships between the brain and its vascular supply represent highly regulated and dynamic processes. Interruption of the supply of metabolic fuels to the brain results in rapid alteration of both behavior and cerebral metabolism. Second, the blood-brain barrier, acting as a filter, regulates the entry and exit of fuels and metabolites. In many instances, compounds that could be utilized by the brain as sources of energy are excluded from entry. Other substances with neurotransmitter and neuromodulatory activity in brain are also excluded; thus, the barrier contributes to regulation of the neuronal microenvironment. Finally, there exists a diverse regional heterogeneity in the populations of neurons, both with regard to their transmitter specificities and their interconnections. *In vitro* biochemical methods that utilize tissue slices, homogenates, or subcellular fractions, are generally unsatisfactory for the study of the human diseases that result from disruption of these metabolic relationships. Positron emission tomography (PET) represents an important bridge between *in vitro* and *in vivo* biochemical measures of cerebral function. It is a noninvasive method in which radiotracers are injected into the bloodstream, and their distribution in the brain is subsequently measured by external detectors. Because of the low radiation doses associated with PET, it can be safely applied in clinical research, allowing the direct study of human neurological disease. This chapter provides an overview of PET methods and their applications (see Phelps et al. [1] for review).

METHODS IN POSITRON EMISSION TOMOGRAPHY

Positron-emitting tracers are used to produce maps of radioactivity distribution in brain

Positron-emitting nuclides share unique physical properties that permit great flexibility and sensitivity in the design of tracer distribution experiments. Isotopes used frequently in PET research allow a variety of radiochemical approaches to ligand synthesis. Of particular importance, isotopes of carbon and nitrogen may be directly substituted, and ^{18}F can be substituted for hydrogen or a hydroxyl substituent in many compounds without loss of bioactivity. Because the isotopes used have short half-lives (Table 1), a cyclotron dedicated for nuclide production and methods for rapid radiochemical synthesis are required. A significant advantage, however, is the limited radiation exposure of patients receiving imaging doses of positron radiopharmaceuticals, since most of the administered activity decays during the study.

Positron decay

The mode of positron decay is particularly advantageous for detection and quantification by external measurement. The decay process involves the nucleus of a neutron-deficient isotope in which there is conversion of a proton to

TABLE 1. Physical properties of positron-emitting nuclides and annihilation photons

Nuclide	Half-life (min)	Energy (meV)	Maximum range (mm H_2O)
^{11}C	20.4	0.97	4.1
^{13}N	9.96	1.20	5.4
^{15}O	2.04	1.74	8.2
^{18}F	110	0.64	2.4
Positron annihilation photons	—	0.511	7,000[a]

[a] Half-value distance.

a neutron with simultaneous emission of a positron from the nucleus [2]. The positron is identical to an electron in physical properties except that it is positively rather than negatively charged. The positron is slowed by loss of energy along its path and ultimately combines with an electron. This reaction, *positron annihilation*, results in disintegration of both the positron and the electron, with the simultaneous emission of energy equivalent to their combined mass of 1.022 meV. The emitted energy is in the form of two γ rays (photons with energies of 511 keV) that travel in opposite directions.

Photons, unlike positrons, undergo relatively little interaction with surrounding materials of low density; they are not deflected from their course and are readily detected at a distance outside the body. Because of the simultaneous emission of the two photons in exactly opposite directions, coincidence-detection algorithms for quantitation of positron decay are employed, resulting in images with a high signal-to-noise ratio.

Detection of positron-emitting tracer and construction of images

Detection of positron decay for brain imaging purposes utilizes multiple detectors arranged in one or more rings surrounding the head. Each ring consists of individual detectors, each of which is paired with an oppositely placed detector by the scanner electronics. Each pair of detectors identifies positron annihilation events along the line (ray) connecting them in space. A transverse section image of the distribution of radioactivity within the head is created from the accumulated coincidence counts from each ring. The pair of detectors registering a coincidence defines the ray along which the positron annihilation occurred. Tomographic techniques analogous to those utilized in X-ray computed tomography are used to reconstruct the image from the rays. Many PET scanners consist of multiple rings, allowing simultaneous acquisi-

tion of data from adjacent levels in the brain. In these cases, pairs of detectors on opposing sides of neighboring rings may be used to identify activity from the tissue between two neighboring rings. These images, termed cross planes, account for the greater number of tissue slices obtained than actual detector rings with multi-ringed scanners. For example, a three-ring scanner can produce five tomographic images simultaneously.

Several correction factors are applied to the PET data during the reconstruction of the images. The photon counts from each detector are corrected for underestimation errors arising from events missed because of detector and electronic limitations at high counting rates. In addition, overestimation errors in coincidence detections due to random coincidence of single counts at high count rates are subtracted. Each detector pair is corrected for sensitivity by scanning a standard source of known activity on a regular basis. Finally, the coincidence counts from each ray are corrected for attenuation of the emitted 511 keV photons within the body. This correction is based either on direct measurement of attenuation with an external radiation source of known activity, or by assuming approximate densities for the tissues within the field of view.

Resolution of PET images

The resulting PET images are spatial maps of radioactivity distribution within tissue slices, and are thus analogous to autoradiograms obtained from brain tissue in animal experiments. The PET method, however, has an important distinction: It is noninvasive and may thus be used in clinical research, including longitudinal studies. A second difference between PET methods and tissue autoradiography is in anatomic resolution. Typical film autoradiographic methods for detection of ^{3}H or ^{14}C provide 50- to 100-μm resolution, allowing clear separation of most brain nuclei from surrounding fiber tracts. The spatial resolution inherent in current PET scans is approximately 7 to 15 mm, resulting from a combination of limitations. The number and geometry of detectors in the scanner as well as the number of counts acquired in the image and their statistical precision, contribute substantially to PET image resolution. These factors vary between tomographs of different design as well as from study to study, due to varying image acquisition times and tissue radioactivity levels. The ultimate theoretical limit of PET resolution, however, is the distance traveled by the positron in tissue before the annihilation reaction. Maximum tissue ranges vary according to the initial energy of the positron (Table 1). As a consequence of limited spatial resolution, small nuclear regions and thin laminar structures such as cortex cannot be completely separated from surrounding tissues and cerebrospinal fluid. Reconstructed PET data thus reflect average isotope concentrations in the imaged tissue volume elements. When the actual tracer distribution is heterogeneous, but below the resolution of the scan, the data underestimate the highest and overestimate the lowest values due to this *partial volume averaging* effect.

PET imaging can generate a pictorial representation of a physiologic or biochemical process as it occurs regionally within the brain

Several basic conceptual elements are shared by the variety of PET methods developed and implemented to date. Most significantly, PET measures generally reflect the functional biochemistry and physiology of the brain in contrast to other imaging methods, such as X-ray computed tomography and magnetic resonance imaging, which excel in the demonstration of tissue structure. The functional nature of PET imaging confers flexibility in the application of PET to neurochemical analysis even though it

imposes constraints on the experimental design and data analysis.

To achieve the generation of functional or parametric images, several conditions must be satisfied by the chosen radiotracer imaging protocol and the data analysis. First, the process of interest must be precisely specified. Successful PET methods generally rely on a body of basic research experience to characterize the process and demonstrate the biochemical and physiologic significance, regulation, and potential pathologic alterations that may be encountered. Next, a tracer appropriate for the application must be identified. Tracer properties, including biochemical and physiologic specificity, ease of synthesis with a positron-emitting nuclide, and metabolic stability, are important factors in the selection of radiotracers. Third, a physiologic compartmental model describing tracer distribution and the factors governing the movement of tracer between compartments must be developed [3]. It is the mathematical representation of this model that ultimately permits calculation of a parametric image from PET data.

Finally, the tracer and model must be tested and validated. Studies in experimental animals are utilized to verify the chemical identity of the radioactivity. Kinetic studies are performed under experimental pathologic situations, i.e., brain lesions and pharmacologic treatments, which have predictable effects on the model and the parameter of interest. At any point along this path of development it may be necessary to revise the model or the method. In some instances, the model must be abandoned altogether or a new tracer selected.

It must be additionally remembered that this preliminary work does not guarantee the accuracy of measurements in clinical research applications. Some diseases may cause unforeseen alterations in brain metabolism that invalidate the model and tracer utilized. Thus, understanding the key assumptions, simplifications, and metabolic relationships involved in

PET tracer methods is essential to the interpretation of images.

PHYSIOLOGIC AND BIOCHEMICAL MEASUREMENTS USING PET

The simplest brain parameter measured with PET is blood volume

The model describing the distribution of blood volume markers consists of a tissue volume element with the intravascular space contained in it representing the only compartment for tracer distribution (Fig. 1B). It is assumed that the tracer enters and leaves the tissue by blood flow, but does not enter the extravascular space and is not metabolized. Carbon monoxide labeled with ^{15}O is inhaled in a single breath. Because of the high specific activity of the [^{15}O]CO, the trace chemical amount of gas administered is nontoxic. Following a brief period of mixing to allow the tracer to bind to hemoglobin and distribute evenly within the blood pool, a PET scan is obtained, and a sample of blood is taken simultaneously for measurement of the tracer concentration. The blood volume in tissue is then determined by dividing the tissue tracer concentration by the blood value.

Normal values for cerebral blood volume (CBV) range from 4 to 6 percent in gray matter and from 2 to 3 percent in white matter (Fig. 1A). Regions containing or adjacent to major arteries or venous sinuses have considerably larger values, owing to partial volume averaging with the vessels. Although the intravascular

FIG. 1. PET measurement of cerebral blood volume in normal human brain. **A**: PET images from adjacent 12-mm horizontal slices between the base of the brain (*upper left*) and the supraventricular level (*lower right*) following inhalation of [^{15}O]CO. Blood volume (ml/g tissue) is displayed according to the gray scale at the right. Major vessels are located on the surface of the brain. Note that extracerebral soft tissue blood volume generally exceeds values within the brain: (C) carotid artery; (J) jugular bulb; (M) middle cerebral artery; (SA) sagittal sinus; (SI) sigmoid sinus; (ST) straight sinus and vein of Galen. **B**: Compartmental model used for calculation of blood volume. Tracer is assumed to remain in the blood pool (B) during the study. The PET scanner views both the intravascular and extravascular tissue compartments, allowing calculation of the intravascular volume. (Images courtesy of L. Junck, Department of Neurology, University of Michigan, Ann Arbor.)

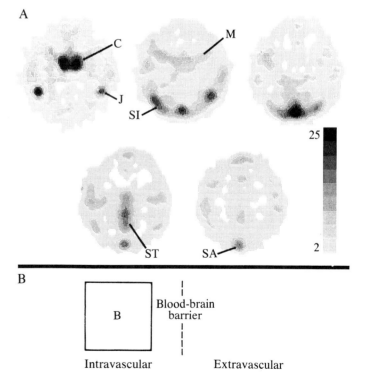

volume itself may occasionally be of interest, the most frequent application is the correction of studies with other tracers for intravascular activity. If the regional intravascular volume and arterial tracer concentrations are known, the measured total tissue activity may be corrected for the intravascular component. This technique is frequently employed in the determination of brain oxygen extraction and metabolism.

Measurement of blood-brain barrier permeability to a test substance utilizes a two-compartment model representing the intravascular and extravascular spaces

The movement of tracer into and out of the tissue volume element occurs by flow of blood, whereas capillary blood exchanges tracer with the tissue (see Chap. 30). Two model parameters are estimated following intravenous injection of the tracer. Arterial blood samples are used to determine the tracer input curve, and serial PET scans of the brain are obtained to define the regional tracer time-activity curves. The first of the parameters, K_1, represents uptake of the tracer by brain from the blood. It is related to both cerebral blood flow, F, and to the regional capillary surface area-permeability product, PS:

$$K_1 = F(1 - e^{-PS/F})$$

The second parameter, k_2, represents the movement of tracer back to the blood from the brain and is equivalent to K_1 divided by the tracer distribution volume in brain. Selection of tracers with appropriate properties allows direct determination of regional permeability using this model. Specifically, for tracers with very low permeability ($F \gg PS$), $K_1 \sim PS$. In addition, tracers with very large distribution volumes in brain allow k_2 to be neglected early, simplifying estimation of K_1. Tracers satisfying

the former condition include ^{82}Rb [4] and [^{68}Ga]EDTA [5]. A tracer satisfying both conditions, aminoisobutyric acid, has been utilized in animal experiments labeled with ^{14}C; however, a positron-labeled analog has yet to be developed.

Determination of regional blood-brain barrier permeability is used primarily when a pathologic increase is anticipated. Measurements in brain tumor and in brain infarction (stroke) have verified the abnormally permeable capillary beds known qualitatively from contrast-enhanced X-ray computerized tomography (CT) scanning. PET methods, however, allow calculation of the permeability coefficient. This allows quantitation of the effects of steroid treatment on blood-brain barrier permeability as well as estimation of regional brain exposure to potential chemotherapeutic agents. Measurement of blood-brain barrier permeability is additionally helpful in excluding potential sources of error from other PET methods, which may be complicated by breakdown of the barrier. Blood-brain barrier permeability to tracers that enter brain readily may be calculated from estimates of their initial uptake combined with independent measurement of regional blood flow according to the relationship given for K_1 above. This may be of benefit in defining the relative flow and permeability contributions to tracer uptake, permitting better understanding of the tracer kinetic model and its sensitivity to pathologic blood flow and blood-brain barrier changes.

Determination of regional cerebral blood flow is a frequently employed PET method

The modeling of cerebral blood flow (CBF) tracer distribution is identical to that presented for blood-brain barrier permeability measurements discussed previously. The tissue volume element consists of two tracer distribution compartments, the intravascular and extravascular spaces (Fig. 2C). The influx rate constant, K_1, is directly proportional to blood flow when the tracer has very high blood-brain barrier permeability, i.e., $PS \gg F$. Under these conditions, two parameters, K_1 and k_2 are estimated for each tissue volume element; K_1 represents regional CBF, whereas K_1/k_2 is the regional tracer distribution volume. The CBF tracer may be introduced into the circulation either by inhalation or by intravenous injection. Data collected consist of serial PET scans of the brain and the arterial input curve to the brain, approximated from measurement of tracer activity in arterial blood samples [6,7].

Several tracers have been employed for CBF measurement, each of which has relative advantages and disadvantages. Initial CBF measurements were made with [^{13}N]NH$_3$ be-

cause of its ease of synthesis; however, NH$_3$ is not inert in cerebral tissue, is restricted from complete equilibration with brain at high normal CBF rates, and its uptake and distribution are affected by tissue and plasma pH and cerebral NH$_3$ metabolism. Thus, newer agents, including [^{15}O]H$_2$O and [^{11}C]butanol have replaced [^{13}N]NH$_3$. Water as a CBF tracer is attractive from the standpoint of easy synthesis, formulation, and injection, but like ammonia it is limited by blood-brain barrier permeability at the upper extremes of physiologic flow rates [11]. Butanol, by comparison, is not diffusion-limited, but is more difficult to synthesize, and the longer half-life of ^{11}C compared to ^{15}O results in greater radiation exposure for an equivalent injected dose.

PET values for CBF in normal individuals

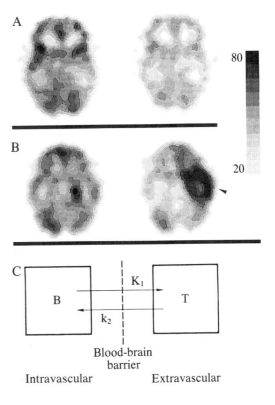

FIG. 2. PET measurement of cerebral blood flow. **A:** CBF determined following injection of [^{15}O]H$_2$O in a subject at rest (*left*) and again during hyperventilation (*right*). The images are at the low ventricular level, corresponding to the third image in Figs. 1, 3, and 4. Note the global reduction in CBF resulting from the decreased arterial CO$_2$ during hyperventilation. **B:** CBF in a subject with partial epilepsy determined at rest (interictal, *left*) and during a seizure (ictal, *right*) at the infraventricular level, corresponding to the second image in Figs. 1, 3, and 4. Note the local increase in CBF at the site of the seizure focus (*arrowhead*). CBF is displayed (ml blood/100 g tissue/min) according to the scale at the right. **C:** Compartmental model for CBF measurement. Two tracer compartments representing blood (B) and tissue (T) tracers are represented. (Images courtesy of B. Abou-Khalil, J. C. Sackellares, and G. J. Siegel, Department of Neurology, University of Michigan, Ann Arbor.)

average approximately 50 ml/min/100 g brain, in agreement with the results of global measures by the Kety-Schmidt arteriovenous difference method (see Chap. 29). Regional CBF values range from 40 to 100 in gray matter and from 15 to 30 in white matter structures (Fig. 2). The average ratio of gray to white matter for CBF in the resting state is approximately three to one with current PET techniques. This is somewhat less than the ratio of five or six to one obtained in autoradiographic animal experiments as a result of partial volume averaging in the PET measurements. The global CBF varies substantially with respiration due to the effect of arterial pCO_2 or pH on the cerebral vasculature (Fig. 2A) (see also Chap. 29). Near the physiologic pCO_2 of 40 mm Hg, CBF increases approximately 1 to 2 percent for each 1 mm Hg increase in pCO_2.

In addition to these global changes, regional CBF changes have been determined both as a result of physiologic activation of the brain and in cerebral pathology. Regional rates of oxidative metabolism are known to be sensitive to changes in neuronal activity (see below). Regional CBF has been reported to vary with metabolic rate in normal brain, presumably based on the need for delivery of metabolic substrates and clearance of metabolites, although the mechanism whereby CBF and metabolism are coupled remains obscure (see Chap. 29). The ease of measuring CBF and the ability to repeat the measure frequently under varying stimulus conditions have thus made CBF studies invaluable in indirectly localizing regions of altered cerebral function. In addition, several neuropathologic conditions are primarily related to altered CBF, and in these cases hypotheses can be tested directly with PET. Finally, CBF measurements contribute to the determination of other physiologic parameters, as in the determination of *PS* values for highly permeable tracers (see above) and in the calculation of the metabolic rate for oxygen (see below).

Regional cerebral glucose metabolism is imaged for the study of brain activity in vivo

Development of the method for determining regional cerebral metabolic rate for glucose (rCMRglu) and its validation in experimental animals [8] are discussed in detail in Chapter 29. The tracer kinetic model for glucose metabolism is more complex than the previously discussed examples due to an additional tissue compartment representing metabolized tracer (Fig. 3B). The model consists of intravascular tracer, a tissue precursor pool in exchange with blood, and a metabolic pool representing tracer that has been chemically transformed. The compartments are interrelated by rate constants K_1 and k_2, representing the exchange of tracer across the blood-brain barrier, and by k_3 and k_4, representing the rate of tracer phosphorylation by hexokinase and dephosphorylation by glucose-6-phosphatase, respectively. The tracers employed for measurement of rCMRglu are 2-deoxy-D-glucoses (2DG), glucose analogs that share transport and phosphorylation processes with the endogenous substrate but that are not appreciably further metabolized following formation of the 6-phosphate derivative. Thus, the 2DG tracers are useful in the determination of the rate of glucose phosphorylation by hexokinase but do not measure subsequent steps in glycolysis or in oxidative metabolism.

At present, two positron-emitting 2DGs are in use: [18F]2-fluoro-2-deoxy-D-glucose ([18F]2FDG) and [11C]2DG. The former tracer has the advantage of a longer half-life and is useful in situations where PET scans of high anatomic resolution and statistical precision at long times following injection are desired. The shorter half-life of [11C]2DG, conversely, is useful when multiple sequential studies on the same experimental subject, e.g., test-retest or baseline and stimulation protocols are planned, since the activity decays quickly enough to

FIG. 3. Regional cerebral glucose utilization in partial epilepsy. **A:** Interictal PET scans following injection of [18F]FDG in a patient with a right temporal lobe seizure focus. Note reduced rCMRglu ipsilateral to the focus (*arrowheads*). Scan levels correspond to those in Figs. 1 and 4. Glucose utilization (mg/100 g brain/min) is displayed according to the scale at the *lower right:* (CB) cerebellum; (CP) caudate and putamen; (F) frontal cortex; (O) occipital cortex; (P) parietal cortex; (PN) pons; (T) temporal cortex; (TH) thalamus; (W) white matter. **B:** Compartmental model for rCMRglu determination. Tracer compartments include DG in plasma (P) and in the extravascular precursor pool (E), as well as in the metabolic product pool (M), representing DG-6-phosphate. (Images courtesy of B. Abou-Khalil, J. C. Sackellares, and G. J. Siegel, Department of Neurology, University of Michigan, Ann Arbor.)

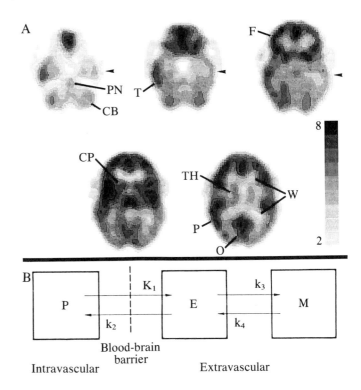

allow repeat tracer injections within 3 to 4 hr intervals.

Measurement of rCMRglu is initiated by the intravenous injection of the labeled DG, followed by the collection of timed arterial blood samples for measurement of the tracer input curve [9,10]. The most commonly employed procedure is to obtain PET brain images beginning 30 to 45 min following the injection, at which time the bulk of the activity represents metabolized tracer. These data, combined with the arterial input function, are analyzed according to a modified version of the operational equation of Sokoloff (see Chap. 29). The calculation of rCMRglu by this procedure relies on the use of population average values of the individual rate constants and the lumped constant. The single-scan protocol is thus analogous to the autoradiographic method employed in the determination of rCMRglu using β-par-

ticle-emitting 2DG tracers in experimental animals.

Under a variety of pathologic conditions, some or all of the assumptions about the rate and lumped constants may be invalidated either globally or regionally, leading to inaccuracies in the estimates of rCMRglu provided by the single scan approach [11,12]. In particular, disruption of the normal relationship and coupling between blood flow and energy metabolism may occur in ischemic states. Wide fluctuations from the normal range of blood glucose concentrations have additionally been demonstrated to produce such alterations. In these circumstances, an alternative experimental protocol involving repeated measurements of tracer distribution may be applied [13]. Serial PET scans are obtained beginning immediately following the injection and ending 45 to 90 min later. The tissue and blood time activity curves are then fitted to the compartmental model by nonlinear least squares approximation, defining optimal values for the rate constants. The rate of 2DG "metabolism" (rCMRdg) is given by

$$rCMRdg = K_1 k_3 / (k_2 + k_3)$$

and the glucose metabolic rate by

$$rCMRglu = C_p \, rCMRdg / LC$$

where C_p represents the arterial plasma glucose concentration, and LC is the lumped constant relating deoxyglucose to glucose metabolism. Using this kinetic approach, the calculated rCMRglu continues to be influenced by the value of LC but is independent of errors introduced by the application of inappropriate rate constants for 2DG transport and metabolism.

Measurements of CMRglu in normal individuals at rest yield average rates for whole brain of approximately 6 mg/100 g brain/min (Fig. 3). This is well within the range of values reported using arteriovenous differences, which is between 4.5 and 6.5 mg/100 g brain/min. The rCMRglu in normal brain varies between 5 and 11 mg/100 g brain/min in gray matter and between 2 and 5 mg/100 g brain/min in white matter. These values demonstrate less range than autoradiographic animal studies in which seven- to eightfold differences between gray and white matter regions are seen. This, again, is a result of inherent volume averaging at the PET level of anatomic resolution.

The measurement of rCMRglu has gained wide application in the study of both normal physiologic activity and pathologic processes, based on the observed relationship between functional neuronal activity and energy metabolism [14]. This relationship has been demonstrated elegantly through a variety of physiologic activation and suppression procedures in both experimental animals and in normal human volunteers. Results of animal studies suggest that the coupling of metabolism to neuronal ac-

tivity is due to the increased transmembrane ionic conductances associated with synaptic transmission (see Chaps. 3 and 29). In general, areas of dense synaptic content within neuropil show the highest regional rates of metabolism and respond most dramatically to alterations in neuronal activity. White matter is less active or reactive when studied at high anatomic resolution by autoradiography in animals. It should be kept in mind that both pre- and postsynaptic terminals participate in functional metabolic responses, and in some instances, the effect of increased neuronal firing may be detected only in distant terminal fields of the activated neurons rather than in the regions of the cell bodies themselves [15]. Thus, under some circumstances, the metabolic response to a change in activity within a particular brain region may be detected in remote brain regions receiving its efferent projections.

Applications of PET rCMRglu measurements include primary investigation of cerebral metabolism and the relationships between glucose and oxygen metabolism. In addition, primary disturbances in substrate delivery, as in ischemia, and in metabolic activity, as in metabolic coma, may be directly investigated. Regional glucose metabolism has most frequently been utilized as a tool for localizing alterations in neuronal activity as a consequence of physiologic stimulation. Here, changes in metabolism reveal the locations of altered neuronal activity resulting from changes in behavioral states or from pathologic processes.

Inhalation of [^{15}O]oxygen allows measurement of regional cerebral oxygen metabolic rate

The regional rate of cerebral oxygen metabolism represents one of two PET methods discussed here that cannot be determined in experimental animals by alternative techniques. The known radioisotopes of oxygen are all extremely short-lived and are thus of little use in conventional biochemical research, since the activity decays too rapidly to allow measurement in dissected tissue samples. The longest-lived oxygen isotope, ^{15}O (half-life, 2.04 min), administered as $[^{15}O]O_2$, has been successfully employed in the measurement of oxygen metabolism by means of PET. Two methods of administration of the agent by inhalation have been described. They rely on a simple two-compartment model of O_2 distribution in which intravascular and extravascular spaces are represented. It is assumed that $^{15}O_2$ in arterial blood is predominantly bound to hemoglobin with a smaller dissolved fraction. During capillary transit, $^{15}O_2$ enters the tissue, where it is rapidly metabolized to $[^{15}O]H_2O$. The labeled water then exchanges with the intravascular compartment. Peripheral metabolism also results in production of $[^{15}O]H_2O$, which recirculates in arterial blood to the brain and must be taken into account. Oxygen metabolism is thus defined as the product of regional oxygen extraction and arterial oxygen delivery:

$$rCMRO_2 = E \times C_a \times rCBF$$

where C_a represents arterial oxygen content; rCBF is regional cerebral blood flow; and E is the fraction of available oxygen extracted during a single capillary transit.

The methods employed are a continuous inhalation protocol with a single-scan determination of regional $^{15}O_2$ extraction [16] or a kinetic multiple scan approach following single-breath inhalation of $^{15}O_2$ [17]. Both methods require arterial blood sampling for determination of O_2 content, $^{15}O_2$, and $[^{15}O]H_2O$. In addition, independent measurement of rCBF, usually with $[^{15}O]H_2O$, is required. Finally, because of the substantial contribution of intravascular activity to the total tissue activity, correction for intravascular volume using $[^{15}O]CO$ is frequently employed.

Results of measurements in normal volunteers indicate resting $CMRO_2$ rates of 1.8 to 5.8 ml O_2/100 g brain/min (70–230 μmol O_2/100 g brain/min) in white and gray matter, respectively. Applications of PET $CMRO_2$ measurements are similar to those discussed above for CMRglu.

The determination of regional ligand binding from *in vivo* tracer distribution has been a long-anticipated development in PET

The kinetic ligand binding model consists of four tracer compartments [18] (Fig. 4). The intravascular compartment communicates with the free ligand pool in the tissue by the rate constants K_1 and k_2, which represent exchange across the blood-brain barrier. The extravascular space contains three tracer compartments: Free ligand; nonspecifically bound ligand; and receptor, or specifically bound ligand. The rate constant k_3 describes specific binding of the ligand to free receptors, and k_4 represents the dissociation of specifically bound ligand. Exchange of free ligand with nonspecific (assumed to be nonsaturable) binding sites in tissue is represented by k_5 and k_6.

The relationship between the kinetic rate constants and the receptor pharmacologic terms k_{on}, k_{off}, K_D, and B_{max} is:

$$k_3 = k_{on}R = k_{on}(B_{max} - RL)$$

$$k_4 = k_{off}$$

where $B_{max} = R + RL$; $K_D = k_{off}/k_{on}$; k_{on} and k_{off} are rate constants for ligand binding to and dissociation from the receptor; B_{max} is the total number of receptor sites; R represents free receptors available for binding; and RL represents receptors occupied by ligand (see also Chap. 9). Even under true tracer conditions in PET studies where radioligand occupies an insignificant number of the total receptor sites, B_{max} and R may be nonidentical, owing to receptor occupancy by endogenous neurotransmitter. Thus,

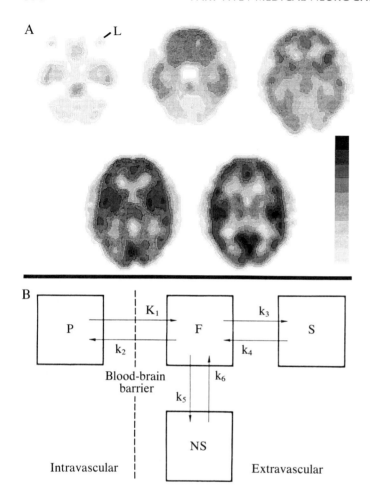

FIG. 4. Muscarinic receptor imaging in normal human brain using [^{11}C]scopolamine. **A**: PET images of scopolamine distribution 90 min following injection are shown at levels corresponding to those in Figs. 1 and 3. Images reflect predominantly specific binding of scopolamine at this time postinjection and are displayed qualitatively with darker areas reflecting higher tracer concentrations. Note that the pattern of receptor labeling differs substantially from CBF and CMRglu (Figs. 2 and 3). The cerebellum demonstrates lower, and the pons greater, binding than their relative metabolic rates. Receptors in the lacrimal glands (L, *upper left*) are visualized. (See Fig. 3 for anatomic correlation.) **B**: Compartmental model describing receptor-ligand distribution. Ligand in plasma (P) exchanges with free tissue ligand (F) across the blood-brain barrier. Extravascular tracer consists of free ligand, nonspecifically bound ligand (NS), and specifically bound ligand (S).

the kinetic receptor binding method determines the product of the binding association rate and the free receptor density ($k_{on}R$) rather than the total receptor number (B_{max}) measured by *in vitro* methods.

In practice, a ligand is injected intravenously, and arterial blood samples are withdrawn for determination of the arterial input function. Unlike most of the previously described PET methods, blood radioactivity measurements must be corrected for the presence of labeled metabolites produced *in vivo* in order to define the input curves properly. Sequential PET scans of the brain are obtained, and the

resulting tracer time courses in tissue and the arterial blood curve are analyzed by nonlinear least squares fitting to provide estimates of the model parameters.

The range of ligand binding sites that may be studied in this way is potentially as varied as the tracers for their study. It is feasible to measure cerebral dopamine, opiate, serotonin, benzodiazepine, and muscarinic cholinergic receptors. In addition, enzyme activity may be determined by using similar modeling assumptions, as demonstrated by the imaging of brain monoamine oxidases [19]. The selection of ligands for receptor measurement is a key step in the successful development of *in vivo* binding techniques, and places greater restriction on the properties of an acceptable tracer than *in vitro* binding situations. First, the selected ligand must have a high specificity for a single receptor type or subtype. In addition, the use of antagonist drugs is preferred, since antagonist binding is more closely described by the simple association and dissociation reactions assumed in the model than is the binding of agonists. Finally, the labeled ligand must not be metabolized within the brain or converted outside the brain to labeled metabolites that enter the brain and complicate interpretation of the tissue activity curves.

Applications of *in vivo* receptor ligand binding methods are potentially diverse, ranging from studies of disease- or therapy-related alterations in the numbers of binding sites to dynamic tests of synaptic function. The latter possibility is based on measurement of changes in free receptor sites caused by altered levels of endogenous neurotransmitter. Thus, either physiologic or pharmacologic challenges that alter presynaptic activity or modify binding of the endogenous transmitter may indirectly produce changes in the radioligand binding to the receptor sites. A baseline receptor scan followed by a repeat study with such an activation procedure may thus serve to identify the integrity of presynaptic terminals. In addition, the regional receptor occupancies accompanying the use of therapeutic doses of direct receptor agonist or antagonist drugs may be determined by repeat ligand binding scans before and after a dose of the unlabeled agent.

CLINICAL APPLICATION OF CEREBRAL PET

The clinical use of cerebral PET techniques has been limited to research protocols because of the expense of PET and the limited number of centers with PET capabilities. The high cost, $1000 per session at most centers, is based on the need for a team of individuals that includes cyclotron operators, radiochemists, nuclear medicine technologists, and physicians to accomplish the study. In addition to the labor-intensive aspects of PET methods, a dedicated cyclotron and computer for image acquisition, reconstruction, and calculation of the parametric images are essential. In recognition of this limitation, PET has been most frequently used to answer fundamental questions about the pathophysiology of human diseases and their regional distribution. These results then have broad implications for other patients with these disorders and may ultimately influence clinical diagnostic and therapeutic decisions without the need for performing PET in each individual. Such studies may additionally localize and characterize physiologic and biochemical abnormalities previously unrecognized, directing subsequent research with more conventional methods.

Many of the degenerative neurological disorders have chronic clinical courses but may respond symptomatically to pharmacological treatment. Thus, postmortem biochemical analysis of the brain in these cases may be influenced by the effect of medication or the effect of chronic systemic disease, or both. PET is of particular value in these instances, providing a noninvasive alternative to brain biopsy or other less direct approaches, such as cerebrospinal fluid analysis. Examples of diseases under study in this manner include Alzheimer's disease, Huntington's disease, and Parkinson's disease. An alternative goal in PET research is the identification of clinical disease markers or responses to therapy that might be extrapolated to the subsequent diagnosis or treatment of an entire patient population. In these instances, we seek predictive correlation between PET measures and results of routinely available and less costly diagnostic tests. Examples of such applications include the study of drug distribution and action, brain tumor response to therapy and studies on the biochemistry and physiology of cerebrovascular disease. Examples of these approaches are presented.

PET studies of epilepsy show the locations of seizure foci

Although idiopathic epilepsy is one of the most frequently encountered human neurologic disorders, the underlying pharmacologic, metabolic and electrophysiologic abnormalities are largely unknown. Medically intractable seizures are frequently associated with epileptogenic foci in the temporal lobes (see Chap. 41).

The first results of PET in partial epilepsy revealed an unanticipated abnormality in the interictal, or between seizure, metabolic pattern [20] (Fig. 3). The presumed site of the seizure focus showed decreased rather than increased blood flow and glucose metabolic rate. In over two-thirds of patients, a well-lateralized zone of hypometabolism is identified. When present, the hypometabolic zone correlates with the location of the seizure focus as determined by ictal depth EEG recording in greater than 90 percent of cases. During ictal discharge the zone of hypometabolism is replaced by a relatively hypermetabolic area that frequently extends beyond the limits of the interictal abnormality.

The etiology of interictal hypometabolism has yet to be established; however, several hypotheses have been proposed that may individually or collectively account for the phenomenon. Hypometabolism may result from active inhibition of neuronal activity; from loss of neurons or simplification of synaptic architecture; or from gross structural atrophy, or partial volume artifact. The frequent finding of mesial temporal sclerosis, consisting of loss of neurons with glial hypertrophy affecting the hippocampus in surgically resected epileptogenic temporal lobes lends support to the proposed structural mechanisms [21]. More recent observations suggest that the lateral temporal neocortex ipsilateral to the seizure focus displays a greater degree of metabolic depression, although histologic abnormalities in these areas are not recognized. Thus, metabolic abnormalities extend beyond known structural pathology to support the involvement of functional connections between the seizure focus and the lateral cortical regions [22].

The coexistence of both hypometabolism and ictal depth EEG localization is a reliable predictor of good surgical response in seizure control. Placement of depth electrodes is an invasive procedure with an associated morbidity. Hence, development of the noninvasive marker for the presence and extent of a unilateral seizure focus that is amenable to surgical resection and for the localization of the focus is a useful advance. Magnetic resonance imaging (MRI) may be preferable when a structural lesion other than mesial temporal sclerosis is present, whereas PET may be more sensitive in detecting sclerotic lesions. Thus, the combination of MRI and PET studies may become routine in the preoperative evaluation of intractable seizures, eliminating the need for invasive monitoring in most cases.

Several aspects of the underlying pharmacology and physiology of the epileptogenic focus remain to be examined by future PET studies. The development of PET receptor binding methods may allow identification of changes in the focus that account for the abnormal excitability of the neurons as well as for the lack of efficacy of conventional anticonvulsants in cases of intractable epilepsy. The studies reported to date have described patients with well-established epilepsy who are generally taking at least one anticonvulsant medication at the time of study. Some of the observed metabolic changes may thus relate either to effects of repeated seizures or medications, or both. Future studies focusing on new-onset seizures in unmedicated patients will allow distinctions among pathogenetic mechanisms, therapeutic effects, and secondary changes resulting from repeated seizures.

PET studies in cerebrovascular disease show the evolution of metabolic and blood flow changes in ischemic brain

The diagnosis and management of patients with cerebrovascular insufficiency is problematic in the clinical neurosciences. The factors that lead to cerebral ischemia are numerous, and there are various methods proposed for its diagnosis and management. Potential therapeutic modalities for ischemic cerebrovascular disease include vascular surgery; anticoagulation, or inhibition of platelet aggregation; and cerebral protection with antioxidant or metabolic inhibiting agents. Prior to the use of PET, the pathophysiologic evolution from ischemic to infarcted brain in human stroke was unknown. Although animal models of stroke have permitted biochemical and physiologic measurements, the relevance to human cerebrovascular disease is controversial (see also Chap. 40).

Several PET studies of completed stroke have examined the evolution of changes in infarcted regions as well as in the surrounding brain. It was demonstrated by using [^{18}F]2FDG and [^{13}N]NH$_3$ that glucose metabolism and blood flow become uncoupled in the course of ischemic infarction [23]. Very early after onset of symptoms, within days, regions of reduced blood flow and relatively preserved metabolic activity are observed. Within the first 2 weeks, these regions become relatively hyperemic with sustained glucose metabolism. In chronic lesions that appear atrophic on CT scans, a relatively matched metabolic and perfusion deficit is observed. A subsequent study of stroke using measures of oxygen metabolism and blood flow [24] revealed an early rise in regional oxygen extraction in the ischemic area that resolves over the first week, becoming hypometabolic, as originally observed with [^{18}F]2FDG. Serial determinations of both oxygen and glucose metabolism in the same patients have identified an abnormal relationship in the infarcted regions. The usual coupling ratio of 6 mol O$_2$/mol glucose

oxidized was found to be reduced to 2/3, indicating that anaerobic glycolysis or oxidation of alternative substrates occurs in recent cerebral infarction [25]. Studies in experimental animals have revealed that the appearance of phagocytic cells in infarcted brain is associated with non-neuronal metabolic activity [15]. Thus, the clinical observation of altered oxygen/glucose stoichiometry in early cerebral infarction may reflect that of inflammatory cells rather than viable brain tissue.

Other PET studies in cerebrovascular disease have focused on the pathophysiologic changes in ischemic but uninfarcted brain [26]. Patients with occlusive disease of the major cerebral arteries have varied blood flow and metabolic abnormalities. Thus, some patients with adequate collateral circulation may demonstrate no abnormality of CBF, CBV, or oxygen extraction. Patients with compensated disease generally show increased CBV but normal flow on the basis of vasodilation distal to the stenotic lesion. Patients with recurrent ischemic symptoms who have inadequate compensatory reserve demonstrate normal oxygen metabolism but have a decreased CBF and increased CBV and oxygen extraction. The latter parameter appears to be the most sensitive and specific marker for inadequate perfusion to meet metabolic demands.

The findings in stroke as well as those in noninfarct cerebrovascular insufficiency suggest a continuum of pathologic alterations with physiologic compensation by vasodilation and collateral circulation. When the metabolic demands of the tissue can no longer be met by increasing the extraction of oxygen and glucose, infarction results. PET studies suggest that cerebral damage occurs rapidly and that possible interventive therapies must therefore be attempted before or soon after the onset of symptoms to be of potential benefit. The application of PET to future studies of cerebrovascular disease will probably focus on prospective monitoring to find changes occurring before or rapidly following onset of symptoms. The diagnostic probes that will distinguish reversible from irreversible ischemic changes and the potential effects of therapeutic intervention remain to be determined.

ACKNOWLEDGMENTS

The assistance of Drs. G. W. Dauth and R. A. Koeppe in the preparation of the figures is deeply appreciated. The author was supported in part by a DOE contract for development of PET techniques during preparation of this chapter.

REFERENCES

1. Phelps, M. E., Mazziotta, J. C., and Schelbert, H. R. (eds.). *Positron Emission Tomography and Autoradiography. Principles and Applications for the Brain and Heart.* New York: Raven Press, 1986.
2. Sorenson, J. A., and Phelps, M. E. *Physics in Nuclear Medicine,* 2nd ed. New York: Grune and Stratton, 1987.
3. Jacquez, J. A. *Compartmental Analysis in Biology and Medicine,* 2nd ed. Ann Arbor: University of Michigan, 1985.
4. Brooks, D. J., Beaney, R. P., Lammertsma, A. A., et al. Quantitative measurement of blood-brain barrier permeability using Rubidium-82 and positron emission tomography. *J. Cereb. Blood Flow Metab.* 4:535–545, 1984.
5. Hawkins, R. A., Phelps, M. E., Huang, S.-C., et al. A kinetic evaluation of blood-brain barrier permeability in human brain tumors with [68Ga]EDTA and positron computed tomography. *J. Cereb. Blood Flow Metab.* 4:507–515, 1984.
6. Huang, S.-C., Carson, R. E., Hoffman, E. J., et al. Quantitative measurement of local cerebral blood flow in humans by positron computed tomography and ^{15}O-water. *J. Cereb. Blood Flow Metab.* 3:141–153, 1983.
7. Herscovitch, P., Markham, J., and Raichle, M. E. Brain blood flow measured with intravenous $H_2^{15}O$. I. Theory and error analysis. *J. Nucl. Med.* 24:782–789, 1983.
8. Sokoloff, L., Reivich, M., Kennedy, C., et al. The [14C]deoxyglucose method for the measurement of local cerebral glucose utilization: Theory, procedure, and normal values in the conscious and anesthetized albino rat. *J. Neurochem.* 28:897–916, 1977.
9. Reivich, M., Kuhl, D., Wolf, A., et al. The [18F]fluorodeoxyglucose method for the measurement of local cerebral glucose utilization in man. *Circ. Res.* 44:127–137, 1979.
10. Phelps, M. E., Huang, S.-C., Hoffman, E. J., et al. Tomographic measurement of local cerebral glucose metabolic rate in humans with (F-18)2-fluoro-2-deoxy-D-glucose: Validation of method. *Ann. Neurol.* 6:371–388, 1979.
11. Hawkins, R. A., Phelps, M. E., Huang, S.-C., and Kuhl, D. E. Effect of ischemia on quantification of local cerebral glucose metabolic rate in man. *J. Cereb. Blood Flow Metab.* 1:37–51, 1981.
12. Crane, P. D., Pardridge, W. M., Braun, L. D., and Oldendorf, W. H. Kinetics of transport and phosphorylation of 2-fluoro-2-deoxy-D-glucose in rat brain. *J. Neurochem.* 40:160–167, 1983.
13. Heiss, W.-D., Pawlik, G., Herholz, K., et al. Regional kinetic constants and cerebral metabolic rate for glucose in normal human volunteers determined by dynamic positron emission tomography of [18F]2-fluoro-2-deoxy-D-glucose. *J. Cereb. Blood Flow Metab.* 4:212–223, 1984.
14. Sokoloff, L. Localization of functional activity in the central nervous system by measurement of glucose utilization with radioactive deoxyglucose. *J. Cereb. Blood Flow Metab.* 1:7–36, 1981.
15. Agranoff, B. W., and Frey, K. A. A regional metabolic contrast method for the study of brain pathology. *Ann. Neurol.* 15:S93–S97, 1984.
16. Frackowiack, R. S., Lenzi, G.-L., Jones, T., and Heather, J. D. Quantitative measurement of regional cerebral blood flow and oxygen metabolism in man using ^{15}O and positron emission tomography: Theory, procedure, and normal values. *J. Comp. Assist. Tomog.* 4:727–736, 1980.

17. Mintun, M. A., Raichle, M. E., Martin, W. R. W., and Herscovitch, P. Brain oxygen utilization measured with O-15 radiotracers and positron emission tomography. *J. Nucl. Med.* 25:17–187, 1984.
18. Frey, K. A., Hichwa, R. D., Ehrenkaufer, R. L. E., and Agranoff, B. W. Quantitative *in vivo* receptor binding III: Tracer kinetic modeling of muscarinic cholinergic receptor binding. *Proc. Natl. Acad. Sci. U.S.A.* 82:6711–6715, 1985.
19. Fowler, J. S., MacGregor, R. R., Wolf, A. P., et al. Mapping human brain monoamine oxidase A and B with ^{11}C-labeled suicide inactivators and PET. *Science* 235:481–485, 1987.
20. Kuhl, D. E., Engel, J., Jr., Phelps, M. E., and Selin, C. Epileptic patterns of cerebral metabolism and perfusion in humans determined by emission computed tomography of [18]FDG and [13]NH₃. *Ann. Neurol.* 8:348–360, 1980.
21. Engel, J., Jr., Brown, W. J., Kuhl, D. E., et al. Pathological findings underlying focal temporal lobe hypometabolism in partial epilepsy. *Ann. Neurol.* 12:518–528, 1982.
22. Abou-Khalil, B. W., Siegel, G. J., Hichwa, R. D., Sackellares, J. C., and Gilman, S. Topography of glucose metabolism in epilepsy of mesial temporal origin. *Ann. Neurol.* 18:151, 1985.
23. Kuhl, D. E., Phelps, M. E., Kowell, A. P., et al. Effects of stroke on local cerebral metabolism and perfusion: Mapping by emission computed tomography of [18]FDG and [13]NH₃. *Ann. Neurol.* 8:47–60, 1980.
24. Wise, R. J. S., Bernardi, S., Frackowiak, R. S. J., et al. Serial observations on the pathophysiology of acute stroke. The transition from ischaemia to infarction as reflected in regional oxygen extraction. *Brain* 106:197–222, 1983.
25. Wise, R. J. S., Rhodes, C. G., Gibbs, J. M., et al. Disturbance of oxidative metabolism of glucose in recent human cerebral infarcts. *Ann. Neurol.* 14:627–637, 1983.
26. Powers, W. J., Press, G. A., Grubb, R. L., et al. The effect of hemodynamically significant carotid artery disease on the hemodynamic status of the cerebral circulation. *Ann. Int. Med.* 106:27–35, 1987.

PART SIX

Behavioral Neurochemistry

CHAPTER 45

Biochemical Aspects of the Psychotic Disorders

Jack D. Barchas, Kym F. Faull, and Glen R. Elliott

Basic Neurochemistry: Molecular, Cellular, and Medical Aspects, 4th Ed., edited by G. J. Siegel et al. Raven Press, Ltd., New York, 1989. Correspondence to Jack D. Barchas, Nancy Pritzker Laboratory, Stanford University School of Medicine, 300 Pasteur Drive, Stanford, California 94305.

Psychosis is a term that has several distinct meanings in the mental health field: It can indicate that a mental illness is especially severe; alternatively, it can signify that a patient is unable to differentiate reliably between objective reality and subjective experience; or it can mean that a patient has a constellation of symptoms, including impaired reality testing, illogical thought processes, hallucinations, and delusions [1]. In this chapter, we discuss mental disorders encompassed by the latter definition, bearing in mind that psychotic disorders have many different forms and a variety of causes.

Psychotic disorders impose a crushing disability on humankind, a burden that would be even greater were it not for the discovery more than 30 years ago of remarkably effective medications that relieved many of the signs and symptoms. Unfortunately, many individuals still do not benefit from the presently available medications, and there remains the problem of undesirable side effects. Furthermore, the causes of most psychoses are still poorly understood.

A few psychotic disorders have known specific causes: Brain tumor, severe hormonal imbalance, and certain toxic chemicals or drugs, such as amphetamine and lysergic acid diethylamide (LSD) that are known to affect the brain. The most common and devastating psychotic disorders, however, are those that have no known cause. In this chapter, we focus on two diagnostic categories: (a) Schizophrenia, a disorder that occurs mainly in adults; and (b) autistic disorder, which typically begins during

infancy [2,3]. Other important psychotic disorders include certain paranoid states and the schizoaffective disorders, which combine aspects of schizophrenia with affective disorders. (As described in Chapter 46 on affective disorders, both depression and mania may also present with psychosis.)

CLINICAL ASPECTS OF SCHIZOPHRENIA

Schizophrenia is a disorder that begins in young persons and affects perception, thought, language, and behavior

Typically, the signs and symptoms of schizophrenia first appear in individuals between the ages of 15 and 35 years [4]. The form of presentation is variable. In some, it starts with a gradual withdrawal and increased introversion. They may begin to lose contact with friends, cease to have goals, and lose interest in prior pursuits that seemed reasonable and appropriate. Only gradually do others become aware that these individuals are also hearing voices; having delusions; and becoming increasingly difficult to understand because of bizarre, illogical thinking. In other cases, the onset of the disorder can be sudden, often following stress, such as the loss of a significant relationship, a transition in school, or entrance into military service. Cases that arise quickly may present a picture of overwhelming deterioration over the course of just a few days.

Most people strongly associate hallucinations with schizophrenia, but neither do they occur exclusively in schizophrenia nor is their presence a requirement for the diagnosis. Hallucinations refer to an inaccurate perception of incoming sensory information, for example, hearing voices when no one is there. Although auditory hallucinations are by far the most common type in schizophrenia, in which case they are usually in the form of voices talking to or about the individual, hallucinations can affect any of the senses. Hallucinations are usually intermittent, and, it is important to note, that they are characteristically perceived by the patient as coming from the outside world.

Delusions are another common component of schizophrenia. They are perhaps the most romanticized aspect of this disorder, forming the basis for many movie thrillers. Delusions, too, are varied but entail an unshakeable belief in something that is improbable or impossible, even in the face of strong contrary evidence. Typical delusions include belief in the possession of magical powers, or manipulation by others for complex but improbable reasons, or having a special destiny or purpose. For instance, an individual may become convinced that he can read the minds of those around him, or that others are reading his mind; or, a patient may insist that she is receiving messages through television commercials, affirming she is going to be the savior of the world. Although some delusions can be gratifying, many are frightening for the patients.

There are also emotional and cognitive changes associated with the schizophrenic state. Most common is a growing sense of confusion and uncertainty about the most routine matters. Although schizophrenics may experience a wide range of intense emotions, such as depression, elation, or anger, most actually have emotional "blunting," a term that refers to a reduced ability to feel and express emotion. As a result, they seem distant. Furthermore, the ability of such individuals to think logically and

convey their thoughts meaningfully can become so impaired that they become increasingly unable to make themselves understood and behave in bizarre and inappropriate ways, even as they become convinced that they hold the keys to vital eternal truths. The latter difficulties are disorders of thought, language, and communication. Rather than reflecting a "split" personality, schizophrenia may better be described as a "fractured" personality.

The possible signs and symptoms of schizophrenia are so numerous and disparate that it is unlikely that all come from a single causal factor. Therefore, biological researchers have attempted to identify clusters of related symptoms. The most common subtypes of the syndrome are defined on the basis of the most prominent symptoms: paranoid, catatonic, disorganized or hebephrenic, undifferentiated, and residual state. The paranoid form tends to start later in life and has a relatively good prognosis, with the personality reasonably intact. The catatonic type is rare, having stereotyped movements and a poor prognosis. The disorganized hebephrenic form is associated with incoherence of speech and silly giggling and also has a poor prognosis. Undifferentiated patients who account for the majority of patients, have a combination of symptoms. The residual state refers to the patient with no active delusions or hallucinations, but with a history of them and continued social dysfunction and strange behavior. Genetic studies have not suggested that specific forms of the disorder are transmitted within a family.

Particular attention recently has turned to the differentiation between type I and type II symptoms. Type I, or positive, symptoms include delusions, hallucinations, and thought disorder; type II, or negative, symptoms include affective flattening, apathy, and poverty of speech. One distinguishing feature between these types is that the former are far more likely to respond to available drug treatments than are the latter. For reasons described later in this chapter, researchers have postulated that type I symptoms are associated with changes in dopamine functioning in the mesolimbic system and that type II symptoms may result from intellectual impairment due to anatomical changes in the brain.

The long-term course of schizophrenia varies. Some patients have only one or a few acute episodes. The hallucinations and delusions that occur in the acute phase tend to disappear, and recovery may be complete. In other patients, acute episodes recur, and in still others, symptoms linger in a chronic condition. It is now clear that the more episodes an individual has, the greater the likelihood of lasting, unfavorable changes. Such changes may be as subtle as a loss of enthusiasm and emotional responsiveness or as pronounced as deteriorated social skills and a complete loss of ambition.

Over the past decade, increasing diagnostic rigor has tended to identify a group of individuals who have many signs and symptoms of schizophrenia and are quite ill. Only about 20 percent of them will have a good outcome; however, if less stringent criteria of psychosis are used to include brief lapses in reality testing and transient hallucinations or delusions, the number of individuals affected increases, and the general overall outcome improves. As a rule, the greater the extent of psychosocial integration prior to a psychotic episode, the greater the likelihood of a good outcome.

The problem in evaluating research is that the definition of schizophrenia has changed, becoming increasingly restrictive

A few decades ago, American psychiatry used a broad definition of schizophrenia. Often, the disorder was diagnosed on the basis of a loosening of associations, a blunting of affect, isolated or withdrawn behavior, and ambivalence, particularly when those symptoms were seen with hallucinations. Now, the American defi-

nition, as described in the *Diagnostic and Statistical Manual*, Third Edition, Revised (DSM-III-R) of the American Psychiatric Association, is much more specific and restrictive [5]. The illness must have been present continuously for at least 6 months, and patients cannot have had manic or depressive symptoms. Using the current definition, perhaps only 10 percent of the persons who a few decades ago were classified as schizophrenic would be so classified now. The American definition is now narrower than that used in Europe—an important consideration when comparing clinical studies from different countries.

A benefit of the current American definition is that it tends to identify a group of severely ill individuals, most of whom will have a progressive disorder; however, there are disadvantages, too. Many disturbed individuals are not included, even though they have clear psychotic symptoms. Unfortunately, the definition is of necessity based on broad observational data rather than on an etiological principle, so that it is unclear whether the current diagnostic criteria identify a group of patients for whom researchers can reasonably search for a single causal agent, or even a few causal factors.

There is evidence for genetic factors in the disorder

The frequency with which schizophrenia occurs in underdeveloped countries is roughly the same as that in the most urbanized societies [6]. It affects males and females about equally, although males tend to have an earlier age of onset. The lifetime prevalence rate of schizophrenia is about 1 percent.

Studies suggest that genetic factors may play a role in schizophrenia [7]. The incidence of the disorder in the parents of schizophrenics is about 4 percent, that in their siblings is about 8 percent, and that in their children, about 12 percent. If both parents are schizophrenic, the chance of an offspring being schizophrenic is about 40 percent. Studies reveal markedly differing rates of twins having schizophrenia, depending on whether they are identical (monozygotic), with a rate of 50 percent, or nonidentical (dizygotic), with a rate of 17 percent. This seems to be true whether or not the twins were raised in the same household or separately. It is equally true that the genetic studies suggest the presence of important nongenetic factors: About half of those who have an identical twin with schizophrenia are not themselves schizophrenic. These poorly understood environmental and psychosocial influences greatly hamper efforts to identify families to which newly emerging techniques in molecular biology can be applied to identify genetic markers of schizophrenia, as is the case for the affective disorders.

Another approach to the study of genetic processes takes advantage of known physiological alterations in schizophrenics. It has been established that a substantial number of schizophrenics and members of their families have changes in eye tracking [8]. The findings raise the possibility of a generalized alteration that may be differentially expressed in some individuals, resulting in schizophrenia. The search for genetic markers using this approach has attracted considerable interest [9].

Brain morphology may be altered in some patients with schizophrenia

In the past 15 years, technical advances have enabled researchers, for the first time, to begin safely studying aspects of brain structure and function in living human beings [10]. For example, X-ray computed tomography (CT) yields detailed cross-sectional images of the brain. Evidence from such studies of schizophrenia suggests that some patients may have a relative increase in the size of their lateral ventricle, although the claim is disputed. The controversy may arise from differences in patient populations, technique, and the control groups that

have been used. Also unclear at present is the clinical significance of the finding, although patients with enlarged ventricles may be less responsive to neuroleptics and may have more negative symptoms. Extensive studies are underway involving magnetic resonance imaging (MRI) and positron emission tomography (PET), which should provide more sensitive information and permit studies of specific brain regions (see also Chap. 44). Direct anatomic studies with postmortem brain have been relatively few but have generally suggested that there may be a decrease in tissue mass. The evidence to date is generally taken to suggest an early developmental injury in some forms of schizophrenia, possibly resulting in, or being the result of, abnormal development of one or more neuroregulatory systems.

The psychosocial environment strongly affects the expression and remission rate of schizophrenia

A variety of social processes have been studied in relation to schizophrenia. For example, it has long been known that the highest rates of the syndrome are found in the lowest socioeconomic group. This may be due to the downward social spiraling of the patients or perhaps to decreased levels of social support or opportunity; however, there is no evidence that social status *per se* is a major factor in the onset of the disorder.

Information about such social factors is of more than merely theoretical interest. For instance, studies of "expressed emotion" led to the interesting hypothesis that individuals with schizophrenia are especially affected by the expression of negative emotion by significant others [11]. When the families of schizophrenics communicate with less negatively expressed emotion, patients tend to have lower rates of relapse. Researchers now have shown that families can be trained to communicate in this fashion, with consequent improvements in the functioning of some patients. Marked improvements in the psychosocial rehabilitation of schizophrenic patients, often an ignored factor, can greatly enhance the daily functioning of this patient population. Evidence suggests that the best treatment today for many patients involves supportive psychosocial treatment together with the use of appropriate medications.

Neuroleptic drugs are an important treatment for schizophrenia, but they are associated with serious side effects, including tardive dyskinesia

Contemporary treatment for schizophrenia began in the early 1950s, with the development of chlorpromazine [12]. Largely by serendipity, clinical investigators found that it had powerful positive effects on patients with schizophrenia. This class of agents came to be termed neuroleptics, or antipsychotics, but they are also called major tranquilizers; however, their pharmacological profiles bear no resemblance to ''minor tranquilizers,'' a term reserved for antianxiety agents such as the benzodiazepines. Several distinct classes of drugs have now been developed, all of which work as antipsychotics and share many other behavioral effects on animals and humans. Research has detailed the ability of these drugs to relieve symptoms of the acute phase of schizophrenia and to decrease the incidence of relapse. The drugs are especially effective against the positive symptoms of schizophrenia, including thought disorder, delusions, and hallucinations.

Unfortunately, all available antipsychotic drugs also share a range of side effects, including those that mimic Parkinson's disease (see Chap. 42). Typical side effects include muscle tremors, rigidity, and spasms. The most worrisome side effect of the antipsychotics is tardive dyskinesia, which usually is associated with long-standing drug treatment. The syndrome includes smacking or sucking movements of the lips and tongue; irregular, involuntary movements may extend to the face and limbs. The movements are associated with supersensitivity of postsynaptic nigrostriatal dopamine receptors (see Chap. 11). For unknown reasons, only about 20 to 40 percent of patients develop tardive dyskinesia. Although there is some correlation with total lifetime antipsychotic dose, there is also evidence that some individuals with schizophrenia who have never received antipsychotic drugs may have similar movement disorders—perhaps a clue to one aspect of the disorder.

DOPAMINE HYPOTHESIS OF SCHIZOPHRENIA

There are many approaches to the neurochemistry of schizophrenia

Although there are a wide range of approaches to the neurochemistry of schizophrenia, most currently focus on neuroregulators, compounds that may function as neurotransmitters or neuromodulators. Hypotheses frequently postulate the relative excess or deficiency of a neuroregulator [13]. Experimental approaches have included investigation of the concentrations of neuroregulators or their metabolites in brain or other available tissues, taking advantage of methods such as high-performance liquid chromatography and mass spectrometry [14,15]. Functional alteration of receptors that interact with neuroregulators has also been under investigation. Studies are also considering other neurochemical systems that may be altered, including such basic processes as glucose metabolism. Pharmacological tools have been important in both basic and clinical neurochemical research. The discovery of antipsychotics (discussed above) that could be used for treatment of schizophrenia, and of drugs that mimic aspects of it, has profoundly altered thinking about schizophrenia.

The pharmacological effects of the antipsychotics formed the basis for a biochemical hypothesis that schizophrenia results from a relative excess of dopamine

This so-called dopamine hypothesis has been the dominant theoretical basis for research in this area over the past two decades [16,17]. Its strongest support is the demonstrated fact that all known antipsychotic agents block dopamine receptors.

The effects of antipsychotics on the dopamine system were noted because some patients receiving antipsychotic agents had movements resembling those occurring in Parkinson's disease, which is thought to be caused by a relative deficiency in dopamine (see Chap. 42). The ability of antipsychotics to bind to postsynaptic dopamine receptors was demonstrated in *in vitro* receptor assays by their competition with radiolabeled dopamine for binding sites (see Chaps. 9 and 11). Potencies of the antipsychotics in these assays closely parallel their clinical efficacy. *In vivo*, antipsychotics have a dramatic effect on the dopamine system. They accelerate the turnover of dopamine, due to a compensatory feedback process resulting from postsynaptic dopamine receptor blockade. Also, they enhance the effects of drugs such as α-methyl-*para*-tyrosine, which inhibit dopamine synthesis, and they antagonize the effects of drugs such as the amphetamines, which stimulate dopamine release.

The dopamine hypothesis postulates that schizophrenia is the result of a relative overstimulation of the dopaminergic system and that inhibition of dopaminergic processes by receptor blockade is therefore an effective means of treatment. The dopamine hypothesis led to the development of a series of compounds that are used to treat psychosis, all of which have as their main mode of action an effect on dopaminergic receptors.

Despite its usefulness, the dopamine hypothesis has three serious limitations:

1. In most patients, the therapeutic effects of antipsychotic drugs occur some time after they actually act on receptors, implying either that there may be other critical components to the drug action or that dopamine overactivity is not the key biochemical defect in the disease.
2. The effects of antipsychotics on schizophrenia do not seem to differ from their effects on other psychoses.
3. Many patients with schizophrenia are resistant to antipsychotic drug therapy.

None of these facts support the concept of a specific dopamine system defect as the sole cause of schizophrenia.

Is there direct evidence for alteration of a dopaminergic system in schizophrenia?

Direct testing of the dopamine hypothesis in patients is difficult [17]. The best available means to assess dopamine activity in human beings is to measure the concentration of dopamine metabolites in either lumbar cerebrospinal fluid (CSF) or plasma. Studies must allow at least 4 weeks, during which the patient is off medication, to obviate direct effects of antipsychotics on dopamine turnover. Homovanillic acid (HVA) is the predominant metabolite measured in these studies, although some attention has been given to minor metabolites, including 3,4-dihydroxyphenylacetic acid (DOPAC) and 3-methoxytyramine. Much of the HVA in the CSF originates in the cortex and probably in the caudate, but considerable amounts may be produced in the spinal cord. There is a gradient in the concentration of HVA from the brain to the lumbar space. Therefore, levels of HVA in the lumbar CSF may not adequately reflect changes in dopamine in areas of the brain where dopamine function is important for emotional behavior, e.g., the limbic centers and regions of cerebral cortex.

In light of the difficulties with measuring metabolites in CSF, it is not surprising that consistency among studies has been low. Seemingly minor differences in technique, including how samples are collected, the amount of physical activity the subject had prior to collection of the sample, and the emotional state of the subject during the interval of a few hours prior to collection, probably can affect results. In addition, as noted earlier, it remains unclear whether HVA concentrations in lumbar CSF are a valid index of dopamine activity in the brain areas of interest. Therefore, a clear picture of altered HVA concentrations in lumbar CSF of schizophrenics has not emerged.

HVA has also been measured in blood plasma, where a substantial fraction, perhaps as much as 25 to 40 percent, is derived from the brain. In addition to the problem of determining the source of the metabolite, certain foods that have precursors to the metabolite can result in alterations in plasma HVA. The relatively limited evidence available suggests that plasma HVA concentrations may be increased in some patient groups. This has been taken to support the hypothesis of a relative increase in dopamine production in schizophrenia.

Researchers have attempted to investigate the dopamine system in tissue obtained at autopsy. Such postmortem studies are not without their own problems, among them accuracy of the diagnosis, which has to be determined retrospectively; the state of the patient at the time of death; changes during the terminal state that are unrelated to the psychiatric diagnosis; the effects of medications that are administered for other illnesses; the amount of antipsychotic given for psychiatric purposes; and problems consequent to the process of obtaining the tissue, including the interval between death and autopsy and the temperature of the specimen

prior to autopsy. Again, the evidence to date has done little to elucidate changes in dopamine concentration or metabolites or in the relative activities of the enzymes involved in the formation of dopamine or other catecholamines.

Particular attention has been focused on studies of receptor number and ligand affinity characteristics in the brains of individuals with schizophrenia. These studies are also complicated by the fact that prior antipsychotic treatment almost certainly affects receptor binding. Still, this has been a prominent area of investigation, and changes have been reported in schizophrenia. It has not been possible to ascertain if the noted increases are primary or due to treatment; but, a few studies in which brains have been obtained from persons who had been unmedicated for sustained periods of time also found an increase in receptor binding.

Methods for studying receptor processes in the intact, living individual have been made possible by the development of positron emission tomography (PET). The development of antipsychotic ligands for this technique may enable researchers to measure regional distribution and relative amounts of neuroactive drugs and dopamine and other receptors (see Chap. 44).

OTHER NEUROREGULATOR SYSTEMS IN SCHIZOPHRENIA

Evidence concerning changes in norepinephrine in schizophrenia has been equivocal

Despite considerable speculation about the role of norepinephrine in schizophrenia, evidence is provocative but equivocal [18]. A number of researchers have suggested that much behavior linked to the dopamine system can also be attributed to the norepinephrine system.

Investigators have examined several parameters, including concentrations of norepinephrine and the activity of enzymes involved in its formation and metabolism. Postmortem brain studies have been inconclusive [19]. The literature suggests a trend toward a slight elevation of norepinephrine in the CSF, but that may be due to a variety of causes; and some studies of drugs thought to act predominantly on norepinephrine systems are intriguing. Clonidine, an agonist of the α_2 receptor (see Chap. 11) has been reported to improve symptoms in some schizophrenics. Early enthusiasm for propranolol, a β-blocker, as a treatment was based on studies that did not have double-blind controls; stronger evidence of its positive effect on schizophrenia is still needed.

The study of hallucinogens three decades ago suggested a role for serotonin in psychosis

Today, evidence relating serotonin to psychosis is viewed in a more guarded manner but with continuing interest. A number of known hallucinogens, including LSD, bind serotonin receptors (see Chap. 12). LSD increases the concentration of brain serotonin and decreases the firing of serotonin-containing neurons in the midbrain [20]. Further, some methylated indoles chemically related to serotonin cause hallucinations, and these compounds also interfere with serotonin functioning. An effort to assess whether such methylated compounds are present endogenously in the brain has been confused by problems of the accuracy of the identification. Even with substantial improvements in analytical techniques, there is still no reliable evidence that they are involved in any form of schizophrenia.

A variety of studies has failed to reveal a consistent pattern of changes in serotonin in schizophrenic patients. Studies of the serotonin metabolite 5-HIAA in CSF suggest that 5-HIAA concentrations may be decreased in persons who have brain atrophy and schizophrenia. An increase in platelet serotonin has been reported

in a number of studies, although the finding is also noted in other illnesses. Some atypical antipsychotics such as clonazepine may act in part through serotonergic mechanisms and bind to a number of receptors, including serotonin receptors; however, none of these findings argue strongly for a central role of serotonin in schizophrenia.

γ-Aminobutyric acid has been postulated to have a role in schizophrenia

γ-Aminobutyric acid (GABA), a major transmitter in the brain (see Chap. 15), is considered to be an inhibitory transmitter on dopaminergic systems, although under some circumstances it may be facilitory [21]. Some investigators have postulated a role for GABA in schizophrenia, hypothesizing that a relative GABA deficiency would mimic a relative dopaminergic excess [22].

Evidence in support of this hypothesis is limited, and results from CSF and plasma studies have been contradictory. Although there are reports of decreased concentrations of GABA in CSF in depression, the results in schizophrenia have been variable. In part, this reflects the many technical problems involved in collecting samples for measurement of GABA.

Another approach to testing the involvement of GABA in schizophrenia has been to study drugs that act on the GABA system. Unfortunately, few such agents are available, and there may be more than one form of GABA receptor, making interpretation difficult (see Chap. 15). The evidence suggests that some agonists of GABA worsen certain cases of schizophrenia. Of interest, some studies suggest that quite high doses of benzodiazepines, which theoretically act through GABA mechanisms, improve the clinical state of selected patients. Thus, it is thought possible that a GABA deficiency may be relevant to the disorder.

Prostaglandin receptors may be altered in schizophrenia

The prostaglandins are neuromodulators that appear to have a wide range of functions (see Chap. 20). Release of prostaglandins is altered by other neuroregulator systems, yet they themselves alter the release of transmitters, especially catecholamines. It has been postulated that either a relative excess or deficiency of prostaglandins might be involved in schizophrenia [23]. The prostaglandin systems are complex and have received relatively little study; however, evidence from a number of studies does suggest a decrease in cyclic AMP (cAMP) production in response to prostaglandin E_1 (PGE_1) in platelets of schizophrenics. Such a change could be due to an alteration at the prostaglandin receptor or its linkage to adenylate cyclase. Measurement of prostaglandins in tissue is difficult and has not yet led to a conclusion with regard to alterations. Investigators have given putative precursors of prostaglandins as an experimental treatment for schizophrenia with no evidence of definitive improvement.

The potential role of various neuropeptides in schizophrenia has been generating increasing interest

Neuropeptides may act directly as transmitters or as modulators of neurotransmitter function and therefore play a key role as neuroregulators. Particularly important to concepts of neuropeptides in relation to schizophrenia has been the emerging view that a given nerve cell may produce several neuroregulators, and that biogenic amines and neuropeptides are often colocalized in the same nerve cells. For example, there is strong evidence that the peptide cholecystokinin (CCK) and dopamine coexist within some cells. It has been difficult to obtain evidence relating the concentrations of peptides to various mental disorders. The same general

problems of postmortem studies mentioned earlier apply, although neuropeptides may have one advantage in these studies in that they seem to be relatively stable in postmortem brain tissue and in CSF [24,25].

Studies of neuropeptide concentrations and enzymatic activity in schizophrenia have yielded an impressive range of results, but no consistent picture has yet emerged. Especially troubling has been the reliance of most studies on assay methods with known problems of specificity. Many assays rely on indirect measures, typically using antibodies. The antigenic determinants are frequently shared by more than one neuropeptide. Consequently, without additional information, including characterization of the peptide and assessment of specificity of the assay, errors can be made. Until the assays are verified, no conclusions should be drawn.

Another approach to the study of peptides has been administration of peptides or derivatives to patients. To be valid, such studies must be conducted in a double-blind fashion in which neither the patient nor the investigators know when the patient is receiving the active substance. Such studies are further complicated, because it is unlikely that many peptides cross the blood-brain barrier, and the behavioral effects of most peptides are still unknown. These arguments do not, of course, rule out the possible effect of the peptides. For example, an administered peptide could act either on peripheral receptors or on receptors at locations where the blood-brain barrier is more permeable. It does, however, strongly argue for the need for caution in interpreting any such reports.

Endorphins in schizophrenia

A number of studies suggest that patients with schizophrenia may have changes in the concentration of endorphins in the CSF (see Chap. 13). Several researchers, using radioreceptor assays, have found increased concentrations of one or more ''endorphin-like'' fractions from the CSF. These promising results have been controversial because the radioreceptor method is nonspecific and the nature of the peptide fractions remains unresolved.

Other measurements have been undertaken using determinations based on radioimmunoassays. Despite efforts by a number of groups, no one has established whether any CSF endorphins are abnormal in schizophrenia. In most studies, the substance measured has not been characterized chemically, meaning that other unsuspected peptides and nonspecific effects may account for the findings. Indeed, in some instances in which antibodies with good specificity were used, what initially seemed to be promising results proved illusory.

Another approach to the study of endorphins in schizophrenia arose from reports that patients with the disorder improved with hemodialysis. The apparent response was attributed to the removal of a specific opioid peptide from the plasma. Repeated studies over the past decade have failed to replicate the results of hemodialysis; at this time, there is no evidence of an opioid peptide in plasma that is altered in schizophrenia.

Nonopioid neuropeptides in schizophrenia

Ongoing studies are dealing with many of the 40 to 50 different neuropeptides that have now been identified in the CNS and are thought to be relevant as neuromodulators or neurotransmitters (see Chap. 14). For some, interesting hypotheses have been developed. For example, neurotensin has been shown to interact with the dopamine systems in the brain, and relative changes in neurotensin have been postulated in relation to schizophrenia. Similarly, there have been hypotheses of changes in CCK based on the colocalization of that neuropeptide with certain dopamine systems. There have been reports of changes in one or another peptide in brain areas, but for none of the peptides is there

the body of literature needed to establish a definitive change.

Neuropeptides and their antagonists used to treat schizophrenia

Episodically, reports suggest that the peripheral administration of one or another neuropeptide can improve the symptoms of schizophrenia. Some studies have provided evidence of central activity that could be due to an action on peripheral receptors or on receptors in a brain area that is not completely protected by the blood-brain barrier. The opioid peptide β-endorphin offers a good case study of such work (see Chap. 13). Initial reports of the effects of β-endorphin on schizophrenia were positive, but further double-blind studies suggested that a single dose did not affect the symptoms of schizophrenia; nor has there been any evidence of a positive effect from endorphin analogues, although some early reports from Europe with des-tyr-γ-endorphin originally claimed potent antipsychotic effects. Negative results have also been obtained with CCK derivatives in controlled studies.

Such studies have enormous problems, not the least of which are the cost of using the substances at pharmacological doses with sufficient numbers of subjects to yield useful results. Failures of replication can have a number of roots, apart from what may be intrinsic inactivity. For example, the subject populations may differ in unsuspected but vital ways. Also, most studies utilize a single dose—a strategy that certainly would not work even for an antipsychotic that is known to be effective. Multiple or sustained doses may be required even if the peptide were effective. Also, the problem of permeability of the blood-brain barrier is substantial and still poorly understood. Undoubtedly, over the coming years, nonpeptide analog agonists and antagonists to peptide systems of interest will become available, at which time studies of this type should be far more informative.

Another strategy for clinical studies of neuropeptide systems involves using peptide antagonists and determining whether they influence the course of schizophrenia. To date, the most notable of such efforts has dealt with the endorphin antagonist naloxone. Double-blind investigations have led to the observation that high doses of naloxone are effective in decreasing chronic hallucinations. The time course of the effect is surprising, for it lasts longer than would be expected on the basis of naloxone's pharmacokinetics; also, the effective dose is far higher than that needed simply to reverse the effects of an opiate overdose. It remains unclear if the decrease in hallucinations is a result of changes in an endorphin system or if naloxone may be acting on some other neurochemical process. The effects do not occur in all patients, and naloxone is not useful clinically as a treatment for auditory hallucinations. Still, the results are of interest in suggesting further hypotheses and experimental approaches.

Phencyclidine and the psychotomimetic σ receptor may provide a new model for the study of psychotic processes

An important new direction for fundamental research that may have direct relevance to mechanisms of psychosis centers on phencyclidine (PCP), a drug with hallucinogenic effects [26]. In some individuals, PCP induces a schizophrenic-like syndrome. The syndrome can be serious and may continue for a substantial period after drug administration; there is therefore interest in determining the mode of action of PCP.

Two sites that bind PCP have been the focus of intense study. One, designated initially as the σ opioid site but now termed the σ site, is differentiated from known opioid sites on pharmacological grounds, although it has an affinity for certain benzomorphan opiates (see Chap. 13). The σ site also binds antipsychotics such as haloperidol, but it is clearly distinct from classical dopamine D_1 and D_2 binding sites

that are ordinarily associated with haloperidol blockade. The σ site may have a role in the release of catecholamines. The second site, designated as the PCP binding site, has a higher affinity for PCP and does not bind haloperidol. Various drugs exhibit extensive cross-reactivity for the two sites, but recent efforts have resulted in ways to distinguish between the two. It is not known which site is most relevant for the action of PCP or whether either is responsible for the psychological effects of the drug.

One action of the PCP group of hallucinogens is believed to be on a subtype of glutamate receptor, the N-methyl-D-aspartate (NMDA) type (see Chap. 15). PCP antagonizes excitation produced by NMDA and is thought to block the ion channel involved in NMDA. This has led to the suggestion that the PCP and NMDA sites may be closely related. The role of PCP in relation to the σ site is also of interest, because the σ site may be involved in increasing catecholamine release, a process affected by certain known psychotogens such as amphetamine. A hypothesis of special interest is that endogenous ligands may exist for the PCP or σ receptor. Such compounds have been reported as further information is being developed about the binding sites.

Positron emission tomography provides new approaches to the study of schizophrenia

Application of positron emission tomography (PET) technology is providing the means of studying neurochemistry in patients (see also Chap. 44). By means of the deoxyglucose method, evidence for a slight decrease in the metabolic activity of the frontal lobe in schizophrenia has been obtained. The normal front-to-back gradient in glucose metabolic activity is maintained but to a lesser degree. These early results suggest a more generalized disorder or one that reflects an alteration in one or more neuroregulator systems [27]. (Other PET studies are discussed in Chap. 44.)

Hypotheses involving a viral or immune etiology have been of interest in the study of schizophrenia

A hypothesis of a viral or immune etiology of schizophrenia would not be inconsistent with neurochemical studies of the disorder [28]. For example, Parkinson's disease is known to involve a profound deficit in the dopamine system, and its current treatment is based on that neurochemical change; yet, viral and environmental toxins, acting through the dopaminergic system, have been shown to cause some cases of Parkinson's disease. Analogous hypotheses have been made for schizophrenia. The frequent occurrence of psychosis was noted in some influenza outbreaks earlier in this century. Two other observations may relate schizophrenia to viral processes. First, an unexpected number of persons with schizophrenia are born in the winter and spring. Second, although the world distribution of the disorder is remarkably even, there are epidemiological pockets with a higher or lower incidence. Still, studies using antibodies to most known viral infections have not shown no consistent change in schizophrenia.

Autoimmune processes also are being examined in schizophrenia. Clinical researchers in this area are trying to assess whether there are changes in immune response in general or to specific antigens involving neuroregulators in the disorder. No consistent pattern has emerged.

CHILDHOOD PSYCHOSES

Although the bulk of research to date has focused on psychotic processes in adults, children also have psychoses. The current diagnostic manual, DSM-III-R [5], does not distinguish between adult and child forms of schizophrenia, and there is no evidence to suggest that the biological processes involved in this disorder differ as a function of age; however, a group of syndromes called the *pervasive developmental disorders* do occur in children, typically before the age of 5 years. These disorders appear to be distinct from schizophrenia, almost always afflict the individual for life, and have no known treatment. A growing body of research has tried to identify possible biological causes [29,30].

Autism is a major pervasive developmental disorder that affects young children

Autism is by far the most extensively and systematically studied of the pervasive developmental disorders [31]. Kanner [3] in 1943 was the first to describe a syndrome he called early infantile autism to emphasize the striking failure of those with this disorder to develop emotional contact and social relationships. Early infantile autism was included as a diagnostic category in DSM-III (1980) as one of the pervasive developmental disorders [32]. Criteria included absent or markedly abnormal social relationships, marked impairment in the production and content of language, bizarre interaction with the environment, the absence of hallucinations or delusions, and onset before age $2\frac{1}{2}$ years. In 1987, DSM-IIIR renamed the diagnosis autistic disorder and provided more detailed criteria that included a developmental perspective and removed the criterion related to age of onset; however, the essential features of the disorder remain the same [5]. Moderate to profound mental retardation is a common but not universal concomitant of autism that complicates both the clinical picture and research efforts. A small fraction of those with autism have normal or even superior intelligence; rare individuals, independent of overall intelligence, have highly unusual abilities in such areas as mathematics.

The social disability of those with autism

is striking and pervasive. Many of these children have minimal social contact with those around them; it is therefore difficult to learn what their world is like. Still, they differ markedly from adults with schizophrenia, and hallucinations and delusions are not a part of the clinical picture. The most severely affected children never exhibit any awareness of others as living beings. As infants, many actively resist human contact and are soothed much more readily if left alone. With advancing age, they usually prefer to be alone and find even the most rudimentary social skills beyond their capabilities.

Communication abnormalities range from severe expressive and receptive deficits to markedly unusual patterns of speech intonation, inflection, rhythm, and content. For example, flat or ''sing-song'' speech is quite common in autism, as is repetition of what is said and poor use of pronouns.

Unusual interaction with the environment typically entails a remarkable attentiveness to trivial detail and an absence of more common forms of interacting with objects. For example, parents often report that the child is fascinated with running water, the edges on objects, or shifting patterns of light and dark. Play characteristically is restricted to repetitively spinning wheels on toy vehicles or compulsively lining up blocks or similar objects in excruciatingly straight lines. Many of these children seem almost completely unaware of their surroundings and yet are exquisitely sensitive to trivial changes in their physical environment. For example, they may go into a rage if a picture is moved from its accustomed place in their room or if a familiar route or routine is changed.

Evidence indicates that autism results from a biological process, probably one with many possible causes

Autism occurs at a rate of one to five per 10,000 in the general population and is at least four times more common in boys than in girls. First-degree relatives of children with autism have an increased prevalence of autism but not of schizophrenia. Furthermore, monozygotic twins are concordant for autism over half the time, with a much lower concordance among dizygotic twins [33].

Several approaches have been taken to study the possible causes of autism. As with schizophrenia, efforts are hampered by the wide range of presentations, which is consistent with the presence of subtypes of autism [34]. Nevertheless, some intriguing clues to the possible causes of autism have emerged. For example, 8 to 10 percent of children exposed to the rubella virus during gestation are autistic, and *in utero* exposure to toxoplasmosis and congenital neurosyphilis also increase the risk of autism. In addition, autism is more common among individuals with phenylketonuria. It is important to emphasize that these conditions are simply risk factors for autism: The majority of individuals exposed to such factors never develop autism, and no causal mechanisms are known [35].

Efforts to identify a problem in either brain anatomy or brain function that is common to children with autism have had little success. To date, few brains of individuals with autism have become available for study, but those that have been studied revealed no specific pathology. Investigators have used X-ray computed tomography (CT) to view aspects of brain anatomy in living subjects with autism. A few reports have suggested specific abnormalities in the left hemisphere or in subcortical structures; however, most concluded that this population has an increased incidence in such nonspecific abnormalities as ventricular enlargement and frontal lobe tissue defects, without evidence of consistent changes in brain structure. Similarly, studies of brain electrophysiology have been inconclusive. Although about 25 percent of individuals with autism develop frank seizure activity by adolescence, no characteristic EEG patterns have been found. Abnormalities have been reported with sensory processing, but such research is greatly complicated by questions about the ability of subjects with autism to cooperate normally.

Despite evidence that autism involves a profound biological change, no research links the disorder to any specific neuroregulator system

Compared with research on schizophrenia, neuroregulator activity in subjects with autism has been little studied, and most research has been exploratory rather than hypothesis oriented. Such studies are especially difficult because of the limitations in obtaining biological samples of any kind from children, hesitations about performing spinal taps on children strictly for research purposes, and the problem of obtaining appropriate controls.

By far the most numerous studies of a neuroregulator in autism involve serotonin, which was noted to be increased in the platelets of children with autism [36]. Numerous subsequent reports using appropriate age- and gender-matched controls have confirmed that one-third of subjects with autism have hyperserotonemia, as do about one-half of nonautistic, severely retarded subjects. The cause of this relative elevation or its relationship, if any, to autism is unknown. In fact, it is unclear that platelet serotonin is a useful indicator of central serotonin activity. One study of CSF 5-HIAA turnover in autistic subjects suggested that central serotonin activity was slightly decreased rather than increased [37]. A study of CSF 5-HIAA concentrations showed a slight increase for subjects with autism. Even if a clear and characteristic pattern of serotonin activity were found in children with autism, no hypothesis has yet been offered to suggest a specific causal role in the disorder.

A few studies have begun to examine the possible role of opioid peptides in autism [38]. These substances are of particular interest be-

cause of their suggested role both in pain systems and in certain aspects of social behavior. Although episodic reports have described decreases in opioid-peptide substances in the blood or CSF of children with autism, the actual identity of the substance being measured is not known; however, the relevance of such research is underscored by recent reports that opiate antagonists such as naloxone and naltrexone may ameliorate certain signs and symptoms of autism.

At present, research on childhood psychoses and autism is at a very early phase. There is almost no information about catecholamines, for example. It can be expected that the study of basic neurochemical mechanisms, combined with improved methods of studying the clinical syndromes, eventually will provide an understanding of these devastating disorders and may lead to improved treatment.

REFERENCES

1. Gelder, M., Gath, D., and Mayou, R. *Oxford Textbook of Psychiatry*. New York: Oxford University Press, 1983.
2. Bleuler, E. *Dementia Praecox or the Group of Schizophrenics*. New York: International Universities Press, 1911. [Translated by Zinkin, J., 1950.]
3. Kanner, L. Autistic disturbances of affective contact. *Nerv. Child.* 2:217–250, 1943
4. Kendell, R. E. Schizophrenia: Clinical features. In R. Michaels and J. O. Cavenar (eds.), *Psychiatry*. Philadelphia: Lippincott, 1985, Vol. 1.
5. American Psychiatric Association. *Diagnostic and Statistical Manual*, 3rd. ed., Washington, DC: American Psychiatric Association, 1987.
6. Helzer, J. E. Schizophrenia: Epidemiology. In R. Michaels and J. O. Cavenar (eds.), *Psychiatry*. Philadelphia: Lippincott, 1985, Vol. 1.
7. Kety, S. S., Rosenthal, D., Wender, P. H., Schulsinger, F., and Jacobsen, F. The biological and adaptive families of adopted individuals who become schizophrenic. In L. C. Wynne, R. L. Corwell, and S. Matthysse (eds.), *The Nature of*

Schizophrenia. New York: John Wiley, 1978, pp. 25–37.

8. Matthysse, S., Holzman, P., and Lange, K. The genetic transmission of schizophrenia: Application of Mendelian latent structure analysis to eye tracking dysfunctions in schizophrenia and affective disorder. *J. Psychiatr. Res.* 20:57–67, 1986.

9. Matthysse, S. The "middle game" in the genetics of schizophrenia. In H. Helmschen and F. A. Henn (eds.), *Biological Perspectives of Schizophrenia.* Chichester: John Wiley, 1987, pp. 7–17.

10. Shelton, R. C., and Weinberger, D. R. Brain morphology in schizophrenia, In H. Y. Meltzer (ed.), *Psychopharmacology: A Second Generation of Progress.* New York: Raven Press, 1987, pp. 773–781.

11. Barchas, P. (ed.). *Sociophysiology of Social Relations.* New York: Oxford Univ. Press (*in press*).

12. Davis, J. M., and Mostert, M. A. Biological treatment of schizophrenic disorders. In P. A. Berger and H. K. H. Brodie (eds.), *American Handbook of Psychiatry.* New York: Basic Books, 1986, Vol. VIII, pp. 466–512.

13. Meltzer, H. Y. Biological studies in schizophrenia. *Schizophr. Bull.* 13:77–111, 1987.

14. Mefford, I. N. Biomedical uses of high performance liquid chromatography with electrochemical selection. In D. Glick (ed.), *Methods of Biochemical Analysis.* New York: John Wiley, 1985, pp. 221–258.

15. Faull, K. F., and Barchas, J. D. Analysis of catecholamines and their metabolites by combined gas chromatography-mass spectrometry. In S. Parvez, I. Nagatsu, T. Nagatsu, and H. Parvez (eds.), *Methods in Biogenic Amine Research.* Amsterdam/New York: Elsevier/North Holland, 1983, pp. 189–236.

16. Carlsson, A., and Lindquist, M. Effect of chlorpromazine and haloperidol on formation of 3-methoxytyramine and normetanephrine in mouse brain. *Acta Pharmacol. Toxocol.* 20:140–144, 1963.

17. Losonczy, M. F., Davidson, M., and Davis, K. L. The dopamine hypothesis of schizophrenia. In H. Y. Meltzer (ed.), *Psychopharmacology: A*

Second Generation of Progress. New York: Raven Press, 1987, pp. 715–726.

18. van Kammen, D. P., and Gelernter, J. Biochemical instability in schizophrenia: The norepinephrine system. In H. Y. Meltzer (ed.), *Psychopharmacology: A Second Generation of Progress.* New York: Raven Press, 1987, pp. 745–751.

19. Kleinman, J. E., Bridge, P., and Karoum, F. Chronic schizophrenia, post-mortem studies. In C. Baxter and T. Melnechuk (eds.), *Perspectives in Schizophrenia Research.* New York: Raven Press, 1980, pp 227–236.

20. Aghajanian, G. K., Foote, W. E., and Sheard, M. H. *Science* 161:706–708, 1968.

21. Roberts, E. Disinhibition as an organizing principle in the nervous system: The role of the GABA system. In E. Roberts, T. Chase, and D. Tower (eds.), *GABA: Nervous System Function.* New York: Raven Press, 1976, pp. 515–539.

22. Garbutt, J. C., and van Kammen, D. P. The interaction between GABA and dopamine: Implications for schizophrenia. *Schizophr. Bull.* 9:336–353, 1983.

23. Rotrosen, J., and Wolkin, A. Phospholipid and prostaglandin hypotheses of schizophrenia. In H. Y. Meltzer (ed.), *Psychopharmacology: A Second Generation of Progress.* New York: Raven Press, 1987, pp. 759–764.

24. Martin, J. B., and Barchas, J. D. (eds.), *Neuropeptides in Neurologic and Psychiatric Disease.* New York: Raven Press, 1986.

25. Nemeroff, C. B., Berger, P. H., and Bissette, G. Peptides in schizophrenia. In H. Y. Meltzer (ed.), *Psychopharmacology: A Second Generation of Progress.* New York: Raven Press, 1987, pp. 727–743.

26. Sonders, M. S., Keana, J. F. W., and Weber, E. Phencyclidine and psychotomimetic sigma opiates: Recent insights into their biochemical and physiological sites of action. *Trends Neurosci.* 11:37–40, 1988.

27. Buchsbaum, M. S. Positron emission tomography in schizophrenia. In H. Y. Meltzer (ed.), *Psychopharmacology: A Second Generation of Progress.* New York: Raven Press, 1987, pp. 783–792.

28. Crow, T. J. Biological basis of mental disorders:

The case of viral etiology. In M. Namba and H. Kaiya (eds.), *Psychobiology of Schizophrenia*. New York: Pergamon Press, 1982.

29. Schopler, E., and Mesibov, G. B. (eds.). *Neurobiological Issues in Autism*. New York: Plenum, 1987.

30. Young, J. G., Leven, L. I., Newcorn, J. H., and Knott, P. J. Genetic and neurobiological approaches to the pathophysiology of autism and pervasive developmental disorders. In H. Y. Meltzer (ed.), *Psychopharmacology: A Second Generation of Progress*. New York: Raven Press, 1987, pp. 825–836.

31. Elliott, G. R., and Ciaranello, R. D. Neurochemical hypotheses of childhood psychoses. In E. Schopler and G. B. Mesibov (eds.), *Neurobiological Issues in Autism*. New York: Plenum, 1987, pp. 245–261.

32. American Psychiatric Association. *Diagnostic and Statistical Manual*, 3rd. ed. Washington, DC: American Psychiatric Association, 1980.

33. Ritvo, E. R., Freeman, B. J., Mason-Brothers, A., Mo, A., and Ritvo, A. M. Concordance for the syndrome of autism in 40 pairs of afflicted twins. *Am. J. Psychiatr.* 142:74–78, 1985.

34. Siegel, B., Anders, T. R., Ciaranello, R. D., Bienenstock, B., and Kraemer, H. C. Empirically derived subclassification of the autistic syndrome. *J. Autism Dev. Disord.* 16:275–293, 1986.

35. Ciaranello, R. D., Vandenberg, S. R., and Anders, T. F. Intrinsic and extrinsic determinants of neuronal development: Relation to infantile autism. *J. Autism Dev. Disord.* 12:115–146, 1982.

36. Schain, R. J., and Freedman, D. X. Studies on 5-hydroxyindole metabolism in autistic and other mentally retarded children. *J. Pediatr.* 58:315–329, 1961.

37. Cohen, D. J., Caparulo, B. K., Shaywitz, B. A., and Bowers, M. B. Dopamine and serotonin metabolism in neuropsychiatrically disturbed children. *Arch. Gen. Psychiatr.* 34:545–550, 1977.

38. Sahley, T. L., and Panksepp, J. Brain opioids and autism: An updated analysis of possible linkages. *J. Autism Dev. Disord.* 17:201–216, 1987.

CHAPTER 46

Biochemical Hypotheses of Affective Disorders and Anxiety

Robert C. Malenka, Mark W. Hamblin, and Jack D. Barchas

Basic Neurochemistry: Molecular, Cellular, and Medical Aspects, 4th Ed., edited by G. J. Siegel et al. Raven Press, Ltd., New York, 1989.
Correspondence to Jack D. Barchas, Nancy Pritzker Laboratory, Stanford Medical School, 300 Pasteur Drive, Stanford, California 94305.

The neurochemistry of psychiatric conditions has been a very active and fruitful field, and despite the limitations of current assumptions, biological hypotheses of mental disorders have been of enormous value in focusing research efforts on the link between psychiatry and the biological sciences. The goal of research has been to identify circumscribed but key portions of biochemical pathways whose alteration is involved in clinical pathology or therapeutic change. For some conditions, progress has been exceedingly slow, for others, key neurochemical events have been described, and the knowledge thus gained offers the potential of direct therapeutic benefit. Two groups of illnesses representing the most common of all psychiatric conditions, the affective and anxiety disorders, are now firmly in the latter category.

AFFECTIVE DISORDERS WITH KNOWN BIOLOGICAL CONCOMITANTS

Two major categories of affective disorders are depression and manic-depressive illness

Affective disorders refer to a group of psychiatric illnesses characterized by disturbances of mood severe enough to alter cognition, judgment, and interpersonal relationships [1]. Appetite, energy level, and sleeping patterns are also profoundly disturbed.

Everyone goes through periods of feeling sad, discouraged, lonely, or disappointed, but these feelings normally pass and do not impair day-to-day functioning. In contrast, patients with clinically significant depression undergo such profound changes in the way they perceive themselves and the world that their lives are greatly disrupted. Attitudes are marked by a pervasive sense of hopelessness and helplessness. Overwhelming feelings of guilt and worthlessness may appear. Attempts at suicide are not uncommon. Depressed patients express little interest or enjoyment in activities previously judged pleasurable. Energy levels plummet to the point where the simple act of speaking becomes slow and labored. A diminished ability to think or concentrate often becomes apparent.

In addition to alterations in mood and perception, a variety of basic physiological parameters are frequently altered in depression. Patients may gain or lose large quantities of weight. Some have great difficulty obtaining a normal night's sleep; others sleep 12 to 18 hr/day. Either agitation or retardation of movement may predominate. Physical symptoms, such as dizziness, headaches, backaches, tightness in the chest, or dry mouth, often accompany depression and can be the presenting complaint, masking the underlying psychiatric illness.

The changes that develop during depression disrupt interpersonal relationships and can exacerbate social losses that may be occurring in the life of the patient. Some depressions seem to be related to obvious social losses; others seem not. Nonetheless, depression can impact on all of the activities of the individual, including employment.

With depression in its most extreme form, patients become psychotic. Such patients distort or misperceive reality, experience hallucinations, or develop bizarre beliefs and behaviors.

Patients that have only recurrent bouts of depression are said to have *unipolar* depression, whereas those having both depression and mania are considered to have *bipolar* disorder. Multiple combinations of these problems are seen: Many patients who experience one depressive episode will unfortunately suffer recurrences. Others will not only experience repeated depressions but will also have episodes of mania or near-mania (also called hypomania) interspersed among their depressions. A few patients experience intermittent bouts of mania without marked depressive episodes.

Although mania can be intuitively thought of as the opposite of depression, the two syndromes share several characteristics. Manic patients initially feel elated, carefree, overconfident, and euphoric. They often overestimate their attractiveness, intelligence, and abilities. They seem to have limitless energy and feel little need for sleep or sustenance. Some feel that they can literally conquer the world; however, euphoria often quickly changes to irritability and hostility. As in depression, cognition and judgment may become significantly impaired, leading to catastrophic consequences. In severe forms, psychosis develops. This is manifested by delusional beliefs of omnipotence and ''flight of ideas''—the occurrence of thoughts so rapid and complex that verbalizations are difficult to follow.

Epidemiological studies indicate that an enormous number of people, three to four percent of the population of the United States, suffer from an affective disorder [2]. Lifetime risk for having at least one major depressive episode is 10 to 15 percent in the general population. There are over 30,000 deaths by suicide each year in the United States, making it a leading cause of death. Understanding the pathophysiological mechanisms underlying mood disturbances is of the utmost importance.

What is the evidence that abnormal biochemical functioning in the brain causes the affective disorders?

The answer can be divided into two categories. The first derives from family and twin studies using epidemiological and, more recently, molecular genetic techniques. These studies have indicated that affective disorders (a) cluster within families; (b) are most likely to occur in first-degree relatives of those with the disorder; and (c) are more prevalent among monozygotic than dizygotic twins [3]. Furthermore, with the use of recombinant DNA techniques, a dominant gene that is inherited along with the dis-

ease-causing gene(s) has been identified in certain families with a high incidence of bipolar disorder [4]. There is thus substantial evidence for a genetic contribution to the affective disorders, although the mode of genetic transmission remains unclear. The penetrance of the predisposing gene(s) is at most 60 to 70%, indicating that the environment also plays a critical etiological role.

The second line of evidence derives from the finding that a variety of pharmacological agents have substantial effects on mood and behavior. A common assumption has been that if an agent modifies a psychiatric symptom for better or worse, then the drug's cellular or neurochemical action may be directly related to the biological dysfunction causing the symptom. This assumption may be flawed. The psychopharmacological agent may act at a site that is independent of the neurochemical abnormality causing the illness yet produce changes in brain function that compensate for the abnormality. Another common assumption underlying much of the work in this area is that all medications useful for the treatment of depression work via a common final mechanism. A related concept inherent in some approaches to the field has been that unipolar depression and bipolar disorder have the same underlying cause; however, clinical studies have shown that unipolar depression and bipolar disorder may each be divided into subtypes.

Patients with affective disorders vary greatly in their responses to medication. Some are markedly improved; others obtain minimal benefit. Some respond equally well to psychosocial treatments, and in many cases there appear to be substantial benefits from combining pharmacological, psychological, and interpersonal treatments [5]. Much effort has gone into attempting to determine variables that predict or explain differences in medication responses among patients, thus far without success. It may be prudent to consider these diagnoses, like schizophrenia, as syndromes that may have a variety of biochemical causes. In terms of the effects of treatment, it is conceivable that different agents and approaches alleviate the symptoms of affective disorders via several distinct mechanisms.

MONOAMINE HYPOTHESES OF AFFECTIVE DISORDERS

The catecholamine hypothesis attempts to explain the etiology of depression and mania

The catecholamine hypothesis states that depression is caused by a functional deficiency of catecholamines, particularly norepinephrine (NE), whereas mania is caused by a functional excess of catecholamines at critical synapses in the brain [6–8]. This hypothesis was based on the correlation of the psychological and cellular actions of a variety of psychotropic agents. Other biogenic amines in brain have also been linked to depression and mania with the development of what are termed monoamine or biogenic amine hypotheses. These have included the indolamine serotonin [5-hydroxytryptamine (5-HT)]; two catecholamines other than NE [dopamine (DA) and epinephrine]; and acetylcholine.

The NE-deficiency hypothesis had several roots: One observation concerned the natural alkaloid, reserpine. This drug had been used in India for centuries as a treatment for mental illness. Beginning in the 1950s, reserpine was used for the treatment of hypertension and schizophrenia. It was noted that in some patients, reserpine caused a syndrome resembling depression. Animals given reserpine also developed a depression-like syndrome consisting of sedation and motor retardation. Subsequently, it was demonstrated that reserpine caused the depletion of presynaptic stores of NE, 5-HT, and DA.

In contrast to reserpine, iproniazid, a compound synthesized in the 1950s for the treatment of tuberculosis, was reported to produce euphoria and hyperactive behavior in some patients. It was found to increase brain concentrations of NE and 5-HT by inhibiting the metabolic enzyme, monoamine oxidase (MAO). Iproniazid as well as other MAO inhibitors were soon shown to be effective in alleviating depression.

The clinical and cellular actions of tricyclic antidepressants such as amitriptyline were considered to support the monoamine hypothesis of affective disorders. These drugs, resulting from a modification of the phenothiazine nucleus, were found to alleviate depression consistently, like the MAO inhibitors. Their major cellular action is to block the reuptake by presynaptic terminals of monoamine transmitters, thereby, presumably, increasing the concentration of monoamines available to interact with synaptic receptors. Thus, the actions of reserpine, MAO inhibitors, and tricyclics were initially thought to be consistent in supporting the monoamine hypothesis.

Inconsistencies arose, however. The pharmacological activities of several other compounds are difficult to reconcile with the monoamine hypothesis. Several clinically effective antidepressant agents, such as iprindole and mianserin, do not significantly inhibit MAO or block the reuptake of monoamines. The antimanic agent, lithium (discussed below), can also be used to treat depression yet does not chronically increase synaptic concentrations of monoamines. Conversely, cocaine, a potent inhibitor of monoamine reuptake, has no antidepressant activity.

More detailed examination of the actions of reserpine, MAO inhibitors, and tricyclics also reveals inconsistencies among their actions. Reserpine induces depression in only about 6 percent of patients, an incidence quite similar to the estimated incidence of depression in the general population. More important, the pharmacologic effects of MAO inhibitors and tricyclic antidepressants on catecholamines are immediate, yet their clinical antidepressant effects develop quite slowly, generally over 2 to 6 weeks.

Dopamine

Although interest in the monoamine hypothesis has centered on the roles of NE and 5-HT, DA may also be involved [8]. Levodopa can induce hypomania in patients with either bipolar disorder or Parkinson's disease, and DA receptor agonists have been reported to have some antidepressant effects. Furthermore, patients in the DA-depleted state of Parkinson's disease often develop a concomitant depression. Antidepressants may interact with central DA receptors. There are problems with postulating a primary role for DA in the affective disorders, however; for example, neuroleptic medications that are known to block DA receptors are not generally associated with the induction of depression.

Acetylcholine

Acetylcholine has also been implicated in the pathogenesis of affective disorders [9]. The cholinergic hypothesis suggests that hyper- and hypocholinergic states induce depression and mania, respectively. Support for this hypothesis comes from the finding that acetylcholinesterase inhibitors and cholinomimetics produce depressive symptoms under certain conditions. Conversely, anticholinergic agents have some antidepressant and euphorigenic properties, and anticholinergic toxicity can induce a state resembling mania. However, agents that act on cholinergic receptors are not very effective in the treatment of affective disorders. In an attempt to reconcile the data on the involvement of cholinergic and monominergic systems in the affective disorders, it has been proposed that an abnormal balance between cholinergic and monoaminergic systems might be critical in the development of depression and mania.

Clinical studies concentrate on measuring monoamines and their metabolites in biological fluids

3-Methoxy-4-hydroxyphenylglycol

Initially, investigators concentrated on measuring 3-methoxy-4-hydroxyphenylglycol (MHPG), a catecholamine metabolite, in urine and cerebrospinal fluid (CSF). Early evidence suggested there was decreased urinary MHPG concentrations in depressed patients and increased levels in mania, but more recent reports are not consistent. This is not entirely surprising, as it is now known that urinary MHPG is a poor indicator of CNS NE turnover because the CNS contributes as little as 20 percent of urinary MHPG. CSF MHPG levels, which may represent a more direct measure of brain NE function, have generally been found to be unaltered in affective disorders, although this remains a controversial area. Antidepressants have been found to decrease MHPG levels consistently in urine and CSF, but the treatment response of patients does not correlate with these changes. (See Chap. 11 for details of the metabolism of catecholamines.)

5-HT and 5-Hydroxyindoleacetic acid

Levels of the 5-HT metabolite, 5-hydroxyindoleacetic acid (5-HIAA), have also been extensively examined in the affective disorders [10] (see Chap. 12). A tentative conclusion from this work is that there is a bimodal distribution of CSF 5-HIAA levels in depressed patients and that patients with low CSF 5-HIAA are more prone to commit suicide. Antidepressants do seem to consistently lower CSF 5-HIAA concentrations, but this occurs whether or not the patient's depression improves.

Homovanillic acid

Like MHPG and 5-HIAA, CSF studies of homovanillic acid (HVA) in the affective disorders have shown no consistent differences between patients with depression or mania and controls (see Chaps. 11 and 42 for metabolic sequences). Many studies report a decrease in HVA levels in depressed patients. The efflux of HVA from the CSF has been inhibited by probenecid. The differences were largest in patients exhibiting psychomotor retardation and insignificant in patients with agitation, suggesting that HVA levels may reflect, at least in part, motor activity.

Acetylcholine

Clinical studies of acetylcholine and its metabolites are limited [9]. It has been reported that patients with depression have altered density of muscarinic receptors compared to controls, but this has been questioned.

There is a lack of consistent abnormalities in the levels of monoamine metabolites in the affective disorders

The lack of consistency is probably due to a variety of factors, the most important being the enormous heterogeneity subsumed under the diagnoses of depression and mania. An example of the evidence for such heterogeneity is provided by the finding that there is probably more than one gene predisposing to the development of bipolar disorder [4,11]. To glean any useful information from metabolite studies it may be necessary to measure and compare a battery of monoamines and their metabolites rather than focusing on single metabolite levels. Further, it will be critical to develop improved methods of studying kinetic processes involving the different neuroregulator systems.

Several alternative strategies have been used to examine the role of monoamines in the affective disorders. Precursor loading entails administering precursors of biogenic amines to subjects to raise monoamine levels in the brain. Administration of the 5-HT precursors, L-tryptophan or 5-hydroxytryptophan (5-HTP), with or without concomitant antidepressant medication, or the catecholamine precursor, levodopa, has been attempted as a therapeutic regimen. None of these compounds are in routine clinical use.

Another approach, used primarily in manic patients, has been to administer inhibitors of enzymes involved in the formation of biogenic amines. In particular, studies have been undertaken of the effects of α-methyl-*para*-tyrosine (AMPT), a competitive inhibitor of tyrosine hydroxylase, to lower levels of catecholamines, or *para*-chlorophenylalanine (PCPA), an inhibitor of tryptophan hydroxylase, to lower levels of 5-HT. AMPT has been reported to improve mania in some manic patients and to worsen depression in some previously depressed patients. PCPA did not decrease symptoms in manic patients but has been noted to reverse the antidepressant effects of imipramine, further suggesting a serotonergic role in the action of that antidepressant. These intriguing findings are the subject of ongoing research.

RECEPTOR HYPOTHESES OF AFFECTIVE DISORDERS

Inconsistencies with the monoamine hypotheses of affective disorders have led some investigators to alternative proposals that attempt to correlate more closely the clinical and cellular actions of antidepressants. These focus particularly on measuring the density and responsiveness of postsynaptic receptors.

β-Adrenergic and, possibly, serotonergic receptors may mediate the clinical effects of antidepressant drugs

During the search for neurochemical events that occur over the same time course as antidepressant actions, investigators found that in experimental animals, long-term (>2 weeks) antidepressant treatment caused a reduction in NE- or isoproterenol-stimulated cyclic AMP (cAMP) accumulation in the brain [12] (see Chaps. 17 and 18 for control of cAMP). Generally, but not uniformly, there is a concomitant decrease in the density of β-adrenergic receptors, that is, a decrease in B_{max}, as defined in Chap. 9. This may be due to the antidepressant-induced increase in synaptic availability of NE and a consequent down-regulation of β-adrenergic receptors. Notably, the decrease in NE-stimulated cAMP accumulation has been shown to occur not only with MAO inhibitors and tricyclic antidepressants but also with iprindole, mianserin, and electroconvulsive therapy (ECT), all of which are effective treatments for depression in humans.

Down-regulation of the 5-HT$_2$ receptor, a subtype of the 5-HT receptor, has also been demonstrated to occur following long-term but not acute antidepressant treatment (see Chap. 12). Lesioning the serotonergic system can prevent down-regulation of β-adrenergic receptors by antidepressants, a finding that suggests that there may be a strong link between serotonergic and noradrenergic systems in mediating the actions of antidepressants [13].

The corollary of the neurotransmitter-receptor hypothesis is that some forms of depression (and mania) may be caused by some abnormality in the regulation of postsynaptic β-adrenergic, and possibly serotonergic, receptors. It has been difficult to test this hypothesis in humans because to do so requires obtaining unfixed brain tissue shortly after death from a large number of affected individuals and controls. Nonetheless, studies using a limited number of autopsy samples tend to show a significant increase in the number of β-adrenergic and 5-HT$_2$ receptors in the brains of suicide victims compared with controls [14]. With the advent of positron emission tomography (PET), which allows *in vivo* quantitation of neurotransmitter receptors, it may be possible to extend these studies more easily (see Chap. 44).

ADDITIONAL BIOCHEMICAL HYPOTHESES OF AFFECTIVE DISORDERS

Other proposed causes for biological dysfunction underlying affective disorders include changes in the levels or activities of the metabolic enzymes, MAO, catechol-*O*-methyltransferase (COMT), or dopamine-β-hydroxylase (DBH) (see Chaps. 11 and 42). Decreased responsiveness to α$_2$-adrenergic agonists in some depressed patients has led to the suggestion that α$_2$-adrenergic receptors are involved in the etiology of depression.

Neuropeptides, such as the opioids, somatostatin, or vasopressin, may play critical roles in the affective disorders; however, neuropeptide systems are particularly difficult to investigate because their assay is complex. There are only limited ways of investigating the kinetics of their turnover and metabolism in humans, and only a fraction of the neuropeptides that may act as critical neuroregulators have been identified [15]. Nevertheless, there is substantial reason to believe that neuropeptides may be coreleased with other neuroregulators and may play important transmitter and regulatory roles (see Chaps. 13 and 14). An example of the interest in neuropeptides is the hypothesis that a relative deficiency or excess of one of the opioid peptides, or an alteration in receptors for opioid peptides, may prove to be important in some forms of depression or mania.

Rather than postulating that simple over-

or underactivity of a neuroregulator system induces depression or mania, some investigators have proposed that dysregulation of one or more neurotransmitter or neuromodulator homeostatic mechanisms is the causative factor [16].

NEUROENDOCRINE DYSFUNCTION IN DEPRESSION

There is substantial evidence for alteration in the hypothalamic-pituitary-adrenal axis in depression

A variety of endocrine disorders have profound psychiatric manifestations. Behavior that is controlled in part by the hypothalamic-pituitary-adrenal axis is disturbed in affective illnesses [17] (see also Chap. 47). It is therefore not surprising that a number of neuroendocrine markers are abnormal in the affective disorders, particularly in depression.

A dysfunction in the hypothalamic-pituitary-adrenal axis is suggested by studies of cortisol secretion and regulation. There is a reasonably consistent finding that during the illness, but not after recovery, a significant percentage of depressed patients hypersecrete cortisol or exhibit an abnormal diurnal variation in cortisol secretion. The additional finding that a majority of depressed patients exhibit decreased sensitivity to the dexamethasone-induced suppression of cortisol secretion suggests that the primary abnormality is hypersecretion of ACTH and/or corticotropin-releasing hormone (CRH). Whether disturbances in the monoaminergic control of hypothalamic or pituitary cells are responsible for these findings is unclear.

Several investigators have reported that stimulation of the secretion of thyroid-stimulating hormone (TSH) by thyrotropin-releasing hormone (TRH) is significantly reduced in some depressed patients. This points again to a dysfunction in the anterior pituitary itself, the hypothalamus, or in the neuronal systems that modulate the activity of these areas (Chap. 14).

Another neuroendocrine abnormality consistently found in depressed patients is decreased growth hormone response to the α_2-adrenergic agonist, clonidine. It is believed that the growth hormone response to clonidine is mediated by hypothalamic α_2-adrenergic receptors.

A new dimension in depression research has come from studies of seasonal affective disorders in which depression may occur in relation to changes in light. There is evidence that this form of depression may be related to the pineal gland and to the secretion of melatonin. It is interesting that this form of depression appears to be treated by exposure to light [18,19].

It should be noted that a significant number of depressed patients exhibit no neuroendocrine abnormalities and that these measurements can be affected by nonspecific factors, such as sex, age, weight, activity level, and stress. Biological rhythms and sleep alterations are also critical factors [20]. The overlap between measurements is unclear. Nevertheless, the multiple links between brain and endocrine organs (see Chap. 47) make it likely that further study of neuroendocrine abnormalities in psychiatric illness will be of value and may facilitate subtyping of forms of affective illness and aid in assessing treatment response.

ACTION OF LITHIUM IN THE TREATMENT OF AFFECTIVE DISORDERS

Lithium is effective in treating mania and depression

Lithium is universally accepted as the treatment of choice for bipolar disorder. Well-controlled clinical studies have shown it to decrease the severity, length, and recurrence of manic episodes. Lithium also has significant antidepressant properties in both bipolar disorder and unipolar depression. The discovery of the clinical effectiveness of lithium in treating mania was serendipitous. In 1949, John Cade, an Australian, injected the urine of manic patients into guinea pigs to test for a toxic substance that might cause illness. The procedure often killed the animals due to the toxicity of urea. While attempting to determine how uric acid modified urea toxicity, he administered lithium urate, the most soluble urate salt, and observed that the animals often became sedated. By performing appropriate controls, Cade discovered that the lithium ion was the sedative. After finding that self-administration produced no significant adverse effects, Cade administered lithium to manic patients, fortuitously in a dose that turned out to be clinically optimal. All of the patients responded positively. Soon after, Mogens Schou, in a series of clinical trials in Denmark, proved that lithium was an effective agent in treating mania and in preventing the recurrence of manic episodes. Lithium was in common use in Europe by the mid-1960s and was finally approved for clinical use in the United States in 1969.

Lithium may alter some biogenic amine systems

Lithium has a wide range of biological actions, including antagonism of enzymes, ion pumps, ion channels, and membrane transport mechanisms. Most of the work attempting to discover the critical cellular site of lithium's therapeutic action has concentrated on its effects on monoaminergic neuronal systems and has paralleled rather closely the study of the mechanism of action of antidepressants [21]. The results of these studies present a complex picture. Initially, lithium increases NE turnover in rat brain, but with long-term administration no significant change occurs. The action of chronic lithium treatment on DA turnover has been inconsistent, with both increases and decreases

as well as no significant change reported. Lithium also initially increases tryptophan uptake, leading to increased 5-HT synthesis; however, with continued administration, tryptophan hydroxylase activity is decreased, resulting in no net change in 5-HT synthesis.

Following the studies of monoamine turnover and in parallel with studies on the mechanism of action of antidepressants, investigators turned their attention to receptor modification as the possible site of lithium action. Lithium was consistently reported to prevent the development of neuroleptic-induced DA receptor supersensitivity. Thus, stabilization of the DA receptor was suggested to be a critical element in controlling mania. Like antidepressants, lithium treatment can also inhibit the β-adrenergic receptor stimulation of adenylate cyclase (see Chap. 17). The relationship between these receptor modifications and the therapeutic activity of lithium remains unclear.

Lithium may act by altering phosphoinositide turnover in the brain

An area of intense research is the effect of lithium on phosphoinositide (PI) turnover in the brain [22] (see Chap. 16). As outlined previously, PI turnover is increased by a variety of putative neurotransmitters and has second-messenger activity analogous to that of the adenylate cyclase-cAMP cascade. Lithium potently inhibits the enzyme *myo*-inositol-1-phosphatase. This blocks the transformation of *myo*-inositol-1-phosphate to *myo*-inositol. The result of chronic lithium treatment is thus an increase in brain levels of *myo*-inositol-1-phosphate and a decrease in the concentration of *myo*-inositol [23]. Since *myo*-inositol is required for the resynthesis of the parent polyphosphoinositides, it has been suggested that lithium may exert its therapeutic actions by damping or altering the cellular responses to those neurotransmitters whose actions are mediated by PI phosphate turnover [24]. There are several attractive aspects to this hypothesis. Lithium commonly takes several days to exert its clinical effects. Similarly, the buildup of *myo*-inositol-1-phosphate and decrease in *myo*-inositol in rat brain does not occur instantaneously, but requires chronic treatment. In addition, the CNS is probably particularly sensitive to decreases in *myo*-inositol levels when compared to peripheral tissues, since cells in the CNS cannot obtain inositol from the plasma, whereas most peripheral cells can.

Perhaps the most important aspect of the hypothesis is the prediction that the ability of lithium to antagonize PI turnover is dependent on activation of the receptor-stimulated PI system. A quiescent cell or one in which PI turnover is low would be relatively unaffected by lithium-mediated inhibition of *myo*-inositol-1-phosphatase, whereas a highly active cell would be expected to accumulate *myo*-inositol-1-phosphate and run out of stores of *myo*-inositol, leading to impaired ability to respond to subsequent stimulation. Thus, the action of lithium would be targeted toward those neuronal systems in which PI turnover is most active. Such a mechanism might explain how lithium is able to treat both mania and depression successfully, behavioral states that probably reflect the activation of distinct neuronal systems. Furthermore, a variety of transmitters, all with the common property of being coupled to PI turnover, would be affected by lithium.

Although both tricyclic antidepressants and lithium alter the sensitivity of the adenylate cyclase-cAMP cascade, only lithium additionally affects PI turnover. These two second-messenger systems are now known to be involved in the actions of a large and growing number of neurotransmitter receptor systems (Chaps. 16 and 19). It is possible that the basic biological defects underlying some affective disorders lie not with neurotransmitter synthesis or metabolism, nor with their receptors, but rather with the regulation of one or both of these intracellular biochemical cascades. Protein kinase A and

C, the kinases activated by cAMP and PI turnover, respectively, can phosphorylate and thereby modulate receptors, synthetic enzymes, and GTP-binding proteins, the proteins that couple receptor to effector. (These phosphorylation reactions are discussed in Chap. 19.)

An abnormality at one step in the second-messenger cascade could have appreciable consequences for a variety of cellular processes and could help explain the diverse results from clinical studies and the variety of reported actions of antidepressants and lithium. Pseudohypoparathyroidism (type 1A) is an example of a well-characterized interruption in the second-messenger cascade. It is an illness caused by a defect in the GTP-binding protein that couples parathyroid hormone receptor to stimulation of adenylate cyclase.

BIOCHEMICAL ASPECTS OF ANXIETY

Anxiety may be a serious illness with several subtypes

Anxiety is the apprehension of danger or something unpleasant. Whereas fear is a response to current, tangible threats, anxiety occurs in anticipation of a threat not yet present and often not clearly defined. Anxiety is a familiar part of everyday human life, and something akin to anxiety probably occurs in most mammals and many other vertebrates. Anxiety has clear adaptive value, and in humans it must certainly be considered normal. Yet in some individuals, anxiety reaches a level that is counterproductive or even incapacitating. There may be several distinct types of anxiety disorders in which the level of anxiety becomes pathological [25].

Anxiety disorders are among the most common of all psychiatric conditions. In addition, anxiety is a prominent symptom in almost all other psychiatric illnesses. Various studies have found that from about 3 to 8 percent of the population has clinically significant anxiety at any one time. This prevalence is surprisingly consistent from culture to culture throughout the world. Because of their tremendous costs to society, anxiety and its disorders have been the subject of intense study. For many years, this study was confined to the psychological realm, and the knowledge gained remains central to a full understanding of anxiety and the treatment of its disorders. In the past three decades, however, a picture of the biology and chemistry of anxiety has begun to emerge; although far from complete, it is changing our perception of anxiety and leading to new approaches for therapy.

The evidence used to determine the neurochemical bases of anxiety has been similar to that for the affective disorders. Most information has come from studying the action of anxiety-reducing, or anxiolytic, drugs. This has been aided by the existence of several animal models of anxiety that are probably closer to the human condition of anxiety than are animal models of affective disorders to their human counterparts. Most of what is known of the biochemistry of anxiety concerns the γ-aminobutyric acid (GABA)-benzodiazepine receptor-Cl^- ionophore system and the serotonergic system.

Benzodiazepines have revolutionized the treatment of anxiety disorders

The introduction of benzodiazepines has also set the stage for greatly increasing our understanding of the biochemistry of anxiety. Anxiolytic drugs were among the earliest effective pharmaceutical agents devised. One of the most prominent effects of ethanol is its tendency to obliterate anxiety, one of the major reasons for its continuing popularity. Opiate alkaloids and belladonna derivatives also have potent anxiolytic activities. Barbiturates and, later, propanediol carbamates such as meprobamate were used extensively for the relief of anxiety in this century. The use of each of these drugs is limited by several side effects, most notably their serious toxicity at high doses and, with the exception of belladonna, their high liability to addiction.

Since the early 1960s, the use of barbiturates and other agents as prescription anxiolytics has been almost entirely superceded by the benzodiazepines, such as chlordiazepoxide and diazepam. The benzodiazepines are very effective for the relief of anxiety. They also have considerably lower potential for addiction than barbiturates and propanediol carbamates and are much less likely to cause death or serious lasting harm when taken in large overdoses. There are now about two dozen different benzodiazepine drugs in clinical use worldwide today. The various compounds appear to differ primarily in their pharmacokinetics—the speed with which they are taken up and eliminated by the body—rather than in their clinical effects. These clinical effects are fourfold: anxiolytic, sedative or sleep-inducing, anticonvulsant, and muscle relaxant. It was thought at first that the benzodiazepines might have a different mechanism of action for each of these effects. For example, it was noted that tolerance to sedation but not anxiolytic action quickly develops in patients taking a benzodiazepine; however, all clinical effects of benzodiazepines appear to be mediated centrally.

In 1977, two groups independently discovered high-affinity binding sites for diazepam in brain [26,27]. The affinities of a variety of benzodiazepines for these sites correlated well with their clinical potency. Correlations with potency in animal models of anxiety were also sought. The most common animal model for anxiety involves pairing a reward for which the animal must perform some behavior, such as lever pressing, with an aversive stimulus, such as a mild electric shock. A conflict is thus produced. Agents that appear to reduce this conflict and increase the rate of responses punished with the shock (punished-responding) generally act as anxiolytics in humans. Benzodiazepines that were most potent in releasing punished-responding behavior had the highest affinity for benzodiazepine binding sites. These binding sites were found in highest density in areas of the brain that developed later in evolution, for example, in cerebral cortex, and are thought to be concerned with the production of emotional responses such as anxiety. The interaction of the benzodiazepines with their receptor appeared to be quite specific: No other classes of compounds known at that time had high affinity for these sites, and benzodiazepines did not demonstrate high affinity for any other neurotransmitter receptors in competitive binding assays. These studies were taken as evidence that it was the binding to these sites that mediated the action of the benzodiazepines [28].

Much effort has gone into determining the nature of benzodiazepine binding sites. For some time it was suspected that benzodiazepine action might be closely associated with GABAergic mechanisms. Electrophysiological studies in the mid-1970s showed that diazepam facilitated GABAergic synaptic transmission.

CNS benzodiazepine binding sites are closely associated with the GABA$_A$ subtype of GABA receptor

The GABA$_A$ subtype of GABA receptor is widely distributed in the CNS, primarily postsynaptically, and mediates changes in neuronal membrane potential by opening a Cl$^-$ channel (see Chap. 15). The GABA$_A$ receptor, the benzodiazepine binding site, and the Cl$^-$ ionophore appear to be part of a single large macromolecular complex because these functions can be copurified in detergent-solubilized preparations [29]. The receptor is a tetramer consisting of two α subunits ($M_r \sim 53,000$) and two β subunits ($M_r \sim 57,000$). The GABA$_A$ receptor has been cloned [30]. GABA and the benzodiazepines each allosterically modulate the binding of the other to this macromolecular complex; the benzodiazepines, by binding to the α subunit, and GABA by binding to the β subunit.

In vitro, Cl$^-$ acts to increase benzodiazepine receptor affinity, and it is necessary for the reciprocal regulation of GABA and benzodiazepine binding. Benzodiazepines facilitate GABAergic transmission primarily by increasing the frequency of Cl$^-$ channel opening in response to occupancy of the GABA$_A$ receptor by GABA. There is also a distinctly different benzodiazepine binding site in the periphery that is unassociated with GABA receptors.

Barbiturates also mediate at least some of their important actions via binding to some portion of this complex closely associated with the Cl$^-$ ionophore (see Chaps. 15 and 41). Like benzodiazepines, they facilitate GABA-dependent Cl$^-$ flux in brain slices and cultured neurons. In addition, barbiturates enhance [^{3}H]benzodiazepine and [^{3}H]GABA agonist binding to their respective sites in *in vitro* binding assays; however, the exact mechanism appears to be somewhat different from that of the benzodiazepines. First, barbiturates are not competitive inhibitors of ligands for either GABA$_A$ or benzodiazepine binding sites. Second, unlike benzodiazepines, barbiturates decrease the frequency of opening of GABA-activated Cl$^-$ channels but still potentiate GABA responses by increasing the mean open time of the ionophore.

GABAergic stimulation with GABA agonists also has an anxiolytic effect

The GABA agonist muscimol has anxiolytic activity in animal models, and picrotoxin, a drug that potently inhibits GABA-promoted Cl$^-$ flux, has the opposite effect. The experimental and clinical utility of GABAergic drugs is limited, however, by their toxicity and in some cases their limited ability to cross the blood–brain barrier. There is growing evidence that ethanol and the propanediol carbamates also produce some of their anxiolytic effects by acting at the GABA-benzodiazepine receptor–Cl^- ionophore complex.

Several classes of compounds act as benzodiazepine antagonists

Compounds that act as benzodiazepine antagonists have also been called inverse agonists because they have behavioral actions opposite to those produced by benzodiazepines—they increase sleeplessness and in higher doses cause seizures. The first type of benzodiazepine antagonists described were esters of β-carbolines. These compounds were first studied as possible endogenous ligands for the benzodiazepine binding site. Although they were subsequently shown not to be present in the body, several other candidate endogenous ligands have since been reported. Peptides that may serve as endogenous ligand candidates have been suggested, one of which appears to be an inverse agonist. The existence and physiological function in humans of any of the endogenous ligands have yet to be established.

Serotonin has also been linked to anxiety processes and may be important in the origin and treatment of anxiety

Aside from the GABA-benzodiazepine receptor complex, no other neurotransmitter system has received so much attention in relation to anxiety as has serotonin (5-HT) [31]. It has long been known that depletion of 5-HT with PCPA or lesioning of the dorsal raphe nucleus, the site of most CNS 5-HT neuronal bodies, with 5,7-dihydroxytryptamine has an anxiolytic-like effect in rodents. Similar suggestive observations were made demonstrating that in some cases serotonergic agonists produced an increase in anxiety; however, some 5-HT antagonists tend to release punished-responding behavior in animals or reduce anxiety in humans, whereas

other 5-HT antagonists have the opposite effect. Confidence in a serotonergic role in anxiety has also been tempered by the fact that the lesioning procedures produce a number of alterations in neurotransmitter systems other than those utilizing 5-HT. It has long been suspected that most serotonergic drugs are nonspecific, and this has been borne out by the demonstration of multiple distinct CNS 5-HT receptors.

It has thus been difficult until very recently to extend studies of serotonin and anxiety to the molecular level. The compound buspirone has been introduced as the first anxiolytic agent whose clinical effects are probably mediated by effects on the 5-HT system. Buspirone and related compounds may both alter the treatment of anxiety and offer new tools for its study, just as the benzodiazepines did a generation ago.

Buspirone actions in humans are different from those of the benzodiazepines. Buspirone, in contrast to the benzodiazepines, has a delayed onset of action—it must be administered for up to several weeks before a significant reduction of anxiety is observed. This is true despite a relatively rapid establishment of steady-state serum drug levels. Buspirone, again unlike the benzodiazepines, has almost no sedative, anticonvulsant, or muscle-relaxant activity. Another distinguishing feature is that buspirone has no significant addiction liability. These last considerations make buspirone a significant advance in the treatment of anxiety in many patients.

Buspirone has no direct effect on the $GABA_A$-benzodiazepine receptor system. Although it has a weak effect on dopamine receptors, its primary effect appears to be mediated by serotonin receptors [32]. Brain serotonin receptors have recently been divided into at least four distinct subtypes based on their pharmacological specificities, anatomical distribution, and function (see also Chap. 12). Buspirone appears to interact preferentially with the $5-HT_{1A}$ subtype [33]. Several additional $5-HT_{1A}$ active compounds have also demonstrated anxiolytic activity in animals. The $5\text{-}HT_{1A}$ receptor is widely distributed as a postsynaptic receptor in the forebrain of rodents, humans, and other mammalian species. It also serves as the autoreceptor on raphe neurons. In rat hippocampal slices it is linked to a K^+ channel shared with the $GABA_B$ receptor, a receptor that is not associated with benzodiazepine action [34]. The $5\text{-}HT_{1A}$ receptor has also been reported to be linked to adenylate cyclase, although this remains controversial, since both stimulation and inhibition of this second-messenger system have been reported. Buspirone has been reported to be a mixed agonist/antagonist at the receptor. It is not yet completely clear whether the anxiolytic actions of this compound are due to its agonist activity or its particular mixed agonist/antagonist character.

REFERENCES

1. Dunner, D. Affective disorders: Clinical features. In R. Michels and J. O. Cavenar (eds.), *Psychiatry*. Philadelphia: Lippincott, 1985, Vol. 1, Chapter 59.
2. Weissman, M. M., and Boyd, J. H. Affective disorders: Epidemiology. In H. I. Kaplan and B. J. Sadock (eds.), *Comprehensive Textbook of Psychiatry IV*. Baltimore: Williams and Wilkins, 1985, Vol. 1, pp. 764–769.
3. Nurnberger, J. I., Jr., and Gershon, E. S. Genetics of affective disorders. In R. M. Post and J. C. Ballenger (eds.), *Neurobiology of Mood Disorders*. Baltimore: Williams and Wilkins, 1984, pp. 76–101.
4. Egeland, J. A., Gerhard, D. S., Pauls, D. L., Sussex, J. N., Kidd, K. K., et al. Bipolar affective disorders linked to DNA markers on chromosome 11. *Nature* 325:783–787, 1987.
5. Klerman, G. L., Weissman, M. M., Rounsaville, B. J., and Chevron, E. S. *Interpersonal Psychotherapy of Depression*. New York: Basic Books, 1984.
6. Schildkraut, J. J. The catecholamine hypothesis of affective disorders: A review of supporting evidence. *Am. J. Psychiatry* 122:509–522, 1965.
7. Bunney, W. E., Jr., and Davis, J. M. Norepinephrine in depressive reactions. *Arch. Gen. Psychiatry* 13:483–494, 1965.
8. Gerner, R. H., and Bunney, W. E., Jr. Biological hypotheses of affective disorders. In P. A. Berger and K. H. Brodie (eds.), *American Handbook of Psychiatry*. New York: Basic Books, 1986, Vol. 8, pp. 265–301.
9. Dilsaver, S. C. Cholinergic mechanisms in depression. *Brain Res. Rev.* 11:285–316, 1986.
10. Van Praag, H. M. Indoleamines in depression and suicide. *Prog. Brain Res.* 65:59–71, 1986.
11. Hodgkinson, S., Sherrington, R., Gurling, H., Marchbanks, R., Reeders, S., et al. Molecular genetic evidence for heterogeneity in manic depression. *Nature* 325:805–806, 1987.
12. Charney, D. S., Menkes, D. B., and Heninger, G. R. Receptor sensitivity and the mechanism of action of antidepressant treatment: Implications for the etiology and therapy of depression. *Arch. Gen. Psychiatry* 38:1160–1180, 1981.
13. Janowsky, A., Okada, F., Manier, D. H., Applegate, C. D., Sulser, F., and Steranka, L. R. Role of serotonergic input in the regulation of the beta adrenergic receptor-coupled adenylate cyclase system. *Science* 218:900–901, 1982.
14. Mann, J. J., Stanley, M., McBride, P. A., and McEwen, B. S. Increased serotonin$_2$ and β-adrenergic receptor binding in the frontal cortices of suicide victims. *Arch. Gen. Psychiatry* 43:954–959, 1986.
15. Martin, J. B., and Barchas, J. D. (eds.). *Neuropeptides in Neurologic and Psychiatric Disease*. New York: Raven Press, 1986.
16. Siever, L. J., and Davis, K. L. Overview: Toward a dysregulation hypothesis of depression. *Am. J. Psychiatry* 142:1017–1031, 1985.
17. Kalin, N. H., and Dawson, G. Neuroendocrine dysfunction in depression: Hypothalamic-anterior pituitary systems. *Trends Neurosci.* 9:261–266, 1986.
18. Lewy, A. J., et al. Light suppresses melatonin secretion in humans. *Science* 210:1267–1269, 1980.
19. Wehr, T. A., and Goodwin, F. K. Biological rhythms and manic-depressive illness. In T. A.

Wehr and F. K. Goodwin (eds.), *Biological Rhythms and Psychiatry*. Pacific Grove, CA: Boxwood Press, 1983.

20. Kupfer, D. A., Monk, T., and Barchas, J. D. (eds.). *Biological Rhythms and Mental Disorders*. New York: Guilford Press, 1988 (*in press*).

21. Bunney, W. E., Jr., and Garland, B. L. Lithium and its possible modes of action. In R. M. Post and J. C. Ballenger (eds.), *Neurobiology of Mood Disorders*. Baltimore: Williams and Wilkins, 1984, pp. 731–743.

22. Drummond, A. H. Lithium and inositol-lipid signalling mechanisms. *Trends Pharmacol. Sci.* 8:129–133, 1987.

23. Sherman, W. R., Gish, B. G., Honchar, M. P., and Munsell, L. Y. Effects of lithium on phosphoinositide metabolism in vivo. *Fed. Proc.* 45:2639–2646, 1986.

24. Berridge, M. J., Downes, C. P., and Hanley, M. R. Lithium amplifies agonist-dependent phosphatidylinositol responses in brain and salivary glands. *Biochem. J.* 206:587–595, 1982.

25. Nemiah, J. C. Anxiety states (anxiety neuroses). In H. I. Kaplan and B. J. Sadock (eds.), *Comprehensive Textbook of Psychiatry IV*. Baltimore: Williams and Wilkins, 1985, Vol. 1, pp. 883–893.

26. Mohler, H., and Okada, T. Benzodiazepine receptor: Demonstration in the central nervous system. *Science* 198:849–851, 1977.

27. Squire, R. F., and Braestrup, C. Benzodiazepine receptors in rat brain. *Nature* 266:732–734, 1977.

28. Paul, S. M., Crawley, J. N., and Skolnick, P. The neurobiology of anxiety: The role of the GABA/benzodiazepine receptor complex. In P. A. Berger and K. H. Brodie (eds.), *American Handbook of Psychiatry*. New York: Basic Books, Inc., 1986, Vol. 8, pp. 581–596.

29. Biggio, G., and Costa, E. (eds.), *GABAergic Transmission and Anxiety*. New York: Raven Press, 1986.

30. Schofield, P. R. Darlison, M. G., Fujita, N., Burt, D. R., Stephenson, F. A., et al. Sequence and functional expression of the $GABA_A$ receptor shows a ligand-gated receptor super-family. *Nature* 328:221–227, 1987.

31. Iversen, S. D. 5-HT and anxiety. *Neuropharmacology* 23:1553–1560, 1984.

32. Dourish, C. T., Hutson, P. H., and Curzon, G. Putative anxiolytics 8-OH-DPAT, buspirone, and TVX Q 7821 are agonists at $5-HT_{1A}$ receptors in the raphe nuclei. *Trends Pharmacol. Sci.* 7:212–214, 1986.

33. Peroutka, S. J. Interactions of novel anxiolytic agents with $5-HT_{1A}$ receptors. *Biol. Psychiatry* 20:971–979, 1985.

34. Andrade, R., Malenka, R. C., and Nicoll, R. A. A G protein couples serotonin and $GABA_B$ receptors to the same channels in hippocampus. *Science* 234:1261–1265, 1986.

Endocrine Effects on the Brain and Their Relationship to Behavior

Bruce S. McEwen

Basic Neurochemistry: Molecular, Cellular, and Medical Aspects, 4th Ed., edited by G. J. Siegel et al. Raven Press, Ltd., New York, 1989.
Correspondence to Bruce S. McEwen, Laboratory of Neuroendocrinology, Rockefeller University, 1230 York Avenue, New York, New
York 10021.

The brain is capable of changes in chemistry and morphology in response to changes in the environment. Hormones play an important role in brain adaptation because they are secreted in response to environmental signals that are processed by the nervous system and then act back on specific brain areas to modify their function. These modifications occur during development, in adult life, in response to neural damage, and during the aging process. Because they can alter genomic activity, steroid hormones give us unique insights into the role of the genome in the control of brain function and behavioral plasticity.

Awareness of endocrine influences on brain function is as old as endocrinology itself. In 1849, Berthold described striking behavioral changes resulting from castration of roosters

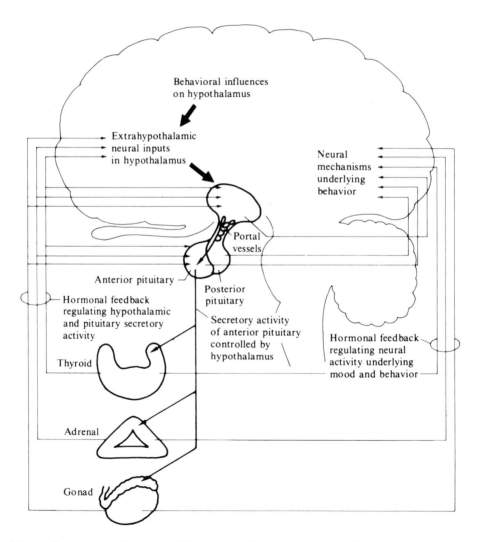

FIG. 1.   Schematic representation of possible reciprocal interactions among hypothalamic, pituitary, thyroid, adrenal, and gonadal hormones.

and the reversal of these changes after testes had been transplanted into the castrated animals [1]. Nearly 100 years later, Beach published *Hormones and Behavior* [2], which has served to instruct recent generations of investigators and motivate them to explore in depth the interactions of hormones and brain. Spectacular growth of the field of neuroendocrinology (see Chap. 14) offers the present generation of neurobiologists unparalleled opportunities to explore with great sophistication the influence of neural activity on endocrine secretion and of endocrine secretion, in turn, on neural activity and behavior.

The nervous system is the medium through which behavioral and endocrine events are related. This chapter focuses on the chemical and molecular aspects of the influences of hormonal secretion on the nervous system and behavior. But before doing so, it is necessary to describe briefly the behavioral events and the accompanying neural activity that can trigger hormone secretion.

BEHAVIORAL CONTROL OF HORMONE SECRETION

The brain produces master hormones, the hypothalamic releasing factors, which regulate release of the anterior pituitary trophic hormones

Neurons in the hypothalamus also produce the hormones oxytocin and vasopressin, which are released by the posterior pituitary into the blood. It is therefore not surprising that behavior and experience, which influence the hypothalamus, sometimes alter the secretion of these hypothalamic releasing factors and hormones (Fig. 1). Consider, for example, the phenomenon of lactation, in which the suckling stimulus to the nipple triggers the release of oxytocin, which facilitates milk ejection, and of prolactin, which helps the mammary gland to replenish the supply of milk [1].

The phenomenon of stress also illustrates the behavioral and emotional control of anterior pituitary hormone secretion. Conditions associated with tissue injury and surgical trauma, as well as the so-called psychic stresses of fear, novelty, and even joy, can activate the release of adrenocorticoid (ACTH), which, in turn, stimulates the secretion of adrenal glucocorticoids. The behavioral-emotional stimuli are mediated by neural pathways that can be modified readily by learning.

Secretion of the gonadotropins is subject to behavioral modification

In the female rabbit, the act of copulation activates spinal reflex pathways that stimulate the secretion of luteinizing hormone (LH) and leads to ovulation [1]. In the male rabbit, the act of copulation also activates the secretion of LH and increases plasma testosterone levels [1]. Social stimuli, too, modify gonadotropin secretion. In mice, olfactory cues from other females can interrupt normal estrous cycles and lead to pseudopregnancies or periods of prolonged diestrus (Lee-Boot effect); olfactory cues from males can shorten the estrous cycle and either cause rapid attainment of estrus (Whitten effect) or terminate pregnancy in a newly impregnated mouse (Bruce effect) [1]. In male rhesus monkeys, sudden decisive defeat by other males leads to prolonged reduction in plasma testosterone levels, which can be reversed in the defeated male by the introduction of a female companion [1]. In men, the anticipation of sexual intercourse has been reported to increase beard growth, a process under the control of circulating androgen [1], although this finding has been disputed.

Hormones secreted in response to behavioral signals act, in turn, on the brain and on other tissues

Functional changes caused by hormones secreted in response to behavioral signals include modifications of behavior. With the sex hormones, these changes act to strengthen and guide the reproductive process. Thus, aggressive encounters between male birds or mammals in defense of territory during the mating period stimulate gonadotropin and testosterone secretion and further increase readiness for sexual activity by enhancing supplies of sperm and seminal fluid. This analysis was taken further by Lehrman [1] who showed that among doves the behavioral sequence of courtship, mating, nest-building, and parenting each involves complex behavioral interplay between the partners that triggers further hormone secretion, which unfolds the next phase of behavior and hormone secretion.

With the adrenal steroids, the behavioral activation of hormonal secretion in stress is part of a mechanism for restoring homeostatic balance. For example, an encounter with a predator may require rapid evasive action in which neural activity and rapidly mobilized hormones such as epinephrine play a role. Adrenal steroid secretion is slower, reaching a peak minutes after the stressful event, and as such is not expected to play a role in coping with the immediate situation. If the evasive action is successful and the animal survives, it will have to re-establish homeostasis; presumably, it will also learn from the experience to minimize the chances of another such encounter. Adrenal steroids act to facilitate such long-term adaptation; that is, they facilitate the extinction of a conditioned avoidance response [2]. Suppose an animal has learned to avoid a certain place where it was previously punished; it later discovers that being in that place no longer results in punishment. If, for example, that place also contains a food or water supply, it is in the best interest of the animal to extinguish the avoidance response in order to take advantage of the available food or water. Adrenal steroids have, in fact, been found to facilitate such extinction and can thus be said to facilitate a form of be-

havioral adaptation [2]. Another aspect of adaptation in which stress-induced secretion of adrenal steroids participate concerns the ability of the organism to cope with a repeated stressful event through a variety of neurochemical changes [3].

Besides stress, adrenal steroids are also secreted in varying amounts according to the time of day, and in this capacity they perform an important role of coordinating daily activity and sleep patterns with food seeking and processing of information [3]. In nocturnally active animals such as the rat, adrenal steroids are secreted at the end of the light period prior to onset of darkness. In humans and in monkeys, adrenal steroid secretion precedes waking in the morning to begin daily activity. Thus, in both rats and primates, adrenal steroid secretion precedes the waking period and appears to contribute, during waking, to optimal synaptic efficacy in the hippocampus for long-term potentiation, a correlate of learning. Moreover, adrenal steroid elevation prior to waking also increases food-seeking behavior and enhances appetite for carbohydrates [3].

Cyclic changes in hormonal secretion, which are under the control of daily and seasonal light-dark rhythms, are important not only for the adrenals but for the gonads as well. Estrous cycles, menstrual cycles, and seasonal breeding patterns represent adaptations of individual species to climatic conditions of their environment. The feedback actions of gonadal and adrenal hormones, which are secreted in response to rhythmic output of hypothalamic and pituitary hormones, prime or activate the nervous system to perform the appropriate behavioral responses. It is important to stress that hormones themselves do not cause behaviors; rather, hormones induce chemical changes in particular sets of neurons, making certain behavioral outcomes more likely as a result of the strengthening or weakening of particular neural pathways.

CLASSIFICATION OF HORMONAL EFFECTS

The principal means of classifying hormone action on target neurons is in terms of cellular mechanisms of action

Hormones act either via the cell surface or via intracellular receptors. Peptide hormones and amino acid derivatives such as epinephrine act on cell surface receptors that may open ion channels to allow exocytosis of hormone from or production of rapid electrical responses in the target cell. Alternatively, they activate second-messenger systems at the cell membrane, such as those involving cyclic AMP (cAMP), Ca^{2+}-calmodulin, or phosphoinositides (see Chaps. 8, 17–19), which lead to phosphorylation of proteins inside various parts of the target cell (Fig. 2A). Steroid hormones and thyroid hormone, on the other hand, act on intracellular receptors in the cell nuclei to regulate gene expression and protein synthesis (Fig. 2B and C).

The various modes of hormone action summarized in Fig. 2 may be distinguished from each other by time course. The fastest effects, both in latency and duration, are those involving direct opening of ion channels and stimulation of exocytosis. Intermediate are those effects involving phosphorylation of enzymes, ion channels, receptors, or structural proteins, which may last for minutes or even hours. Slowest and most enduring are those effects which alter gene expression and lead to induction or repression of enzyme or receptor proteins, growth responses, and even the structural remodeling of tissues.

Second-messenger systems, through phosphorylation of nuclear proteins, can influence gene expression; however, the purest examples of genomic regulation of neuronal function stem from the actions of gonadal and adrenal steroids and thyroid hormone, and many of these actions are involved in the plasticity of behavior that results from hormone secretion, such as changes in aggressive and reproductive behavior and adaptation to repeated stress. In fact, hormone actions that involve the genome are pervasive throughout the life cycle, and we can distinguish four major types of hormone actions on the nervous system:

1. Developmental actions, such as are involved in sexual differentiation
2. Reversible effects on the functioning of neurons and glial cells that are responsible for cyclical changes in behavior and adaptation to stress
3. Actions that occur during response to neural damage and promote repair
4. Effects that promote or potentiate neural damage and cell death

BIOCHEMISTRY OF STEROID HORMONE ACTION

Steroid hormones are divided into six classes, based on physiological effects: estrogens, androgens, progestins, glucocorticoids, mineralocorticoids, and vitamin D

Steroid hormone action on the brain and on other target tissues involves intracellular receptor sites that interact with the genome [4] (Fig. 2). There are also important metabolic transformations of certain steroids, occurring in the nervous system, that either generate more active metabolites or result in the production of less active steroids. Such transformations are particularly important for the actions of androgens, of lesser importance for estrogens and progestins, and of practically no importance for glucocorticoids and mineralocorticoids. For vitamin D, the principal transformation to an active metabolite occurs in the kidney and liver [5].

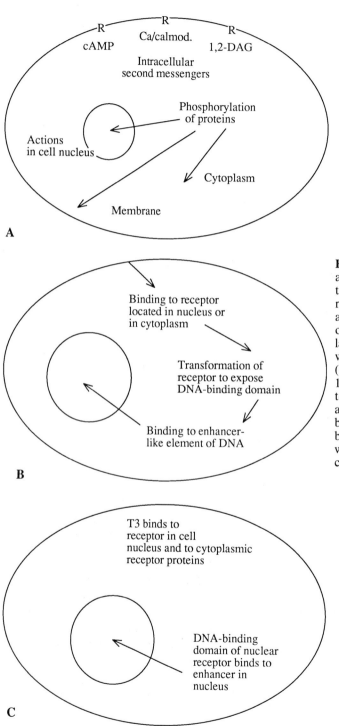

FIG. 2. Schematic representation of interaction of hormones with target cells. **A:** Peptide, protein, and other surface-acting hormones interact with cell surface receptors to activate second-messenger systems. The second messengers activate protein phosphorylation, among which are proteins that interact with the genome: (cAMP) cyclic 3′5′AMP; (Ca/calmod) calcium/calmodulin; (1,2-DAG) 1,2-diacyl-glycerol. **B:** Steroid hormones interact with intracellular receptors that can be activated or transformed to expose DNA binding domain. **C:** Thyroid hormone T_3 binds to cell nuclear receptor, which interacts with DNA in a manner similar to steroid receptor.

Metabolism of steroid hormones in brain tissue

The brain, like the seminal vesicles, is able to convert testosterone to 5 α-dihydrotestosterone (DHT) [Fig. 3 (a)] and, like the placenta, converts testosterone to estradiol (Fig. 3). Neither conversion occurs equally in all brain regions. Regional distribution of 5α-reductase activity toward testosterone in rat brain is found in midbrain and brain stem; intermediate activity in hypothalamus and thalamus; and lowest activity in cerebral cortex [6]. The pituitary has higher

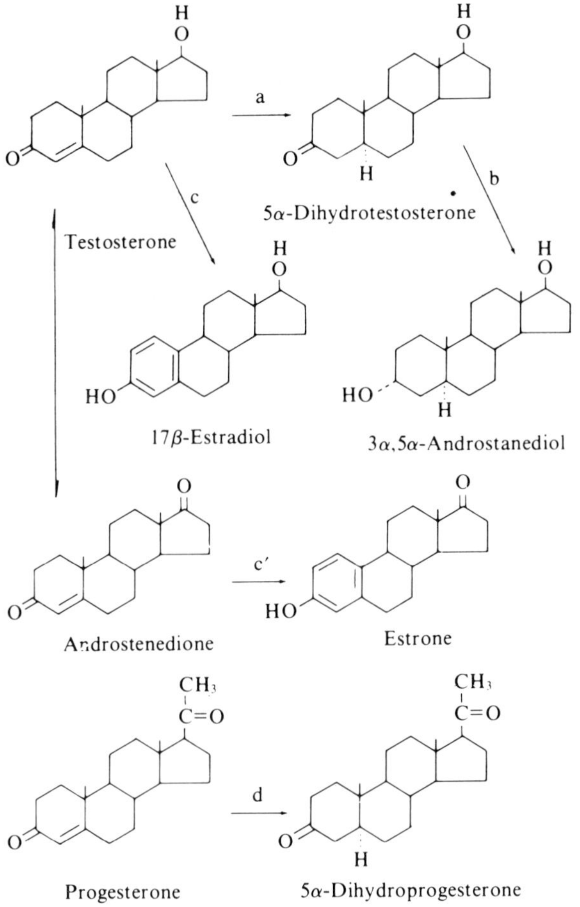

FIG. 3. Some steroid transformations that are carried out by neural tissue.

5α-reductase activity than any region of the brain, and its activity is subject to changes as a result of gonadectomy, hormone replacement, and postnatal age [1,6]. 5α-DHT has been implicated in the hypothalamus and pituitary as a potent regulator of gonadotropin secretion but it is relatively inactive toward male rat sexual behavior [1]. Labeled metabolites with the R_f value of 5α-DHT have been detected in extracts of hypothalamic and pituitary tissue after [³H]testosterone administration in both adult and newborn rats. It is interesting that progesterone inhibits 5α-reductase activity toward [³H]testosterone and that [³H]progesterone is itself converted to [³H]5α-dihydroprogesterone [Fig. 3 (d)]. Progesterone competition for 5α-reductase may explain some of the antiandrogenicity of this steroid [1,6]. 5β-DHT is a metabolite of testosterone formed in the bird CNS, as is 5α-DHT; 5β-DHT is inactive toward sexual behavior and is believed to represent an inactivation pathway for testosterone [7].

The aromatization of testosterone to form estradiol, and of androstenedione to form estrone [Fig. 3 (c) and (c'), respectively], has been described in brain tissue *in vitro* and *in vivo* [6]. Aromatization is higher in hypothalamus and limbic structures than in cerebral cortex or pituitary gland and, in noncastrated animals, is higher in male than in female brains. Aromatization has been found in brains of reptiles and amphibia as well as in brains of mammals [6]. The capacity to aromatize testosterone and related androgens may therefore be a general property of vertebrate brains. The functional role of aromatization has been studied most extensively in the rat: Male sexual behavior is facilitated by estradiol [7], and testosterone facilitation of male sexual behavior can be blocked by a steroidal inhibitor of aromatization [1,6,7]. There are indications that a similar situation exists in birds, amphibia, and reptiles; that is, testosterone and estradiol can stimulate heterotypical sexual behavior in males and females. Curiously, not all mammals are like the rat; for example, male sexual behavior of the guinea pig and rhesus monkey is restored by the nonaromatizable androgens androstenedione and dihydrotestosterone [1,7].

Both aromatization and 5α-reductase are regulated by gonadal steroids. In mammals such as the rat, it is principally the neural aromatase activity that is upregulated by androgens acting via neural androgen receptors [8]. In birds, neural aromatase and 5α-reductase are both induced by testosterone, and this regulation provides a way by which androgens can regulate CNS hormone sensitivity without regulating receptor number [9].

Both estrogens and glucocorticoids appear to act on brain cells without being first metabolized because both [3H]estradiol and [3H]corticosterone are recovered unchanged from their cell nuclear binding sites in brain [1]. However, estradiol is subject to conversion to the catecholestrogen 2-hydroxyestradiol, and this metabolite is both a moderately potent estrogen via intracellular estrogen receptors as well as an agent capable of interacting with cell surface receptors such as those for catecholamines, albeit at fairly high concentrations [10]. Vitamin D, prior to acting in the brain, is converted to an active metabolite, 1,25-dihydroxy vitamin D_3, by enzymes in liver and kidney [5].

There is evidence that steroid hormone receptor sites exist in brain and pituitary

The availability in the early 1960s of tritium-labeled steroids of high specific activity (20–25 Ci/mmol at each labeled position) permitted the measurement of specific binding sites of low capacity that had previously escaped detection when [14C]-labeled steroids were used [1]. In the brain, high-resolution autoradiographic methods utilizing [3H]-labeled steroids have permitted mapping of steroid-hormone target cells in specific brain regions (Fig. 4). It should be noted that tritium permits a high degree of spatial resolution (particle range 1–2 μm in light micro-

scope autoradiography), owing to the low energy of the β-particle released [1].

Cell fractionation procedures are basic to the biochemical identification and study of steroid hormone binding sites

Isolation of highly purified cell nuclei from small amounts of tissue from discrete brain regions is generally accomplished with the aid of a nonionic detergent such as Triton X-100 (see McEwen [1], for example). Cytosol fractions of brain tissue (prepared by centrifugation of homogenates at $105,000 \times g$ for 60 min) contain the soluble steroid hormone binding proteins, and a variety of methods intended to separate bound from unbound steroid have been used for measuring their binding activity [1]. The most commonly employed are gel filtration chromatography and sucrose density gradient centrifugation. Dextran-coated charcoal is frequently used because it effectively absorbs unbound steroid and leaves intact the complexes between steroid and putative receptor. Other methods, such as gel electrophoresis and precipitation of putative receptor material by protamine sulfate, have more restricted uses.

The objective of such studies is to measure the affinity, capacity, and specificity of the hormone-receptor interaction [1]. Measurements of affinity and capacity are accomplished by kinetic analysis (Fig. 5). Specificity is based on competition between the labeled and various unlabeled ligands for binding sites. (These methods are described in Chap. 9.)

Several criteria determine whether a steroid hormone binding site is a putative receptor

First, the steroid hormone binding site must be present in hormone-responsive tissues (or brain regions) and absent from nonresponsive ones. Second, it should bind steroids that are either active agonists or effective antagonists of the

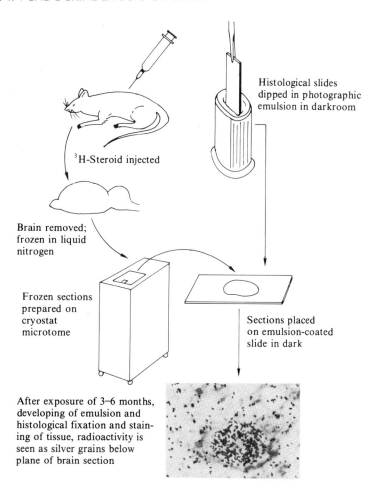

FIG. 4. Flow diagram of a frequently used procedure for autoradiographic localization of ³H-steroid hormones in neural tissue.

Histological slides dipped in photographic emulsion in darkroom

³H-Steroid injected

Brain removed; frozen in liquid nitrogen

Frozen sections prepared on cryostat microtome

Sections placed on emulsion-coated slide in dark

After exposure of 3–6 months, developing of emulsion and histological fixation and staining of tissue, radioactivity is seen as silver grains below plane of brain section

hormone effect and not bind steroids that are inactive in either sense.

A final methodological point concerns the true subcellular location of steroid receptors whether in the cytoplasm or nucleus, or both. Cell fractionation studies reveal so-called cytosol receptors in the absence of steroid whereas binding to nuclei is found after steroid is taken up by the cells [1]. Yet, there is information suggesting that the cytosol estrogen receptor may have leaked from cell nuclei after breaking the cell in that the estrogen receptor antibodies show a nuclear localization of this receptor even in the absence of steroid [11]. In contrast, antibodies to glucocorticoid receptors reveal cytoplasmic receptor in the absence of steroid and nuclear receptor in the presence of steroid [12]. There is presently no resolution of the dilemma, and it appears likely that the intracellular locus of unoccupied steroid receptors varies.

Properties and topography of steroid receptors in brain

Steroid hormone receptors are proteins of 55 to 120 kilodaltons (kDa) in apparent molecular weight that are similar to each other in that they

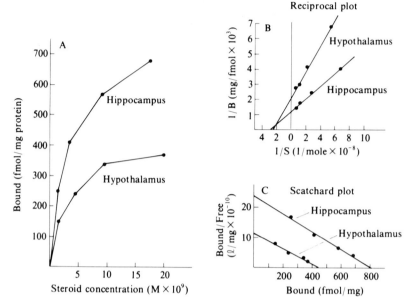

FIG. 5. **A**: Concentration-dependence curve for binding of [³H]dexamethasone by cytosols from hippocampus and hypothalamus. **B**: Expression of data in **A** in the form of a reciprocal plot: 1/bound (B) vs. 1/steroid (S) concentration. **C**: Scatchard plot of same data: bound/free steroid vs. bound; (fmol) 10^{-15} mol; (*l*) liters.

all have a DNA binding domain and a steroid binding domain [4,13]. They are also phosphoproteins, for which the state of phosphorylation appears to influence functional activity [14].

Estradiol

The first neural steroid receptor type to be recognized was that for estradiol (Fig. 3) [1]. *In vivo* uptake of [³H]estradiol (Fig. 6) and binding to cell nuclei isolated from hypothalamus, pituitary, and other brain regions revealed steroid specificity that closely resembles that of the uterus, where steroid receptors were first discovered [1]. Cytosol estrogen receptors isolated from pituitary and brain tissue resemble closely those found in uterus and mammary tissue. A hallmark of the estrogen receptor is its existence as an aggregate of subunits that dissociate during steroid-induced transformation to the DNA-binding nuclear form of the receptor. This part

of the estrogen receptor complex was recently cloned from human breast cancer cells [16] and consists of a 65 to 70 kDa hormone and DNA binding subunit [16]. The dissociation constant of estradiol binding is approximately 0.2 nM. Approximately 12,000 estradiol molecules are bound per cell in uterus and pituitary, where at least 80 percent of cells have receptors; in hypothalamus, where fewer cells have receptors, the figure is only 2,000 to 3,000 molecules per cell on the average.

Progesterone

Detection of progesterone receptors in brain was made possible by the use of the synthetic progestin R5020 (promegestrone; 17-α, 21-dimethyl, 19-nor-pregna-4,9-diene-3,20-dione), which has a high affinity for the progestin receptor (K_D = 0.4 nM) [17] (Fig. 3). The progestin receptor has been cloned from chick oviduct

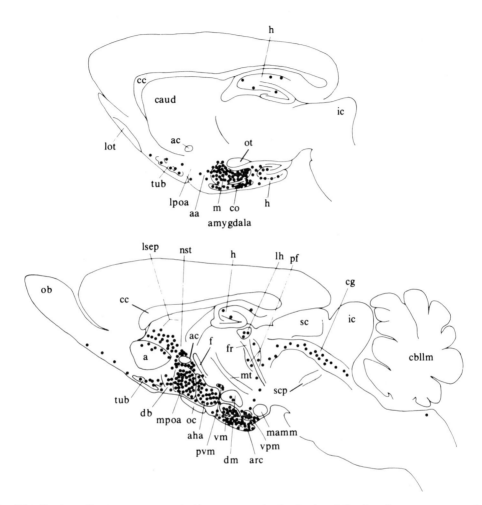

FIG. 6. Distribution of estrogen-concentrating neurons in the brain of the female rat represented schematically in two sagittal sections. Most labeled neurons can be represented in a medial plane (**bottom**). Estradiol-concentrating neurons in the amygdala and hippocampus are represented in a more lateral plane (**top**). Locations of estradiol-concentrating neurons are represented by *solid circles*. [From Pfaff and Keiner (15).] (a) Nucleus accumbens; (aha) anterior hypothalamic area; (arc) arcuate nucleus; (cbllm) cerebellum; (cc) corpus callosum; (cg) central grey; (dm) dorsomedial nucleus of the hypothalamus; (db) diagonal band of Broca; (fr) fasciculuc retroflexus; (h) hippocampus; (ic) inferior colliculus; (lh) lateral habenula; (lsep) lateral septum; (mamm) mammillary bodies; (mpoa) medial preoptic area; (mt) mammillothalamic tract; (nst) bed nucleus of the stria terminalis; (ob) olfactory bulb; (oc) optic chiasm; (pf) nucleus parafascicularis; (pvm) paraventricular nucleus; (sc) superior colliculus; (scp) superior cerebellar peduncle; (tub) olfactory tubercle; (vm) ventromedial nucleus; (vpm) ventral premammillary nucleus.

and consists of a steroid and DNA binding sub-unit of 108 kDa, although a 79 kDa subunit has also been described [16]. Progestin receptors of similar physical chemical properties are found in pituitary, reproductive tract, and in most es-trogen-receptor-containing brain regions, and these receptors are inducible by estrogen treat-ment [17]. There are also progestin receptor sites in brain areas lacking estrogen receptors, such as the cerebral cortex of the rat, and these receptors are not induced by estradiol treat-ment; such receptors nevertheless resemble those which are induced by estradiol [17]. An-other inducer of progestin receptors in brain is testosterone, which works through its conver-sion to estradiol via aromatization [17]. Proges-terone works rapidly to induce feminine sexual behavior in female rats that have been primed with estradiol to induce progestin receptor sites [17]. The principal site of action is the ventro-medial nucleus of the hypothalamus [18]. De-spite the rapidity of the induction (within 1 hr), progesterone induction of lordosis is dependent on protein synthesis [18].

Androgen

Androgen receptors have a steroid binding sub-unit estimated to be 120 kDa [13] (Fig. 3). The estimated K_D for active androgens is on the order of 1 to 2 nM [1]. Androgen receptors are found widely distributed in brain and pituitary tissue, although highest concentrations are found in hypothalamus, preoptic area, and lim-bic brain tissue [1]. Androgen receptors are de-ficient in the androgen-insensitivity (Tfm) mu-tation, and such animals show defects in sexual behavior, juvenile rough-and-tumble play be-havior, and certain aspects of neuroendocrine function, thus indicating the actions of testos-terone that are mediated by androgen receptors, as opposed to those mediated by aromatization of testosterone to estradiol (see above) and es-trogen receptors [1,16].

Glucocorticoid

Adrenal steroid receptors have been subdivided into two categories, one of which is the classical glucocorticoid receptor (Fig. 7) [3]. This recep-tor has been cloned from human and rat sources and consists of a steroid and DNA binding sub-unit of 95 kDa [13,16]. Such receptors, which have dissociation constants for glucocorticoids of 4 to 5 nM, are widely distributed across brain regions and are found in neurons and glial cells [2].

The other type of glucocorticoid receptor is similar to the mineralocorticoid receptor orig-inally described in the kidney [2]. In the brain, receptors of this type bind the glucocorticoid, corticosterone, with high affinity ($K_D \sim 1$ nM) and they are responsible for the high uptake of tracer levels of [^{3}H]corticosterone by the hip-pocampus [2] (Fig. 8). These corticosterone re-ceptors may be involved in mediating effects of the diurnally varying levels of corticosterone [3].

Mineralocorticoid

Mineralocorticoid receptors (Fig. 7) with phys-icochemical properties and sequence similar to the corticosterone receptor of the hippocampus are known to exist in kidney. Uptake of [^{3}H]aldosterone by brain tissue reveals two types of binding sites: those in the hippocampus that can be preferentially occupied by corticos-terone; and sites that are more diffusely dis-tributed in the brain and that appear to retain [^{3}H]aldosterone preferentially in the presence of the normally higher levels of corticosterone [2]. The exact nature of these elusive brain mineralocorticoid receptors remains to be de-termined.

Vitamin D

Vitamin D is a steroid hormone (Fig. 7), pro-duction of which by the body requires the action of light, so that it is often necessary to ingest a

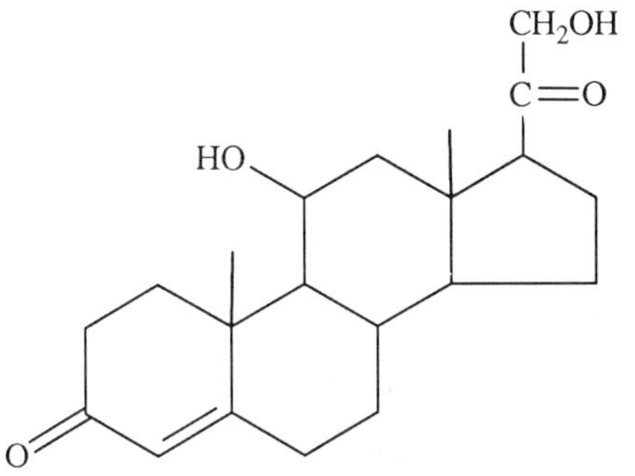

Corticosterone

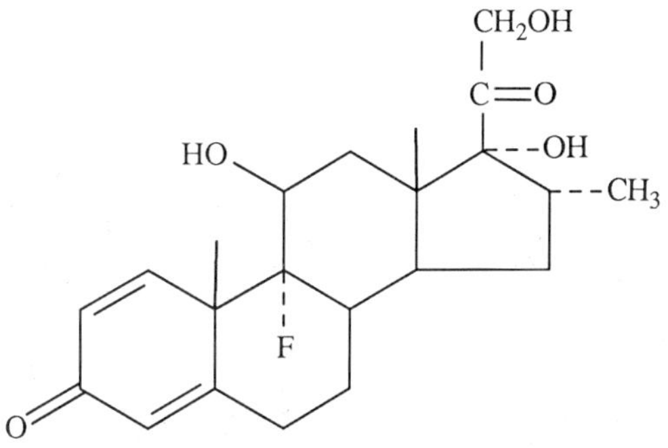

Dexamethasone

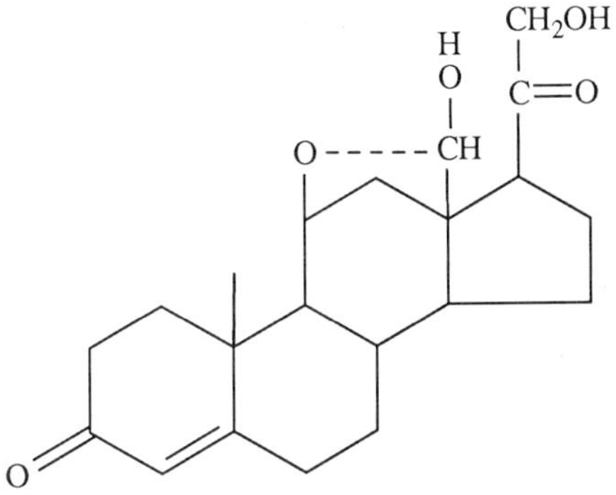

Aldosterone

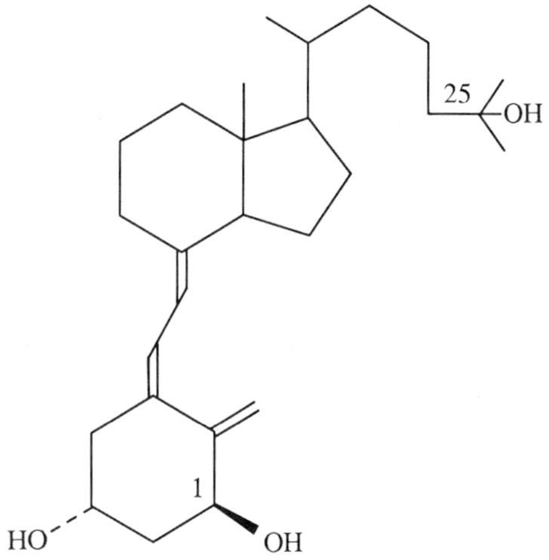

1α25(OH)$_2$ Vitamin D$_3$

FIG. 7. Formulas of four steroid hormones.

certain amount of it as a vitamin in the diet [5]. Moreover, vitamin D is converted by kidney and liver to the active metabolite, 1,25-dihydroxy vitamin D_3 [5]. Vitamin D_3 receptors consist of a hormone and DNA binding subunit of 55 kDa [13]. Receptor sites for 1,25-dihydroxy vitamin D_3 are found in pituitary and in brain, especially in the forebrain, hindbrain, and spinal cord neurons [21]. In the brain, one site containing vitamin D_3 receptors, the bed nucleus of the stria terminalis, responds to exogenous 1,25-dihydroxy vitamin D_3 with an induction of choline acetyltransferase, even though the calcium-binding protein that is regulated by vitamin D_3 in intestine is not regulated by this hormone in brain [22]. Moreover, vitamin D_3 also corrects deficiencies in serum testosterone and LH in vitamin D-deficient male rats [22]. It is not clear, however, whether this represents a major effect of vitamin D_3 in the pituitary gland or brain, or both.

Diversity of steroid hormone action in brain

Steroid hormone effects on the brain link the environment surrounding the organism with the genome of target brain cells through the process

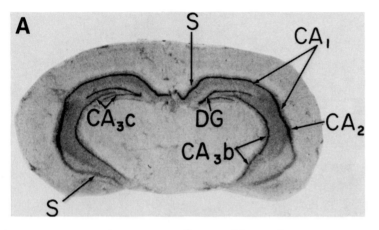

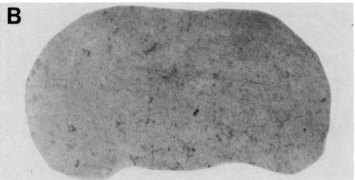

FIG. 8. **A:** Autoradiograph showing presence of radioactivity injected as [³H]corticosterone in hippocampal formation of adrenalectomized rat. **B:** shows lack of specific uptake in brain from rat injected with excess unlabeled corticosterone. (From Sapolsky et al. [20].) (S) subiculum; (DG) dentate gyrus; (CA₁, CA₂, CA₃b, and CA₃c) pyramidal cell layers of Ammon's horn; (B) nonspecific binding.

of variable genomic activity [23]. By this we mean that an organism experiences light, dark, heat, cold, fear, and sexual excitement. These experiences influence hormone secretion and these hormones in turn act on the genome of receptor-containing brain cells to alter their functional state. The genome of brain cells, like those of other cells of the body, is continually active from embryonic life until death and is continually responsive to intra- and extracellular signals. This activity can be seen from the high levels of RNA metabolism in neurons. The differential influence of steroid hormones on variable genomic activity is evident from studies showing rapid and brain region-specific induction of ribosomal and messenger RNA, as well as changes in cell nuclear diameter and chromatin structure [17,23]. However, variable genomic activity changes qualitatively with the state of differentiation of the target cells: Embryonic neurons show growth responses that result in permanent changes in circuitry, whereas adult neurons show impermanent responses. Under other circumstances, the same hormonal signals can promote damage and even neuronal loss; under still other conditions, adult neurons can be stimulated to grow and repair damage by treatment with hormones.

Developmental actions

Steroid hormone receptors become evident in target neurons of the brain within several days of final cell division [7]. Whether some receptors are also present in dividing neuronal precursors is not clear. After they have appeared, these receptors mediate a variety of developmental actions. For example, glucocorticoids direct differentiation of adrenergic/cholinergic neurons of the autonomic nervous system to develop in the adrenergic direction [2], and they increase the number of epinephrine-containing small, intensely fluorescent cells in autonomic ganglia [2]. Glucocorticoids are also required for the normal postnatal ontogeny of serotonin neurons in the forebrain [2].

Gonadal hormones, on the other hand, are involved in the sexual differentiation of the brain. The presence of testosterone during a critical period of pre- or postnatal development in birds and mammals leads to the permanent masculine development of neural circuits mediating sexual and aggressive behaviors (in mammals) and song (in birds). In mammalian males, testicular activity and testosterone secretion during this critical period is the natural signal leading to masculine sexual differentiation [7,24]. Sexual behavior in birds is determined in the reverse manner; females produce either estradiol or testosterone, either of which feminizes the brain, which would otherwise develop a masculine pattern in the absence of gonadal steroids [7,23].

As for the mechanism of sexual differentiation, we must consider the metabolism of the hormone, receptor types involved, and the primary receptor-mediated events. Testosterone, as noted above, is a prohormone that is converted into either 5-α-DHT or estradiol within the brain; these products exert effects on brain sexual differentiation via androgen and estrogen receptors, respectively [7,24]. Masculinization of sexual and aggressive behavior involves either 5α-DHT alone or a combination of 5α-DHT plus estradiol acting on different cells. Besides masculinization, there is in some mammals a process called defeminization, in which feminine responses that would develop in the absence of testosterone are suppressed by its presence during the critical period. Conversion to estradiol appears to be involved in this process [7,24]. Progesterone plays no major role in brain sexual differentiation, but it does have the ability to antagonize actions at both androgen and estrogen receptors and thus is an agent that can moderate the degree of masculinization and defeminization.

As to the primary developmental actions of testosterone, growth and differentiation appear to be involved. Testosterone or estradiol stimulates outgrowth of neurites from developing hypothalamic neurons that contain estrogen receptors [25]. This is believed to be the basis of testosterone action that increases the number of neurons and the size of neurons within specific hypothalamic nuclei in males, compared to females [26]. 5α-DHT may have a similar effect on androgen-sensitive neurons. Differentiation of target neurons also occurs; hormones like estradiol can evoke responses in adult brain tissue that differ between adult male and female rats.

Activation and adaptation

Hormone secretion by the adrenals and gonads is controlled by endogenous oscillators that can be entrained by environmental cues such as light and dark. The actions of hormones secreted cyclically on behavior and brain function are referred to as activational effects. In addition to the cyclic mode, there is another mode of secretion initiated by such experiences as stress, fear, and aggressive and sexual encounters. In this case, actions of hormones secreted in response to experience lead to adaptive responses by the brain, which, in the case of adrenal steroids, help the animal cope with stressful situations [2,3]. The activational and adaptational effects are largely reversible and involve a variety of neurochemical changes, most of which appear to be initiated at the genomic level. For example, estradiol is secreted cyclically during the estrous cycle in the female rat and triggers the surge of LH, which induces a surge of progesterone from the ovary. Progesterone in turn stimulates sexual responsiveness to the male rat (Fig. 9).

Estradiol action to promote feminine sexual behavior in the rat involves a cascade of induced protein synthesis in specific hypothalamic neurons accompanied by morphological changes indicative of increased genomic activity [18]. Among the induced proteins are: receptors for progesterone (see above) crucial for activating sexual behavior; receptors for acetylcholine and oxytocin that are active in enabling the hypothalamic neurons to respond to afferent input; and proteins that are axonally transported from the hypothalamus to the midbrain, where they may be involved in neurotransmission [18].

Adrenal steroids secreted in the diurnal cycle are responsible for reversibly activating exploratory activity, food-seeking behavior, carbohydrate appetite, and synaptic efficacy; they appear to do this by acting on the hippocampus, where there are many corticosterone receptors (see above). Adaptational effects of adrenal steroids that result from single or repeated stress appear to operate via the classical glucocorticoid receptor found not only in hippocampus but also in other brain regions [2]. Changes in synaptic vesicle proteins, high-affinity γ-aminobutyric acid (GABA) transport, neurotransmitter-stimulated cAMP formation, and central serotonin and noradrenergic sensitivity are known to accompany repeated glucocorticoid elevation [2]. One view of these changes induced by glucocorticoids is that they counteract some of the immediate and persistent neural effects of stress and are therefore part of the mechanism of adaptation [2,3].

Repair of neural damage

The response of neural tissue to damage involves some degree of collateral growth and

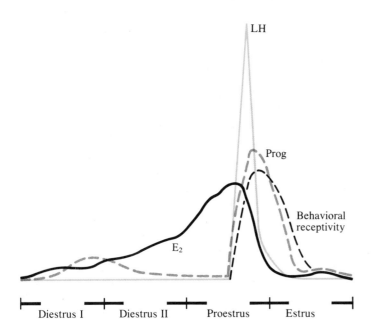

FIG. 9. Schematic representation of the secretion pattern of estradiol (E_2), progesterone (Prog), and luteinizing hormone (LH) during the 4-day estrous cycle of the female rat. Estradiol secretion primes the neuroendocrine system to deliver the LH surge on the afternoon of proestrus, which in turn induces the progesterone surge. Progesterone secretion, coming after the estradiol priming effects on the brain, induces behavioral receptivity (dashed line), which coincides temporally with the period of maximum fertility. (From Davis and McEwen [27].)

reinnervation of vacant synaptic sites, a process facilitated in some cases by steroid hormones [23]. In the hypothalamus, estrogen treatment promotes increases in the number of synapses following knife cuts that destroy certain inputs. In the hippocampus, glucocorticoid treatment promotes homotypical sprouting of serotonin fibers to replace damaged serotonin input. It has also been noted that androgens enhance the regrowth of the severed hypoglossal nerve [23]. One interpretation of these steroid effects is that they represent the reactivation, by damage, of developmental programs of genomic activity that normally operate during the phase of synaptogenesis in early development [23].

Enhancement of neural damage

Steroid hormones can also promote neural damage. High-dose estrogen treatment of adult female rats induces the hypothalamic disconnection syndrome by activating low-level persistent ovarian estrogen secretion. This persistent secretion induces morphological changes in the hypothalamus associated with dysfunction of the cyclic gonadotropin-releasing mechanism [23]. Persistent effects of estrogen secretion occurring naturally throughout life span are believed to facilitate termination of cyclic hypothalamic function with regard to ovulation [23].

Glucocorticoids can promote neural damage as well. Treatment of adult rats with corticosterone for 12 weeks induces loss of pyramidal neurons in hippocampus, which mimics the loss of such neurons in aging rats. The presence of elevated glucocorticoids at the time of hypoxic damage (Chap. 40) or kainic acid lesions (Chap. 15) to the brain potentiates the necrosis. Adrenalectomy reduces such damage and also retards loss of neurons with age [28]. Thus, adrenal steroids operate in conjunction with neural excitability to promote damage, and it has been suggested that they do so by compromising the ability of the brain to obtain nutrients to support ATP generation [28]. It should

be noted, however, that damage is not a primary or an immediate consequence of elevated glucocorticoid levels and that glucocorticoid secretion in conjunction with stress has the beneficial influence of protecting the body from overreacting to stress and thereby destroying itself.

Membrane effects of steroids

The rapid effect of some steroid hormones on neuronal excitability is difficult to explain in terms of genomic action [29]. Instead, some type of membrane receptor is inferred [30]. Indeed, several types of interactions with neural membranes have been described. Direct binding assays have revealed membrane sites for glucocorticoids and gonadal steroids [2]; indirect binding assay results have implied interaction of the catecholestrogens with dopamine and with adrenergic receptors [10]. Studies of release of luteinizing-hormone releasing-hormone (LHRH) from hypothalamic slices have revealed rapid, direct effects of estradiol and progesterone that are unlikely to involve genomic mediation [31]. There are now indications for the interaction of progesterone metabolites with the chloride ionophore of the GABA-benzodiazepine receptor complex [32]. None of the findings undermine the importance of the intracellular genomic actions of steroids. Rather, they increase the richness of the cellular actions of steroid hormones and raise the possibility that there may be connections between genomic and nongenomic actions of steroids. For example, genomic action may induce receptors that mediate nongenomic effects.

BIOCHEMISTRY AND FUNCTIONAL SIGNIFICANCE OF THYROID HORMONE ACTION ON BRAIN

Like steroid hormones, thyroid hormones interact with receptors to alter genomic activity and affect the synthesis of specific proteins during development [33], and like testosterone and progesterone, metabolic transformation of thyroxine (T_4) is critical to its action [33]. Moreover, like steroid hormones, thyroid hormones alter brain functions in adult life in ways that both resemble and differ from their action during development [33,34].

The initial step after cellular uptake of T_4 is metabolic transformation to 3,5,3'-tri-iodothyronine (T_3) (Fig. 10), which interacts with cytosolic and nuclear receptors, as well as with synaptosomal membrane binding sites of unknown function [33]. Cytosolic receptors are proteins of 70 kDa that do not appear to undergo translocation to cell nuclei, nor do they appear to be nuclear proteins that have leaked out of cell nuclei during cell rupture; nuclear receptors are proteins of 50 to 70 kDa that have both DNA and hormone binding domains [33]. Evidence points to homology between the nuclear T_3 receptor and the *c-erb-A* gene, cellular counterpart of the viral oncogene, *v-erb-A* [35].

Nuclear T_3 receptors are present in higher levels during stages of neural development than they are in adult life [33]. In human fetal brain, nuclear T_3 receptors increase in concentration from 10 weeks of gestation up to the sixteenth week, when neuroblast multiplication is high [36]. Glial cells as well as neurons contain nuclear T_3 receptors [36]. Functionally, many neurons develop prior to the appearance of significant T_3 receptor levels and therefore appear to be independent of large-scale thyroid influence. Other neurons, such as those in cortex and cerebellum, show a more profound dependence on thyroid function. Although thyroid hormone affects the number of replicating cells in the external granular layer of the developing cerebellum, it is not possible to conclude that T_3 directly affects the mechanism of cell replication [33]. Rather, the most pronounced effect of hypothyroidism is a hypoplastic neuropil, with shorter dendrites and fewer spines, and it has been shown that a major effect of T_3 involves the development of the neuronal cytoskeleton [33]. Proteins such as microtubule-associated protein (MAP2) and *tau* (see Chap. 24), which

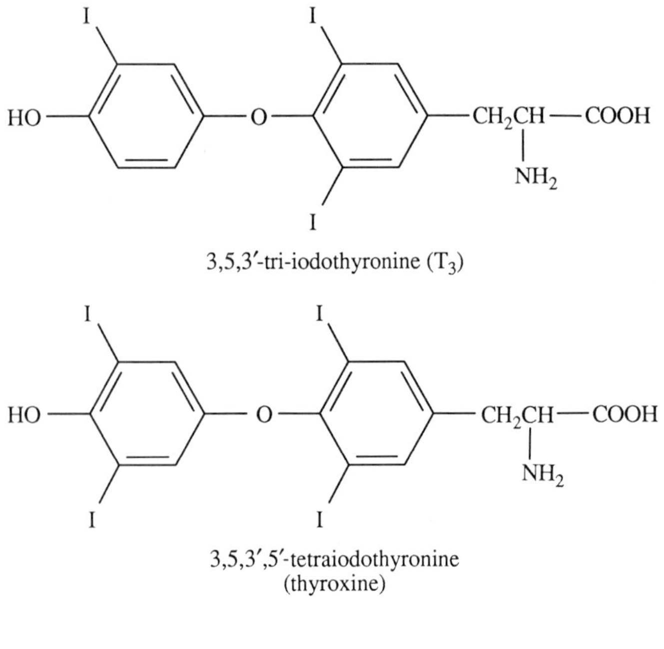

3,5,3'-tri-iodothyronine (T_3)

3,5,3',5'-tetraiodothyronine
(thyroxine)

FIG. 10. Formulas for thyroxine (T_4) and tri-iodothyronine (T_3).

are polymorphic and which affect microtubular assembly, are differentially affected by T_3 absence or excess [33].

Developmentally, thyroid hormones interact with sex hormones in that hypothyroidism prolongs the critical period for testosterone-induced defeminization (see above) [1]; in contrast, the hyperthyroid state terminates the sensitivity to testosterone prematurely [1]. Undoubtedly, an important link in these and other effects is synapse formation. Hypothyroidism decreases synaptic density, and hyperthyroidism increases synaptic density, at least transiently [1]. Interesting parallels with synapse formation are reported for learning behavior in rats: Neonatal hypothyroidism impairs learning ability, whereas hyperthyroidism accelerates learning initially, followed by a decline later in life [1].

The adult brain is endowed with nuclear as well as cytosol and membrane T_3 receptors that have been visualized by autoradiography and studied biochemically [33]. Both neurons and neuropil are labeled by $[^{125}I]T_3$, and the labeling is selective across brain regions. Functionally, one of the most prominent features of neural action of thyroid hormone in adulthood is subsensitivity to norepinephrine as a result of a hypothyroid state [34]. These changes may be reflections of loss of dendritic spines in at least some neurons of the adult brain (see Nunez [33]). Clinically, thyroid hormone deficiency increases the probability of depressive illness, whereas thyroid excess increases the probability of mania in susceptible individuals [34].

ACKNOWLEDGMENTS

Research in the author's laboratory is supported by NIH Grant NS07080 and NIMH Grant MH41256. The author thanks Ms. Inna Perlin for editorial assistance and Ms. Maryse Aubourg for help with illustrations.

REFERENCES

1. McEwen, B. S. Endocrine effects on the brain and their relationship to behavior. In G. J. Siegel, R. W. Albers, B. W. Agranoff, and R. Katzman (eds.), *Basic Neurochemistry*, 3rd. ed. Boston: Little Brown & Co., 1981, pp. 775–799.
2. McEwen, B. S., DeKloet, E. R., and Rostene, W. Adrenal steroid receptors and actions in the nervous system. *Physiol. Rev.* 66:1121–1188, 1986.
3. McEwen, B. S., and Brinton, R. E. Neuroendocrine aspects of adaptation. In E. R. Dekbet, V. Wiegant, and D. DeWied (eds.), *Progress in Brain Research*. Amsterdam: Elsevier, 1987 pp. 11–26.
4. Yamamoto, K. Steroid receptor regulated transcription of specific genes and gene networks. *Annu. Rev. Genet.* 19:209–252, 1985.
5. Norman, A., and Henry, H. Vitamin D to 1,25-dihydroxycholecalciferol: Evolution of a steroid hormone. *Trends Biochem. Sci.* 414–418, 1979.
6. Celotti, F., Naftolin, F., and Martini, L. (eds.) *Metabolism of Hormonal Steroids in Neuroendocrine Structures*. New York: Raven Press, 1984.
7. Goy, R. W., and McEwen, B. S. (eds.) *Sexual Differentiation of the Brain*. Cambridge: MIT Press, 1980.
8. Roselli, C., Horton, L., and Resko, J. Distribution and regulation of aromatase activity in the rat hypothalamus and limbic system. *Endocrinology* 117:2471–2477, 1985.
9. Schumacher, M., and Balthazart, J. Testosterone-induced brain aromatase is sexually dimorphic. *Brain Res.* 370:285–293, 1986.
10. Merriam, J., and Lipsett, M. (eds.) *Catechol Estrogens*. New York: Raven Press, 1983.
11. King, W. J., and Greene, G. L. Monoclonal antibodies localize estrogen receptor in nuclei of target cells. *Nature* 307:745–747, 1984.
12. Fuxe, K., Wikstrom Okret, S., Agnati, L. F., Harfstrand, A., Yu, Z.-Y., Granholm, L., Zoli, M., Vale, W., and Gustafsson, J.-A. Mapping of glucocorticoid receptor immunoreactive neurons in the rat tel- and diencephalon using a monoclonal antibody against rat liver glucocorticoid receptor. *Endocrinology* 117:1803–1812, 1985.
13. Danielson, M., Northrop, J., and Ringold, G.

The mouse glucocorticoid receptor: Mapping of functional domains by cloning, sequencing and expression of wild-type and mutant receptor proteins. *EMBO J.* 5:2513–2522, 1986.

14. Baldi, A., Boyle, D., and Wittliff, J. Estrogen receptor is associated with protein and phospholipid kinase activities. *Biochem. Biophys. Res. Commun.* 135:597–606, 1986.

15. Pfaff, D. W., and Keiner, N. Atlas of estradiol-concentrating cells in the central nervous system of the female rat. *J. Comp. Neurol.* 151:121–158, 1973.

16. King, R. Receptor structure: A personal assessment of the current status. *J. Ster. Biochem.* 25:451–454, 1986.

17. McEwen, B. S., Davis, P., Gerlach, J. L., Krey, L. C., MacLusky, N., McGinnis, M., Parsons, B., and McEwen, B. S. Progestin receptors in the brain and pituitary gland. In C. W. Bardin, P. Mauvais-Jarvis, and Milgrom (eds.), *Progesterone and Progestin.* New York: Raven Press, 1983, pp. 59–76.

18. McEwen, B. S., Jones, K., Pfaff, D. W. Hormonal control of sexual behavior in the female rat: Molecular, cellular and neurochemical studies. *Biol. Reprod.* 36:37–45, 1987.

19. Meaney, M. J., Stewart, J., Poulin, P., and McEwen, B. S. Sexual differentiation of social play in rat pups is mediated by the neonatal androgen receptor system. *Neuroendocrinology* 37:85–90, 1983.

20. Sapolsky, R. M., McEwen, B. S., and Rainbow, T. C. Quantitative autoradiography of ^{3}H-corticosterone receptors in rat brain. 271:331–335, 1983.

21. Stumpf, W., Sar, M., and Clark, S. Brain target sites for 1,25-dihydroxy Vitamin D$_3$. *Science* 215:1403–1405, 1982.

22. Sonnenberg, J., Luine, V. N., Krey, L. C., and Christakos, S. 1,25-dihydroxyvitamin D$_3$ treatment results in increased choline acetyltransferase activity in specific brain nuclei. *Endocrinology* 118:1433–1439, 1986.

23. McEwen, B. S. Steroid hormones and the brain: Linking "nature and nurture." *Neurochem. Res.* 13:663–669, 1988.

24. Adler, N. (ed.) *Neuroendocrinology of Reproduction, Physiology and Behavior.* New York: Plenum Press, 1981.

25. Toran-Allerand, C. D. On the genesis of sexual differentiation of the central nervous system: Morphogenetic consequences of steroidal exposure and possible role of alpha-fetoprotein. In G. De Vries et al (eds.), *Progress in Brain Research*, Amsterdam: Elsevier, 1984, Vol. 61, pp. 63–98.

26. Arnold, A. P., and Gorski, R. A. Gonadal steroid induction of structural sex differences in the central nervous system. *Annu. Rev. Neurosci.* 7:413–442, 1984.

27. Davis, P., and McEwen, B. S. Neuroendocrine regulation of sexual behavior. In R. Friedman (ed.), *Behavior and Menstrual Cycle.* New York: Marcel Dekker, 1982, pp. 43–64.

28. Sapolsky, R. M., Krey, L. C., and McEwen, B. S. The neuroendocrinology of stress and aging: The glucocorticoid cascade hypothesis. *Endocrinol. Rev.* 7:284–301, 1986.

29. McEwen, B. S., Krey, L. C., and Luine, V. N. Steroid hormone action in the neuroendocrine system: When is the genome involved? In S. Reichlin, R. J. Baldessarini, and J. B. Martin (eds.), *The Hypothalamus.* New York: Raven Press, 1978, pp. 255–268.

30. Dufy, B., Vincent, J.-D., Fleury, H., DuPasquier, P., Gourdji, D., and Tixier-Vidal, A. Membrane effects of thyrotropin-releasing hormone and estrogen shown by intracellular recording from pituitary cells. *Science* 204:509–510, 1979.

31. Drouva, S. V., Laplante, E., and Kordon, C. Progesterone-induced LHRH release *in vitro* is an estrogen as well as Ca^{2+}- and calmodulin-dependent secretory process. *Neuroendocrinology* 40:325–331, 1985.

32. Majewska, M. D., Harrison, N., Schwartz, R., Barker, J., and Paul, S. M. Steroid hormone metabolites are barbiturate-like modulators of the GABA receptor. *Science* 232:1004, 1986.

33. Nunez, J. Effects of thyroid hormones during brain differentiation. *Mol. Cell. Endocrinol.* 37:125–132, 1984.

34. Whybrow, P., and Prange, A. A hypothesis of thyroid-catecholamine-receptor interaction. *Arch. Gen. Psychiatry* 38:106–113, 1981.

35. Sap, J., Munoz, A., Damm, K., Goldberg, Y., Ghysdael, J., Leutz, A., Beug, H., and Vennstrom, B. The c-erb-A protein is a high-affinity receptor for thyroid hormone. *Nature* 324:635–640, 1986.

36. Bernal, J., and Pekonen, F. Ontogenesis of the nuclear 3,5,3'-triiodothyronine receptor in the human fetal brain. *Endocrinology* 114:677–680, 1984.

37. Comb, M., Birnberg, N., Seasholtz, A., Herbert, E., and Goodman, H. A cyclic AMP and phorbol ester-inducible DNA element. *Nature* 323:353–356, 1986.

CHAPTER 48

Learning and Memory

Bernard W. Agranoff

No aspect of the brain sciences can so quickly conjure up both interest and controversy than the subject of the biological basis of learning and memory—the encoding and storage of behavioral information. Some of the controversy stems from disagreement among investigators with regard to definitions of learning and memory and acceptable experimental criteria. The complexity of the problem to a great extent reflects the structural and functional complexity of the brain itself—biochemical correlates of learning and memory are generally highly in-

Basic Neurochemistry: Molecular, Cellular, and Medical Aspects, 4th Ed., edited by G. J. Siegel et al. Raven Press, Ltd., New York, 1989.
Correspondence to Bernard W. Agranoff, Neuroscience Laboratory, University of Michigan, 1103 East Huron, Ann Arbor, Michigan, 48104-1687.

ferential and involve compromise, either in the behavioral model and paradigm used or in the precision of the experimental probe employed. For example, a behavioral scientist might consider the study of long-term potentiation in a rat hippocampal slice preparation a far cry from Pavlovian conditioning, even though, for the neurochemist, it provides a highly accessible preparation for studying synthesis and post-translational modification of neuronal proteins. On the other hand, using inhibitors of macromolecular synthesis permits an investigator to study the effects of disruption of DNA or RNA or of protein synthesis on the behavior of the otherwise intact experimental animal. While the behavioral aspect of this *in vivo* approach may be highly acceptable, it can be anticipated that such massive interventions will produce multiple metabolic effects, which will complicate interpretation of the results at the molecular level. The ultimate value of these divergent experimental approaches may prove to be greatest when they can be integrated into a single consistent model. They may also prove to be of value by leading to more critical experimental models, or by adding constraints to extant theoretical models of how the brain processes information.

Although the answer to the question of how memory is stored continues to prove elusive, significant progress is nevertheless being made, with ever-increasing momentum. It can be attributed to the following factors: (a) increased knowledge of neurotransmitter action within the nervous system, particularly the role of excitatory amino acids; (b) a better understanding of neural development and regeneration, including the availability of molecular biological technology; (c) improved methods for measurement of regional metabolism of brains of experimental animals (see Chap. 29), as well as noninvasive probes for the study of the human brain (see Chap. 44); (d) continued progress in the genetic dissection of behavior in species well suited to this approach; (e) a growing body of information with regard to altered behavior in invertebrate species in which there is evidence that the observed changes are mediated by circuitry confined to a relatively small number of identified cells.

The history of neurochemical research on learning and memory up to the 1980s has been summarized in Chapter 40 of the third edition of this book [1]. This chapter is intended to convey to the reader a sense of the current status of this rapidly evolving field. The issue is no longer whether, but rather when, definitive mechanisms will be elucidated and which approach(es) will ultimately prove most useful to the experimentalist.

SOME DEFINITIONS

Learning can be broadly defined as an adaptive change on the part of an organism in response to an environmental input. Models outside the nervous system, e.g., immunological or bacterial ''learning,'' have been proposed, but are not considered here. Learning is quantified experimentally as the probability that an organism will respond to the same stimulus differently on retesting. This altered probability is based on the organism's *memory* of what it has learned. It is thus not possible to consider learning without memory or, conversely, memory without learning. We can, however, distinguish between the memory necessary for acquisition, which we term *short-term memory*, from that required to demonstrate a learned behavior over longer periods of time. For example, an animal might demonstrate acquisition of a conditioned response during a 30-min training session, indicating learning and the attendant short-term memory of the training task. Evocation of the newly learned behavior in a second training session, hours to weeks later, constitutes evidence for *long-term memory* formation. Thus, during and shortly after a training session, demonstration by the subject of a learned behavior is considered to be based on short-term memory; at later times, it is believed to be mediated by long-term memory [1] (Fig. 1). It is important to remember that although we conceive of learning and memory as intrinsic biological processes or states, our behavioral measures are based entirely on the experimental subject's performance. When a previously trained animal does not demonstrate an acquired behavior under a specified set of conditions, such as a drug-induced state, it will then depend on the skill of the experimenter to determine whether the absent behavior is suppressed or whether the subject is truly amnesic. Although Pavlovian, or *classical conditioning*, as described below is the most universally accepted behavioral paradigm, there are more complex and simpler ones [1]. Among the simpler are habituation and sensitization, in which the same repetitive stimulus produces a decreased or augmented behavioral response, respectively.

It may be useful at this point to distinguish "memory" and "memories". Although there is considerable evidence that specific brain regions, such as the hippocampus and amygdala, play a key role in memory formation, there is equally good evidence that the stored memory itself is broadly distributed in the brain. Given the capacity of the brain to store seemingly limitless quantities of detailed information, a distributed network, in which combinations of neuronal ensembles are employed [2], would seem more likely than a point-by-point "one association per cell" system. Thus, in approaches such as the search for metabolic correlates of memory, described below, we do not seek the locus of a specific memory but of the memory-producing process.

CORNERSTONES OF MEMORY RESEARCH

Current hypotheses on the neurochemical basis of memory are based on a number of premises

that are enumerated here. The remainder of this chapter relies on their validity.

Behavioral information is ultimately stored in synaptic connections

This concept can be traced to Ramón y Cajal, who first recognized the enormous complexity of the brain's neuronal network. Although it may seem self-evident that an organism's most complex function resides in its most complex structures, the proof is indirect. It is supported by the many indications that synaptic complexity increases with development and environmental input ([3]; see also Greenough and Bailey [4]). Alternative hypotheses, such as proposals that memory resides in glia, have not been pursued sufficiently to warrant further consideration here. It has been proposed that memory is not based on altered chemical states but rather in reverberating circuits or in charge distributions. Neurochemists generally adopt the premise that long-lived biological phenomena are ultimately preserved and protected in the form of covalent chemical bonds, be they in nucleic acids, in structural proteins, or in both.

The behavioral unit of learning is the conditioned response

Pavlov's characterization [5] has served as a template for cellular and subcellular models of learning and memory. He emphasized temporal requirements for optimal learning: The conditioned, or neutral, stimulus (CS) such as a tone, must precede the unconditioned stimulus (US), such as food presentation that results in salivation, a punishing electrical shock that results in altered heart rate, or a puff of air that results in an eye blink. Direct application of these characteristics to a two- or three-neuron model may have extremely limited applicability to the mammalian brain, in which the stimulus specificity of a learned behavior may reside in a relatively large population of cells. The cellular

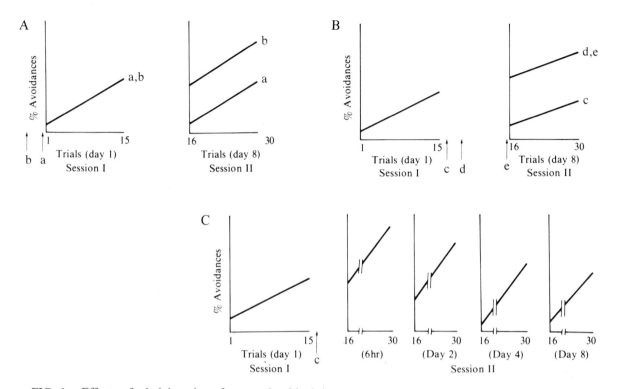

FIG. 1.   Effects of administration of agents that block long-term memory of a multitrial task—the goldfish shuttle box shock-avoidance paradigm—at various times before or after a training session (times a–e). Goldfish are transferred from home tanks to one side of a training apparatus termed a shuttle box, which is divided into halves by a submerged barrier. A trial begins with the onset of a light signal (the CS) on the end of the shuttle box nearest the fish. This is followed 20 sec later by a mild electrical shock (the US) administered through the water. Naive fish respond to the US by swimming over the barrier on onset of shock to the dark, and presumably safe, end of the shuttle box. This escape response is eventually replaced after many trials by the learned avoidance response, in which the fish swims over the barrier before the onset of the punishing shock. Whether the fish demonstrates the conditioned response or the unconditioned response, it will end up on the side of the shuttle box opposite its position at the beginning of the trial. The next trial begins with a light signal at the fishes' end of the apparatus. The location of the fish in the shuttle box is determined by photodetectors, and its avoidance or escape scores are recorded automatically. Figure 1A shows that the probability of an avoidance response during 15 trials (session I) increases progressively, indicating that short-term memory is formed. Fish returned immediately to their home tanks and retrained 1 week later indicate their prior learning and show additional improvement in session II. If an amnestic agent is injected intracranially just before the session (time a), normal acquisition is seen, but there is a profound deficit in performance on retraining 1 week later. If the agent is administered sufficiently in advance of session I (time b), normal retention is seen on day 8, since the effects of the injection will have worn off by the time of the training session. By varying the time of injection before training, the duration of a given agent's amnestic effect can be established. Intracranial injection of the protein synthesis inhibitor puromycin is effective when given 24, but not 72 hr before session I. Figure 1B shows the effects of amnestic agents administered after training. An injection immediately after session I (c) results in profound deficits on retraining 1 week later. The process is time-dependent, since fish return to their home tanks and, given the injection a few hours later (d), show no deficit on retraining in session II, 1 week later. In fact, fish not treated previously and given the amnestic agent just before retraining on day 8 (e) show a learned response. This time-dependence of the treatment rules out both chronic (lingering) and acute toxic effects of the amnestic agents as possible explanations for the observed

model may be highly relevant to studies of learning in invertebrates in which identified neurons appear to mediate behavior [6,7]. The contingency criteria, i.e., that the CS precede the US and that there be an optimal latency (CS–US interval), must be met in true associative learning.

The formation of long-term memory of a newly acquired behavior requires ongoing brain protein synthesis; memory required for acquisition, or learning, does not

Studies over the past 25 years in fish, rodents, birds, and invertebrates (most recently, *Aplysia* [8,9]) have all indicated that the formation of short-term and long-term memory can be distinguished on the basis of susceptibility to agents that block brain protein synthesis (see Agranoff [1] for review). An example of such experimental evidence is shown in Fig. 1. Typical agents used are shown in Fig. 2. Consideration of the temporal aspects of learning and memory and knowledge of the temporal scale of biochemical processes have led to the prediction that learning and short-term memory formation, which can occur within milliseconds and last for minutes to hours, are mediated by post-translational modification at the synapse [10]. Long-term memory, which can form within hours to days, and can last a lifetime, is predicted to be mediated by a process that requires *de novo* protein synthesis and is therefore dependent on the neuronal genome and requires that there be communication between the cell surface and nucleus, presumably by retrograde axonal transport (see Chap. 24).

These three assumptions will then serve as a framework for evaluating the following diverse experimental neurochemical approaches to the understanding of learning and memory.

Do excitatory neurotransmitters mediate learning?

For some time, the rat hippocampus has served as a model system for the study of memory formation. When afferent fibers to the CA1 region are stimulated electrically in close temporal proximity to depolarization of the postsynaptic neurons, a long-lasting increase in sensitivity of these cells develops, which may persist for weeks. It is referred to as long-term potentiation (LTP) [11]. LTP also can be demonstrated in hippocampal slice preparations, providing a convenient preparation for *in vitro* studies. There is considerable evidence to indicate that glutamate plays a key role as the excitatory neurotransmitter in LTP formation and that the postsynaptic receptor activated is of the *N*-methyl-D-aspartate (NMDA) type (see Chap. 15). When stimulation conditions are optimal for LTP formation, there appears to be a resultant increase in intracellular Ca^{2+}, but it is uncertain how the elevation of postsynaptic Ca^{2+} leads to LTP. Hypotheses include (a) the activation of the Ca^{2+}-activated protease, calpain [12], which in turn is proposed to degrade cytoskeletal elements and thereby to reorganize cell shape and receptor distribution; and (b) the activation of calmodulin-dependent enzymes, phospholipase A_2 or protein kinase C, which is also activated by Ca^{2+} as well as by diacylglycerol released in the breakdown of the phosphoinositides (see Chap. 16). NMDA does not, however, stimulate phosphoinositide turnover in the hippocampus. It is at present not known

reduced responding rates and indicates that the agent produces a specific memory loss. The decay of short-term memory is shown in Fig. 1C. Injection of a blocking agent just after (or before) session 1 results in failure to form long-term memory. In this experiment, individual groups of animals so treated and retrained at various times earlier than 8 days, e.g., 6, 48 or 96 hr after session I, demonstrate the learned response. The experiments thus constitute evidence for the decay of short-term memory (see text) (from Agranoff [10].)

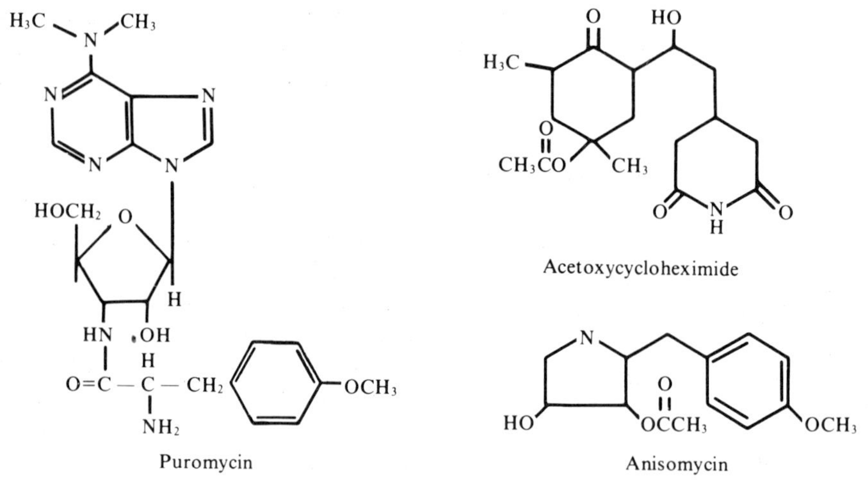

FIG. 2. Three classes of eukaryotic protein synthesis inhibitors that block long-term memory formation and do not affect short-term memory formation. Because they bear little structural similarity and block different steps in protein synthesis, it is concluded that their common amnestic action is by inhibition of protein synthesis, rather than by side effects. Replacement of the acetoxy group by H of acetoxycycloheximide (AXM) results in the structure of cyclohex   imide (CXM), whereas substitution with OH gives the structure of streptovitacin A.

whether NMDA receptors are also important in memory formation. LTP has also been proposed as a suitable model of epilepsy (see Chap. 41).

Does neural development or regeneration provide a useful model for studies on memory?

The brain at birth is far from a clean slate. For example, an animal may respond with fear to a visual presentation of a nonspecific predator, even though it has had no prior exposure. It seems likely that, as we propose for learned behavior, the information subserving inborn behavior is coded in synaptic connections. Although the synaptic connections that subserve instinctual behavior form during development, those mediating neuroplasticity—(an all-encompassing term that includes the brain's response to learning conditions as well as to

trauma; see also Chap. 26)—have a low probability of forming in the absence of an external input.

It is generally held that there is little or no neurogenesis after infancy, and since learning and memory formation go on into adulthood, one looks to the complexity of neuronal branching and synapse formation as the site most likely to reflect neuroplasticity. This view has some experimental support. Regeneration of the CNS occurs in amphibia and in fishes, and the study of regeneration of the axotomized optic nerve in these genera is relevant in that, like learning, they involve neuronal process growth and eventual synapse formation within the scaffolding of an adult brain.

This optic nerve preparation was used to identify the growth-associated proteins (GAPs) synthesized during regeneration and in development, but not by the intact mature neuron. One of these, GAP 43, has been identified as a component of growth cones. It is identical to F1, a substrate for protein kinase C, the phosphorylation of which is selectively enhanced under conditions of LTP formation in the rat hippocampus [13]. This same protein, also known as B50, was identified by W. Gispen as a component of synaptic membranes, the phosphorylation of which is believed to regulate PIP kinase, an enzyme that is part of the phosphoinositide second-messenger system (see Chap. 16). It is relevant that inhibitors of protein synthesis block the sustained LTP. The GAPs represent a class of proteins, the synthesis and regulation of which may be necessary for memory formation.

Can memory processes be localized on the basis of their metabolic activity?

The [^{14}C]2-deoxyglucose (2DG) method of Sokoloff (see Chap. 29) would seem ideally suited to establishing whether a specific brain region is activated under conditions in which an imposed behavioral procedure results in an altered state of an animal that fulfills the criteria of a learned behavior. That there have been few such reports can be attributed to a number of technical problems and limitations. First, there is no assurance that the putative metabolic changes in the brain that accompany learning and/or memory formation will be measurable. Although one can distinguish the differences between simple and complex sensory inputs by examining the altered metabolic patterns of appropriate cortical regions by the [^{14}C]2DG technique, it does not necessarily follow that the method possesses the requisite spatial or temporal resolution to address the question. Indications that this approach may indeed prove successful have been reported in the rat, using a classical conditioning paradigm in which the US is cardiac slowing produced by stimulation of the reticular formation. Coupling this stimulation to an auditory tone, which serves as the CS, leads to classical conditioning. Presentation of the tone after learning [14] is correlated with increased labeling of the molecular layer of the hippocampus.

The utility of the 2DG method in behavioral experiments is greatly increased by a technique that permits two experiments to be performed in the same animal, instead of one. For example, [^{14}C]2DG can be injected while the experimental animal is at rest or engaged in a behavioral task that does not result in detectable learning, e.g., random presentations of CS and US. After 20 to 30 min, either ^{3}H- or ^{18}F-labeled DG is injected. After the second incorporation period, equal in duration to the first, the brain is removed for autoradiographic analysis. As originally described, discrete tissue samples are analyzed quantitatively in a scintillation counter, and the ratio of the two isotopes is computed [15].

Adaptation to an autoradiographic approach requires the development of two images in the presence and absence of film interposed between tissue section and the image film. The interposed film absorbs the weaker isotope: ^{3}H in the ^{3}H/^{14}C pair and ^{14}C in the ^{14}C/^{18}F pair. Removal of the contribution of the higher energy isotope to the image produced by the weaker isotope is a more difficult problem but can be addressed successfully by a variety of strategies [16–18]. The use of ^{18}F is attractive, since it has a short half-life (see Chap. 44), and after its decay, the remaining nuclide, i.e., ^{14}C, can be easily measured [16]. This isotopic pair was used in a study on learning and memory in the cat [18]. Although John et al. [18] argue that the results support the hypothesis that memory is not localized in the brain, a number of technical aspects of the study have been questioned [19]. The problems are all experimentally addressable, and we may anticipate greater application of the double-label 2DG method to behavioral studies in the future.

The concept that higher brain function can be localized receives support from studies on human learning and memory employing positron emission tomography (PET). It has long been known that local cerebral blood flow (LCBF), usually measured in PET with ^{15}O-H_2O, and local metabolism, measured either by [^{18}F]2DG uptake or by ^{15}O-O_2 fixation, are highly correlated in all brain regions (see Chap. 44). The great advantage of ^{15}O-H_2O for studies of LCBF is that it has a 2-min half-life. It therefore becomes possible to perform multiple studies in the same subject. The advantage of being able to perform such test-retest paradigms for behavioral studies in human subjects is as described above for the sequential double-label studies in animals. There is a limit of six to eight PET studies in a single session imposed by both the minimum counts needed for imaging the brain and the maximal acceptable radiation dose limit for the subject. Using this method, Peterson et al. [20] have reported distinctive regional patterns in cortical LCBF resulting from visual presentation of words, depending on whether or not the word was simply read or was also spoken by the subject and, further, whether there was semantic processing; i.e., the subject indicated a use for the word. These reports confirm and to some degree extend results obtained earlier with single-photon studies under more invasive and often heroic circumstances.

Although the degree of localization with PET is at least two orders of magnitude less than can be achieved in animals with the autoradiographic approach, its noninvasive nature carries enormous advantages: first, the possibility of performing repeated studies in the same subject and second, applicability to the human brain. Since we are most interested in human memory, and since human learning and memory involve ideational processes such as the use of language and symbolic manipulation, there is in this sense no alternative experimental subject.

Can genetic models be used to probe memory mechanisms?

The concept of neurogenetic dissection of behavior is exemplified by work of the laboratory of S. Benzer and his associates on *Drosophila*. It has been possible to identify a number of mutant strains that are seemingly normal except for the inability to learn or to store memory of a training task. Sensitization, habituation, and classical conditioning paradigms, as well as behavioral screens for the detection of defective strains, have been devised [21,22]. In some instances, temperature-sensitive mutants have been developed so that an otherwise lethal gene can be suppressed until the behavioral training and/or retrieval sessions. Phototaxis, attractant and repellent odors, and mating behavior frequently serve as the basis of behavioral input.

Mutants in neurotransmitter metabolism, such as in DOPA decarboxylase have been reported. In insects, this enzyme is important not only for the synthesis of dopamine and serotonin, but also for the decarboxylation of tyrosine to octopamine (see Chap. 11). Dopamine is essential for cuticle formation, so that development is impaired in deficient mutants. This can be overcome by the use of temperature-sensitive alleles.

The best documented behavioral mutant is Dunce (*dnc*), in which a deficiency in the structural gene for cyclic AMP (cAMP) phosphodiesterase has been established. How this becomes translated into a behavioral deficit is not known, but some effect on a K^+ channel via failure of a cAMP-dependent protein kinase is a favored possibility. Three cAMP phosphodiesterases have been identified in *Drosophila*. The *dnc* mutant appears to be deficient in PDE II, which form accounts for 70 percent of the total cAMP-hydrolyzing activity of fly homogenates. It differs from PDE I and III by a low K_m for its substrate, but not for cyclic GMP (cGMP), and by its insensitivity to calmodulin. Predictably, *dnc* mutants have elevated cAMP levels. Genes for various *dnc* subtypes have been cloned; *dnc* is on the X chromosome.

A related behavioral mutant is rutabaga (*rut*). Memory forms in this mutant, but decays rapidly. Although the biochemistry and molecular genetics of *rut* are not as well worked out as those of *dnc*, it is clear that it is also on the X chromosome and involves cAMP. In the case of *rut*, the defect appears to be in the synthetic enzyme AMP cyclase. The affected cyclase accounts for only 30 percent of the body total and is primarily in the abdomen. It is forskolin-sensitive.

Another species subjected to genetic analysis is the nematode *Caenorhabditis elegans*. Its behavioral repertoire is less impressive than that of the fruit fly, but it has the anatomical advantage of having only a few hundred neurons. Thus, altered phenotypic expression in the morphology of the nervous system can be more readily correlated with altered behavior.

What has been learned from simple systems in which identified neurons mediate learned behavior?

The sea snail *Aplysia californica* has a relatively small number of large, easily impaleable, identified neurons. The laboratory of E. Kandel has been instrumental in mapping the circuitry of *Aplysia* in considerable detail. Nonassociative learning paradigms, sensitization and habituation, have been applied using mantle and siphon-mediated gill withdrawal as end-points, as well as escape responses following noxious stimuli. These phenomena appear to be mediated presynaptically, and increased and decreased synaptic release zones are reported in sensitization and habituation, respectively. Sensitization appears to be heterosynaptic; habituation appears to be homosynaptic. The altered states appear to be mediated by serotonin, and facilitation can be demonstrated on addition of serotonin to dissociated cell cultures. Anisomycin, an inhibitor of protein synthesis, blocks this action of serotonin, and the observation has been argued to militate in favor of the hypothesis that long-term memory is dependent on protein synthesis [8,9].

At the short-term level of temporal resolution, serotonin is proposed to increase cAMP, which in turn activates kinases that regulate a K^+ channel. This latter action is antagonized by the neuroactive peptide FMRFamide (Phe-Met-Arg-Phe-NH_2), the action of which is believed to be mediated by a lipoxygenase metabolite of arachidonate [23].

Classical conditioning has also been studied in *Aplysia*. In this case, a mild stimulus to the siphon serves as CS and is coupled to a US, tail shock, which triggers the escape response. The facilitory effect of the US is mediated presynaptically, much as in sensitization. The biochemical nature of the signal appears to be Ca^{2+} release, and the message is carried via cAMP. The combination of elevated Ca^{2+} and neurotransmitter-activated cyclase is the presumed site of convergence needed for a molecular model of classical conditioning.

Conditioning has also been studied in another invertebrate, *Hermissenda crassicornis*. In this case, the CS is a positive phototaxis that is paired with high-speed rotation, the US, which leads to suppression of the unconditioned response. Daily sessions of 50 to 100 pairings for a few days result in retention of the learned response for over 2 weeks. Of a number of cellular changes found following conditioning, a reduced K^+ current in the type B photoreceptors has been pursued experimentally [24]. From experiments involving various drugs and microinjections of enzymes, it has been inferred that Ca^{2+} and calmodulin-activated protein kinases mediate associative learning both in *Hermissenda* and in *Aplysia*. A major difference is that in *Hermissenda*, Ca^{2+} influx is the result of depolarization, as is proposed in hippocampal LTP, whereas in *Aplysia*, it is neurotransmitter-mediated. Inhibitors of protein synthesis prolong the altered biophysical correlates of conditioning in *Hermissenda*. It has been speculated that this seemingly paradoxical result is related to short-term rather than long-term memory formation [25]. Microinjection experiments and the application of phorbol esters indicate that protein kinase C and the phosphoinositide pathway may play an important role in associative learning, as is further discussed below.

OTHER MODELS OF LEARNING AND MEMORY

Imprinting

Newborn chicks and ducklings will follow a moving object to which they are first exposed following hatching. Neurochemical correlates have been investigated over a number of years in the laboratory of S. Rose [26]. Changes in macromolecular synthesis in the roof of the telencephalon are correlated with successful imprinting.

Kindling

Repeated subeffective electrical stimulation of a brain region can ultimately lead to the development of a seizure focus. Kindling has been used as a model of seizure disorders as well as of learning. The latter stems from the lack of gross anatomical or physiological changes in the kindled tissue despite the growing increase in sensitivity to the stimulus.

Enhancement of memory

Loss of the ability to form new memory as a function of age in humans is well known. In addition to the severe forms of this deficiency associated with the dementias (see Chap. 43), milder forms abound. Pharmaceutical development of cognition enhancers has not yet proven successful. Animal models are generally inadequate in that human brain structure and function differ from those of the experimental animal more than does any other organ. Many screening programs for cognition activators employ animals in which a behavioral decrement produced by one agent is reversed by the test drug. For example, scopolamine-induced amnesia can be relieved by cholinergic agonists in a screening assay. Because of the artifactual nature of the approach, results of such studies must be interpreted cautiously.

The claims in the 1960s of memory transfer via injection of RNA or of protein have long since subsided for want of evidence. An interesting footnote is the retrospective suggestion that the "memory transfer" peptide scotophobin was actually an enkephalin-like molecule [27]. For further information on other systems used for the study of memory, the interested reader is referred to an earlier review [1] and the general references found at the end of this chapter.

COMMON FEATURES IN BIOCHEMICAL APPROACHES

There are diverse approaches to the biochemical basis of learning and memory, but there is increasing "cross-talk." Common threads are the implications of second-messenger systems in learning and short-term memory and of protein synthesis in long-term memory formation. Both require a better understanding of the brain's languages: the neurotransmitters and neuromodulators that are used for signal transduction between cells, and the cell's intracellular language. The intracellular language is that of the second messengers and has at least two vital functions. These are the integration of multiple inputs, such as Ca^{2+} entry and membrane-bound enzyme activation, and activation of the genome [28,29].

Caution should be exerted before jumping on the bandwagon of a given neurotransmitter or second messenger as the crucial intermediate that links behavior and molecules. It should be kept in mind that there may be large differences in memory mechanisms between species and even within the same brain. For example, although the optimal CS-US interval in classical conditioning in the rat is usually measured in seconds or less, it can be much longer. In the phenomenon of bait shyness, the animal is given an emetic agent (the US) several hours after the presentation of a novel food (the US). This results in avoidance of the novel food. It is easy to understand the survival value of the long CS-US interval, but it would be difficult to include this example in distinguishing short- and long-term memory on the basis of underlying biochemical mechanisms.

A major unanswered question is how learning is conserved, or is converted, to long-term memory. It is well-known that brain proteins turn over at rates no different than those of other organs. Altered synaptic relationships that underlie stored memory must then depend on feedforward loops generated in the cell nucleus. There is ample independent evidence that the genome regulates phenotypic expression throughout the lifetime of the cell, and in the case of neurons, the lifetime of the individual. How then are the events at the membrane surface that occur during learning, or acquisition, communicated to the nucleus? A possible model is furnished by progress in our knowledge of the phosphoinositide second-messenger system (see also Chap. 16). A number of growth factors exert their mitogenic effects at the cell surface from which the message to the cell nucleus proceeds via stimulated breakdown of PIP_2. Both elevated intracellular Ca^{2+} and protein kinase C activation result from PIP_2 breakdown and may convey their message to the genome in a number of ways. For example, they activate the Na^+/H^+ exchanger, raising intracellular pH, which can lead to cell proliferation [28]. It has additionally become apparent that several oncogene products participate in the inositide-linked second-messenger system. It is also of interest in this regard that intracellular injection of protein kinase C mimics LTP in the rat hippocampus [30] and that classical conditioning of the rabbit eyelid is reported to lead to protein kinase C activation in the CA1 region of the hippocampus [31]. Whether protein kinase C, Ca^{2+}, or still other intracellular chemical messengers mediate communication between the synaptic receptor site and genomic regulation within the cell nucleus, it is apparent that there exists an intracellular language that links these loci in development as well as in neuroplastic events relevant to behavioral change.

REFERENCES

1. Agranoff, B. W. Learning and memory: Biochemical approaches. In G. J. Siegel, R. W. Albers, B. W. Agranoff, and R. Katzman (eds.), *Basic Neurochemistry*, 3rd ed. Boston: Little, Brown and Company, 1981, pp. 801–820.
2. McNaughton, B. L., and Morris, R. G. M. Hippocampal synaptic enhancement and information storage within a definitive memory system. *Trends Neurosci.* 10:408–415, 1987.
3. Bailey, C. H., and Chen, M. Long-term memory in *Aplysia* modulates the total number of varicosities of single identified sensory neurons. *Proc. Natl. Acad. Sci. U.S.A.*, 85:2373–2377, 1988.
4. Greenough, W. T., and Bailey, C. H. The anatomy of a memory: Convergence of results over a diversity of tests. *Trends Neurosci.* 11:142–146, 1988.
5. Pavlov, I. P. In G. V. Anrep (ed.) *Conditioned Reflexes*. London: Oxford University Press, 1927.
6. Kandel, E. R. *Cellular Basis of Behavior*. San Francisco: Freeman, 1976.
7. Kandel, E. R., and Schwartz, J. H. Molecular biology of learning: Modulation of transmitter release. *Science* 218:433–443, 1982.
8. Montorolo, P. G., Goelet, P., Castellucci, V. F., Morgan, J., Kandel, E. R., and Schacher, S. A critical period for macromolecular synthesis in long-term heterosynaptic facilitation in *Aplysia*. *Science* 234:1249–1254, 1986.
9. Dale, N., Kandel, E. R., and Schacher, S. Serotonin produces long-term changes in the excitability of *Aplysia* sensory neurons in culture that depend on new protein synthesis. *J. Neurosci.* 7:2232–2238, 1987.
10. Agranoff, B. W. Biochemical events mediating the formation of short- and long-term memory. In Y. Tsukada and B. W. Agranoff (eds.), *Neu-*

robiological Basis of Learning and Memory. New York: Wiley, 1980, pp. 135–147.

11. Bliss, T. V. P., and Lømo, T. Long-lasting potentiation of synaptic transmission in the dentate gyrus of the rat following selective depletion of monoamines. *J. Physiol. London* 232:331–356, 1973.

12. Lynch, G., and Baudry, M. The biochemistry of memory: A new and specific hypothesis. *Science* 224:1057–1063, 1984.

13. Routtenberg, A., Lovinger, D. M., and Steward, O. Selective increase in phosphorylation of a 47 kDa protein (F1) is directly related to long-term potentiation. *Behav. Neural Biol.* 43:3–11, 1986.

14. Gonzalez-Lima, F., and Scheich, H. Classical conditioning of tone-signaled bradycardia modifies 2-deoxyglucose uptake patterns in cortex, thalamus, habenula, caudate-putamen and hippocampal formation. *Brain Res.* 363:239–255, 1986.

15. Agranoff, B. W., Boast, C. A., Frey, K. A., and Altenau, L. L. Evaluation of regional brain metabolism by a sequential double label 2-deoxyglucose method. In J. V. Passonneau, R. A. Hawkins, W. D. Lust, and F. A. Welsh (eds.), *Cerebral Metabolism and Neural Function.* Baltimore: Williams & Wilkins, 1980, pp. 331–337.

16. Olds, J. L., Frey, K. A., Ehrenkaufer, R. L., and Agranoff, B. W. A sequential double-label autoradiographic method that quantifies altered rates of regional glucose metabolism. *Brain Res.* 361:217–224, 1985.

17. Friedman, H. R., Bruce, C. J., and Goldman-Rakic, P. S. A sequential double-label 14C- and 3H-2-DG technique: Validation by double dissociation of functional states. *Exp. Brain Res.* 66:543–554, 1987.

18. John, E. R., Tang, Y., Brill, A., Young, R., and Ono, K. Double-labeled maps of memory. *Science* 233;1167–1175, 1986.

19. McEacheron, D. L., Gallistel, C. R., and Hand, P. J. Do 15 million cat neurons mediate the memory of a circle and a star? *Science* 238:1586–1587, 1987.

20. Peterson, S. E., Fox, P. T., Posner, M. I., Mintun, M., and Raichle, M. E. Positron emission tomographic studies of the cortical anatomy of single word processing. *Nature* 331:585–589, 1988.

21. Dudai, Y. Cyclic AMP and Learning in *Drosophila. Adv. Cyclic Nucleotide Protein Phosphorylation Res.* 20:343–361, 1986.

22. Dudai, Y. Neurogenetic dissection of learning and short-term memory in *Drosophila. Annu. Rev. Neurosci.* 11:1988.

23. Piomelli, D., Volterra, A., Dale, N., Siegelbaum, S. A., Kandel, E. R., and Belardetti, F. Lipoxygenase metabolites of arachidonic acid as second messengers for presynaptic inhibition of *Aplysia* sensory cells. *Nature* 328:38–43, 1987.

24. Alkon, D. L. Calcium-mediated reduction of ionic currents. A biophysical memory trace. *Science* 226:1037–1045, 1984.

25. Alkon, D. L., Bank, B., Naito, S., Chung, C., Ram, J. Inhibition of protein synthesis prolongs Ca^{2+}-mediated reduction of K^+ currents in molluscan neurons. *Proc. Natl. Acad. Sci. U.S.A.* 84:6948–6952, 1987.

26. Rose, S. P. R. Neurochemical correlates of early learning in the chick. In Y. Tsukada and B. W. Agranoff (eds.), *Neurobiological Basis of Learning and Memory.* New York: Wiley, 1980, pp. 179–191.

27. Wilson, D. Scotophobin resurrected as a neuropeptide. *Nature* 320:313–314, 1986.

28. Berridge, M. Second messenger dualism in neuromodulation and memory. *Nature* 323:294–295, 1986.

29. Goelet, P., Castelluci, V. F., Schacher, S., and Kandel, E. R. The long and short of long-term memory—a molecular framework. *Nature* 322:419–422, 1986.

30. Hu, G.-Y., Hvalby, O., Walaas, S. I., Albert, K. A., Skjeflo, P., Andersen, P., and Greengard, P. Protein kinase C injection into hippocampal pyramidal cells elicits features of long term potentiation. *Nature* 328:426–429, 1987.

31. Bank, B., Dewer, A., Kuzirian, A. M., Rasmussen, H., and Alkon, D. L. Classical conditioning induces long-term translation of protein kinase C in rabbit hippocampal CA1 cells. *Proc. Natl. Acad. Sci. U.S.A.* 85:1988–1992, 1988.

General References

Changeux, J.-P., and Konishi, M. (eds.). *The Neural and Molecular Bases of Learning* (Dahlem Konferenzen). Chichester, England: John Wiley and Sons, 1987.

Edelman, G. M., Gall, W. E., and Cowan, W. M. (eds.). *Synaptic Function.* New York: Wiley, 1987.

Trends Neurosci. 11(4), 1988. [Special issue on learning and memory]

Tsukada, Y., and Agranoff, B. W. (eds.). *Neurobiological Basis of Learning and Memory.* New York: Wiley, 1980.

Glossary

A	Adenosine
AADC	Aromatic amino acid decarboxylase
AC	Adenylate cyclase
ACh	Acetylcholine
AChE	Acetylcholinesterase
AChR	Acetylcholine receptor
ACTH	Adrenocorticotropic hormone
ADP	Adenosine 5'-diphosphate
aFGF	Acid fibroblast growth factor
ALD	Adrenoleukodystrophy
AMD	Acidic maltase deficiency
AMP	Adenosine 5'-monophosphate
AMPT	α-Methyl-*p*-tyrosine
ANP	Atrial natriuretic peptide
AP4	2-Amino-4-phosphonobutyric acid
AP5	2-Amino-5-phosphonovaleric acid
AP7	2-Amino-7-phosphonoheptanoic acid
ARAS	Ascending reticular activating system
Asp-T	Aspartate transaminase
ATP	Adenosine 5'-triphosphate
BAR	β-Adrenergic receptor
BARK	β-Adrenergic receptor kinase
BBB	Blood-brain barrier
BCDHC	Branched-chain dehydrogenase complex
BCH	2-Aminononbornane-2-carboxylic acid
bFGF	Basic fibroblast growth factor
BTX	Batrachotoxin
α-BTX	α-Bungarotoxin
β-BTX	β-Bungarotoxin
CAM	Cell adhesion molecule
cAMP	Cyclic AMP; adenosine 3',5'-cyclic phosphate
CBF	Cerebral blood flow
CBV	Cerebral blood volume
CCK	Cholecystokinin
cDNA	Complementary deoxyribonucleic acid
CDP	Cytidine 5'-diphosphate
CDP-DG	Cytidine diphosphodiacylglycerol
CDPC	Cytidine diphosphocholine
CDPE	Cytidine diphosphoethanolamine
CG	Chorionic gonadotropin
cGMP	Cyclic GMP; guanosine 3',5'-cyclic phosphate
CGRP	Calcitonin gene-related peptide
ChAT	Choline acetyltransferase
CK	Creatinine kinase
CMP	Cytidine 5'-monophosphate
CMRGl	see CMRGlc

CMRGlc	Cerebral metabolic rate for glucose
CMRO$_2$	Cerebral metabolic rate for oxygen
CNPase	2',3'-Cyclic nucleoside-3'-phospho-diesterase
CNS	Central nervous system
CoA	Coenzyme A
COMT	Catechol-*O*-methyltransferase
COX	Cytochrome oxidase
CPT	Carnitine palmitoyltransferase
CRF	Corticotropin-releasing factor (see CRH)
CRH	Corticotropin-releasing hormone (same as CRF)
CSF	Cerebrospinal fluid
CT	Computed tomography
CTP	Cytidine 5'-triphosphate
CVA	Cerebrovascular accident (cerebral infarction)
D	Dextro isomer
Da	Dalton (unit of molecular mass)
DAG	Diacylglycerol (same as DG)
DBH	Dopamine-β-hydroxylase
DDC	Dopa decarboxylase
2-DG	2-Deoxy-D-glucose
DG	Diacylglycerol (see DAG)
DHAP	Dihydroxyacetone phosphate
DHT	Dihydrotestosterone
DNA	Deoxyribonucleic acid
DNase I	Deoxyribonuclease I
L-DOPA	3,4-dihydroxy-L-phenylalanine
DOPAC	3,4-Dihydroxyphenylacetic acid
DPN$^+$, DPHN	See NAD$^+$, NADH
DSM-III-R	*Diagnostic Statistical Manual*, 3rd. ed., revised
dT	Deoxythymidine
EAE	Experimental allergic encephalomyelitis
EAMG	Experimental autoimmune myasthenia gravis
EAN	Experimental allergic neuritis
ECF	Extracellular fluid
ECG	Electrocardiogram
ECS	Electroconvulsive shock
ECT	Electroconvulsive shock therapy
EDTA	Ethylenediaminetetraacetic acid
EEG	Electroencephalogram
EGF	Epidermal growth factor
EGTA	Ethyleneglycol-bis-(β-amino-ethylether)-N,N,N',N',-tetra-acetic acid
ELISA	Enzyme-linked immunosorbent assay

EM	Electron microscopy
EMG	Electromyography
EPA	Eicosapentaenoic acid
EPP	End-plate potential
EPSP	Excitatory postsynaptic potential
ER	Endoplasmic reticulum
FAD	Flavin-adenine dinucleotide
FAP	Familial amyloidotic polyneuropathy
FDG	2-Fluoro-2-deoxy-D-glucose
FFA	Free fatty acid
FGF	Fibroblast growth factor (a, acidic; b, basic)
FSH	Follicle-stimulating hormone
G proteins	Family of homologous guanine nucleotide-binding proteins involved in signal transduction
G_i	G protein involved in inhibition of adenylate cyclase
G_s	G protein involved in stimulation of adenylate cyclase
GABA	γ-Aminobutyric acid
GABA-T	GABA: α-oxyglutarate transaminase
GAD	Glutamic acid decarboxylase
galC	Galactocerebroside
GAP	i) Gonadotropin-releasing hormone associated protein; ii) growth-associated protein
GDP	Guanosine 5'-diphosphate
GFAP	Glial fibrillary acidic protein
GHRH	Growth hormone-releasing hormone
GLC	Gas-liquid chromatography
GnRH	Gonadotropin-releasing hormone (formerly called LHRH)
GO	G protein (other) found in brain and retina (see transducin)
GTP	Guanosine 5'-triphosphate
GTPase	Guanosine triphosphatase
5-HIAA	5-Hydroxyindoleacetic acid
HIOMT	Hydroxyindole-*O*-methyltransferase
HLA	Human leukocyte antigen system
HMG	β-Hydroxy-β-methylglutaryl
HMM	Heavy meromysin
HMSN	Hereditary motor and sensory neuropathy
hnRNA	Heterogeneous nuclear RNA
HPLC	High-performance liquid chromatography
HSPG	Heparan sulfate proteoglycan
5-HT	5-Hydroxytryptamine (serotonin)
5-HTP	5-Hydroxytryptophan
HVA	Homovanillic acid (4-hydroxy-3-methoxyphenylacetic acid)

IAP	Islet activating protein
ICAMs	Intracellular cell adhesion molecules
IM	Intermediate protein
INH	Isonicotonic hydrazide
IP_1	Inositol-1-phosphate
IP_2	Inositol-1,4-bisphosphate
IP_3	Inositol-1,4,5-trisphosphate
IP_4	Inositol-1,3,4,5-tetratrisphosphate
IPSP	Inhibitory postsynaptic potential
IQ	Intelligence quotient
KA	Kainic acid
kb	Kilobase
K_d	Dissociation constant
kDa	Kilodalton (see Da)
KGDHC	α-Ketoglutarate dehydrogenase complex
KSS	Kearns-Sayre syndrome
L	Levo isomer
LCAM	Liver cell adhesion molecule
LCMRGl	Local cerebral metabolic rate for glucose (also rGMRGlc)
LD_{50}	Mean lethal dose
LDH	Lactate dehydrogenase
LDL	Low-density lipoprotein
LEMS	Lambert-Eaton myasthenic syndrome
LH	Luteinizing hormone
LHRH	Luteinizing hormone-releasing hormone (see GnRH)
LPH	Lipotropic hormone
LMM	Light meromysin
LSD	Lysergic acid diethylamide
LT	Leukotriene
LTP	Long-term potentiation
M_r	Molecular weight (relative molecular mass)
M1,M2	Subtypes of muscarinic receptors
MAG	Myelin-associated glycoprotein
MAO	Monoamine oxidase
MAP_2 (MAP-2)	Microtubule-associated protein
MBP	Myelin basic protein
MeAIB	2-methylamino-isobutyric acid
MELAS	Myopathy, encephalopathy, lactic acidosis, and stroke-like episodes
MEPP	Miniature end-plate potential
MERRF	Myoclonus epilepsy with ragged red fibers
MHPG	3-Methoxy-4-hydroxyphenylglycol
MLD	Metachromatic leukodystrophy
MPP	*N*-Methyl-4-phenylpyridine
MPTP	*N*-Methyl-4-phenyl-1,2,3,6-tetrahydropyridine
MRI	Magnetic resonance imaging

mRNA	Messenger RNA
MSH	Melanocyte-stimulating hormone
mtDNA	Mitochondrial DNA
N-CAM (NCAM)	Neural (neuronal) cell adhesion molecule
Na,K-ATPase	$Na^+ + K^+$-stimulated adenosine triphosphatase
NAD^+	Oxidized nicotinamide-adenine dinucleotide
NADH	Reduced nicotinamide-adenine dinucleotide
$NADP^+$	Oxidized nicotinamide-adenine dinucleotide phosphate
NADPH	Reduced nicotinamide-adenine dinucleotide phosphate
NE	Norepinephrine
NF	Neurofilament
NFT	Neurofibrillary tangles
NgCAM	Neuronal-glial cell adhesion molecule
NGF	Nerve growth factor
NMDA	*N*-Methyl-D-aspartate
NMJ	Neuromuscular junction
NMP	Nucleoside monophosphate
NMLA	*N*-Methyl-L-aspartic acid
NMR	Nuclear magnetic resonance
NPY	Neuropeptide Y
P_i	Inorganic phosphate
P5C	Δ^1-Pyrroline-5-carboxylic acid
PA	Phosphatidic acid
Pao_2	Partial pressure of ambient arterial oxygen
PAPS	3'-Phosphoadenosine 5'-phosphosulfate
PAS	Periodic acid-Schiff
PC	Pyruvate carboxylase
PCP	Phencyclidine
PCPA	*para*-Chlorophenylalanine
PCr	Phosphocreatine
PDE	Phosphodiesterase
PDGF	Platelet-derived growth factor
PDHC	Pyruvate dehydrogenase complex
PE	Phosphatidylethanolamine
PEPCK	Phosphoenolpyruvate carboxykinase
PET	Positron emission tomography
PFK	Phosphofructokinase
PG	Prostaglandin
PGE (F)	Prostaglandin E (or F)
PGG_2	Prostaglandin G_2
PGH_2	Prostaglandin H_2
PGK	Phosphoglycerate kinase
PHF	Paired helical filament
PI	Phosphatidylinositol
PIP	Phosphatidylinositol-4-phosphate
PIP_2	Phosphatidylinositol-4,5-bisphosphate

PK-C	Protein kinase C
PKU	Phenylketonuria
PLA	Phospholipase A_2
PLC	Phospholipase C
PLP	Proteolipid protein
PML	Progressive multifocal leukencephalopathy
PNMT	Phenylethanolamine-*N*-methyltransferase
PNS	Peripheral nervous system
POMC	Pro-opiomelanocortin
PP_i	Pyrophosphate
PS	Phosphatidylserine
PSEP	Postsynaptic excitatory potential
PTH	Parathyroid hormone
PZ	Pirenzepine
rCMRGlc	Regional cerebral metabolic rate for glucose (also LCMRGl)
REM	Rapid eye movement stage of sleep
RER	Rough endoplasmic reticulum
RFLP	Restriction fragment-length polymorphism
RIA	Radioimmunoassay
RNA	Ribonucleic acid
RQ	Respiratory quotient
RRF	Reiterated DNA restriction fragment (of DNA)
SC	Slow components of axoplasmic transport (SCa, SCb)
scDNA	Single-copy DNA
SDS-PAGE	Sodium·dodecylsulfate-polyacrylamide gel electrophoresis
SER	Smooth endoplasmic reticulum
SIF	Small, intensely fluorescent (cells in sympathetic ganglia)
SM	Sphingomyelin
SNE	Subacute necrotizing encephalomyopathy
SR	Sarcoplasmic reticulum
SRP	Signal recognition particle
SSADH	Succinic semialdehyde dehydrogenase
STX	Saxitoxin
T_3	Triiodothyronine
T_4	Thyroxine
TBX	Thromboxane
TCA	Tricarboxylic acid (see Krebs cycle, citric acid cycle)
TDP	Thiamine diphosphate (same as TPP)
TH	Tyrosine hydroxylase
ThPP	see TPP
TK	(i) Transketolase; (ii) thymidine kinase

TLC	Thin-layer chromatography	TTP	Thiamine triphosphate
TnC;TnI;TnT	Protein components of troponin	TTX	Tetrodotoxin
TPA	Tetradecanoyl phorbol acetate		
TPN$^+$, TPNH	see NADP$^+$, NADPH		
TPP	Thiamine pyrophosphate (cocarboxylase)	UDP	Uridine 5'-diphosphate
TRH	Thyrotropin-releasing hormone (or factor)	VIP	Vasoactive intestinal peptide
tRNA	Transfer ribonucleic acid	VMA	Vanillymandelic acid

Amino acids in proteins

Symbol		Name	Codons					
One letter	Three letter							
A	Ala	Alanine	GCA	GCC	GCG	GCU		
C	Cys	Cysteine	UGC	UGU				
D	Asp	Aspartate	GAC	GAU				
E	Glu	Glutamate	GAA	GAG				
F	Phe	Phenylalanine	UUC	UUU				
G	Gly	Glycine	GGA	GGC	GGG	GGU		
H	His	Histidine	CAC	CAU				
I	Ile	Isoleucine	AUA	AUC	AUU			
K	Lys	Lysine	AAA	AAG				
L	Leu	Leucine	UUA	UUG	CUA	CUC	CUG	CUU
M	Met	Methionine	AUG					
N	Asn	Asparagine	AAC	AAU				
P	Pro	Proline	CCA	CCC	CCG	CCU		
Q	Gln	Glutamine	CAA	CAG				
R	Arg	Arginine	AGA	AGG	CGA	CGC	GCG	GCU
S	Ser	Serine	AGC	AGU	UCA	UCC	UCG	UCU
T	Thr	Threonine	ACA	ACC	ACG	ACU		
V	Val	Valine	GUA	GUC	GUG	GUU		
W	Trp	Tryptophan	UGG					
Y	Tyr	Tyrosine	UAC	UAU				

Subject Index

Page numbers in *italics* refer to illustrations; page numbers followed by t refer to tables

hnRNA, nonpolyadenylated, mental retardation and, 446
RNase protection, gene expression analysis by, 439–440
Rod cell(s), 138
  disk membranes of, 139–140
  function of, rhodopsin phosphorylation and, 388–389
  light response of, 139
  lipids of, 140
  rhodopins of, 140–143, *141–143*
Rotational behavior
  dopamine receptor density and, 249
  dopaminergic tissue transplants in, 517–518
Rubella, autism and, 872
Rutabaga *Drosophila* mutant, 922–923

S-100, as developmental cell marker, 483t
S-1 nuclease, in cDNA cloning, 432
Saccharopine dehydrogenase, *735*
Saccharopinemia and lysinemia, *735*, 744t
Sandhoff's disease, 716, 719t, 723–724
  infantile form of, 723
Sanfilippo's disease, 725t, 726
Sarcomeres, 610
Sarcoplasmic reticulum, 616–618, *617*
  abnormalities of, periodic paralysis and, 618
  Ca^{2+} pump of, 616–618, *617*
    in Duchenne dystrophy, 619
    lipid modulation of, 617–618
  Ca^{2+} release from, excitation-contraction coupling and, 616, *617*
  Ca^{2+} uptake of, 616–617
Sarcosine, disorders of, 746t
Sarcosine dehydrogenase deficiency, 743, 746t
Sarcosinemia, 746t
Saxitoxin, ionic channel function study with, *81*, 83
Scatchard plot, 186–188, *187*, 196, *197*
SCH-23390, dopamine receptor characterization with, 244
Scheie's syndrome, 724–726, 725t
Schizophrenia
  age and, 860
  γ-aminobutyric acid in, 867
  benzodiazepines in, 867
  brain morphology in, 863
  catatonic, 861

cerebral metabolism in, 587, 587t
chlorpromazine for, 864
cholecystokinin in, 868, 869
clinical aspects of, 860–864
confusion in, 861
course of, 862
definition of, 862
delusions in, 861
des-tyr-γ-endorphin in, 869
3,4-dihydroxyphenylacetic acid in, 865
disorganized, 861
dopamine hypothesis of, 864–866
emotional blunting in, 861
endorphins in, 868–869, 869
eye tracking in, 863
genetic factors in, 862–863
hallucinations in, 861
  naloxone and, 870
hebephrenic, 861
homovanillic acid in, 865–866
immune etiology in, 871
3-methoxytyramine in, 865
neuroleptic drugs for, 864
neuropeptide antagonists for, 869–870
neuropeptides in, 868
neurotensin in, 869
nonopioid neuropeptides in, 869–870
norepinephrine in, 866–867
paranoid, 861
PET of, 870–871
prostaglandin receptors in, 868
psychosocial environment in, 863–864
receptor ligand affinity in, 866
receptor number in, 866
residual state, 861
serotonin in, 867
subtypes of, 861
tardive dyskinesia in, 864
type I symptoms of, 861–862
type II symptoms of, 861–862
undifferentiated, 861
viral etiology in, 871
Schmidt-Lantermann clefts, 27, *117*, 118
Schwann cell(s), 7, 687–688
  cell markers for, 483t
  Corynebacterium diphtheriae toxin binding to, 691
  cytoplasm of, 28, 30
  fingers of, 28, *30*, *31*
  galactocerebroside expression by, 687
  Hansen's bacilli growth in, 691
  myelin production of, 27–30, *29*, 687
  nonmyelinating, 687

onion bulb formation of, 690, 692
phenotypes of, 687
PNS myelination and, 118, *119*
in remyelination, 712
satellite, 687
structure of, 28, *29*
trauma response of, 30, 690
tube formation by, 30
tubular aggregates of, 687
visceral neuroglia and, 687
Schwann cell tumor, 694
Scopolamine, receptor binding of, PET of, 849–851, *850*
Scorpion toxin, ionic channel function study with, *81*, 83
Scurvy, 683
Sea snake toxin, acetylcholine receptor effects of, 637–639
Second-messenger system(s), *375*, *376*
  adenylate cyclase, 349–362
  in affective disorders, 886
  cyclic nucleotide, 349–363
    criteria for, 350–351
  histamine receptor binding and, 260–262
  hormone activation of, 897, *898*
  neuronal integration and, 343
  phosphoinositide, 333–347
  protein phosphorylation and, 394–396
  in pseudohypoparathyroidism, 886
  in seizures, 803–804
Second-wind phenomenon, 648
Secretor gene, 445
Secretory proteins, fast axonal transport of, 464–465, *465*
Sedation, prostaglandin E effect of, 411
Seizure(s), 797–810
  ADP:ATP ratio in, 802
  amino acid activity and, 327, 560
  amino acid changes in, 560
  γ-aminobutyric acid levels and, 560
  ATP levels in, 801
  in autism, 872
  blood flow in, 805–806
  brain damage in, 805–808
  cerebral blood flow in, 800–801, 801t
  cerebral metabolic rate in, 801, 801t
  CSF 5-HIAA in, 818t
  CSF homovanillic acid in, 818t
  drug prevention of, 799–800
  energy metabolism in, 587t, 588, 805–806
  experimental, 798–799
  foci localization in, 852
  GDP:GTP ratio in, 802, *804*